Clinical Aspects of Immunology

CLINICAL ASPECTS OF IMMUNOLOGY

EDITED BY

P. J. LACHMANN
ScD FRCP PRCPath FRS
Sheila Joan Smith Professor of Immunology
and Honorary Director of MRC Molecular Immunopathology Unit
University of Cambridge, UK

SIR KEITH PETERS
MD(Hon) MB FRCP FRCPath
Regius Professor of Physic
University of Cambridge School of Clinical Medicine
Addenbrooke's Hospital, Cambridge, UK

F. S. ROSEN
MD
James L. Gamble Professor of Pediatrics
Harvard Medical School, Boston, USA

M. J. WALPORT
PhD FRCP MRCPath
Professor of Rheumatology
Royal Postgraduate Medical School
Hammersmith Hospital, London, UK

IN THREE VOLUMES
VOLUME 2

FIFTH EDITION

BOSTON
BLACKWELL SCIENTIFIC PUBLICATIONS
OXFORD LONDON EDINBURGH
MELBOURNE PARIS BERLIN VIENNA

Editorial offices:
238 Main Street, Cambridge
Massachusetts 02142, USA
Osney Mead, Oxford OX2 0EL, England
25 John Street, London WC1N 2BL
England
23 Ainslie Place, Edinburgh EH3 6AJ
Scotland
54 University Street, Carlton
Victoria 3053, Australia

Other Editorial Offices:
Librairie Arnette SA
2, rue Casimir-Delavigne
75006 Paris
France

Blackwell Wissenschafts-Verlag
Meinekestrasse 4
D-1000 Berlin 15
Germany

Blackwell MZV
Feldgasse 13
A-1238 Wien
Austria

First published 1963
Revised reprint 1964
Second edition 1968
Third edition 1975
Fourth edition 1982
Fifth edition 1993

Set by Setrite Typesetters, Hong Kong
Printed and bound in the USA
by The Maple-Vail Book
Manufacturing Group, New York

93 94 95 96 5 4 3 2 1

DISTRIBUTORS

USA
Blackwell Scientific Publications, Inc.
238 Main Street
Cambridge, Massachusetts 02142
(*Orders*: Tel: 617 876-7000
800 759-6102)

Canada
Times Mirror Professional Publishing, Ltd
130 Flaska Drive
Markham, Ontario L6G 1B8
(*Orders*: Tel: 416 470-6739
800 268-4178)

Australia
Blackwell Scientific Publications Pty Ltd
54 University Street
Carlton, Victoria 3053
(*Orders*: Tel: 03 347-5552)

Outside North America and Australia
Marston Book Services Ltd
PO Box 87
Oxford OX2 0DT
(*Orders*: Tel: 0865 791155
Fax: 0865 791927
Telex: 837515)

Library of Congress
Cataloguing-in-Publication Data

Clinical aspects of immunology/
edited by P.J. Lachmann . . . [*et al.*].
—5th ed.
p. cm.
Includes bibliographical references and index.
ISBN 0-86542-297-4
1. Clinical immunology. 2. Immunology.
I. Lachmann, P.F. (Peter Julius)
[DNLM: 1. Hypersensitivity. 2. Immunity.
WD 300 C641]
RC582.C52 1993
616.07'9—dc20
DNLM/DLC
for Library of Congress

Contents

List of Contributors

C.L.Anderson MD, *Department of Internal Medicine, The Ohio State University College of Medicine, Columbus, USA*

B.M.Ansell MB ChB, FRCP, MRCS, *Consultant Rheumatologist, Stoke Poges, UK*

M.A.Arnaout MD, *Director, Leukocyte Biology and Inflammation Program, Associate Physician, Renal Unit and Department of Medicine, Massachusetts General Hospital, Charlestown and Associate Professor of Medicine, Harvard Medical School, Boston, USA*

J.-F.Bach MD, DSc, *Professor and Director, Département d'Immunologie Clinique, Hospital Necker, Paris, France*

J.I.Bell DM, FRCP, *Nuffield Professor of Clinical Medicine, John Radcliffe Hospital, Oxford, UK*

R.M.Bernstein MA, MD, FRCP, *Consultant Rheumatologist, Manchester Royal Infirmary, University of Manchester, UK*

K.Berzins PhD, *Associate Professor, Department of Immunology, Stockholm University, Stockholm, Sweden*

J.M.Blackwell PhD, *Glaxo Professor of Molecular Parasitology, Departments of Pathology and Medicine, University of Cambridge, UK*

E.Bonifacio PhD, *Lecturer, Department of Immunology, London Hospital Medical College, UK*

L.K.Borysiewicz MB, PhD, FRCP, *Professor of Medicine, University of Wales College of Medicine, Cardiff, UK*

G.F.Bottazzo MD, FRCP, FRCPath, *Professor of Immunology and Clinical Immunology, Department of Immunology, London Hospital Medical College, UK*

D.L.Brown MD, FRCPath, *Consultant Immunologist, Addenbrooke's Hospital, Cambridge, UK*

A.E.Butterworth MB BChir, PhD, *Medical Research Council External Scientific Staff and Honorary Reader in Medical Parasitology, University of Cambridge, UK*

Sir Roy Calne MA, MS, FRCS, FRS, *Professor of Surgery, Department of Surgery, University of Cambridge Clinical School, Addenbrooke's Hospital, Cambridge, UK*

T.A.Calvelli PhD, *Associate Professor, Departments of Pediatrics, Microbiology and Immunology, Albert Einstein College of Medicine, Bronx, USA*

R.D.Campbell BSc, PhD, *Senior Scientist, MRC Immunochemistry Unit, Department of Biochemistry, University of Oxford, UK*

D.A.Carson MD, *Professor, Department of Medicine, University of California, San Diego, USA*

R.K.Chandra OC, MD, PhD, DSc(Hon), DPhil(Hon), FRCPC, *Professor of Pediatrics, Medicine and Biochemistry, Memorial University of Newfoundland and Director, WHO Center for Nutritional Immunology, St. John's, Newfoundland, Canada*

T.A.Chatila MD, *Assistant Professor of Pediatrics, Harvard Medical School, Division of Immunology, The Children's Hospital, Boston, USA*

P.M.S.Clark PhD, MRCPath, *Principal Biochemist, Addenbrooke's Hospital, Cambridge, UK*

S.C.Clark PhD, *Vice President, Discovery Research, Genetics Institute Inc., Cambridge, USA*

J.Cohen MB BS, MSc, FRCP, *Professor and Director of Department of Infectious Diseases and Bacteriology and Honorary Consultant Physician, Royal Postgraduate Medical School, Hammersmith Hospital, London, UK*

P.J.Cole BSc, MB BS, FRCP, MRCS, *Professor, National Heart and Lung Institute, Brompton Hospital, London, UK*

D.H.Conrad PhD, *Department of Microbiology and Immunology, Medical College of Virginia, Richmond, USA*

A.Cooke BSc, DPhil, *Lecturer in Immunology, Department of Pathology, University of Cambridge, UK*

R.S.Cotran MD, *F.B. Mallory Professor of Pathology, Harvard Medical School, and Chairman, Department of Pathology, Brigham and Women's Hospital, Boston, USA*

C.A.Dinarello MD, *Professor of Medicine and Pediatrics, Tufts University School of Medicine, New England Medical Center, Boston, USA*

W.F.Doe MSc, FRACP, FRCP, *Professor of Medicine and Clinical Science, John Curtin School of Medical Research, Australian National University, Canberra, Australia*

R.M.du Bois MA, MD, FRCP, *Consultant Physician, Royal Brompton National Heart & Lung Hospital and Honorary Senior Lecturer, National Heart & Lung Institute, London, UK*

I.Dunham BA, DPhil, *Postdoctoral Research Fellow, Paediatric Research Unit, Guy's Hospital, London, UK*

A.L.W.F.Eddleston DM, FRCP, *Professor of Liver Immunology, Institute of Liver Studies, King's College School of Medicine and Dentistry, London, UK*

G.I.Evan MA, PhD, *Senior Scientist, Imperial Cancer Research Fund Laboratories, London, UK*

P.W.Ewan MB, FRCP, MRCPath, *MRC Clinical Scientist and Honorary Consultant in Allergy and Clinical Immunology, MRC Molecular Immunopathology Unit, University of Cambridge School of Clinical Medicine and Addenbrooke's Hospital, UK*

J.M.Farrant MD, MRCP, *Wellcome Clinical Research Fellow, Institute of Liver Studies, King's College School of Medicine and Dentistry, London, UK*

A.J.Frew MA, MD, MB BChir, MRCP, *Senior Lecturer, Department of University Medicine, Southampton General Hospital, UK*

R.S.Geha MD, *Professor of Pediatrics, Harvard Medical School, and Chief, Division of Immunology, The Children's Hospital, Boston, USA*

I.Gigli MD, *Professor of Medicine and Chief, Division of Dermatology, University of California, San Diego, USA*

S.Gordon MB ChB, PhD, *Glaxo Professor of Cellular Pathology, Sir William Dunn School of Pathology, University of Oxford, UK*

C.D.Gregory PhD, *Senior Lecturer, Department of Immunology, University of Birmingham Medical School, UK*

E.C.Guinan MD, *Assistant Professor of Pediatrics, Division of Pediatric Oncology, Dana–Farber Cancer Institute, Harvard Medical School, Boston, USA*

A.G.Hadley BSc, DPhil, *Manager, Antibody Function Laboratory, International Blood Group Reference Laboratory, Bristol, UK*

C.N.Hales MD, PhD, FRCP, FRCPath, FRS, *Professor and Head of Department of Clinical Biochemistry, Addenbrooke's Hospital, Cambridge, UK*

F.C.Hay BTech, PhD, *Professor of Immunology, and Head of Department of Cellular and Molecular Sciences,*

P.G.Hellewell PhD, *Senior Lecturer, Department of Applied Pharmacology, National Heart & Lung Institute, London, UK*

B.Henderson BSc, PhD, *Senior Lecturer in Biochemistry, Institute of Dental Surgery, University of London, UK*

P.M.Henson PhD, *Professor of Pathology and Medicine, National Jewish Center for Immunology and Respiratory Medicine, Denver, USA*

G.A.Higgs BSc, PhD, *Head of Inflammation Biology, Celltech Ltd, Slough, UK*

T.Hirano MD, PhD, *Professor, Division of Molecular Oncology, Biomedical Research Centre, Osaka University Medical School, Japan*

S.T.Holgate MD, DSc, FRCP, *MRC Clinical Professor of Immunopharmacology, Medicine 1, Southampton General Hospital, UK*

N.Holmes PhD, *Division of Immunology, Department of Pathology, University of Cambridge, UK*

J.Hopkins BSc, PhD, MIBiol, *Senior Lecturer in Veterinary Pathology, Royal (Dick) School of Veterinary Studies, University of Edinburgh, UK*

N.C.Hughes-Jones DM, PhD, FRCP, FRS, *Honorary Member, Scientific Staff, MRC Molecular Immunopathology Unit, MRC Centre, Cambridge, UK*

The Late J.H.Humphrey FRS, *Latterly of the Department of Immunology, Royal Postgraduate Medical School, London, UK*

G.Husby MD, *Professor of Rheumatology, Department of Rheumatology, The University of Tromsø, Norway*

J.Ivanyi MD, PhD, *Director of MRC Tuberculosis and Related Infections Unit, Hammersmith Hospital, London, UK*

H.H.Jabara *Chief Technologist, The Children's Hospital, Boston, USA*

N.D.James BSc, MRCP, FRCR, *Lecturer in Oncology, Ludwig Institute for Cancer Research, St. Mary's Hospital Medical School, London, UK*

E.Jenkinson BSc, PhD, *Department of Anatomy, University of Birmingham Medical School, UK*

J.P.Johnson PhD, *Senior Scientist, Institute for Immunology, University of Munich, Republic of Germany*

P.M.Johnson MA, PhD, DSc, MRCPath, *Professor of Immunology, University of Liverpool, UK*

R.B.Johnston, Jr MD, *Adjunct Professor of Pediatrics, Yale University School of Medicine, New Haven, USA*

D.L.Kasper MD, *William Ellery Channing Professor of Medicine, Harvard Medical School, Co-Director, Channing Laboratory, Brigham and Women's Hospital, and Chief, Division of Infectious Diseases, Beth Israel Hospital, Boston, USA*

A.B.Kay PhD, DSc, FRCP, *Professor and Director, Department of Allergy and Clinical Immunology, National Heart & Lung Institute, London, UK*

D.M.Kenney PhD, *Assistant Professor of Pediatrics, Harvard Medical School and Investigator, The Center for Blood Research, Boston, USA*

T.Kishimoto MD, PhD, *Professor, Department of Internal Medicine III, Osaka University Medical School, Japan*

G.G.B.Klaus PhD, MS, BVSc, *Laboratory of Cellular Immunology, National Institute for Medical Research, London, UK*

S.C.Knight PhD, FIBiol, *Head, Antigen Presentation Research Group, MRC Clinical Research Centre, Harrow, UK*

R.R.Kretschmer MD, FAAP, FAAAI, *Head, Division of Immunology, Unidad de Investigación Biomédica CMN-IMSS and Subdivisión de Medicina Experimental Universidad Nacional Autónoma de Mexico, Mexico DF*

P.J.Lachmann ScD, FRCP, PRCPath, FRS, *Sheila Joan Smith Professor of Immunology and Honorary Director of MRC Molecular Immunopathology Unit, MRC Centre, Cambridge, UK*

R.I.Lechler PhD, FRCP, *Professor of Molecular Immunology and Honorary Consultant in Medicine, Department of Immunology, Royal Postgraduate Medical School, Hammersmith Hospital, London, UK*

T.H.Lee MD, MRCPath, FRCP, *Professor of Allergy and Allied Respiratory Disorders, Guy's Hospital, London, UK*

P.F.Lehmann MA, MSc, PhD, *Associate Professor of Microbiology, Medical College of Ohio, Toledo, USA*

T.Lehner MD, BDS, PhD (Hon), FRCPath, FDS RDS, *Head, Division of Immunology, United Medical and Dental Schools of Guy's and St. Thomas's Hospitals, London, UK*

M.H.Lessof MA, MD, FRCP, *Emeritus Professor of Medicine, United Schools of Guy's and St. Thomas's Hospitals, London, UK*

C.M.Lockwood MB BChir, FRCP, *Wellcome Reader in the School of Clinical Medicine, University of Cambridge, Addenbrooke's Hospital, Cambridge, UK*

T.T.MacDonald PhD, MRCPath, *Reader in Gut Immunology and Wellcome Senior Lecturer, Department of Paediatric Gastroenterology, St. Bartholomew's Hospital, London, UK*

I.C.M.MacLennan MB BS, PhD, MRCP, FRCPath, *Head of Department of Immunology, University of Birmingham Medical School, UK*

P.D.Mason BSc, MRCP, *Squibb Lecturer in Renal Medicine, Department of Medicine, Royal Postgraduate Medical School, Hammersmith Hospital, London, UK*

I.McConnell MA, PhD, BVMS, MRCVS, MRCPath, FRSE, *Professor of Veterinary Pathology, Royal (Dick) School of Veterinary Studies, University of Edinburgh, UK*

I.G.McFarlane PhD, MRCPath, *Consultant Biochemist, Institute of Liver Studies, King's College School of Medicine and Dentistry, London, UK*

A.M.McGregor MA, MD, FRCP, *Professor of Medicine, King's College School of Medicine, London, UK*

A.J.McMichael PhD, MB BChir, MRCP, FRS, *MRC Clinical Research Professor of Immunology, Institute of Molecular Medicine, University of Oxford, UK*

P.A.R.Meyer MA, MB BChir, MRCP, *Wellcome Research Fellow, Department of Ophthalmology, Addenbrooke's Hospital, Cambridge, UK*

N.A.Mitchison BSc, DPhil, FRS, *Scientific Director, Deutsches Rheuma — Forschungszentrum Berlin, Republic of Germany*

S.Moncada PhD, DSc, *Research Director, Wellcome Research Laboratories, Beckenham, UK*

P.J.Morris PhD, FRCS, FACS(Hon), FRACS *Nuffield Professor of Surgery, University of Oxford, UK*

J.B.Natvig MD, PhD, *Professor, Institute of Immunology and Rheumatology, University of Oslo, Norway*

P.E.Newburger MD, *Associate Professor of Pediatrics and Molecular Genetics/Microbiology, Department of Pediatrics, University of Massachusetts Medical School, Worcester, USA*

A.Newman Taylor MSc, FRCP, FFOM, *Consultant Physician, Royal Brompton National Heart & Lung Hospital and Honorary Senior Lecturer, National Heart & Lung Institute, London, UK*

J.Newsom-Davis MA, MD, FRCP, FRS, *Professor of Clinical Neurology, Neurosciences Group, Institute of Molecular Medicine, University of Oxford, John Radcliffe Hospital, Oxford, UK*

G.J.V.Nossal MD, PhD, FRCP, FRS, *Director, The Walter and Eliza Hall Institute of Medical Research, Melbourne, Australia*

D.B.G.Oliveira PhD, MRCP, *Lister Institute Research Fellow and Honorary Consultant Physician, Department of Medicine, University of Cambridge School of Clinical Medicine, Addenbrooke's Hospital, Cambridge, UK*

W.H.Ouwehand MD, PhD, *Consultant Haematologist, Lecturer in Transfusion Medicine, Division of Transfusion Medicine, University of Cambridge, UK*

M.J.Owen BA, PhD, *Principal Scientist, Imperial Cancer Research Fund, Lincoln's Inn Fields, London, UK*

J.L.Pace PhD, *Research Associate Professor, Departments of Pathology/Oncology and Microbiology/Molecular Genetics/Immunology, Wilkinson Laboratory for Cancer Research, University of Kansas Medical Center, Kansas City, USA*

D.C.Parker PhD, *Professor, Department of Molecular Genetics and Microbiology, University of Massachusetts Medical School, Worcester, USA*

D.M.V.Parrott PhD, DSc, FRS(Edin), *Visiting Professor, Department of Paediatric Gastroenterology, St. Bartholomew's Hospital, London, UK*

T.W.Pearson PhD, *Professor, Department of Biochemistry and Microbiology, University of Victoria, Canada*

P.Perlmann PhD, *Professor Emeritus, Department of Immunology, Stockholm University, Sweden*

D.K.Peters MD(Hon), MB FRCP, FRCPath, *Regius Professor of Physic, University of Cambridge School of Clinical Medicine, Addenbrooke's Hospital, Cambridge, UK*

E.R.Pettipher BSc, PhD, *Senior Research Scientist, Pfizer Central Research, Groton, USA*

A.J.Pinching DPhil, FRCP, *Louis Freedman Professor of Immunology, Medical College of St. Bartholomew's Hospital, London, UK*

T.A.E.Platts-Mills MD, PhD, FRCP, *Oscar Swineford Jr. Professor of Medicine and Microbiology, and Head, Division of Allergy and Clinical Immunology, University of Virginia, Charlotsville, USA*

J.H.L.Playfair MB BChir, DSc, PhD, *Professor of Immunology, University College Medical School, London, UK*

J.S.Pober MD, PhD, *Professor of Pathology, Immunobiology and Biology, and Director, Molecular Cardiobiology, Boyer Center for Molecular Medicine, Yale University School of Medicine, New Haven, USA*

E.R.Podack MD, *Professor of Microbiology, Immunology and Oncology, Department of Microbiology and Immunology, University of Miami School of Medicine, USA*

R.Pujol-Borrell MD, PhD, *Associate Professor of Immunology, Hospital Universitari Germans Trias I, Barcelona, Spain*

C.D.Pusey MSc, FRCP, *Reader in Renal Medicine and Honorary Consultant Physician, Department of Medicine, Royal Postgraduate Medical School, Hammersmith Hospital, London, UK*

T.H.Rabbitts BSc, PhD, FRS, *Joint Head of Protein and Nucleic Acid Division, MRC Laboratory of Molecular Biology, Cambridge, UK*

A.J.Rees MSc, FRCP, *Professor of Nephrology, Department of Medicine, Royal Postgraduate Medical School, Hammersmith Hospital, London, UK*

J.R.Regueiro PhD, *Senior Registrar, Department of Immunology, Hospital 12 de Octubre, Madrid, Spain*

G.Reimer MD, *Assistant Professor (Privatdozent) of Dermatology, University of Erlangen-Nürnberg, Republic of Germany*

G.Riethmüller MD, *Director, Institute for Immunology, University of Munich, Republic of Germany*

A.B.Rickinson PhD, *Head of Department of Cancer Studies, Cancer Research Campaign Laboratories, The Medical School, University of Birmingham, UK*

F.S.Rosen MD, *James L. Gamble Professor of Pediatrics, Harvard Medical School, Boston, USA*

G.D.Ross PhD, *Professor and Chairman, Department of Microbiology and Immunology, University of Louisville, USA*

A.Rubinstein MD, *Professor, Departments of Pediatrics, Microbiology and Immunology, Albert Einstein College of Medicine, Bronx, USA*

C.O.S.Savage PhD, MRCP, *Clinical Scientist and Honorary Consultant Physician, Clinical Research Centre, Northwick Park Hospital, Harrow, UK*

L.B.Schwartz MD, PhD, *Charles and Evelyn Thomas Professor of Medicine, Medical College of Virginia, Virginia Commonwealth University, Richmond, USA*

J.P.Scott MD, *Associate Professor, Mayo Clinic, Rochester, USA*

M.Seligmann MD, FRCPath, *Professor of Immunology and Head of Department of Immunohaematology, Hospital Saint-Louis, Paris, France*

D.W.Shaw MD, *Clinical Fellow, Division of Dermatology, Department of Medicine, University of California, San Diego, USA*

M.J.Sicklick MD, *Department of Pediatrics, Albert Einstein College of Medicine, Bronx, USA*

K.Sikora MA, PhD, FRCP, FRCR, *Department of Clinical Oncology, Royal Postgraduate Medical School, Hammersmith Hospital, London, UK*

G.J.Silverman MD, *Assistant Professor, Division of Rheumatology, Department of Medicine, University of California, San Diego, USA*

J.G.P.Sissons MD, FRCP, *Professor of Medicine, University of Cambridge School of Clinical Medicine, UK*

The Late T.F.Slater MSc, PhD, DSc, MD(Hon), D.Univ(Paris), *Latterly Professor of Biochemistry, Brunel University, Uxbridge, UK*

T.A.Springer PhD, *Latham Family Professor, Harvard Medical School, Boston, USA*

C.J.F.Spry DPhil, FRCP, FRCPath, *British Heart Foundation Professor of Cardiovascular Immunology, St. George's Hospital Medical School, London, UK*

G.T.Stevenson MD, DPhil, *Professor of Immunochemistry, University of Southampton, UK*

R.Storb MD, *Professor of Medicine, University of Washington and Member, Fred Hutchinson Cancer Research Center, Washington, USA*

T.B.Strom MD, DSc(Hon), *Professor of Medicine, Harvard Medical School and Head, Division of Immunology, Beth Israel Hospital, Boston, USA*

Q.A.Summers MB BS, FRACP, *Research Fellow, Medicine 1, Southampton General Hospital, UK*

E.M.Tan MD, *W.M. Keck Autoimmune Disease Center, The Scripps Research Institute, La Jolla, USA*

C.Terhorst PhD, *Chief, Division of Immunology, Beth Israel Hospital, Harvard Medical School, Boston, USA*

H.C.Thomas BSc, PhD, FRCP, FRCPath, *Professor of Medicine, St. Mary's Hospital Medical School, Imperial College of Science, Technology and Medicine, University of London, UK*

J.Trowsdale PhD, *Head, Human Immunogenetics Laboratory, Imperial Cancer Research Fund, Lincoln's Inn Fields, London, UK*

M.W.Turner DSc(Med), FRCPath, *Professor of Molecular Immunology, Institute of Child Health, University of London, UK*

E.R.Unanue MD, *Professor and Chairman, Department of Pathology, Washington University School of Medicine, St. Louis, USA*

H.Valdimarsson MD, FRCPath, *Professor and Chairman, Department of Immunology, Landspitalinn, The National University Hospital, Reykjavik, Iceland*

P.J.W.Venables MD, MRCP, *Senior Lecturer in Rheumatology, Kennedy Institute of Rheumatology, London, UK*

D.Vercelli MD, *Assistant Professor of Pediatrics, Harvard Medical School, Boston, USA*

A.C.Vincent MB BS, MSc, MRCPath, *University Lecturer in Clinical Neoroimmunology, Neurosciences Group, Institute of Molecular Medicine, University of Oxford, John Radcliffe Hospital, Oxford, UK*

M.Wahlgren MD, PhD, *Associate Professor, Department of Immunology, Stockholm University, Sweden*

B.H.Waksman MD, *Adjunct Professor of Pathology, New York University and Visiting Scientist in Neurology, Harvard University, Boston, USA*

H.Waldmann FRS, *Kay Kendall Professor of Therapeutic Immunology, University of Cambridge, UK*

T.A.Waldmann MD, *Chief, Metabolism Branch, National Cancer Institute, National Institute of Health, Bethesda, USA*

J.Wallwork MB ChB, FRCS Ed, *Consultant Cardiothoracic Surgeon, Department of Cardiothoracic Surgery, Papworth Hospital, Cambridge, UK*

M.J.Walport PhD, FRCP, MRCPath, *Professor of Rheumatology, Royal Postgraduate Medical School, Hammersmith Hospital, London, UK*

S.Ward PhD, *Assistant Professor, Department of Microbiology, The University of Texas Southwestern Medical Center at Dallas, USA*

J.A.Warner PhD, *Lecturer in Allergy and Immunology, Child Health, University of Southampton, Southampton General Hospital, UK*

J.O.Warner MD, FRCP, DCH, *Professor of Child Health, University of Southampton, Southampton General Hospital, UK*

A.H.Waters PhD, FRCP, FRCPath, *Head of Department of Haematology, St. Bartholomew's Hospital and Medical College, London, UK*

R.J.Wedgwood MD, *Professor Emeritus, Department of Pediatrics, University of Washington, USA*

A.P.Weetman MD, FRCP, *Professor of Medicine, University of Sheffield Clinical Sciences Centre, Northern General Hospital, Sheffield, UK*

M.R.Wessels MD, *Assistant Professor of Medicine, Harvard Medical School, Associate Physician, Channing Laboratory, Brigham and Women's Hospital and Associate Physician, Division of Infectious Diseases, Beth Israel Hospital, Boston, USA*

J.R.W.Wilkinson MD, MRCP, *Lecturer in Medicine, University of Southampton, UK*

H.N.A.Willcox MA, MB BChir, PhD, *University Research Lecturer, Neurosciences Group, Institute of Molecular Medicine, University of Oxford, John Radcliffe Hospital, Oxford, UK*

R.C.Williams Jr MD, *Eminent Scholar, Marcia Whitney Schott Chair in Rheumatoid Arthritis, Department of Medicine, University of Florida School of Medicine, Gainesville, USA*

G.Winter PhD, FRS, *Member, MRC Laboratory of Molecular Biology, Cambridge, UK*

R.P.Witherspoon MD, *Associate Professor of Medicine, University of Washington and Associate Member, Fred Hutchinson Cancer Research Center, Washington, USA*

P.Woo PhD, FRCP, *Head, Section of Molecular Rheumatology, Clinical Research Centre, Northwick Park Hospital, Harrow, UK*

K.J.Wood PhD, *University Lecturer in Immunology, Royal Postgraduate Medical School, Hammersmith Hospital, London, UK*

Preface to the Fifth Edition

Eleven years have gone by since the Fourth Edition of *Clinical Aspects* was published. These years have seen no slackening in the rate of progress of immunology or of its clinical aspects and the book has again required major restructuring and almost total rewriting. For this task two further editors have been recruited and Peter Lachmann and Keith Peters warmly welcome Fred Rosen, from the Center for Blood Research at Harvard University, and Mark Walport, from the Royal Postgraduate Medical School, as co-editors. Together with an American editor we have for this edition recruited authors from further afield, particularly from the United States, but also from Australia, Canada, France, Germany, Iceland, Japan, Mexico, Norway and Sweden. The book has again grown substantially. This edition has 109 chapters compared with the 64 of the Fourth Edition. The editors have discovered that as the number of authors increases linearly the difficulty of obtaining chapters on time rises exponentially and we are only too aware that this edition has had a longer incubation period than we had either hoped or expected. Nevertheless, with the help of contributors in updating their chapters, we are confident that the book is a timely overview of the subject for the rest of the millennium.

The editors would like to express their sincere thanks to those contributors to the Fourth Edition who are not contributing this time. We would also like to welcome all those contributing to this edition for the first time.

We were greatly saddened by the death of several of the contributors to the Fourth Edition: Ed Franklin, Mavis Gunter, John Humphrey, Henry Kunkel and Tony Waterson. All are a sadly felt loss to immunology, to medicine and to this book. The chapter written in the Fourth Edition by Gerry Klaus and John Humphrey has been revised for this edition by Gerry Klaus alone and is published as a tribute to John. We were also greatly saddened by the death of one of the contributors to this edition, Trevor Slater, while the book was in press. Trevor was a major British authority on oxygen radicals and a wonderfully enthusiastic scientist.

The new layout of the book reflects the great changes that have occurred in immunology in the past 10 years. There are new chapters on newly characterized molecules: adhesion molecules, Fc receptors and various cytokines. The mystery of the T cell receptors has now been solved and their genes are considered alongside those for immunoglobulins which they closely resemble. Understanding of the complement system has expanded to such an extent that there are now two additional chapters on complement receptors and complement deficiencies. Antigens have been joined by superantigens. The new techniques section contains chapters on molecular biology and on transgenic animals as well as on antibody engineering; and monoclonal antibody therapy has advanced to the stage where it is well worthy of its own chapter. Allergy is promoted to having its own section as is connective tissue disease, immunodeficiency and the acquired immune deficiency syndrome. The AIDS epidemic is indeed the greatest change that has occurred in the clinical aspects of immunology. The organ-specific section contains similar chapter titles to earlier editions but the contents reflect the great changes that have occurred with changes in the basic science.

P.J.L., D.K.P.
F.S.R., M.J.W.

Section 4
Advances in Technology

41: Molecular Biology Techniques in Immunology

I. Dunham and R.D. Campbell

Introduction

In recent years the application of recombinant deoxyribonucleic acid (DNA) techniques has revolutionized the study of the molecular and genetic aspects of immunology. For instance, the solution of the genetic basis of antibody diversity (Tonegawa 1987), the identification of the T cell receptor genes (Kronenberg *et al.* 1986) and the engineering of monoclonal antibodies of novel specificity (Riechmann *et al.* 1988) have provided vivid demonstrations of the power of the methodology. In the future it is expected that the technology will continue to play an increasing role in the study of the molecular basis of immune phenomena. Applications range from investigation of molecular interactions in immune regulation and tolerance (Davis and Bjorkman 1988) to possible therapeutic use of recombinant monoclonal antibodies (Riechmann *et al.* 1988) and lymphokines/cytokines. Tissue typing will continue to benefit from recombinant DNA methods (Parham 1988). Furthermore, analysis of genetic and other elements involved in autoimmune disease (Todd *et al.* 1988) should facilitate identification of individuals at risk so that they can be monitored and early treatment given if necessary. On a different tack, the development of rapid recombinant DNA-based diagnostic procedures will assist in the identification of infectious agents, including the discrimination of strains.

The purpose of this review is to describe some of the more important techniques which are available and to illustrate their use. Detailed protocols are not given here but can be found in the references cited and also in a number of texts/laboratory manuals (Davis *et al.* 1986; Ausubel *et al.* 1987; Berger and Kimmel 1987; Sambrook *et al.* 1989). In addition, because of the rapid development of techniques, protocols and reagents, no attempt has been made to critically assess or recommend particular examples. Rather the emphasis is on giving a broad outline of the principles and illustrating how specific questions can be approached.

The basic tools of molecular biology

The recombinant DNA revolution has been built on three simple foundations: first, the ability to detect the presence of a specific nucleotide sequence within a sample of DNA or ribonucleic acid (RNA); secondly, the availability of a range of purified enzymes that allow the manipulation of nucleic acids; and finally the ability to produce sufficient quantities of a specific DNA region of interest. All recombinant DNA experiments involve at least one, and usually all, of these elements and it is wise to dwell on these before discussing particular techniques.

Hybridization and labelling of nucleic acids

HYBRIDIZATION

Detection of specific DNA or RNA species utilizes the property of complementary nucleic acid strands to anneal or hybridize and form a base-paired duplex. The ability of two, single-stranded nucleic acids to hybridize is dependent on a number of experimental variables (temperature, salt concentration, concentration of nucleic acid samples, amount of formamide in the buffer), but also on the length and degree of homology of the nucleic acid sequences and the proportion of guanine–cytosine (G–C) to adenine–thymine (A–T) pairs (Hames and Higgins 1985). Thus the hybridization reaction provides a test for the presence of complementary sequences.

In most hybridizations, one nucleic acid sample contains the target sequence which is to be detected, while the other nucleic acid species involved is a DNA fragment of known sequence, the probe, which may be a synthetic oligonucleotide or a specific DNA fragment. In many applications, for instance Southern blot analysis, the sample containing the target sequence is denatured and immobilized on a nitrocellulose or nylon membrane. This prevents the target DNA from renaturing to itself and competing with the probe in the hybridization, while also conferring useful positional information (see below).

In practice, the conditions of hybridization and subsequent washing to remove non-specifically bound probe are chosen according to the length, G–C content and degree of homology expected between the complementary regions of the probe and the target sequence (Hames and Higgins 1985). Briefly, as the length, G–C content and homology of the hydrogen-bonded region increase, the stability of the resulting double-stranded hybrid also increases and hence the stringency of hybridization and washing may be increased (i.e. higher temperature, increased formamide concentration, lower NaCl concentration). Thus, the hybridization and washing conditions can be adjusted to optimize detection of specific nucleotide sequences above non-specific background hybridization.

LABELLING

The probe DNA may be labelled with one of a variety of reporter groups including biotin, enzymes such as alkaline phosphatase, or, most commonly, radio-isotopes, chiefly ^{32}P or ^{35}S (Sheldon *et al.* 1986; Cunningham and Mundy 1987; Sambrook *et al.* 1989). The label is incorporated into the nucleic acid probe by one of a number of enzymatic techniques (Sambrook *et al.* 1989):

1 Single- and double-stranded oligonucleotides and DNA fragments that have 5′ OH groups can be end-labelled using T4 polynucleotide kinase, which transfers the γ-^{32}P group from a ribonucleoside 5′-triphosphate donor (usually ^{32}P-adenosine triphosphate (^{32}P-ATP)) to the free 5′ OH moiety (Maxam and Gilbert 1977). Double-stranded DNA fragments generated from restriction enzyme digests that yield 5′ protruding ends can be end-filled using the Klenow fragment of DNA polymerase I in the presence of the appropriate α-^{32}P-deoxynucleotide triphosphate (α-^{32}P-dNTP) (Sambrook *et al.* 1989). These two methods provide probes of a defined length, but with only 1–6 ^{32}P groups per molecule. However, for most filter and *in situ* hybridizations, greater sensitivity is required and methods which incorporate label at higher density are used.

2 Double-stranded DNA can be labelled by nick translation (Rigby *et al.* 1977), which involves the simultaneous action of two enzymes, pancreatic deoxyribonuclease (DNase) I and *Escherichia coli* DNA polymerase I (Fig. 41.1). In this reaction partial DNase I digestion generates nicks with free 3′ OH groups in a DNA duplex. The 5′ to 3′ exonuclease activity of DNA polymerase I removes nucleotides starting at these nicks, while at the same time its 5′ to 3′ polymerase activity successively adds nucleotides to the free 3′ OH groups using the complementary DNA as template. The newly synthesized DNA is radiolabelled since one or more of the four nucleotide triphosphates present in the reaction mixture contains a radioisotope in the α position. Since the DNase I introduces nicks randomly a uniformly labelled population of molecules is produced.

3 An alternative uniform labelling protocol is the random primer method (Feinberg and Vogelstein 1983, 1984) (Fig. 41.1). Here the template is single-stranded DNA so double-stranded DNA must be denatured by boiling prior to the start of the reaction. The reaction mixture contains a series of random hexanucleotides which anneal to the template DNA in many positions and serve as primers for initiation of DNA synthesis by the Klenow fragment of *E. coli* DNA polymerase I, thereby incorporating labelled nucleotides into the nascent strand. Both random primer labelling and nick translation result in a double-stranded probe which must be denatured before used in hybridization. Random primer labelling yields probes with slightly higher specific activities than nick translation, which can facilitate the detection of rare sequences but the mean probe length is shorter (~200 bp vs. ~500 bp) (Cunningham and Mundy 1987). The random primer method is relatively insensitive to impurities in the template DNA preparation, unlike nick translation, and hence fragments with agarose still present can be efficiently labelled (Feinberg and Vogelstein 1984).

4 A number of methods have been developed recently which utilize transcription of cloned DNA sequences from appropriate promoters by RNA polymerases derived from bacteriophages such as SP6, T3 or T7 (Krieg and Melton 1984; Melton *et al.* 1984). The template DNA is cloned into one of a range of suitable vectors containing the bacteriophage promoter, and the double-stranded construct is used directly in the synthesis reaction. The resulting probe is an RNA of defined length and high specific activity which does not contain the competing strand.

Additional information on the relative merits of labelling techniques and choice of labels is provided in Hames and Higgins (1985). A number of other labelling methods, including protocols for end-labelling the various termini generated by restriction enzyme cleavage, are available (Sambrook *et al.* 1989).

Enzymes used in molecular biology

RESTRICTION ENDONUCLEASES

Type II restriction endonucleases (REs) cleave double-stranded DNA at or near specific sequences. The recognition sites are typically palindromic sequences of 4–6 bp in length. For instance, the enzyme *Bam*HI recognizes the sequence

5′ – G.GATCC – 3′
3′ – CCTAG.G – 5′

and cleaves the DNA strands at positions four nucleotides apart, to generate DNA fragments with overhanging, 'sticky' ends capable of annealing to other fragments with the same cohesive ends. Hence different restriction fragments generated with the same enzyme or with enzymes that produce complementary termini (e.g. *Bam*HI G.GATCC and *Mbo*I .GATC) can join to produce novel recombinant molecules. A large number of REs have now been isolated and are available commercially, including enzymes which generate 5′ overhangs (e.g. *Bam*HI), 3′ overhangs (e.g. *Kpn*I – GGTAC.C) or blunt ends (e.g. *Pvu*II – CAG.CTG) (Roberts 1987).

The sequence-specific cleavage properties of REs provide a means to generate and manipulate precise DNA fragments, but are also used to provide landmarks in DNA of unknown sequence by RE site mapping. A restriction map depicts the physical distances between RE sites (Fig. 41.2). Such a map is generated by analysis, using a combination of gel electrophoresis and Southern blotting, of the sizes of restriction fragments generated by single, double and partial digestion with various REs. Production of a restriction map is the first step in any analysis of a particular stretch of DNA as the information obtained enables appropriate strategies to be adopted for further investigation. Obviously the presence of an RE site at a particular point on a piece of DNA is indicative of the nucleotide sequence at that point. The presence or absence of an RE site can also be used as a genetic marker (Botstein *et al.* 1980; Donis-Keller *et al.* 1987; Nakamura *et al.* 1987).

The size of restriction fragments produced by RE digestion is dependent on the length and nucleotide sequence of the enzyme recognition

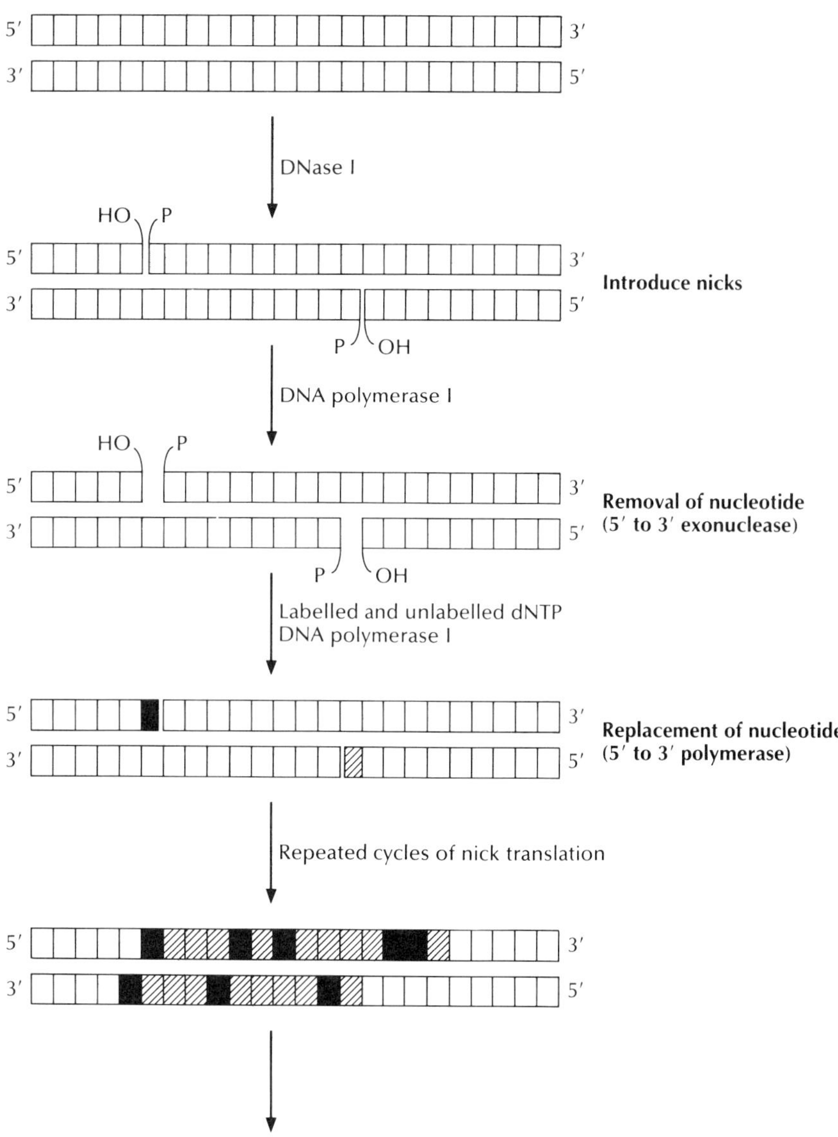

Fig. 41.1(a). Schematic diagram of nick translation.

site and also on the source of the DNA analysed. Assuming that the composition and distribution of nucleotides in a given DNA sample is random, sites for an RE with a tetranucleotide target (e.g. *Mbo*I) should occur every 4^4 (256) bp. Similarly hexanucleotide target sequences should occur every 4^6 (4096) bp. Therefore REs with tetranucleotide recognition sequences are useful for generating small DNA fragments suitable for fine mapping or nucleotide sequencing. Restriction endonucleases with hexanucleotide recognition sequences are more useful for mapping larger regions of DNA, for instance when analysing gene structure.

This simple picture is sufficient when dealing with most REs and is only slightly affected by the base composition of the DNA sample. However, for DNA from many sources, nucleotides and dinucleotides are not randomly distributed and, furthermore, neither are the frequencies of all dinucleotides the same (Josse *et al.* 1961; Swartz *et al.* 1962). Thus sites for certain REs occur more or less frequently than would be expected. For instance, there is a class of REs which cut mammalian geno-

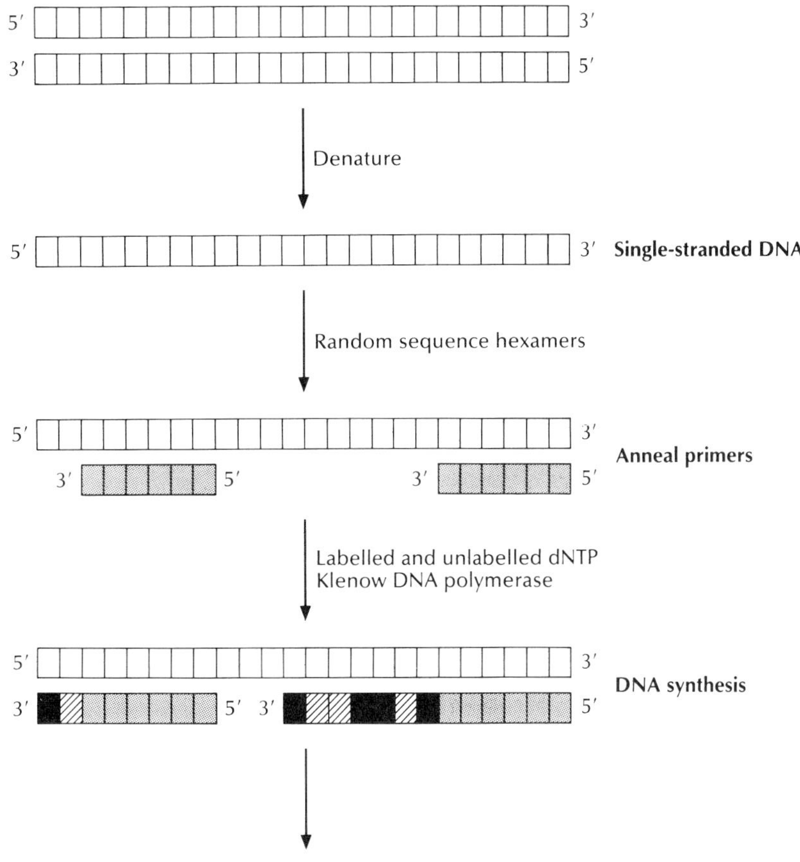

Fig. 41.1(b). Schematic diagram of primer extension.

mic DNA very infrequently (Table 41.1). These 'rare-cutter' enzymes have 6 or 8 bp recognition sequences which contain one or more CpG dinucleotides. They cleave infrequently since the CpG dinucleotide is under-represented in the mammalian genome, occurring at only one-fifth of the expected frequency in bulk DNA. In addition CpG dinucleotides are frequently methylated in vertebrate DNA at the 5 position in the cytosine ring and many of these REs are sensitive to methylation of their recognition sequences (Bird 1986; Brown and Bird 1986; Lindsay and Bird 1987). Hence digestion of uncloned mammalian DNA with these REs produces large restriction fragments (20–1000 kb) and is therefore useful in long-range mapping of regions of mammalian genomes in conjunction with pulsed field gel electrophoresis (PFGE) (Brown and Bird 1986; see also below). Interestingly there is now considerable evidence that unmethylated CpG dinucleotides

Table 41.1. Restriction enzymes that cleave infrequently in the mammalian genome

Enzyme	Recognition site	Enzyme	Recognition site
*Not*I	GCGGCCGC	*Nar*I	GGCGCC
*Mlu*I	ACGCGT	*Sal*I	GTCGAC
*Nru*I	TCGCGA	*Xho*I/*Pae*R71	CTCGAG
*Pvu*I	CGATCG	*Cla*I	ATCGAT
*Bss*HII	GCGCGC	*Rsr*II	CGGWCCG
*Sac*II	CCGCGG	*Sma*I	CCCGGG
*Eag*I	CGGCCG	*Sfi*I	GGCCN$_5$GGCC
*Nae*I	GCCGGC		

N = any nucleotide; W = adenine or thymine.

and consequently sites for rare-cutter REs are clustered in so-called HTF (*Hpa*II tiny fragment) islands at the 5′ ends of many genes (Bird 1986). This means that the position of candidate gene sequences can be identified by detecting clusters

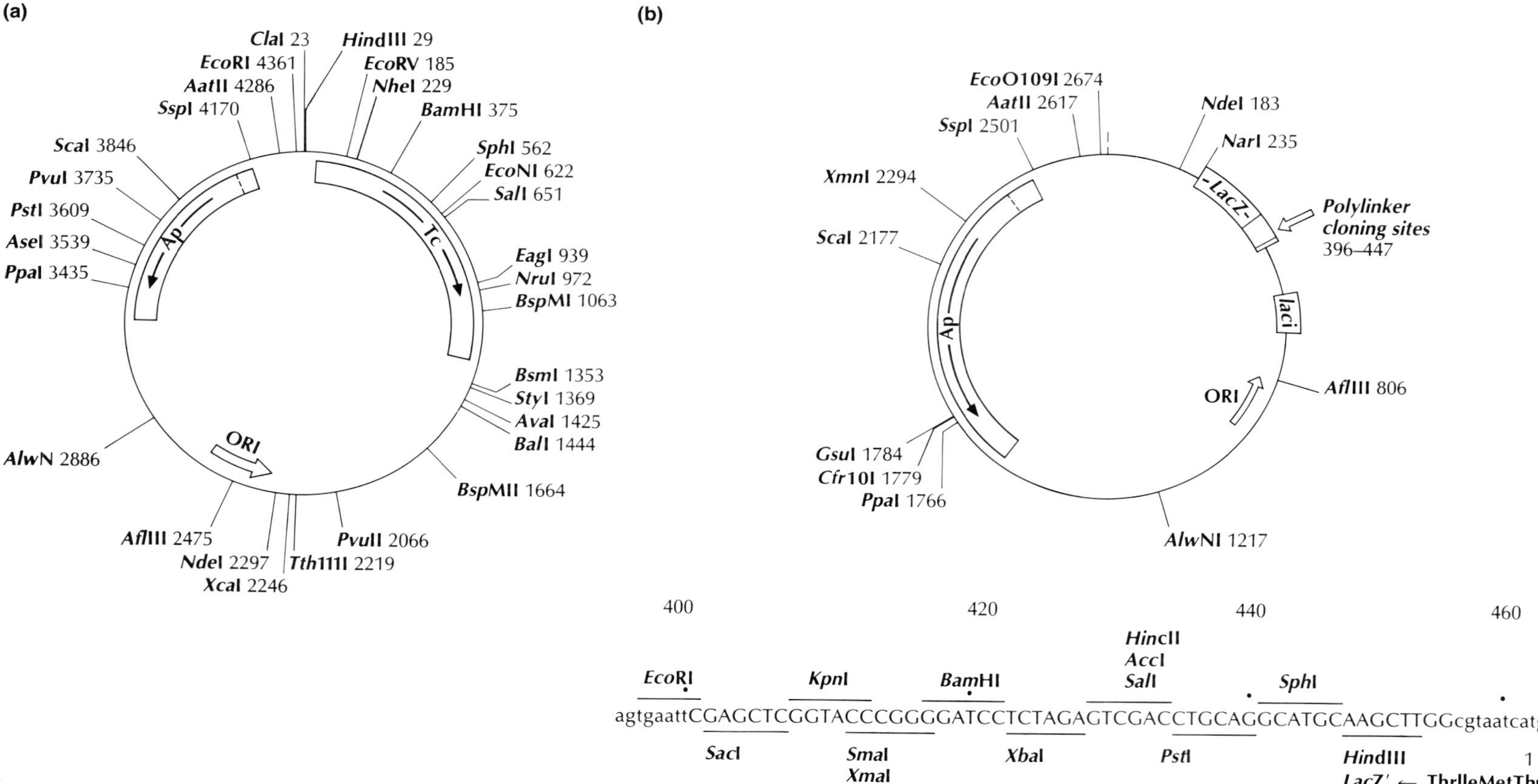

Fig. 41.2. Restriction maps of (a) pBR322 and (b) pUC19. (a) pBR322, which is an *E. coli* plasmid cloning vehicle, is a double-stranded DNA circle 4363 bp in length. Numbering of the sequence begins within the unique *Eco*RI site; the first T in the sequence GAATTC is designated as nucleotide number 1. Numbering then continues around the molecule in a clockwise direction. The map shows the restriction sites of those enzymes that cut the DNA once. Tc is the tetracycline resistance gene, Ap is the ampicillin resistance gene and ORI is the origin of DNA replication. (b) pUC19 is also an *E. coli* plasmid cloning vehicle, but is only 2686 bp in length. Numbering starts at the first T in the sequence TCGCGCGTTT and proceeds in a clockwise direction. The map shows the restriction sites of those enzymes that cut the DNA once. The polylinker, which contains sites for 13 different 6 bp specific restriction enzymes, is shown below the map. Ap is the ampicillin resistance gene, *lac*Z encodes β-galactosidase and ORI is the origin of DNA replication.

of rare-cutter RE sites (Lindsay and Bird 1987; Sargent *et al*. 1989a).

OTHER ENZYMES

Table 41.2 summarizes the properties and uses of some of the other enzymes frequently used in molecular biology. All of these enzymes are readily available from commercial suppliers.

Cloning vectors

In order to obtain large quantities of a specific DNA molecule, the DNA is introduced into a

Table 41.2. Properties of some enzymes frequently used in molecular biology

RE methylase	Methylates RE site to render it resistant to cleavage by the RE	Taq polymerase	DNA polymerase which can synthesize DNA at high temperatures
T4 DNA ligase	Catalyses the formation of a phosphodiester bond between juxtaposed 5′ phosphate and 3′ hydroxyl termini in double-stranded DNA	Alkaline phosphatase	Removes the 3′ phosphate from the ends of DNA fragments
T4 RNA ligase	Catalyses the ligation of 5′ phosphoryl-terminated single-strand RNA or DNA to a 3′ hydroxyl-terminated RNA or DNA acceptor	Terminal transferase	Incorporates oligodeoxynucleotide tails on to the 3′ ends of DNA fragments
T4 polynucleotide kinase	Catalyses the transfer of γ-PO_4 group from γ-ATP to the 5′ hydroxyl terminus of DNA fragments	DNase 1	Digests single- and double-stranded DNA to oligodeoxyribonucleotides
Reverse transcriptase	Synthesizes a complementary DNA strand from either a single-stranded RNA or a DNA template	S1 nuclease	Single-strand specific endonuclease which hydrolyses single-strand RNA or DNA into 5′ mononucleotides
DNA polymerase 1	Synthesizes a complementary DNA strand from a single-stranded DNA template. Also used to convert 5′ overhangs on RE fragments to blunt ends. Also possesses 3′–5′ and 5′–3′ exonuclease activity	Nuclease BAL-31	Single-strand specific endodeoxyribonuclease. Also has 3′ and 5′ exonuclease activity that simultaneously degrades both the 3′ and 5′ termini of duplex DNA
DNA polymerase 1 large fragment (Klenow fragment)	Has polymerase and 3′–5′ exonuclease activity, but lacks 5′–3′ exonuclease activity	Ribonuclease A	Endoribonuclease that cleaves RNA at the 3′-adjacent phosphodiester bond of pyrimidine nucleotides
SP6 or T7 RNA polymerase	Synthesizes RNA copy of DNA cloned into vectors which contain the SP6 or T7 phage promoters	Ribonuclease H	Endoribonuclease which specifically degrades the RNA strand of an RNA–DNA hybrid to produce 5′ phosphate-terminated oligoribonucleotides and single-strand DNA

suitable host in a form which can replicate within the host. By suitable selection, a line of genetically identical organisms is obtained containing the DNA of interest, which may be propagated in bulk, i.e. the DNA molecule has been cloned. An obvious prerequisite is the ability to easily re-isolate the cloned DNA from the host. Cloning vectors are DNA molecules which allow replication and reisolation of a DNA molecule in an appropriate host. It should be pointed out, however, that the advent of the polymerase chain reaction (PCR) makes it possible to obtain large quantities of a particular DNA sequence without the need for cloning in many circumstances (see below).

Escherichia coli has been the traditional host of choice for molecular cloning experiments. However, the many advantages of cloning in the yeast, *Saccharomyces cerevisiae*, mean that it is an increasingly attractive system for certain applications. Initially the discussion will be confined to *E. coli*-based cloning vectors.

Escherichia coli cloning vectors utilize the functional elements of natural bacteriophages and plasmids, which possess their own DNA replication origins. The original phage or plasmid DNA molecules have been engineered to possess a number of desirable features such as convenient restriction sites into which to insert foreign DNA fragments, selectable phenotypes to distinguish recombinants, and optimization of cloning capacity and copy number. Descriptions of the biology of *E. coli* plasmids and phage can be found in Hardy (1981, 1987) and Hendrix *et al*. (1983). Restriction maps of commonly used vectors can be found in the catalogues of many commercial suppliers.

PLASMID VECTORS

A large number of plasmid vectors are available for cloning in *E. coli*, most of which are based on the *Col*E1 replication origin. The prototypic plasmid cloning vector is pBR322 (Bolivar *et al*. 1977). In addition to the replication origin, pBR322 contains genes for resistance to ampicillin and tetracycline, and a number of unique restriction sites (Fig. 41.2). For cloning, pBR322 is cleaved with an RE that cuts at a unique site, for instance *Pst*I. The resulting linear molecule may be treated with phosphatase, which prevents recircularization of the vector during ligation, and restriction fragments with compatible ends are ligated into the cloning site (Fig. 41.3). The recombinant molecules are used to transform competent *E. coli* cells. The most widely used transformation protocol involves precipitation of the recombinant plasmid DNA on to cells that have been treated with $CaCl_2$ and gives $\sim 10^7$ transformants/μg of DNA (Mandel and Higa 1970). However, Hanahan (1983) has made a detailed study of transformation conditions and has developed protocols which yield higher transformation efficiencies. These methods should be considered when the desired clone may be rare. Competent cells giving high transformation efficiencies are available from a number of commercial sources.

Depending on the cloning strategy, bacteria containing the recombinants may be selected for antibiotic resistance, inactivation of antibiotic resistance if the foreign DNA fragment is inserted into a restriction site within one of the antibiotic resistance genes, hybridization with a probe complementary to the inserted DNA or restriction analysis of DNA isolated from a number of transformants (Sambrook *et al*. 1989). Deoxyribonucleic acid from positive clones can be readily isolated away from *E. coli* chromosomal DNA by caesium chloride gradient centrifugation (Radloff *et al*. 1967) or more frequently and conveniently by a rapid 'miniprep' method (Birnboim and Doly 1979).

Another commonly used vector is pAT153, which also encodes ampicillin and tetracycline resistance but grows at a slightly higher copy number than pBR322 (Twigg and Sherratt 1980). The pUC line of vectors (Yanisch-Perron *et al*. 1985) contain only an ampicillin resistance gene and are correspondingly smaller giving higher copy number. In addition pUC plasmids contain the *E. coli lac*Z gene, which expresses the α-peptide of β-galactosidase, as well as the lac regulatory gene (Fig. 41.2). Presence of the pUC plasmid will complement a lacΔM15 mutation in the host to produce functional β-galactosidase, giving blue colonies when grown on medium containing isopropyl-β-D-thiogalactoside (IPTG), 5-bromo-4-chloro-3-indolyl-β-D-galactoside (X-gal) and ampicillin. Insertion of foreign DNA into a restriction site within the multipurpose cloning site disrupts the α-complementation and results in white plaques. Hence there is a colour assay for detecting recombinants.

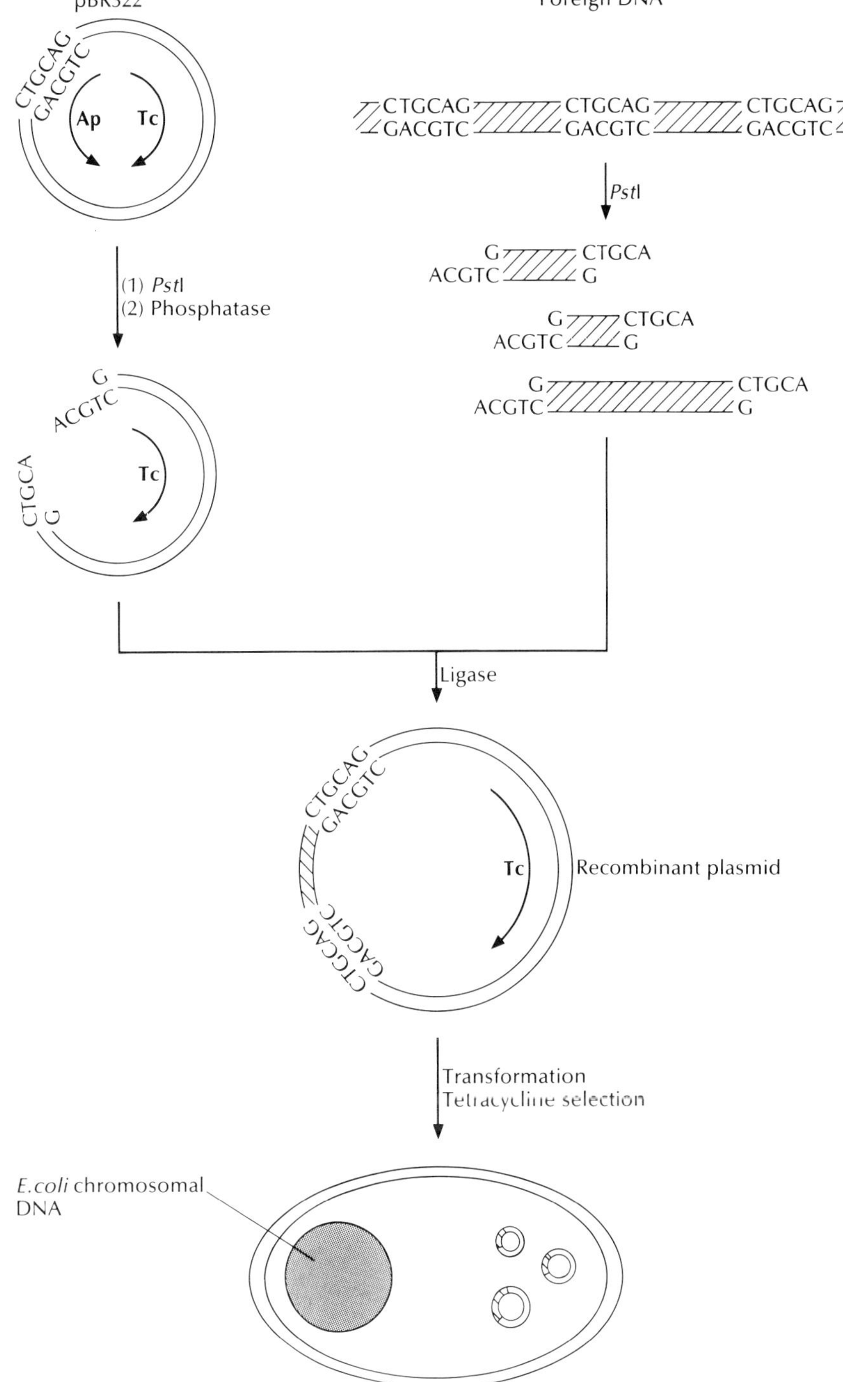

Fig. 41.3. Steps involved in cloning a restriction fragment into a plasmid. In this example pBR322 is cleaved with *Pst*I at the unique *Pst*I site within the Ap gene. The DNA is treated with phosphatase, which removes the 5′ phosphate group and prevents T4 DNA ligase from recircularizing the DNA. The foreign DNA is digested to completion with *Pst*I. The restriction fragments are incubated with the vector in the presence of ligase, which joins a DNA fragment to the vector to reform a closed, circular molecule that can be propagated in an *E. coli* strain such as MC1061. *Escherichia coli* containing the recombinant plasmids are selected for on agar plates containing tetracycline.

Several recently developed vectors based on the pUC vectors also contain an f1 phage replication origin, so-called phagemids (Short *et al.* 1988). These vectors can be used to directly rescue single-stranded DNA suitable for sequencing via infection with helper phage. Other vectors contain promoters for the T3, T7 or SP6 phage polymerases so that single-stranded RNA hybridization probes can be produced from the cloned insert, e.g. the pSP vectors (Melton *et al.* 1984). Obviously the appropriate choice of vector depends on the anticipated application.

BACTERIOPHAGE VECTORS

Bacteriophage lambda (λ) is the most intensively studied *E. coli* phage and has formed the basis for a number of widely used vectors (Hendrix *et al.* 1983). The major advantage of the use of λ vectors is that the recombinant DNA is packaged into phage particles and hence can be introduced into *E. coli* by the normal phage infection pathway (Hohn and Murray 1977); this circumvents the need for transformation and results in higher cloning efficiency.

Lambda vectors can be classified as either insertion or replacement vectors. Insertion vectors have single cloning sites and may accept fragments up to 10 kb. Replacement vectors are used to clone larger fragments (9–23 kb) by replacing non-essential regions of λ (the stuffer fragment) by the foreign DNA fragment. The λ packaging system requires that the recombinant molecules are 78–106% of the size of wild-type λ DNA. A number of genetic systems are available to ensure the presence of recombinant molecules and DNA is isolated from positive clones by methods which purify the intact phage away from *E. coli* chromosomal DNA (Hohn 1979).

COSMIDS

Cosmids are small plasmid vectors which, in addition to a replication origin and antibiotic resistance gene, contain a λ *cos* site (Collins and Hohn 1978; Ish-Horowicz and Burke 1981). Deoxyribonucleic acid may be packaged into λ phage particles using *in vitro* packaging extracts, if it contains *cos* sites separated by 35–50 kb. Therefore, if foreign DNA fragments of 30–45 kb are ligated into cosmid vectors, the recombinants may be packaged into phage particles and used to infect *E. coli*. Inside the bacteria the cosmid DNA replicates as a large circular plasmid. Thus cosmid vectors have a large DNA cloning capacity, of use in chromosome walking experiments (Bender *et al.* 1983; Hood *et al.* 1983; see also below).

M13 VECTORS

The M13mp series of vectors are derived from the filamentous coliphage, M13 (Messing 1983; Yanisch-Perron *et al.* 1985). This phage contains single-stranded DNA that infects F′ bacteria. Double-stranded replicative form (RF) intermediates arise during replication and the infected cells extrude phage particles containing single-stranded DNA. The M13 system has, therefore, provided a convenient means to clone DNA fragments and obtain single-stranded DNA for dideoxy-DNA sequencing (Sanger *et al.* 1977, 1982; see also below). Single-stranded DNA can also be used for site-directed mutagenesis (Kunkel *et al.* 1987). The M13mp vectors contain various arrays of cloning sites, 'polylinkers', within the 5′ end of the *lacZ* gene. To use as a cloning vector, the RF form of the vector is isolated and cleaved with an appropriate RE. The vector is treated with phosphatase, and foreign DNA fragments are ligated into the cloning site. Recombinants may be transformed into competent *E. coli* and identified as colourless plaques, since insertion disrupts the *lacZ* gene. Although M13 infection does not lyse the bacteria, growth is significantly inhibited, producing turbid plaques. Single-stranded DNA is isolated from the medium after culturing cells from a single plaque.

Techniques

Electrophoresis of deoxyribonucleic acid

Deoxyribonucleic acid can be separated on the basis of size by electrophoresis through both agarose and polyacrylamide gels (Sambrook *et al.* 1989), with mobility being inversely proportional to the logarithm of molecular weight. The relative mobility of a given DNA molecule is also affected by the concentration of the agarose or polyacrylamide in the gel, with higher concentrations resulting in increased resolution of smaller DNA fragments. It should be noted, however, that circular and supercoiled DNA molecules migrate anomalously. Generally electrophoresis in agarose gels is used to separate DNA fragments in the 0.5–30 kb size range, while polyacrylamide gel electrophoresis (PAGE) is used for DNA fragments <1.0 kb in size (Sambrook *et al.* 1989), although sieving agaroses are available which will separate small DNA fragments (FMC Bioproducts). Deoxyribonucleic acid molecules of known size, for instance restriction fragments of λ DNA, are typically electrophoresed as size markers. The positions of the DNA fragments can be detected

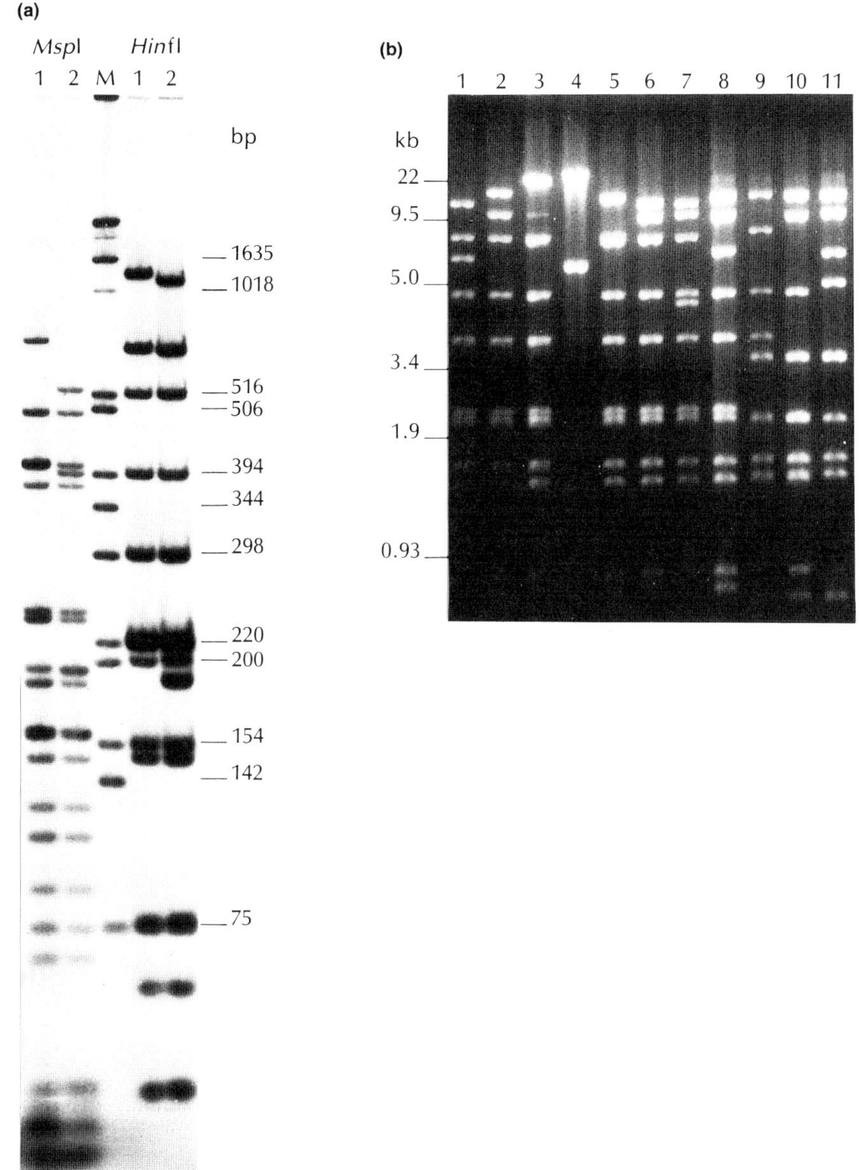

Fig. 41.4. Separation of DNA restriction fragments by (a) polyacrylamide gel electrophoresis and (b) agarose gel electrophoresis. (a) Two different DNA samples have been digested with *Msp*I or *Hin*fI and then electrophoresed on a 4% polyacrylamide gel. The useful separation of these gels is from a few base pairs to ~2000 bp. The marker fragments whose sizes are given on the right are from a *Hin*f1 digest of pBR322. (b) *BamHI* digests of a number of cosmids from the Class III region of the human MHC, which contain the C2 and factor B genes. The digests have been electrophoresed on a 0.8% agarose gel. The useful separation of these gels is from ~0.1 kb to ~30 kb. The marker fragments whose sizes are given on the left are from an *Eco*RI/*Hin*dIII double digest of λ DNA.

by staining the gel with the intercalating dye, ethidium bromide, and observing fluorescence in UV light (Sharpe *et al.* 1973). For PAGE DNA fragments may also be end-labelled radioactively and separation visualized by autoradiography. Figure 41.4 shows examples of electrophoretic separations of DNA fragments. Thus, gel electrophoresis can be used to determine the size of fragments produced by RE digestion of DNA molecules, so that restriction maps can be constructed, and can be used to purify a specific RE fragment from a complex mixture.

Southern and Northern blotting

Often it is desirable to localize particular nucleotide sequences to a specific restriction fragment, for instance to establish the position of a sequence on the restriction map of a clone or to identify sequences within digests of complex source DNA. Southern blotting is a powerful technique that allows DNA fragments separated by agarose gel electrophoresis to be analysed by hybridization methods (Southern 1975, 1979).

After agarose gel electrophoresis, the gel is stained and photographed to record the positions of the DNA fragments. The DNA is then denatured within the gel and transferred to a membrane. In this way the relative positions of the DNA fragments in the gel are preserved. The immobilized DNA is then hybridized with the labelled probe of interest, and the positions of hybridizing sequences are detected by appropriate means, usually autoradiography.

Figures 41.5 and 41.6 show two examples of Southern blot experiments. In Fig. 41.5 *Bam*HI RE digests of DNA from a set of overlapping cosmid clones covering ~300 kb of the Class III region of the human major histocompatibility complex (MHC) were fractionated on a 0.8% agarose gel (Sargent *et al.* 1989b). The gel was Southern-blotted and the membrane hybridized with a radiolabelled oligonucleotide complementary to part of the human heat-shock protein 70 (hsp70) gene sequence. After washing and autoradiography, hybridization to a 7 kb (which turned out to be a doublet) and a 4.8 kb *Bam*HI fragment in

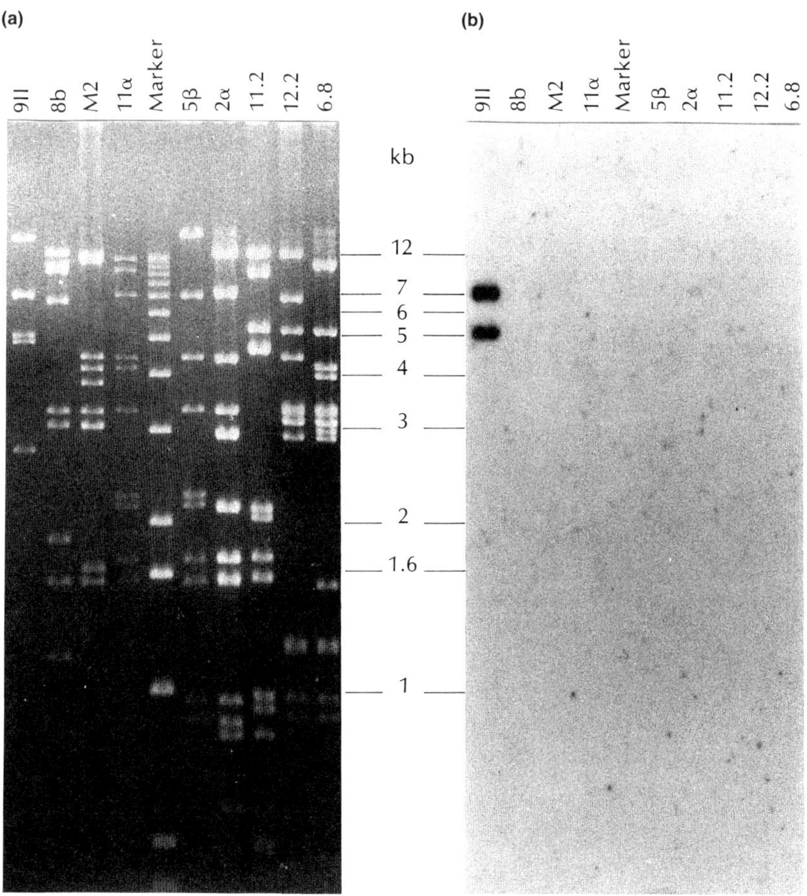

Fig. 41.5. Southern blot hybridization analysis showing that an HSP70 oligonucleotide hybridizes only to fragments from cosmid 9II. Cosmid DNA containing ~300 kb of genomic DNA from the HLA Class III region was digested with *Bam*HI, and the digests were fractionated on a 0.8% agarose gel. After straining the gel with ethidium bromide (a) to visualize the position of the DNA fragments, the fragments were transferred by Southern blotting to nitrocellulose and hybridized with a 26 base long oligonucleotide corresponding to nucleotides 31–56 of the human HSP70 gene. After autoradiography for 5 hours (b) the HSP70 oligonucleotide was found to hybridize only to 4.8 and 7 kb *Bam*HI fragments from the cosmid 9II. The marker is the BRL 1 kb ladder.

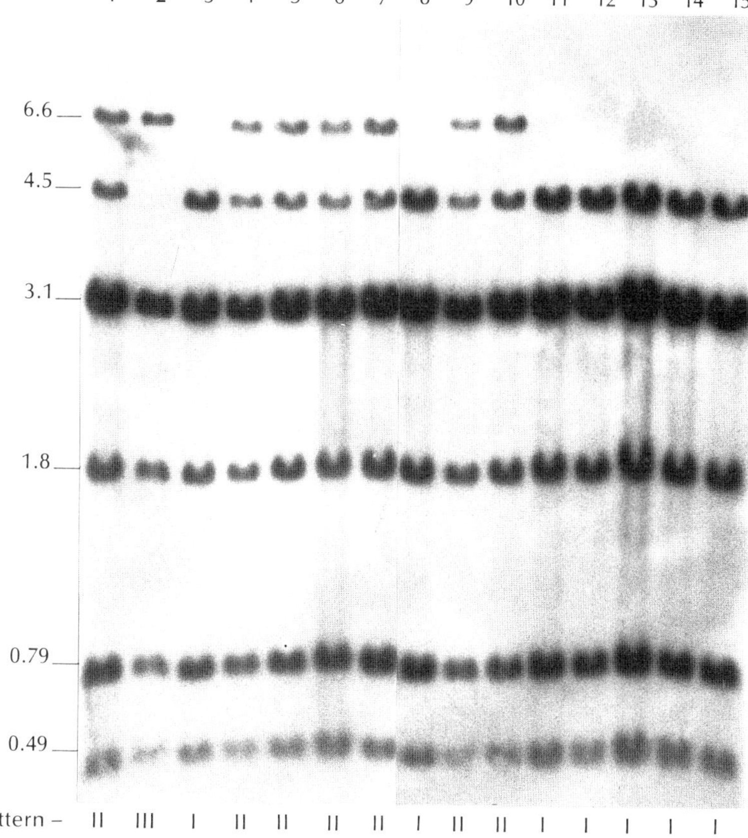

Fig. 41.6. Southern blot hybridization analysis. *Taq* I-digested genomic DNA from 15 individuals was fractionated on a 0.7% agarose gel and transferred by Southern blotting to a nitrocellulose membrane. The blot was hybridized with the full-length factor B cDNA probe. After washing the blot and autoradiography three different patterns of fragments were visualized. Pattern I is illustrated in lanes 3, 8 and 11–15 and has fragments at 4.5 kb, 3.1 kb, 1.8 kb, 0.79 kb and 0.49 kb, pattern II is illustrated in lanes 1, 4–7 and 9–10 and has fragments at 6.6 kb, 4.5 kb, 3.1 kb, 1.8 kb, 0.79 kb and 0.49 kb, while pattern III is illustrated in lane 2 and has fragments at 6.6 kb, 3.1 kb, 1.8 kb, 0.79 kb and 0.49 kb.

the DNA from cosmid clone 9II was observed. This result provided strong evidence that genes for human hsp70 were located within the Class III region of the human MHC (Sargent *et al.* 1989b). In Fig. 41.6 total genomic DNA isolated from several individuals was digested with the RE *Taq*I, Southern-blotted and hybridized with a full-length factor B complementary DNA (cDNA) (see below) probe. Three different patterns of fragments were observed. Four fragments (3.1 kb, 1.8 kb, 0.79 kb and 0.49 kb) are common to all the samples. However, the 4.5 kb fragment in pattern I was absent in pattern III, which had a 6.6 kb fragment, while pattern II had both of these fragments. Individuals with both the 4.5 kb and 6.6 kb fragments are heterozygous while individuals with patterns I and III are homozygous for the 4.5 kb and 6.6 kb *Taq*I fragments, respectively (Cross *et al.* 1985). This is an example of a restriction fragment length polymorphism (RFLP), where a mutation has resulted in the loss or gain of a particular RE site such that the size of the fragment that hybridizes to the probe is altered. Restriction fragment length polymorphisms associated with coding regions or anonymous DNA probes can be used as genetic markers for linkage analysis (Donis-Keller *et al.* 1987; Nakamura *et al.* 1987).

A number of variations are available for Southern blotting protocols. If the DNA to be transferred is large (>5–10 kb), it is necessary to partially nick the DNA to facilitate transfer. This may be achieved either by acid depurination (Wahl *et al.* 1979) or by prolonged exposure of ethidium bromide-stained DNA to UV light. Nitrocellulose has been the most widely used membrane, but it is fragile and does not readily survive multiple hybridizations. Additionally, the DNA is not covalently bound to the membrane, resulting in loss of signal intensity with repeated use. Nylon-backed nitrocellulose membranes are more robust while retaining the binding characteristics of nitrocellulose. Nylon and activated nylon membranes have the advantage that the DNA can be covalently cross-linked to the membrane (Church and Gilbert 1984). Using nylon membranes it is also possible to transfer the DNA from the gel under denaturing conditions, so-called alkaline blotting (Reed and Mann 1985), which produces stronger signals and sharper bands. In the classic Southern blot protocol, transfer is by capillary action, although faster transfer can be achieved by vacuum suction or electroblotting.

The blot transfer technique can be adapted to analyse sequences present in RNA samples, 'Northern' blotting (Lehrach *et al.* 1977; Fourney *et al.* 1988). Ribonucleic acid is isolated from fresh or frozen tissue and may be enriched for polyadenylated messenger RNA (mRNA) by chromatography on oligo-dT cellulose (Aviv and Leder 1972; Wahl *et al.* 1979; Sambrook *et al.* 1989). The RNA is separated by electrophoresis in agarose gels containing a denaturing agent such that mobility is inversely proportional to the logarithm of molecular weight. Denatured single-stranded DNA fragments or specially prepared RNA molecules are electrophoresed as markers, although the positions of the intensely staining 28S and 18S ribosomal RNA (rRNA) bands in total RNA may also serve this purpose. The RNA may be visualized by staining with ethidium bromide although some believe this inhibits transfer (Sambrook *et al.* 1989). The RNA is transferred on to an appropriate membrane and hybridized as above. Figure 41.7 shows an autoradiograph of a Northern blot filter which has been hybridized with the full-length factor B cDNA. The 2.6 kb mRNA is detected in liver and in the human hepatoma cell line HepG2. However, the factor B mRNA is not detected in two cell lines known not to synthesize factor B, the human epithelial cell line HeLa and the mouse fibroblast cell line Ltk −ve (Wu *et al.* 1987).

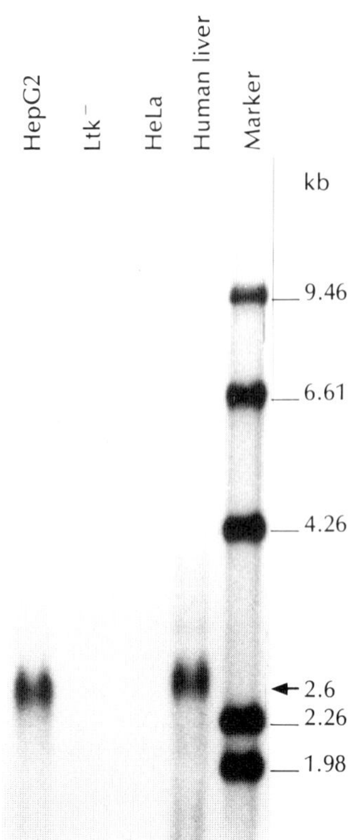

Fig. 41.7. Northern blot analysis. Total cytoplasmic RNA (20 μg), isolated from human liver, from the human cell lines HepG2 and HeLa, and from the mouse cell line Ltk$^-$, was fractionated in a 0.8% agarose formaldehyde gel, transferred by blotting on to a nylon membrane and hybridized with the nick-translated full-length factor B cDNA probe. The marker (M) was an end-filled *Hin*dIII digest of λ DNA.

Pulsed field gel electrophoresis

Many genes encoding proteins involved in immunity are large or are arranged in large gene complexes covering hundreds of kilobases such as the MHC (Dunham *et al.* 1987), the immunoglobulin heavy chain variable region genes (Matsuda *et al.* 1988), the T cell receptor genes (Davis and Bjorkman 1988) and the regulators of complement activation (RCA) cluster (Carroll *et al.* 1988; Rey-Campos *et al.* 1988). When analysing the genomic organization of these regions, it would be useful to be able to separate large DNA fragments. However, conventional agarose gel electrophoresis will separate DNA up to only 30–50 kb in size. Gel electrophoresis using very low agarose concentration can increase this upper size limit, but is impractical for routine use. Schwartz and Cantor (1984) realized that, if DNA molecules were subjected to electric fields of alternating orientation, a novel mechanism of separation would result. Thus the technique of PFGE was developed, and it is now possible to separate DNA molecules up to 10 000 kb. A number of improvements to and variations on the original concept have been developed, making the technique routinely applicable (Carle *et al.* 1986; Chu *et al.* 1986; Gardiner *et al.* 1986; Southern *et al.* 1987; Clark *et al.* 1988).

The mobility of DNA molecules during PFGE is more or less linearly dependent upon molecular weight within the size range of optimal resolution. The size range of molecules that can be resolved is dependent upon the time interval between switching the alternating fields (Schwartz and Cantor

1984; Birren *et al.* 1988). In general, the longer the switching interval, the larger the size of DNA that can be separated. The mechanism for the separation is still unclear but several papers have recently appeared on this subject (Deutsch 1988; Schwartz and Koval 1989; Smith *et al.* 1989).

In order to apply PFGE to analysis of the mammalian genome, it is necessary to prepare DNA of high molecular weight and to be able to generate large restriction fragments. High-molecular-weight DNA can be prepared by encapsulating cells in agarose blocks (van Ommen and Verkerk 1986) and treating the cells with protease and detergent. The DNA in agarose blocks can then be digested with REs that cut infrequently in the mammalian genome (Brown and Bird 1986; see also above). Digested DNA is separated by PFGE, using concatemers of λ DNA (Waterbury and Lane 1986) or yeast chromosomes (Schwartz and Cantor 1984) as size markers, and then may be subjected to conventional Southern blot analysis.

Figure 41.8 shows typical PFGE separations of RE-digested high-molecular-weight human DNA on the crossed field gel electrophoresis system of Southern *et al.* (1987). Figure 41.9 shows the result of Southern blot analysis of *Not*I-digested DNA that had been separated on the orthogonal field alternation gel electrophoresis (OFAGE) system (Carle *et al.* 1986). The same Southern blot filter was hybridized successively with DQA, DRA and C4 gene probes, stripping the filter of signal between each hybridization. Autoradiography revealed that each probe hybridized to a 980 kb *Not*I fragment, implying physical linkage of the DR and DQ subregions of the human MHC with the C4 gene (Dunham *et al.* 1987). Hybridization of the same filter with a DPA probe identified a 340 kb *Not*I fragment. A complete analysis of gene organization in this way requires the construction of a conventional restriction map (see, for example, Brown and Bird 1986; Hardy *et al.* 1986; Dunham *et al.* 1987).

Pulsed field gel electrophoresis can also be used in conjunction with Southern blotting to compare the genomic organization between DNA isolated from different individuals (Dunham *et al.* 1989) or

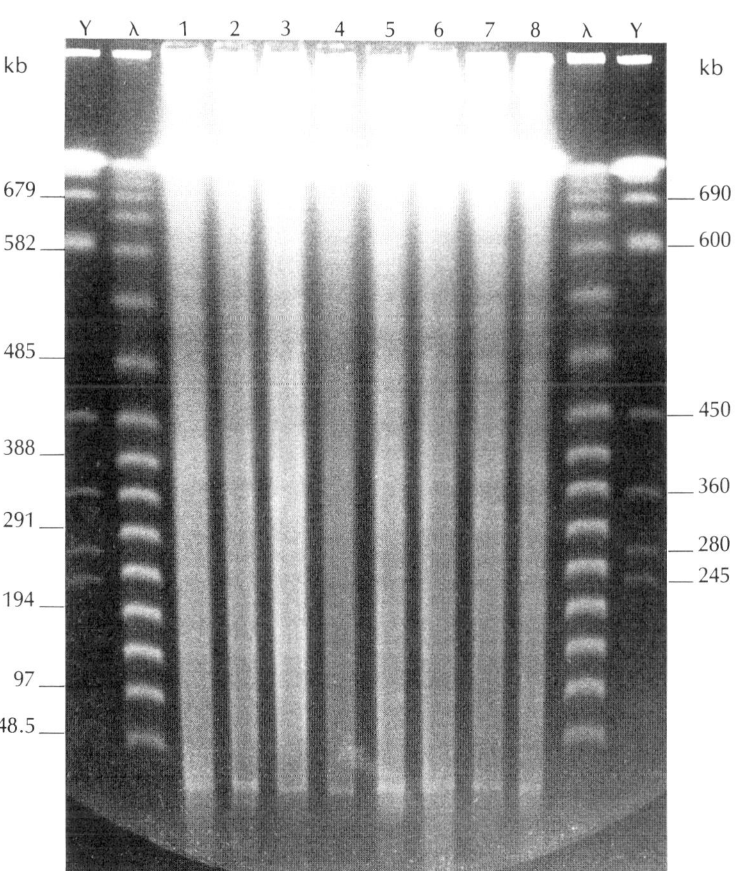

Fig. 41.8. Separation of restriction digests of genomic DNA by pulsed field gel electrophoresis. *Mlu*I-digested genomic DNA was fractionated on the crossed-field gel electrophoresis system of Southern *et al.* (1987) at a 30 second switching interval. Note that the tracks are straight, allowing easy comparison between lanes. The marker sizes on the left correspond to concatemers of λ DNA, while the marker sizes on the right correspond to yeast chromosomes.

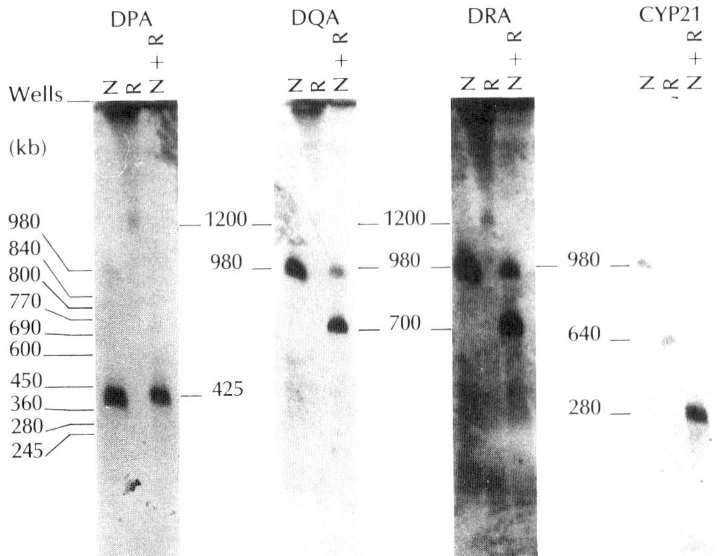

Fig. 41.9. Southern blot hybridization analysis of genomic DNA separated by OFAGE. Fragments generated by *Not*I (N), *Nru*I (R) and *Not*I + *Nru*I digests of genomic DNA were fractionated using a 65 second pulse interval, and transferred by Southern blotting to a nylon membrane which was hybridized sequentially with the probes shown. Yeast chromosomes were electrophoresed as size markers and are indicated on the left. Fragment sizes are given in kb.

to isolate specific DNA fragments for cloning experiments (Michiels *et al.* 1987).

Complementary deoxyribonucleic acid cloning

Complementary DNA cloning refers to the isolation of a cDNA copy of a specific mRNA. Complementary DNA cloning allows the study of the sequences comprising an mRNA transcript, double-stranded cDNA being far easier to handle and manipulate than mRNA. The information contained in a cDNA clone predicts the protein sequence. Therefore isolation of a cDNA clone is the obvious course if protein sequence is required, if expression of the protein in prokaryotic or eukaryotic systems is planned, for site-directed mutagenesis and for study of the sites and levels of expression of the mRNA.

Having decided to isolate a cDNA clone, there are two major issues to address. The first is to devise an appropriate screening procedure, since the correct clone may only be present at one copy in 10^5 or 10^6. Secondly, it is essential to choose the correct library to screen. The method of screening depends on the information that is available. If the mRNA of interest comprises a high percentage of the polyadenylated mRNA in a particular tissue, it may be possible to pick clones at random and sequence the cloned cDNA (Sambrook *et al.* 1989). However, in the vast majority of current applications the desired species is present at low levels in a complex population of mRNA and it is necessary to screen a large number of clones.

The preferred methods are either hybridization to the cloned DNA immobilized on filters or identification of expression of a particular antigen or biological activity (Huynh *et al.* 1985). Hybridization probes may be oligonucleotides based on available protein sequence (Suggs *et al.* 1981), other cDNA probes if homology is predicted (for instance if the cDNA has been cloned in another species or if it encodes a highly related protein) or a genomic DNA probe that is thought to contain coding sequence. In the case of oligonucleotides a region of the protein that would be encoded by the least degenerate DNA sequence and that is at the C-terminal end of the protein should be chosen, cDNA libraries generally being enriched for the 3′ ends of mRNA. When using an antibody-based screening procedure, it is necessary that the antibody does not cross-react with other antigenic determinants.

The choice of cDNA library is based on finding a tissue that expresses the desired mRNA at high levels, since the number of clones that must be screened is determined by its abundance. It is quite possible that the appropriate library has already been made and is available either from other investigators, the American Type Culture Collection (12301 Perlawn Drive, Rockville, Maryland 20852, USA) or commercial sources. It is also desirable that the library should contain a high proportion of true 5′ ends rather than truncated or rearranged cDNAs. For large mRNAs the chance of this is increased if the insert DNA is large.

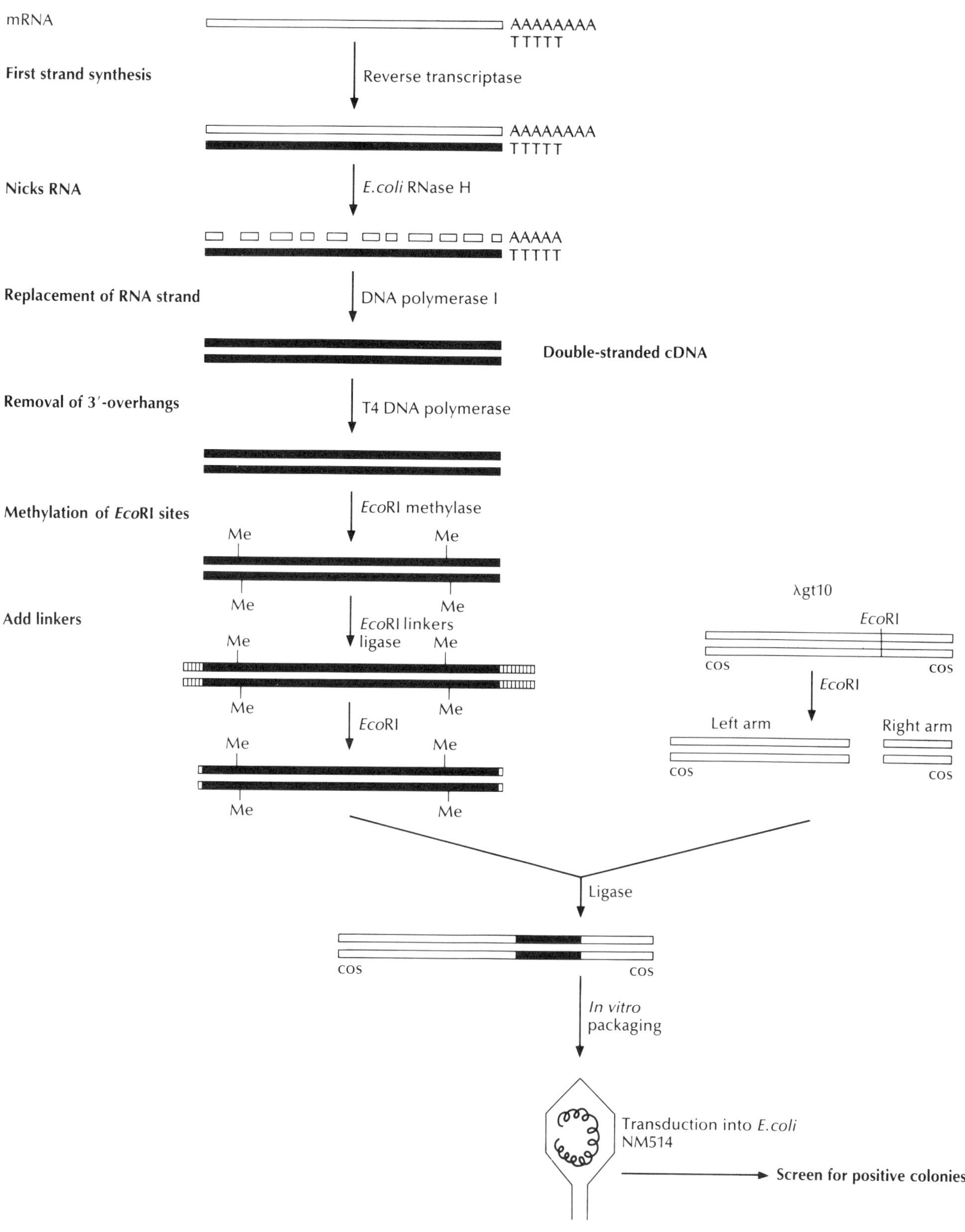

Fig. 41.10. Preparation of a cDNA library. Oligo-dT hybridizes to the poly (A) tail and serves as a primer for reverse transcriptase, which synthesizes a cDNA copy of the mRNA. Ribonuclease H creates nicks in the mRNA strand and then DNA polymerase I catalyses replacement of the RNA strand. The double-stranded DNA is made blunt-ended by the action of T4 DNA polymerase. The cloning strategy involves the ligation of the cDNA into *Eco*RI-cut λgt10 (or λgt11). This is achieved by the methylation of *Eco*RI sites in the cDNA by *Eco*RI methylase and the ligation of *Eco*RI linkers to the cDNA, followed by cleavage of the linkers to a single site using *Eco*RI. After ligation of the cDNA to the λgt10 (or λgt11) arms, the mixture is packaged *in vitro*, using λ packaging extracts prior to the transduction of a suitable *E. coli* strain such as NM514.

A number of schemes have been devised for producing cDNA libraries. The approach that is currently considered optimal is outlined in Fig. 41.10 (Gubler and Hoffmann 1983). Using this method, full-length cDNAs of 5–8 kb are obtainable. It is essential to start with high-quality mRNA, free from contaminating nuclease, and generally selected for polyA + mRNA. The first step is to synthesize a DNA strand complementary to the mRNA, using reverse transcriptase primed by oligo-dT, thereby producing an mRNA–DNA hybrid (Sambrook *et al.* 1989). A second DNA strand is then synthesized by replacement synthesis of the RNA by *E. coli* DNA polymerase I, initiated at nicks introduced in the RNA by ribonuclease (RNase) H (Okayama and Berg 1982). Second-strand synthesis is completed by ligation to repair the nicks, filling single-stranded overhangs with dNTPs to produce blunt ends. The *Eco*RI sites within the cDNA are methylated by *Eco*RI methylase to render them resistant to cleavage. Synthetic *Eco*RI linkers are ligated to the cDNA and digested with *Eco*RI, and cDNA that is ready to be cloned is finally purified away from free linkers (Ausubel *et al.* 1987). The cDNA may be size fractionated at this point to select for large inserts. If the mRNA is large or clones from the 5′ end are not present in the library, the first-strand synthesis can be primed by oligonucleotides of random sequence or a sequence specific to the desired mRNA.

The cDNA may be cloned into either plasmid or λ insertion vectors. If the cDNA is expected to be rare and many recombinants are to be screened, λ vectors are recommended since they give higher cloning efficiencies. The cDNA is ligated into the λ vector and the recombinants packaged into phage heads *in vitro* and infected into *E. coli*. The two vectors commonly in use, λgt10 and λgt11, are both insertion vectors designed for cloning *Eco*RI fragments up to 7 kb (Huynh *et al.* 1985). In both cases left and right vector arms are prepared from purified vector DNA and dephosphorylated. In λgt10, cDNA with cleaved *Eco*RI linkers is ligated into the *Eco*RI site in the repressor cI gene, allowing recombinants to form plaques on Hfl *E. coli* strains while non-recombinants lysogenize and do not form plaques. The recombinant library is screened by plating phage, taking replica plaque lifts on to filter membranes, and then lysing the phage *in situ* and hybridizing with the DNA probe. Insertion of cDNA into the *Eco*RI site in λgt11 interrupts the β-galactosidase gene in the vector and hence recombinant plaques are colourless in the presence of IPTG and X-gal. λgt11 libraries may be screened by DNA hybridization or using antibodies since the peptide-coding regions of the cDNA are fused to the 5′ end of the β-galactosidase gene. It should be noted that many more clones must be screened with an antibody since the cDNA is only fused in the correct reading-frame one time out of every six.

When a positive clone is identified in a primary library screen, it is usually contaminated with other undesired clones. Thus the positive area of the plated library is removed, replated and rescreened. Characterization of positive clones includes RE mapping and DNA sequencing.

Novel approaches to cDNA cloning utilize the PCR (see below) to generate probes based on predicted protein sequence, or to clone allelic variants from cDNA libraries or total RNA using conserved primary sequence.

Deoxyribonucleic acid sequencing

There are two methods to rapidly determine the DNA sequence of a cloned DNA molecule, the chemical cleavage method (Maxam and Gilbert 1977, 1980) and the enzymatic chain terminator method (Sanger *et al.* 1977, 1982). The principle of both methods is broadly similar. A set of labelled DNA fragments is generated which possess one fixed end and which differ in length by single nucleotides. The sequence is determined by four separate partial reactions, each specific to one or two bases, which produce sets of molecules some of which terminate at every occurrence of that base in the DNA sequence. The single-stranded products of the four reactions are separated side by side on a high-resolution denaturing acrylamide gel which can resolve single base size differences. The sequence is read from the ladder of fragments visualized on the gel, as illustrated in Figs 41.11 and 41.12.

MAXAM AND GILBERT CHEMICAL CLEAVAGE

In the Maxam and Gilbert chemical cleavage sequencing method (Maxam and Gilbert 1977, 1980), purified 3′ or 5′ end-labelled single-stranded, or

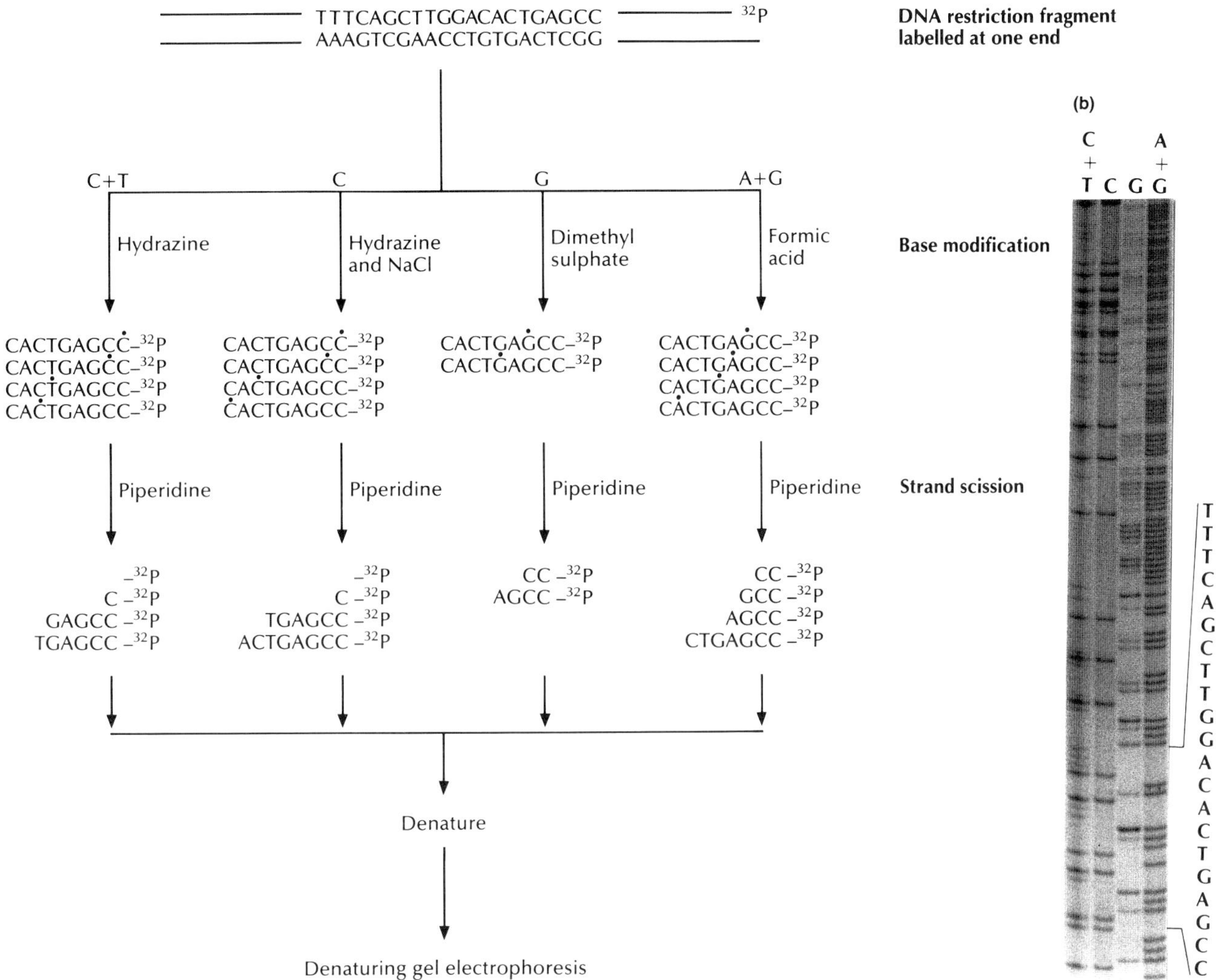

Fig. 41.11. Maxam–Gilbert sequence analysis. (a) A uniquely end-labelled restriction fragment, which can be either single- or double-stranded, is reacted with the base-modifying reagent in a limited reaction. Piperidine then displaces the modified base from its sugar, and catalyses β-elimination of both phosphates from that sugar to break the DNA. Partial chemical cleavage produces a nested set of end-labelled products, each specific for different bases, which are electrophoresed in parallel on a polyacrylamide/urea denaturing gel. (b) Autoradiography of a sequencing gel, exhibiting the four vertical ladders of staggered horizontal bands. The four different nested sets of end-labelled fragments produced after partial cleavage at cytosines and thymines (C+T), cytosines (C), guanines (G) and guanines and adenines (A+G), using the chemical reactions summarized in (a), were electrophoresed after denaturation on a 10% polyacrylamide/7 M urea sequencing gel. A portion of the sequence is shown to the right of the autoradiograph.

uniquely end-labelled double-stranded, DNA is partially reacted with base-specific chemical reagents which modify the bases. Dimethylsulphate modifies G residues, formic acid reacts with G and A, hydrazine with T and C and hydrazine in the presence of NaCl reacts with C residues. Piperidine is then used to cleave the DNA strand at the modified bases and the products separated on sequencing gels. Only the end-labelled fragments are visualized and the sequence is read as shown in Fig. 41.11.

Chemical cleavage sequencing has become less popular in recent years because of the ease of generating large amounts of sequence information by the dideoxy method. However, it is not subject to problems in determining certain kinds of

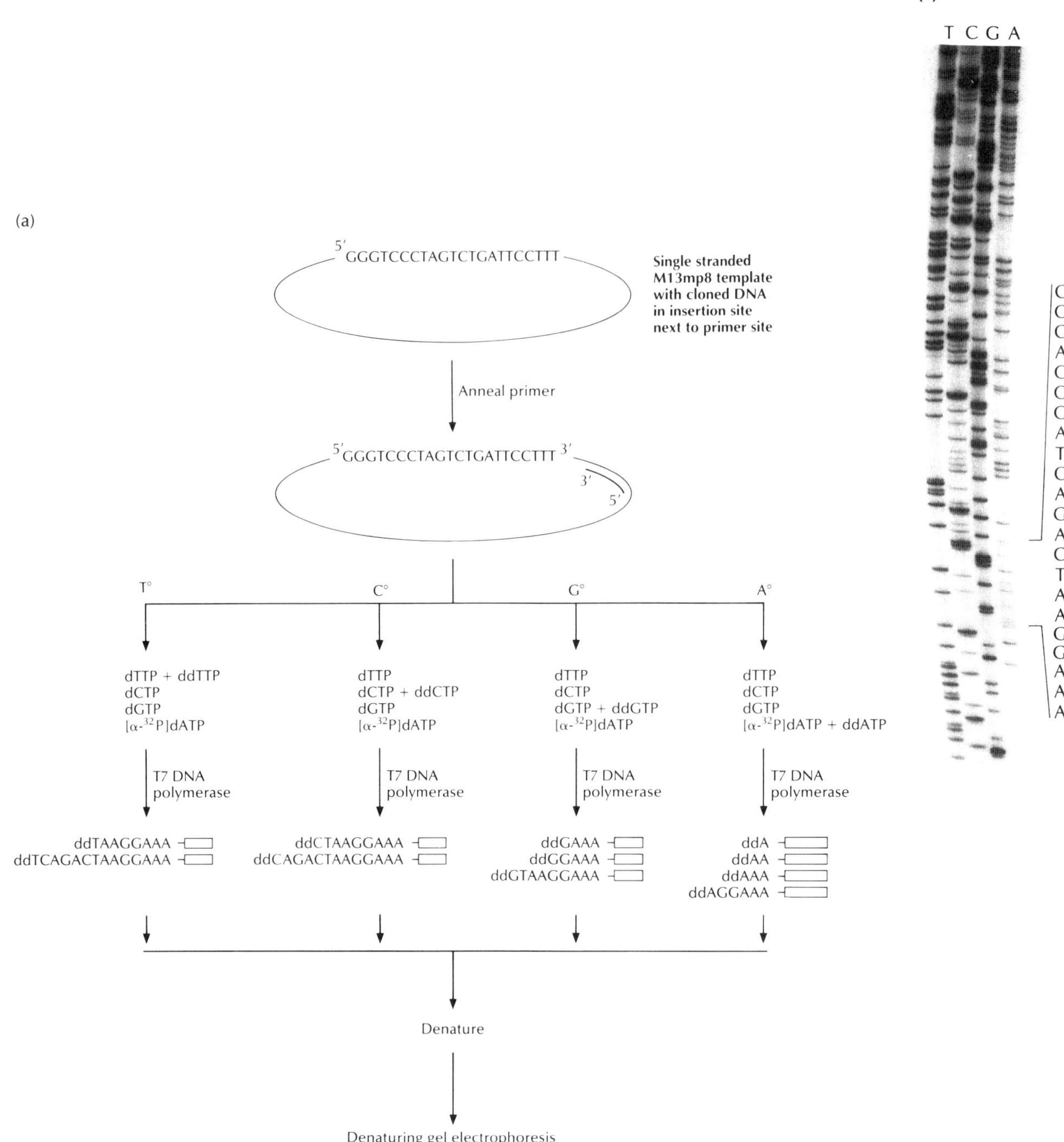

Fig. 41.12. A suitable primer, in the case of M13 the universal primer (5′GAAAACCCAGTCACGAC3′), is annealed to a single-stranded DNA template with cloned DNA in the insertion site next to the primer site. A DNA polymerase (in this case T7 DNA polymerase) synthesizes a copy of the insert DNA by extension from the primer in the presence of all four dNTPs and one of the 2′,3′-dideoxynucleotide (ddNTP) base analogues. The polymerase is able to incorporate the ddNTP into the nascent chain but incorporation of the analogue prevents further extension since it does not possess a 3′ OH group. The concentration of the ddNTP in each reaction is adjusted to give a partial synthesis reaction with fragments terminating at each occurrence of the particular base. After denaturation the four base-specific reactions are electrophoresed in parallel on a polyacrylamide/urea denaturing gel.
(b) Autoradiograph of a sequencing gel exhibiting the four vertical ladders of staggered horizontal bands. The four different partial synthesis reactions specific for thymine (T), cytosine (C), guanine (G) and adenine (A) were electrophoresed after denaturation on a 6% polyacrylamide/7 M urea sequencing gel. A portion of the sequence is shown to the right of the autoradiograph.

sequence associated with DNA polymerase and is useful for these difficult areas. In addition, vectors are now available that facilitate production of DNA suitable for chemical sequencing (Eckert 1987).

DIDEOXYNUCLEOTIDE CHAIN TERMINATION SEQUENCING

The dideoxy sequencing method of Sanger (Sanger *et al.* 1977, 1982) utilizes a DNA polymerase (initially the Klenow fragment of *E. coli* DNA polymerase I) to synthesize a copy of single-stranded DNA by extension from a primer that is annealed to the 3′ end of the template (Fig. 41.12). The template DNA can be isolated from M13 vectors (Sanger *et al.* 1982; Messing 1983), rescued from phagemids (Short *et al.* 1988) or produced by denaturing plasmid DNA in alkali (Chen and Seeburg 1985). Appropriate sequencing primers are available for commonly used vectors and enzymes. The synthesis reaction includes all four dNTPs and one of the 2′,3′-dideoxynucleotide (ddNTP) base analogues. The polymerase is able to incorporate the ddNTP into the nascent chain, but incorporation of the analogue prevents further extension since it does not possess a 3′ OH (Fig. 41.12). The concentration of the ddNTP in each reaction is adjusted to give a partial synthesis reaction with fragments terminating at each occurrence of the particular base. The products of the reaction are labelled either by incorporation of a labelled nucleotide into the nascent chain or by use of a labelled primer.

The four base-specific reaction products are denatured and separated on denaturing PAGE gels. If radiolabelled dNTPs are used the gels are thin and are dried down after electrophoresis to give greater resolution by autoradiography. Use of $\alpha^{35}S$ deoxyadenosine triphosphate (dATP) (Biggin *et al.* 1983) also increases resolution of fragments. The extent of readable sequence may be increased by running buffer gradient (Biggin *et al.* 1983) or wedge-shaped gels (Chen and Seeburg 1985). Figure 41.12 shows an example of a dideoxy sequencing gel.

There are two major problems associated with DNA sequencing by this method: (1) the enzyme sometimes terminates prematurely at regions of DNA secondary structure, particularly in long stretches of G and C nucleotides; and (2) 'compressions' occur where two or more fragments of different size run at the same place in the gel due to secondary structure in the synthesized product. A number of variations on the method have been developed to deal with these problems. The sequencing reactions can be performed with reverse transcriptase, which gives more faithful synthesis in GC-rich regions, modified T7 DNA polymerase (Tabor and Richardson 1987), which synthesizes more nucleotides without leaving the template and has higher affinity for ddNTPs, or *Taq* DNA polymerase at high temperature (Innis *et al.* 1988), which minimizes secondary structure in the template. In addition the nucleotide analogues deoxyinosine triphosphate (dITP) (Mills and Kramer 1979) 7-deaza-deoxyguanosine triphosphate (7-deaza-dGTP) (Mizusawa *et al.* 1986) can be used in place of dGTP to prevent secondary structure forming in the products. It is also essential to sequence fragments in both orientations since compressions may occur only in the products generated from one strand.

When sequencing regions of DNA greater than a few hundred base pairs a suitable strategy should be devised. With detailed restriction mapping, restriction fragments can be chosen that give overlapping coverage of the region (Messing 1983). An alternative is to clone fragments generated by random breakage (Sanger *et al.* 1982) and to analyse overlaps by computer. A third popular strategy is to generate a series of clones containing fragments successively deleted from one end, so that sequencing different clones extends progressively into the region of interest (Heinkoff 1984; Dale *et al.* 1985; Hoheisel and Pohl 1986). In all cases some form of computer-assisted analysis is required to generate restriction maps, recognize overlaps, identify open reading-frames and run homology searches for structural and functional information (*Nucleic Acids Res.* 1986; Ausubel *et al.* 1987; Bishop and Rawlings 1987). Strategies are also available for much larger-scale sequencing projects but these are beyond the scope of this review (*Nucleic Acids Res.* 1986; Bishop and Rawlings 1987; Church and Kieffer-Higgins 1988).

Cloning of genomic deoxyribonucleic acid

The purpose of cloning genomic DNA is to isolate clones that contain the gene encoding a particular mRNA. The gene structure and information about sequences that regulate the expression of that mRNA can be studied using clones that contain the gene. A second aim might be to clone a particular region of the genome, for instance the region containing the immunoglobulin heavy chain locus (Edgell *et al.* 1979; Matsuda *et al.* 1988) or the MHC (Sargent *et al.* 1989a). This is accomplished by isolating a series of genomic clones, each of which contains DNA that partially overlaps the DNA in the next clone, to generate a 'contig'. This process is called chromosome walking.

There are essentially two ways to isolate genomic clones. The first is to isolate restriction fragments of a specific size and to clone them into a plasmid vector to create a subgenomic library (Frischauf *et al.* 1984), i.e. a library that contains a portion of the genome. The clone of interest is then isolated by DNA hybridization. This method requires information on the appropriate restriction fragment and is not useful for isolating large regions of DNA. The second, more frequently used, method entails constructing a library of clones that contains large DNA fragments representing as closely as possible the whole genome (Sambrook *et al.* 1989).

The two common approaches for construction of genomic libraries utilize either cosmid (Collins and Hohn 1978; Ish-Horowicz and Burke 1981) or λ replacement (Sambrook *et al.* 1989; Frischauf *et al.* 1984) (e.g. λEMBL3) vectors. The high cloning efficiency of both types of vector, due to the use of *in vitro* packaging into λ phage heads, is advantageous, since a large number of clones must be generated to represent the whole genome. The methods for generating libraries are essentially the same for cosmid and λ vectors, but the difference lies in the size of DNA insert that may be accommodated by the vector. This cloning capacity is dictated by the size of DNA that can be packaged into the phage heads. Thus λ vectors have a cloning capacity of ~20 kb, whereas cosmids can accept fragments of 30–45 kb.

The size of a library of essentially random clones required to ensure representation of a particular sequence is determined by the size of the genome and the size of the cloned insert DNA. The number of clones (N) that must be screened to isolate a sequence with a probability P is given by

$$N = \ln(1 - P)/\ln[1 - (I/G)]$$

where I is the average size of cloned DNA insert and G is the size of the genome (Clarke and Carbon 1976). For a 99% chance of isolating a clone containing a human gene the number of clones that must be screened for a typical λ vector is 690 000. For a cosmid vector with an average insert size of 40 kb it is 345 000. Obviously the advantage of using cosmids is that fewer clones have to be screened, combined with the fact that larger steps can be taken in a walking experiment (see below).

We shall consider cloning in cosmids, but the steps for λ cloning are essentially similar (outlined in Fig. 41.13). An essential prerequisite is the isolation of high-molecular-weight DNA as this increases the chances of generating molecules of the right size for cloning with two clonable ends. Care must be taken during DNA isolation to avoid shearing of the DNA molecules. The high-molecular-weight DNA is used to generate large segments of DNA distributed at random through the genome. The only way to generate completely random fragments, so that there is no systematic exclusion of sequences, is to use mechanical shearing (Clarke and Carbon 1976). However, shearing produces DNA termini that are difficult to clone and require repair so that cloning efficiencies are low. An alternative is to use partial digestion with an RE that has a tetranucleotide recognition site (Maniatis *et al.* 1982; Seed *et al.* 1982). This results in a population of fragments that are close to random, although certain sequences may be under-represented and may not be easy to clone into an appropriate vector. Suitable REs are *Sau*3A

Fig. 41.13. Genomic DNA is partially digested with an RE (in this case *Mbo*I) to generate a random selection of fragments, which are size-selected by sucrose gradient ultracentrifugation. Fragments of 35–50 kb are ligated to the cosmid vector arms. Preparation of the arms is dependent upon the particular cosmid being used. In the example shown using the cosmid vector pTCF two separate double digests are carried out. One involves the RE *Cla*I followed by treatment with calf intestinal alkaline phosphatase to remove the 3′ phosphate group and prevent religation of the vector. The second involves the RE *Hpa*I, followed by treatment with alkaline phosphatase. The linearized vectors are then cleaved with the RE *Bam*HI, which generates the cloning sites that are compatible with the genomic fragments generated using the RE *Mbo*I. After ligation only those molecules which have two cos sites in the same orientation and at the correct distance apart will be packaged *in vitro*, using λ packaging extracts, prior to transduction of a suitable *E. coli* strain such as ED8767.

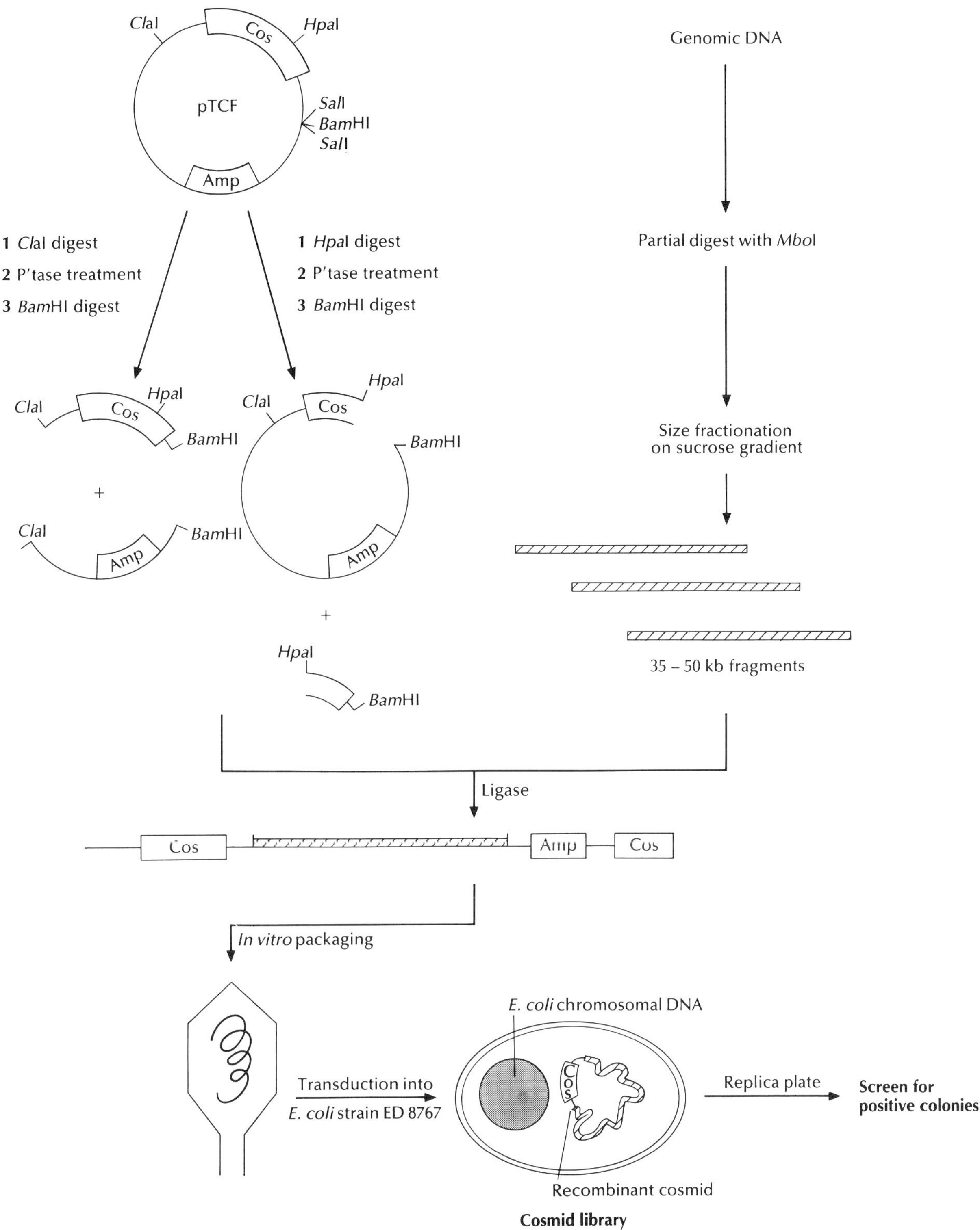
Preparation of cosmid library
ClaI
Cos
HpaI
pTCF
SalI
BamHI
SalI
Amp
Genomic DNA
1 ClaI digest
2 P'tase treatment
3 BamHI digest
1 HpaI digest
2 P'tase treatment
3 BamHI digest
Partial digest with MboI
ClaI
Cos
HpaI
BamHI
+
ClaI
Amp
BamHI
ClaI
Cos
HpaI
BamHI
Amp
Size fractionation
on sucrose gradient
+
HpaI
BamHI
35 – 50 kb fragments
Ligase
Cos
Amp
Cos
In vitro packaging
E. coli chromosomal DNA
Transduction into
E. coli strain ED 8767
Cos
Replica plate
Screen for
positive colonies
Recombinant cosmid
Cosmid library

and *Mbo*I. Partial digestion is achieved by optimizing the time of digestion and the amount of enzyme used.

Appropriate partial digests of the insert DNA are pooled and fractionated either on sucrose density gradients or by agarose gel electrophoresis. After analysis of sucrose gradient fractions of partially digested DNA by electrophoresis on a 0.4% agarose gel, the fractions that contain DNA of the right size for cloning are pooled and treated with phosphatase. These two steps of size fractionation and dephosphorylation are necessary to prevent small genomic DNA fragments from ligating together to form erroneous clones. The insert DNA is then ligated into the cosmid vector.

An important consideration in cosmid cloning is the prevention of multimer formation where several vector molecules can ligate together. This is usually achieved by the use of REs that cleave the cosmid vector on a different side of the cos site. The resulting fragments are treated with phosphatase and then cleaved with the cloning site enzyme (Fig. 41.13). The fragments are then ligated to the genomic DNA. The only packageable molecules that can be formed will consist of one donor fragment linked to a cosmid fragment on either end, preventing the formation of multimers. Only those ligated molecules which have two cos sites in the same orientation and at the proper distance apart will be packaged.

The transduction of the ligated cosmid DNA molecules is based on an *in vitro* DNA packaging system (Hohn and Murray 1977). This involves the preparation of complementary extracts from two defective *E. coli* lysogens. For example, the strains BHB2690 and BHB2688 are lysogenic for λ phage with nonsense mutations in the λ genes D and E, respectively. An extract from the E strains contains all the λ head proteins in soluble form, except the major capsid protein E. This extract can therefore complement the second extract from the D strain which contains empty precursor particles. Once packaged into phage particles, the recombinant DNA can be introduced into *E. coli* by the normal phage infection pathway. High-quality packaging extracts are now widely available from commercial suppliers.

The recombinants are grown at high density on filter membranes on selective medium, and replicas are taken. The membranes may be screened with DNA hybridization probes, and positives are picked from the master plates and rescreened as for cDNA clones. Deoxyribonucleic acid from positive clones is prepared by a plasmid miniprep procedure and can be analysed by restriction mapping and Southern blotting. Figure 41.5 shows restriction digests of cloned cosmid DNA.

Unfortunately, a library constructed in this way may not contain all the sequences in the genome. The basis for this is not entirely clear, though certain sequences such as long inverted repeats, strong prokaryotic promoter homologies, operator homologies and repressor binding sites may all make the DNA difficult to clone in *E. coli*.

CHROMOSOME WALKING

In order to chromosome-walk, it is necessary to isolate probes from the ends of one cosmid clone. These probes are used to screen the cosmid library, obtaining new clones that overlap existing clones and expand the cloned locus. In many organisms this process is complicated by the presence of dispersed repetitive sequences throughout the genome. Therefore, in order to obtain 'walking probes', cosmid insert restriction fragments that are free from repetitive sequences must be identified. This may be done by identifying restriction fragments that do not hybridize with labelled total genomic DNA (Shen and Maniatis 1980). The single-copy nature of the potential probe is confirmed by detecting the appropriate restriction fragments in Southern blot hybridization with RE-digested genomic DNA. The walking probe is then used to screen the cosmid library and the overlap of positive clones with existing clones is confirmed by restriction enzyme analysis.

Because chromosome walking in cosmids can be a slow and labour-intensive process, other types of libraries, such as chromosome jumping and linking libraries (Poustka and Lehrach 1986), have been constructed in an attempt to bridge the large physical distances separating markers and genes in mammalian genomes.

CLONING IN YEAST ARTIFICIAL CHROMOSOMES

Recently Burke *et al*. (1987) have developed a novel system that allows cloning of large DNA fragments in yeast artificial chromosomes (YACs). The YAC system makes use of the natural elements required to form a functional chromosome in yeast, all of which have been isolated and characterized (Blackburn and Szostak 1984). These are autonomous replication sequence (ARS) elements, required for autonomous replication of any exogenous DNA, centromeres, required for stable segregation of the chromosomes, and telomeres, needed to maintain the ends of linear chromosomes. The YAC vector plasmid contains each of of these elements along with various yeast and *E. coli* selectable markers and a cloning site (Fig. 41.14). The vector is cleaved to produce two arms, each of which contains a telomere at one end and a selectable marker. These arms are ligated to large DNA fragments that have been size-fractionated, and the recombinants are transformed into yeast. Non-recombinants are selected against by selection for insertional inactivation of the yeast *sup*4 gene, Deoxyribonucleic acid hybridization screening protocols are available

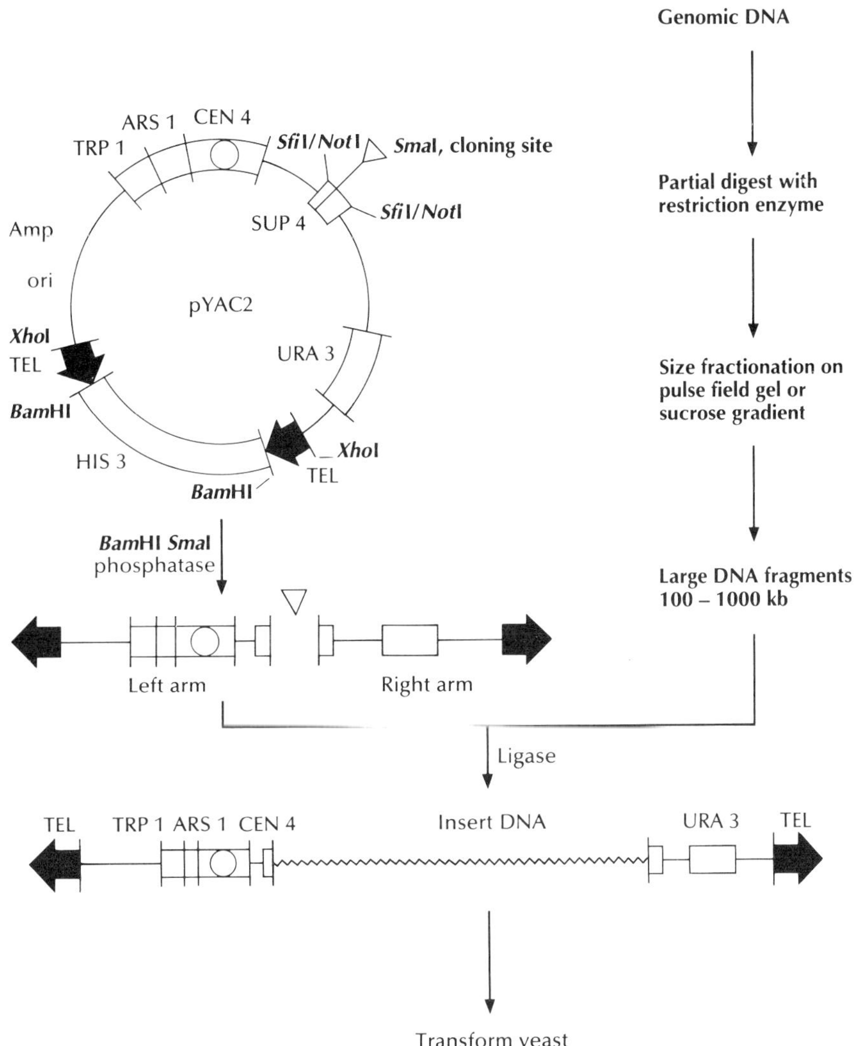

Fig. 41.14. In the pYAC2 vector illustrated above the sequences derived from the plasmid pBR322 are shown by a thin line; SUP4 is an ochre-suppressing allele of a tyrosine transfer RNA gene, which is interrupted when exogenous DNA is cloned into the *Sma*I cloning site; TRP1 and URA3 are selectable markers that allow selection for recombinant molecules that have acquired both chromosome arms from the vector; ARS1 is an autonomous replication sequence; CEN4 provides centromere function; and the two TEL sequences allow telomere formation *in vivo*. The cloning protocol involves double digestion of the YAC vector with *Bam*HI and *Sma*I. The two arms are treated with calf intestinal alkaline phosphatase to prevent religation and then ligated to large DNA fragments that have blunt ends and that have been size-selected on pulsed-field gels or sucrose gradients. The ligation products are then transformed into yeast spheroplasts.

(Brownstein *et al.* 1989) and the cloned DNA can be examined directly by PFGE (Burke *et al.* 1987). The ability to clone fragments of DNA at least 10 times larger than it is possible to clone in cosmids provides major advantages for walking and mapping projects (Coulson *et al.* 1988). It is also possible that sequences that are unclonable in *E. coli* may be stably propagated in yeast.

Gene mapping by physical methods

Having cloned a cDNA or gene, it is often extremely informative to determine the chromosomal location of that gene. The two most powerful physical methods for gene mapping are somatic cell genetics (Tunnacliffe *et al.* 1983, 1984) and *in situ* hybridization (Buckle and Craig 1986).

The technique of somatic cell genetics relies upon the fact that when human and rodent cells in culture are fused the resulting heterokaryons are unstable and tend to lose only the human chromosomes, but in a more or less random way. Thus it is possible to assemble a panel of hybrid cell lines that contain different numbers and distributions of human chromosomes. By analysing these hybrid cell lines for the presence of the gene or the gene product, in relation to the human chromosomes also present in the hybrids, it is possible to assign the gene to a particular human chromosome. A number of indirect methods have been employed in gene mapping including enzymatic assays specific for the human gene product, detection of the electrophoretic variants of the human protein, and the use of monoclonal and polyclonal antibodies which react with human cell surface antigens or with the human protein in Western blot analysis. However, mapping at the DNA level is by far the most direct approach in gene mapping (Ruddle 1981). This method relies on the sequence differences and/or the RFLPs between human and rodent genes and has the advantage that the gene under investigation does not need to be expressed in the hybrids used for mapping. Southern blot hybridization analysis is carried out and the chromosomal assignment can be made based upon the presence of the human RE fragments in relation to the human chromosomes contained in the hybrids. This procedure can sometimes fail and an alternative approach exploiting the PCR has been developed (Iggo *et al.* 1989). In this case primers flanking introns were used to identify species-specific differences in PCR products due to variation in intron length. Again the presence of the human PCR product in the hybrids was correlated with the human chromosomes present, allowing chromosomal assignment of the gene under investigation. More refined mapping to a particular chromosomal region is possible as hybrids are available which contain chromosomes with naturally occurring deletions, translocation chromosomes or chromosomal fragments generated by gamma irradiation of human cells (Goss and Harris 1977) or by chromosome-mediated gene transfer (Porteous 1987).

In situ hybridization involves the hybridization of a ^{3}H-labelled single-stranded DNA probe directly to human metaphase chromosomes which have been fixed and spread on microscope slides. After hybridization the slides are coated with photographic emulsion and left in the dark before developing. The slides are examined under the microscope and the position of the silver grains in the emulsion noted. A large number of spreads have to be analysed to generate a statistically significant result. The chromosomal location of the gene corresponds to the position of the greatest number of silver grains.

Transfection and expression

Genes can be introduced into mammalian cells either transiently or stably (Spandidos and Wilkie 1984; Gorman 1985). In transient gene expression the DNA introduced into cells in culture does not necessarily need to be integrated into the chromosomal DNA in order to be expressed. Expression of incoming DNA can be monitored within 12 hours of uptake and can continue for up to 80 hours. Alternatively, the incoming DNA can be incorporated into the chromosomal DNA to form stably transformed cell lines.

The most commonly used method for introducing cloned genes into mammalian cells is the calcium phosphate ($CaPO_4$) method (Graham and van der Eb 1973). This involves forming a fine precipitate of the DNA to be introduced into the cells in buffer containing $CaPO_4$, and incubating the cells with the precipitate, some of which is taken up by the cells. This method can be used for either transient expression or stable transformation. An alternative method, which is much better for studying the transient expression of transferred genes, involves the use of DEAE-dextran (Sompayrac and Danna 1981). A third method for introducing DNA into cells is electroporation (Potter *et al.* 1984). A high-voltage pulse is generated in a foil-lined cuvette containing the mammalian cells and DNA. The cells become permeable to DNA and take up the exogenous DNA. One of the advantages of transient expression is that it is quick and relatively easy and can give information regarding expression of a particular coding sequence, the nature of the control sequences at the 5′ end of a gene required for its expression, and agents which modulate expression of that gene.

In order to generate stably transformed cell lines it is necessary to have a genetic marker in the transfected exogenous DNA that produces a selectable change in the phenotype of the transfected cells. This is because only a small fraction of cells stably integrate the exogenous DNA into their genome. One such selectable marker is the thymidine kinase gene, which is based upon the expression of exogenously added thymidine kinase (tk) gene in mutant cells (tk −ve) which lack this activity (Wigler *et al.* 1987). However, of more general applicability is the use of dominant selectable markers such as expression of the *E. coli* genes hypoxanthine phosphoribosyltransferase (gpt) (Mulligan and Berg 1981) or aminoglycoside 3′ phosphotransferase [APH(3′) II (*neo*)] (*neo*^{R}) (Southern and Berg 1982). The mechanism for selection in the case of *neo*^{R} is based upon the cell's sensitivity to the aminoglycoside antibiotic G418. G418 can be inactivated by the *neo*^{R} enzyme APH(3′) II (*neo*). When the *neo* gene is linked to or co-integrated with another gene whose stable integration is desired in the transformed cell, selection for resistance to G418 also selects for stable integration and expression of the desired gene.

A number of different plasmid vectors are available which can be used in gene transfer experiments (Gorman 1985; Bebbington and Hentschel 1987). These include different promoter and enhancer elements which control initiation of transcription once the construct has been introduced into mammalian cells. In addition they contain sequences which are necessary for efficient processing of the transcripts. These include a polyadenylation signal and also an intron. These elements are invariably isolated from mammalian retroviruses such as simian virus type 40 (SV40) or respiratory syncytial virus (RSV), and utilize strong promoters and enhancers, or cell-specific promoters and enhancers isolated from mammalian genes. The choice of vector is usually based upon the particular mammalian cell lines being used in the transfection experiments.

In addition it is possible to analyse in detail the sequences which constitute mammalian gene promoters and enhancers by placing them in vectors which contain readily assayable protein-coding regions such as the chloramphenicol acetyl transferase (cat) gene (Gorman *et al.* 1982), the luciferase gene (Nguyen *et al.* 1988) and the β-galactosidase gene (Hall 1983). This allows quantitation of the strength of sequences derived from a eukaryotic promoter by enzyme assay after transient expression (Walker *et al.* 1983; Israël *et al.* 1986; Wu *et al.* 1987).

Mutagenesis

Oligonucleotide-directed *in vitro* mutagenesis is a powerful technique which can be used to generate site-specific mutations in any cloned DNA segment of interest (Fritz 1985; Kunkel *et al.* 1987). This makes it possible to substitute different amino acids into a protein in order to define the contribution that particular amino acids play in the function of that protein.

Several methods have been developed for carrying out *in vitro* mutagenesis, each of which generally involves the use of single-stranded target DNA. The target DNA is made single-stranded either by subcloning into a single-stranded phage vector, such as M13 (Yanisch-Perron *et al.* 1985), or into phagemids (Short *et al.* 1988), plasmids which can be obtained in single-stranded form with the aid of helper phage. An alternative to the above is the 'gapped duplex' method (Kramer 1984), which involves annealing double-stranded vector DNA, which is linearized beforehand with the RE used for cloning the inserted fragment, to an excess of circular single-stranded recombinant DNA containing an insert. Thus the annealed fragment is double-stranded at the portion that is derived from the vector DNA and single-stranded at the insert.

The desired mutation is generated using an oligonucleotide containing the base(s) to be modified, but which is otherwise identical to the insert DNA. This primes for DNA synthesis using

DNA polymerase, and ligation completes the second strand. After transformation of a suitable bacterial strain, phage or plasmids containing the desired mutation(s) are screened for.

The power of the methodology has recently been demonstrated in two papers describing experiments designed to define the binding sites in the Fc domain of immunoglobulin G (IgG) for complement and for cell receptors. In one case a single amino acid substitution in a mouse IgG-2b antibody (Glu 235 — Leu) was engineered and this change enabled the antibody to bind to the Fc receptor I (FcRI) (high-affinity receptor) on human monocytes with a 100-fold improvement in affinity (Duncan and Winter 1988). This indicates that the Leu at position 235 is a major determinant in the binding of antibody to FcRI. In order to define the binding site for the first component of complement (C1) surface residues in the C_H2 domain of the mouse IgG-2b isotype were systematically altered (Duncan *et al.* 1988). This localized the binding site for C1q to three side-chains, Glu 318, Lys 320 and Lys 322.

The polymerase chain reaction

The PCR allows *in vitro* amplification of a specific sequence present in a small amount in complex DNA, resulting an enrichment of that sequence by $>10^6$-fold (Saiki *et al.* 1985; Erlich 1989). Such amplification greatly eases subsequent steps such as DNA sequencing or cloning.

The PCR uses two oligonucleotides that flank the DNA segment to be amplified (Fig. 41.15). The primers anneal to opposite strands oriented tail to tail (3′ end towards 3′ end) and are able to prime synthesis of DNA complementary to the region between hybridization sites. The newly synthesized DNA can serve as template for DNA synthesis primed by the other oligonucleotide. Successive cycles of denaturation of the double-stranded DNA template, annealing of primers and *de novo* DNA synthesis result in an exponential increase in the target DNA sequence. The product is a fragment of discrete length which can be analysed and purified on PAGE or sieving agarose gels. (Fig. 41.15). The present incarnation of the PCR makes use of *Taq* DNA polymerase, which is thermostable and can survive multiple cycles through the DNA denaturation step (Saiki *et al.* 1988). This makes the process suitable for automation using a programmable cycling heating block. In addition, the specificity and yield of the reaction are optimized since the synthesis step occurs at high temperature (the optimal temperature of *Taq* polymerase is 70–75°C) which causes poorly matched primer–template hybrids to dissociate (Saiki *et al.* 1988).

The PCR makes it feasible to rapidly sequence many allelic variants (Saiki *et al.* 1986; Todd *et al.* 1987; Scharf *et al.* 1988) and has found applications in assaying for infectious agents, detecting carriers of genetic disease (Embury *et al.* 1987; Montandon *et al.* 1989; Roberts *et al.* 1989a) and cloning of genomic DNA (Scharf *et al.* 1986; Stoflet *et al.* 1988) and cDNA (Lee *et al.* 1988) without the construction of complex libraries. A number of innovative adaptations of the technique allow amplification of DNA regions outside known sequence (inverted PCR (Ockman *et al.* 1988; Triglia *et al.* 1988; Silver and Keerikatte 1989)), of mRNA where only one end of the sequence is known (Loh *et al.* 1989) or of cDNA using mixed oligonucleotides designed from protein sequence (Lee *et al.* 1988). Finally it has proved possible to apply PCR to amplify single-copy sequences from single cells (Li *et al.* 1988).

Detection of nucleotide sequence differences

Determination of DNA sequence differences among allelic variants, between functional and defective genes, among viral strains or within a cell population is becoming increasingly important to the understanding of many immune phenomena. A number of methods are now available which can rapidly provide this information (Cotton 1989). The first approach involves using the PCR to amplify the region of interest, followed by direct sequencing (Todd *et al.* 1987; Scharf *et al.* 1988), hybridization with allele-specific oligonucleotides (Saiki *et al.* 1986) or application of one of the

Fig. 41.15. The two primers anneal to the opposite strands flanking the DNA segment to be amplified and are able to prime *de novo* DNA synthesis by *Taq* DNA polymerase. The newly synthesized DNA can serve as template for DNA synthesis primed by the other oligonucleotide. Successive cycles of denaturation of the double-stranded DNA template, annealing of primers and extension using *Taq* DNA polymerase can result in an enrichment of the sequence by $>10^6$-fold.

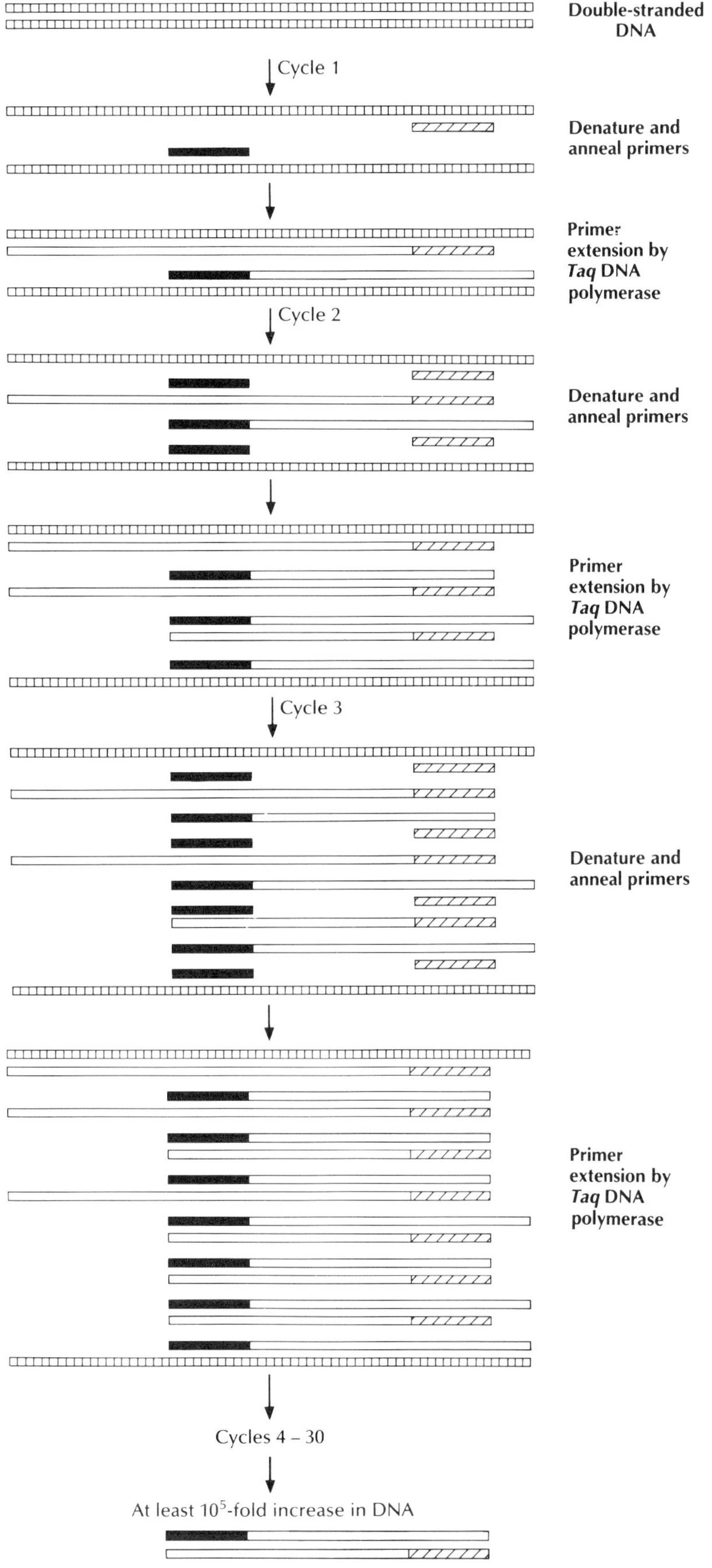
Double-stranded DNA
Cycle 1
Denature and anneal primers
Primer extension by *Taq* DNA polymerase
Cycle 2
Denature and anneal primers
Primer extension by *Taq* DNA polymerase
Cycle 3
Denature and anneal primers
Primer extension by *Taq* DNA polymerase
Cycles 4 – 30
At least 10^5-fold increase in DNA

methods mentioned below. If the sequencing path is taken, a large amount of DNA sequence can be rapidly generated. The *Taq* polymerase has no 'proof-reading' mechanism and so nucleotide incorporation errors occur at a significant frequency and it is advisable to sequence the products of separate amplifications.

Alternative methods do not involve direct determination of the DNA sequence, but rather detect the presence of single-base mismatches in heteroduplexes between a labelled probe strand whose sequence is known and the target sequence. Heteroduplexes of several hundred base pairs can be analysed. In the denaturing gradient gel electrophoresis technique (Myers *et al.* 1985a), the heteroduplex is electrophoresed in a denaturing gradient of increasing strength. Mismatched duplexes denature more quickly than perfectly matched homoduplexes, causing a decrease in migration rate. However, this method gives no information on the position of the mismatch.

The RNase A cleavage assay (Myers *et al.* 1985b) is based on cleavage by RNase A of some single-base mismatches in heteroduplexes between a labelled RNA probe and a DNA or RNA target. The probe and target sequence are annealed and treated with RNase A, and the products are separated by denaturing PAGE to identify the position of cleavage. It is estimated that only 50% of all single-base mismatches are detected.

The HOT method (Cotton *et al.* 1988) is based on chemical cleavage of the DNA at mismatched bases in the heteroduplex. The method uses single-stranded or double-stranded DNA probes which are annealed to the target DNA. The resulting heteroduplexes are treated with either osmium tetroxide or hydroxylamine to modify mismatched thymine (and cytosine) or cytosine bases, respectively. Subsequent treatment with piperidine cleaves the DNA at the modified base and the products are electrophoresed on denaturing PAGE to identify the position of cleavage. In a manner similar to Maxam–Gilbert sequencing a partial reaction can be produced that gives the position of all mismatches in a single heteroduplex (Cotton *et al.* 1988; Cotton and Campbell 1989). Use of both sense and antisense strands as probes allows all possible mismatches to be identified. This method has been applied directly to mRNA in the study of mutant collagen genes (Dahl *et al.* 1989; Lamande *et al.* 1989) and to viral RNA isolated from infected cells (Cotton and Wright 1989). In combination with PCR the HOT mismatch analysis can be used to determine the position of mutations in cDNA synthesized from total RNA (Grompe *et al.* 1989) and in genomic DNA samples (Montandon *et al.* 1989; Roberts *et al.* 1989b).

Summary

The research into the understanding of the molecular basis of immune phenomena has required the application of many different techniques. The recent advances in the study of the molecular and genetic aspects of immunology have been due to a very large extent to the revolution which has taken place in molecular biology in the last 5–10 years. The ability to easily clone and characterize genes and the corresponding mRNAs (through cDNA) and to manipulate these genes has given us valuable new insights into the structures and functions of immunologically important molecules. A wide range of methods are available for the cloning, analysis and manipulation of DNA and RNA. Although not a complete summary, this review illustrates some of the more commonly used methods which form the basis for much of the work involving the use of recombinant DNA technology described elsewhere in this volume. The choice of methods depends largely on the application which is anticipated. Several excellent molecular biology manuals are available which contain detailed protocols, in addition to giving advice on equipment, reagents and precautions that are appropriate to establishing recombinant DNA methods in a laboratory.

Addendum

Since the time of writing this review the use of the PCR in molecular biology has increased dramatically [see Erlich, H.A., Gelfand, D. and Snisky, J.J. (1991) *Science* **252**, 1643]. In addition the use of YAC cloning (see Schlessinger, D. (1990) *Trends Genet.* **248**, 255) and non-radioactive methods for *in situ* hybridization (see Trask, B.I. (1991) *Trends Genet.* **7**, 149) have also increased.

References

Ausubel, F.M., Brent, R., Kingston, R.E. *et al.* (eds) (1987). *Current Protocols in Molecular Biology*. J. Wiley, New York.

Aviv, H. and Leder, P. (1972). *In vitro* synthesis of ribosomal RNA by *Bacillus Subtilis* RNA polymerase. *Proc. Nat. Acad. Sci. (USA)* **69**, 407–11.

Bebbington, C.R. and Hentschel, C.C.G. (1987). The use of vectors based on gene amplification for the expression of cloned genes in mammalian cells. In *DNA Cloning*, vol. III, ed. D.M. Glover, pp. 163–88, IRL Press, Oxford.

Bender, W., Spierer, P. and Hogness, D.S. (1983). Chromosomal walking and jumping to isolate DNA from the Ace and rosy loci and the bithorax complex in *Drosophila melangoster*. *J. Mol. Biol.* **168**, 17–23.

Berger, S.L. and Kimmel, A.R. (eds) (1987). Guide to Molecular Cloning Techniques. *Methods Enzymol.* **152**, 1–812 (whole volume).

Biggin, M.D., Gibson, T.J. and Hong, G.F. (1983). Buffer gradient gels and ^{35}S label as an aid to rapid DNA sequence determination. *Proc. Nat. Acad. Sci. (USA)* **80**, 3963–5.

Bilofsky, H.S., Burks, C., Fickett, J.W. *et al.* (1986). The GenBank genetic sequence databank. *Nucleic Acids Res.* **14**, 1–4.

Bird, A.P. (1986). CpG-rich islands and the function of DNA methylation. *Nature* **321**, 209–13.

Birnboim, H.C. and Doly, J. (1979). A rapid alkaline extraction procedure for screening recombinant plasmid DNA. *Nucleic Acids Res.* **7**, 1513–23.

Birren, B.W., Lai, E., Clark, S.M., Hood, L. and Simon, M.I. (1988). Optimized conditions for pulsed field gel electrophoretic separations of DNA. *Nucleic Acids Res.* **16**, 7563–82.

Bishop, M.J. and Rawlings, C.J. (eds) (1987). *Nucleic Acid and Protein Sequence Analysis: a Practical Approach*. IRL Press, Oxford.

Blackburn, E.M. and Szostak, J.W. (1984). The molecular structure of centromeres and telomeres. *Ann. Rev. Biochem.* **53**, 163–94.

Bolivar, F., Rodriguez, R.L. Greene, M.C. *et al.* (1977). Construction and characterization of new cloning vehicles. II. A multipurpose cloning system. *Gene* **17**, 95–113.

Botstein, D., White, R.L., Skolnick, M. and Davis, R.W. (1980). Construction of a genetic linkage map in man using restriction fragment length polymorphisms. *Am. J. Hum. Genet.* **32**, 314–31.

Brown, W.R.A. and Bird, A.P. (1986). Long-range restriction site mapping of mammalian genome DNA. *Nature* **322**, 477–81.

Brownstein, B.H., Silverman, G.A., Little, R.D. *et al.* (1989). Isolation of single-copy human genes from a library of yeast artificial chromosome clones. *Science* **244**, 1348–51.

Buckle, V. and Craig, I. (1986). *In situ* hybridization. In *Human Genetic Diseases*, ed. K.E. Davies, pp. 85–100, IRL Press, Oxford.

Burke, D.T., Carle, G.F. and Olson, M.V. (1987). Cloning of large segments of exogenous DNA into yeast by means of artificial chromosome vectors. *Science* **236**, 806–11.

Carle, G.F., Frank, M. and Olson, M.V. (1986). Electrophoretic separations of large DNA molecules by periodic inversion of the electric field. *Science* **232**, 65–8.

Carroll, M.C., Alicot, E.M., Katzman, P.J., Klickstein, L.B., Smith, J.A. and Fearon, D.T. (1988). Organization of the genes encoding complement receptors type 1 and 2, decay-accelerating factor, and C4-binding protein in the RCA locus on human chromosome 1. *J. Exp. Med.* **167**, 1271–80.

Chen, E.Y. and Seeburg, P.H. (1985). Supercoil sequencing: A fast and simple method for sequencing plasmid DNA. *DNA* **4**, 165–70.

Chu, G., Vollrath, D. and Davis, R.W. (1986). Separation of large DNA molecules by contour-clamped homogeneous electric fields. *Science* **234**, 1582–5.

Church, G.M. and Gilbert, W. (1984). Genomic sequencing. *Proc. Nat. Acad. Sci. (USA)* **81**, 1991–5.

Church, G.M. and Kieffer-Higgins, S. (1988). Multiplex DNA sequencing. *Science* **240**, 185–8.

Clark, S.M., Lai, E., Birren, B.W. and Hood, L. (1988). A novel instrument for separating large DNA molecules with pulsed homogeneous electric fields. *Science* **241**, 1203–5.

Clarke, L. and Carbon, J. (1976). A colony bank containing synthetic Col El hybrid plasmids representative of the entire *E. coli* genome. *Cell* **9**, 91–9.

Collins, J. and Hohn, B. (1978). Cosmids: A type of plasmid gene-cloning vector that is packageable *in vitro* in bacteriophage λ heads. *Proc. Nat. Acad. Sci. (USA)* **75**, 4242–6.

Cotton, R.G.H. (1989). Detection of single base changes in nucleic acids. *Biochem. J.* **263**, 1–10.

Cotton, R.G.H. and Campbell, R.D. (1989). Chemical reactivity of matched cytosine thymine bases near mismatched and unmatched bases in a heteroduplex between DNA strands with multiple differences. *Nucleic Acids Res.* **17**, 4223–33.

Cotton, R.G.H. and Wright, P.J. (1989). Rapid chemical mapping of dengue virus variability using RNA isolated directly from cells. *J. Virol. Methods* **26**, 67–76.

Cotton, R.G.H., Rodrigues, N.R. and Campbell, R.D. (1988). Reactivity of cytosine and thymine in single-base-pair mismatches with hydroxylamine and osmium tetroxide and its application to the study of mutations. *Proc. Nat. Acad. Sci. (USA)* **85**, 4397–401.

Coulson, A., Waterston, R., Kiff, J., Sulston, J. and Kohara, Y. (1988). Genome linking with yeast artificial chromosomes. *Nature* **335**, 184–6.

Cross, S.J., Bentley, D.R., Edwards, J.E. and Campbell, R.D. (1985). DNA polymorphism of the C2 and factor B genes. *Immunogenetics* **21**, 39–48.

Cunningham, M.W. and Mundy, C.R. (1987). Labelling nucleic acids for hybridization. *Nature* **326**, 723–4.

Dahl, H.-H.M., Lamande, S.R., Cotton, R.G.H. and Bateman, J.F. (1989). Detection and localization of base changes in RNA using a chemical cleavage method. *Anal. Biochem.* **183**, 263–8.

Dale, R.M.K., McClure, B.A. and Houchins, J.P. (1985). A rapid single-stranded cloning strategy for producing a sequential series of overlapping clones for use in DNA sequencing: Application to sequencing the corn mitochondrial T8 S rDNA. *Plasmid* **13**, 31–40.

Davis, L.G., Dibner, M.D. and Battey, J.F. (1986). *Basic Methods in Molecular Biology*, Elsevier, New York.

Davis, M.M. and Bjorkman, P.J. (1988). T-cell antigen receptor genes and T-cell recognition. *Nature* **334**, 395–402.

Deutsch, J.M. (1988). Theoretical studies of DNA during gel electrophoresis. *Science* **240**, 922–4.

Donis-Keller, H., Green, P., Helms, C. *et al.* (1987). A genetic linkage map of the human genome. *Cell* **51**, 319–37.

Duncan, A.R. and Winter, G. (1988). The binding site for Clq on IgG. *Nature* **332**, 738–40.

Duncan, A.R., Woof, J.M., Partridge, L.J., Burton, D.R. and Winter, G. (1988). Localization of the binding site for the human high-affinity Fc receptor on IgG. *Nature* **332**, 563–64.

Dunham, I., Sargent, C.A., Trowsdale, J. and Campbell, R.D. (1987). Molecular mapping of the human major histocompatibility complex by pulsed-field gel electrophoresis. *Proc. Nat. Acad. Sci. (USA)* **84**, 7237–41.

Dunham, I., Sargent, C.A., Dawkins, R.L. and Campbell, R.D. (1989). An analysis of variation in the long-range genomic organization of the human major histocompatibility complex class II region by pulsed-field gel electrophoresis. *Genomics* **5**, 787–96.

Eckert, R.L. (1987). New vectors for rapid sequencing of DNA fragments by chemical degradation. *Gene* **51**, 247–54.

Edgell, M.H., Weaver, S., Haigwood, N. and Hutchinson, C.A. (1979). In *Genetic Engineering*, ed. J.K. Setlow and A. Hollaender, vol. I, p. 37, Plenum, New York.

Embury, S.H., Scharf, S.J., Saiki, R.K. *et al.* (1987). Rapid prenatal diagnosis of sickle cell anemia by a new method of DNA analysis. *N. Engl. J. Med.* **316**, 656–61.

Erlich, H.A. (ed.) (1989). *PCR Technology*, pp. 1–244. Stockton Press, New York.

Feinberg, A.P. and Vogelstein, B. (1983). A technique for radiolabeling DNA restriction endonuclease fragments to high specific activity. *Anal. Biochem.* **132**, 6–13.

Feinberg, A.P. and Vogelstein, B. (1984). A technique for radiolabeling DNA restriction endonuclease fragments to high specific activity. *Anal. Biochem.* **137**, 266–7.

FMC Bioproducts Technical Bulletins T-14, T-19.

Fourney, R.M., Miyakoski, J., Day, R.E. and Patterson, M.C. (1988). *Focus (BRL)* **10**, 5.

Frischauf, A., Lehrach, H., Poustka, A. and Murray, N. (1984). Lambda replacement vectors carrying polylinker sequences. *J. Mol. Biol.* **170**, 827–42.

Fritz, H.J. (1985). The oligonucleotide-directed construction of mutations in recombinant filamentous phage. In *DNA Cloning*, ed. D.M. Glover, vol. I, pp. 151–63, IRL Press, Oxford.

Gardiner, K., Laas, W. and Patterson, D. (1986). Fractionation of large mammalian DNA restriction fragments using vertical pulsed-field gradient gel electrophoresis. *Som. Cell Mol. Genet.* **12**, 185–95.

Gorman, C. (1985). High efficiency gene transfer into mammalian cells. In *DNA Cloning: a Practical Approach*, ed. D.M. Glover, vol. II, pp. 143–90, IRL Press, Oxford.

Gorman, C., Moffat, L. and Howard, B. (1982). Recombinant genomes which express chloramphenicol acetyltransferase in mammalian cells. *Mol. Cell. Biol.* **2**, 1044–51.

Goss, S.J. and Harris, H. (1977). Gene transfer by means of cell fusion. *J. Cell. Sci.* **25**, 17–37.

Graham, F. and van der Eb, A. (1973). A new technique for the assay of infectivity of human adenovirus 5 DNA. *Virology* **52**, 456–67.

Grompe, M., Muzny, D.M. and Caskey, C.T. (1989). Scanning detection of mutations in human ornithine transcarbamoylase by chemical mismatch cleavage. *Proc. Nat. Acad. Sci. (USA)* **86**, 5888–92.

Gubler, U. and Hoffmann, B.J. (1983). A simple and very efficient method for generating cDNA libraries. *Gene* **25**, 263–9.

Hall, C. (1983). Expression and regulation of *Escherichia coli lac-Z* gene fusions in mammalian cells. *J. Mol. Appl. Genet.* **2**, 101–9.

Hames, B.D. and Higgins, S.J. (1985). *Nucleic Acid Hybridisation: a Practical Approach*. IRL Press, Oxford.

Hanahan, D. (1983). Studies on transformation of *Escherichia coli* with plasmids. *J. Mol. Biol.* **166**, 557–80.

Hardy, D.A., Bell, J.I., Long, E.O., Lindsten, T. and McDevitt, H.O. (1986). Mapping of the class II region of the human major histocompatibility complex by pulsed-field gel electrophoresis. *Nature* **323**, 453–5.

Hardy, K. (1981). *Bacterial Plasmids*. American Society of Microbiology, Washington, D.C.

Hardy, K. (1987). *Plasmids: a Practical Approach*. IRL Press Oxford.

Heinkoff, S. (1984). Unidirectional digestion with exonuclease III creates targeted breakpoints for DNA sequencing. *Gene* **28**, 351–7.

Hendrix, R.W., Roberts, J.W., Stahl, F.W. and Weisberg, R.A. (1983). *Lambda II*, CSH, New York.

Hoheisel, J. and Pohl, F.M. (1986). Simplified preparation of unidirectional deletion clones. *Nucleic Acids Res.* **14**, 3605.

Hohn, B. (1979). *In vitro* packaging of λ and cosmid DNA. *Methods Enzymol.* **68**, 299–309.

Hohn, B. and Murray, K. (1977). Packaging recombinant DNA molecules into bacteriophage particles *in vitro*. *Proc. Nat. Acad. Sci. (USA)* **74**, 3259–68.

Hood, L., Steinmetz, M. and Malissen, B. (1983). Genes of the major histocompatibility complex of the mouse. *Ann. Rev. Immunol.* **1**, 529–68.

Huynh, T.V., Young, R.A. and Davis, R.W. (1985). Constructing screening cDNA libraries in λgt 10 and λgt 11. In *DNA Cloning: a Practical Approach*, ed. D.M. Glover, pp. 49–78, IRL Press, Oxford.

Iggo, R., Gough, A., Xu, W., Lane, D.P. and Spurr, N.K. (1989). Chromosome mapping of the human gene encoding the 68-kDa nuclear antigen (p68) by using the polymerase chain reaction. *Proc. Nat. Acad. Sci. (USA)* **86**, 6211–14.

Innis, M.A., Myambo, K.B., Geltard, D.H. and Brow, M.A.D. (1988). DNA sequencing with Thermus aquaticus DNA polymerase & direct sequencing of polymerase chain reaction-amplified DNA. *Proc. Nat. Acad. Sci. (USA)* **85**, 9436–40.

Ish-Horowicz, D. and Burke, J.F. (1981). Rapid & efficient cosmid cloning. *Nucleic Acids Res.* **9**, 2989–98.

Israël, A., Kimura, A., Fournier, A., Fellows, M. and Kourilsky, P. (1986). Interferon response sequence potentiates activity of an enhancer in the promoter region of a mouse H-2 gene. *Nature* **322**, 743–6.

Josse, J., Kaiser, A.D. and Kornberg, A. (1961). Enzymatic synthesis of deoxyribonucleic acid VIII. Frequencies of nearest neighbor base sequences in deoxyribonucleic acid. *J. Biol. Chem.* **236**, 864–75.

Kramer, W. (1984). The gapped duplex DNA approach to oligonucleotide-directed mutation construction. *Nucleic Acids Res.* **12**, 9441–56.

Krieg, P. and Melton, D. (1984). Functional messenger RNAs are produced by SP6 *in vitro* transcription of cloned cDNAs. *Nucleic Acids Res.* **12**, 7057–70.

Kronenberg, M., Siu, G., Hood, L.E. and Shastri, N. (1986). The molecular genetics of the T-cell antigen receptor and T-cell antigen recognition. *Ann. Rev. Immunol.* **4**, 529–91.

Kunkel, T.A., Roberts, J.D. and Zakour, R.A. (1987). Rapid

and efficient site-specific mutagenesis without phenotypic selection. *Methods Enzymol.* **154**, 367–82.

Lamande, S.R., Dahl, H.-H.M., Cole, W.G. & Bateman, J.F. (1989). Characterization of point mutations in the collagen COL1A1 and COL1A2 genes causing lethal perinatal osteogenesis imperfecta. *J. Biol. Chem.* **264**, 15809–12.

Lee, G.C., Wu, X., Gibbs, R.A., Cook, R.G., Muzny, D.M. and Caskey, C.T. (1988). Generation of cDNA probes directed by amino acid sequence: cloning of urate oxidase. *Science* **239**, 1288.

Lehrach, H., Diamond, D., Wozney, J.M. and Boedtker, H. (1977). RNA molecular weight determinations by gel electrophoresis under denaturing conditions, a critical reexamination. *Biochemistry* **16**, 4743–51.

Li, H., Gyllensten, U.B., Cui, X., Saiki, R.K., Erlich, H.A. and Arnheim, N. (1988). Amplification and analysis of DNA sequences in single human sperm and diploid cells. *Nature* **335**, 414–17.

Lindsay, S. and Bird, A.P. (1987). Use of restriction enzymes to detect potential gene sequences in mammalian DNA. *Nature* **327**, 336–8.

Loh, E.Y., Elliot, J.F., Cwirla, S., Lanier, L.L. and Davis, M.M. (1989). Polymerase chain reaction with single-sided specificity. Analysis of T cell receptor δ chain. *Science* **243**, 217–20.

Mandel, M. and Higa, A. (1970). Calcium-dependent bacteriophage DNA infection. *J. Mol. Biol.* **53**, 159–62.

Matsuda, F., Lee, K.H., Nakai, S. *et al.* (1988). Dispersed localization of D segments in the human immunoglobulin heavy-chain locus. *EMBO J.* **7**, 1047–51.

Maxam, A.M. and Gilbert, W. (1977). A new method for sequencing DNA. *Proc. Nat. Acad. Sci. (USA)* **74**, 560–64.

Maxam, A.M. and Gilbert, W. (1980). Sequencing end-labeled DNA with base-specific chemical cleavages. *Methods Enzymol.* **65**, 499–560.

Melton, D., Krieg, P.A., Rebagliati, M.R., Maniatis, T., Zinn, K. and Green, M.R. (1984). Efficient *in vitro* synthesis of biologically active RNA and RNA hybridization probes from plasmids containing a bacteriophage SP6 promoter. *Nucleic Acids Res.* **12**, 7035–56.

Messing, J. (1983). New M13 vectors for cloning. *Methods Enzymol.* **101**, 20–78.

Michiels, F.M., Burmeister, M. and Lehrach, H. (1987). Derivation of clones close to met by preparative field inversion gel electrophoresis. *Science* **236**, 1305–08.

Mills, D.R. and Kramer, F.R. (1979). Structure-independent nucleotide sequence analysis. *Proc. Nat. Acad. Sci. (USA)* **76**, 2232–35.

Mizusawa, S., Nishimura, S. and Seela, F. (1986). Improvement of the dideoxy chain termination method of DNA sequencing by use of deoxy-7-deazaguanosine triphosphate in place of dGTP. *Nucleic Acids Res.* **14**, 1319–24.

Montandon, A.J., Green, P.M., Gianelli, F. and Bentley, D.R. (1989). Direct detection of point mutations by mismatch analysis: application to haemophilia B. *Nucleic Acids Res.* **17**, 3347–58.

Mulligan, R. and Berg, P. (1981). Selection for animal cells that express the *Escherichia coli* gene coding for xanthine-guanine phosphoribosyltransferase. *Proc. Nat. Acad. Sci. (USA)* **78**, 2072–6.

Myers, R.M., Lumelsky, N., Lerman, L.S. and Maniatis, T. (1985a). Detection of single base substitutions in total genomic DNA. *Nature* **313**, 495–98.

Myers, R.M., Larin, Z. and Maniatis, T. (1985b). Detection of single base substitutions by ribonuclease cleavage at mismatches in RNA:DNA duplexes. *Science* **230**, 1242–6.

Nakamura, Y., Leppert, M., O'Connell, P. *et al.* (1987). Variable number of tandem repeat (VNTR) markers for human gene mapping. *Science* **235**, 1616–22.

Nguyen, V.T., Morange, M. & Bensaude, O. (1988). Firefly luciferase luminescence assays using scintillation counters for quantitation in transfected mammalian cells. *Anal. Biochem.* **171**, 404–8.

Ockman, H., Gerber, A.S. and Harth, D.L. (1988). Genetic applications of an inverse polymerase chain reaction. *Genetics* **120**, 621–3.

Okayama, H. and Berg, P. (1982). High-efficiency cloning of full-length cDNA. *Mol. Cell. Biol.* **2**, 161–30.

Parham, P. (1988). Histocompatibility typing: Mac is back in town. *Immunol. Today* **9**, 127–30.

Porteous, D.J. (1987). Chromosome mediated gene transfer: a functional assay for complex loci and an aid to human genome mapping. *Trends Genet.* **3**, 177–82.

Potter, H., Weir, L. and Leder, P. (1984). Enhancer-dependent expression of human K immunoglobulin genes introduced into mouse pre-B lymphocytes by electroporation. *Proc. Nat. Acad. Sci. (USA)* **81**, 7161–5.

Poustka, A. and Lehrach, H. (1986). Jumping libraries and linking libraries: the next generation of molecular tools in mammalian genetics. *Trends Genet.* **2**, 174–9.

Radloff, R., Bauer, W. and Vinograd, J. (1967). A dye-buoyant-density method for the detection and isolation of closed circular duplex DNA: The closed circular DNA in hela cells. *Proc. Nat. Acad. Sci. (USA)* **57**, 1514–21.

Reed, K.C. and Mann, D.A. (1985). Rapid transfer of DNA from agarose gels to nylon membranes. *Nucleic Acids Res.* **13**, 7207–21.

Rey-Campos, J. Rubenstein, P. and Rodriguez de Cordoba, S. (1988). Physical map of the human regulator of complement activation gene cluster linking the complement genes CR1, CR2, DAF and C4BP. *J. Exp. Med.* **167**, 664.

Riechmann, L., Clark, M., Waldmann, H., Winter, G. (1988). Reshaping human antibodies for therapy. *Nature* **332**, 323–7.

Rigby, P.W.J., Dieckmann, M., Rhodes, C. and Berg, P. (1977). Labeling deoxyribonucleic acid to high specificity activity *in vitro* by nick translation with DNA polymerase I. *J. Mol. Biol.* **113**, 237–51.

Roberts, R.G., Cole, C.G., Hart, K.A., Bobrow, M. and Bentley, D.R. (1989a). Rapid carrier and prenatal diagnosis of Duchenne and Becker muscular dystrophy. *Nucleic Acids Res.* **17**, 811.

Roberts, R.G., Montandon, A.J., Bobrow, M. and Bentley, D.R. (1989b). Detection of novel genetic markers by mismatch analysis. *Nucleic Acids Res.* **17**, 5961–71.

Roberts, R.J. (1987). Restriction enzymes and their isoschizomers. *Nucleic Acids Res.* **15** (suppl.), r189–r217.

Ruddle, F.H. (1981). A new era in mammalian gene mapping: somatic cell genetics and recombinant DNA methodologies. *Nature* **294**, 115–20.

Saiki, R.K., Scharf, S.J., Faloona, F. *et al.* (1985). Enzymatic amplification of β-globin genomic sequences and restriction site analysis for diagnosis of sickle cell anemia. *Science* **230**, 1350–4.

Saiki, R.K., Bugawan, T.L., Horn, G.T., Mullis, K.B. and Erlich, H.A. (1986). Analysis of enzymatically amplified β-globin and HLA-DQα DNA with allele-specific oligonucleotide probes. *Nature* **324**, 163–6.

Saiki, R.K., Gelford, D.H., Stoffel, S. *et al.* (1988). Primer-directed enzymatic amplification of DNA with a thermostable DNA polymerase. *Science* **239**, 487–91.

Sambrook, J., Fritsch, E.F. and Maniatis, T. (1989). *Molecular Cloning: a Laboratory Manual*. (2nd edn.), CSH, New York.

Sanger, F., Nicklen, S. & Coulson, A.R. (1977). DNA sequencing with chain-terminating inhibitors. *Proc. Nat. Acad. Sci. (USA)* **74**, 5463–7.

Sanger, F., Coulson, A.R., Barrell, B.G., Smith, A.J.H. and Roe, B.A. (1982). Cloning in single-stranded bacteriophage as an aid to rapid DNA sequencing. *J. Mol. Biol.* **143**, 161–78.

Sargent, C.A., Dunham, I. and Campbell, R.D. (1989a). Identification of multiple HTF-island associated genes in the human major histocompatibility complex class III region. *EMBO J.* **8**, 2305–12.

Sargent, C.A., Dunham, I., Trowsdale, J. and Campbell, R.D. (1989b). Human major histocompatibility complex contains genes for the major heat shock protein HSP70. *Proc. Nat. Acad. Sci. (USA)* **86**, 1968–72.

Scharf, S.J., Horn, G.T. and Erlich, H.A. (1986). Direct cloning and sequence analysis of enzymatically amplified genomic sequences. *Science* **233**, 1076–8.

Scharf, S.J., Friedmann, A.F., Brauttner, C. *et al.* (1988). HLA Class II allelic variation and susceptibility to pemphigus vulgaris. *Proc. Nat. Acad. Sci. (USA)* **85**, 3504–8.

Schwartz, D.C. and Cantor, C.R. (1984). Separation of yeast chromosome-sized DNAs by pulsed fixed gradient gel electrophoresis. *Cell* **37**, 67–75.

Schwartz, D.C. and Koval, M. (1989). Conformational dynamics of individual DNA molecules during gel electrophoresis. *Nature* **338**, 520–21.

Seed, B., Parker, B.C. and Davidson, N. (1982). Representation of DNA sequences in recombinant DNA libraries prepared by restriction enzyme partial digestion. *Gene* **19**, 201–9.

Sharpe, P.A., Sugden, B. and Sambrook, J. (1973). Detection of two restriction endonuclease activities in Haemophilus parainfluenzae using analytical agarose-ethidium bromide electrophoresis. *Biochemistry* **13**, 3055–63.

Sheldon, E.L., Kellogg, D.E., Watson, R., Levenson, C.H. and Erlich, H.A. (1986). Use of nonisotopic M13 probes for genetic analysis: Application to HLA class II loci. *Proc. Nat. Acad. Sci. (USA)* **83**, 9085–89.

Shen, J.C.K. and Maniatis, T. (1980). The organization of repetitive sequences in a cluster of rabbit β-like globin genes. *Cell* **19**, 379–91.

Short, J.M., Fernandez, J.M., Sorge, J.A. and Huse, W.D. (1988). λ ZAP: a bacteriophage λ expression vector with *in vivo* excision properties. *Nucleic Acids Res.* **16**, 7583–600.

Silver, J. and Keerikatte, V. (1989). Novel use of polymerase chain reaction to amplify cellular DNA adjacent to an integrated protovirus. *J. Virol.* **63**, 1924–28.

Smith, S.B., Aldridge, P.K. and Callis, J.B. (1989). Observation of individual DNA molecules undergoing gel electrophoresis. *Science* **243**, 203–6.

Sompayrac, L. and Danna, K. (1981). Efficient infection of monkey cells with DNA simian virus 40. *Proc. Nat. Acad. Sci. (USA)* **12**, 7575–8.

Southern, E.M. (1975). Detection of specific sequences among DNA fragments separated by gel electrophoresis. *J. Mol. Biol.* **98**, 503–17.

Southern, E.M. (1979). Gel electrophoresis of restriction fragments. *Methods Enzymol.* **68**, 152–76.

Southern, E.M., Anand, R., Brown, W.R.A. and Fletcher, D.S. (1987). A model for the separation of large DNA molecules by crossed field gel electrophoresis. *Nucleic Acids Res.* **15**, 5925–43.

Southern, P. and Berg, P. (1982). Transformation of mammalian cells to antibiotic resistance with a bacterial gene under control of the SV40 early region promoter. *J. Mol. Appl. Genet.* **1**, 327–41.

Spandidos, D.A. and Wilkie, N.M. (1984). In *Transcription and Translation: a Practical Approach*, ed. B.D. Hames and S.J. Higgins, p. 1–48, IRL Press, Oxford.

Stoflet, E.S., Koeberl, D.D., Sarker, G. and Sommer, S.S. (1988). Genomic amplification with transcript sequencing. *Science* **239**, 491–4.

Suggs, S.V., Wallace, R.B., Hirose, T., Kawoshima, E.H. and Hakura, K. (1981). Use of synthetic oligonucleotides as hybridization probes: isolation of cloned cDNA sequences for human β_2-microglobulin. *Proc. Nat. Acad. Sci. (USA)* **78**, 6613–17.

Swartz, M.N., Trautner, T.A. and Kornberg, A. (1962). Enzymatic synthesis of deoxyribonucleic acid. *J. Biol. Chem.* **237**, 1961–7.

Tabor, S. and Richardson, C.C. (1987). DNA sequence analysis with a modified bacteriophage T7 DNA polymerase. *Proc. Nat. Acad. Sci. (USA)* **84**, 4767–71.

Todd, J.A., Bell, J.I. and McDevitt, H.O. (1987). HLA-DQβ gene contributes to susceptibility and resistance to insulin-dependent diabetes mellitus. *Nature* **329**, 599–604.

Todd, J.A., Acha-Orbea, H., Bell, J.I. *et al.* (1988). A molecular basis for MHC Class II-associated autoimmunity. *Science* **240**, 1003–09.

Tonegawa, S. (1987). Somatic generation of antibody diversity. *Nature* **302**, 575–81.

Triglia, T., Peterson, M.G. and Kemp, D.J. (1988). A procedure for *in vitro* amplification of DNA segments that lie outside the boundaries of known sequences. *Nucleic Acids Res.* **16**, 8186.

Tunnacliffe, A., Jones, C. and Goodfellow, P. (1983). Somatic cell genetics, immunogenetics and gene mapping. *Immunol. Today* **4**, 230–3.

Tunnacliffe, A., Benham, F. and Goodfellow, P. (1984). Mapping the human genome by somatic cell genetics. *Trends Biochem. Sci.* **9**, 5–7.

Twigg, A.J. and Sherratt, D. (1980). Trans-complementable copy-number mutants of plasmid CO1E1. *Nature* **283**, 216–18.

van Ommen, G.J.B. and Verkerk, J.M.H. (1986). Restriction analysis of chromosomal DNA in a size range up to two million base pairs by pulsed field gradient electrophoresis. In *Human Genetic Disease: a Practical Approach*, ed. K.E. Davies, pp. 113–33, IRL Press, Oxford.

Wahl, G.M., Stern, M. and Stark, G.R. (1979). Efficient transfer of large DNA fragments from agarose gels to diazobenzyloxymethyl-paper and rapid hybridization by using dextran sulfate. *Proc. Nat. Acad. Sci. (USA)* **76**, 3683–7.

Walker, M.D., Edlund, T., Bourlet, A.M. and Rutter, W.J. (1983). Cell-specific expression controlled by the 5′-flanking region of insulin and chymotrypsin genes. *Nature* **306**, 557–61.

Waterbury, P.G. and Lane, M.J. (1986). Generation of lamda phage concatemers for use as pulsed field electrophoresis size markers. *Nucleic Acids Res.* **15**, 3930.

Wigler, M., Silverstein, S., Lee, L.-S., Pellicer, A., Cheng, Y.-C. and Axel, R. (1987). Transfer of purified herpes virus thymidine kinase gene to cultured mouse cells. *Cell* **11**, 223–32.

Wu, L.C., Morley, B.J. and Campbell, R.D. (1987). Cell-specific expression of the human complement protein factor B gene: evidence for the role of two distinct 5′-flanking elements. *Cell* **48**, 331–42.

Yanisch-Perron, C., Vieira, J. and Messing, J. (1985). Improved M13 phage cloning vectors and host strains: nucleotide sequences of the M13 mp18 and pUC19 vectors. *Gene* **33**, 103–19.

42: Transgenic Animals as Tools for Immunology Research

N. Holmes

The ability to alter the germline deoxyribonucleic acid (DNA) of the mouse by artificial manipulation has become a powerful and important tool in the understanding of complex biological systems and has been used extensively to study the genes, gene products and cellular interactions of the immune system. Mice whose genome has been altered by specific procedures are termed transgenic. There are two distinct types of transgenic mice which have had an impact on investigations of the immune system. These may be called insertional transgenics and mutational transgenics respectively. Insertional transgenics are animals into whose germline new genetic material has been introduced without intentionally altering any of the pre-existing endogenous genes. This can be achieved by several techniques but is almost invariably done by microinjecting the DNA to be inserted into the male pronucleus of a single-cell fertilized embryo, which is subsequently introduced into a suitable pseudopregnant female recipient and allowed to develop.

Mutational transgenics, by contrast, deliberately alter a normal endogenous gene, usually involving disrupting it so as to prevent expression of the normal gene product. This is made possible by the use of embryonic stem (ES) cells, which can be cultured under special conditions *in vitro* so as to retain totipotency, including the ability to contribute to the germline, while permitting manipulation in culture. It is now possible to introduce homologous DNA which has been altered, e.g. by the introduction of an in-frame stop codon or other disruptive event, into these ES cells, and to select for the integration of the DNA. Subsequently it is necessary to screen clones or pools of clones of the transformed ES cells for one which has undergone site-specific recombination, in which one copy of the homologous normal gene has been modified in the desired way. The process is referred to as gene targeting. The targeted ES cells must then be reintroduced into a genetically marked blastocyst-stage embryo, which is implanted into suitable recipient animals to produce live offspring.

It may be noted that, while insertional transgenic founder mice are usually pure heterozygotes for the insertion (occasionally chimerism can result from the integration event occurring after some number of cell divisions), mutational transgenic founders are always chimeric. In both cases it is possible for the founder animals to fail to transmit the transgene to their offspring, although this is more frequent in ES-cell-derived animals. The mutational transgenic experiment will almost always rely on producing homozygotes by breeding first pure heterozygotes and then intercrossing these.

It is neither practical nor desirable to examine in this chapter all the immunologically relevant transgenic experiments performed to date. The author's intention is to try to outline the areas within immunology in which transgenic technology has had the most impact and to briefly look forward to possible future applications.

Regulation of gene expression

It has become apparent that the transcriptional regulation of gene expression is an exceptionally complex process. Deoxyribonucleic acid elements defined as enhancers by *in vitro* assays, even using transfection into appropriate tissue culture cell lines, may not be either necessary or sufficient to direct cell-type-specific, developmentally regulated transcription *in vivo*. Transgenic studies of gene expression have therefore become the state-of-the-art method for defining the necessary DNA elements required to give correct spatial and temporal expression of a specific gene.

In some cases it appears that a single major regulatory element (which nevertheless may contain binding sites for multiple factors and which will certainly require the presence of other non-specific transcriptional elements) may be sufficient to define the proper expression pattern. This type of element has been called a dominant control region (DCR), and was originally described by Grosveld *et al*. 1987 in the β-globin gene system. Immunoglobulin (Ig), T cell receptor (TCR), CD2 and CD3 genes apparently have DCRs. It is tempting to generalize and suggest that genes which are expressed at high levels only by a single cell lineage are likely to be regulated in this way.

Immunoglobulin gene regulation

The Ig genes were one of the earliest gene systems of the immune system to be subjected to transgenic experiments. They also present an excellent example of the usefulness of transgenic animals in the study of gene regulation. Certain sequence elements have been defined as required for correct transcription of Ig genes in transfected cell lines (reviewed by Calame 1985). The two most prominent are a conserved octanucleotide just upstream of the TATA box and an intron enhancer, distinct forms of which are found in both the κ and the IgH loci. Early transgenic experiments, using quite small rearranged κ or μ DNA inserts, seemed to show cell-type-specific expression in lymphoid cells and, in the case of some κ transgenes, B cells only (Storb *et al*. 1984). Several experiments have examined the importance of the intron enhancer element in transgene regulation, either by constructing an IgH 'gene' which lacks this region (Yamamura *et al*. 1984) or by attaching the heavy chain enhancer to a reporter gene (e.g. Gerlinger *et al*. 1986; Reik *et al*. 1987). These studies suggested that the IgH intron enhancer was sufficient (in the latter cases) and necessary (in the former experiment) for correct Ig gene transcription. Other transgenic experiments suggest that neither the IgH (e.g. Yamamura *et al*. 1986) nor the κ (Meyer *et al*. 1990) intron enhancer is sufficient to ensure the correct level of expression in B cells. Constructs including these enhancers do not produce sufficient Ig ribonucleic acid (RNA) to prevent rearrangement of the appropriate endogenous chains, although in some cases high copy number can overcome this inefficiency. More recent analysis has revealed the presence of a further enhancer downstream of both κ and IgH loci. Neuberger's group isolated a region of DNA 3′ of κ which, when included with the introduced DNA segment, dramatically increased the level of transcription both in transfected cell lines and in transgenic mice (Meyer *et al*. 1990). Transgenic constructs including this sequence are transcribed at normal high levels. They also essentially prevent endogenous κ rearrangement and permit somatic hypermutation of the transgenes (O'Brien *et al*. 1987; Sharpe *et al*. 1991). It seems probable that these downstream enhancers are the major 'DCR' of the κ and IgH loci and that they might not have been discovered but for the relative inability of short transgenes to reproduce the behaviour of endogenous Ig genes.

T-cell-specific genes

Genetic control elements with properties of T-cell-specific DCRs have been isolated from the TCR α and β loci, the CD2 and the CD3 genes. As with Ig genes, the TCR locus elements are also located 3′ of the constant-region segments and are also obligatory for proper high-level expression and allelic exclusion (e.g. Uematsu *et al.* 1988). The CD3 genes are to some extent distinct in that all three core CD3 chains (γ, δ ε) are encoded by closely linked loci, apparently regulated by a single DCR.

Major histocompatibility complex genes

Transgenic analysis has contributed substantially to our understanding of the regulation of Class II major histocompatibility complex (MHC) gene expression. This subject was reviewed recently by Benoist and Mathis (1990). These genes differ from those discussed above in that they are expressed in several different cell types and are under both constitutive and inducible control. Essentially, the production of transgenic lines with distinct altered (deleted or mutated) gene constructs has allowed the delineation of several important regulatory elements, some of which function in specific cell types, e.g. B cells or thymic epithelial cells. Further analysis of this highly complex system is still proceeding. Somewhat less attention has been given to Class I MHC gene regulation in transgenic animals. Several groups have produced transgenic lines with Class I MHC genes from a number of species with apparently normal expression patterns. Apart from being consistent with the *in vitro* transfection data that all the necessary sequence elements reside within a few hundred base pairs 5′ of the RNA start site, these experiments reveal little new information. However, recent work in this laboratory has shown that a human Class I MHC transgene is not expressed on thymic epithelium until 14–21 days after normal endogenous expression begins. Subsequent analysis has shown that the early-onset high-level expression of Class I MHC genes in this specialized epithelial tissue must require some sequence other than the previously characterized 5′ regulatory regions (M. Osmond *et al.*, in preparation). Transgenic studies are uniquely suited to the elucidation of this type of developmental cell-type-specific regulatory element.

T cell development

The area of T cell development and T cell subset function is perhaps the topic which has been most actively pursued through transgenic animal models, certainly over the past 3 years. The first publication describing an experiment designed to investigate the effect of transgenic expression (of a rearranged TCR β chain in that case) on thymocyte development appeared in March 1988 (Uematsu *et al.* 1988). Since that time, literally dozens of reports have appeared and we now have transgenic animals with TCR αβ and TCR γδ genes, as well as mutational transgenics lacking Class I MHC (β-2-microglobulin), CD8, CD4 and Class II MHC genes, plus several other transgene experiments approaching the same problems. Although few truly new ideas have emerged from these numerous studies, they have provided solid foundations for understanding the mysterious processes of thymic development and have permitted tests of hypotheses, some more than 10 years old, previously impervious to straightforward experimental evaluation.

Several groups have produced transgenic mice with rearranged TCR genes. Von Boehmer, Steinmetz and their colleagues developed mice containing either the β or both α and β chains encoding the TCR from a cytotoxic T cell clone, B6.2.16, which recognizes the male H-Y antigen when presented by the Class I MHC molecule H-$2D^b$ (reviewed by von Boehmer 1990). The β-chain-only mice showed initially that the 30+ kb of genomic DNA injected gave high-level tissue-specific expression and that this inhibited, almost completely, endogenous TCR β-chain rearrangements (Uematsu *et al.* 1988). The double-transgenic mice were of great functional importance since they permitted direct testing of the generally held hypothesis that developing T cells pass through two stages of selection during thymic ontogeny, namely positive selection for self-MHC-restricted T cells and negative selection against self-MHC-plus self-peptide (antigen)-reactive T cells. Indeed, their results showed that, in H-2^b male mice carrying the rearranged αβ transgenes, the thymus was grossly abnormal — very small and containing a mere fraction (2–3%) of the normal number of the dominant CD4 +ve, CD8 +ve thymocytes (Kisielow *et al.* 1988). These autoreactive cells had apparently been deleted by a negative selection process. In H-2^b female mice, by contrast, the thymus was of normal size with more or less normal numbers of CD4 +ve, CD8 +ve (double-positive) cells. These female mice provided a test for the reality of positive selection since the majority (even if not all) of their developing T cells expressed a receptor which was known to be capable of self MHC (D^b) restriction. The data showed that such transgenic mice had a dramatic increase in the numbers of CD4 −ve, CD8 +ve mature thymocytes. However, these TCR transgenic females did not have a noticeable difference in the ratio of CD4 +ve and CD8 +ve single-positive mature T cells in their peripheral lymphoid organs, despite the fact that almost all lymph node T cells expressed the transgenic β chain. This result appeared to contradict the idea that T cell precursors which express a Class I MHC-restricted receptor will develop into CD4 −ve, CD8 +ve mature cells. However, it soon became apparent that, although 'all' the peripheral T cells expressed the transgenic β chain, only the CD8 +ve cells expressed the transgenic TCR α chain (Teh *et al.* 1988). Indeed, it has become clear that endogenous α-chain rearrangement can and does occur in TCR α transgenic mice (Blüthmann *et al.* 1988).

Further clarification of the process known as positive selection was achieved by breeding the TCR αβ transgenic mice with severe combined immunodeficiency diseases (SCID) mice carrying a genetic defect in TCR and Ig gene rearrangement. The TCR−SCID mice are now expected to be monoclonal with respect to T cell receptor expression (although actually this turns out to be not quite true in practice). Von Boehmer and his colleagues then used female TCR−SCID mice, which were $H\text{-}2^{b/d}$ (expected to select the TCR αβ T cells and develop only CD8 +ve cells) or $H\text{-}2^{d/d}$ (expected to fail to positively select the transgenic αβ T cells due to lack of the appropriate restriction element), to test whether positive selection was an essential requirement for T cell development and whether a Class I MHC-restricted receptor determined a CD4 −ve, CD8 +ve phenotype. The results provided strong evidence for the hypothesis that positive selection is required for the development of CD8 +ve mature T cells and that thymocytes bearing Class I MHC-restricted receptors only mature into CD8 +ve cells (Scott *et al.* 1989). This experiment also provided a number of less well-predicted results. Firstly, SCID mice bearing a rearranged TCR β chain can productively rearrange their endogenous α chain, albeit at low frequency. Second, such cells can mature and form part of the peripheral lymphoid system, either as CD4 +ve, CD8 −ve (presumably Class II MHC-restricted) T cells or as CD4 −ve, CD8 +ve transgenic α −ve cells. Finally, in both $H\text{-}2^{b/d}$ and $H\text{-}2^{d/d}$ animals, CD4 −ve, CD8 −ve cells expressing transgenic TCR αβ receptors form a major class of T cells in the lymph node. These cells do not apparently require positive selection by self MHC within the thymus.

Many other TCR αβ double-transgenic animals have since been produced and their evaluation has reinforced and extended these conclusions. In particular, mice harbouring rearranged TCR transgenes specifying Class II MHC-restricted receptors positively select those cells in the presence of appropriate self MHC molecules to develop into CD4 +ve, CD8 −ve T cells (Berg *et al.* 1989; Kaye *et al.* 1989). These experiments with TCR αβ transgenic mice have confirmed the hypotheses that T cell precursors undergo both positive and negative selection and that MHC class restriction determines the CD4, CD8 phenotype of the resulting mature T cells.

Non-T cell receptor transgenics

The TCR αβ transgenic experiments have not addressed related questions of whether the CD4 and CD8 molecules are required for either or both selective events and how the binding of the TCR to its MHC ligand influences expression of the CD4, CD8 molecules. These last two issues have been and are being tackled with other transgenic models. Essentially, we can now say that CD8 is required for both positive and negative selection. Transgenic mice expressing altered Class I MHC genes which no longer bind CD8 (at least operationally) fail to either positively or negatively select the appropriate transgenic Class I MHC-restricted T cells (Aldrich *et al.* 1991; Ingold *et al.* 1991). Even more cogently, if mice expressing a CD8-deficient D^b molecule are intercrossed with the TCR αβ transgenics of von Boehmer *et al.*, specific for D^b plus H-Y, they behave as D^b −ve animals (N. Killeen and D. Littman, unpublished results). In addition, genetically CD8-deficient mice have been produced by mutational transgenesis and apparently lack Class I MHC-restricted T cells (Fung-Leung *et al.* 1991). Correspondingly, β-2-microglobulin- (and hence Class I MHC-) deficient transgenic mice lack CD8 +ve T cells (Koller *et al.* 1990; Zjilstra *et al.* 1990).

Genetic deficiencies of CD4 (Rahemtulla *et al.* 1991) and Class II MHC (Cosgrove *et al.* 1991) have also been recently reported. All of these 'gene knock-out' experiments support the view that CD4–Class II MHC and CD8–Class I MHC interactions are essential in the normal selection of thymocytes. These studies go further and provide important evidence about the function of the two subsets of T cells in both thymus and periphery. They show that neither CD4 nor Class II MHC molecules are required for the development of CD8 +ve cells and conversely that neither CD8 nor Class I MHC molecules are needed for the normal development of CD4 +ve T cells. CD8-deficient mice are defective in generating allogeneic or virus-specific cytotoxic T cells and cannot proliferate in response to Class I MHC alloantigen; they do, however, make a normal antiviral antibody, response, including isotype switching from IgM to IgG. CD4-deficient mice, by contrast, do generate virus-specific cytotoxic T lymphocytes (CTL), showing that CD4 +ve T cells are not absolutely required to help CTL generation, but do not make antigen-specific antibody responses. Class II MHC-deficient mice provide further information: these lack all but a few CD4 +ve cells, which seem to be of a specialized subset also seen in normal mice in small numbers. Such mice possess a normal B cell compartment, showing that neither Class II MHC antigen nor the 'normal' CD4 +ve T cell complement is needed for B cell development. Functionally, the Class II MHC –ve animals behave like mice lacking helper T cells, in that they make little or no antibody response to T-dependent antigens.

Class II MHC transgenic mice with cell-type-specific expression defects, also generated by Benoist and Mathis, have assisted in the understanding of which cell types present self MHC to developing T cells during selection. Experiments with irradiation chimeras and thymic-grafted animals had suggested that the interaction of thymocytes with thymic cortical epithelial cells leads to positive selection while interaction with bone marrow-derived thymic dendritic cells led to negative selection. Transgenic mice expressing the Class II MHC molecule H-2E on thymic epithelium but not dendritic cells achieve both positive and negative selection. Conversely, mice expressing H-2E on dendritic cells but not thymic epithelium only accomplish negative selection (van Ewijk *et al.* 1988; Benoist and Mathis 1989). These data therefore confirm that positive selection occurs through the interaction of TCR molecules on thymocytes with self MHC on thymic epithelium but demonstrate that either epithelial or dendritic cells are able to tolerize the T cell compartment through negative selection.

T cell receptor gamma-delta transgenic mice

Since the demonstration several years ago of the existence of a second minor population of T cells which express a distinct clonally variable receptor, TCR $\gamma\delta$, there has been both interest and controversy as to the relationship between the two types of T cell. Mice transgenic for rearranged TCR γ and δ genes have largely answered these questions. Essentially, the $\alpha\beta$ and $\gamma\delta$ lineages are separate. If mice are made transgenic for rearranged γ and δ genes using a large γ transgene of 40 kb, then these animals develop normal numbers of $\alpha\beta$ +ve thymocytes and T cells from birth (Ishida *et al.* 1990). If, however, a shorter γ transgene of 15–17 kb is used, then transgene expression blocks $\alpha\beta$ T cell development, apparently at the $V\beta \rightarrow D\beta J\beta$ stage (Bonneville *et al.* 1989). In such mice, $\alpha\beta$ +ve T cells do develop but some weeks after birth and only in cell clones which have down-regulated or lost expression of the γ transgene (Bonneville *et al.* 1989; Dent *et al.* 1990). Dent *et al.*'s results also showed that $\gamma\delta$ T cells are subject to negative selection in the thymus, in a similar fashion to $\alpha\beta$ T cells. Taken together, these data show that in normal T cell development the $\alpha\beta$ lineage does not express γ chain, so that, even if γ rearrangement occurs, it does not effect β- and subsequent α-chain rearrangement. Clearly, there is a silencer element present, some distance 3′ of the $C\gamma$ segment, which is 'on' in cells destined to become $\alpha\beta$ +ve T cells and 'off' in cells destined to become $\gamma\delta$ +ve T cells. It is still possible that cells which fail to make a productive rearrangement of γ, or perhaps δ, could go on to become $\alpha\beta$ T cells by default, as proposed by Pardoll *et al.* (1987). However, this remains to be demonstrated and seems likely to contribute only a small fraction of the $\alpha\beta$ +ve T cells at best.

Peripheral tolerance

Transgenic mice have also made an important contribution to the study of extrathymic tolerance of T cells and B cell tolerance. The transgenic method is especially useful in the study of peripheral tolerance, party because of the ability to produce mice with a dominant clonal receptor, either T or B cell, as referred to previously, and partly because transgene expression can be manipulated to make neo-self antigens appear at different times during development and in distinct locations. As we have seen already, animals become tolerant of MHC molecules expressed on antigen-presenting cells in the thymus through the deletional process of negative selection. If specific constructs are prepared so that MHC transgenes are expressed only in extrathymic peripheral tissues, this does not occur. Several types of such peripheral MHC transgenic mice have been produced and in all cases the transgenic animals remain tolerant of their transgenes, despite having T cells capable of recognizing the peripherally expressed allo-MHC (Lo *et al.* 1988, 1989; Morahan *et al.* 1989; Murphy *et al.* 1989). In some cases this peripheral tolerance does not extend to *in vitro* culture (Morahan *et al.* 1989; Böhme *et al.* 1989), although in other cases it apparently does (Lo *et al.* 1988, 1989). In common with non-transgenic models of peripheral tolerance, the tolerant state is not easily broken, for example by injection of normal, i.e. non-tolerant, T cells (e.g. Lo *et al.* 1989).

More recently, this type of experiment has been extended to look at the effects of crossing peripheral MHC transgenics with transgenic mice expressing rearranged T cell receptor genes specific for the relevant MHC antigen (Schönrich *et al.* 1991). In this case, mice expressing the Class I MHC molecule K^b apparently only in certain neuroectodermal cells, primarily in the brain, were produced using a glial fibrillary acidic protein (GFAP) gene promoter. The GFAP$-K^b$ mice are tolerant *in vivo*, not only of their endogenous K^b-expressing cells but also of skin grafts differing only at K^b. Furthermore, this peripheral MHC expression was sufficient to effectively tolerize the TCR transgenic cells in double-transgenic mice. The mechanism of tolerance appeared to be a down-regulation of both CD8 and TCR $\alpha\beta$ on peripheral T cells. Interestingly, this particular TCR $\alpha\beta$ transgenic line produces approximately equal numbers of CD4 and CD8 mature T cells expressing transgenic TCR, and only the CD8 +ve TCR $\alpha\beta$ +ve cells are affected by the peripheral antigen expression. *In vitro* culture restored both antigen expression and functional competence. It should be noted, however, that this receptor/accessory molecule down-regulation is only one way in which peripheral tolerance may occur and probably does not account for all or even most situations.

Peripheral expression of soluble antigens as transgenes leads to tolerance to the peptide fragments of these antigens presented on normally expressed self MHC molecules, even when the soluble antigens are themselves (engineered) MHC molecules (Arnold *et al.* 1990), but not in the latter case to tolerance to the membrane-bound form of the MHC molecule itself.

B cell tolerance has also been examined using the specific Ig transgene approach. Goodnow and co-workers made transgenic mice expressing IgM and IgD anti-hen egg lysozyme (HEL) and examined the effect of introducing HEL transgenes into the same animals. They found that, providing the serum level of HEL was above a certain threshold, the otherwise hyper-responsive IgM/D anti-HEL transgenic B cells were tolerized (Goodnow *et al.* 1988, 1989). The double-transgenic mice still contained a high proportion of anti-HEL B cells, but these had only low levels of IgM anti-HEL on their surface, in contrast to the Ig-only transgenics. The B cells remained tolerant, even on adoptive transfer with appropriate helper T cells. This represents peripheral tolerance of B cells and is probably the normal mechanism of B cell tolerance to serum antigens present in sufficient amounts. Low-level soluble antigens probably do not tolerize B cells but rely on T cell tolerance only.

Cell surface antigens, however, probably tolerize B cells by clonal deletion. This is suggested by the data of Nemazee and Bürki (1989), who made transgenic animals with IgM anti H-$2K^k$ expression. When the transgenic B cells developed in H-2^k mice, no transgenic IgM expression was seen in peripheral B cells, even when the transgenic B cells were derived from bone marrow chimeras, in which the B cells themselves did not express the target antigen. This deletion mechanism is probably not specific to MHC antigens but depends on the ability of the toleragen to cross-link antigen-specific IgM and/or IgD molecules on the surface of pre-B cells.

Autoimmunity

Transgenesis has also proved a fruitful technique for studying autoimmunity. However, as with all transgenic experiments, the complex nature of the experiment means that the results obtained may be unexpected and/or difficult to interpret. For example, a number of different groups attempted to test the hypothesis that aberrant expression of Class II MHC molecules by the β islet cells of the endocrine pancreas was in itself sufficient to cause autoimmune diabetes. The result of directing expression of self or allo-Class II MHC molecules to the β cells, using rat insulin promoter-driven constructs, was indeed diabetes (Lo *et al.* 1988; Sarvetnick *et al.* 1988). Nevertheless, the hypothesis is incorrect; the results showed that the diabetes did not result from an autoimmune response. Indeed, other investigators found no diabetes in mice expressing Class II MHC molecules on β islet cells (Böhme *et al.* 1989). Others had shown that Class I MHC expression directed to β islet cells also caused non-immune destruction of the β cells and hence diabetes (Allison *et al.* 1988). It seems that the level of expression may be an important factor; possibly over-expression of many proteins, particularly perhaps membrane proteins, could disrupt the cell's metabolism.

Two other types of transgenic experiments have been directed at understanding the pathogenesis of autoimmune diabetes. In the first kind of experiment, viral proteins have been targeted to the β islet cells. These experiments have had several different outcomes. Hanahan and colleagues looked at a number of different lines of transgenic mice expressing simian virus type 40 (SV40) T antigen. They found that there was an integration site-specific variation in the timing of onset of T antigen expression in the different lines. When T antigen expression occurred early in development (before birth), it produced tolerance and the mice were normoglycaemic. When T antigen was only turned on several weeks after birth, a histologically observable immune infiltrate (insulitis) occurred and autoimmune antibodies developed (Adams *et al.* 1987). Further development of this type of model has involved the infection of mice expressing a viral transgene with the cognate virus. Using this type of approach, Ohashi *et al.* (1991) found that infection with lymphocytic choriomeningitis virus (LCMV) of mice expressing LCMV glycoprotein (LCMV-GP) only in their β cells produced insulitis and diabetes. Similarly, Oldstone *et al.* (1991) produced a number of transgenic mouse lines expressing either LCMV-GP or LCMV-NP (nucleoprotein) in their β islet cells; these mice were also healthy and became diabetic after LCMV infection. These experiments have been interpreted as showing that the relevant antigen-specific T cells are indifferent to β islet cell-expressed antigen but not tolerant of the same antigen when presented by antigen-presenting cells. An alternative explanation is that the animals are tolerant of the transgenic antigen alone but that this tolerance can be broken by live whole-virus infection: this is difficult to test directly. Ohashi *et al.* (1991) went further in crossing their LCMV-GP transgenic mice with TCR αβ transgenics whose receptor is specific for self MHC plus LCMV-GP. These double-transgenic animals were, like their parents, normally healthy until infected with LCMV. It would be interesting to try to stimulate the potentially autoreactive T cells in these mice with the LCMV-GP peptide for which they are specific. This might provide a way of testing whether they were in any sense tolerant.

The other approach makes use of non-obese diabetic (NOD) strain mice, which spontaneously develop an autoimmune diabetes. This mouse strain does not express the H-2E molecule, and its other Class II MHC antigen (H-2A) is rather unusual in sequence. It was initially shown that introduction of an H-2Eα chain restores H-2E expression and protects the Eα transgenics from diabetes (Nishimoto *et al.* 1987). Subsequent experiments introduced the expression-variant transgenes of Mathis and Benoist and showed that only the wild-type expression pattern produced protection (Böhme *et al.* 1990). These results suggest that protection does not arise from H-2E-induced deletion of cross-reactive T cell clones but requires both positive selection of H-2E-restricted T cells in thymus and antigen presentation by one or more H-2E-expressing cell types in the periphery. Further work has shown that normal expression of H-$2A^k$ will protect the animals (Miyazaki *et al.* 1990; Slattery *et al.* 1990). Two additional experiments have been directed to examining the importance of the unique sequence of the $A\beta^{NOD}$ gene. Miyazaki *et al.* (1990) showed that simply changing residue 57 of $A\beta^k$ from aspartic acid to the NOD-specific serine made no difference to the ability of the modified molecule to protect transgenic NOD mice from insulitis and diabetes, whereas Lund *et al.* (1990) showed that NOD mice can be protected by a modified $A\beta^{NOD}$ transgene with the change of histidine to proline at position 56. Taken together, these data show the crucial role played by MHC genes in autoimmune diseases, and emphasize the subtle sequence-specific effects of MHC allelic polymorphism on immune response phenotype.

Although the importance of Class II MHC molecules in autoimmunity is widely recognized, the links with Class I MHC molecules are somewhat tenuous. The single exception is human leucocyte antigen (HLA)-B27, which is very prominently involved in a number of reactive arthopathies, for which no good animal models exist. Initial attempts to produce such a model by making B27 transgenic mice failed: the B27 mice are quite healthy (Krimpenfort *et al.* 1987; Taurog *et al.* 1988). Hammer, Taurog and colleagues have recently produced a series of rat transgenic lines with the human β-2-microglobulin and HLA-B27 genes (Hammer *et al.* 1990). Of seven independent lines produced, one shows a spontaneous autoimmune syndrome with a striking resemblance to various B27-associated (human) diseases. However, only one other line seems abnormal, exhibiting an apparently autoimmune diarrhoea, while the other five are seemingly quite healthy. Clearly, further investigation is required, but the first line may produce a valuable model for B27-associated diseases or may prove, like the first Class II MHC-expressing pancreatic islets, to be a red herring. The very close resemblance of the pathology of the autoimmune B27 rats to the human appearance engenders some optimism.

Summary

Transgenic animals have had a substantial impact on immunological research in the past several years. At the time of writing, many dozens of transgenic experiments are in progress. The manipulation of CD4 and CD8 expression in developing thymocytes should reveal how the apparent silencing of the non-required accessory molecule is achieved. Animals lacking appropriate kinases, phosphatases or other signalling proteins, produced through gene targeting, will help establish the roles of the various candidates in effecting the different outcomes of cell stimulation. Unpublished experiments in which the TCR α, β and δ genes have been inactivated have already been performed. Many other genes, some only discovered a year ago or less, are already being subjected to gene targeting. It seems probable that before very long mutational transgenics will exist for most of the known immunologically important molecules. One major advantage of these is that they are almost all from the same inbred strain, which will unable multiple mutations to be assembled without creating the need for laborious back-crossing. Natural genetic deficiencies have already played a vital part in understanding biological systems in general and the immune system in particular. Combining these mutational transgenics with the ability to introduce complementing genes carrying defined mutations will certainly be a powerful and essential tool in the continuing investigation of how the immune system works.

References

Adams, T.E., Alpert, S. and Hanahan, D. (1987). Non-tolerance and autoantibodies to a transgenic self antigen expressed in pancreatic β cells. *Nature* **326**, 223–8.

Aldrich, C.J., Hammer, R.E., Jones-Youngblood, S. *et al.* (1991). Negative and positive selection of antigen-specific cytotoxic T lymphocytes affected by the α3 domain of MHC molecules. *Nature* **352**, 718–21.

Allison, J., Campbell, L., Morahan, G., Mandel, T.E., Harrison, L.C. and Miller, J.F.A.P. (1988). Diabetes in transgenic mice resulting from over-expression of class I histocompatibility molecules in pancreatic β cells. *Nature* **333**, 529–33.

Arnold, B., Messerle, M., Jatsch, L., Kublbeck, G. and Koszinowski, U. (1990). Transgenic mice expressing a soluble foreign H-2 class I antigen are tolerant to allogeneic fragments presented by self class I but not to the whole membrane-bound alloantigen. *Proc. Nat. Acad. Sci. (USA)* **85**, 2269–73.

Benoist, C. and Mathis, D. (1989). Positive selection of the T cell repertoire: where and when does it occur? *Cell* **58**, 1027–33.

Benoist, C. and Mathis, D. (1990). Regulation of major histocompatibility complex class II genes: X, Y and other letters of the alphabet. *Ann. Rev. Immunol.* **8**, 681–715.

Berg, L., Pullen, A.M., De St Groth, B.F., Mathis, D., Benoist, C. and Davis, M.M. (1989). Antigen/MHC specific T cells are preferentially exported from the thymus in the presence of their MHC ligand. *Cell* **58**, 1035–46.

Blüthmann, H., Kisielow, P., Uematsu, Y. *et al.* (1988). T-cell-specific deletion of T-cell receptor transgenes allows functional rearrangement of endogenous α- and β-genes. *Nature* **334**, 156–9.

Böhme, J., Haskins, K., Stecha, W. *et al.* (1989). Transgenic mice with I-A on islet cells are normoglycaemic but immunologically intolerant. *Science* **244**, 1179–83.

Böhme, J., Schuhbaur, B., Kanagawa, D., Benoist, C. and Mathis, D. (1990). MHC-linked protection from diabetes dissociated from clonal deletion of T cells. *Science* **249**, 293–5.

Bonneville, M., Ishida, I., Mombaerts, P. *et al.* (1989). Blockage of αβ T-cell development of TCR γδ transgenes. *Nature* **342**, 931–4.

Calame, K.L. (1985). Mechanisms that regulate immunoglobulin gene expression. *Ann. Rev. Immunol.* **3**, 159–95.

Cosgrove, D., Gray, D., Dierich, A. *et al.* (1991). Mice lacking MHC class II molecules. *Cell* **56**, 1051–66.

Dent, A.L., Matis, L.A., Hooshmand, F., Widacki, S.M., Bluestone, J.A. and Hendrick, S.M. (1990). Self-reactive $\alpha\delta$ T cells are eliminated in the thymus. *Nature* **343**, 714–19.

Fung-Leung, W.P., Schilham, M.W., Rahemtulla, A. *et al.* (1991). CD8 is needed for development of cytotoxic T cells but not helper T cells. *Cell* **65**, 443–9.

Gerlinger, P., LeMeur, M., Irrmann, C. *et al.* (1986). B lymphocyte targeting of gene expression in transgenic mice with the immunoglobulin heavy chain enhancer. *Nucleic Acids Res.* **14**, 6565–77.

Goodnow, C.C., Crosbie, J., Adelstein, S. *et al.* (1988). Altered immunoglobulin expression and functional silencing of self-reactive B lymphocytes in transgenic mice. *Nature* **334**, 676–82.

Goodnow, C.C., Crosbie, J., Brink, R.A. and Basten, A. (1989). Induction of self-tolerance in mature peripheral B lymphocytes. *Nature* **343**, 385–91.

Grosveld, F., van Assendelft, G.B., Greaves, D.R. and Kollias, G. (1987). Position-independent, high-level expression of the human β-globin genes in transgenic mice. *Cell* **51**, 975–85.

Hammer, R.E., Maika, S.D., Richardson, J.A., Tang, J.P. and Taurog, J.D. (1990). Spontaneous inflammatory disease in transgenic rats expressing HLA-B27 and human β2 M: an animal model of HLA-B27-associated human disorders. *Cell* **63**, 1099–112.

Ingold, A.L., Landel, C., Knall, C., Evans, G.A. and Potter, T.A. (1991). Co-engagement of CD8 with the T cell receptor is required for negative selection. *Nature* **353**, 721–3.

Ishida, I., Verbeek, S., Bonneville, M., Itohara, S., Berns, A. and Tonegawa, S. (1990). T-cell receptor $\gamma\delta$ and γ transgenic mice suggest a role of a γ gene silencer in the generation of $\alpha\beta$ T-cells. *Proc. Nat. Acad. Sci. (USA)* **87**, 3067–71.

Kaye, J., Hsu, M.L., Sauron, M.E., Jameson, S., Gascoigne, N.R.J. and Hedrick, S.M. (1989). Selective development of CD4+ T cells in transgenic mice expressing a class II MHC-restricted receptor. *Nature* **341**, 746–9.

Kisielow, P., Blüthmann, H., Staerz, U.D., Steinmetz, M. and von Boehmer, H. (1988). Tolerance in T-cell receptor transgenic mice involves deletion of nonmature CD4$^+$ 8$^+$ thymocytes. *Nature* **333**, 742–6.

Koller, B.H., Marrack, P., Kappler, J.W. and Smithies, O. (1990). Normal development of mice deficient in β2m, MHC class I protein and CD8 T cells. *Science* **248**, 1227–30.

Krimpenfort, P., Rudenko, G., Hochstenbach, F., Güssow, D., Berns, A. and Ploegh, H. (1987). Crosses of two independently derived transgenic mice demonstrate complementation of the genes encoding heavy (HLA-B27) and light (β_2-microglobulin) chains of HLA class-1 antigens. *EMBO J.* **6**, 1673–6.

Lo, D. Burkly, L.C., Widera, G., Cowing, C., Flavell, R.A., Palmiter, R.D. and Brinster, R.L. (1988). Diabetes and tolerance in transgenic mice expressing class II MHC molecules in pancreatic beta cells. *Cell* **53**, 159–68.

Lo, D., Burkly, L.C., Flavell, R.A., Palmiter, R.D. and Brinster, R.L. (1989) Tolerance in transgenic mice expressing class II MHC on pancreatic acinar cells. *J. Exp. Med.* **170**, 87–104.

Lund, T., O'Reilly, L., Hutchings, P. *et al.* (1990). Prevention of insulin-dependent diabetes mellitus in non-obese diabetic mice by transgenes encoding modified I-A β-chain or normal I-E α-chain. *Nature* **345**, 727–9.

Meyer, K., Sharpe, M.J., Surani, M.A. and Neuberger, M.S. (1990). The importance of the 3′-enhancer region in immunoglobulin κ gene expression. *Nucleic Acids Res.* **18**, 5609–15.

Miyazaki, T., Uno, M., Uehira, M. *et al.* (1990). Direct evidence for the contribution of the unique I-A^{NOD} to the development of insulitis in non-obese diabetic mice. *Nature* **345**, 722–4.

Morahan, G., Allison, J. and Miller, J.F.A.P. (1989). Tolerance of class I histocompatibility antigens expressed extrathymically. *Nature* **339**, 623–4.

Murphy, K.M., Weaver, C.T., Elish, M., Allen, P.M. and Lo, D.Y. (1989). Peripheral tolerance to allogeneic class II histocompatibility antigens expressed in transgenic mice: evidence against a clonal-deletion mechanism. *Proc. Nat. Acad. Sci. (USA)* **86**, 10034–8.

Nemazee, D. and Bürki, K. (1989). Clonal deletion of autoreactive B lymphocytes in bone marrow chimaeras. *Proc. Nat. Acad. Sci. (USA)* **86**, 8039–43.

Nishimoto, H., Kikutani, H., Yamamura, K. and Kishimoto, T. (1987). Prevention of autoimmune insulitis by expression of I-E molecules in NOD mice. *Nature* **328**, 432–4.

O'Brien, R.L., Brinster, R.L. and Storb, U. (1987). Somatic hypermutation of an immunoglobulin transgene in κ transgenic mice. *Nature* **326**, 405–9.

Ohashi, P.S., Oehen, S., Buerki, K. *et al.* (1991). Ablation of 'tolerance' and induction of diabetes by virus infection in viral antigen transgenic mice. *Cell* **65**, 305–17.

Oldstone, M.B.A., Neremberg, M., Southern, P., Price, J. and Lewicki, H. (1991). Virus infection triggers insulin-dependent diabetes in a transgenic model: role of anti-self (virus) immune response. *Cell* **65**, 319–31.

Pardoll, D.M., Fowlkes, B.J., Bluestone, J.A. *et al.* (1987). Differential expression of two distinct T-cell receptors during thymocyte development. *Nature* **326**, 79–82.

Rahemtulla, A., Fung-Leung, W.P., Schilham, W. *et al.* (1991). Normal development and function of CD8$^+$ cells but markedly decreased helper cell activity in mice lacking CD4. *Nature* **353**, 180–4.

Reik, W., Williams, G., Barton, S., Norris, M., Neuberger, M. and Surani, M.A. (1987). Provision of the immunoglobulin heavy chain enhancer downstream of a test gene is sufficient to confer lymphoid-specific expression in transgenic mice. *Eur. J. Immunol.* **17**, 465–9.

Sarvetnick, N., Liggitt, D., Pitts, S.L., Hansen, S.E. and Stewart, T.A. (1988). Insulin-dependent diabetes mellitus induced in transgenic mice by ectopic expression of class II MHC and interferon-gamma. *Cell* **52**, 773–82.

Schönrich, G., Kalinke, U., Momburg, F. *et al.* (1991). Down-regulation of T-cell receptors on self-reactive T-cells as a novel mechanism for extrathymic tolerance induction. *Cell* **65**, 293–304.

Scott, B., Blüthmann, H., Teh, H.S. and von Boehmer, H. (1989). The generation of mature T-cells requires an interaction of the $\alpha\beta$ T-cell receptor with MHC antigens. *Nature* **338**, 591–3.

Sharpe, M.J., Milstein, C., Jarvis, J.M. and Neuberger, M.S. (1991). Somatic hypermutation of immunoglobulin κ may depend on sequences 3′ of Cκ and occurs on passenger transgenes. *EMBO J.* **10**, 2139–45.

Slattery, R.M., Kjer-Nielsen, L., Allison, J., Charlton, B., Mandel, J.M. and Miller, J.F.A.P. (1990). Prevention of diabetes in non-obese diabetic I-A^k transgenic mice. *Nature* **345**, 724–6.

Storb, U., O'Brien, R.L., McMullen, M.D., Gollahon, K.A.

and Brinster, R.L. (1984). High expression of cloned immunoglobulin κ gene in transgenic mice is restricted to B lymphocytes. *Nature* **310**, 238–41.

Taurog, J.D., Lowe, L., Forman, J. and Hammer, R.E. (1988). HLA-B27 in inbred and non-inbred transgenic mice: cell surface expression and recognition as an alloantigen in the absence of human β2-microglobulin. *J. Immunol.* **141**, 4020–3.

Teh, H.S., Kisielow, P., Scott, B. *et al.* (1988). Thymic major histocompatibility complex antigens and the αβ T-cell receptor determine the CD4/CD8 phenotype of T cells. *Nature* **335**, 229–33.

Uematsu, Y., Ryser, S., Dembic, Z. *et al.* (1988). In transgenic mice the introduced functional T-cell receptor β gene prevents expression of endogenous β genes. *Cell* **52**, 831–41.

van Ewijk, W., Ron, Y., Monaco, J. *et al.* (1988). Compartmentalization of MHC class II gene expression in transgenic mice. *Cell* **53**, 357–70.

von Boehmer, H. (1990). Developmental biology of T cells in T cell receptor transgenic mice. *Ann. Rev. Immunol.* **8**, 531–56.

Yamamura, K., Kikutani, H., Takahashi, N. *et al.* (1984). Introduction of human γ1 immunoglobulin genes into fertilized mouse eggs. *J. Biochem. (Japan)* **96**, 357–63.

Yamamura, K., Kudo, A., Ebihara, T. *et al.* (1986). Cell-type-specific and regulated expression of a human γ1 heavy-chain immunoglobulin gene in transgenic mice. *Proc. Nat. Acad. Sci. (USA)* **83**, 2152–6.

Zjilstra, M., Bix, M., Simister, N.E., Loring, J.M., Raulet, D.H. and Jaenisch, R. (1990). β2 microglobulin deficient mice lack $CD4^{-}8^{+}$ cytolytic T cells. *Nature* **344**, 742–6.

43: Antibody Engineering

G. Winter and S. Ward

Introduction

Antibodies can be regarded as natural therapeutic agents which bind to a foreign antigen and mark it for clearance by a variety of mechanisms, ranging from phagocytosis and antibody-dependent cell-mediated cytotoxicity (ADCC) to complement-dependent lysis. In the clinic, horse antiserum has been used since the turn of the century, proving effective, for example, in the treatment of diphtheria and pneumococcal pneumonia, but with complications of immune complex disease and anaphylaxis. Although serotherapy was superseded by antibiotics in the 1940s for treatment of bacterial infections, the discovery of monoclonal antibodies (Köhler and Milstein 1975) may herald its renaissance. For example, monoclonal antibodies directed against cell surface antigens have been used to target and to kill T and B lymphocytes (Hale *et al.* 1983): these antibodies have potential in the treatment of bone marrow transplantation, lymphoma and autoimmune disease.

Recombinant deoxyribonucleic acid (DNA) technology adds a further dimension (for reviews see Morrison 1985; Neuberger 1985; Verhoeyen and Riechmann 1988; Williams 1988). It allows us to build better antibodies, and to dissect antibody binding and effector functions. For example, antibody–enzyme conjugates have been constructed (Neuberger *et al.* 1984), antigen-binding sites have been transplanted from mouse to human antibodies (Jones *et al.* 1986; Riechmann *et al.* 1988a; Verhoeyen *et al.* 1988) and the binding sites for complement 1q (C1q) (Duncan and Winter 1988) and the human high-affinity receptor, FcRI, (Duncan *et al.* 1988) have been localized in the constant domains of the antibody. Such protein engineering studies imply a detailed knowledge of the three-dimensional structure of the antibody and the underlying gene structure.

The antibody molecule consists of four chains: two identical heavy chains and two identical light chains (Fig. 43.1) (Porter 1973). Each chain consists of a string of domains and each domain consists of a β-sheet sandwich, held together by an internal buried disulphide bond. In the assembled molecule, the chains pack together through non-covalent interactions between domains. The two heavy chains are also linked by one or more disulphide bonds in the hinge region, and the heavy and light chains are also held together by a

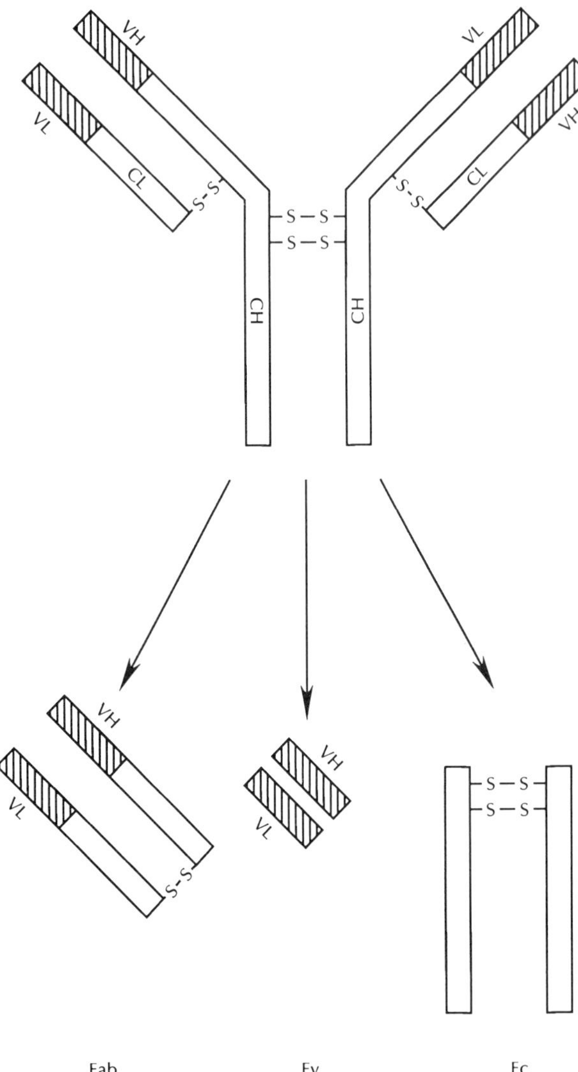

Fig. 43.1. Schematic diagram of the structure of an antibody molecule, showing two heavy and light chains joined by sulphhydryl bonds. The Fab, Fv and Fc fragments are also shown.

disulphide bond in the same region. The antigen-binding site and effector functions are localized in different regions of the antibody molecule, and historically were separated by cleavage of the antibody hinge with papain, to generate the Fab and the Fc fragments (Porter 1973).

The Fab fragment carries the antigen-binding site and is composed of the heavy chain variable domain, first constant domain and part of the hinge, and the entire light chain. The chains are covalently joined by a disulphide bond between the constant domains. Rarely, the antibody has been cleaved into an Fv fragment, which carries the antigen-binding site and consists only of non-covalently associated heavy and light chain variable domains (Inbar *et al.* 1972; Kakimoto and Onoue 1974; Sharon and Givol 1976). The fc fragment carries binding sites for C1q and Fc receptors (Davies and Metzger 1983; Duncan and Winter 1988; Duncan *et al.* 1988) and consists of part of the hinge, and the second and third constant domains of the heavy chain. The chains are covalently joined by one or more disulphides in the hinge.

The domain structure of an antibody is mirrored at the gene level, as the protein domains are arranged as a series of individual exons. The genes encoding an antibody are assembled by DNA rearrangements during the differentiation of antibody-secreting cells (Fig. 43.2). The variable region itself is assembled from the union of germline V elements with separate genetic elements (D segment, and J_H elements for the heavy chain, and $J\kappa$ or $J\lambda$ elements for the light chain). In the heavy chain assembly, first the D and J_H are joined, followed by the V and DJ_H (Alt *et al.* 1984). A large component of antibody variable region diversity is combinatorial: for example in mouse there are about 500–1000 germline V_H genes (Livant *et al.* 1986), at least 15 D segments and 4 J_H elements. The rearranged V_H genes are brought together with constant region genes: for example in mouse there are several classes of immunoglobulin (Ig) genes, IgG (isotypes $\gamma 1$, $\gamma 2a$, $\gamma 2b$, $\gamma 3$), IgA (α), IgM (μ), IgD (δ) and IgE (ε). During early differentiation of a B lymphocyte, a given V_H region is expressed as a μ chain. Recombination by class switching (Shimuzu and Honjo 1984) allows immunoglobulins with different isotypes, and therefore effector functions with distinct biological roles, to be produced during differentiation to a plasma cell.

A toolkit for antibody engineering

The domains are the building-blocks for antibody engineering, and their arrangement in individual exons facilitates cutting and pasting by recombinant DNA techniques, allowing assembly of complete antibodies or of groups of domains (for example Fab, Fv or Fc) or fusions with domains from other proteins. A toolkit for antibody engineering requires sets of domains and vectors for expression. The genes encoding the rearranged

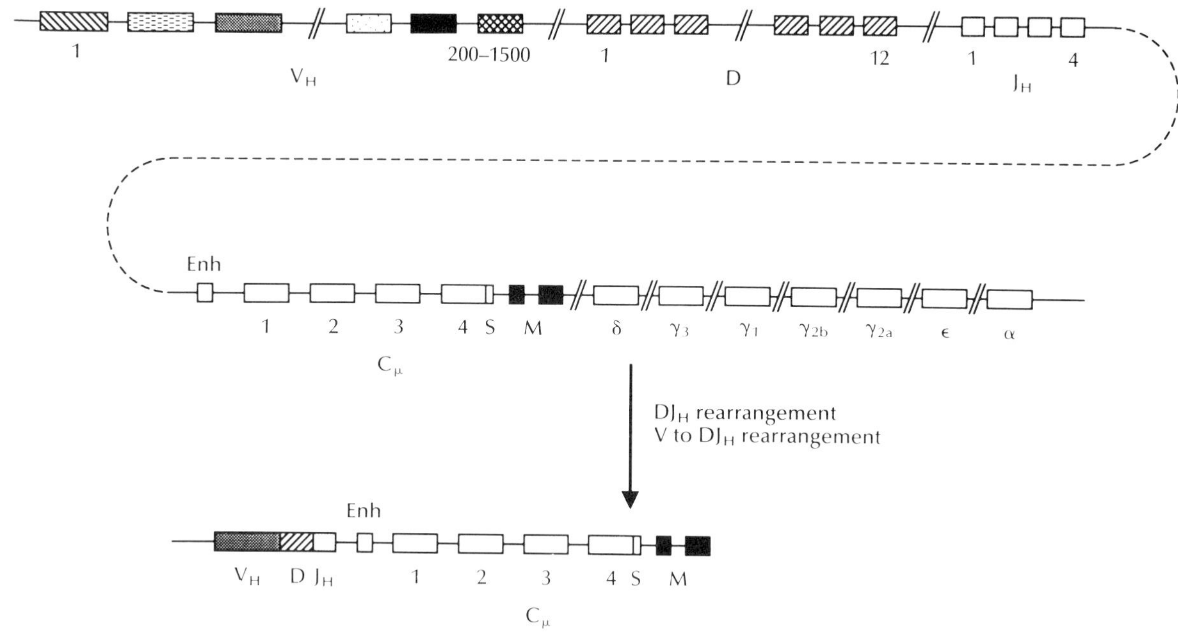

Fig. 43.2. Recombination of mouse Ig germline segments to produce functionally rearranged antibody gene.

variable domains are usually derived from a hybridoma of the required antigenic specificity, and the constant region genes from genomic or complementary DNA (cDNA) libraries. At its simplest, for Ig genes cloned from genomic DNA, the expression of antibody can be driven in cells of lymphoid origin by the Ig promoter and enhancer. Synthetic oligonucleotides are also required, as probes for Ig genes, for gene synthesis, as primers for cDNA synthesis, for sequencing, for mutagenesis and for the polymerase chain reaction (Saiki *et al.* 1985, 1988).

Cloning and sequencing

The sequence of the Ig variable regions is usually derived by direct sequencing of the hybridoma messenger ribonucleic acid (mRNA), or by sequencing cloned DNA. The mRNA can be sequenced directly using primers based at the 5′ end of the constant region if the class or isotype of constant region is known (for example κ or λ light chain). Alternatively the mRNA can be sequenced with reverse transcriptase using primers based in the conserved J regions of either heavy or light chains. Two methods are available for the sequencing reactions: (i) chain termination with dideoxynucleotide triphosphates and α-^{32}P or α-^{35}S nucleotide triphosphates (Sanger *et al.* 1977), or (ii) chemical cleavage of a cDNA transcript derived from primer labelled at its 5′ end with γ-^{32}P adenosine triphosphate (ATP) (Maxam and Gilbert 1977). It is usually desirable, however, to clone the gene.

Rearranged variable regions have been cloned from the cDNA by tailing with homopolymeric tails, attaching linkers or blunt-end cloning, and from genomic DNA by screening λ-phage libraries with probes based at the 3′ end of the J regions. The polymerase chain reaction (PCR) offers new avenues for cloning variable regions from cDNA or genomic DNA. Polymerase chain reaction amplification involves repeated rounds of extension from two primers specific for regions at each end of the gene. Since conserved necleotide sequences are present at both ends of most mouse variable region genes, they are readily amplified and cloned (Chiang *et al.* 1989; Larrick *et al.* 1989a, b; Orlandi *et al.* 1989). However, the primers need not match the gene sequence exactly, and restriction sites can be incorporated within the primers to allow the forced cloning of the amplified DNA (Orlandi *et al.* 1989). By this means the gene can be cloned directly for expression (Fig. 43.3). Immunoglobulin constant region genes have been cloned from the cDNA and from the genomic

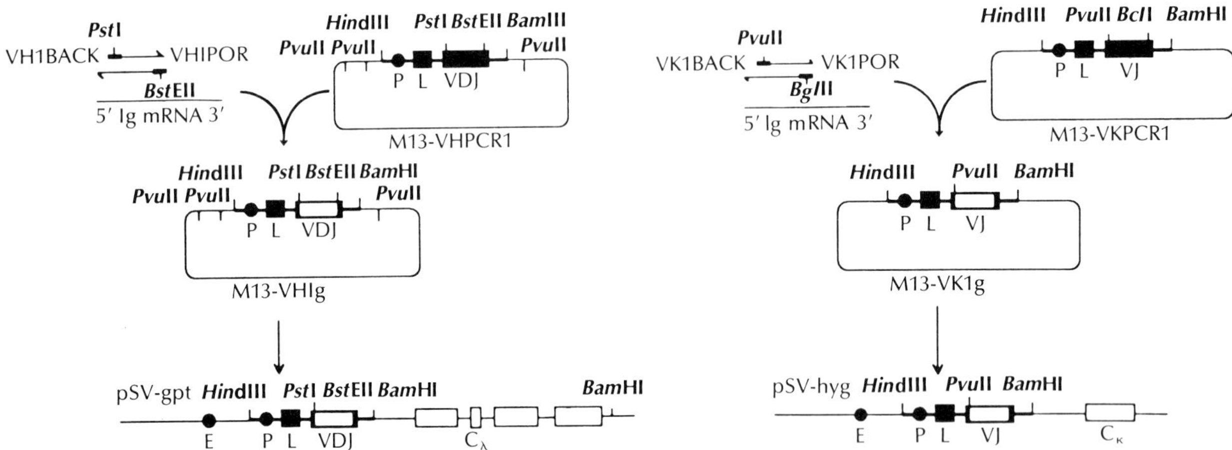

Fig. 43.3. Scheme for the amplification of cDNA and cloning into phage M13 vectors to link up V region genes for expression (Orlandi *et al.* 1989). The vectors M13-VHPCR1 and M13-VKPCR1, for cloning the amplified DNA, contain introns: transcription is driven from the Ig heavy chain promoter (P), and the signal sequence (L) and leader intron are taken from the mouse V47 unrearranged V_H gene (Neuberger 1983). The non-coding sequences to the 3′ ends of the V_H and $V\kappa$ genes have been previously described (Neuberger 1983; Riechmann *et al.* 1988a).

DNA by screening λ-phage libraries with Ig cDNA probes (same species or even cross species).

Vectors for expression in eukaryotic cells

Vectors for stable expression and secretion of antibodies from eukaryotic cells have several elements: a promoter and enhancer to drive Ig gene expression, a dominant marker for selection of transfected eukaryotic cells, and a colE1 origin of replication and antibiotic resistance gene for a selection in *Escherichia coli*.

The Ig promoter and enhancer have been used to drive transcription of Ig genes in lymphoid cells (for review see Neuberger and Cook 1988). The promoter and enhancer elements are functional in these cells only (see, for example, Neuberger 1983), and are known to bind to a lymphoid-specific transcription factor (Müller *et al.* 1988; Scheidereit *et al.* 1988). Furthermore for the Ig enhancer/promoter there is an intron requirement for expression of the cloned genes (Neuberger and Williams 1988), and therefore genomic constructs are used. Other promoters and enhancers, for example human cytomegalovirus (HCMV) (Boshart *et al.* 1985), heat-shock protein (HSP)-70 promoter (Pelham 1982) or simian virus 40 (SV40) (Okayama and Berg 1983), have also been used to drive expression of genomic or cDNA constructs in lymphoid cells (Liu *et al.* 1987), COS cells (Whittle *et al.* 1987), Chinese hamster ovary (Weidle *et al.* 1987) and neuroglioma cells (Cattaneo and Neuberger 1987) (Fig. 43.4).

For selection of transfected myeloma cells, three dominant markers under the control of the viral SV40 early promoter are currently available. These markers, the *E. coli* xanthine-guanine phosphoribosyltransferase gene, the transposon Tn5 phosphotransferase gene and the hygromycin resistance gene, are derived from the pSV*gpt* (Mulligan and Berg 1981), pSV*neo* (Southern and Berg 1981) and pSV*hygro* (Smith, Miyajima and Strehlow, pers. comm.) vectors respectively. As these markers function in different pathways (Fig. 43.3), they can be used, for example, for independent selection of heavy and light chain expression from two different plasmids. Amplification of the transfected genes in myeloma cells is possible by including a methotrexate-resistant dihydrofolate reductase on the plasmid (Schmike 1984; Dorai and Moore 1987). Vectors devised recently for cloning antibody variable domains by the PCR and the expression of mouse–human chimeric antibodies in myeloma cells are described in Figs 43.3 and 43.4.

The cloned Ig genes are now usually introduced into myeloma cells by electroporation (Potter *et al.* 1984), which has proved more effective than spheroplast fusion (Oi *et al.* 1983) or calcium phosphate co-precipitation (Graham and Van der Eb 1973).

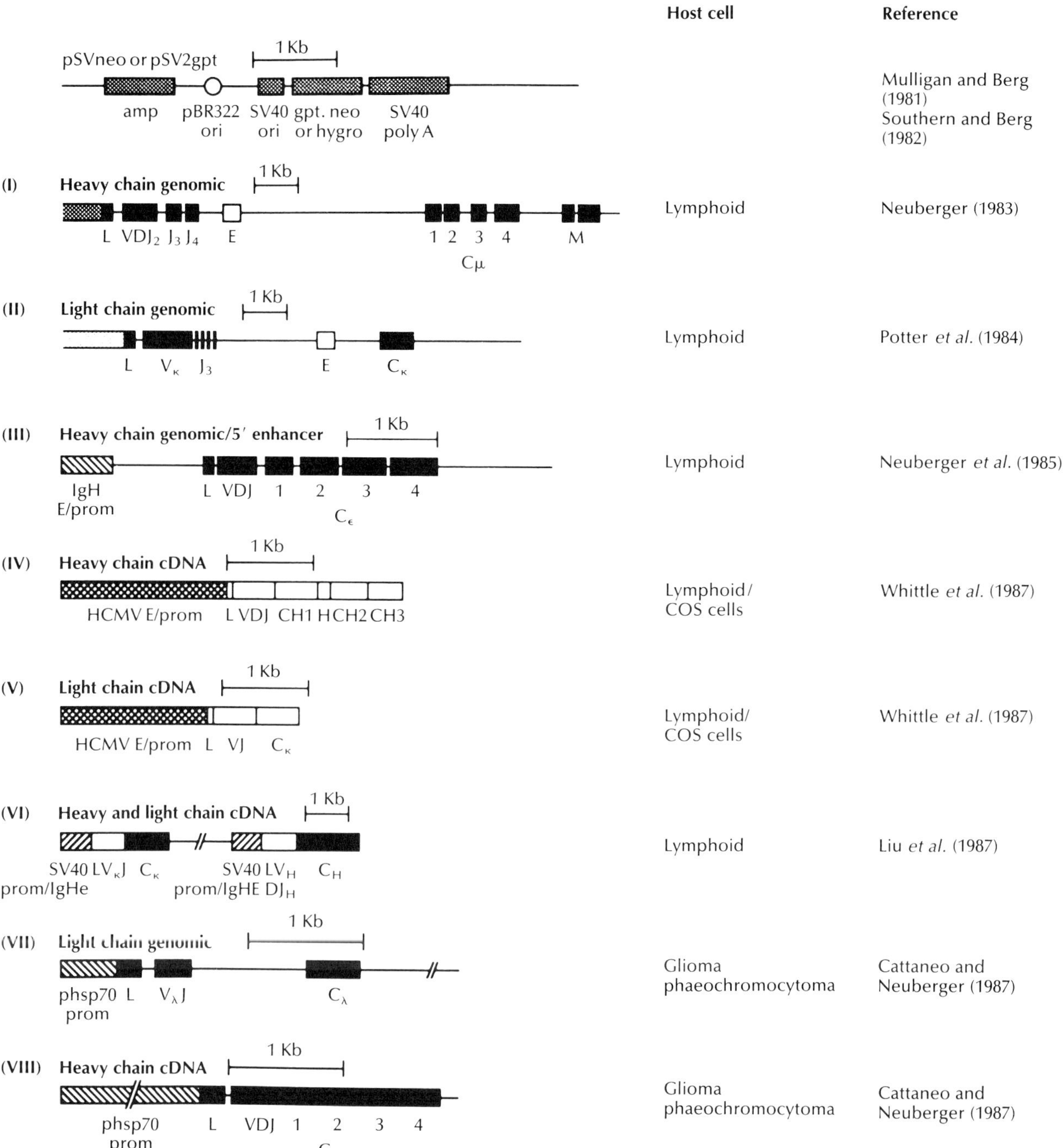

Fig. 43.4. Plasmid constructions for the expression of recombinant antibodies in mammalian cells. promp=promoter, IgH E=immunoglobulin heavy chain enhancer; HCMV E=human cytomegalovirus enhancer, phsp70=heat-shock protein 70. For further details, see references cited in the illustration.

Vectors for expression in *Escherichia coli*

At first sight, the expression of antibody in *E. coli* seems unpromising. Expressed antibody (Boss *et al*. 1984; Cabilly *et al*. 1984) or antibody fragments (Kurokawa *et al*. 1983; Liu *et al*. 1984; Ishizaka *et al*. 1986) accumulate in the cytoplasm as inclusion bodies. It is possible to refold the isolated protein from denaturing buffers but yields of functional antibody are poor (Boss *et al*. 1984; Cabilly *et al*.

1984). Furthermore, *E. coli* is not suitable for the production of glycosylated constant domains, which is necessary for function of IgG isotypes. In contrast, IgE constant domains can be produced in functional form in *E. coli* (Liu *et al*. 1984; Coleman *et al*. 1985; Ishizaka *et al*. 1986) as glycosylation is not necessary for function. Single-chain Fv fragments, however, in which the heavy and light chain variable domains are connected by a peptide linker, show improved yields on refolding from inclusion bodies (Bird *et al*. 1988; Huston *et al*. 1988) (Fig. 43.5). In addition, by attaching N-signal sequences (ompA, phoA or pelB) for export into the periplasm to antibody genes, Fv or Fab fragments have been secreted in an active form, in yields ranging from 0.3 to 10 mg/l (Better *et al*. 1988; Skerra and Plückthun 1988; Ward *et al*. 1989a) (Fig. 43.5). Single (V_H)-domain antibodies have also been expressed and secreted in *E. coli* in yields of 0.2–0.5 mg/ml (Ward *et al*. 1989a). The use of Fv fragments and V_H domains from *E. coli* should permit the rapid alteration and screening of new antigen-binding specifities.

Applications of antibody engineering

Antibody fragments: V_H, Fv, Fab, $(Fab)_2'$, Fc

Perhaps the simplest form of antibody engineering is the expression of individual domains or sets of domains. Antigen-binding fragments based on the Fv fragment (V_H and V_L domains) have been expressed and secreted in *E. coli* (Skerra and Plückthun 1988) and in myeloma cells (Riechmann *et al*. 1988), and have been refolded from *E. coli* inclusion bodies (Boss *et al*. 1984; Cabilly *et al*. 1984). For the secreted Fv fragments, the signal sequence was cleaved on secretion to reveal the N-terminal amino acid of the 'mature' variable domains. The V_H and V_L domains of the Fv fragments can associate non-covalently (Riechmann *et al*. 1988b; Skerra and Plückthun 1988; Ward *et al*. 1989a), and the packing between V_H and V_L domains is highly conserved (Chothia *et al*. 1985). Some interchain contacts are made between the antigen-binding loops of both chains (Chothia *et al*. 1985; Saul *et al*. 1987) and it is therefore difficult to predict whether Fv fragments in general will prove stable. The V_H and $V\kappa$ domains of an Fv fragment with antilysozyme specificity are in dynamic equilibrium (Riechmann *et al*. 1988b), and it is possible that a chemical cross-link or disulphide bond introduced between the two domains could be advantageous. Recently the generation of single-chain antibodies, in which a V_H is linked by a peptide linker to a $V\kappa$, has been reported (Bird *et al*. 1988; Huston *et al*. 1989). Repertoires of V_H domains have recently been expressed and secreted in *E. coli* (Ward *et al*. 1989a). These repertoires of V_H domains were generated using the PCR to amplify and then clone the rearranged V_H genes directly from mouse spleen DNA. Such single domains can have reasonable affinities for antigens (approximately 20 nM). These single V_H domains have been termed 'single-domain antibodies' and they represent a

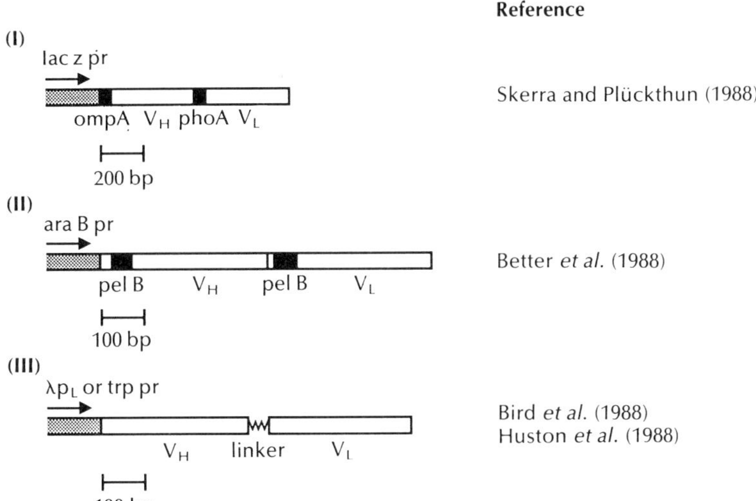

Fig. 43.5. Plasmid constructions for the expression of antibody Fv (I), Fab (II) or single chain Fvs (III) in *E. coli*. Plasmids (I) and (II) have prokaryotic sequences (ompA, phoA and pelB) for secretion of the expressed protein into the periplasm. pr=promoter. For further details, see references cited in the illustration.

new class of recombinant antibody fragments and may be of use in therapy and diagnostics. In addition, it is expected that they could be used as building-blocks for Fv and Fab fragments or complete antibodies. The small size of the Fv fragment and single-domain antibody should facilitate the determination of the three-dimensional structure of the antigen-binding site by both X-ray crystallography and nuclear magnetic resonance (NMR) analyses.

Fab fragments have been secreted from *E. coli* (Better *et al.* 1988). $(Fab)_2'$ fragments (Neuberger *et al.* 1984) and a Fab-like fragment, with V_H and V_L domains each joined to Cκ domains (Sharon *et al.* 1984), have been secreted from myeloma cells. Also a range of fragments containing parts of the Fc region of IgE have been expressed in *E. coli* as inclusion bodies and refolded. This expression system has been used to localize the binding site for the IgE receptor, $Fc_{\varepsilon}RI$, on the Cε2 and Cε3 domains (Helm *et al.* 1988).

Antibody fragments joined to other proteins: enzymes, toxins and receptors

At its simplest, making a gene fusion with antibody may provide a handle for its detection and purification (Neuberger *et al.* 1984). Furthermore, enzyme activities, such as alkaline phosphatase or horse-radish peroxidase linked directly to Fab fragments could be invaluable for enzyme-linked immunosorbent assay (ELISA) and other diagnostic tests. Genes encoding staphylococcal nuclease and Klenow polymerase (Neuberger *et al.* 1984) were linked to antibody Fab genes as a model system for such antibody fusions. The enzymes, which are monomeric, were attached to the N-terminal portion of the IgG C_H2 domain. This region of the antibody, which leads from the hinge, is disordered in the crystallographic structure, and may provide a flexible link. Both Fab–enzyme and $(Fab)_2'$–enzyme constructs were expressed (the hinge sulph-hydryl groups are present), and the constructs shown to possess both antigen-binding activity and enzyme activity.

Fab–enzyme fusions may also have therapeutic potential, although the enzyme moiety is likely to be immunogenic. For example, tissue plasminogen activator (TPA) has been linked to an anti-fibrin Fab, which should direct the TPA to the vicinity of blood clots, where it can locally activate plasminogen (Schnee *et al.* 1987). Likewise for pro-drug therapy, an enzyme capable of cleaving the pro-drug could be linked to a suitable Fab or $(Fab)_2'$ fragment. Yet another possibility lies in linking a toxin, such as ricin, diphtheria toxin or *Pseudomonas* exotoxin, to the Fab or Fv fragment, to create an immunotoxin (Chaudhary *et al.* 1989; for review, see Ahmad and Law 1988). Here the strategy is different: such toxins must be delivered inside the target cell, where, for example, they catalyse the ribosylation of EFTu. A single molecule of toxin can kill the cell. However the entry of the Fab/Fv–toxin into the target cells is likely to prove difficult, as well as its expression and secretion from myeloma cells.

Other kinds of antibody fusions have been made, for example in which the antibody variable domains have been replaced by a T cell receptor Vα domain, on either the Ig heavy chain (Gascoigne *et al.* 1987) or the Ig light chain (Mariuzza and Winter 1989) constant domains. Likewise CD4, which binds to the acquired immune deficiency syndrome (AIDS) human immunodeficiency virus (HIV)-1 gp(glycoprotein)120 coat protein, has been assembled with Ig heavy chain constant regions to create an 'immunoadhesin'. The fusion enhances the serum half-life of CD4 and the antibody effector functions may prove effective in killing AIDS virus-infected cells (Capon *et al.* 1989).

Simple chimeric antibodies

During the maturation of the immune response, the class of Ig heavy chain is switched from IgM to IgG (for review see Shimizu and Honjo 1984). Likewise the isotype of IgG can be switched and involves bringing the rearranged V_H gene into the proximity of a new set of constant region genes, with deletion of the intervening DNA (Davis *et al.* 1980; Maki *et al.* 1980; Kataoka *et al.* 1981; Obata *et al.* 1981). As expected from the Ig domain structure, class switching does not seem to alter the affinity of the antibody for antigen (Neuberger and Rajewsky 1981). Class switching underlies the concept of simple chimeric antibodies: the variable regions from one source are attached to constant regions from another. This allows the species, class and isotype of constant regions to be selected for the antibody, which in turn dictates its immunogenicity and effector functions.

A variety of simple chimeric antibodies have been made (Boulianne *et al.* 1987; Morrison *et al.* 1984; Neuberger *et al.* 1985; Sun *et al.* 1987). The most extensive collection is based on the mouse B1-8 heavy chain with mouse λ light chain (Brüggeman *et al.* 1987). The heavy chain variable region has been attached to a variety of mouse, rat and human constant regions. These antibodies have a specificity for the haptens NP (and NIP (Neuberger and Rajewsky 1981)), and are readily purified on columns of hapten–Sepharose. Cell surfaces are readily derivatized using NIP-succinimide ester (which reacts with protein cell surface markers) or NIP-cephalin (which inserts into the membrane lipid), and this facilitates the assay of effector functions such as complement lysis and cell-mediated killing (for reviews see Winkelhake *et al.* 1978; Burton 1987). Such 'matched sets' of chimeric antibodies have proved invaluable for comparing effector functions (Brüggeman *et al.* 1987; Stepelewski *et al.* 1988) and segmental flexibility (Oi *et al.* 1984; Dangl *et al.* 1988) of different antibody isotypes. For example, it emerges that the human γ1 isotype is the most active in complement lysis and ADCC, indicating that it is the most suitable for therapy (Brüggeman *et al.* 1987; Riechmann *et al.* 1988a).

Reshaped antibodies

The antigen-binding site is localized to the loops at the tips of the variable region, and correlates with the regions of hypervariable sequence (or complementarity-determining regions, CDRs) in each of the V_H and V_L domains (Kabat *et al.* 1987). Reshaped antibodies, in which the antigen-binding site only is derived from another antibody, have been constructed by transplanting the CDRs (Jones *et al.* 1986; Riechmann *et al.* 1988a; Verhoeyen *et al.* 1988). This not only allows the choice of constant region, as with the simple chimeric antibodies, but also the choice of variable region β-sheet 'framework' and loops adjacent to the constant domains. Such human antibodies, in which only the antigen-binding site is derived from a mouse antibody, may prove less immunogenic in humans than a simple chimeric antibody, in which the entire variable region is taken from a mouse antibody. However, there are several assumptions underlying this approach. In particular, certain structural features of both antibodies must be matched for the graft to 'take' on its new framework: the packing of the heavy and light chain variable domains; the packing of the two β-sheets within a domain; the packing of the CDRs on to the β-sheet framework; and the contact of the antigen only with CDR residues (or conserved residues in the β-sheet). Inspection of the available crystallographic structures suggests that the packing of domains, sheets and loops are relatively conserved (Lesk and Chothia 1982; Chothia and Lesk 1987) and that the vast majority of contacts between antibody and antigen are made via CDR residues (Amit *et al.* 1986; Sheriff *et al.* 1987; Padlan *et al.* 1989). Nevertheless, in reshaping the anti-lymphocyte antibody, CAMPATH-1, to avoid loss of binding activity the framework region of the human antibody had to be adapted to accommodate the CDRs of the rat antibody (Riechmann *et al.* 1988a).

Dissecting antibody affinity and effector functions

The diversity of antibody-binding sites is not only based on the recombinatorial diversity of the genetic elements (V_H, D, J_H; Vκ, Jκ; Vλ, Jλ) and diversity at the junctions, but also on somatic mutation during the muturation of the immune response (for review see Tonegawa 1983). Point mutations in antibody variable regions are sufficient to alter antibody affinity and specificity (Rudikoff *et al.* 1982; Roberts *et al.* 1987). For example, higher-affinity antibodies derived from a V_H gene family which expresses antibodies directed against the hapten NP appear to be determined by a replacement of tryptophan 33 by leucine (Allen *et al.* 1988). It should also be possible to construct higher-affinity antibodies by design: mutations constructed in the hypervariable regions of an anti-lysozyme antibody were shown to increase its affinity for antigen (Roberts *et al.* 1987). Enhancing the affinity and specificity of antibodies has important practical applications, for example in increasing the sensitivity of ELISA or of *in vivo* imaging and therapy.

The binding of antibody to a cell receptor has been illuminated by construction of a single mutant. Binding of antigen–antibody complexes to specialized cells via three receptors, FcRI, FcRII and FcRIII (Anderson and Looney 1986), can trigger ADCC. The high-affinity receptor FcRI appears to interact via the C_H2 domain of the antibody (Burton 1987) and studies with human myeloma proteins in which the hinge was deleted had indicated that the top of the C_H2 domain must be accessible (Klein *et al.* 1981). Sequence comparisons of several antibodies and their properties led to the proposal that the monocyte-binding site was located mainly in the hinge link, and possibly associated with Leu 235 (Woof *et al.* 1986). This proposal was confirmed by site-directed mutagenesis. The mouse IgG-2b isotype has a glutamic acid residue at position 235 and does not bind to the human FcRI receptor and by mutagenesis binding activity was conferred on this isotype by replacing glutamic acid 235 by leucine (Duncan *et al.* 1988).

The interaction of antibody with C1q has also been dissected by making a range of mutants. The site of interaction of C1q for antibody had been localized to the C_H2 domain. Based on chemical modification studies, inhibition of complement lysis by synthetic peptides and oligosaccharides, and sequence comparisons of antibody isotypes, a wide variety of proposals had been made. Taken together, these residues cover most of the solvent accessible surface of the C_H2 domain. An engineering approach, 'surface scanning' (Bedouelle and Winter 1986) was used, in which side-chains of the antibody were removed systematically and scored for C1q binding. This approach identified three polar side chains, Glu 318, Lys 320 and Lys 322, as essential for C1q binding (Duncan and Winter 1988), confirming aspects of an earlier proposal by Dwek and colleagues (Burton *et al.* 1980). Since these features are conserved in isotypes which do not bind C1q or are non-lytic, there must also be other factors involved, for example steric blocking of the Fc by the Fab arms (Isenman *et al.* 1975) or segmental flexibility (Oi *et al.* 1984).

Future directions

At present, the raw material of antibody engineering is the hybridoma. Although it has proved difficult to derive human monoclonal antibodies by hybridoma technology (Carson and Freimark 1986; Borrebaeck *et al.* 1988; Thompson 1988), antibody engineering offers an indirect route of 'humanizing' rodent monoclonal antibodies, by making simple chimeric antibodies or by reshaping human antibodies. Preliminary clinical results are promising: simple chimeric antibodies have an extended serum half-life compared with the mouse antibodies (LoBuglio *et al.* 1989) and a reshaped human antibody directed against lymphocytes was effective in clearing a large mass of tumour in two patients (Hale *et al.* 1988). Whether such chimeric antibodies or reshaped antibodies will prove much more immunogenic than genuine human monoclonal antibodies and whether this will curtail therapy are open questions. In a mouse model, it seems that the immune response is directed mainly against constant regions, although a significant part of the response is mounted against the framework regions of the variable region.

The ability to tailor effector functions may help define the routes of clearance of pathogen in clinical situations. For example, the construction of a human $\gamma 1$ antibody which does not activate complement lysis but does bind to receptors could help identify the role of complement-dependent lysis and ADCC in cell killing.

In future, antigen-binding activities may be derived by approaches other than hybridoma technology (Ward *et al.* 1989a), for example: using the PCR to clone variable regions for expression directly from mRNA (Orlandi *et al.* 1989; Sastry *et al.* 1989) or from genomic DNA of spleen (Ward *et al.* 1989a) or of peripheral blood lymphocytes; the mutation of antigen-binding sites with mutagenic primers (Ward *et al.* 1989b); the building of antigen-binding sites by structure prediction (Chothia and Lesk 1987). Furthermore, by tinkering with the antigen-binding site, it may prove possible to enhance antibody affinity (Roberts *et al.* 1987). Finally, the ability to derive catalytic antibodies by immunization with transition state analogues (Pollack *et al.* 1986; Tramontano *et al.* 1986; Napper *et al.* 1987) opens a new avenue for antibody engineering, for example by building in side-chains to selectively stabilize the transition state or by introducing attachment sites for co-factors (Pollack *et al.* 1988; Baldwin and Schulz 1989).

References

Ahmad, A. and Law, K. (1988). Strategies for designing antibody-toxin conjugates. *Trends Biotechnol.* **6**, 246–8.

Allen, D., Simon, T., Sablitzky, F., Rajewsky, K. and Cumano, A. (1988). Antibody engineering for the analysis of affinity maturation of an anti-hapten response. *EMBO J.* **7**, 1995–2001.

Alt, F.W., Yancopoulos, G.D., Blackwell, T.K. *et al.* (1984). Ordered rearrangement of immunoglobulin heavy chain variable region segments. *EMBO J.* **3**, 1209–19.

Amit, A.G., Mariuzza, R.A., Phillips, S.E.V. and Poljak, R.J. (1986). Three-dimensional structure of an antigen–antibody complex at 2.8 Å resolution. *Science* **233**, 747–54.

Anderson, C.L. and Looney, R.J. (1986). Human leukocyte IgG Fc receptors. *Immunol. Today* **7**, 264–6.

Baldwin, E. and Schulz, P.G. (1989). Generation of a catalytic antibody by site-directed mutagenesis. *Science* **245**, 1104–7.

Bedouelle, H. and Winter, G. (1986). A model of synthetase/transfer RNA interaction as deduced by protein engineering. *Nature* **320**, 371–3.

Better, M., Chang, C.P., Robinson, R.R. and Horwitz, A.H. (1988). *Escherichia coli* secretion of an active chimeric antibody fragment. *Science* **240**, 1041–3.

Bird, R.E., Hardman, K.D., Jacobson, J.W. *et al.* (1988). Single-chain antigen-binding proteins. *Science* **423**, 423–6.

Borrebaeck, C.A.K., Danielsson, L. and Möller, S.A. (1988). Human monoclonal antibodies produced by primary *in vitro* immunization of peripheral blood lymphocytes. *Proc. Nat. Acad. Sci. (USA)* **85**, 3995–9.

Boshart, M., Weber F., Jahn, G., Dorsch-Häsler, K., Fleckenstein, B. and Schaffner, W. (1985). A very strong enhancer is located upstream of an immediate early gene of human cytomegalovirus. *Cell* **41**, 521–30.

Boss, M.A., Kenten, J.H., Wood, C.R. and Emtage, J.S. (1984). Assembly of functional antibodies from immunoglobulin heavy and light chains synthesised in *E. coli*. *Nucleic Acids Res.* **12**, 3791–806.

Boulianne, G.L., Isenman, D.E., Hozumi, N. and Shulman, M.J. (1984). Biological properties of chimeric antibodies: interaction with complement. *Mol. Biol. Med.* **4**, 37–49.

Brüggemann, M., Williams, G.T., Bindon, C.I. *et al.* (1987). Comparison of the effector functions of human immunoglobulins using a matched set of chimeric antibodies. *J. Exp. Med.* **166**, 1351–61.

Burton, D.R. (1987). Structure and function of antibodies. In *Molecular Genetics of Immunoglobulins*, ed. F. Calabi and M.S. Neuberger, pp. 1–50, Elsevier, Amsterdam.

Burton, D.R., Boyd, J., Brampton, A.D. *et al.* (1980). The C1q receptor site on immunoglobulin G. *Nature* **288**, 338–44.

Cabilly, S., Riggs, A.D., Pande, H. *et al.* (1984). Generation of antibody activity from immunoglobulin polypeptide chains produced in *Escherichia coli*. *Proc. Nat. Acad. Sci. (USA)* **81**, 3273–7.

Capon, D.J., Chamow, S.M., Mordenti, J. *et al.* (1989). Designing CD4 immunoadhesions for AIDS therapy. *Nature* **337**, 525–9.

Carson, D.A. and Freimark, B.D. (1986). Human lymphocyte hybridomas and monoclonal antibodies. *Adv. Immunol.* **38**, 275–311.

Cattaneo, A. and Neuberger, M.S. (1987). Polymeric immunoglobulin M is secreted by transfectants of non-lymphoid cells in the absence of immunoglobulin J chain. *EMBO J.* **6**, 2753–8.

Chaudhary, V.K., Queen, C., Junghans, R.P., Waldmann, T.A., Fitzgerald, D.J. and Pastan, I. (1989). A recombinant immunotoxin consisting of two antibody variable domains fused to *Pseudomonas* exotoxin. *Nature* **339**, 394.

Chiang, Y.L., Sheng-Dong, R., Brow, M.A. and Larrick, J.W. (1989). Direct cDNA cloning of the rearranged immunoglobulin variable regions. *BioTechniques* **7**, 360–6.

Chothia, C. and Lesk, A.M. (1987). Canonical structures for the hypervariable regions of immunoglobulins. *J. Mol. Biol.* **196**, 901–17.

Chothia, C., Novotny, J. and Bruccoleri, R. (1985). Domain association in immunoglobulin molecules: the packing of variable domains. *J. Mol. Biol.* **186**, 651–63.

Coleman, J.W., Helm, B.A., Stanworth, D.R. and Gould, H.J. (1985). Inhibition of mast cell sensitization *in vitro* by a human immunoglobulin ε-fragment synthesised in *Escherichia coli*. *Eur. J. Immunol.* **15**, 966–9.

Dangl, J.L., Wensel, T.G., Morrison, S.L., Stryer, L., Herzenberg, L.A. and Oi, V.T. (1988). Segmental flexibility and complement fixation of genetically engineered chimeric human, rabbit and mouse antibody. *EMBO J.* **7**, 1989–94.

Davies, D.R. and Metzger, H. (1983). Structural basis of antibody function. *Ann. Rev. Immunol.* **1**, 87–117.

Davis, M.M., Calame, K., Early, P.W. *et al.* (1980). An immunoglobulin heavy-chain gene is formed by at least two recombinational events. *Nature* **283**, 733–9.

Dorai, H. and Moore, G.P. (1987). The effect of dihydrofolate reductase-mediated gene amplification on the expression of transfected immunoglobulin genes. *J. Immunol.* **139**, 4232–41.

Duncan, A.R. and Winter, G. (1988). The binding site for C1q on IgG. *Nature* **332**, 738–40.

Duncan, A.R., Woof, J.M., Partridge, L.J., Burton, D.R. and Winter, G. (1988). Localisation of the binding site for the human high-affinity Fc receptor on IgG. *Nature* **332**, 563–4.

Gascoigne, N.R.J., Goodnow, C.C., Dudzik, K.I., Oi, V.T. and Davis, M.M. (1987). Secretion of a chimeric T-cell receptor-immunoglobulin protein. *Proc. Nat. Acad. Sci. (USA)* **84**, 2936–40.

Graham, F.L. and van der Eb, A.J. (1973). A new technique for the assay of infectivity of human adenovirus 5 DNA. *Virology* **52**, 456–67.

Hale, G., Swirsky, D.M., Hayhoe, F.G.J. and Waldman H. (1983). Effects of monoclonal anti-lymphocyte antibodies *in vivo* in monkeys and humans. *Mol. Biol. Med.* **1**, 321–34.

Hale, G., Dyer, M.J.S., Clark, M.R. *et al.* (1988). Remission induction in non-Hodgkin lymphoma with reshaped human monoclonal antibody CAMPATH-1H. *Lancet* 17 December, 1394–9.

Helm, B., Marsh, P., Vercelli, D., Padlan, E., Gould, H. and Geha, R.S. (1988). The mast cell binding site on human immunoglobulin E. *Nature* **331**, 180–3.

Huston, J.S., Levinson, D., Mudgett-Hunter, M. *et al.* (1988). Protein engineering of antibody binding sites: recovery of specific activity in an anti-digoxin single-chain Fv analogue produced in *Escherichia coli*. *Proc. Nat. Acad. Sci. (USA)* **85**, 5879–83.

Inbar, D., Hochman, J. and Givol, D. (1972). Localisation of antibody-combining sites within the variable portions of heavy and light chains. *Proc. Nat. Acad. Sci. (USA)* **69**, 2659–62.

Isenman, D.E., Dorrington, K.J. and Painter, R.H. (1975). The structure and function of immunoglobulin domains. *J. Immunol.* 1726–9.

Ishizaka, T., Helm, B., Hakimi, J., Niebyl, J., Ishizaka, K. and Gould, H. (1986). Biological properties of a recombinant human immunoglobulin ε-chain fragment *Proc. Nat. Acad. Sci. (USA)* **83**, 8323–7.

Jones, P.T., Dear, P.H., Foote, J., Neuberger, M.S. and Winter, G. (1986). Replacing the complementarity-determining regions in a human antibody with those from a mouse. *Nature* **321**, 522–4.

Kabat, E.A., Wu, T.T., Reid-Miller, M., Perry, H.M. and Gottesmann, K.S. (1987). *Sequences of Proteins of Immunological Interest.* US Department of Health and Human Services, US Government Printing Office.

Kakimoto, K. and Onoue, K. (1974). Characterisation of the Fv fragment isolated from a human immunoglobulin M. *J. Immunol.* **112**, 1373–82.

Kataoka, T., Miyata, T. and Honjo, T. (1981). Repetitive sequences in class-switch recombination regions of immunoglobulin heavy chain genes. *Cell* **23**, 357–68.

Klein, M., Haeffner-Cavallon, N., Isenman, D.E. *et al.* (1981). Expression of biological effector functions by immunoglobulin G molecules lacking the hinge region. *Proc. Nat. Acad. Sci (USA)* **78**, 524–8.

Köhler, G. and Milstein, C. (1975). Continuous culture of fused cells secreting antibody of predefined specificity. *Nature* **256**, 495–7.

Kurokawa, T., Seno, M., Sasada, R. *et al.* (1983). Expression of human immunoglobulin E ε chain cDNA in *E. coli. Nucleus Acids Res.* **11**, 3077–84.

Larrick, J.W., Danielsson, L., Brenner, C.A. *et al.* (1989a). Polymerase chain reaction using mixed primers: cloning of human monoclonal antibody variable region genes from single hybridoma cells. *Biotechnology* **7**, 934–8.

Larrick, J.W., Danielsson, L., Brenner, C.A., Abrahamson, M., Fry, K.E. and Borrebaeck, C.A.K. (1989b). Rapid cloning of rearranged immunoglobulin genes from human hybridoma cells using mixed primers and the polymerase chain reaction. *Biochem. Biophys. Res. Comm.* **160**, 1250–5.

Lesk, A.M. and Chothia, C. (1982). Evolution of proteins formed by beta sheets. II. The core of the immunoglobulin domains. *J. Mol. Biol.* **160**, 325–42.

Liu, A.Y., Mack, P.W., Champion, C.I. and Robinson, R.R. (1987). Expression of mouse:: human immunoglobulin heavy-chain cDNA in lymphoid cells. *Gene* **54**, 33–40.

Liu, F., Albrandt, K.A., Bry, C.G. and Ishizaka, T. (1984). Expression of a biologically active fragment of human IgE ε chain in *Escherichia coli. Proc. Nat. Acad. Sci. (USA)* **81**, 5369–73.

Livant, D., Blatt, C. and Hood, L. (1986). One heavy chain variable region gene segment subfamily in the BALB/c mouse contains 500–1000 or more members. *Cell* **47**, 461–70.

LoBuglio, A.F., Wheeler, R.H., Trang, J. *et al.* (1989). Mouse/human chimeric monoclonal antibody in man; kinetics and immune response. *Proc. Nat. Acad. Sci. (USA)* **86**, 4220–4.

Maki, R., Traunecker, A., Sakano, H., Roeder, W. and Tonegawa, S. (1980). Exon shuffling generates an immunoglobulin heavy chain gene. *Proc. Nat. Acad. Sci. (USA)* **77**, 2138–42.

Mariuzza, R.A. and Winter, G. (1989). Secretion of a homodimeric VαCκ T-cell receptor-immunoglobulin chimeric protein. *J. Biol. Chem.* **264**, 7310–16.

Maxam, A.M. and Gilbert, W. (1977). A new method for sequencing DNA. *Proc. Nat. Acad. Sci. (USA)* **74**, 560–4.

Morrison, S.L. (1985). Transfectomas provide novel chimeric antibodies. *Science* **229**, 1202–7.

Morrison, S.L., Johnson, M.J., Herzenberg, L.A. and Oi, V.T. (1984). Chimeric human antibody molecules: mouse antigen-binding domains with human constant region domains. *Proc. Nat. Acad. Sci. (USA)* **81**, 6851–5.

Müller, M.M., Ruppert, S., Schaffner, W. and Matthias, P. (1988). A cloned octamer transcription factor stimulates transcription from lymphoid-specific promoters in non-B cells. *Nature* **336**, 544–51.

Mulligan, R.C. and Berg, P. (1981). Selection for animal cells that express the *Escherichia coli* gene coding for xanthine-guanine phosphoribosyl transferase. *Proc. Nat. Acad. Sci. (USA)* **78**, 2072–6.

Napper, A.D., Benkovic, S.J., Tramontano, A. and Lerner, R.A. (1987). A stereospecific cyclisation catalysed by an antibody. *Science* **237**, 1041–3.

Neuberger, M.S. (1983). Expression and regulation of immunoglobulin heavy chain gene transfected into lymphoid cells. *EMBO J.* **2**, 1373–8.

Neuberger, M.S. (1985). Making novel antibodies by expressing transfected immunoglobulin genes. *Trends. Biochem.* **10**, 347–9.

Neuberger, M.S. and Cook, G.P. (1988). The expression of immunoglobulin genes. *Immunol. Today* **9**, 278–81.

Neuberger, M.S. and Rajewsky, K. (1981). Switch from hapten-specific immunoglobulin M to immunoglobulin D secretion in a hybrid mouse cell line. *Proc. Nat. Acad. Sci. (USA)* **78**, 1138–42.

Neuberger, M.S. and Williams, G.T. (1988). The intron requirement for immunoglobulin gene expression is dependent upon the promoter. *Nucleic Acids Res.* **16**, 6713–24.

Neuberger, M.S., Williams, G.T. and Fox, R.O. (1984). Recombinant antibodies possessing novel effector functions. *Nature* **13**, 602–8.

Neuberger, M.S., Williams, G.T., Mitchell, E.B., Jouhal, S.S., Flanagan, J.G. and Rabbitts, T.H. (1985). A hapten-specific chimaeric IgE antibody with human physiological effector function. *Nature* **314**, 268–70.

Obata, M., Kataoka, T., Nakai, S. *et al.* (1981). Structure of a rearranged γ1 chain gene and its implication to immunoglobulin class-switch mechanism. *Proc. Nat. Acad. Sci. (USA)* **78**, 2437–41.

Oi, V.T., Morrison, S.L., Herzenberg, L.A. and Berg, P. (1983). Immunoglobulin gene expression in transformed lymphoid cells. *Proc. Nat. Acad. Sci. (USA)* **80**, 825–9.

Oi, V.T., Vuong, T.M., Hardy, R. *et al.* (1984). Correlation between segmental flexibility and effector function of antibodies. *Nature* **307**, 136–40.

Okayama, H. and Berg, P. (1983). A cDNA cloning vector that permits expression of cDNA inserts in mammalian cells. *Mol. Cell. Biol.* **3**, 280–9.

Orlandi, R., Gussow, D.H., Jones, P.T. and Winter. G, (1989). Cloning immunoglobulin variable domains for expression by the polymerase chain reaction. *Proc. Nat. Acad. Sci. (USA)* **86**, 3833–7.

Padlan, E.A., Silverton, E.W., Sheriff, S., Cohen, G.H., Smith-Gill, S.J. and Davies, D.R. (1989). Structure of an antibody-antigen complex: crystal structure of the HyHEL-10 Fab-lysozyme complex. *Proc. Nat. Acad. Sci. (USA)* **86**, 5938–42.

Pelham, H.R.B. (1982). A regulatory upstream promoter element in the *Drosophila* Hsp 70 heat-shock gene. *Cell* **30**, 517–28.

Pollack, S.J., Jacobs, J.W. and Schultz, P.G. (1986). Selective chemical catalysis by an antibody. *Science* **234**, 1570–3.

Pollack, S.J., Nakayama, G.R. and Schultz, P.G. (1988). Introduction of nucleophiles and spectroscopic probes into antibody combining sites. *Science* **242**, 1038–40.

Porter, R.R. (1973). Structural studies of immunoglobulins. *Science* **180**, 713–16.

Potter, H., Weir, L. and Leder, P. (1984). Enhancer-dependent expression of human κ immunoglobulin genes introduced into mouse pre-B lymphocytes by electroporation. *Proc. Nat. Acad. Sci. (USA)* **81**, 7161–5.

Riechmann, L., Clark, M., Waldmann, H. and Winter, G. (1988a). Reshaping human antibodies for therapy. *Nature* **332**, 323–7.

Riechmann, L., Foote, J. and Winter, G. (1988b). Expression of an antibody Fv fragment in myeloma cells. *J. Mol. Biol.* **203**, 825–8.

Roberts, S., Cheetman, J.C. and Rees, A.R. (1987). Generation of an antibody with enhanced affinity and specificity for its antigen by protein engineering. *Nature* **328**, 731–4.

Rudikoff, S., Giusti, A.M., Cook, W.D. and Scharff, M.D. (1982). Single amino acid substitution altering antigen-binding specificity. *Proc. Nat. Acad. Sci. (USA)* **79**, 1979–83.

Saiki, R.K., Scharf, S., Faloona, F. *et al.* (1985). Enzymatic amplification of β-globin genomic sequences and restriction site analysis for diagnosis of sickle cell anemia. *Science* **230**, 1350–4.

Saiki, R.K., Gelfand, D.H., Stoffel, S. *et al.* (1988). Primer-directed enzymatic amplification of DNA with a thermostable DNA polymerase. *Science* **239**, 487–91.

Sanger, F., Nicklen, S. and Coulson, H.R. (1977). DNA sequencing with chain-terminating inhibitors. *Proc. Nat. Acad. Sci. (USA)* **74**, 5463.

Sastry, L., Alting-Mees, M., Huse, W.D. *et al.* (1989). Cloning of the immunological repertoire in *Escherichia coli* for generation of monoclonal catalytic antibodies: construction of a heavy chain variable region-specific cDNA library. *Proc. Nat. Acad. Sci. (USA)* **86**, 5728–32.

Saul, F.A., Amzel, L.M. and Poljak, R.J. (1987). Preliminary refinement and structural analysis of the Fab fragment from human immunoglobulin New at 2.0 Å resolution. *J. Biol. Chem.* **253**, 585–97.

Scheidereit, C., Cromlish, J.A., Gerster, T. *et al.* (1988). A human lymphoid-specific transcription factor that activates immunoglobulin genes is a homoeobox protein. *Nature* **336**, 551–7.

Schmike, R.T. (1984). Gene amplification in cultured animal cells. *Cell* **37**, 705–13.

Schnee, J.M., Runge, M.S., Matsueda, G.R. *et al.* (1987). Construction and expression of a recombinant antibody-targeted plasminogen activator. *Proc. Nat. Acad. Sci. (USA)* **84**, 6904–8.

Sharon, J. and Givol, D. (1976). Preparation of Fv fragment from the mouse myeloma XRPC-25 immunoglobulin possessing anti-dinitrophenyl activity. *Biochemistry* **15**, 1591–4.

Sharon, J., Gefter, M.L. Manser, T., Morrison, S.L., Oi, V.T. and Ptashne, M. (1984). Expression of a VH Cκ chimaeric protein in mouse myeloma cells. *Nature* **309**, 364–7.

Sheriff, S., Silverton, E.W., Padlan, E.A. *et al.* (1987). Three-dimensional structure of an antibody–antigen complex. *Proc. Nat. Acad. Sci. (USA)* **84**, 8075–9.

Shimizu, A. and Honjo, T. (1984). Immunoglobulin class switching. *Cell* **36**, 801–3.

Skerra, A. and Plückthun, A. (1988). Assembly of a functional immunoglobulin Fv fragment in *Escherichia coli*. *Science* **240**, 1038–40.

Southern, P.J. and Berg, P. (1981). Transformation of mammalian cells to antibiotic resistance with a bacterial gene under control of the SV40 early region promoter. *J. Mol. Appl. Genet.* **1**, 327–41.

Stepelewski, Z., Sun, L.K., Shearman, C.W., Ghrayeb, J., Daddona, P. and Koprowski, H. (1988). Biological activity of human-mouse IgG1, IgG2, IgG3, and IgG chimeric monoclonal antibodies with antitumour specificity. *Proc. Nat. Acad. Sci. (USA)* **85**, 4852–6.

Sun, L.K., Curtis, P., Rakowicz-Szulczynska, E. *et al.* (1987). Chimeric antibody with human constant regions and mouse variable regions directed against carcinoma-associated antigen 17-1A. *Proc. Nat. Acad. Sci. (USA)* **84**, 214–18.

Thompson, K.M. (1988). Human monoclonal antibodies. *Immunol. Today* **9**, 113–16.

Tonegawa, S. (1983). Somatic generation of antibody diversity. *Nature* **302**, 575–81.

Tramontano, A., Janda, K.D. and Lerner, R.A. (1986). Catalytic antibodies. *Science* **234**, 1566–9.

Verhoeyen, M. and Riechmann, L. (1988). Engineering of antibodies. *Bioessays* **8**, 74–8.

Verhoeyen, M., Milstein, C. and Winter, G. (1988). Reshaping human antibodies: grafting an antilysozyme activity. *Science* **239**, 1534–6.

Ward, E.S., Gussow, D.H., Griffiths, A.D., Jones, P.T. and Winter, G. (1989a). Binding activities of a repertoire of single immunoglobulin variable domains secreted from *Escherichia coli*. *Nature* **341**, 544–6.

Ward, E.S., Gussow, D.H., Griffiths, A.D., Jones, P.T. and Winter, G.G. (1989b). Expression and secretion of repertoires of VH domains in *Escherichia coli*: isolation of antigen binding activities. In *Progress in Immunology*, ed. F. Melcher *et al.* pp. 1144–51. Springer-Verlag, Berlin.

Weidle, H., Borgya, A., Mattes, R., Lenz, H. and Buckel, P. (1987) Reconstitution of functionally active antibody directed against creatine kinase from separately expressed heavy and light chains in non-lymphoid cells. *Gene* **51**, 21–9.

Whittle, N., Adair, J., Lloyd, C. *et al.* (1987). Expression in COS cell of a mouse–human chimaeric B72.3 antibody. *Protein Eng.* **1**, 499–505.

Williams, G. (1988). Novel antibody reagents: production and potential. *Trends Biotechnol.* **6**, 36–42.

Winkelhake, J.L. (1978). Immunoglobulin structure and effector functions. *Immunochemistry* **15**, 695–714.

Woof, J.M., Partridge, L.J., Jefferis, R. and Burton, D.R. (1986). Localisation of the monocyte-binding region on human immunoglobulin G. *Mol. Immunol.* **23**, 319–30.

44: Immunoassays

P.M.S. Clark and C.N. Hales

Introduction

Antigen recognition and binding by antibody represent a reaction of great specificity and often of high affinity. The potential of this reaction for use as an assay technique was recognized over 50 years ago. However, it was the use of a high specific activity radio-isotope (^{131}I) to monitor the reaction at very low concentrations of antigen which realized its applicability to assay problems requiring extremely high sensitivity. Yalow and Berson (1971) have described their early research which led to the introduction of the first of such assays — radio-immunoassay. In this chapter we summarize the present state of development of immunoassays applicable to the measurement of very low concentrations of substances in biological fluids.

Radio-immunoassay is a method in which an antigen is labelled with radioactivity. Subsequently it was suggested that immunoassays involving the use of antibodies labelled with radioisotopes, enzymes or even viruses might be advantageous for assays of high sensitivity (Miles and Hales 1968). The introduction of a method of producing monoclonal antibodies (Kohler and Milstein 1975) greatly increased the practicability of the labelled antibody approach. Over the years a bewildering variety of methods, depending on labelling either antigen or antibody, the use of different labels, and various ways of separating antigen from antibody and of detecting the final signal, have been introduced. Many of these have come to be known by an equally confusing array of acronyms. In Table 44.1 we list a number of those most commonly used at present.

Underlying all these methods are a few basic principles which simplify the understanding of the procedures. There are also a limited number of criteria against which their performance can be judged.

Principles

Immunoassay methods employing labelled antigen rely on competition between the labelled antigen and the substance to be measured for binding to an antibody binding site. They are thus one

Table 44.1. Table of the commonly used acronyms in immunoassay

Acronym	Full name	Distinguishing features
RIA	Radio-immunoassay	Radioisotope-labelled antigen; requires separation of bound and free fractions
IRMA	Immunoradiometric assay	Radioisotope-labelled antibody; requires separation, requires use of immunoadsorbent
RAST	Radioallergosorbent test	Radioisotope-labelled antibody, specifically for measuring IgE antibodies in serum
EIA	Enzyme immunoassay	Enzyme label: this is a general term for immunoassays using enzyme labels
ELISA	Enzyme-linked immunosorbent assay	Enzyme-labelled solid-phase assay requiring separation, chiefly notable for its delightful acronym
IEMA	Immunoenzymometric assay	Enzyme-labelled equivalent of IRMA
EMIT	Enzyme-mediated immunoassay technique	Trademark of Syva Co.: refers solely to their homogeneous enzyme-labelled assays
FIA	Fluoroimmunoassay	Fluorescent label: this is a general term for immunoassays using fluorescent labels
LIA	Luminescent immunoassay	Luminescent label

example of a broader type of assay procedure known as 'competitive binding assays'. The essence of competitive binding assays is the use of a highly specific binding reaction such that the substance to be measured competes with a related but labelled molecule for binding to a limited number of binding sites. In principle, a number of protein binding reactions, including hormone-binding proteins and allosteric protein binding sites, could be exploited in this way. In order that effective competition takes place at the very low concentrations of the substance to be measured, it is necessary to work with very low concentrations of ligand, which in an immunoassay would be an antibody. Hence the antibody affinity is particularly important in immunoassays. The binding sites of individual antibodies have definable specificities and affinities determined by the amino acids which constitute the area of contact between antigen and antibody. When monoclonal antibodies are used, the properties of the reaction are relatively simple. The properties of polyclonal antisera, on the other hand, reflect the sum of the properties of the individual antibodies and are therefore often complex. Nevertheless, in either assay situation, as the concentration of unlabelled substance or standard is increased, less labelled antigen may be bound by the antibody. In order to determine the amount of antigen bound to antibody, it is usually necessary to separate free from bound antigen and determine the amount of either. A typical standard curve for such an assay, in which the bound antigen has been measured, is shown in Fig. 44.1. Immunoassay methods which do not depend upon the separation of free from bound antigen or antibody have been described and are termed 'homogeneous' assays.

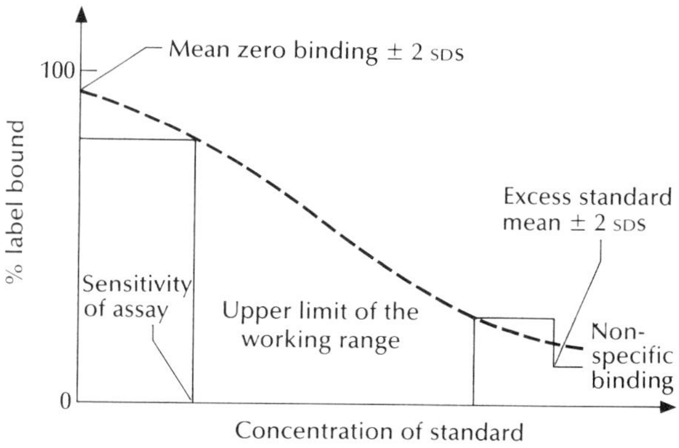

Fig. 44.1. Standard curve for radio-immunoassay.

Immunoassays using labelled antibodies do not depend upon competition but rather on the reaction of as much as possible of the antigen with the labelled antibody. The latter is therefore usually present in considerable molar excess. Under these conditions, satisfactory assays can be produced using antibodies whose affinity for antigen is too low to make them suitable for use in labelled antigen assays of similar sensitivity. Labelled antibody assays are now most frequently used in the 'two-site' (Addison and Hales 1971) format (Fig. 44.2). This configuration is also sometimes known as a 'sandwich' assay. In this assay, the antigen is bound between two antibodies. The two antibodies are usually directed against different epitopes on the antigen. The diagram in Fig. 44.2 has been drawn to illustrate the possibility of the formation of cyclic complexes involving two molecules each of antigen and antibody. It has been proposed that such complexes are very stable and confer high avidity on the reaction system (Moyle *et al.* 1983). This feature of two-site assays may provide an additional explanation as to why satisfactory assays can be obtained in this format with two antibodies whose affinities for antigen would render them unsuitable for use in a labelled antigen assay.

Criteria of assay performance

In establishing immunoassays applicable to research and clinical problems, there are a number of criteria against which they may be judged, and these are defined below.

Sensitivity: the precision at zero analyte concentration.

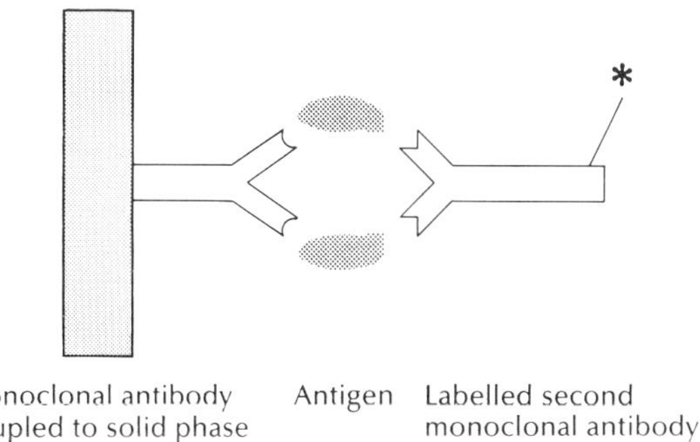

Fig. 44.2. Two-site immunometric assay: formation of cyclic antigen–antibody complexes.

Detection limit: the ability to distinguish a low analyte concentration as being statistically different from zero.

Working range: the concentration range of analyte over which the precision of the assay is acceptable — commonly taken as the range over which the coefficient of variation is less than 10%.

High-dose hook effect: effect whereby increasing analyte concentration beyond a certain point (the 'hook') causes a reduction in the measured signal due to an excess of antigen over antibody.

Precision: the agreement between replicate measurements.

Accuracy: the extent to which a result is close to the true value.

Specificity: the degree to which a binding protein(s) binds its particular ligand and does not bind structurally similar compounds.

In order to compare the performance of various assays each must be determined by standard laboratory methods.

The following sections describe the recent advances in the three major components of an immunoassay — the antibody, the label and the solid phase — and the development of biosensors based on immunoassays.

Antibodies

Polyclonal

In recent years the widespread development of monoclonal antibodies has meant that fewer assays are now based on polyclonal antisera. The production of antisera is still somewhat unpredictable; factors such as choice of species, purity of antigen, adjuvant, site of injection and time course may all have a significant influence on the possibility of obtaining suitable antisera (Hurn and Landon 1971).

Monoclonal

There is now a wealth of advice on the procedures for raising monoclonal antibodies and their applications to immunoassay (see Siddle 1985; French *et al.* 1986; Samoilovich *et al.* 1987). The outcome of immunization for the production of monoclonal antibodies may be improved by coupling the antigen to other larger proteins, enriching the B cells making the desired antibody, optimization of media, stringent screening and other such manoeuvres.

The hybridoma technology allows the production of an unlimited amount of homogeneous antibody, with single epitope specificity, which is easy to purify but which does not require pure antigen for its generation. A number of disadvantages have been identified. Often the affinity of a monoclonal antibody is low, the antibody may be more specific than is required and precipitation techniques may not be possible. There are high costs involved in their production and identifying the right monoclonal antibody is labour-intensive.

Some particular problems with their use in immunoassays are detailed below.

SPECIFICITY

Assays which depend upon the antigen linking two antibodies together may be complicated by other molecules (e.g. anti-immunoglobulins) which can also cross-link the two antibodies used in the assay. It has now been shown that a number of different types of endogenous antibody may cause falsely elevated results in immunometric assays. Those that have been identified include anti-mouse antibodies (if mouse monoclonal antibodies are used), autoantibodies, e.g. rheumatoid factor, anti-idiotypic antibody and anti-label antibodies. The addition of non-immune mouse serum to reagent buffers and the use of Fab′ conjugates may overcome some of these problems.

In contrast, the use of monoclonal antibody in two-site immunometric assays may result in a very narrow range of specificity such that normal variants of the antigen, e.g. different degrees of glycosylation, may not contain the recognized epitopes or may only bind weakly. This has been a particular problem for assays of the polypeptide hormones (Biggart *et al.* 1985).

LABELLING

The activity of an antibody may be reduced if the label is attached to the binding site. Since this site does not contain carbohydrate, a label attached to the antibody carbohydrate region may preserve the binding site activity. However, this approach is limited by the small carbohydrate content of antibodies. Simonson and co-workers (1988) overcame this problem by treating a hybridoma with a mannosidase inhibitor, leading to a monoclonal with a higher carbohydrate content, which could be labelled by the periodate reaction, followed by reaction with, for example, iodinated glycyltyrosylglycylglycylarginine in the presence of cyanoborohydride (Rodwell *et al.* 1986) with no loss of immunoreactivity.

New developments in monoclonal antibody technology relevant to immunoassays

BISPECIFIC ANTIBODIES

Enzyme labelling of antibodies for immunoassay is usually carried out by covalent bonding. However, the procedure does result in a poorly defined mixture of simple and complex, active and inactive species. Not all monoclonal antibodies retain function when chemically modified. There have been assays described where an enzyme-labelled antibody is connected to the antigen-specific antibody by an anti-immunoglobulin ‘bridge’ antibody. An alternative approach is to covalently link an antigen–antibody and an anti-enzyme label antibody. Such paired antibodies have been used to measure immunoglobulin M (IgM) and alphafetoprotein (AFP), the latter in a homogeneous assay format (Porstmann *et al.* 1984; Ashihara *et al.* 1987).

Another approach is to use bispecific monoclonal antibodies produced by hybrid hybridomas. The resulting cells secrete hybrid antibodies showing the binding characteristics of the two parental hybridomas in a single molecule. These bispecific monoclonal antibodies are structurally bivalent but functionally univalent for each combining site (Milstein and Cuello 1983; Suresh *et al.* 1986). Although the techniques for ‘quadroma’ production have yet to be fully explored, they have been applied to enzyme immunoassays, for example for human chorionic gonadotrophin (HCG).

IDIOTYPES AND ANTI-IDIOTYPES

The determinants making up the antibody variable region are termed ‘idiotopes’. Some are located in the combining site (also known as the 'paratope') and others occur outside the combining site. The full set of variable region determinants is called the 'idiotype' of the antibody molecule.

Monoclonal antibodies are homogeneous and are potentially antigenic, so that antibodies can be derived to the idiotypes and these new antibodies are known as anti-idiotypic antibodies. There are several types of anti-idiotypic antibodies with different binding characteristics. Antibodies to the paratope (combining site) inhibit ligand binding and are ligand-inhibited. They may act as molecular mimics of the ligands and thus may be used as substitutes for them in competitive binding assays. This has the advantage that the antigen does not need to be purified, labelled or stored under specialized conditions. Such antibodies have been applied to an assay for the drug haloperidol (Linthicum *et al.* 1988a, b).

ANTIBODY DESIGN

The production of monoclonal antibodies with higher affinities, unusual specificities and of a required class or subclass may come with improvements in current methodologies. It seems increasingly likely that both somatic cell genetics and genetically engineered antibodies will be used to generate tailor-made antibodies. Examples of these approaches are the selection of somatic mutants and the production of genetically engineered antibodies.

Somatic mutants

Class and subclass switching and somatic mutants both occur spontaneously *in vitro* in cultured myeloma and hybridoma cells. More useful monoclonal antibodies may be generated by identifying those subclones that contain a particular class switch or higher-affinity variants. A number of techniques have been developed to do this (Aguila *et al.* 1986).

Genetically engineered antibodies

In 1983 Oi and colleagues reported that lymphoid cells can express cloned, transfected immunoglobulin genes, and since then there has been much effort put into genetically engineering antibodies, from cloning the variable regions of the antibody to replacement of the complementarity-determining regions (Morrison *et al.* 1988; Moore 1989). The reader is referred to Chapter 43 for full details, but there are a number of possible implications for immunoassay, namely isotype switching, increasing affinity or avidity, using gene fusion to generate bispecific antibodies, and altering effector functions, such as Fc receptor binding and complement activation.

Interestingly, Winter and colleagues (Ward *et al.* 1989) have been able to clone immunoglobulin heavy-chain variable (V_H) genes and express them in *Escherichia coli*. The V_H domains bind antigen with good affinity in the absence of the light-chain (V_L) domains. These single-domain antibodies have a number of potential advantages (see Chapter 43), for example the need for tissue culture is avoided. The advantages of their use in immunoassays have yet to be established.

AVIDIN/STREPTAVIDIN—BIOTIN

Avidin binds to biotin with a very high affinity (10^{-15} M/l) and has four biotin-binding sites. Avidin and its binding to biotin have been used extensively in immunoassays by labelling the avidin and biotinylating antibodies or antigen. Biotin labelling of antibodies has been shown to be simple and reproducible. Streptavidin is a four-subunit 60 kD protein with similar binding properties to avidin. It is not glycosylated, however, and has a lower pI, factors which may decrease the non-specific binding to solid phases and proteins compared with labelled avidin (Wilchek and Bayer 1984). The avidin/streptavidin-biotin system has been used to increase the sensitivity and speed of colorimetric and luminometric immunoassays (Hart and Taffe 1987; Vilja *et al.* 1988).

Labels

Radio-immunoassays were developed three decades ago and represented an important milestone in analytical biochemistry. ^{125}Iodine is probably the most commonly used radioactive label (Thompson 1984), but the last few years have seen a major research effort in developing non-isotopic labels. The aim has been to improve sensitivity, to lengthen reagent shelf-life, and in particular to overcome the health hazards and regulations associated with handling ionizing radiation. Non-isotopic labels may indeed also facilitate automation and allow the development of visual detection systems. It must be remembered, though, that with respect to sensitivity there is a dependence of sensitivity on antibody affinity, thus making absolute comparisons of label sensitivity impossible unless the same antibody is used. The array of non-isotopic labels is bewildering but well reviewed (Schall and Tenoso 1981; Howanitz 1988). Some of the more widely used and sensitive approaches are described in the following sections. For further details of other techniques, such as particle labels and liposomes, the reader is referred to the above-mentioned reviews.

Luminescence

Chemiluminescence is the phenomenon observed when the vibrationally excited product of a chemical reaction reverts to the ground state with the emission of photons. It can thus be distinguished, for example, from fluorescence, where the absorption of light brings about an excited state. The term bioluminescence is used in those luminescent systems where a catalytic protein increases the efficiency of the luminescent reaction. The quantum yields (i.e. the number of photons emitted per molecule of reactant) of bioluminescent reactions may approach unity, although those of simple chemiluminescent reactions rarely exceed 0.2.

Luminescent reactions can be employed in immunoassays in several ways — for example, by direct use of a chemiluminescent substance as label, by using a catalyst or co-factor for a luminescent reaction as label or by monitoring the products of labels luminescently (Kricka and Carter 1982; Kricka 1985). In practice, luminescent immunoassays have been most widely developed using luminol, isoluminol or acridinium compounds as labels (Weeks *et al.* 1986), and these are now commercially available. Assays based on the luminescent monitoring of enzyme labels, for example peroxidase and alkaline phosphatase (Fig. 44.3), have been developed (Geiger and Miska 1987; Miska and Geiger 1987).

The luminescent reaction has several advantages: sensitivity, wide range, longer shelf-life of reagents and safety. However, its physical characteristics impose requirements on instrument design. The basic elements of a luminometer are a light-tight detection chamber and a light detector. Photomultiplier tubes and silicon photoelectrodes are most widely used with appropriate spectral response and sensitivity, though photographic film has also been used. Because of the speed of the luminescent reaction (1–60 s), it is necessary to add reagents whilst the reaction tube is in front of the detector in the light-tight box and to mix rapidly. These problems have been overcome with peroxidase/luminol systems, where the addition of phenols, e.g. *p*-iodophenol and *p*-phenylphenol, to the reaction system both enhances and prolongs the light output (Thorpe *et al.* 1985).

Fluorescence

Fluorescence is the emission of light that occurs when molecules, excited from their ground state to an electronically excited singlet state by incident radiation, decay back to their ground state. Fluorescence emission occurs at a longer wavelength than the incident radiation, the difference between excitation and emission wavelengths being known as the Stokes' shift. The intensity of fluorescence is directly proportional to the intensity of the incident radiation, the molar extinction coefficient and the fluorescence quantum yield.

Fluorescent labels have been widely used in immunoassays with either direct fluorescent labelling or indirect labelling with substrate, co-factor or enzyme. Widely used fluorescent labels include fluorescein, rhodamine, umbelliferone and, more recently, the phycobiliproteins (Kricka 1985; Kronick 1986).

Fluorescence detection has particular advantages in terms of stability of the label and hence long shelf-life, and theoretically in terms of sensitivity. However, in practice difficulties may arise due to interference by the sample. Endogeneous fluorophores such as drugs and bilirubin can produce a background fluorescence or absorb the excitation or fluorescence emission. In addition, turbidity due to lipids causes Rayleigh and Raman scattering. These factors all limit sensitivity and will be greatest for the homogeneous fluoroimmunoassays. They may be minimized by sample dilution or solvent extraction. For analytes where sensitivity is not a problem these approaches may be adequate, but for many assays, for example the peptide hormone assays, greater sensitivity is required. In these assays a separation step, as in the two-site immunometric assays, and also time-resolved fluorescence detection have been used to

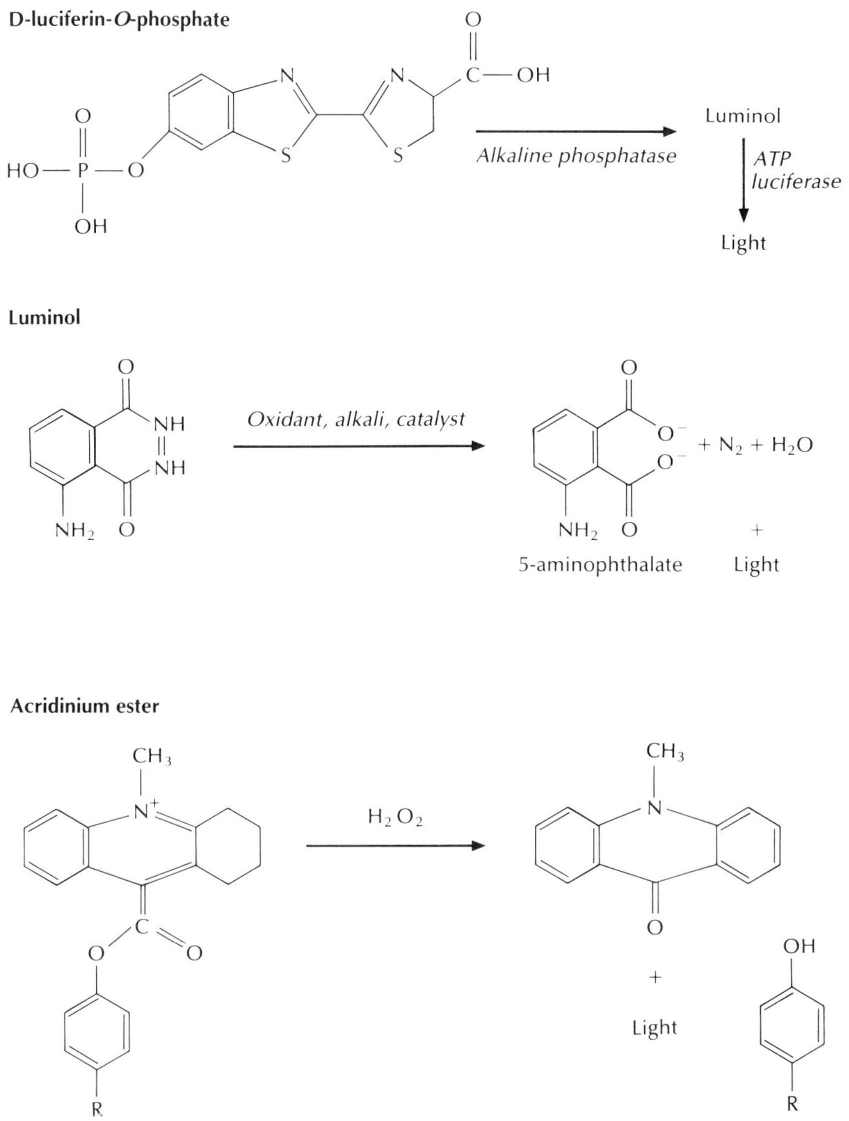

D-luciferin-*O*-phosphate

Alkaline phosphatase → Luminol; *ATP luciferase* → Light

Luminol

Oxidant, alkali, catalyst → 5-aminophthalate $+ N_2 + H_2O$ + Light

Acridinium ester

H_2O_2 → + Light

Fig. 44.3. Luminescent labels for immunoassays.

improve sensitivity. Examples of some of the more widely used fluoroimmunoassays are detailed below.

TIME-RESOLVED FLUORESCENCE

Time-resolved fluorescence is a method where the fluorescence emission is counted with a certain time delay after pulsed excitation (Jackson and Ekins 1986; Hemmilä 1988). The background, non-specific fluorescence decays rapidly and with the appropriate choice of label the specific signal has a longer decay time (100–1000 μs) and a large Stokes' shift (250 nm). In these methods the fluorescence is measured after a period of time (Fig. 44.4). The tervalent lanthanide ions, especially Eu^{3+} and Tb^{3+}, show a fluorescence with narrow-banded emission lines and long fluorescence decay time (more than 40-fold longer than the average background decay time). When chelated with suitable ultraviolet (UV) light-absorbing ligands, for example β-diketones, the fluorescence is enhanced by several orders of magnitude, in addition to having a longer decay time. This has meant that relatively simple instrumentation, using for example N_2 laser or pulsed xenon discharge lamps as the excitation source, can be used (Hemmilä 1985). The quenching and dissociative properties of water on Eu^{3+} can be overcome by dissociation of the cations from the antibody-bound complex

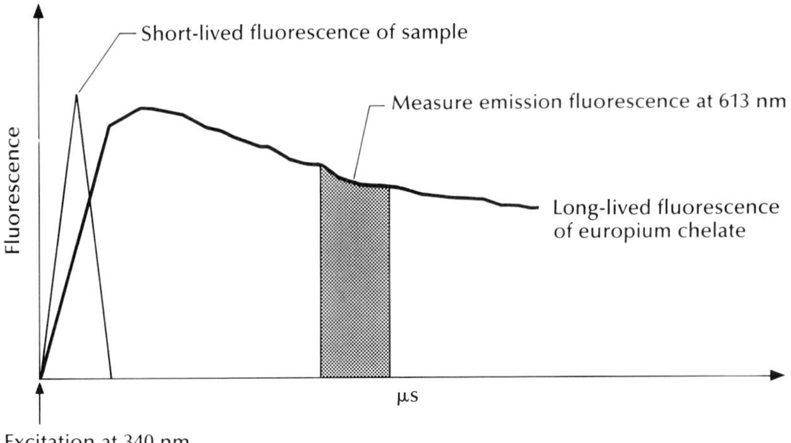

Fig. 44.4. Principles of time-resolved fluorescence, using europium chelates.

ones prior to the formation of the fluorescent chelates. Water molecules can be replaced by the addition of a synergistic compound (tri-*n*-octylphosphine oxide (TOPO)) and micelle-forming detergents. The chelate Ln^{3+}(β-diketone)$_3$ ($TOPO_{2-3}$) is then solubilized by the micelles. This dissociative fluorescent enhancement also overcomes the optical problems encountered when measuring at surfaces. Double-labelled assays using Eu^{3+} and Tb^{3+} have also been developed.

FLUORESCENCE POLARIZATION ASSAYS

If a fluorescent molecule is excited with polarized light, the emitted fluorescence will be polarized if the fluorescence is emitted in such a short time that the molecules have not rotated significantly, i.e. if the rotational relaxation time is long compared with the decay time of the excited state. This situation obtains, for example, in crystalline solids and may obtain in viscous fluids. If the physical rotation of a fluorescent label is sterically hindered by the binding of antigen to antibody, then there will be a change in the degree of polarization of the emitted fluorescence consequent on antigen–antibody binding. Measurement of the polarization allows the estimation of the extent of this binding without separation of bound and free fractions. This assay principle has been applied to a number of analytes, including cortisol, gentamicin, insulin, phenytoin and thyroxine, and has been applied commercially (e.g. TDX kits by Abbott Laboratories). Although there are advantages of small sample volume (1–2 μl) and speed of assay, the major disadvantage of this technique is that it is restricted to molecules with a molecular weight of less than 20 000, as the assay depends on a significant increase in size when labelled antigen and antibody bind.

FLUORESCENCE QUENCHING AND ENHANCEMENT ASSAYS

Just as the rotational relaxation time of a fluorescent molecule may be altered by the alteration in environment consequent on antigen–antibody binding, so the amount of fluorescence (the quantum yield) may be altered. Probes which alter their quantum yield when the polarity of their environment changes are widely used in the study of membranes and of conformational changes in enzymes. In many cases, the quantum yield increases as the environment becomes less polar.

Fluorescent quenching and enhancement assays have been described, for example, for gentamicin and cortisol.

FLUORESCENCE ENERGY-TRANSFER IMMUNOASSAY

The formation of antigen–antibody complexes can be monitored if a pair of labels that interact in some measurable way are used. In fluorescence energy-transfer immunoassay, two different fluorescent dyes (a donor and an acceptor) are chosen such that the fluorescence spectrum of the donor overlaps the excitation spectrum of the acceptor (Ullman *et al.* 1976). Several fluorescence derivatives have been used as acceptors, and the phycobiliproteins have been used as both donors and acceptors. Assays using antigen labelled with donor (e.g. fluorescein) and antibody labelled with acceptor dye (e.g. tetramethylrhodamine) rely on the measurement of the fluorescence quenching on immune complex formation, as the fluorescence of the donor undergoes energy transfer with the nearby acceptor molecule on the antibody. Competition between sample antigens and antigen–donor conjugate for antibody–acceptor reduces the quenching. Fluorescence is therefore directly proportional to antigen concentration. This technique has also been adapted using fibre optics to develop an immunochemical sensor for phenytoin.

Enzyme labels

Enzymes have been widely used as detection systems for immunoassays. They may be used in both labelled antibody (immunometric) assays and competition assays and either directly as label or as reagents with the enzyme substrate, co-enzyme or inhibitor as label. Enzyme immunoassays may be either heterogeneous (requiring a separation step) or homogeneous (no separation stage necessary). When used in immunoassays, enzyme activity may be measured by spectrophotometry, fluorescence or luminescence. Commonly used enzymes are peroxidase (EC 1.11.1.7; indicator H_2O_2/chromagen or H_2O_2/luminol), alkaline phosphatase (EC 3.1.3.1; indicator 4-nitrophenol or 4-methylumbelliferone), and β-D-galactosidase (EC 3.2.1.23; indicator 2-nitrophenol or 4-methylumbelliferone) (Oellerich 1984; Kricka 1985). The preferred enzyme labels have a high turnover number and are easy to assay. Though expensive, enzyme conjugates are relatively stable, having a longer shelf-life than isotopic labels.

There have been two major areas of development in enzyme immunoassays: firstly enzyme amplification to improve assay sensitivity and secondly the use of hybrid antibodies in homogeneous assays. These will be discussed in subsequent sections.

A further interesting development is the amperometric determination of the activity of an enzyme label. This approach has been used in immunoassays with alkaline phosphatase as the label and phenyl phosphate or [*N*-ferrocenoyl]-4-aminophenyl phosphate as substrate. The phenol or ferrocene produced is then measured amperometrically (Wehmeyer *et al.* 1985; Doyle *et al.* 1986; McNeil *et al.* 1987–8).

A foretaste of the impact of genetic engineering on immunoassays is illustrated by a new homogeneous immunoassay, CEDIA. Using recombinant deoxyribonucleic acid (DNA) techniques, Henderson and co-workers (1986) constructed enzyme acceptors and enzyme donors of β-galactosidase (EC 3.2.1.23). The enzyme acceptors are large polypeptides with missing sequences in the encoded protein. In solution, these polypeptides are inactive monomer chains. The enzyme donors are small polypeptides containing some of the missing sequences in the enzyme acceptors and they are also enzymatically inactive. The enzyme acceptors and donors associate spontaneously to form enzymatically active tetramers. In the assay, antigen coupled to enzyme donor is prevented from combining with the enzyme acceptor by an antigen-specific antibody. Antigen in the serum sample competes with the antigen-enzyme donor for antibody, thus modulating the amount of β-galactosidase formed. The signal generated with enzyme substrate is directly proportional to analyte concentration (Fig. 44.5).

Enzyme amplification

The sensitivity of conventional enzyme immunoassays has been restricted by the detection of the limited number of coloured product molecules generated by the enzyme label. Sensitivity can be improved by 'amplification', where the primary enzyme label produces a second catalyst for a secondary enzyme–substrate system. The second catalyst may be another enzyme, a modulator of enzyme activity or a substance or co-factor taking part in a cyclic sequence of reactions (Johannsson and Bates 1988). There are a number of enzyme amplification systems that could be used, for example based on two zymogens from the blood coagulation cascade (factor X and prothrombin) and the fructose-6-phosphate/fructose-bis-phosphate substrate cycle. An amplification system that has been widely applied to assays of clinical importance is that based on the dephosphorylation of nicotinamide adenine dinucleotide phosphate (NADP) to NAD by alkaline phosphatase coupled to antibody, which then catalytically activates a specific redox cycle involving alcohol dehydrogenase and diaphorase. During each cycle one molecule of a tetrazolium salt is reduced to an intensely coloured formazan. To optimize the sensitivity and working range of the amplification

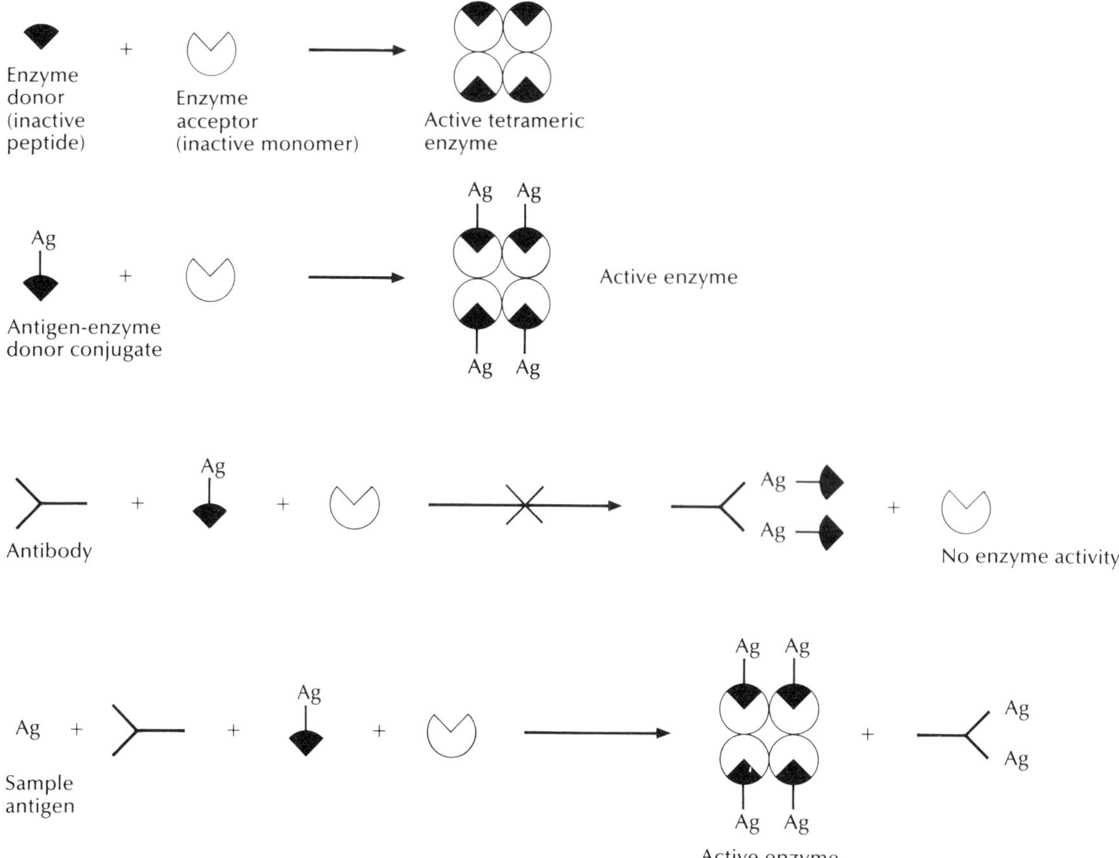

Fig. 44.5. CEDIA homogeneous immunoassay.

systems, the rate of colour formation is usually determined, i.e. kinetic rather than end-point determinations. This necessitates the use of microtitre plate readers capable of measuring the absorbance of solutions in 96 wells repeatedly within a matter of minutes. The use of fibre optics in plate readers and appropriate data handling facilitated this advance. Alternatively, the detection of cycling systems may be adapted to electrometric determinations.

Solid phases

Binding of antigen or antibody to a solid-phase reagent may be via a covalent bond or by adsorption. The requirements of a solid phase for use in immunoassay are that antigen or antibody should be bound stably to the solid phase, which should have a high capacity for binding, and immunological activity should be retained on binding with low non-specific binding (Kemeny and Challacombe 1988). Those solid phases of high capacity include agarose, Sephadex, cellulose and nitrocellulose and those of low capacity include polystyrene, polyvinyl chloride and nylon. The forms in which these are used as solid phases include tubes, microtitre plates, beads and pegs, and directly influence the type of automation, if any, that is used. The adsorption of antigen or antibody to solid phases is still poorly understood, although a number of modifications of the solid phase, such as treatment with glutaraldehyde or protein A, may improve reproducibility of binding. One of the major limitations of the surface solid phases (tubes, microtitre plates) as compared with mobile solid phases (cellulose particles) is the slower reaction kinetics of the antibody–antigen reaction, which will in part be determined by the rates of diffusion. Surfaces in contact with solution are thought to be surrounded by the 'Nernst layer', which restricts diffusion and mass transport across the liquid/solid interface. In addition, there may be a reduction in the apparent affinity constant of the antibody on binding to a solid phase and significant non-specific binding, both of which will reduce assay sensitivity (Jacobs 1981; Kemeny and Challacombe 1988).

There have been a number of approaches to overcome these problems. Firstly, exposure of sample and reagents to ultrasound for 5 minutes has been used as this has been found to accelerate interfacial mass transfer, probably by reducing the thickness of the unstirred layer (Chen *et al.* 1984). Secondly, immunometric assays have been developed where both labelled and 'capture' antibodies are in solution (Rattle *et al.* 1984). The 'capture' antibody is labelled with fluorescein isothiocyanate (FITC) and separation is achieved by incubation with anti-FITC antibodies coupled to magnetic particles. Using a magnet, the solid phase is then separated. Several different magnetic particle-based assays have now been described.

Another approach to improving the reaction kinetics of immunoassays is to generate the solid phase *in situ* after the specific antigen–antibody reaction has occurred. This can be achieved, for example, by using an antibody labelled with a polymerizable organic monomer. After the antigen–antibody reaction has taken place, polymerization of the monomer is initiated by a reaction generating free radicals or by a change in temperature. The resulting insoluble polymer particles and antigen–antibody complex can then be separated (Auditore–Hargreaves *et al.* 1987).

Dry-phase technology

Dry-phase chemistry systems, in which the assay reagents are incorporated into a dry matrix and are activated on addition of the sample, were developed in the 1970s, in the first instance for relatively simple analytes such as glucose. They have notable advantages in ease of use and access and stability of reagents. This type of technology has been applied to immunoassays in two ways. One approach has been to use homogeneous assay principles and to incorporate all the reagents into a single dry-phase matrix, using, for example, an enzyme substrate as label with fluorescence detection as the end-point. The second approach is to use the different assay components separated into different layers, so that the reactions occur in the correct sequence as fluid diffuses through the system (Morris *et al.* 1987). In practice most assays are based on liquid reagents and solid-phase detection systems, such as multilayer elements (Fig. 44.6) or enzyme immunochromatography (Zuk *et al.* 1985). In the latter case, capillary migration of analyte along a strip is combined with enzyme detection to produce a colour. The height of the developed colour is directly proportional to analyte concentration (Fig. 44.7). Lastly, in 'immunoconcentration' assays (Valkirs and Barton 1985) the immobilized antibody layer is positioned about an absorbent bed which acts as a reservoir for excess reagents and wash solution. Sample is added to the device and excess allowed to drain to the absorbent bed. Wash solution is added, followed by enzyme-labelled antibody, wash solution and then enzyme substrate. The colour generated is proportional to analyte concentration. The development and commercialization of such a variety of these 'single-unit' assay systems reflect the large potential market for extralaboratory testing. One must add a note of caution that the problems of

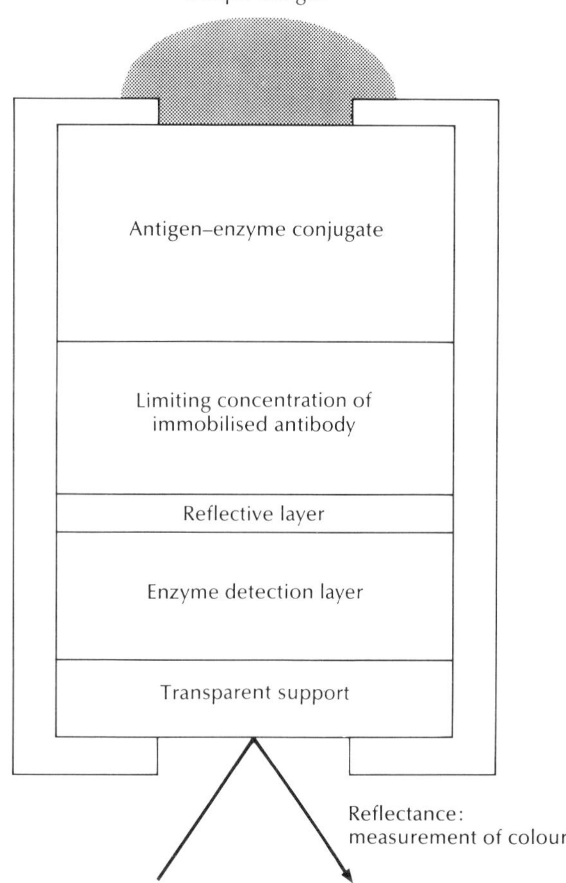

Fig. 44.6. Multilayer element for enzyme-labelled immunoassay.

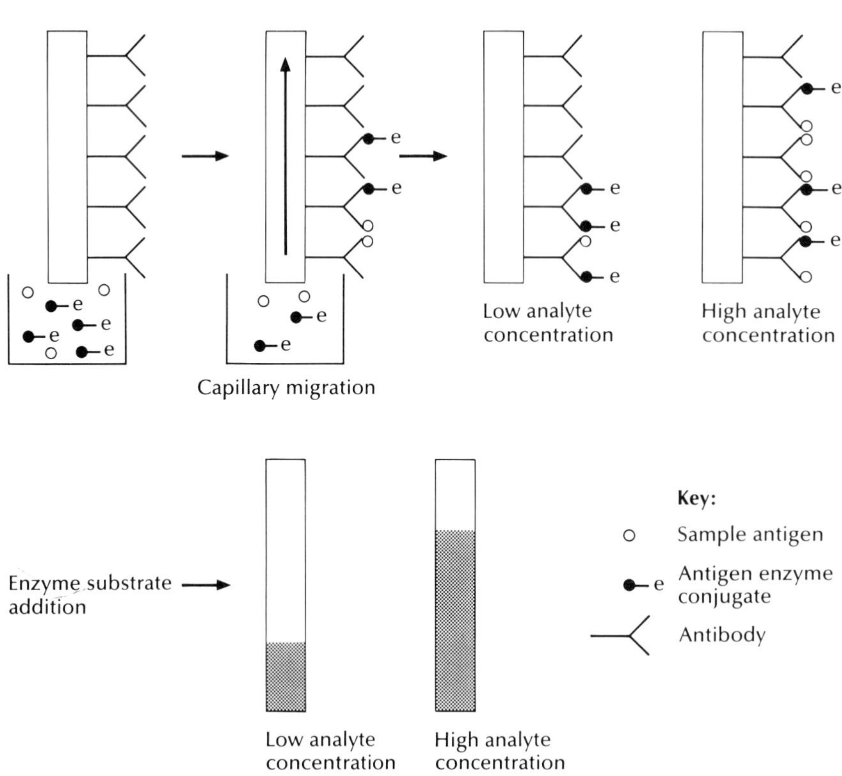

Fig. 44.7. Principles of immunochromatography.

assuring the quality of results and the high costs of the conventional chemistry dry-phase systems are also likely to be found with the dry-phase immunoassays.

Biosensors

A biosensor consists of a biological material that is responsive to the substance being sensed, in contact with a suitable transducing element that converts the signal sensed into a signal that can easily be processed. Thus immunosensors detect the immunological reaction between the antibody and the antigen via one of the immunological components attached to the transducer. A number of transducing mechanisms have been used, including metal or semiconductor electrodes, ion-selective electrodes, thermistors, piezo-electric crystals, field-effect transistors (FETs) and opto-electronic devices (Place *et al.* 1985; Badley *et al.* 1987; Ekins 1987).

The attraction of this type of immunoassay is the potential of small size, continuous measurement and simplicity of instrumentation, allowing non-laboratory use. Although this field of research has attracted much attention, a number of problems have to be addressed. For example, antigen–antibody complexes show relatively slow dissociation rates such that, unless this can be changed, the lag time between separate measurements is likely to be prohibitively long. Alternatively, the immunosensor would have to be cheap enough to be disposable after a single measurement.

Currently most transducers rely on a non-specific change in the electrical or optical properties of the surface, as in immunofield-effect transistors and potentiometric and optical systems. The potentiometric techniques for detecting antigen/antibody reaction on antibody-coated electrodes have been used to measure, for example, HCG in urine from pregnant women. The approach has also been applied to conventional enzyme immunoassays by detecting the products of the enzyme reaction with a conventional potentiometric electrode (Aizawa 1987; Green 1987). However, non-specific effects, due to, for example, buffer ions, have been found and this problem has also been found to bedevil the development of the immunofield-effect transistors.

Piezo-electric systems are based on the ability of certain crystals and plastics to respond to mechanical stress by the generation of electrical signals. The binding of antigen to bound antibody results in a change in mass which can be detected electronically. This can be done by measuring the changes in the propagation velocity of acoustic waves across the crystal surface or by measuring the change in the resonance frequency of the crystal in an appropriate oscillator circuit. Both approaches have been used, though sensitivity remains a problem.

There are only a limited number of optical techniques applicable to monitoring immunological reactions on the continuous surface of a sensor, partly due to the thinness of the immunological monolayer (20–40 nm) and due to the fact that the main changes on antigen–antibody binding affect size and refractive index. The main optical techniques used have been ellipsometry, internal reflection spectroscopy (IRS) methods, including 'evanescent wave' immunosensors, and surface plasmon resonance. Ellipsometry is a technique for the measurement of thickness and refractive indices of very thin films and is a polarimetric technique. A collimated, linearly polarized monochromatic light beam is reflected from the sample surface. After reflection the light beam is no longer linear but elliptically polarized; the ellipticity can be related to the change in film thickness. The technique has been used to study a range of analytes including albumin, fibrinogen, factor VIII, growth hormone and streptococcal proteins, but it is apparent that the specific and non-specific reactions are influenced by many factors, including the relative concentrations of the binding pair and other plasma proteins. Internal reflection spectroscopy involves a sample material being in contact with an optically denser but transparent medium. Light is introduced into the denser medium and the wavelength dependence (spectrum) of the reflectivity at the interface is measured. The IRS system can be designed to allow multiple internal reflections and thus multiple interactions of the light beam with the sample film, which should improve sensitivity. The 'evanescent wave' immunosensor falls into this category. Lastly, surface plasmon resonance has been used to detect immunological reactions on glass/metallic surfaces (Cullen *et al.* 1987–8). Light of a defined wavelength, incident angle and polarization is reflected at the interface. With a certain thickness of layer, electromagnetic coupling occurs in the metal layer and the light beam is attenuated at a specific angle. The major limitations of the immunosensors currently are the non-specific effects of the sample. Only when these problems are overcome can they become analytically useful tools for clinical investigation.

Conclusions

With the wider availability of monoclonal antibodies, the last few years have seen a rapid development of immunometric assays, in particular for the polypeptides of clinical interest. Monoclonal antibodies have also been used in reagent-limiting format for assay of low-molecular-weight analytes. There is now a wide variety of non-isotopic labels which are used in immunoassays, reflecting the ingenuity of the chemists and the large commercial market. As yet there appears to be no clear winner in terms of assay performance. There is a growing tendency for assay reagents to be tied commercially to 'black-box' instrumentation. This has the unfortunate effect of limiting the scope for method and equipment adaptation and development within research and hospital laboratories. Whilst there have been undoubted benefits to the immunoassayist in the development of non-isotopic, immunometric assays, the shadow of patent law and litigation is never far away (Ekins 1989).

References

Addison, G.M. and Hales, C.N. (1971). The immunoradiometric assay In *Radioimmunoassay Methods*, ed. K.E. Kirkham and W.M. Hunter, pp. 447–61, Churchill Livingstone, Edinburgh.

Aguila, H.L., Pollock, R.R., Spira, G. and Scharff, M.D. (1986). The production of more useful monoclonal antibodies. 1. The use of somatic-cell genetic and recombinant-DNA technology to tailor-make monoclonal antibodies. *Immunol. Today* **7**, 380–3.

Aizawa, M. (1987). Immunosensors. *Phil. Trans. Roy. Soc. (London)* **B316**, 121–34.

Ashihara, Y., Nishizono, I., Suzuki, H. and Kasahara, Y. (1987). Homogeneous enzyme immunoassay for macromolecular antigens using hybrid antibody. *J. Clin. Lab. Anal.* **1**, 77–9.

Auditore-Hargreaves, K., Houghton, R.L., Monji, N. *et al.* (1987). Phase-separation immunoassays. *Clin. Chem.* **33**, 1509–16.

Badley, R.A., Drake, R.A.L., Shanks, I.A., Smith, A.M. and Stephenson, P.R. (1987). Optical biosensors for immunoassays: the fluorescence capillary-fill device. *Phil. Trans. Roy. Soc. (London)* **B316**, 143–60.

Biggart, E.M., Paterson, N., Gillespie, S. *et al.* (1985). Potency differences in immunometric assays for serum TSH. *J. Endocrinol.* **104** (suppl.), 125 (abstract).

Bullock, D.G. and Wheeler, M.J. (1989). Presentation of performance characteristics of immunological assay systems. *ACB News Sheet* **319**, 9–12.

Chen, R., Weng, L., Sizto, N.C. *et al.* (1984). Ultrasound-accelerated immunoassay, as exemplified by enzyme immunoassay of chorio-gonadotropin, *Clin. Chem.* **30**, 1446–51.

Cullen, D.C., Brown, R.G.W. and Lowe, C.R. (1987–8). Detection of immuno-complex formation via surface plasmon resonance on gold-coated diffraction gratings. *Biosensors* **3**, 211–25.

Doyle, M.J., Halsall, H.B. and Heineman, W.R. (1986). Enzyme-linked immunosorbent assay with electrochemical detection for α_1-acid glycoprotein. *Analyt. Chem.* **56**, 2355–60.

Ekins, R.P. (1987). An overview of present and future ultrasensitive non-isotopic immunoassay development. *Clin. Biochem. Rev.* **8**, 12–23.

Ekins, R.P. (1989). A shadow over immunoassay. *Nature (London)* **340**, 256–8.

French, D., Fischberg, E., Buhl, S. and Scherff, M.D. (1986). The production of more useful monoclonal antibodies. *Immunol. Today* **7**, 344–6.

Geiger, R. and Miska, W. (1987). Bioluminescence enhanced enzyme immunoassay. *J. Clin. Chem. Clin. Biochem.* **25**, 31–8.

Green, M.J. (1987). Electrochemical immunoassays. *Phil. Trans. Roy. Soc. (London)* **B316**, 135–42.

Hart, R.C. and Taaffe, L.R. (1987). The use of acridinium ester-labelled streptavidin in immunoassays. *J. Immunol. Method.* **101**, 91–6.

Hemmilä, I. (1985). Fluoroimmunoassay and immunofluorometric assays. *Clin. Chem.* **31**, 359–70.

Hemmilä, I. (1988). Lanthanides as probes for time-resolved fluorometric immunoassays. *Scand. J. Clin. Lab. Invest.* **48**, 389–400.

Henderson, D.R., Friedman, S.B., Harris, J.D., Manning, W.B. and Zoccoli, M.A. (1986). CEDIA^{TM}, a new homogeneous immunoassay system. *Clin. Chem.* **32**, 1637–41.

Howanitz, J.H. (1988). Immunoassay innovations in label technology. *Arch. Pathol. Lab. Med.* **112**, 775–9.

Hurn, B.A.L. and Landon, J. (1971). Antisera for radioimmunoassay. In *Radioimmunoassay Methods*, ed. K.E. Kirkham and W.M. Hunter, pp. 121–42, Churchill Livingstone, Edinburgh.

Jackson, T.M. and Ekins, R.P. (1986). Theoretical limitations on immunoassay sensitivity: current practice and potential advantages of fluorescent Eu^{3+} chelates as non-radioisotopic tracers. *J. Immunol. Methods* **87**, 13–20.

Jacobs, P.M. (1981). Separation methods in immunoassay. *Ligand Quart.* **4**, 23–33.

Johannsson, A. and Bates, D.L. (1988). Amplification by second enzymes. In *ELISA and Other Solid Phase Immunoassays*, ed. D.M. Kemeny and S.J. Challacombe, pp. 85–106, John Wiley & Sons, Chichester.

Kemeny, D.M. and Challacombe, S.J. (1988). Microtitre plates and other solid phase supports. *In Elisa and Other Solid Phase Immunoassays*, ed. D.M. Kemeny and S.J. Challacombe, pp. 31–55, John Wiley & Sons, Chichester.

Kohler, G. and Milstein, C. (1975). Continuous cultures of fused cells secreting antibody of predefined specificity. *Nature (London)* **256**, 495–7.

Kricka, L.J. (1985). *Ligand–Binder Assays: Labels and Analytical Strategies*. Marcel Dekker, New York.

Kricka, L.J. and Carter, T.J.N. (1982). Luminescent immunoassays. In *Clinical and Biochemical Luminescence*, ed. L.J. Kricka and T.J.N. Carter, pp. 153–78, Marcel Dekker, New York.

Kronick, M.N. (1986). The use of phycobiliproteins as fluorescent labels in immunoassay. *J. Immunol.* **92**, 1–13.

Linthicum, D.S., Bolger, M.B., Kussie, P.H. *et al.* (1988a). Analysis of idiotypic and anti-idiotypic antibodies as models of receptor and ligand. *Clin. Chem.* **34**, 1676–80.

Linthicum, D.S., Kussie, P.H., Combs, S. and Yatko, D. (1988b). Idiotypes and anti-idiotypes: significance in immunoassays. *J. Clin. Immunoassay* **11**, 31–6.

McNeil, C.J., Higgin, I.J. and Bannister, J.V. (1987–8). Amperometric determination of alkaline phosphatase activity: application to enzyme immunoassay. *Biosensors* **3**, 199–209.

Miles, L.E.M. and Hales, C.N. (1968). Labelled antibodies and immunological assay systems. *Nature (London)* **219**, 186–9.

Milstein, C. and Cuello, A.C. (1983). Hybrid hybridomas and their use in immunohistochemistry. *Nature (London)* **305**, 537–40.

Miska, W. and Geiger, R. (1987). Synthesis and characterization of luciferin derivatives for use in bioluminescence enhanced enzyme immunoassays. *J. Clin. Chem. Clin. Biochem.* **25**, 23–30.

Moore, G.P. (1989). Genetically engineered antibodies. *Clin. Chem.* **35**, 1849–53.

Morris, D.L., Ledden, D.J. and Bogusiaski, R.C. (1987). Dry-phase technology for immunoassay. *J. Clin. Lab. Anal.* **1**, 243–9.

Morrison, S.L., Canfield, S., Porter, S., Tan, L.K., Tao, M. and Wims, L.A. (1988). Production and characterization of genetically engineered antibody molecules. *Clin. Chem.* **34**, 1668–75.

Moyle, W.R., Anderson, D.M. and Ehrlich, P.H. (1983). A circular antibody–antigen complex is responsible for increased affinity shown by mixtures of monoclonal antibodies to human chorionic gonadotropin. *J. Immunol.* **131**, 1900–5.

Oellerich, M. (1984). Enzyme-immunoassay: a review. *J. Clin. Chem. Clin. Biochem.* **22**, 895–904.

Oi, V.T., Morrison, S.L., Herzenberg, L.A. and Berg, P. (1983). Immunoglobulin gene expression in transformed lymphoid cells. *Proc. Nat. Acad. Sci. (USA)* **80**, 825–9.

Place, J.F., Sutherland, R.M. and Dähne, C. (1985). Opto-electronic immunosensors: a review of optical immunosensors at continuous surfaces. *Biosensors* **1**, 321–53.

Porstmann, B., Avrameas, S., Ternynck, T., Portsmann, T., Micheel, B. and Guesdon, J.L. (1984). An antibody chimera technique applied to enzyme immunoassay for human alpha-1-fetoprotein with monoclonal and polyclonal antibodies. *J. Immunol. Methods* **66**, 179–85.

Rattle, S.J., Purnell, D.R., Willams, P.I.M., Siddle, K. and Forrest, G.C. (1984). New separation method for monoclonal immunoradiometric assays and its application to assays for thyrotropin and human chorionic gonadotropin. *Clin. Chem.* **30**, 1457–61.

Rodwell, J.D., Alvarez, V.L., Lee, C. *et al.* (1986). Site-specific covalent modification of monoclonal antibodies — *in vitro* and *in vivo* evaluations. *Proc. Nat. Acad. Sci. (USA)* **83**, 2632–6.

Samoilovich, S.R., Dugan, C.B. and Macario, A.J.L. (1987). Hybridoma technology: new developments of practical interest. *J. Immunol. Methods* **101**, 153–70.

Schall, R.F. and Tenoso, H.J. (1981). Alternatives to radioimmunoassays: labels and methods. *Clin. Chem.* **27**, 1157–64.

Siddle, K. (1985). Monoclonal antibodies in clinical biochemistry. *Recent Adv. Clin. Biochem.* **3**, 63–102.

Simonson, R.B., Ultea, M.E., Long, C.G., Gillette, R.W., McKearn, T.J. and Rodwell, J.D. (1988). Inhibition of mannosidase in hybridomas yields monoclonal antibodies with greater capacity for carbohydrate labelling. *Clin. Chem.* **34**, 1713–16.

Suresh, M.R., Cuello, A.C. and Milstein, C. (1986). Advantages of bispecific hybridomas in one-step immunocytochemistry and immunoassays. *Proc. Nat. Acad. Sci. (USA)* **83**, 7989–93.

Thompson, S.G. (1984). Competitive-binding assays. In *Clinical Chemistry: Theory, Analysis and Correlation*, ed. L.A. Kaplan and A.J. Pesce, pp. 211–31, CV Mosby, St Louis.

Thorpe, G.H.G., Kricka, L.J., Moseley, S.B. and Whitehead, T.P. (1985). Phenols as enhancers of the chemiluminescent horseradish peroxidase–luminol–hydrogen peroxide reaction: application in luminescence monitored enzyme immunoassays. *Clin. Chem.* **31**, 1335–41.

Ullman, E.F., Schwarzber, M. and Rubenstein, K.E. (1976). Fluorescent excitation energy transfer immunoassay. *J. Biol. Chem.* **251**, 4172–8.

Valkirs, G.E. and Barton, R. (1985). Immuno Concentration™ — a new format for solid-phase immunoassays. *Clin. Chem.* **31**, 1427–31.

Vilja, P., Wichmann, L., Isola, J. and Tuohimaa, P. (1988). Monoclonal antibody-based noncompetitive avidin–biotin assay for lutropin in urine. *Clin. Chem.* **34**, 1585–90.

Ward, E.S., Güssow, D., Griffiths, A.D., Jone, P.T. and Winter, G. (1989). Binding activities of a repertoire of single immunoglobulin variable domains secreted from *Escherichia coli*. *Nature (London)* **341**, 544–6.

Weeks, I., Sturgess, M.L. and Woodhead, J.S. (1986). Chemiluminescence immunoassay: an overview. *Clin. Sci.* **70**, 403–8.

Wehmeyer, H.R., Halsall, H.B. and Heineman, W.B. (1985). Heterogenous enzyme immunoassay with electrochemical detection: competitive and 'sandwich'-type immunoassays. *Clin. Chem.* **31**, 1546–9.

Wilchek, M. and Bayer, E.A. (1984). The avidin–biotin complex in immunology. *Immunol. Today* **5**, 39–43.

Yalow, R.S. and Berson, S.A. (1971). Introduction and general considerations In *Principles of Competitive Protein Binding Assays*, ed. W.D. O'Dell and W.H. Doughaday, pp. 1–21, Lippincott, Philadelphia.

Zuk, R.F., Ginsberg, V.K., Houts, T. *et al.* (1985). Enzyme immunochromotography — a quantitative immunoassay requiring no instrumentation. *Clin. Chem.* **31**, 1144–50.

45: The Interpretation of Tests of T Cell and Natural Killer Cell Function in Man

D.L. Brown

Introduction

In this chapter are reviewed the many tests of lymphocyte and natural killer (NK) function which may be used to dissect the basis of abnormalities of function of these cells in patients with disturbances of immune function. Several developments in recent years have allowed the design of increasingly specific tests of lymphocyte function, notably: (i) an increasingly detailed understanding of the cell surface molecular architecture; (ii) identification of cytokines and their receptors; and (iii) knowledge of intracellular signalling pathways. The application of this knowledge to tests of cell function will be reviewed. In the future many of the assays described in this chapter may be replaced by tests of the activity of populations of lymphocytes bearing defined antigen-specific receptors, now that it is possible to analyse the T cell receptor repertoire in health and disease.

T lymphocytes

Activation of T lymphocytes by lectins

Plant lectins, notably phytohaemagglutinin (PHA), concanavalin A (Con A) and pokeweed mitogen (PWM), have been used to study lymphocyte function *in vitro* for many years. They are still the most widely used and most accessible reagents for activating patients' lymphocytes in routine diagnostic work. Despite wide usage, their mode of action at a molecular level is not fully understood and to some extent they have been replaced as T cell activators in research by more precise reagents, particularly by monoclonal antibodies directed at the CD3 (T3)/Ti receptor and the CD2 (T11, sheep red blood cell (SRBC)) receptor. Nevertheless, the available evidence suggests that, provided the stimulus is of sufficient magnitude, it does not matter whether the initial stimulus is via ill-defined lectin receptors or via defined functional lymphocyte receptors. Both can trigger T cells into similar pathways of activation, which eventually lead to proliferation and differentiation. Recent evidence suggests that at least one binding site, that for PHA-P, is on or very close to the CD2 molecule, since CD2 −ve T cells do not respond to PHA-P and normal T cells can be blocked in their responsiveness to PHA-P by anti-CD2 (O'Flynn *et al.* 1986). However, this is not the only binding site for PHA on T lymphocytes and several membrane glycoproteins may fulfil this role. Plant lectins are powerful agglutinators of cells and bind to cell membrane glycopeptides by multiple binding sites. The interaction between the lectin and the glycopeptide is inhibitable by oligosaccharides, which are characteristic for each lectin. For example, oligosaccharides containing *N*-acetyl-D-galactosamine inhibit the binding of PHA, while those containing α-methyl mannoside and other α-D-gluco- and mannopyranosides inhibit the binding of Con A. It is likely that several different membrane glycopeptides can express similar terminal oligosaccharide groups and so bind and cross-link lectins. Phytohaemagglutinin immobilized on Sepharose can induce the blast transformation of lymphocytes, suggesting that the internalization of lectins is not necessary for the trigger mechanism.

Highly purified T cells require factors additional to receptor binding in order to trigger optimal activation. The response to PHA is no exception. Thus pure T cell preparations are poorly responsive to PHA. If exogenous recombinant interleukin 2 (IL-2) is added to cultures, the T cells will proliferate and express Ia and IL-2 receptors (IL-2R); however, no endogenous IL-2 secretion occurs unless adherent cells are present in the initial cultures (Katzen *et al.* 1985; Vine *et al.* 1988). Two important cytokines derived from macrophages, IL-1β and tumour necrosis factor (TNF)-α, will enhance the responsiveness of purified T cells to PHA, although IL-1β is the more powerful and specific of the two and, in addition to augmenting proliferation, will also increase the expression of IL-2 messenger ribonucleic acid (mRNA) and IL-2 secretion (Hackett *et al.* 1988).

Activation of T lymphocytes via the CD3 (T3) complex

Normal peripheral blood T cells and T cell clones which express the CD3 complex can be activated by anti-CD3 monoclonal antibodies. The technique has been successfully used in attempts to explore the trigger mechanism for the CD3-Ti receptor complex, but at present is not widely used for routine diagnostic studies. The activation of T cell clones via the Ti clonotypic receptor (the T cell antigen receptor) is largely a research procedure (Acuto and Reinherz 1985).

Different anti-CD3 monoclonals vary greatly in their ability to activate T cells and in a soluble form will only activate purified T cells if accessory cells are included in the cultures. The precise role of accessory cells is still obscure and likely to be multifactorial. They probably provide a cytophilic cell membrane for presenting an array of CD3 molecules, but also provide Fc/Fc receptor interactions (Ceuppens *et al.* 1985; Clement *et al.* 1985; Geppert and Lipsky 1986) and secrete macrophage/monocyte-dependent cytokines, such as IL-1 and TNF, both of which enhance mitogen-induced lymphocyte proliferation (Scheurich *et al.* 1987; Hackett *et al.* 1988). Because of the uncertainties concerning the mechanism by which adherent cells contribute to the activation step, attempts have been made to bypass it. This has been achieved by immobilizing anti-CD3 monoclonals on solid support media. Anti-CD3 linked to Sepharose beads partly fulfils this requirement, although individual monoclonal anti-CD3 antibodies vary greatly in their ability to activate T cells, presumably because of variables such as specificity, affinity and stability of cross-linking. Additional activating agents, such as phorbolesters, are often added to optimize the stimulus (Davis and Lipsky 1986). Immobilization of anti-CD3 in plastic microtitre wells seems to be particularly effective and virtually, if not actually, accessory cell-independent. Geppert and Lipsky (1986) induced the proliferation of purified CD4 lymphocytes and endogenous IL-2 release by this technique, although the anti-CD3 used (64.1) seems to be an unusually powerful mitogen.

Activation of T lymphocytes via the CD2 (T11, sheep red blood cell) molecule

The CD2 molecule is a 55 kD glycoprotein which appears on thymocytes as one of the earliest markers of intrathymic maturation and remains throughout the ontogeny of the T lymphocyte. Its inclusion as an activation molecule of potential importance in the study of T lymphocyte function is justified by the observation that two selected non-cross-reacting anti-CD2 monoclonal antibodies will bind to the CD2 molecule in strict sequence and trigger an 'alternative pathway' of T cell activation. Anti-T11$_2$ binds to CD2 and apparently alters the conformation of a critical activation epitope. This altered epitope then binds anti-T11$_3$ and triggers T cell activation. The combination of anti-T11$_2$ and anti-T11$_3$ is powerfully mitogenic and induces T cell proliferation (Meuer *et al*. 1984). The significance of this CD2 activation pathway, especially in relation to T cell responses *in vivo*, is still unknown, but some clues may be contained in the observations that the natural ligands for the CD2 molecule include the lymphocyte function-associated antigen (LFA)-3, SRBC and possibly PHA-P (see above). At present, one attractive view is that the CD2 molecule somehow contributes a 'second-site' signal required for an optimal response following binding of antigen to the CD3—Ti complex. In support of this view is the growing evidence that the CD2 and CD3—Ti sites are functionally linked. Thus, stimulating T cells with mitogenic concentrations of anti-T11$_2$ and anti-T11$_3$ causes phosphorylation of the γ-peptide of the three-peptide complex of CD3. The same γ-chain is also phosphorylated following activation via the CD3—Ti complex. If CD3 is modulated or capped off by a non-mitogenic anti-CD3, then anti-T11$_2$ plus anti-T11$_3$ are unable to induce calcium mobilization and mitogenesis (Breitmeyer *et al*. 1987). At present there seems to be no clinical relevance in testing the integrity of the CD2-triggered pathway or any reason for using anti-T11$_2$ plus anti-T11$_3$ as a T cell mitogen in preference to the more readily available plant lectins or anti-CD3. Nevertheless, available evidence suggests that CD2-triggered mitogenesis is analogous to the better-known forms and it sets in motion the same autocrine cycle of increased IL-2R expression, endogenous IL-2 release and T cell proliferation (Meuer *et al*. 1984).

Intracellular events and protein kinase C activation by phorbol myristate acetate

Following the mitogen-induced trigger events at the T lymphocyte surface, a complex train of intracellular metabolic events is set in motion which eventually lead to IL-2 secretion and IL-2R expression. The key events are a steep rise in intracellular ionic calcium, probably derived from intracellular stores and by influx from the surrounding medium via postulated calcium ion channels, the activation of the phosphatidyl inositol cycle, translocation of protein kinase C from the cytosol to the cell membrane and phosphorylation of cell membrane receptor peptides. The precise interactions between the various components of the systems have still to be unravelled (Nel *et al*. 1987), and it is far from clear which, if any, of these measures of intracellular activation will turn out to have a practical clinical application. Changes in calcium flux show some promise. For example, it is possible to continuously monitor intracellular free calcium in T cells during activation by anti-CD3, anti-CD2 or ionomycin by flow cytometry, utilizing changes in the calcium-sensitive fluorescence emission spectrum of the dye indo-1-acetoxymethyl ester (Breitmeyer *et al*. 1987; Ledbetter *et al*. 1987; Hayward *et al*. 1988).

Protein kinase C activation is a key early event in T cell triggering and one which must be sustained if the T cells are going to express the high-affinity IL-2R and secrete endogenous IL-2. Protein kinase C is probably a direct ligand for phorbol myristate acetate (PMA) and combined treatment with PMA and ionomycin to raise intracellular calcium will cause sustained protein kinase C activation and redistribution. This in turn leads to phosphorylation and down-regulation of the T3/Ti receptors (Cantrell *et al*. 1985). In effect PMA and ionomycin can bypass all the steps required to activate T cells via the CD3 and CD2 receptor system (Truneh *et al*. 1985). This is in contrast to simulation of T cells with immobilized anti-CD3, which will only induce temporary protein kinase C activation and down-regulation of the T3/Ti complex, unless accessory cells and early lymphokines are present. If PMA is used to trigger T cells in functional assays, then its potency as a direct activator and its limitations as a true representation of physiological events need to be borne in mind.

Assays of lymphocyte activation based on deoxyribonucleic acid synthesis and cell cycle analysis

The earliest assays were based on the morphological appearance of blast transformation, which takes place when lymphocytes are cultured with plant mitogens. Differences from resting lymphocytes are seen as early as 12—24 hours, when a proportion of cells enlarge through increases in volume of both cytoplasm and nucleus. One or more nucleoli appear. The nuclear staining becomes lighter with a more open reticulate pattern due to the fragmentation of euchromatin, and the cytoplasm becomes more basophilic due to an increase in polyribosomes and endoplasmic reticulum. A prominent Golgi apparatus can sometimes be seen adjacent to the nucleus. This phase, which corresponds approximately to G_1 of the cell cycle, merges imperceptibly into the S phase as the nucleus increases still further in size and the deoxyribonucleic acid (DNA) content doubles. Up to 50% of the cells in a lymphocyte culture stimulated by PHA will show these changes on thin films or cytocentrifuge preparations stained with May Grunwald/Giemsa or Wright's stain. Although the changes are striking, they are difficult to quantitate and it is impossible to tell which cells are in the G_1 or S phase because of many intermediate forms. A further difficulty in using blast transformation as a possible end-point is that some lymphocyte activators fail to trigger the release of endogenous IL-2 or other autocrine growth factors, so that the cells never progress beyond the G_1 phase of the cell cycle.

More objective methods for detecting events in the cell cycle and linking these to the role of activators are required. The first of these assays to be introduced, the uptake of tritiated thymidine, has remained the mainstay of activation and proliferation studies up to the present time, but it too has potentially serious limitations as a quantitative measure of lymphocyte proliferation. These have been reviewed in detail by Ashman (1984). Thymidine will freely enter lymphocytes under normal conditions of culture, although some drugs can interfere with cell uptake. Within the cell, thymidine is phosphorylated stepwise to the triphosphate before incorporation into DNA. If phosphorylation is inhibited because of some metabolic block, e.g. adenosine deaminase deficiency, or via the action of analogue drugs, or if thymidine triphosphate is diverted to DNA repair, apparently substantial uptake values by the cells may not reflect S phase DNA synthesis. Incorporation into nucleotides can be distinguished from simple uptake of thymidine into cells by demonstrating the acid insolubility of the complexed forms of the molecule.

Correlations between DNA synthesis, as measured by cell cycle analysis in flow cytometers, and the uptake of tritiated thymidine are less than perfect. At least one confounding process is the ability of intranuclear tritium to produce detectable delays in entry into the G_2 and M phase of the cell cycle, probably because β particles emitted by the tritium cause strand breaks in the DNA (Pollack *et al.* 1979). Here again, the simple uptake of tritiated thymidine may seriously overestimate apparent DNA synthesis.

Flow cytometry

Flow cytometry is the best available method at present for relating cell cycle progression, an objective indicator of cell activation, to the temporal appearance of activation markers on or in lymphocytes during blast transformation (Cotner *et al.* 1983). The flow cytometer must be capable of measuring the DNA content of cells simultaneously with the activation marker of choice. All modern single-argon laser-powered instruments are capable of this type of dual-parameter analysis and use appropriate colour filters and dichroic mirrors to separate the distinctive colour emissions from fluorescein isothiocyanate (FITC)-labelling the marker monoclonal and propidium iodide-labelling the DNA. The principle of the technique for preparing lymphocytes for flow cytometry involves a preliminary lymphocyte or whole-blood fixation step, usually with methanol or paraformaldehyde/methanol, depending on whether cell surface or intracellular markers are under investigation (Levitt and King 1987; Kurki *et al.* 1988), and then staining for the activation marker with the appropriate FITC-labelled monoclonal antibody, followed by staining of the DNA with a stoichiometrically intercalating dye, such as propidium iodide or Hoechst 33342 (Cotner *et al.* 1983). The flow cytometer is set to discriminate lymphocytes from other nucleated blood cells by their light scatter characteristics. The FITC light emission from the activation marker and the propidium iodide light emission from the DNA are then collected from 5000–20 000 lymphocytes and correlated with each other in a two-dimensional plot.

The basic technique of dual-parameter flow cytometry has many further applications which are independent of direct cell cycle analysis. It can also be used to compare the rate of appearance of a combination of activation markers on both T and B lymphocytes in culture. Here, two monoclonal antibodies are required, one labelled with FITC, the other labelled with phycoerythrin (PE) (Kikutani *et al.* 1986; Creemers 1987). More prosaically, dual-parameter studies of surface markers are widely used to study extended series of double-staining combinations in the subtype or 'phenotype' analysis of T cells (Morimoto *et al.* 1980; Blue *et al.* 1985; Stites *et al.* 1986; Creemers 1987; De Paoli *et al.* 1988). In a strict sense, simple delineation of lymphocyte subtypes, even when expressed in absolute values, does not constitute a functional assay, although in clinical practice this distinction is sometimes blurred or overlooked when changes in subtype numbers, particularly in the direction of deficiency, are known to correlate well with alterations of function.

Assays with potential as measures of lymphocyte activation are those detecting cell cycle nuclear activation antigens by monoclonal antibodies. One of these, Ki-67 (Gerdes *et al.* 1984), has been adapted for flow cytometry, but only at the slight inconvenience of using isolated nuclear suspensions. A second monoclonal antibody, anti-PCNA/cyclin (Ogata *et al.* 1987), may be more suited for clinical work since it can be used to directly label whole lymphoblasts after paraformaldehyde/methanol fixation. The antigen PCNA is a 36 kD polypeptide thought to be functionally associated with DNA polymerase delta. Flow cytometry of lymphoblasts which have been dual-labelled for PCNA and DNA has successfully recorded a PCNA signal which rises in G_1, peaks in the S phase and declines in the G_2 and M phase of the proliferation cell cycle (Kurki *et al.* 1988). Lymphoblasts containing PCNA can also be identified as single cells by indirect fluorescence microscopy. Monitoring PCNA concentrations may possibly prove to be a more precise indicator of T cell activation than blast transformation.

Yet another technique, the incorporation of the nucleoside bromodeoxyuridine, has similarities to both uptake of thymidine and detection of activation markers such as PCNA. The discovery of monoclonal antibodies to bromodeoxyuridine made it possible to detect the uptake of this nucleoside into S phase cells by flow cytometry (Dolbeare *et al.* 1983). Thus, the first step of the assay resembles thymidine uptake, but without the risk of a radioactive isotope, and the second phase is the detection of the bromodeoxyuridine incorporated into DNA, as though it were an intranuclear activation marker (Vanderlaan and Thomas 1985).

Final mention should be made in this section of a rapid assay of cell growth as a measure of T cell activation, especially where cell proliferation is the dominant event of interest, for example by the action of lymphokines such as IL-2. The MTT assay was first described by Mosmann in 1983 and has been subsequently modified and improved (Mosmann and Fong 1989). It is based on the principle that mitochondrial succinic dehydrogenase in viable cells will metabolize the tetrazolium salt, 3-(4,5-dimethylthiazol-2-yl)-2-5-diphenyltetrazolium bromide (MTT) to a coloured formazan product. In effect it is measuring energy metabolism rather than DNA synthesis and therefore must be a quantitative index of viable cell mass. Nevertheless, it is claimed that there are no major differences between the results obtained from this assay and those based on DNA synthesis. It is relatively cheap, rapid and suitable for handling large numbers of samples and has been adapted to an automated microculture technique using the related salt XTT (R.H. Shoemaker quoted in Mosmann and Fong 1989).

Assays for interleukin 2 and related lymphokines

It is over a decade since Gillis and Smith (1977) demonstrated that long-term cultures of murine cytolytic T cell lines (CTCL) could readily be established in 'conditioned' medium derived from the supernatants of PHA-stimulated T cells. A bioassay for the 'conditioning' factor which sustained growth soon followed (Gillis *et al.* 1978) and the factor is now recognized as IL-2.

It was not recognized at the time that several lymphokines are present in conditioned medium, including IL-1α, IL-1β, IL-2, IL-4, IL-6 and interferon-γ, nor was it recognized that most lymphokines act on more than one type of cell and that each cell type responds to a range of lymphokines in a characteristic manner. It is therefore perhaps fortunate that the CTCL cells and other long-term murine T cell lines are very sensitive to the growth-promoting activity of human IL-2 but insensitive to human IL-4. Their value as a substrate for measuring functional IL-2 activity remains undisputed provided some safeguards are incorporated. Mosmann and Fong (1989) have discussed at some length the controls required to establish that cytokine bioassays are monospecific. The most valuable agents for controlling monospecificity are monoclonal antibodies which block cytokine activity. They can be used to test for and to block the effects of unwanted lymphokines or to block the specific activity under investigation. Pure recombinant lymphokines can be added to see whether they enhance the specific activity under investigation. Further controls are provided by the comparative performance of internationally accepted standard preparations in different laboratories. An international standard for IL-2 has been evaluated and selected in a multicentre collaborative study (Gearing and Thorpe 1988). This is freeze-dried material derived from Jurkat cell cultures (86/504) with a nominal potency of 100 u. A second recombinant IL-2 standard (86/564) is also available as a National Institute for Biological Standards and Controls (UK) reference reagent with a value of 202 u/ampoule. The CTCL assay remains the gold standard for measuring IL-2 functional activity, although several other murine cell lines and mitogen-activated preparations are satisfactory. For clinical work the need to maintain murine cell lines is a significant drawback, and attempts have been made to use human peripheral blood T cells as the cellular substrate for functional IL-2 assays. A technique of potential clinical application is one whereby human T cells are isolated from blood by magnetic beads coated with anti-CD3 and exposed to IL-2 in a single-step procedure (Leivestad *et al.* 1988). The authors claim a level of sensitivity and specificity for the assay comparable to the CTCL assay. All functional IL-2 assays rely on ^{3}H-thymidine incorporation to measure T cell proliferation.

Several enzyme-linked immunosorbent assays (ELISA) and radio-immunoassays have been developed to measure immunochemical IL-2. These are highly specific but rather less sensitive than functional assays and cannot distinguish between free IL-2 and IL-2 functionally inactivated by binding to soluble IL-2R. Most are double-antibody sandwich assays, usually employing monoclonals, where one antibody in the solid phase captures IL-2 via one epitope while the second antibody binds to a different epitope on IL-2. A labelled antiglobulin then completes the reaction (Gehman and Robb 1984; Cardenas *et al.* 1986). A potentially interesting variant of this procedure is to use IL-2R derived from activated blast cells as the 'capture antibody' in the first stage of an ELISA assay (Igietseme and Herscowitz 1988).

Evaluation of lymphocyte activation by the intracellular induction of lymphokine messenger ribonucleic acid

During the complex process of lymphocyte activation a necessary preliminary to the exogenous secretion of lymphokines is the expression of the appropriate genes and the induction of the corresponding mRNA. This induction can be monitored within a population of cells or at the single-cell level by the application of radiolabelled sense and antisense complementary DNA (cDNA), RNA or other oligonucleotide probes. Messenger RNA from a large number of cells (>5000) can be detected by Northern blotting or dot blotting. *In situ* hybridization can be used for single cells. In principle, there is no limit to the number and type of activated gene products which can be detected by these techniques, provided the probes are available and are well characterized. In addition to the lymphokines IL-2, interferon-γ and granulocyte–macrophage colony-stimulating factor (GM-CSF), success has been achieved with the oncogenes c-fos, c-myc and c-myb (Granelli-Piperno *et al.* 1986; Shaw *et al.* 1987; Shipp and Reinherz 1987). The assays are highly specific and in the simplified dot-blot procedure, can provide detailed semi-quantitative data about the temporal appearance of lymphokine mRNA during cell cycle activation.

A more elaborate extension of this technique is the demonstration of mRNA in single dispersed cells by *in situ* hybridization. This allows the monitoring of the appearance of mRNA cell by cell in a semi-quantitative manner, based on grain counts in the coating emulsion (Granelli-Piperno 1988). The study of IL-2 mRNA has been particularly rewarding, firstly in demonstrating the ability of cyclosporin A to inhibit the induction of IL-2 mRNA (and interferon-γ and GM-CSF mRNA) while not affecting the induction of mRNA for the α chain (p55) of the IL-2R (Granelli-Piperno *et al.* 1986) and secondly in demonstrating the transient nature of the expression of IL-2 mRNA during the T cell activation cycle (Shaw *et al.* 1988). The Northern blotting and dot blotting procedures are still too exacting and time-consuming to have wide clinical application but they are likely to be invaluable in elucidating the actions of new immunosuppressive drugs, particularly analogues of cyclosporin or unrelated drugs which inhibit lymphokine generation at the level of mRNA transcription.

The interleukin 2 receptor as a measure of T cell activation

Information about the T cell receptor for IL-2 has accumulated steadily since 1981, when Uchiyama *et al.* demonstrated that a monoclonal antibody, anti-Tac, reacted with an antigen induced on the surface of T cells activated by mitogens or allogeneic cells. The antigen was induced at a stage which preceded DNA synthesis. Shortly afterwards, it was directly demonstrated that the Tac antigen was identical to a protein which bound the recently discovered T cell growth factor (Robb and Greene 1983). We now call the T cell growth factor IL-2 and know that the Tac antigen is the α-peptide of the IL-2R complex. The historical development of an understanding of the IL-2R and its interactions with IL-2 has been reviewed recently by Smith (1988).

Interleukin 2 binds to its receptor in an unusual reaction which generates a ternary complex between IL-2 and two peptide chains which are independently assembled and presented at the T cell surface. The p70–75 β-peptide is present on normal resting T cells and can bind IL-2 directly with intermediate affinity. The p55 α-peptide is rapidly induced on activated T cells and, at maximum induction, its numbers exceed the β-peptide by about 10-fold. The p55 α-peptide binds IL-2 with low affinity and this complex in turn is then able to bind the β-peptide to form a high-affinity complex. This stepwise conversion to a high-affinity receptor must be important in the efficient functioning of the receptor, and a mathematical kinetic explanation for it has been offered (Saito *et al.* 1988). Both the α- and β-peptide genes have been identified and fully sequenced and the primary gene products have been cloned (Hatakeyama *et al.* 1989). Only the β-peptide has a large intracellular domain, which presumably interacts with a signal transduction pathway. It is therefore no surprise that the β-peptide acts to internalize IL-2 (Robb and Greene 1987; Tanaka *et al.* 1988; Hatakeyama *et al.* 1989). The p55 α-chain is expressed early in the T cell activation cycle following mitogenic stimulation, at a time when the cells are progressing from G_0 to G_1. Its expression appears to be concurrent with an increase in mRNA, and occurs slightly before the expression of the transferrin receptor. It can therefore be used as a reliable marker of early T cell activation (Konttinen *et al.* 1986; Poulton *et al.* 1988; Schauer *et al.* 1989). This can be contrasted with the ability of the authentic growth factor for T cells, IL-2 itself, to induce progression through G_1 to S (Stern and Smith 1986).

Anti-Tac is the prototype monoclonal antibody for detecting the IL-2R through an epitope on the α-peptide, and has been widely used to detect the induction of IL-2R in flow cytometric studies. A soluble form of the IL-2R α-chain is present in small amounts in serum. It is approximately 10 kD smaller than the p55 peptide but shares most of its epitopes and is presumably derived from the parent molecule by proteolysis which releases it from cell membranes. Recently several monoclonal antibodies have been raised to epitopes which are different from the original 'Tac' epitope. In suitable combinations they can be used in 'sandwich' ELISA assays to measure soluble IL-2R in serum (Rubin *et al.* 1985; Honda *et al.* 1988). Several clinical applications for these assays are emerging and the most important seem to be in the area of lymphoid neoplasia. Soluble IL-2R concentrations are elevated, sometimes grossly, in the sera of patients with hairy cell leukaemia, adult (Japanese) T cell leukaemia, childhood acute lymphocytic leukaemia (ALL) and adult chronic lymphocytic leukaemia (CLL). Values can be 20–60 times higher than normal and in some diseases fall with anti-tumour therapy (Green *et al.* 1986; Kay *et al.* 1988; Steis *et al.* 1988; Yasuda *et al.* 1988).

Elevations of soluble IL-2R in body fluids are unlikely to be specifically diagnostic but may simply reflect intense lymphocyte activation. On this basis predictable elevations are found in Epstein–Barr virus (EBV) infections (Tomkinson *et al.* 1987) and in rheumatoid arthritis, where they correlate with disease activity (Symons *et al.* 1988). Monoclonal antibodies to the p75, IL-2R β-peptide have only recently been isolated, but their use should enable a systemic survey of the constitutive expression of the intermediate-affinity receptor on various cell types. Anti-p75 monoclonals are of great potential interest because they are mitogenic for T cells and probably bind to an epitope on the p75 peptide which facilitates signal transduction via the intracellular domain (Nakamura *et al.* 1989).

Natural killer cells

Functional characteristics

Natural killer cells were identified in the early 1970s as lymphocytes with the capacity to kill some leukaemic cell lines, haemopoietic precursors and virally infected cells. They did this directly and non-specifically, unlike T cells or K cells, which required specific ligands. This spontaneous cytotoxicity is demonstrated by cells which are morphologically large granular lymphocytes (LGL) with an expanded cytoplasm containing azurophilic granules. Although it is accepted that not all LGL are NK cells by precise phenotypic definitions, it is likely that LGL are functionally related cells, all capable of non-major histocompatibility complex (MHC)-restricted 'natural' cytotoxicity. There have been several excellent reviews of the development of knowledge about the biology of NK cells, particularly in attempting to define their phenotypic and functional characteristics in relation to non-MHC-restricted cytotoxicity mediated by T cells (Trinchieri and Perussia 1984; Lanier *et al.* 1986b; Jondal 1987).

Natural killer cells express the CD16 antigen recognized by the Leu 11a monoclonal antibody of Lanier *et al.* (1983, 1986a), an antigen which is an epitope on the low-affinity immunoglobulin G (IgG) FC receptor $FcR_{\gamma}III$ (Perussia *et al.* 1984). Although CD16 is not present on T cells, it is not unique to NK cells. However, its presence on other very distinctive cells, for example neutrophils, is not a confusion, since these cells are readily distinguished from NK cells by morphological and functional criteria (Lanier *et al.* 1988a). The $FcR_{\gamma}III$ receptor binds human IgG-1 and IgG-3, and it is the binding of this receptor to its ligands on sensitized target cells which mediates antibody-dependent cell cytotoxicity (ADCC). Thus NK and ADCC activities are expressed by phenotypically similar cells by what is likely to be a common lytic mechanism, although the initial triggering pathways may be different (Abrams and Brahmi 1988). A further example of a direct relationship between NK and cytotoxicity and ADCC is the ability of CD16 +ve cells to lyse hybridomas expressing monoclonal antibodies to CD16 (Lanier *et al.* 1988a), and yet another is the ability of anti-CD16 to 'arm' NK cells so that they mediate killing of target cells possessing $FcR_{\gamma}II$ receptors for IgG-1 in a 'reverse orientation' ADCC reaction (Uggla *et al.* 1989).

Several other surface markers are expressed consistently in association with CD16, particularly CD56 (Leu 19) (NKH-1), CD11a/18 (LFA-1) and CD2. Natural killer function seems to be most active within the CD16 +ve, Leu-19 +ve subtype rather than CD16 +ve, Leu-19 −ve (Schmidt *et al.* 1987), and this view is supported by evidence from CD16 +ve lymphoproliferative disorders where CD16 +ve, Leu-7 −ve, Leu-19 +ve cells rather than CD16 +ve, Leu-7 +ve, Leu-19 −ve cells contain the principal NK activity (Bray *et al.* 1987). In addition, the CD2 molecule and the CD11a/18 LFA complex are involved in NK activation and adhesion respectively, although the exact mechanism of involvement in each case is not yet clear. Antibodies to CD18 and CD11a appear to block LGL adherence and cytotoxicity against the NK targets, K562 and Molt-4 (Timonen *et al.* 1988; Werfel *et al.* 1989). A distinctive characteristic of NK cells is their ability to respond directly to IL-2, without a requirement for mitogens, adherent cells or other lymphokines. They express the intermediate affinity IL-2R 70 kD β-peptide in the unstimulated state. Interaction with IL-2 or with CD16 ligands rapidly induces the transcription of the 55 kD α-peptide of the IL-2R and assembly of the high-affinity receptor (Trinchieri *et al.* 1984; London *et al.* 1986; Anegón *et al.* 1988). Activated NK cells express transferrin receptors and human leucocyte antigen (HLA)-DR and HLA-DQ. They also exhibit enhanced cytotoxicity within 4 hours and will kill cell lines which are resistant to unstimulated NK cells (Lanier *et al.* 1988b). Lymphokine-activated killer (LAK) cells are generated from unfractionated peripheral blood or spleen mononuclear cells by incubation with IL-2. The great majority of cells with enhanced tumour cell cytotoxicity produced by this technique are phenotypically CD16 +ve, Leu-19 +ve, CD3 −ve, DR +ve, DQ +ve, i.e. are activated NK cells. Very few cells are CD3 +ve, Leu-19 +ve (Phillips and Lanier 1986). A T cell subtype with weak NK-like activity is CD8 +ve, Leu-7 +ve. Elevations of these cells are seen in chronic or reactivation virus infections, especially when caused by cytomegalovirus (CMV). CD8 +ve, Leu-7 +ve cells will mediate mitogen-induced or anti-CD3-induced cytotoxicity, and they may represent a set of primed cytotoxic T cells (Rüthlein *et al.* 1988). An actual role for NK cells as *in vivo* cytotoxic effectors has not yet been formally demonstrated in a clinical context. By analogy with the mechanisms by which murine NK cells increase resistance to mouse herpesvirus infections, it seems likely that human NK cells respond very early in viral infections to reduce viral replication before specific MHC-restricted T cell cytotoxicity can be generated.

Qualitative deficiencies of NK cell function have been demonstrated in a wide range of diseases, though most convincingly in systemic lupus erythematosus (SLE), acquired immune deficiency syndrome (AIDS) and the X-linked lymphoproliferative syndrome. However, in each of these diseases the NK dysfunction is only part of a much wider immunological aberration and is unlikely to be the principal defect leading to increased susceptibility to viral infections or to the emergence of lymphoid tumours. More convincing and understandable as deficiencies of NK function are those occurring in Chediak–Higashi syndrome and CD11/CD18 leucocyte adhesion molecule deficiencies. At the time of writing, there is only one description of a complete and specific lack of CD16 +ve, Leu-19 +ve cells in a patient with a corresponding failure of NK, ADCC and LAK function. A 19-year-old woman had three severe attacks of herpesvirus infections over a period of 5 years. The first was a varicella pneumonia, the second a CMV interstitial pneumonia and the third a primary herpes simplex infection with a generalized rash. On each occasion the patient recovered after a protracted illness and after treatment with antiviral drugs. T cell, B cell and neutrophil function were apparently intact (Biron *et al.* 1989).

Purification of natural killer cells

Two major practical problems confront anyone attempting to study NK activity in a clinical setting. The first is the need to find a method which will allow the isolation of lymphocytes of an acceptable NK phenotype in sufficient quantities, and the second is to devise NK functional assays which are consistent and quantitative. Neither of these ideals has so far been fully realized. Percoll density centrifugation has been widely used to isolate LGL and successive refinements have reduced to a minimum contamination with other mononuclear cells, particularly monocytes (Timonen *et al.* 1982; Pohajdak *et al.* 1984; Schlesinger *et al.* 1984). The weakness of the technique is the variability of distribution of LGL, including CD16 +ve cells, within the gradient fractions. Since NK cells only constitute 5–15% of the peripheral blood mononuclear cells, an alternative approach to gradient centrifugation is a series of selection steps with mononuclear antibodies. Ideally these should include a primary adherence phase to remove monocytes and B cells, and then one or more panning, rosetting or cell sorting steps to remove CD3 +ve T cells (Cosentino and Cathcart 1987). Techniques which remove T cells via the CD2 receptor should be avoided, since there is growing evidence that CD2 is functionally active on CD16 +ve NK cells (Schmidt *et al.* 1987).

It would appear easy to cell-sort peripheral blood lymphocytes directly on the CD16 marker, but the limitation here is the long sorting period required to obtain sufficient NK cells. However, pure NK cells obtained by this first step can be plated in limiting dilution and cultured to establish clonal cell lines. Cells grown in this manner will maintain the NK phenotype but, following exposure to growth factors, are in an activated state (DR +ve) (Windebank *et al.* 1988). A somewhat similar approach is to grow NK cells out of bulk preparations of adherence −ve mononuclear cells as 10-day cultures in the presence of irradiated B lymphoblastoid cells (RPMI 8866 or Daudi cells). A 10-fold increase in what are, in effect, activated killer cells occurs, with a predominance of CD16 +ve cells. These are then separated by negative selection from the minor CD3 +ve subtypes (Perussia *et al.* 1987; Anegón *et al.* 1988).

Functional assays

The standard NK assay is a 3–4-hour cytotoxicity assay in which the NK effector cells are incubated with ^{51}Cr-labelled target cells. The assay can only be performed with NK-sensitive targets, and these are usually tumour cell lines, which can be readily grown and maintained in culture. The two most commonly used are K562, a cell line derived from a chronic myeloid leukaemia in blast crises, and MOLT-4, from a T-cell-derived ALL. Ideally the target cells should not express Class I or II MHC glycoproteins. There are many variations of the standard ^{51}Cr-labelled cytotoxicity assays performed at different effector/target ratios (Lanier *et al.* 1983; Trinchieri and Perussia 1984). Attempts have been made from time to time to replace the radioactive chromium in the target cells with a non-isotopic marker, although none has so far successfully replaced it. A method of promise is to use fluorochrome-labelled cells, utilizing the principle of flurochromasia, where a non-polar fluorogenic substrate is taken up by target cells and converted to a polar and fluorescent molecule. The labelled cells can then be used in a standard cytotoxicity assay but the residual viable targets need to be harvested and the fluorescence measured in an automated fluorescence concentration analyser (Wierda *et al.* 1989).

Epstein–Barr virus-infected B cell lymphoblastoid cell lines, for example Daudi or Raji cells, are resistant to direct NK cytotoxicity and can act as negative controls. However, these cells become variably sensitive to NK killing as do other resistant tumour cell lines when NK cells are activated with IL-2. They will also take part as targets in ADCC assays when opsonized with IgG-1 subclass antibodies.

The standard lytic assays provide information about mass NK lytic activity but no information at the single-cell level. Further information can be obtained from cell conjugation killing assays in agarose, where conjugate pairs of effectors and targets can be examined directly by phase-contrast microscopy and dead targets identified by uptake and staining with trypan blue. These assays give information about the distribution of NK cells in an effector population (Bonavida *et al.* 1983). If the conjugate assay is combined with the ^{51}Cr release assay, then a more systemic analysis of the kinetics of single-cell cytotoxicity and the recycling of effector cells can be obtained (Ullberg and Jondal 1981). Conjugate formation, as opposed to killing, can also be informative. Of potential clinical value when evaluating NK activity in pathological states is the computation of maximum conjugation frequency (α_{max}) (Garcia-Penarrubia *et al.* 1989). A plot of $1/\alpha$ versus the effector/target (E/T) ratio, but with the effectors kept constant, is always linear with an intercept of $1/\alpha_{max}$. The authors claim that α_{max} is a constant for all E/T ratios and effector numbers and, at least for normal NK donors, is close to 60% for highly purified NK cells and 26% for unpurified but monocyte-depleted peripheral blood lymphoid cells. A major limitation of conjugate-based assays is that they depend on multiple and rather laborious counts by light microscopy.

Automated lytic NK assays capable of analysis by flow cytometry hold considerable potential for future clinical use. The key to the successful development of assays of this type is the ability to discriminate between live and dead K562 target cells by gating on forward and perpendicular light scatter (Vitale *et al.* 1989). One particular advantage of this approach is that the K562 cells are unlabelled and require the minimum number of *in vitro* manipulations.

Intradermal skin testing for delayed hypersensitivity

This long-standing technique is at present the only practical *in vivo* test of cell-mediated immunity, although in the not too distant future it may be possible to obtain more specific and detailed information about the *in vivo* immune response by injecting purified lymphokines or 'cocktails' and detecting changes in lymphocyte populations and levels of activation to them.

Single antigens are made up to the desired strength in sterile saline and are injected in 0.1 ml volumes intradermally into the volar aspect of the forearm at a site free of visible veins. A fine-gauge needle is used bevel-up at a depth sufficient to raise a 6–8 mm weal. Ideally, antigens should be selected with known frequencies of positive responses in the type of individual being tested at the antigenic strength employed. Although this technique is desirable for tailor-made or unusual antigens, there has been a major swing towards the use of a preloaded multipuncture device where the antigens are driven into the skin to a preset depth on acrylic tines (Multitest CMI, Merieux). The device uses a fixed range of seven microbial antigens at high concentrations, suitable for prick testing. Its advantage is the high degree of standardization and ease of use; its disadvantage is the fixed, albeit carefully selected, range of antigens and the need for sufficient technical skill to ensure that all the multipuncture heads penetrate to the full depth.

The multitest procedure elicits recall delayed hypersensitivity, whereas injection of the lectin

PHA will elicit a direct response. Primary skin test reactions can be produced by sensitizing with dinitrochlorobenzene (DNCB) (Catalonia 1972) and rechallenging 6 weeks later. The long wait for an answer makes this inconvenient in clinical work. There are also a greater risk of a severe reaction on rechallenging and the worry about the possible carcinogenic effects of DNCB.

Delayed hypersensitivity reactions should be inspected for induration at 48 hours rather than 24 hours. This is to ensure that the period of maximum cellular infiltrate is recorded rather than the earlier mixed cellular and oedematous phase. Erythema is ignored. A small-vessel perivascular accumulation of mononuclear cells commences at 6 hours and continues to 48–96 hours. The cells are mainly activated blast-like lymphocytes and a variable lesser proportion of macrophages. Marked dermal and epidermal oedema appears, due to damage to the vascular endothelium, and this is accompanied by some red cell leakage and deposition of large amounts of dermal fibrin at intravascular sites (Dvorak *et al.* 1974). The majority of the mononuclear cells are T cells, with CD4+ve cells predominating at 6 hours, but with CD4/8 ratios approximately like those in peripheral blood at 15–48 hours. By 15 hours T cells bearing transferrin receptors and IL-2 receptors and the activation markers DR and Ta_1 appear and these continue to increase in number up to 48 hours (Platt *et al.* 1983; Fullmer *et al.* 1987). By 96 hours keratinocytes expressing DR are present and this has been interpreted as demonstrating a role for interferon-γ in cell migration and activation in the lesions. This is supported by direct evidence that interferon-γ is the principal lymphokine in promoting the migration of lymphocytes through the high endothelium of venules in the dermis (Issekutz *et al.* 1988).

The percentage of positive reactions to common delayed-hypersensitivity antigens rises progressively from birth and reaches adult proportion at rates which vary for the antigens. The major rise in range and intensity occurs in the 2nd year of life (Kniker *et al.* 1985). In 5-year-old children, 65–75% give positive reactions to *Candida* and streptokinase–streptodornase (SKSD) (Shannon *et al.* 1966; Munoz and Limbert 1977). As might be expected, positive reactions to tetanus toxoid develop early, presumably following active immunization. Nevertheless, about 15% of healthy children are still 'hypoergic' at 7 years, although this proportion has fallen to 3% at 16 years (Corriel *et al.* 1985). It is likely that the positive profile to a range of antigens like those in the Multitest applicator will vary with race, geographical location and sex (Moesgaard *et al.* 1987). The question of fall-off in reactivity with old age is debatable, although it does not seem to occur in strictly healthy elderly populations.

Anergy is associated with a wide range of diseases and pathological states. The list is so extensive that the isolated finding of skin anergy is of limited diagnostic value. Anergy occurs in measles, in mumps and following vaccination with live attenuated viruses. It probably occurs in many viral infections where viral dissemination occurs during a viraemic phase. It also occurs in miliary tuberculosis (TB), disseminated mycotic infections, lepromatous leprosy, typhoid, scarlet fever and sarcoidosis. As might be expected, primary and secondary T cell deficiencies, cyclosporin and high-dose steroid therapy usually result in the anergic state. More non-specifically, fever, uraemia, leucocytosis and anaemia in hospitalized patients are significantly associated with the anergic state (Palmer and Reed 1974). Similarly, anergy is found in surgical patients, where it is associated with an increased incidence of sepsis and mortality (Christou 1985).

References

Abrams, S.I. and Brahmi, Z. (1988). Target cell directed NK inactivation: concomitant loss of NK and antibody-dependent cellular cytotoxic activity. *J. Immunol.* **140**, 2090.

Acuto, O. and Reinherz, E.L. (1985). The human T cell receptor: structure and function. *N. Engl. J. Med.* **312**, 1100.

Anegón, I., Cuturi, M.C., Trinchieri, G. and Perussia, B. (1988). Interaction of Fc receptor (CD16) ligands induces transcription of interleukin 2 receptor (CD25) and lymphokine genes and expression of their products in human natural killer cells. *J. Exp. Med.* **167**, 452.

Ashman, R.F. (1984). Lymphocyte activation. In *Fundamental Immunology*. ed. W.E. Paul, p. 267, Raven Press, New York.

Biron, C.A., Byron, K.S. and Sullivan, J.L. (1989). Severe herpes virus infections in an adolescent without natural killer cells. *N. Engl. J. Med.* **320**, 1731.

Blue, M.-L., Daley, J.F., Levine, H. and Schlossman, S.F. (1985). Coexpression of T4 and T8 on peripheral blood T cells demonstrated by two color fluorescence flow cytometry. *J. Immunol.* **134**, 228.

Bonavida, B., Bradley, T.P. and Grimm, E.A. (1983). The single cell assay in cell mediated cytotoxicity. *Immunol. Today* **4**, 196.

Bray, R.A., Gottschalk, L.R., Landay, A.L. and Gebel, H.M.

(1987). Differential surface marker expression in patients with CD16+ lymphoproliferative disorders: *in vivo* model for NK differentiation. *Hum. Immunol.* **19**, 105.

Breitmeyer, J.B., Daley, J.F., Levine, H.B. and Schlossman, S.F. (1987). The T11 (CD2) molecule is functionally linked to the T3/Ti T cell receptor in the majority of T cells. *J. Immunol.* **139**, 2899.

Cantrell, D.A., Davies, A.A. and Crumpton, M.J. (1985). Activators of protein kinase C down-regulate and phosphorylate the T3/T cell antigen receptor complex of human T lymphocytes. *Proc. Nat. Acad. Sci. (USA)* **82**, 8158.

Cardenas, J.M., Marshall, P., Henderson, B. and Altman, A. (1986). Human interleukin 2: quantitation by a sensitive radioimmunoassay. *J. Immunol. Methods* **89**, 181.

Catalonia, W.J. (1972). A method for dinitrochlorobenzene contact sensitization: a clinicopathological study. *N. Engl. J. Med.* **286**, 399.

Ceuppens, J.L., Bloemmen, F.J. and Van Wauwe, J.P. (1985). T cell unresponsiveness to the OKT3 antibody results from a deficiency of monocyte Fc γ receptors for murine IgG2a and inability to crosslink the T3-Ti complex. *J. Immunol.* **135**, 3882.

Christou, N.V. (1985). Host-defence mechanisms in surgical patients: a correlative study of the delayed hypersensitivity skin test response, granulocyte function and sepsis. *Can. J. Surg.* **28**, 39.

Clement, L.T., Tilden, A.B. and Dunlap, N.E. (1985). Analysis of the monocyte Fc receptors and antibody-mediated cellular interactions required for the induction of T cell proliferation by anti-T3 antibodies. *J. Immunol.* **135**, 165.

Corriel, N.R., Kniker, W.T., McBryde, J.L. and Lesourd, B.M. (1985). Cell-mediated immunity in schoolchildren assessed by Multitest skin testing: normal values and proposed scoring system for healthy children. *Am. J. Dis. Child.* **139**, 141.

Cosentino, L.M. and Cathcart, M.K. (1987). A multistep isolation scheme for obtaining CD16+ human natural killer cells. *J. Immunol. Methods* **103**, 195.

Cotner, T., Williams, J.M., Christenson, L., Shapiro, H.M., Strom, T.B. and Strominger, J. (1983). Simultaneous flow cytometric analysis of human T cell activation antigen expression and DNA content. *J. Exp. Med.* **157**, 461.

Creemers, P.C. (1987). Determination of co-expression of activation antigens on proliferating CD4+, CD4+CD8+ and CD8+ lymphocyte subsets by dual parameter flow cytometry. *J. Immunol. Methods* **97**, 165.

Davis, L. and Lipsky, P. (1986). Signals involved in T cell activation. II. Distinct roles of accessory cells, phorbol esters and interleukin 1 in activation and cell cycle progression of resting T lymphocytes. *J. Immunol.* **136**, 3588.

De Paoli, P., Battista, S., Crovatto, M. *et al.* (1988). Immunologic abnormalities related to antigenaemia during HIV-1 infections. *Clin. Exp. Immunol.* **74**, 317.

Dolbeare, F., Gratzner, H., Pallavincini, M.G. and Gray, J.W. (1983). Flow cytometric measurement of total DNA content and incorporated bromodeoxyuridine. *Proc. Nat. Acad. Sci. (USA)* **80**, 5573.

Dvorak, H.F., Mihm, M.C., Dvorak, A.M. *et al.* (1974). Morphology of delayed type hypersensitivity reaction in man. 1. Quantitative description of the inflammatory response. *Lab. Invest.* **31**, 111.

Fullmer, M.A., Shen, J.-Y., Modlin, R.L. and Rea, T.H. (1987). Immunohistological evidence of lymphokine production and lymphocyte activation antigens in tuberculin reactions. *Clin. Exp. Immunol.* **67**, 383.

Garcia-Penarrubia, P., Koster, F.T. and Bankhurst, A.D. (1989). The maximum conjugate frequency (α_{max}) characterizes killer cell populations. *J. Immunol. Methods* **118**, 199.

Gearing, A.J.H. and Thorpe, R. (1988). The international standard for human interleukin-2: calibration by international collaborative study. *J. Immunol. Methods* **114**, 3.

Gehman, L.O. and Robb, R.J. (1984). An ELISA-based assay for the quantitation of human interleukin-2. *J. Immunol. Methods* **74**, 39.

Geppert, T.D. and Lipsky, P.E. (1986). Accessory cell T-cell interaction involved in anti-CD3-induced T4 and T8 cell proliferation: analysis with monoclonal antibodies. *J. Immunol.* **137**, 3065.

Gerdes, J., Lemke, H., Baisch, H., Wacker, H.H., Schwab, U. and Stein, H. (1984). Cell cycle analysis of a cell proliferation-associated human nuclear antigen defined by the monoclonal antibody Ki-67. *J. Immunol.* **133**, 1710.

Gillis, S. and Smith, K.A. (1977). Long term culture of tumour-specific cytotoxic T cells. *Nature* **268**, 154.

Gillis, S., Ferm, M.M., Ou, W. and Smith, K.A. (1978). T cell growth factor parameters of production of a quantitative microassay for activity. *J. Immunol.* **120**, 2027.

Granelli-Piperno, A. (1988). *In situ* hybridization for interleukin 2 and interleukin 2 receptor mRNA in T cells activated in the presence or absence of cyclosporin A. *J. Exp. Med.* **168**, 1649.

Granelli-Piperno, A., Andrus, L. and Steinman, R.M. (1986). Lymphokine and non-lymphokine mRNA levels in stimulated human T cells: kinetics, mitogen requirements and effects of cyclosporin A. *J. Exp. Med.* **163**, 922.

Green, W.C., Leonard, W.J., Depper, J.M., Nelson, D.L. and Waldmann, T.A. (1986). The human interleukin-2 receptor: normal and abnormal expression in T cells and in leukaemia induced by the human T-lymphotropic retroviruses. *Ann. Intern. Med.* **105**, 560.

Hackett, R.J., Davis, L.S. and Lipsky, P.E. (1988). Comparative effects of tumor necrosis factor-α and IL-1β on mitogen-induced T cell activation. *J. Immunol.* **140**, 2639.

Hatakeyama, M., Tsudo, M., Minamoto, S. *et al.* (1989). Interleukin-2 receptor β chain gene: generation of three receptor forms by cloned human α and β chain cDNAs. *Science* **244**, 551.

Haynes, B.F., Hemler, M.E., Mann, D.L. *et al.* (1981). Characterization of a monoclonal antibody (4F2) that binds to human monocytes and to a subset of activated lymphocytes. *J. Immunol.* **126**, 1409.

Hayward, A., Laszlo, M., Turman, M., Vafai, A. and Tedder, D. (1988). Non-productive infection of human newborn blood mononuclear cells with herpes simplex virus: effect on T cell activation, IL-2 production and proliferation. *Clin. Exp. Immunol.* **74**, 196.

Honda, M., Nagao, S., Yamamoto, N., Tanaka, Y., Tozawa, H. and Tokunaga, T. (1988). Fluorescence sandwich enzyme-linked immunosorbent assay for detecting human interleukin-2 receptors. *J. Immunol. Methods* **110**, 129.

Igietseme, J.U. and Herscowitz, H.B. (1988). A modified in-situ enzyme-linked immunosorbent assay for quantitating interleukin-2 activity employing monoclonal anti-IL2 receptor antibody. *J. Immunol. Methods* **108**, 145.

Issekutz, T.B., Stoltz, J.M. and Van der Meide, P. (1988). The recruitment of lymphocytes into the skin by T cell lymphokines: the role of γ-interferon. *Clin. Exp. Immunol.* **73**, 70.

Jondal, M. (1987). The human NK cell — a short over-view and an hypothesis on NK recognition. *Clin. Exp. Immunol.* **70**, 255.

Katzen, D., Chu, E., Terhorst, C. *et al.* (1985). Mechanisms of human T cell response to mitogens: IL2 induces IL2 receptor expression and proliferation but not IL2 synthesis in PHA-stimulated T cells. *J. Immunol.* **135**, 1840.

Kay, N.E., Burton, J., Wagner, D. and Nelson, D.L. (1988). The malignant B cells from B-chronic lymphocytic leukaemia patients release TAC-soluble interleukin-2 receptors. *Blood* **72**, 447.

Kikutani, H., Kimura, R., Nakamura, H. *et al.* (1986). Expression and function of an early activation marker restricted to human B cells. *J. Immunol.* **136**, 4019.

Kniker, W.T., Lesourd, B.M., McBryde, J.L. and Corriel, R.N. (1985). Cell-mediated immunity measured by Multitest CMI skin testing in infants and preschool children. *Am. J. Dis. Child.* **139**, 840.

Konttinen, Y.T., Bergroth, V., Nordström, D., Segerberg-Konttinen, M. and Toluanen, E. (1986). Expression of MHC Class II antigen, interleukin-2 receptor, transferrin receptor and gp40/80 glycoprotein during different phases of normal PHA-driven lymphocyte activation *in vitro*. *Acta Pathol. Microbiol. Immunol. Scand. C* **94**, 181.

Kurki, P., Ogata, K. and Tan, E.M. (1988). Monoclonal antibodies to proliferating cell nuclear antigen (PCNA)/cyclin as probes for proliferating cells by immunofluorescence microscopy and flow cytometry. *J. Immunol. Methods* **109**, 49.

Lanier, L.L., Le, A.M., Phillips, J.H., Warner, N.L. and Babcock, G.F. (1983). Subpopulations of human natural killer cells defined by expression of the Leu-7 (HNK-1) and Leu-II (NK-15) antigens. *J. Immunol.* **131**, 1789.

Lanier, L.L., Le, A.M., Civin, C.I., Loken, M.R. and Phillips, J.H. (1986a). The relationship of CD16 (Leu-II) and Leu-19 (NKH-1) antigen expression on human peripheral blood NK cells and cytotoxic T lymphocytes. *J. Immunol.* **136**, 4480.

Lanier, L.L., Philips, J.H., Hackett, J., Tutt, M. and Kuman, V. (1986b). Natural killer cells: definition of a cell type rather than a function. *J. Immunol.* **137**, 2735.

Lanier, L.L., Ruitenberg, J.J. and Phillips, J.H. (1988a). Functional and biochemical analysis of CD16 antigen on natural killer cells and granulocytes. *J. Immunol.* **141**, 3478.

Lanier, L.L., Buck, D.W., Rhodes, L. *et al.* (1988b). Interleukin 2 activation of natural killer cells rapidly induces the expression and phosphorylation of the Leu-23 activation antigen. *J. Exp. Med.* **167**, 1572.

Ledbetter, J.A., June, C.H., Grosmaire, L.S. and Rabinovitch, P.S. (1987). Crosslinking of surface antigens causes mobilization of intracellular ionized calcium in T lymphocytes. *Proc. Nat. Acad. Sci. (USA)* **84**, 1384.

Leivestad, T., Gaudernack, G., Halvorsen, R. and Thorsby, E. (1988). A simple and sensitive bioassay for the detection of IL-2 activity. *J. Immunol. Methods* **114**, 95.

Levitt, D. and King, M. (1987). Methanol fixation permits flow cytometric analysis of immunofluid stained intracellular antigens. *J. Immunol. Methods* **96**, 233.

London, L., Perussia, B. and Trinchieri, G. (1986). Induction of proliferation *in vitro* of resting human natural killer cells: IL-2 induces into cell cycle most peripheral blood NK cells, but only a minor subset of low density T cells. *J. Immunol.* **137**, 3845.

Meuer, S.C., Hussey, R.E., Fabbi, M. *et al.* (1984). An alternative pathway of T cell activation, a functional role for the 50 kD T11 sheep erythrocyte receptor protein. *Cell* **36**, 897.

Moesgaard, F., Nielsen, M.L., Larsen, P.N., Christophersen, S. and Mosbech, H. (1987). Cell-mediated immunity assessed by skin testing (Multitest). *Allergy* **42**, 591.

Morimoto, C., Reinherz, E.L., Schlossman, S.F., Schur, P.H., Mills, J.A. and Steinberg, A.D. (1980). Alterations in immunoregulatory T cell subsets in active systemic lupus erythematosus. *J. Clin. Invest.* **66**, 1171.

Mosmann, T.R. (1983). Rapid colorimetric assay for cellular growth and survival: application to proliferation and cytotoxicity assays. *J. Immunol. Methods* **65**, 55.

Mosmann, T.R. and Fong, T.A.T. (1989). Specific assays for cytokine production by T cells. *J. Immunol. Methods* **116**, 151.

Munoz, A.I. and Limbert, D. (1977). Skin reactivity to *Candida* and streptokinase–streptodornase antigens in normal paediatric subjects: influence of age and acute illness. *Pediatrics* **91**, 565.

Nakamura, Y., Inamoto, T., Sugie, K. *et al.* (1989). Mitogenicity and down-regulation of high affinity interleukin-2 receptor by YTA-1 and YTA-2 monoclonal antibodies that recognize 75-kDa molecules on human large granular lymphocytes. *Proc. Nat. Acad. Sci. (USA)* **86**, 1318.

Nel, A.E., Wooten, M.W. and Galbraith, R.M. (1987). Molecular signaling mechanisms in T-lymphocyte activation pathways: a review and future prospects. *Clin. Immunol. Immunopathol.* **44**, 167.

O'Flynn, K., Russul-Saib, M., Ando, I. *et al.* (1986). Different pathways of human T cell activation revealed by PHA-P and PHA-M. *Immunology* **57**, 55.

Ogata, K., Kurki, P., Celis, J.E., Nakamura, R.M. and Tan, E.M. (1987). Monoclonal antibodies to a nuclear protein (PCNA/cyclin) associated with DNA replication. *Exp. Cell. Res.* **168**, 475.

Palmer, D.L. and Reed, W.P. (1974). Delayed hypersensitivity skin testing. 1. Response rates in a hospitalized population. *J. Infect. Dis.* **130**, 132.

Perussia, B., Trinchieri, G., Jackson, A. *et al.* (1984). The Fc receptor for IgG on human natural killer cells: phenotypic, functional and comparative studies using monoclonal antibody. *J. Immunol.* **133**, 180.

Perussia, B., Ramoni, C., Anegón, I., Cuturi, M.C., Faust, J. and Trinchieri, G. (1987). Preferential proliferation of natural killer cells among peripheral blood mononuclear cells cocultured with B lymphoblastoid cell lines. *Nat. Immunol. Cell Growth Regulation* **6**, 171.

Phillips, J.H. and Lanier, L.L. (1986). Dissection of the lymphokine activated killer phenomenon. *J. Exp. Med.* **164**, 814.

Platt, J.L., Grant, B.W., Eddy, A.A. and Michael, A.F. (1983). Immune cell populations in cutaneous delayed type hypersensitivity. *J. Exp. Med.* **158**, 1227.

Pohajdak, B., Gomez, J., Wilkins, J. and Greenberg, A. (1984). Tumor-activated NK cells trigger monocyte oxidative metabolism. *J. Immunol.* **133**, 2430.

Pollack, A., Bagwell, C.B. and Irvin, G.L. (1979). Radiation from tritiated thymidine perturbs the cell cycle progression of stimulated lymphocytes. *Science* **203**, 1025.

Poulton, T.A., Gallagher, A., Potts, R.C. and Swanson Beck, J. (1988). Changes in activation markers and cell marker receptors on human peripheral blood T lymphocytes during cell cycle progression after PHA stimulation. *Immunology* **64**, 419.

Robb, R.J. and Greene, W.C. (1983). Direct demonstration of the identity of T cell growth factor binding protein and the TAC antigen. *J. Exp. Med.* **158**, 1332.

Robb, R.J. and Green, W.C. (1987). Internalization of interleukin-2 is mediated by the β-chain of the high affinity interleukin 2 receptor. *J. Exp. Med.* **165**, 1201.

Rubin, L.A., Kurman, C.C., Fritz, M.E. *et al.* (1985). Soluble interleukin 2 receptors are released from activated human lymphoid cells *in vitro*. *J. Immunol.* **135**, 3172.

Rüthlein, J., James, S.P. and Strober, W. (1988). Role of CD2 in activation and cytotoxic function of CD8/Leu7+ T cells. *J. Immunol.* **141**, 3791.

Saito, Y.S., Sabe, H., Suzuki, N. *et al.* (1988). A larger number of L chains (Tac) enhance the association rate of interleukin 2 to the high affinity site of the interleukin 2 receptor. *J. Exp. Med.* **168**, 1563.

Schauer, U., Krolikowski, I. and Rieger, C.H.L. (1989). Detection of activated lymphocyte subsets by fluorescence and MTT staining. *J. Immunol. Methods* **116**, 221.

Scheurich, P., Thoma, B., Ücer, U. and Pfizenmaier, K. (1987). Immunoregulatory activity of recombinant human tumor necrosis factor (TNF)-α; induction of TNF receptors on human T cells and TNF-α-mediated enhancement of T cell responses. *J. Immunol.* **138**, 1786.

Schlesinger, M., Lew, F. and Bekesi, J. (1984). Surface antigen determinants in subpopulations of peripheral blood NK- and T-cells separated by Percoll density fractionation. *J. Clin. Lab. Immunol.* **13**, 195.

Schmidt, R.E. Michon, J.M., Woronicz, J., Schlossman, S.F., Reinherz, E.L. and Ritz, J. (1987). Enhancement of natural killer function through activation of the T11 E rosette receptor. *J. Clin. Invest.* **79**, 305.

Shannon, D.C., Johnson, G., Rosen, F.S. and Austen, K.F. (1966). Cellular reactivity to *Candida albicans* antigen. *N. Engl. J. Med.* **275**, 690.

Shaw, J., Meerovitch, K., Elliott, J.F., Bleackley, R.C. and Paetkau, V. (1987). Induction, suppression and superinduction of lymphokine mRNA in T lymphocytes. *Mol. Immunol.* **24**, 409.

Shaw, J., Meerovitch, K., Bleackley, R.C. and Paetkau, V. (1988). Mechanisms regulating the level of IL-2 mRNA in T lymphocytes. *J. Immunol.* **140**, 2243.

Shipp, M.A. and Reinherz, E.L. (1987). Differential expression of nuclear proto-oncogenes in T cells triggered with mitogenic and nonmitogenic T3 and T11 activation signals. *J. Immunol.* **139**, 2143.

Smith, K.A. (1988). Interleukin-2: inception, impact and implications. *Science* **240**, 1169.

Steis, R.G., Marcon, L., Clark, J. *et al.* (1988). Serum soluble IL-2 receptor as a tumor marker in patients with hairy cell leukaemia. *Blood* **71**, 1304.

Stern, J.B. and Smith, K.A. (1986). Interleukin-2 induction of T-cell G1 progression and c-myh expression. *Science* **233**, 203.

Stites, D.P., Casavant, C.H., McHugh, T.M. *et al.* (1986). Flow cytometric analysis of lymphocyte phenotypes in AIDS using monoclonal antibodies and simultaneous dual immunofluorescence. *Clin. Immunol. Immunopathol.* **38**, 161.

Symons, J.A., Wood, N.C., DiGiovine, F.S. and Duff, G.W. (1988). Soluble IL-2 receptor in rheumatoid arthritis: correlation with disease activity, IL-1 and IL-2 inhibition. *J. Immunol.* **141**, 2612.

Tanaka, T., Saiki, O., Doi, S., Shigeru, N. and Kishimoto, S. (1988). Interleukin 2 functions through novel interleukin 2 binding molecules in T cells. *J. Immunol.* **140**, 470.

Timonen, T., Reynolds, C., Ortaldo, J. and Herberman, R. (1982). Isolation of human and rat natural killer cells. *J. Immunol. Methods* **51**, 269.

Timonen, T., Patamoyo, M. and Gahmberg, C.G. (1988). CD11a-c/CD18 and gp84 (LB-2) adhesion molecules on human large granular lymphocytes and their participation in natural killing. *J. Immunol.* **141**, 1041.

Tomkinson, B.E., Wagner, D.K., Nelson, D.L. and Sullivan, J.L. (1987). Activated lymphocytes during acute EB virus infection. *J. Immunol.* **139**, 3802.

Trinchieri, G. and Perussia, B. (1984). Human natural killer cells: biological and pathological aspects. *Lab. Invest.* **50**, 489.

Trinchieri, G., Matsumoto-Kabayashi, M., Clark, S.C., Sechra, J., London, L. and Perussia, B. (1984). Response of resting human peripheral blood natural killer cells to interleukin 2. *J. Exp. Med.* **160**, 1147.

Truneh, A., Albert, F., Golstein, P. and Schmitt-Verhulst, A.-M. (1985). Early steps of lymphocyte activation bypassed by synergy between calcium ionophores and phorbol esters. *Nature* **313**, 318.

Uchiyama, T., Broder, S. and Waldmann, T.A. (1981). A monoclonal antibody (anti-Tac) reactive with activated and functionally mature T cells. *J. Immunol.* **126**, 1313.

Uggla, C.K., Geisberg, M., Jondal, M. and Knowles, R.W. (1989). Agonistic effects of anti-CD2 and anti-CD16 antibodies on human natural killer killing. *Scand. J. Immunol.* **29**, 507.

Ullberg, M. and Jondal, M. (1981). Recycling and target binding capacity of human natural killer cells. *J. Exp. Med.* **153**, 615.

Vanderlaan, M. and Thomas, C.B. (1985). Characterization of monoclonal antibodies to bromodeoxyuridine. *Cytometry* **6**, 501.

Vine, J.B., Geppart, T.D. and Lipsky, P.E. (1988). T4 cell activation by immobilized phytohaemagglutinin: differential capacity to induce IL-2 responsiveness and IL-2 production. *J. Immunol.* **141**, 2593.

Vitale, M., Neri, L.M., Comani, S. *et al.* (1989). Natural killer function in flow cytometry. II. Evaluation of NK lytic activity by means of target cell morphological changes detected by right angle light scatter. *J. Immunol. Methods* **121**, 115.

Werfel, T., Uciechowski, P., Tetterlo, P.A.T., Kurle, R., Deicher, H. and Schmidt, R.E. (1989). Activation of classical human natural killer cells via Fc_{γ}RIII. *J. Immunol.* **142**, 1102.

Wierda, W.G., Mehr, D.S. and Kim, Y.B. (1989). Comparison of fluorochrome-labelled and ^{51}Cr-labelled targets for natural killer cytotoxicity assay. *J. Immunol. Methods* **122**, 15.

Windebank, K.P., Abraham, R.T., Powis, G., Olsen, R.A., Barna, T.J. and Leibson, P.J. (1988). Signal transduction during human natural killer cell activation: inositol phosphate generation and regulation by cyclic AMP. *J. Immunol.* **141**, 3951.

Yasuda, N., Lai, P.K., Ip, S.H. *et al.* (1988). Soluble interleukin-2 receptors in sera of Japanese patients with adult T cell leukaemia mark activity of disease. *Blood* **71**, 102.

Section 5
Immunological Intervention

46: Graft Rejection and Immunosuppression in Kidney Transplantation

T.B. Strom

The success of kidney transplantation, the treatment of choice for many patients with end-stage renal diseases, is limited primarily by allograft rejection. Direct manipulation of the host's immune response provides a practical means of achieving engraftment even when tissue matching of donor and recipient is less than optimal. Although several highly efficacious immunosuppressive agents have been developed, acute rejection occurring within days or months after a transplant operation or chronic rejection occurring months or years later are the major obstacles to the success of organ replacement.

Immunosuppressive protocols for organ transplantation are in a state of flux. Although immunosuppressive therapies to abrogate host reactivity to allografts have been applied since the early days of clinical transplantation, immunosuppressive agents and protocols are constantly evolving. Treatment regimens may vary from unit to unit even though the same agents are used. No attempt will be made to discuss the fine details of protocols developed at different centres.

During the early 1970s there was little improvement in graft survival, but a steady improvement in patient survival was seen as experience with monitoring and management of infectious complications improved (Tilney *et al.* 1978). Clinical immunosuppression has advanced from the use of steroids and antimetabolites such as azathioprine, which provide a generalized modulation of the immune and inflammatory response, through the more finely targeted antilymphocyte sera, cyclosporin and, more recently, monoclonal antibodies and FK-506.

Immunotherapy should, preferably, be donor-specific and targeted to minimize the risks of non specific immunosuppression. An ideal immunosuppressant would specifically block the activities of only the small population of antigen-specific cells actually engaged in the events of rejection. In order to understand the mechanisms by which currently applied therapies dampen rejection, a brief description of the molecular events of T cell activation and rejection follows.

T cell activation and graft rejection

Each of the agents used in the clinic to suppress rejection blocks certain aspects of T cell activation. It is therefore important to understand the mechanisms of rejection in order to deduce the mode of action of immunosuppressive drugs. Rejection is affected by a diverse assembly of white blood cells, including CD4+ve helper T cells, CD8+ve cytotoxic T cells, antibody-forming B cells and accessory cells such as macrophages. It is likely that cytokine-activated kidney cells can also be recruited into the process. However, the rejection process is ultimately dependent upon a small population of T cells that bear recognition units, or receptors, for the histocompatibility antigens of the donor graft (Strom 1984).

The T cell antigen recognition complex is a seven-peptide chain structure that includes two immunoglobulin-like chains encoded in cassette-like fashion by genes that undergo recombination during intrathymic T cell maturation, akin to the well-described recombination events involved in the generation of antibody specificity in B cells (Kronenberg *et al* 1986). These are the alpha and beta T cell receptor chains. A very small population of mature T cells express kindred gamma and/or delta T cell receptor chains but lack the alpha and beta receptor proteins. The other five chains, called CD3 proteins, are non-covalently linked to the alpha and beta T cell receptor chains and are involved in the transmembrane signal produced by interaction of the alpha and beta T cell receptor proteins with antigen (Weiss *et al*. 1986; Clevers *et al*. 1988).

As a result of the encounter of donor-specific T cell clones with graft antigens, T cell activation and proliferation occur (Fig. 46.1). The cascade of activation-associated events culminates in a remarkable amplification of immune activity by attracting a large number and wide variety of activated white blood cells into the graft. These events can now be described in a molecular context.

The cascade is initiated by the presentation of incompatible graft antigens to the host. Helper cells bearing the distinctive CD4 protein are activated by donor human leucocyte antigen (HLA) Class II molecules such as HLA-DR (Fig. 46.1). The incompatible, i.e. antigenic, portion of the Class II molecule is recognized by the T cell receptor. The CD4 protein binds to a separate non-polymorphic region of HLA Class II, thereby giving further strength to the attachment of the CD4 +ve T cell to the Class II +ve donor cell. The Class II-activated CD4 +ve molecule activates an intracellular tyrosine kinase, which provides another T cell activation signal. In contrast, cytotoxic T cells bearing the CD8 protein are activated primarily via recognition of HLA Class I molecules of the graft. The T cell receptor recognizes the incompatible (polymorphic) portion of the Class I molecule while the CD8 protein binds to non-polymorphic domains of the Class I molecule, adding strength to the attachment as well as providing activation of CD8 +ve-linked tyrosine kinase.

T cell activation is initiated when those few clones of T cells bearing cell surface receptors specific for the graft antigens actively bind to these graft antigens. However, while antigen is the first external signal required for initiating T cell activation, antigen recognition is not itself sufficient to bring about T cell proliferation (Fig. 46.1). Activated accessory cells, e.g. dendritic cells or macrophages, are also required (Fig. 46.2). Direct

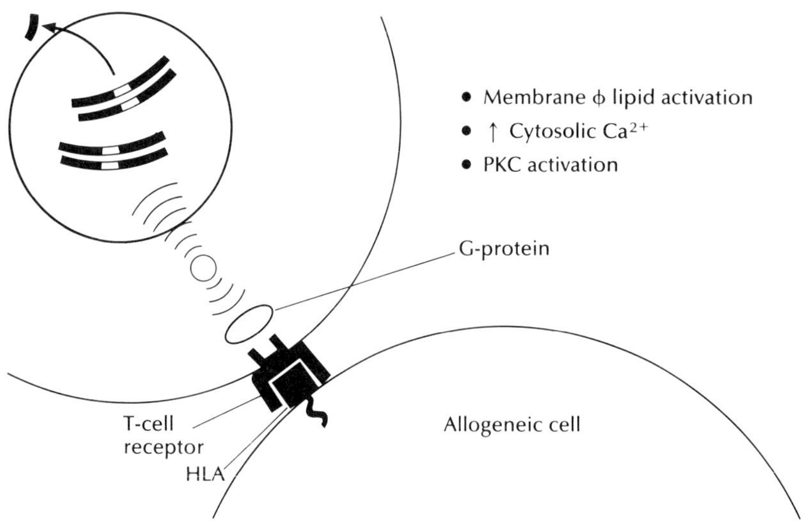

Fig. 46.1. The immune response to allogeneic tissues is initiated as T cells bearing antigen-specific receptor recognition units bind to alloantigen-bearing transplanted tissues. T cell activation signals initiated through engagement of antigen receptors are transduced via intracellular messengers.

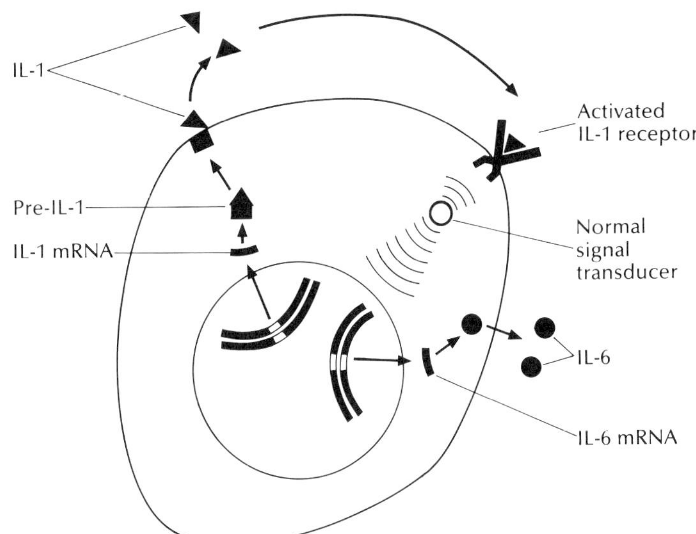

Fig. 46.2. Immune activation of alloantigen-specific T cells also results in activation of macrophages. Activated macrophages manufacture pro-inflammatory cytokines that support T cell activation.

cell–cell contact between T cells and macrophages or stimulation of macrophages by soluble T cell products causes macrophage activation (Fig. 46.3), which is required for full T cell activation (Williams *et al.* 1985). Engagement of T cell receptors with antigen causes the formation of intracellular second messengers that transduce signals from the cell membrane to the T cell nucleus (see Fig. 46.1) (Meuer *et al.* 1984; Weiss *et al.* 1985).

The cytoplasmic second messengers formed in T cells in response to antigen stimulation result from activation of T-cell-specific tyrosine kinases and formation of diacylglycerol from phosphatidylinositol biphosphate (Nisbet–Brown *et al.* 1985; Shapiro *et al.* 1985), which activates protein kinase C, and formation of inositol triphosphate, which causes a precipitous rise in free cytosolic calcium (reviewed in Gardner 1989) (see Fig. 46.1). Some of the increased free cytosolic calcium is also mobilized from extracellular sources. Direct cell-to-cell interaction of T cells and antigen-bearing target cells or stimulation of antigen-activated T cells by certain cytokines provides co-stimulatory signals — signals that trigger antigen-stimulated

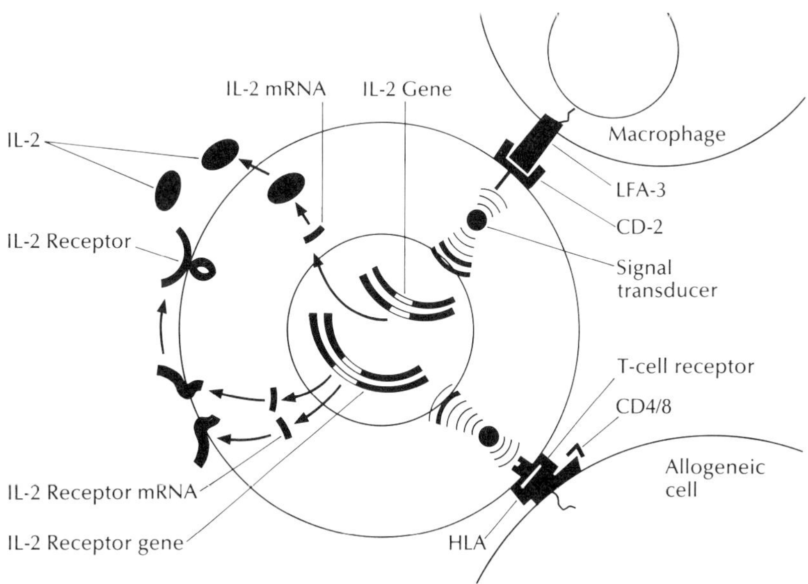

Fig. 46.3. At least two signals are required to stimulate T cell proliferation. Engagement of the T cell antigen receptor by antigen is necessary but not sufficient for T cell activation. Full T cell activation requires stimulation by antigen and accessory cells or their products.

T cells into an autocrine pathway of T cell activation (Fig. 46.4). Attachment of T cell CD4 or CD8 proteins to non-polymorphic domains of HLA Class I or Class II molecules upon target cells activates CD4 or CD8 tyrosine kinase activity (Fig. 46.3). Attachment of T cell surface CD2 molecules to target cell lymphocyte function-associated antigen (LFA)-3 proteins on target cells stimulates a sharp rise in T cell cytosolic calcium flux (Fig. 46.3). In macrophages and other accessory cells activation by T cells or their products elicits the formation of second messengers, which, in turn, activate the interleukin 1 (IL-1) gene (see Fig. 46.2). Transcription of messenger ribonucleic acid (mRNA) encoding IL-1 proceeds, followed by translation of large alpha and beta pro-IL-1 molecules (Auron *et al*. 1987). Precursor molecules are cleaved intracellularly, and the considerably smaller mature forms of IL-1 are secreted (see Fig. 46.2). Interleukin 1 is an autocrine factor that activates transcription of the IL-6 gene in murine macrophages (Pankewycz *et al*. 1990).

T cells are stimulated by antigen and IL-1/IL-6 or by direct cell-to-cell contact to secrete the T cell growth factor, IL-2 (Pankewycz *et al*. 1990), and express *de novo* cell surface IL-2 receptors (Fig. 46.4) (Cantrell and Smith 1984; Williams *et al*. 1984; Weiss *et al*. 1986). Formation of IL-2 receptors and release of IL-2 is of central importance in the events of T cell activation for several reasons (Weiss *et al*. 1985; Auron *et al*. 1987). Interleukin 2 is not only a growth factor; it also stimulates antigen-activated T cells to release several other lymphokines that are critical to the events of rejection (Fig. 46.4) (Howard *et al*. 1983; Inaba *et al*. 1983; Ythier *et al*. 1985). Antigen-activated, IL-2-stimulated T cells release B cell activation factors (Inaba *et al*. 1983), such as IL-4 and IL-5, which enable antigen-activated B cells to elaborate high-affinity, high-titre anti-graft antibodies. Interleukin 2 causes helper cells to release factors that permit the cytotoxic capacity of cytotoxic T cells to develop. It stimulates, too, the release of interferon gamma (IFN-γ) (Farrar *et al*. 1981), which in turn activates the cytodestructive activities of macrophages. Further, this lymphokine stimulates cells of the transplant, e.g. tubular and endothelial cells, that normally do not express Class II HLA molecules to express such molecules (Pober *et al*. 1983; Kelley *et al*. 1984). The interaction of soluble IL-2 and cellular IL-2 receptors stimulates clonal proliferation (Fig. 46.4) of both antigen-activated helper and cytotoxic T cells (Cantrell and Smith 1984). Interleukin 2 is also an anabolic factor essential for the viability of activated T cells (Maddock *et al*. 1985). Thus IL-2-dependent mechanisms result in the activation of B cells, helper cells, cytotoxic cells and macrophages. Moreover, the allograft displays new HLA molecules induced by the actions of IL-2-dependent secretion of IFN-γ thus initiating a vicious circle of rejection-associated events. The initial response of a small number of donor-specific T cell clones orchestrates the activation of a critical mass of clonally expanded, antigen-activated T cells and other cells required for rejection.

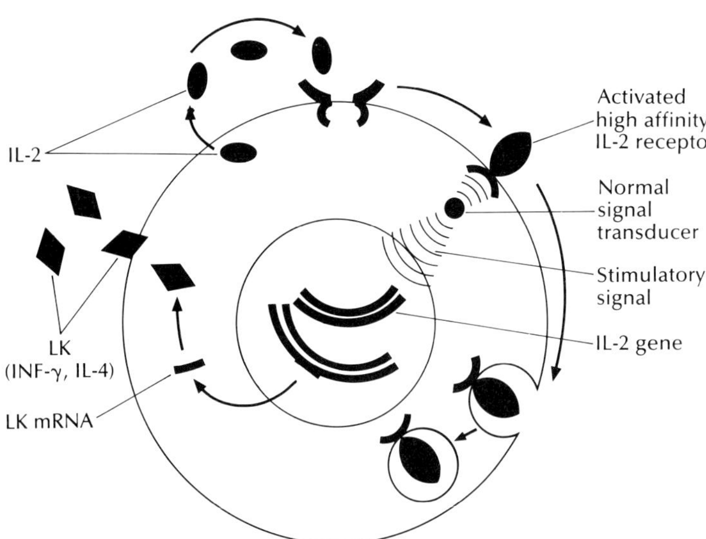

Fig. 46.4. While activation of T cells by antigen and accessory cells initiates T cell activation, IL-2 plays a central role in T cell activation. Interleukin 2 receptor-bearing, antigen-activated lymphocytes can be stimulated to secrete lymphokines by IL-2.

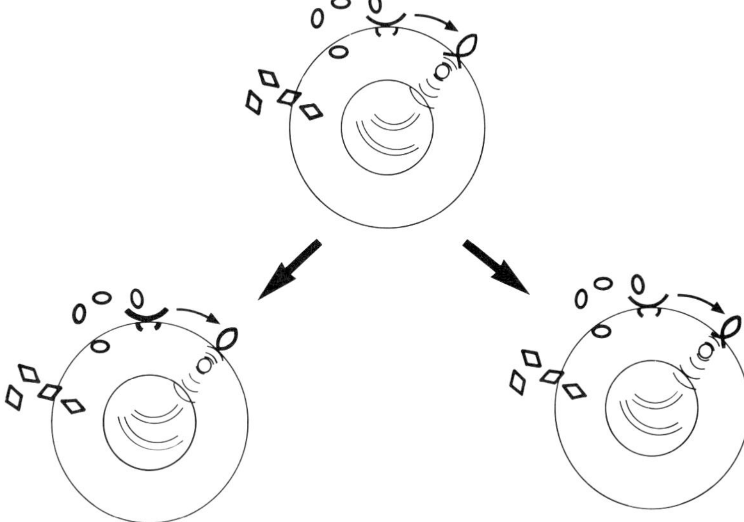

Fig. 46.5. The interaction of IL-2 (a T cell growth factor) with antigen-activated T cells bearing high-affinity IL-2 receptors stimulates proliferation of these IL-2 receptor-responsive cells. The IL-2-responsive population includes cytotoxic T cells and lymphokine-secreting cells. As a consequence, the small population of donor-specific alloreactive cells propagates and becomes instrumental in rejecting the allograft.

Nature has, fortunately, ensured that antigen-stimulated T cell lymphoproliferation can eventually be halted. As time passes following antigen activation, transcription of mRNA encoding lymphokines and IL-2 receptor proteins wanes and the remaining transcripts, which possess adenine-uracil (AU)-rich, ribonuclease (RNase)-sensitive domains in the flanking regions, are inherently labile molecules, and degenerate. In the absence of IL-2 and IL-2 receptors, T cell proliferation ceases, and T cells revert, in the main, to the functional status of resting cells. Active intervention by crudely defined, albeit real, suppressor immune phenomena may contribute to regulation of the immune response.

Immunosuppression in graft rejection

Immunosuppressive therapy to prevent or reverse acute rejection attempts to abrogate selectively the patient's reactivity to the allograft, while sparing as much as possible the host immune response to other foreign antigens. Although this ideal immunosuppression has not been fully achieved, great strides have been made.

Three drugs have gained wide acceptance in the prevention of renal allograft rejection. The success of azathioprine and corticosteroids in the control of acute graft rejection was the breakthrough that allowed kidney transplantation to become a routinely applicable clinical reality. Cyclosporin, developed in the 1970s and widely used in the 1980s, proved to be a boon to transplantation: one-year cadaver kidney graft survival improved by 15–20%. Each of these drugs blocks T cell proliferation, albeit at a slightly different step in the activation cascade. However, none of these agents inhibits the initial engagement of T cells by antigen.

Corticosteroids

Most immunosuppressive drug regimens employ an adrenal corticosteroid such as prednisolone or prednisone in combination with other immunosuppressive agents. Corticosteroids provide a block in the T cell activation cascade; they interfere with T cell proliferation through their ability to block activation of the IL-1 and IL-6 genes in accessory cells (Fig. 46.6) (Knudsen *et al.* 1987; Zanker *et al.*, submitted for publication) and the IL-2 gene in T cells (Crabtree 1989). Corticosteroid-treated macrophages do not produce IL-1-encoding mRNA, even when subsequently cultured in the presence of powerful macrophage stimulants. Interleukin 1 was previously called endogenous pyrogen, because one of the major activities of this protein is to stimulate the thermoregulatory centres of the central nervous system and thereby to cause fever. The ability of steroids to prevent fever in septic states almost certainly derives from the blocking of the release of IL-1 and IL-6. The fever associated with allograft rejection is probably caused by the secretion of pyrogenic cytokines

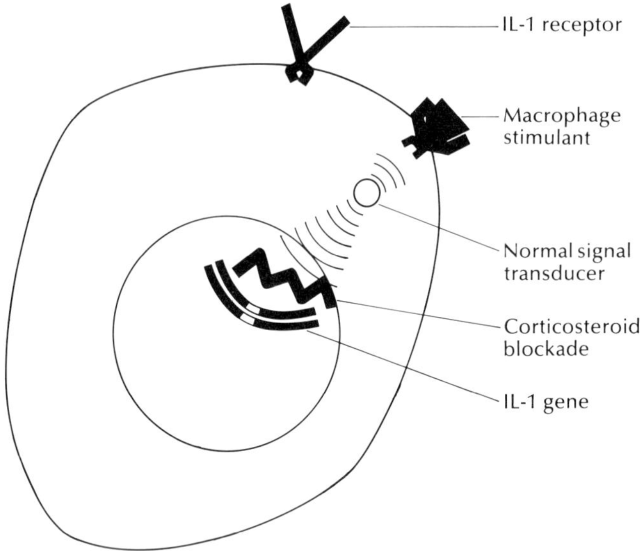

Fig. 46.6. Corticosteroids block activation of the IL-1 (and IL-6) genes.

such as IL-1 and IL-6. Febrile renal transplant recipients experiencing rejection generally do not respond unless steroid treatment first abolishes fever. Because IL-2 release is dependent upon IL-1 and/or IL-6 release (see Fig. 46.2), corticosteroids also indirectly block IL-2 through this mechanism (Table 46.1). Corticosteroids also directly block activation of the IL-2 gene in T cells. It is likely, but not certain, that these effects are produced via the capacity of activated glucocorticoid receptors, which are deoxyribonucleic acid (DNA)-binding proteins, to bind directly to glucocorticoid response elements possessed by the IL-1, IL-6 and IL-2 genes and thereby interfere with gene transcription (Almawi *et al.* 1991).

Conventional therapies for the treatment of acute renal allograft rejection include high-dose pulses of glucocorticoids. Glucocorticoids have broad, non-specific immunosuppressive and anti-inflammatory effects. Besides their effects on lymphokines, glucocorticoids reduce the migration of monocytes to sites of inflammation (Bach and Strom 1986). A major drawback to the use of glucocorticoids in the treatment of acute rejection is that they inhibit the entire immune and inflammatory systems and alter many other steroid-responsive systems as well. This use of high doses of glucocorticoids can thus produce severe undesirable side-effects. These include decreased inflammatory and phagocytic capacity, resulting in increased susceptibility to infection, hyperglycaemia, hyperkalaemia, osteoporosis, increased capillary fragility and growth suppression in children.

Table 46.1. Steroids in immunosuppression

Mode of action	Side-effects
Blocks IL-1 release directly Blocks IL-6 release directly Blocks IL-2 release directly and indirectly Non-specific immunosuppressive and anti-inflammatory effects Inhibits migration of immune cells to site of inflammation	Increased susceptibility to infection Impaired wound healing Growth suppression in children Aseptic necrosis of bone Depression, sleep disturbances with high dose Hyperglycaemia Oedema Hypertension

Azathioprine

Although useful for inhibiting primary immune responses, azathioprine has little effect on secondary responses or in the reversal of acute allograft rejections. It blocks T cell activation at the most distal point compared with the other two drugs discussed here. This antimetabolite (Bach and Strom 1986) is the imidazole derivative of 6-mercaptopurine and other antimetabolites. It does not prevent initial gene activation, but instead powerfully inhibits gene replication and T cell activation (Fig. 46.7; Table 46.2).

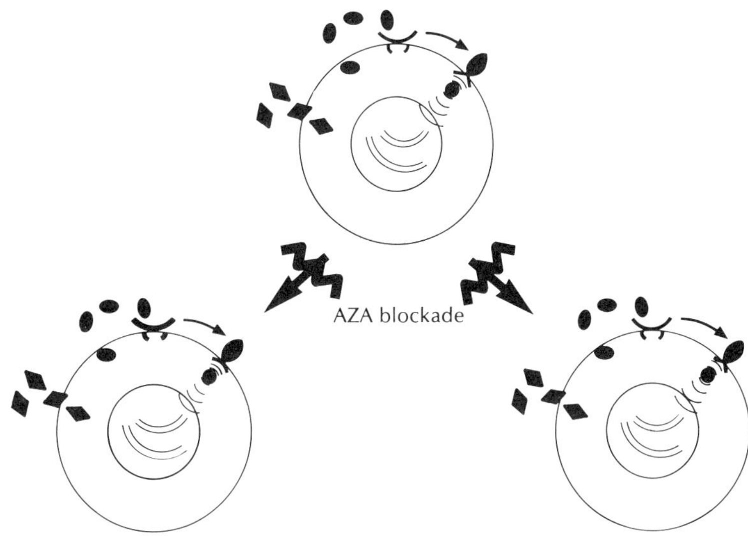

Fig. 46.7. Azathioprine is a classic antimetabolite and blocks cell proliferation.

Moreover, azathioprine decreases the number of migratory mononuclear cells and granulocytes whilst inhibiting the proliferation of promyelocytes within bone marrow. As a result, the number of circulating monocytes capable of differentiating into macrophages is decreased. The documented deleterious effects of azathioprine administration include occasional severe leucopenia and/or thrombocytopenia, gastrointestinal disturbances, fever, hepatotoxicity and an increased risk of neoplasia (see also Chapter 51).

Cyclosporin and FK-506

The more recent introduction of cyclosporin, a small cyclic peptide of fungal origin, has played a major role in preventing early irreversible rejection episodes, resulting in improved graft survival rates

Table 46.2. Azathioprine in immunosuppression

Mode of action	Side-effects
Inhibits DNA and RNA synthesis	Myelocyte suppression
Decreases the number of migratory mononuclear and granulocytic cells	Dose-related leucopenia, thrombocytopenia
Inhibits promyelocyte proliferation	Gastrointestinal disturbances
	Hepatotoxicity
	Increased risk of certain neoplasia
	Increased susceptibility to infection

in treated patients. Due to its mode of action, cyclosporin (like azathioprine) is of limited value in the treatment of acute allograft rejection.

Cyclosporin blocks T cell activation although certain elements of T cell activation proceed in an unimpeded fashion in the presence of cyclosporin (Fig. 46.8). Cyclosporin does not totally prevent activation of the IL-2 receptor gene and does not completely interfere with IL-2 receptor expression on the surface of antigen-stimulated T cells. Its primary action is to block the activation of the c-myc gene and the IL-2 and other lymphokine genes so that c-myc- and IL-2-encoding mRNA is not transcribed and IL-2 is not secreted (Granelli-Piperno *et al*. 1984) In the absence of IL-2, T cells are arrested in the G_{1b} cell cycle phase and do not proliferate, macrophage-activating IFN-γ is not released, B cell activating factors are not released, and the events of T cell activation are sharply curtailed. The c-myc gene product is vital for progression of proliferating cells from the G_{1b} into the DNA synthetic phase of the cell cycle. Thus, blockade of c-myc transcription arrests T cell activation at the G_{1b} phase of the cell cycle. It now appears likely that cyclosporin blocks activation of these T cell activation genes by inactivating cyclosphilin — an enzyme with peptidyl-propyl isomerase activity that alters the conformation of various proteins. The mechanism by which inhibition of cyclophilin leads to a failure to transcribe the c-myc and various cytokine genes remains uncertain; however, I will suggest that the isomerase proves to be

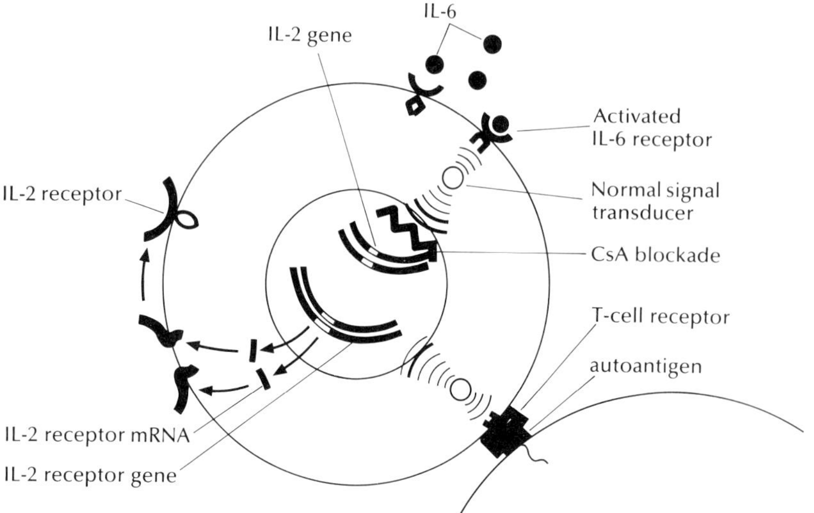

Fig. 46.8. Cyclosporin blocks activation of the IL-2 and other lymphokine genes. CsA: cyclosporin.

important in properly folding a transcriptional factor important in activation of these various genes. Cyclosporin is probably the most powerful of the available drugs used to prevent rejection, with the best risk–benefit ratio.

FK-506, an experimental drug of considerable promise, appears to block activation of T cell activation genes in an inhibitory effect upon another peptidyl-propyl isomerase. This agent, which appears to block *in vitro* T cell activation at lower concentrations than cyclosporin, may prove to have a 'larger therapeutic window' than cyclosporin.

It is ironic that nephrotoxicity should be a major side effect of cyclosporin because the clinical features distinguishing cyclosporin kidney toxicity from other causes of graft dysfunction are not clearly established. Signs of rejection, such as an increase in serum creatinine level or oliguria, may be due to cyclosporin toxicity, too, making the diagnosis difficult, even with biopsy, in so far as rejection and drug toxicity can coexist. Concern about the potentiation of early acute nephrotoxicity by cyclosporin has led to the development of regimens that avoid its use in the first few days after transplantation, and the use of other strong immunosuppressive agents such as monoclonal or polyclonal anti-thymocyte/lymphocyte globulin to supplement immunosuppression in the immediate post-transplant period (Hourmant *et al*. 1985).

Individual patients have remarkably different pharmacokinetic profiles after cyclosporin administration. Further definition of this variability, with the assessment of each patient's pharmacokinetic profile at the time of transplantation, might considerably improve this agent's risk–benefit ratio. A more fundamental hope is that a non-nephrotoxic derivative may soon be produced. However, initial concern about the delayed severe kidney damage and extreme hypertension caused by cyclosporin has been alleviated by the gradual recognition that major reductions in cyclosporin dosage still provide excellent immunosuppression during the post-transplant months (Table 46.3) (see also Chapter 51).

Multiple drug protocols

A regimen of azathioprine and corticosteroids in combination was the standard treatment for recipients of organ allograft prior to the introduction of cyclosporin. The widespread use of cyclosporin

Table 46.3. Cyclosporin in immunosuppression

Mode of action	Side-effects
Blocks activation of the IL-2 gene	Nephrotoxicity
Blocks activation of the c-myc gene	Hepatotoxicity
Inhibits proliferation of T cells	Hyperkalaemia
Prevents IFN-γ release	Hypertension
Prevents release of B cell activating factors	Hirsutism
	Breast fibroadenomas
	Gingival hypertrophy
	Increased susceptibility to infection
	Tremors of seizures

has significantly improved both patient and graft survival; however, nephrotoxicity and the occurrence of rejection episodes remain drawbacks when high-dose cyclosporin is used as the sole drug. Although cyclosporin alone has been used with modest success in Europe, the results have not been as good in the United States. Accordingly most European and North American transplant centres have evolved protocols using various combinations of drugs to reduce adverse drug reactions while maintaining improved patient and graft survival.

To date, almost all such protocols have included adjunctive steroid treatment. Corticosteroids appear to provide a synergistic effect with cyclosporin, and this double drug regimen allows frequent kidney engraftment to patients who are HLA-mismatched, are strong immune-responders or have received no pre-transplantation transfusions.

Different schedules of cyclosporin, corticosteroids and/or azathioprine have been adopted to reduce the potential cyclosporin-induced nephrotoxicity (Simmons *et al*. 1985). Each of the drugs blocks T cell proliferation, albeit at a slightly different step in the activation cascade. For that reason, triple drug therapy protocols may provide more effective immunosuppression than double drug protocols. Further, the complications associated with any one drug could be minimized or even avoided in protocols employing lower doses of all three drugs. One practical advantage of triple drug therapy is that it permits more flexible immunosuppression. The dosage of the individual components can be altered to minimize complications or adverse effects (e.g. leucopenia, cyclosporin-induced nephrotoxicity, liver dysfunction) while maintaining adequate overall immunosuppression. Long-term studies are needed to evaluate multiple drug protocols and to determine the optimal dosages.

Despite the encouraging results achieved thus far with multiple drug protocols, the shortcomings of current conventional immunosuppressive regimens cannot be ignored. These agents exert potent side-effects on non-lymphoid tissues. They impair the function of all T cells, not only the small proportion of donor or sensitized T cells that mediate rejection; infection, therefore, remains a hazard. The well-documented modest increase in certain malignancies (Penn 1978, 1987) remains a valid concern, but no one agent seems to produce a particular predisposition to malignancies. The magnitude of overall immunosuppression and the presence of Epstein–Barr virus infection are important in predisposing certain recipients to malignant disease processes.

Toward selective immunosuppression

Polyclonal immune globulins

Polyclonal antilymphocyte globulin (ALG) or antithymocyte globulin (ATG) preparations, available for use in organ transplantation since the 1960s, have proved to be more effective than steroids alone for reversing acute renal allograft rejection (Burdick 1986; Cosimi and Delmonico 1986). Such polyclonal immune globulins are obtained by immunizing animals (e.g. horses, rabbits) with human lymphoid cells (e.g. B cell lymphoblasts, peripheral T cell lymphocytes or thymus lymphocytes), and then separating the resulting immune sera to obtain purified gamma globulin fractions.

Many types of cells have been evaluated as immunogens. Cultured lymphoblasts (to produce ALG) and human thymocytes (to produce ATG) are commonly used (Table 46.4). Cultured lymphoblasts are readily available, and are free of contaminating blood cells and stromal tissue, which could otherwise stimulate the production of many unwanted antibodies. One possible disadvantage of cultured lymphoblasts arises from the fact that lymphoblasts are B cells rather than T cells (Burdick 1986; Cosimi and Delmonico 1986). Human thymus tissue, an excellent source of T cell antigens,

Table 46.4. Polyclonal immune globulins in immunosuppression

Mode of action	Side-effects
Clearance of lymphocytes due to reticuloendothelial uptake	Thrombocytopenia, granulocytopenia
Complement-mediated lysis of lymphocytes	Antigen–antibody-induced glomerulonephritis
Blocking of lymphocyte function	Complex-mediated hypersensitivity (serum sickness)
Possible expansion of suppressor cell populations	Leucopenia
	Increased susceptibility to infection
	Fever, chills

may not always be available in adequate amounts. With thymus cell preparations, absorption of anti-erythrocyte and anti-platelet antibodies is required, yielding relatively pure anti-sera. Polyclonal immune globulins represent a heterogeneous group of antibodies, only a minority of which are specific to T cells. Non-T-cell-specific antibodies, in fact, account for the greatest binding activity of these preparations; some of them may react inappropriately with B cells and/or non-lymphoid tissue, even following absorption procedures to remove unwanted antibodies.

There are several possible mechanisms by which polyclonal immune globulin may exert its immunosuppressive effect. These include classic complement-mediated lysis of lymphocytes, opsonization of lymphocytes, expansion of suppressor cell populations, or the masking of functionally important T cell surface antigens, which may result in the blocking of lymphocyte function. T-cell-specific antibodies bind to lymphocytes, and this usually results in a prompt and profound lymphopenia. Following cessation of treatment, lymphopenia soon abates, and the number of circulating T cells gradually increases, although the proliferative response of T cells continues to be impaired. In short, the resolution of cell-mediated graft rejection results from the elimination of circulating T cells, and the subsequent positive inhibition of proliferative responses maintains the immunosuppressive effect (Burdick 1986; Cosimi and Delmonico 1986).

Each polyclonal immune globulin preparation varies in its constituent antibodies. Due to the unpredictable nature of the antibody mixture, treatment is associated with variable efficacy as well as with adverse reactions. Batch standardization and assessments of immunosuppressive potency are therefore difficult. Unwanted antibodies can cause thrombocytopenia, granulocytopenia, serum sickness or glomerulonephritis. Owing to the development of host antibodies to the polyclonal immune globulin, anaphylactoid reactions are common (Burdick 1986; Cosimi and Delmonico 1986).

One early concern focuses on the potential for over-immunosuppression, not infrequently resulting in opportunistic infections. Caution is necessary when combining ATG with other immunosuppressive agents. The risk of over-immunosuppression has been related to the dosage and duration of therapy rather than the specific polyclonal immune globulin selected for treatment. If the effect on T cell levels is monitored, the dosage can be altered and the agent administered every other, or every third, day instead of daily, to achieve a level of T cells roughly 10% of that pre-treatment. The total treatment period for ATG is usually 10–14 days, antibody formation against the foreign protein being the limiting factor. It is prudent to administer polyclonal immune globulin through a central catheter because ATG tends to have an irritative sclerosing effect on peripheral veins. Intermittent fever, chills and rash are ameliorated with administration of acetaminophen and diphenhydramine. Anaphylactic shock may have occurred in a few cases due to the formation of xenogeneic serum protein antibodies, but this is extremely rare.

Recent studies have demonstrated: a 10–15% improvement in renal graft survival with polyclonal immune globulin prophylaxis compared with conventional immunosuppression; that prophylactic use may reduce the number and severity of rejection episodes; and that those which do occur may be delayed and may be more easily reversible. In addition, polyclonal immune globulin is used at certain transplant centres during the initial period after allografting, before administration of cyclosporin is begun, in an effort to avoid early post-transplant nephrotoxicity without sacrificing protection from rejection (Hourmant *et al*. 1985).

Monoclonal antibodies (see also Chapter 47)

Monoclonal antibodies hold great promise for a more sophisticated approach to immunosuppressive protocols. The constant domains of the T cell antigen receptor–CD3 complex can now be directly targeted for therapy by the use of monoclonal antibodies. An early objective was to develop a pan-T cell monoclonal antibody that would function in the same way as a polyclonal antibody. However, the OKT3 monoclonal antibody does not remove all T cells, although it has been found to block T cell function by specific interaction with molecules of the T cell receptor–CD3 complex (Goldstein 1987a, b). To date, OKT3 is the only commercially available monoclonal antibody for therapeutic use.

Six non-covalently linked T cell surface proteins

constitute the T cell antigen recognition complex (Weiss *et al.* 1985, 1986; Kronenberg *et al.* 1986). These six proteins are expressed on essentially every functionally active T cell. The alpha and beta chains are the antigen-binding proteins; their distal portions are unique and complementary for each antigen. As noted previously, the other four CD3 proteins appear to play a key role in transducing signals from the antigen-binding alpha and beta chains to the interior of the T cell (Weiss *et al.* 1985; Kronenberg *et al.* 1986). OKT3 antibody binds to a T-cell-specific 20 kD CD3 molecule. Hence, OKT3 binds to a constant or non-varying component of the T cell antigen recognition complex. Immunosuppression with OKT3 monoclonal antibody blocks cytotoxic T-lymphocyte-mediated cell lysis and other T cell functions (Van Wauwe *et al.* 1980; Landegran *et al.* 1982).

The clone that generated OKT3 was produced by sensitizing a mouse with human T lymphocytes, and then fusing the mouse's spleen cells with mouse myeloma cells to immortalize them. The resulting hybridomas were screened to select those producing the desired antibody — in this case, one uniquely reactive against a specific target site on human T cells. The hybridoma was then cloned to produce a strain of cells that produce a monoclonal antibody directed only against CD3. Because the stable hybridomas can provide a virtually limitless supply of specific antibodies that can be purified to complete homogeneity, the biological variability that complicates the use of polyclonal antibodies is eliminated.

Whenever allograft rejection occurs despite maintenance drug therapy, OKT3 is remarkably effective in reversing cellular rejection (Goldstein 1987a). When this agent binds to the T cell antigen recognition complex, each of the latter's six proteins is stripped from the cell surface, either by shedding or by internalization. OKT3-treated T cells therefore become literally blinded to the antigens of the allograft, and the rejection process comes to a halt. Other monoclonal antibodies that react with T cells and cause their removal from the circulation have not yielded comparable rejection reversal rates (Goldstein 1987b). Although OKT3 is a potent T cell mitogen (Chang *et al.* 1981) in short-term cultures, it blocks all known T cell functions *in vivo*. The advent of the pan-T cell monoclonal antibody OKT3 therefore represents an important refinement in therapy, for the broad reactivity of conventional drugs with non-lymphoid tissues has been avoided.

The efficacy and safety of OKT3 as therapy for acute renal allograft rejection is substantiated by the results of controlled trials and widespread clinical experience. In a major, randomized, multicentre trial in the United States, it was shown that acute rejection episodes in cadaveric renal transplants were reversed in 94% of cases with OKT3, compared with a 75% reversal with conventional high-dose corticosteroid treatment ($p = 0.009$) (Ortho Multicenter Transplant Study Group 1985). This difference in efficacy was reflected in a 17% greater graft survival 1 year after transplantation in patients treated with OKT3 than in those treated with high-dose steroids (Ortho Multicenter Transplant Study Group 1985).

OKT3 therapy is not without adverse effects (Table 46.5). Nearly all patients develop severe flu-like symptoms following administration of the first or second dose, consisting of fever, shaking and chills and which may include nausea, vomiting, diarrhoea, headache, anorexia and weakness. These symptoms are likely to be due to an effect on T cells, for they are not seen once the CD3 antigen has been capped (Ortho Multicenter Transplant Study Group 1985). It is now certain that these effects are related to the transient mitogen-like properties of OKT3 and directly linked to the capacity of the agent to provoke cytokine release. Adverse reactions may be dampened by the administration of corticosteroids with the first dose, and this is now done routinely. However, because of the severity of these symptoms, and because some patients become hypotensive

Table 46.5. OKT3 monoclonal antibody in immunosuppression

Mode of action	Side-effects
Clearance of T lymphocytes due to reticuloendothelial uptake	Influenza-like symptoms following administration of first or second dose
Blocks T cell effector function	Fever, chills, tremors, headache
Modulation of antigen receptor–CD3 molecular complex	Respiratory symptoms (i.e. dyspnoea)
Postulated to block sessile T cells in the allograft	Increased susceptibility to infection
	Hypotension

because of diarrhoea and vasodilation, patients should be monitored carefully in the hospital during the first 2 or 3 days of therapy. As with polyclonal antibody, the period of treatment is limited by the formation of neutralizing anti-mouse antibodies. One precaution that must be carefully observed is that the patient is not volume-overloaded prior to the initiation of OKT3 therapy. Owing to a capillary leak syndrome produced by OKT3, severe pulmonary oedema has been reported in patients who were volume-overloaded prior to the first injection of OKT3.

Currently, there are multicentre trials under way to assess the use of OKT3 perioperatively. The objective of these studies is to determine whether OKT3 may be used prophylactically, instead of polyclonal ATG, to delay the initiation of cyclosporin therapy. The approach uses OKT3 to provide a window of immunosuppression until graft function is established, followed by the introduction of cyclosporin into the therapeutic protocol. The results of early trials in allograft recipients are encouraging; however, long-term follow-up is needed.

Experimental solutions

The ideal goal of blocking the activities of only those T cell clones that recognize the allograft could be realized by breaking the lock-and-key arrangement that intimately engages the graft antigens with those T cells bearing receptors that recognize them. This approach would be ideal because the overwhelming majority of immune cells involved in protective host defence mechanisms would not be targeted, and undesirable broad or pan-immunosuppression would be avoided. In theory, a perfect solution would be obtained by developing antibodies that react with the antigen-combining site of T cell antigen receptors for donor graft antigens. However, this has been confounded, at least temporarily, by the great genetic diversity of the HLA system, as well as by the substantive genetic repertoire of the T cell receptor for antigen. As predicted by knowledge of the extensive gene shuffling rearrangements of the T cell receptor, at least 1 million forms of this receptor exist. Clearly, too many reagents would be required to bring about clone-specific immunosuppressive therapy.

If the antigen-binding domains of individual T cell receptors cannot be easily targeted, can other structures be used to target selectively the small population of T cells actually engaged in rejection? Activated T cells express a variety of plasma membrane receptors that are absent from the surface of resting cells. One of these receptors, the IL-2 receptor, is not found on non-lymphoid tissues. One approach therefore being explored is to target IL-2 receptor +ve cells, as only newly activated cells bear this important protein. The IL-2 receptor is only transiently expressed during the brief proliferative burst of lymphocytes triggered in response to antigen. As the receptor is not expressed on either resting or long-term memory cells, it was postulated that administration of anti-IL-2 receptor monoclonal antibodies in the early post-transplant period might provide selective immunosuppression. Could a single antibody directed against a receptor protein expressed in the common pathway of T cell activation be used in every recipient and donor combination?

In the mouse model, cardiac grafts transplanted across major transplantation barriers are permanently engrafted following a 10-day course of rat anti-mouse anti-IL-2 receptor monoclonal antibody (Kirkman *et al.* 1985a). Even delayed application of the antibody can totally reverse ongoing cardiac graft rejection (Kirkman *et al.* 1985b). Dramatic effects have also been noted with mouse anti-rat antibodies in a rat heart transplant model (Kupiec-Weglinski *et al.* 1986). Despite cessation of therapy, graft rejection does not occur. Passive transfer experiments indicate that, while donor-specific alloreactive helper cells are destroyed (Kupiec-Weglinski *et al.* 1987), donor-specific suppressor T cells (Kupiec-Weglinski *et al.* 1986) are spared the effects of activated IL-2 receptor-directed therapy. These data demonstrate the significance of activated IL-2 receptor-bearing lymphocytes in graft rejection. In several models, the combined effects of anti-IL-2 receptor antibody and cyclosporin have been found to be synergistic. Early clinical experience with anti-IL-2 receptor monoclonal antibodies is highly promising (Soulillou *et al.* 1987; Cantorovich *et al.* 1989; Kirkman *et al.* 1989).

Other future prospects

It is to be hoped that the future of immunosuppressant therapy will include the development of additional monoclonal antibodies, or other T-cell-specific 'magic bullets' of low toxicity. For example, it may be possible to use genetic engineering strategies to produce 'fully' humanized anti-T cell monoclonal antibodies or to target the IL-2 receptor with IL-2 toxin fusion proteins. The great variety of agents and of the antigens against which they can be directed renders this a promising but complex field for investigation over the next few years.

References

Almawi, W.Y., Lipman, M.L., Stevens, A.C., Zanker, B., Hadro, E.T. and Strom, T.B. (1991). Abrogation of glucocorticoid-mediated inhibition of T cell proliferation by the synergistic action of IL-1, IL-6, and IFN-gamma. *J. Immunol.* **146**, 3523–7.

Auron, P.E., Warner, S.N. *et al.* (1987). Studies on the molecular nature of human interleukin-2. *J. Immunol.* **138**, 1447–56.

Bach, J.F. and Strom, T.B. (1986). *The Mode of Action of Immunosuppressive Agents*, 2nd edn., pp. 105–58. Elsevier, Amsterdam.

Burdick, J.F. (1986). The biology of immunosuppression mediated by antilymphocyte antibodies. In *Kidney Transplant Rejection: Diagnosis and Treatment*, ed. G.M. Williams, J.F. Burdick and K. Solez, pp. 307–10, Marcel Decker, New York.

Cantrell, P.A. and Smith, K.A. (1984). The interleukin-2 T cell system: a new cell growth model. *Science* **224**, 1312.

Cantarovich, D., LeMauff, J., Hourmant, M. *et al.* (1989). Anti-IL-2 receptor monoclonal antibody (33B3.1) in prophylaxis of early kidney rejection in humans: a randomized trial vs. rabbit antithymocyte globulin. *Transplant. Proc.* **21**, 1769–71.

Chang, T.W., Kung, P.C., Gingras, S.P. *et al.* (1981). Does OKT3 monoclonal antibody react with an antigen-recognition structure on human T cells? *Proc. Nat. Acad. Sci. (USA)* **78**, 1805–8.

Clevers, H., Alarcon, B., Wileman, T. *et al.* (1988). The T-cell receptor/CD3 complex: a dynamic protein ensemble. *Ann. Rev. Immunol.* **6**, 629–62.

Cosimi, A.B. and Delmonico, F.L. (1986). Antilymphocyte antibody immunosuppressive therapy. In *Kidney Transplant Rejection: Diagnosis and Treatment*, ed. G.M. Williams, J.F. Burdick and K. Solez, pp. 335–41, Marcel Decker, New York.

Crabtree, G.R. (1989). Contingent genetic regulatory events in T lymphocyte activation. *Science* **243**, 355–63.

Farrar, W.L., Johnson, H.M. and Farrar, J.J. (1981). Regulation of the production of immune interferon and cytotoxic T lymphocytes by interleukin-2. *J. Immunol.* **126**, 1120–5.

Gardner, P. (1989). Calcium and T lymphocyte activation. *Cell* **59**, 15–20.

Goldstein, G. (ed.) (1987a). Therapeutic use of the monoclonal antibody Orthoclone OKT3. *Transplant. Proc.* **19** (suppl. 1), 1–57.

Goldstein, G. (ed.) (1987b). Overview of the development of Orthoclone OKT3: monoclonal antibody for therapeutic use in transplantation. *Transplant. Proc.* **19** (suppl. 1), 1–6.

Granelli-Piperno, A., Inaba, K. and Steinman, R.M. (1984). Stimulation of lymphokine release from T lymphoblasts: requirement for mRNA synthesis and inhibition by cyclosporin A. *J. Exp. Med.* **160**, 1792–802.

Hourmant, M., Soulillou, J.P., Remi, J.P. *et al.* (1985). Use of cyclosporin A after antilymphocyte serum in renal transplantation. *Presse Med.* **145**, 2093–6.

Howard, M., Matis, L, Malek, T.R. *et al.* (1983). Interleukin-2 induces antigen-reactive T cell lines to secrete BCGF-1. *J. Exp. Med.* **158**, 2024–39.

Inaba, K., Granelli-Piperno, A. and Steinman, R.M. (1983). Dendritic cells induce T lymphocytes to release B cell-stimulating factors by an interleukin-2 dependent mechanism. *J. Exp. Med.* **158**, 2040–57.

Kahan, B.D. (1984). Immunopharmacodynamic evaluation of cyclosporine-treated renal allograft recipients. *Transplantation* **38**, 657–64.

Kelley, V.E., Fiers, W. and Strom, T.B. (1984). Cloned human interferon-gamma, but not interferon-beta or -alpha, induces expression of HLA-DR determinants by fetal monocytes and myeloid leukemic cell lines. *J. Immunol.* **132**, 240–5.

Kirkman, R.L., Barret, L.V. *et al.* (1985a). Administration of an anti-interleukin-2 receptor monoclonal antibody prolongs cardiac allograft survival in mice. *J. Exp. Med.* **162**, 358–62.

Kirkman, R.L., Barret, L.V. *et al.* (1985b). The effect of anti-interleukin-2 receptor monoclonal antibody on allograft rejection. *Transplantation* **40**, 719–22.

Kirkman, R.L., Shapiro, M.E., Carpenter, C.B. *et al.* (1991). A randomized prospective trial of anti-Tac monoclonal antibody in human renal transplantation. *Transplantation* **51**, 107–13.

Knudsen, P.J., Dinarello, C.A. and Strom, T.B. (1987). Glucocorticoids inhibit transcription and post-transcriptional expression of interleukin-1. *J. Immunol.* **139**, 4129–34.

Kronenberg, M., Siu G., Hood, L.E. *et al.* (1986). The molecular genetics of the T cell antigen receptor and T cell antigen recognition. *Ann. Rev. Immunol.* **4**, 593–621.

Kupiec-Weglinski, J.W., Diamantstein, T., Tilney, N.L. *et al.* (1986). Therapy with monoclonal antibody to interleukin-2 receptor spares suppressor T cells and prevents or reverses acute allograft rejection in rats. *Proc. Nat. Acad. Sci. (USA)* **83**, 2624–7.

Kupiec-Weglinski, J.W., Padberg, W. *et al.* (1987). Selective immunosuppression with anti-interleukin-2 receptor targeted therapy: helper and suppressor cell activity in rat recipients of cardiac allografts. *Eur. J. Immunol.* **17**, 313–19.

Landegran, U., Ranstedt, U., Axberg, I. *et al.* (1982). Selective inhibition of human T cell cytotoxicity at levels of target recognition or initiation of lysis by monoclonal OKT3 and leu IIa antibodies. *J. Exp. Med.* **155**, 1579–684.

Maddock, E.O., Maddock, S.W., Kelley, V.E. *et al.* (1985). Rapid stereospecific stimulation of lymphocyte metabolism by interleukin-2. *J. Immunol.* **135**, 4004–8.

Meuer, S.C., Hussey, R.E., Cantrell, D.A. *et al.* (1984). Triggering of the T3–T1 antigen-receptor complex results in clonal T cell proliferation through an interleukin-2 dependent autocrine pathway. *Proc. Nat. Acad. Sci. (USA)* **81**, 1509–13.

Nisbet-Brown, E., Cheung, R.K. and Grinstein, S. (1985). Antigen-dependent increase in cytosolic free calcium in specific human T-lymphocyte clones. *Nature* **316**, 545–7.

Ortho Multicentre Transplant Study Group (1985). A randomized clinical trial of Orthoclone OKT3 monoclonal antibody for acute rejection of cadaveric renal transplants. *N. Engl. J. Med.* **313**, 337–42.

Pankewycz, O.G., Yui, M., Kelley, V.E. and Strom, T.B. (1990). The cascading interrelated roles of interleukin-1, interleukin-2, and interleukin-6 in anti-CD3 driven T-cell proliferation. *Clin. Immunol. Immunopath.* **55**, 67–85.

Penn, I. (1978). Malignancies associated with immunosuppressive or cytotoxic therapy. *Surgery* **83**, 492.

Penn, I. (1987). Cancers following cyclosporine therapy. *Transplantation* **43**, 32–5.

Pober, I.S., Gimbrone, M.A., Cotran, R.S. *et al.* (1983). Ia expression by vascular endothelium is inducible by activated T cells and by human gamma interferon. *J. Exp. Med.* **157**, 1339.

Shapiro, D.N., Adams, B.J. and Niederhaber, J.E. (1985). Antigen specific T cell activation results in an increase in cytosolic free calcium. *J. Immunol.* **135**, 2256–61.

Simmons, R.L., Canafax, D.M., Strand, M. *et al.* (1985). Management and prevention of cyclosporine nephrotoxicity after renal transplantation: use of low doses of cyclosporine, azathioprine, and prednisone. *Transplant. Proc.* **17** (suppl. 1), 266–75.

Soulillou, J.P., Peyronnet, P., LeMauff, J. *et al.* (1987). Prevention of rejection of kidney transplant by monoclonal antibody directed against interleukin-2 (receptors). *Lancet* **i**, 1339–42.

Strom, T.B. (1984). Immunosuppressive agents in renal transplantation. *Kidney Int.* **26**, 353–65.

Tilney, N.L., Strom, T.B., Vineyard, G.C. and Merrill, J.P. (1978). Factors contributing to the declining mortality rate in renal transplantation. *N. Eng. J. Med.* **299**, 1321–5.

Van Wauwe, J.P., DeMey, J.R. and Grossend, J.G. (1980). A monoclonal anti-human T lymphocyte antibody with potent mitogenic properties. *J. Immunol.* **124**, 2708.

Weiss, A., Imboden, J. *et al.* (1985). The role of T3 antigen/receptor complex in T cell activation. *Ann. Rev. Immunol.* **4**, 593–620.

Williams, J.M., Loertscher, R., Cotner, T. *et al.* (1984). Dual parameter flow cytometric analysis of DNA content, activation antigen expression, and T cell subset proliferation in the human mixed lymphocyte reaction. *J. Immunol.* **132**, 2330–7.

Williams, J.M., DeLoria, D., Hansen, J.A. *et al.* (1985). The events of primary T cell activation can be staged by use of Sepharose-bound anti-T3 (64.1) monoclonal antibody and purified interleukin-1. *J. Immunol.* **135**, 2249–55.

Ythier, A.A., Abbud-Filho, M., Williams, J.M. *et al.* (1985). Interleukin-2-dependent release of interleukin-3 activity by T4 human T-cell clones. *Proc. Nat. Acad. Sci. (USA)* **82**, 7020–4.

Zanker, B., Walz, G., Wieder, K.J. *et al.* (1990). Evidence that glucocorticosteroids block expression of human interleukin-6 gene by accessory cells. *Transplantation* **49**, 198–201.

47: Monoclonal Antibodies as Immunosuppressive Agents

H. Waldmann

Introduction

It is fair to say that virtually all immune responses depend on collaboration between lymphocytes. T lymphocytes (T cells) are necessary participants in these collaborative events. This is true for protective responses to foreign antigens, as well as for the destructive reponses that can inflict damage on body tissues. For successful transplantation of a foreign organ and bone marrow grafts, and for reversal of autoimmune diseases, one would like to control those T cells responsible for the damage, without penalizing the whole immune system. Current immunosuppressive strategies interfere with the function of the whole immune system, rely on long-term drug administration and risk infection and drug toxicity. There is therefore a need for a more sophisticated approach to immunosuppression.

The special attraction of monoclonal antibodies is that their target antigens can be so precisely defined and that one should be able to target the cells of choice, with minimal toxicity. As T cells need to collaborate with many other cell types in order for the immune system to operate, interruption of those collaborative events should result in therapeutic immunosuppression (Waldmann 1989). The drawback of antibodies as immunosuppressants is that they have to be given systemically. At best, therefore, they can only be considered for short courses of therapy. That may be sufficient in allogeneic bone marrow transplantation (BMT), where depletion of T cells from donor marrow and from recipient as a one-off may be all that is necessary for control of graft-versus-host disease (GVHD) and marrow rejection (Waldmann *et al.* 1990a). It is not obvious, however, that one-off treatments would be sufficient to prevent organ graft rejection or induce prolonged remissions in diseases like rheumatoid arthritis or multiple sclerosis, unless used to enhance the benefits of other immunosuppressive drugs. It is not obvious because we tend to assume that the adult immune system is not capable of contributing to the immunosuppressive process in its own right. If we knew that it could, and if we understood the mechanisms by which it did so, then short-term therapies designed to activate those mechanisms would be appropriate.

I propose, in this chapter, to discuss the experimental basis for short-term antibody therapy as a novel way to achieve antigen-specific long-term immunosuppression. Operationally, that is the same as achieving immunological tolerance (Cobbold *et al.* 1990a; Qin *et al.* 1990). I will review experimental studies in rodents that show that an adult animal with a mature immune system can be tolerized to a range of foreign antigens. I will then discuss the mechanisms by which antibodies could both induce and maintain the tolerant state. Finally, I will briefly consider the present position and future prospects of tolerance therapy in man.

Guidance of an adult immune system towards tolerance

I here summarize experiments that demonstrate the ease with which the immune system of a mouse can be tolerized to simple proteins and skin, heart and bone marrow grafts. These studies were initiated to look at the long-term effects of single short-term courses of therapy with immunosuppressive antibodies. As CD4 monoclonal antibodies proved to be amongst the most effective (Cobbold *et al.* 1984, 1986a, b; Cobbold and Waldmann 1986), most of the discussion below concerns them.

Tolerance to a simple protein antigen

Mice injected with the foreign protein antigen HGG, under the umbrella of CD4 monoclonal antibody therapy, became tolerant of that antigen (Benjamin and Waldmann 1986; Benjamin *et al.* 1986, 1988; Gutstein *et al.* 1986; Qin *et al.* 1987, 1990; Carteron *et al.* 1988) while remaining responsive to other antigens. Tolerant animals remained unresponsive to HGG for at least 4 months. Further injections of HGG given before tolerance had been lost extended the tolerant state indefinitely. Clearly, whereas antibody therapy had induced the tolerant state, antigen was necessary to maintain it. In the absence of antigen, tolerance was lost as new T cells from the thymus replaced those in the periphery.

In order to get an understanding of the possible mechanisms involved, it is worth considering the following features of the model:

1 Both antigen (HGG) and the CD4 monoclonal antibody had to be injected within a limited time frame of each other (i.e. antigen had to be given under the antibody umbrella). Neither was sufficient alone.

2 Loss of tolerance with time was due to the disappearance of antigen from the animal and the export of fresh T cells from the thymus (Qin *et al.* 1990).

3 Tolerance could be induced in mice whose thymus had been removed in adult life, and could therefore be truly classified as peripheral in nature (Qin *et al.* 1990).

4 CD8 T cells were not required at any stage in the induction, maintenance or expression of tolerance.

5 T cell depletion was not necessary, as tolerance could be elicited with fragments or non-depleting subclasses of the CD4 antibody.

6 Adoptive transfer studies of tolerant cells into fresh hosts showed that the CD4 T cells had become tolerized (Benjamin *et al.* 1988).

7 Tolerance could not be broken by the injection of naïve T cells. However, depletion of host CD4 T cells abrogated that resistant state, showing that host CD4 T cells were responsible for resistance. As resistance seems to be a common feature of antibody-induced tolerance (see later), we conclude that it probably plays a critical role in maintaining the tolerant state.

Tolerance to tissue grafts

We reasoned that, if, once induced, tolerance could be maintained by persistent antigen, then tissue allografts and autoantigens ought to be able to provide that persistent antigen once tolerance had been generated. By combining CD4 and CD8 monoclonal antibodies, we have demonstrated that tolerance can be easily induced to skin and bone marrow grafts that differ from the recipient in multiple minor antigens (Qin *et al.* 1989, 1990). T cell depletion is not required. We have observed that tolerance, once induced, is permanent, requiring no further extrinsic antigen to maintain it. It is interesting to note that, although the recipient seems to be tolerant from the outset, the recipient T cells may not become tolerant for some time. In a skin graft model Qin *et al.* (in preparation) have shown that, although tolerance can be induced with only a week of non-depleting antibody therapy, T cells do not become fully tolerant until at least 4 weeks after therapy has been terminated. This tends to rule out explanations such as negative signalling via CD4, because any such signalling should be maximal in the period of antibody therapy. We favour the explanation that the immune system takes time to be guided into tolerance. It may be that this is the time required for resistance to develop.

Tolerance to skin grafts is accompanied by a state of antigen-specific resistance, in that normal spleen cells from an immunocompetent donor are unable to break the tolerance to the inducing graft, although they will reject a third-party graft. As before, resistance is determined by recipient T cells, and can be abrogated by knocking out host T-cells with depleting antibodies (Qin *et al.* 1992, in preparation).

In order to determine the fate of transfused T-cells that failed to break tolerance, we looked at the consequences of mixing normal T cells with 'marked' tolerant T cells within the tolerant host. We observed that coexistence of normal T cells with tolerant T cells within the skin-graft-tolerant host results in the normal T cells themselves becoming tolerant (Qin *et al.* 1992). Not only is tolerance infectious, but so is resistance, as the originally normal T cells in turn resist fresh infusions of naïve T cells. This clearly demonstrates the pervasiveness and apparent infectivity of the tolerant state. All the phenomena outlined, namely tolerance induction, maintenance, resistance and infectious tolerance, seem to be generated in the peripheral T cell system, as all are demonstrable in adult-thymectomized mice (Qin *et al.* 1992).

We can now propose an explanation of how peripheral tolerance can be maintained, once it has been induced. We suggest that the first cohort of tolerant T cells is used to educate or influence subsequent cohorts emerging from the thymus, and these too act to educate further cohorts lifelong. As long as antigen is available to bring T cells (both normal and tolerant) to sites of its own (antigen) presentation, tolerance can be organized as an antigen-specific and self-sustaining process.

Tolerance induced in memory cells

Tolerance to skin allografts could also be induced in mice previously primed to the donor minor antigens (Cobbold *et al.* 1990a). The tolerant state generated is sustained long-term even after regrafting, and grafts remain healthy and viable even after prompt rejection of a third-party graft. Again, all this could be brought about with antibodies that were relatively ineffective at T cell depletion. This shows that a sensitized immune system is eminently tolerizable—a point critical to the concept of tolerance therapy in autoimmune disease.

Antibody therapy was also capable of tolerizing mice that were actively rejecting their skin grafts. Again, T cell depletion was not necessary as half the mice became tolerant with non-depleting antibody therapy. However, the best results were achieved with initial debulking of host T cells before the CD4/CD8 antibody therapy began. Under these circumstances, even mice that had rejected their first graft could be rendered tolerant to a second graft (Cobbold *et al.* 1990a).

Tolerance induced across major histocompatibility barriers

We have extended our studies of monoclonal antibody-mediated tolerance to the transplantation of major histocompatibility complex (MHC)-incompatible heart, bone marrow and skin (Cobbold *et al.* 1990a; Chen *et al.* 1992; Leung *et al.* 1992). Tolerance to vascularized heart grafts, both allogeneic and xenogeneic, could be induced by simple low-impact monoclonal antibody therapies (Wood 1990; Chen *et al.* 1992). In contrast, aggressive T-cell-depleting protocols were necessary to guarantee acceptance of MHC-mismatched bone marrow grafts. Transplantation tolerance (i.e. to donor skin) induced by BMT required sufficient donor haemopoietic chimerism (Leung *et al.* 1992). Adequate chimerism could only be achieved by creating haemopoietic space within the bone marrow by agents like dimethyl myeleran (DMM). Non-lethal regimens of conditioning with DMM enabled us to achieve classical-type transplantation tolerance in a number of MHC-incompatible combinations (see also Sykes and Sachs 1990).

Perhaps most difficult of all the transplant systems is that of MHC-mismatched skin. Again, by combining T cell debulking with CD4/CD8 non-depleting monoclonal antibody therapy, it has been possible to achieve tolerance in some, but not all, strain combinations (Cobbold *et al.* 1990a).

From all this we can conclude that the peripheral T cell system of a mouse is tolerizable at all stages of its development (immature, naïve, primed and effector). Short-course one-off therapy has permitted the antigen or graft to induce and sustain a prolonged tolerant state in the immune system. Certain principles of Immunology can be generalized across species. We have no reason to think that the peripheral tolerance mechanisms that we have uncovered are unique to the mouse. If one could understand more about the mechanisms operating, one could hope to harness them for control of human autoimmune disease and transplantation rejection.

Anergic T cells

So far we have not discussed what happens to the tolerized T cells. Do they die or do they become anergic (i.e. alive but impotent (Qin *et al.* 1989, Schwartz 1990))? By use of strain combinations that differed in their expression of Mls alleles (a retroviral-encoded 'self-superantigen'), we were able to follow the fate of a set of T cells bearing well-defined receptors preoccupied with Mls recognition. In a BMT model, we observed tolerance accompanied by persistence of T cells bearing those receptors. The T cells were viable, and yet non-stimulable *in vitro*. In this case, then, tolerance was associated with T cell anergy (Qin *et al.* 1989; Waldmann *et al.* 1990a).

If we assume that T cell recognition of Mls is not, in principle, different from recognition of other antigens, then we would expect that anergy to minor and major transplantation antigens might also underlie T cell tolerance in the various models we have studied. Clonal anergy, like clonal deletion, seems to be a natural mechanism operating in self-tolerance (Morahan *et al.* 1989). We assume that our experimental manipulations with antibodies are not doing something novel to the immune system. Rather, we imagine that we are guiding T cells to take an option naturally open to them.

Possible mechanisms underlying tolerance induced with antibody therapy (Waldmann 1989; Cobbold *et al.* 1990b)

We have proposed that therapy with CD4 and CD8 monoclonal antibodies guides the immune system to tolerance by initially hindering collaborative events between T cells themselves and with other cells (e.g. antigen-presenting cells (APC)). In the absence of collaboration, T cells are somehow directed towards tolerance. We know that process takes time, and must assume that this reflects some aspect of antibody pharmacology, where T cells would not be able to register antigen until their surface CD4 monoclonal antibody had decayed to some critical level. Alternatively, it may have taken time for resistor-type T cells to emerge, and perhaps these cells were responsible for imposing tolerance on any potentially antigen-reactive cells. As anergic T cells possess receptors for antigen and still express the full range of adhesion molecules, what would stop them accumulating at sites of antigen presentation? If they did accumulate at those sites, perhaps they could hinder the formation of useful collaborative units. As impotent contributors within an attempted collaborative unit, they would exhibit their presence as resistor-type cells and ensure that T cell collaborations failed. We have proposed that T cells need collaborations with other T cells to mount any immune response, and to rescue them from tolerance induction by antigen (Waldmann *et al.* 1990b). If anergic cells interfere with collaboration, then so, by default, could they impose tolerance on other uncommitted T cells that bound antigen. Such tolerance would arise by default, i.e. from a T cell contacting antigen but failing to get help.

It could be, however, that anergic cells are irrelevant to the resistance phenomenon and simply represent the garbage or ghosts of tolerogenic encounters. If so, then we are left with T-cell-mediated suppression as the only other explanation for the above data. In that case, we need to understand the mechanism underlying suppression, and in time find simpler routes to harnessing them to achieve tolerance for therapeutic purposes.

Can monoclonal antibodies be used to achieve tolerance in man?

If tolerance therapy were to be applicable to humans, then one would need antibodies that could deplete T cells and T cell subsets; antibodies that could block the functions of those cells; and antibodies that could inactivate APC, say, for example, to reduce the immunogenicity of a transplanted organ. As rodent antibodies are foreign to humans, it is also essential to render them invisible to the human immune system. Antibody engineering to humanize therapeutic antibodies has reduced the risk of immunogenicity (Reichmann *et al.* 1988; Gorman *et al.* 1991; Routledge *et al.* 1991). Having said this, much of the clinical experience with antibodies has been empirical, with monoclonal antibodies being used in addition to available immunosuppressive drugs. It is only in BMT, where antibodies have been used to deplete donor marrow of T cells *ex vivo*, that antibodies have been used to replace conventional immunosuppressants (Waldmann *et al.* 1990a). In this arena, the control of GVHD has been achieved but new problems of marrow rejection and leukaemia relapse have temporarily obviated the benefit.

Antibody selection

EMPIRICISM

For obvious reasons, it has not been easy to get many monoclonal antibodies properly evaluated as therapeutic agents. The production of therapeutic-grade antibody is no simple matter, especially for academic institutions. In order for the pharmaceutical industry to provide antibodies, substantial investment and development time are required, based on very very little preclinical information to minimize risk. Although some monoclonal antibodies to human lymphocyte antigens cross-react with non-human primate cells, the only real test of efficacy is the clinical experiment.

There have been relatively few antibodies evaluated in organ transplantation. Of these, OKT3 has been the most widely used. It has been shown to be effective in reversal of acute cellular rejection episodes (Ortho Multicentre Transplant Study Group 1985; Ponticelli *et al.* 1987; Renlund *et al.* 1989; Chatenoud and Bach 1990; Conti and Cosimi 1990), both as a rescue therapy for patients unresponsive to high-dose steroids and as a first-line treatment. Some studies have suggested value in its use as an additional prophylactic agent given peritransplant (Renlund *et al.* 1989; Chatenoud and Bach 1990). However, OKT3 and other CD3 monoclonal antibodies are potent T-cell-activating agents *in vivo*. In so doing, they activate the release of a variety of cytokines, which can provoke the unacceptable side-effects often seen in the first dose (Chatenoud and Bach 1990). This makes it difficult to dissect the mechanisms relevant to OKT3 therapy. Is activation valuable? Are any of the cytokines contributing to the immunosuppression? We do not know. In addition, OKT3 is a murine antibody and evokes antiglobulin responses in the majority of patients (Chatenoud and Bach 1990; Conti and Cosimi 1990). It should now be the goal, in using any therapeutic antibody, to avoid sensitizing the patient. Therefore, it is probably appropriate that CD3 monoclonal antibodies should be investigated as engineered antibodies with a number of alternative properties:

1 Fully humanized (Routledge *et al.* 1991) to prevent sensitization.

2 Modified to render them more efficient at activating host effector mechanisms (such as complement) to achieve a better T cell kill (Clark *et al.* 1989; Routledge *et al.* 1991).

3 Modified to prevent binding to Fc receptors. This should render them less able to activate T cells and release cytokines, and yet, by binding to CD3, they should still retain their ability to immunosuppress. These ideas are currently being developed in Cambridge and elsewhere.

There has been interest in targeting activated T cells on the argument that these must include the antigen-reactive cohort. The interleukin 2 (IL-2) receptor (IL-2R) is an obvious choice. Rodent studies, using somewhat weak antigenic graft systems (cardiac allografts), suggest that anti-IL-2R antibodies were immunosuppressive and could synergize with cyclosporin A (Kupiec-Weglinski *et al.* 1988). The anti-human IL-2R monoclonal antibodies anti-Tac (murine) (Reed *et al.* 1989) and CAMPATH 6 (rat) (Tighe *et al.* 1988), directed to the 55 kD chain, both prolonged kidney allograft survival in cynomolgus monkeys and baboons respectively. Limited clinical studies using prophylactic IL-2R antibodies have given mixed results. Modest effects were seen with anti-Tac in a small patient group; a randomized study in liver transplant recipients could show no significant benefit from CAMPATH 6 (Friend *et al.* 1991a); but a randomized study by Soulillou and colleagues (1990) suggested that the murine monoclonal antibody 33B3.1 was as effective as antithymocytic globulin (ATG) in the prophylactic regimen. Although one cannot at this stage make a compelling case for a role for naked IL-2R antibodies as immunosuppressants, it is always possible that they could be combined in a synergistic combination with other agents. An alternative way of targeting high-affinity IL-2R through engineered chimeric toxins seems a more promising way to ensure cell destruction (see Chapter 46).

Rather than quoting further examples of antibodies tried in this empirical way, I recommend the reader to the excellent reviews by Conti and Cosimi (1990) and Jonker (1990), which list many of the clinical and non-human primate studies. It may be that the empirical approach will be rewarding in time. However, with the knowledge that we already have about the immune system, it should be possible to investigate antibody immunosuppression in a more rational way.

RATIONAL INTERVENTION

Cell lysis with antibodies

Antibodies can kill cells through activation of the complement system, through binding to Fc receptors on a range of effectors capable of delivering killing signals, and by signalling cells to undergo apoptosis. Some effort has gone into defining the rules underlying complement lysis and Fc receptor binding. Antibody-mediated apoptosis has not yet been exploited in immunosuppression. Surprisingly little is known about the factors that influence the ability of a monoclonal antibody to kill its target cell through determining the natural effector systems. The target antigen seems to be critical in this, and not just on the basis of antigen density. For example, antibodies to CDw52 (the CAMPATH 1™) antigen are very effective at activating lysis by human complement, unlike most other antibodies to T cell surface antigens (Bindon *et al.* 1988, 1990). The CD45 pan-leucocyte antigen is probably expressed at levels equivalent to CAMPATH-1 (Bindon *et al.* 1985), and yet CD45 monoclonal antibodies tend to be poorly complement-lytic. We have suggested that the critical issue might be whether antibody binds close to the cell membrane (Meng-Qi *et al.* 1991), as it is bound to do in the case of CAMPATH-1™. One of the benefits of understanding the constraints to cell lysis will be the possibility of improving antibody therapy to overcome them. For example, we have found that a pair of antibodies to two non-overlapping epitopes of CD45 are very efficient at complement lysis in comparison with the individual parent antibodies (Bindon *et al.* 1985). The synergistic pair have proved effective in purging cadaveric kidneys of passenger leucocytes peritransplant. In a randomized study performed in one centre (Brewer *et al.* 1989), the incidence of acute rejection episodes was substantially reduced (6/36 patients) in the antibody-purged group compared with the group whose kidneys were purged with albumin solution (23/36 patients).

In an equally informative study, we observed that a rat CD3 monoclonal antibody was ineffective at complement lysis. By replacing one of its two light chains with an irrelevant light chain, we produced a univalent monoclonal antibody, capable of activating human complement (Clark *et al.* 1989). A genetically engineered, humanized, univalent version of the same CD3 antibody has a similar capacity to kill T cells with complement (Routledge *et al.* 1991).

There are obviously many other antigen-related factors (modulation, shedding, density, heterogeneity, etc.) that can affect lytic potency. However, the demonstration that a pan-lympocyte monoclonal antibody (CAMPATH-1G) can bring about substantial lymphocyte depletion in humans (Hale *et al.* 1987; Dyer *et al.* 1989; Friend *et al.* 1991b), and its conversion to a humanized form (CAMPATH-1H) (Reichmann *et al.* 1988; Hale *et al.* 1988) should allow evaluation of the potency of immunosuppression achieved by lymphocyte debulking.

Of the antibody-related factors, isotype (class and subclass) is clearly important, as shown in rodent studies (Cobbold *et al.* 1989) and in humans (Dyer *et al.* 1989). For rodent antibodies, there are clear differences in the ability of the various antibody subclasses to activate complement and bind to Fc receptors (Hale *et al.* 1985; Kipps *et al.* 1985; Bruggemann *et al.* 1989). To some extent this is consistent with *in vivo* efficacy (Dyer *et al.* 1989). The human subclasses do exhibit differences *in vitro* (Bruggemann *et al.* 1987; Routledge *et al.* 1991), but there are no data on the ability of the different human subclasses to clear target cells *in vivo*. Such information will not be easily derived, for both logistic and ethical reasons. Recently Isaacs *et al.* (1992) observed that human immunoglobulin G (IgG) subclasses can exploit rodent effector systems *in vivo*. As mouse effector systems are able to use critical motifs on human IgG, it may be possible to define these effector systems more clearly, and in so doing to extrapolate their human counterpart. In addition, it should be possible to monitor the efficacy of any genetically engineered, improved forms.

Although antibody class is important, unique features of individual antibodies are also relevant, in that some antibodies kill better than others of the same isotype. It is not clear what these unique features are.

In summary, individual antibodies to defined cellular antigens vary in their lytic potential. It is a hope of antibody engineering that one could endow the individual monoclonal antibody Fc region with a substantially improved effector function so as to lessen the unique features of monoclonal antibody and target antigen.

Antibodies to block function

As so many antibodies fail to kill cells, one would expect that those binding to critical surface receptors or adhesion molecules should be able to block (or interfere with) function. As already discussed, the hope that blocking antibodies can be used to harness internal regulatory mechanisms for immunosuppression is a real one. As T cells have to migrate extensively in the course of targeting a diseased tissue, there are many adhesion events open to intervention. As T cells need constant inductive encounters with antigen to sustain their involvement in an immune response, intervention at the level of the T cell and the APC could be sufficient to interrupt the process, albeit temporarily. We need to know how crucial any known adhesion interactions of T cells are to the disease process we are interested in. Is there redundancy in the system that would permit other receptor–ligand combinations to replace the one we have interrupted? If we are to interrupt these complex processes with single blocking agents, do we need to create complex multifunctional antibodies that could bind simultaneously to multiple distinct receptors on T cells?

It is encouraging that in non-human primates a prophylactic course of CD54 (intercellular adhesion molecule 1 (ICAM-1)) monoclonal antibody could prolong renal graft survival (Cosimi *et al.* 1990) and that it reversed rejection induced by withdrawal of cyclosporin A. This suggests that ICAM-1 is a critical molecule in the pathogenesis of renal allograft rejection, and that there cannot be too much redundancy to allow other adhesive molecules to replace its role.

There have been many attempts to use CD4 and CD8 monoclonal antibody therapy to simulate the rodent data, without real success so far. It is probably unproductive to speculate as to why tolerance has been so hard to achieve clinically thus far. Rather, I would emphasize the need for a better understanding of the mechanisms underlying tolerance in rodents. In this way, we can aspire to direct therapy to harness such mechanisms in whatever way is necessary.

Antibody therapy in autoimmunity

ANIMAL MODELS

A range of rodent models of autoimmunity have demonstrated that immunosuppressive antibodies given prior to the onset of clinical disease could in turn prevent disease onset. In murine lupus (Wofsy and Seaman 1987; Wofsy and Carteron 1990), therapy could be started after disease onset and still be effective. Resolution once disease has started has not, however, been a universal finding. In most animal models CD4 monoclonal antibodies given alone were effective, although in some cases added CD8 monoclonal antibodies gave an improved therapeutic effect (Kantwerk *et al.* 1987; Hutchings *et al.* 1990). There are now good examples of long-term disease control extending well beyond the period of immunosuppression (Kipps *et al.* 1985; Shizuru *et al.* 1988; Hutchings *et al.* 1992).

Attempts at selective inactivation of T cells have used monoclonal antibodies to IL-2R or to particular T cell receptor (TCR) β chains. In murine experimental allergic encephalomyelitis (EAE) TCR usage was shown to be heavily restricted amongst the pathogenic T cell clones (Acha-Orbea *et al.* 1988), leading to selective ablation of T cells involved. If restricted TCR usage were found in human autoimmunity, then the case for TCR-restricted monoclonal antibodies would be strong. At the time of writing, there is still uncertainty on the issue of restricted TCR usage in the major autoimmune diseases—rheumatoid arthritis, juvenile diabetes or multiple sclerosis.

HUMAN DISEASE

Given the success of antibody therapy in rodent autoimmunity, it is appropriate that clinical studies have been undertaken with T-cell-biased monoclonal antibodies in human autoimmunity. Rheumatoid arthritis, as a common, debilitating disease, where many patients become refractory to conventional therapy, has been an obvious target area. Short-term responses have been documented with a wide selection of antibodies, including CD5-ricin (Byers *et al.* 1989), CAMPATH-6 (anti-IL-2R) (Kyle *et al.* 1989), a range of CD4 monoclonal antibodies (e.g. Herzog *et al.* 1989; Homeff *et al.* 1991) and CAMPATH-1H (J. Isaacs *et al.* in preparation). It is encouraging that monoclonal antibodies can halt active disease, albeit for short periods. For there to be long-term value in such treatment, it is essential that one builds on the present findings to design strategies to achieve longer-term remissions. This may involve antibody combinations, or synergy with other immunosuppressive agents. A good example of long-term benefit from a monoclonal antibody combination has been seen in a patient with a refractory vasculitic disease treated here in Cambridge (Mathieson *et al.* 1990). CAMPATH-1H^{TM} was used to achieve a series of clinical remissions, all short-lived. After the fourth course of CAMPATH-1H^{TM}, the patient was injected with a rat CD4 monoclonal antibody and has remained well for nearly 3 years. Individual patient studies of this kind may be most valuable in designing the best immunosuppressive protocols of the future.

Conclusion

Tolerance therapy (i.e. reprogramming the immune system to induce tolerance) is still some way off, but monoclonal antibodies have provided an impetus for targeting old problems with a plethora of new anti-inflammatory, immunosuppressive antibodies. With the knowledge accumulating from animal studies and from ever-increasing clinical investigations, we can hope to witness a major transformation in the selection of immunosuppressive drugs in the future, where T-cell-directed humanized antibodies will figure prominently.

Acknowledgements

The author acknowledges the support of the Medical Research Council, Arthritis and Rheumatism Council and Gilman Trust. CAMPATH-1 is a trademark of the Wellcome Foundation.

References

Acha-Orbea, H., Mitchell, D., Timmerman, L. *et al.* (1988). Limited heterogeneity of T-cell receptors from lymphocytes mediating autoimmune encephalomyelitis allows specific immune intervention. *Cell* **54**, 263–73.

Benjamin, R.J. and Waldmann, H. (1986). Induction of tolerance by monoclonal antibody therapy. *Nature* **320**, 449.

Benjamin, R.J., Cobbold, S.P., Clark, M.R., Waldmann, H. (1986). Tolerance to rat monoclonal antibodies: implications for serotherapy. *J. Exp. Med.* **163**, 1539–52.

Benjamin, R.J., Qin, S., Wise, M. and Cobbold, S.P., Waldmann, H. (1988). Mechanisms of monoclonal antibody-facilitated tolerance induction: a possible role for the CD4 (L3T4) and CD11a (LFA-1) molecules in self–non-self discrimination. *Eur. J. Immunol.* **18**, 1079–88.

Bindon, C.I., Hale, G., Clark, M.R. and Waldmann, H. (1985). Therapeutic potential of monoclonal antibodies to the human leucocyte common antigen (CD45): synergy and interference in complement-mediated lysis. *Transplantation* **40**, 538–44.

Bindon, C.I., Hale, G. and Waldmann, H. (1988). Importance of antigen specificity for complement mediated lysis by antibodies. *Eur. J. Immunol.* **18**, 1507–14.

Bindon, C.I., Hale, G. and Waldmann, H. (1990). Complement activation by immunoglobulin does not depend solely on C1q binding. *Eur. J. Immunol.* **20**, 277–81.

Brewer, Y., Palmer, A., Taube, D. *et al.* (1989). Effect of graft perfusion with two CD45 monoclonal antibodies on incidence of kidney allograft rejection. *Lancet* **ii**, 935–7.

Bruggemann, M., Williams, G.T., Bindon, C.I. *et al.* (1987). Comparison of the effector functions of human immunoglobulins using a matched set of chimeric antibodies. *J. Exp. Med.* **166**, 1351–61.

Bruggemann, M., Teale, C., Clark, M., Bindon, C.I. and Waldmann, H. (1989). A matched set of rat/mouse chimeric antibodies. *J. Immunol.* **142**, 3145–50.

Byers, V.S., Scannon, P.J., Fishwild, D. *et al.* (1989). Patients with rheumatoid arthritis treated with a pan-T-lymphocyte immunotoxin: phase II studies. *FASEB J.* **4**, A1855.

Carteron, N.L., Wofsy, D. and Seaman, W.E. (1988). Induction of immune tolerance during administration of monoclonal antibody to L3T4 does not depend upon depletion of L3T4 cells. *J. Immunol.* **140**, 713–16.

Chatenoud, L. and Bach, J.-F. (1990). Monoclonal antibodies to CD3 as immunosuppressants. *Semin. Immunol.* **2**, 437–47.

Chen, Z., Cobbold, S.P., Metcalfe, S. and Waldmann, H. (1992). Tolerance in the mouse to MHC mismatched heart allografts, and to rat heart xenografts, using monoclonal antibodies to CD4 and CD8. *Eur. J. Immunol.* **22**, 805–10.

Clark, M., Bindon, C.I., Friend, P. and Dyer, M. (1989). The improved lytic function and *in vivo* efficacy of monovalent monoclonal CD3 antibodies. *Eur. J. Immunol.* **19**, 381–8.

Cobbold, S.P. and Waldmann, H. (1986). Skin allograft rejection by L3T4 and Lyt2 T-cell subsets. *Transplantation* **41**, 634–9.

Cobbold, S.P., Jayasuriya, A; Nash, A., Prospero, T.D. and Waldmann, H. (1984). Therapy with monoclonal antibodies by elimination of T-cell subsets. *Nature* **312**, 548–51.

Cobbold, S.P., Martin, G. and Waldmann, H. (1986a). Monoclonal antibodies for prevention of graft versus host disease and marrow graft rejection. *Transplantation* **42**, 239–47.

Cobbold, S.P., Martin, G. and Waldmann, H. (1986b). Monoclonal antibodies to promote marrow engraftment and tissue graft tolerance. *Nature* **323**, 164–6.

Cobbold, S.P., Martin, G. and Waldmann, H. (1990a). The

induction of skin-graft tolerance in MHC mismatched or primed recipients: primed T-cells can be tolerized in the periphery with CD4 and CD8 antibodies. *Eur. J. Immunol.* **20**, 2747–55.

Cobbold, S.P., Qin, S.-X. and Waldmann, H. (1990b). Reprogramming the immune system for tolerance with monoclonal antibodies. *Semin. Immunol.* **2**, 377–87.

Cobbold, S.P., Barel, D. and Waldmann, H. (1989). Manipulating the immune system with monoclonal antibodies. In *T-cell Activation and Disease*, ed. M. Feldmann and J. Lamb, pp. 147–69, Wiley, New York.

Conti, D.J. and Cosimi, B.A. (1990). Effect of monoclonal antibodies on primate allograft rejection. *Crit. Rev. Immunol.* **10**, 113–30.

Cosimi, B.A., Conti, D., Delmonico, F.L. *et al.* (1990). *In vivo* effects of monoclonal antibodies to ICAM1 (CD54) in non-human primates with renal allografts. *J. Immunol.* **144**, 4604–12.

Dyer, M.J.S., Hale, G., Hayhoe, F.G.J. and Waldmann, H. (1989). Effects of CAMPATH-1 antibodies *in vivo* in patients with lymphoid malignancies: influence of antibody isotype. *Blood* **73**, 1431–9.

Friend, P.J., Waldmann, H., Cobbold, S.P. *et al.* (1991a). The anti-IL2 receptor monoclonal antibody YTH 906 in liver transplantation. *Transplant. Proc.* **23**, 1390–2.

Friend, P.J., Waldmann, H., Hale, G. *et al.* (1991b). Reversal of allograft rejection using the monoclonal antibody CAMPATH-1G. *Transplant. Proc.* **23**, 2253.

Gorman, S.D., Clark, M.R., Routledge, E.R., Cobbold, S.P. and Waldmann, H. (1991). Re-shaping a therapeutic CD4 antibody. *Proc. Nat. Acad. Sci. (USA)* **88**, 4181–5.

Gutstein, N.L., Seaman, W.E., Scott, J.H. and Wofsy, D. (1986). Induction of tolerance by administration of monoclonal antibody to L3T4. *J. Immunol.* **137**, 1127–32.

Hale, G., Clark, M. and Waldmann, H. (1985). Therapeutic potential of rat monoclonal antibodies: isotype specificity of antibody-dependent cell-mediated cytotoxicity with human lymphocytes. *J. Immunol.* **134**, 3056–61.

Hale, G., Cobbold, S.P., Waldmann, H., Easter, G., Matejtschuk, P. and Coombs, R.R.A. (1987). Isolation of low-frequency class-switch variants from rat hybrid myelomas. *J. Immunol. Methods* **103**, 59–67.

Hale, G., Clark, M.R., Marcus, R. *et al.* (1988). Remission induction in non-Hodgkin lymphoma with reshaped human monoclonal antibody CAMPATH-1H. *Lancet* **ii**, 1394–6.

Herzog, C., Walker, C., Pilcher, W.J. *et al.* (1989). Anti-CD4 antibody treatment of patients with rheumatoid arthritis: 1. Effect on clinical course and circulating T-cells. *J. Autoimmunity* **2**, 627–42.

Horneff, G., Burmester, G.R., Emmrich, F. and Kalden, J.R. (1991). Treatment of rheumatoid arthritis with an anti-CD4 monoclonal antibody. *Arthritis Rheum.* **34**, 129–40.

Hutchings, P.R., Simpson, E., O'Reilly, L.A., Lund, T., Waldmann, H. and Cooke, A. (1990). The involvement of Lyt2+ cells in beta cell destruction. *J. Autoimmunity* **3** (suppl. 1), 101–9.

Hutchings, P.R., O'Reilly, L.A., Waldmann, H. *et al.* (1992). The use of non-depleting anti-CD4 monoclonal antibody to re-establish tolerance to β cells in NOD mice. *Eur. J. Immunol.* (in press).

Isaacs, J., Clark, M., Greenwood, J. *et al.* (1992). Therapy with monoclonal antibodies: an *in vivo* model for the assessment of therapeutic potential. *Eur. J. Immunol.* (in press).

Jonker, M. (1990). The importance of non-human primates for preclinical testing of immunosuppressive monoclonal antibodies. *Semin. Immunol.* **2**, 427–36.

Kantwerk, G., Cobbold, S.P., Waldmann, H. and Kolb, H. (1987). L3T4 and Lyt2 cells are both involved in the generation of low dose streptozotocin diabetes in mice. *Clin. Exp. Immunol.* **70**, 585–92.

Kipps, T.J., Parham, P., Punt, J. and Herzenberg, L.A. (1985). Importance of immunoglobulin isotype in human antibody-dependent cell-mediated cytotoxicity directed by murine monoclonal antibodies. *J. Exp. Med.* **161**, 1–17.

Kupiec-Weglinski, J.W., Diamenstein, T. and Tilney, N.L. (1988). Interleukin 2 receptor-targeted therapy — rationale and application in organ transplantation. *Transplantation* **46**, 785–92.

Kyle, V, Coughlan, R.J., Tighe, H., Waldmann, H. and Hazleman, B.L. (1989). Beneficial effect of monoclonal antibody to interleukin 2 receptor on activated T-cells in rheumatoid arthritis. *Ann. Rheum. Dis.* **48**, 428–9.

Leong, L., Qin, S.-X., Cobbold, S.P. *et al.* (1992). Classical transplantation tolerance in the adult: the interaction between haemopoietic space and immunosuppression in the induction of tolerance across major histocompatibility barriers. *J. Exp. Med.* (in press).

Mathieson, P.W., Cobbold, S.P., Hale, G. *et al.* (1990). Monoclonal antibody treatment in systemic vasculitis. *N. Engl. J. Med.* **323**, 250–4.

Meng-Qi, Xia, Tone, M., Packman, L. *et al.* (1991). Characterisation of the CAMPATH-1 (CDw52) antigen: biochemical analysis and cDNA cloning reveal an unusually small peptide backbone. *Eur. J. Immunol.* **21**, 847.

Morahan, G., Allison, J. and Miller, J.F.A.P. (1989). Tolerance of Class I histocompatibility antigens expressed extrathymically. *Nature* **339**, 622–4.

Ortho Multicenter Transplant Study Group (1985). A randomised clinical trial of OKT3 antibody for acute rejection of cadaveric renal transplants. *N. Engl. J. Med.* **313**, 337–42.

Ponticelli, C., Rivolta, E., Tarantino, A., De Vecchi, A. and Vegeto, A. (1987). Rescue of severe steroid-resistant rejection with OKT3. *Transplant. Proc.* **19**, 1908–9.

Qin, S., Cobbold, S.P., Tighe, H., Benjamin, R. and Waldmann, H. (1987). CD4 monoclonal antibody pairs for immunosuppression and tolerance induction. *Eur. J. Immunol.* **17**, 1159–65.

Qin, S., Cobbold, S.P., Benjamin, R. and Waldmann, H. (1989). Induction of classical transplantation tolerance in the adult. *J. Exp. Med.* **169**, 779–94.

Qin, S., Wise, M., Cobbold, S.P. *et al.* (1990). Induction of tolerance in peripheral T-cells with monoclonal antibodies. *Eur. J. Immunol.* **20**, 2737–45.

Qin, S., Franks, H., Cobbold, S.P. *et al.* (1992). Pervasive transplantation tolerance. (Submitted.)

Qin, S., Cobbold, S.P. and Waldmann, H. Induction and maintenance of adult transplantation tolerance. (In preparation.)

Reed, M.H., Shapiro, M.E., Strom, T.B. *et al.* (1989). Prolongation of primate renal allograft rejection survival by anti-tac, an anti-human IL2 receptor monoclonal antibody. *Transplantation* **47**, 55–9.

Reichmann, L.M., Clark, M., Waldmann, H. and Winter, G.

(1988). Reshaping human antibodies for therapy. *Nature* **332**, 323–7.

Renlund, D.G., O'Connell, J.B., Gilbert, E.M. *et al.* (1989). A prospective comparison of murine monoclonal CD3 (OKT3) antibody-based and equine anti-thymocyte antibody-based rejection prophylaxis in cardiac transplantation. *Transplantation* **47**, 599–605.

Routledge, E.G., Lloyd, I., Gorman, S.D., Clark, M.R. and Waldmann, H. (1991). A humanized monovalent CD3 antibody which can activate homologous complement. *Eur. J. Immunol.* **21**, 2717–25.

Schwartz, R.H. (1990). A cell culture model for T-lymphocyte clonal anergy. *Science* **248**, 1349–56.

Shizuru, J.A., Taylor-Edwards, C., Banks, B.A., Gregory A.K. and Fathman, C.G. (1988). Immunotherapy of the non-obese diabetic mouse: treatment with an antibody to helper T-cells. *Science* **240**, 659–62.

Soulillou, J.P., Cantarovitch, D., Le Mauff, B. *et al.* (1990). Randomized control trial of a monoclonal antibody against the interleukin-2 receptor (33B3.1) as compared to rabbit anti-thymocyte globulin for prophylaxis against rejection of renal allografts. *N. Engl. J. Med.* **322**, 1175–82.

Sykes, M. and Sachs, D.H. (1990). Bone marrow transplantation as a means of inducing tolerance. *Semin. Immunol.* **2**, 401–17.

Tighe, H, Friend, P.S., St J. Collier, J. *et al.* (1988). Delayed allograft rejection in patients treated with anti-IL2 receptor monoclonal antibody CAMPATH-6. *Transplantation* **45**, 226–8.

Waldmann, H. (1989). Manipulation of T-cell responses with monoclonal antibodies. *Ann. Rev. Immunol.* **7**, 407–44.

Waldmann, H., Hale, G., Cobbold, S.P. *et al.* (1990a). Monoclonal antibody therapy for the prevention of graft versus host disease. *Hematology* **12**, 277.

Waldmann, H., Cobbold, S.P., Clark, M. *et al.* (1990b). The generation of immunological tolerance as a therapeutic procedure: horizons in medicine. *Transmed. Eur.* **2**, 229.

Wofsy, D. and Carteron, N.L. (1990). CD4 therapy in systemic lupus erythematosus. *Semin. Immunol.* **2**, 419–25.

Wofsy, D. and Seaman, W.E. (1987). Reversal of advanced murine lupus in NZB/NZW F1 mice with monoclonal antibody to L3T4. *J. Immunol.* **138**, 3247–53.

Wood, K.J. (1990). Transplantation tolerance with monoclonal antibodies. *Semin. Immunol.* **2**, 389–99.

48: Plasma Exchange

P.D. Mason and C.D. Pusey

Introduction

The term plasmaphaeresis (from the Greek meaning 'withdrawal') was first used by Abel *et al.* in 1914, who separated plasma and cells from a dog's blood, returning the latter to the animal. The technique was used for the collection of plasma from human volunteers during World War II, and therapeutically for the treatment of myeloma and macroglobulinaemia in the 1950s. More efficient blood cell separators, developed in the 1960s, allowed larger volumes of plasma to be removed, but therapeutic application to a wide range of disorders only occurred following reports of the beneficial effect in anti-glomerular basement membrane (GBM) disease in the mid-1970s. Removal of large volumes of plasma requires replacement with a colloid solution to prevent a fall in oncotic pressure; the term 'plasma exchange' is therefore more appropriate.

This chapter addresses the evidence supporting the use of plasma exchange in immunologically mediated diseases. In addition, there is evidence that plasma exchange is valuable in conditions such as hyperviscosity syndrome, homozygous familial hypercholesterolaemia and Refsum's disease, but these will not be discussed.

Mechanisms of action of plasma exchange

Plasma exchange was first used therapeutically to treat hyperviscosity with macroglobulinaemia (Skoog and Adams 1959; Soloman and Fahey 1963). In this situation it is clear that removal of plasma containing high levels of paraprotein and replacement with albumin will immediately reduce viscosity and alleviate symptoms. The early use of plasma exchange in the treatment of anti-GBM disease (Lockwood *et al.* 1975) was justified by the presence of antibodies that had been shown to be pathogenic and the rapidity with which renal damage occurred in these patients. The more widespread use in immune disorders was similarly justified by the implication that antibodies or immune complexes were important in pathogenesis.

Plasma exchange obviously results in the removal of all plasma components in addition to antibodies and immune complexes. It is possible that the removal of these other components may be relevant to the mechanism of action of plasma exchange (see below). The effectiveness of plasma exchange in removing individual constituents depends partly on their synthetic and catabolic rates, but to a greater extent on their distribution in intravascular and extravascular compartments. Disappearance curves for several plasma proteins have been determined in a normal subject and several patients (Derksen *et al.* 1984) and, as predicted, immunoglobulin M (IgM) (predominantly intravascular) is more effectively cleared than proteins with more widespread distribution (Fig. 48.1). However, some components equilibrate with the intravascular compartment more readily than others, resulting in a greater than predicted removal, and removal rates vary in different patients (Derksen *et al.* 1984). Consequently, the actual removal rates for each component can only reliably be determined by direct measurement, although for most (including immunoglobulins and immune complexes) diminishing fractional removal with continuing plasma exchange makes exchange beyond 1–1.5 plasma volumes inefficient.

There has been little work on the mechanisms by which plasma exchange has beneficial effects in immunological disorders in man, although there are several hypotheses which are not mutually exclusive.

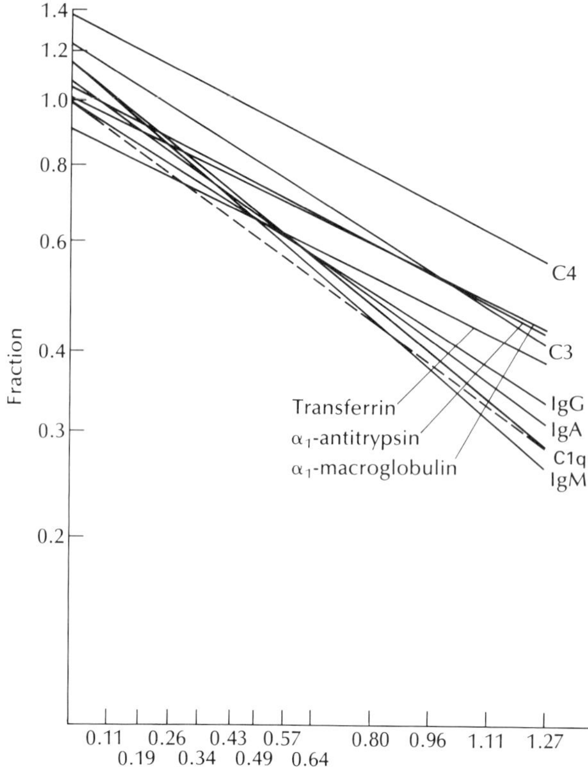

Fig. 48.1. The disappearance of various plasma proteins from the intravascular compartment during plasma exchange, in a healthy volunteer, expressed as a fraction of pre-exchange intravascular amount. The interrupted line represents that predicted from a model assuming a closed intravascular compartment. Fractions >1 imply protein influx, from extravascular to intravascular compartments, increasing predicted removal. From Derksen *et al.* 1984.

Removal of autoantibodies

The removal of autoantibodies would seem a reasonable explanation in conditions where antibodies clearly have a pathogenic role. Diseases in this category include anti-GBM disease, myasthenia gravis, Eaton–Lambert syndrome, haemolytic anaemia (including cold agglutinin disease), pemphigus vulgaris and Graves' disease. Even when such antibodies are present, plasma exchange alone only transiently reduces levels and benefit is not inevitable. There are many other organ-specific and non-specific diseases, associated with circulating autoantibodies, in which there is little evidence that removal benefits the clinical condition and in which the presence of autoantibodies may be an epiphenomenon.

Removal of immune complexes

Many diseases are associated with immune deposits in tissues and/or detectable circulating complexes, of which mixed essential cryoglobulinaemia (MEC) and systemic lupus erythematosus

(SLE) are good examples (see Chapters 99 and 61). It has been suggested that such complexes are pathogenically important (Theofilopoulos and Dixon 1979), but there is no direct proof of this in man. However, it was their presence which initially stimulated the use of plasma exchange in a variety of conditions. There is now increasing evidence that immune deposits in glomerulonephritis may result from *in situ* reactions between glomerular autoantigens or foreign antigens planted in the glomerulus, and circulating antibody. Thus, although removal of circulating complexes by plasma exchange may not be relevant, removal of the antibody concerned could have effects on the immune deposits.

Effects on reticuloendothelial system

Clearance of isotope-labelled, antibody-coated, senescent red blood cells is impaired in patients with primary vasculitis (Lockwood *et al.* 1979), SLE and MEC (Frank *et al.* 1979; Walport *et al.* 1985). Improvement in reticuloendothelial system (RES) function has been shown to occur following plasma exchange (Lockwood *et al.* 1979; Walport *et al.* 1985), and this finding was supported by the observation in some patients that levels of circulating immune complexes continued to fall after the procedure. Clearance of micro-aggregated albumin has also been shown to be improved after plasma exchange in SLE (Law *et al.* 1985).

Other effects

Data relating to other possible effects of plasma exchange are poor. Apart from occasional case reports, studies assessing lymphocyte numbers and function have failed to demonstrate consistent changes after plasma exchange. Tsokos *et al.* (1982) studied various lymphocyte functions before and after sham or real plasma exchange in a small double-blind randomized trial. No significant differences between the two groups were seen, even though some patients' tests were abnormal as compared with healthy controls. Plasma exchange has also been claimed to enhance monocyte killing of bacteria (Steven *et al.* 1981), but this study was uncontrolled and alternative explanations of the data are possible. Another suggestion is that removal of antibody by plasma exchange stimulates the B cells concerned, thus sensitizing them to the effect of cytotoxic drugs. Rebound synthesis of depleted antibody is known to be associated with increased B cell proliferation (Sturgill and Worzniak 1970), and the synchronized use of cyclophosphamide and plasma exchange has been reported to be effective in uncontrolled studies (Schroeder *et al.* 1987).

It has been suggested that depletion of complement components, clotting factors or other plasma proteins may play a role in limiting tissue injury, but there are no convincing data to support these claims. Furthermore, clotting factors generally return to normal within 48 hours of discontinuation of plasma exchange, even in immunosuppressed patients (Lockwood *et al.* 1979). Similar suggestions that removal of inflammatory mediators, such as cytokines and eicosanoids, plays a role are also unsubstantiated. Finally, non-specific effects such as reduction in plasma viscosity with improved blood flow in diseased microcirculations may be important.

Techniques of plasma exchange

Whilst cell separators are used by most haematologists and units specializing in plasmaphaeresis, the introduction of hollow fibre plasma filters has led to wider use of the technique, particularly by nephrologists. It should not be assumed that both devices have equivalent biological effects, although the sieving coefficient of modern hollow fibre membrane devices approaches one for immunoglobulins (150 kD) and even β-lipoprotein (2400 kD) (Gurland *et al.* 1984). The techniques required for vascular acccess and potential complications of the procedure are similar for both types of device. We shall consider the use of replacement fluids in this section, but consider the 'dose' — i.e. volume and frequency of exchange — under the various clinical applications.

Separation devices

Plasma may be removed with centrifugal or membrane separators. Two centrifugal designs are in use, the discontinuous flow and the continuous flow cell centrifuge. In the discontinuous flow system, blood is pumped into a centrifuge bowl, which allows withdrawal of plasma into a collection bag during rotation, until the bowl contains only packed cells. The centrifuge is then stopped, and the cells are pumped into a reinfusion bag for return to the patient, together with the substitution fluid. This cycle is then repeated, and during each cycle approximately 500 ml of blood are processed (depending on the patient's haematocrit). The continuous flow system allows the simultaneous removal of plasma and of cellular components from separation ports within the centrifuge. It is therefore possible to perform the exchange without stopping the centrifuge, permitting a faster procedure and lower extracorporeal volume.

Plasma may also be separated from cells by microporous membranes. Plasma passes across the membrane (pore size normally 0.2–0.5 μm) and is removed, while the cells continue through the separator and return to the patient with replacement fluid. The efficiency of this process depends upon the characteristics of the membrane and the device used, but in general all immunoglobulins and most immune complexes cross the membrane, and the procedure is rapid with adequate two-site access. Large immune complexes (several million kD) may not be cleared as effectively, but although this has been suggested to be a disadvantage no practical differences have been demonstrated.

In attempting to make plasma exchange more selective and safer by eliminating the need for replacement colloid, several variations have been devised, but none are used widely. Most involve prior separation of plasma (usually by filtration), followed by secondary treatment of the filtered plasma before return to the patient. Initial efforts used a series of secondary filters of different pore sizes, allowing removal of immune complexes, immunoglobulins or cryoglobulins and this became known as 'cascade filtration'. However, although useful for selectively removing IgM in macroglobulinaemia or β-lipoproteins in familial hypercholesterolaemia, no commercially available membrane allows sufficiently good separation of IgG and albumin. Immunoglobulin G may be removed using columns of protein A which bind, to a varying extent, most IgG subclasses. This technique of immunoadsorption has been used for removal of antibodies to factor IX in haemophilia (Nilsson *et al.* 1981), GBM (Bygren *et al.* 1985) and human leucocyte antigens (HLA) (Palmer *et al.* 1989). Antigen-coated columns have been used experimentally to remove antibodies against GBM (Pusey *et al.* 1985), and clinically to remove anti-deoxyribonucleic acid (DNA) antibodies (El-Habib *et al.* 1984), anti-factor IX antibodies (Nilsson *et al.* 1984) and anti-blood group antibodies (Bensinger *et al.* 1985). The latter two reports described adsorption from whole blood, obviating the need for prior plasma separation.

Complications and replacement fluids

Complications of plasma exchange have a low incidence when careful attention is paid to fluid and electrolyte balance, vascular access sites to prevent infection, and use of anticoagulation, particularly in patients at risk of haemorrhage. Many 'incidents' on plasma exchange and the occasional death have been associated with the use of fresh frozen plasma (FFP) as replacement fluid (Huestis 1983), and so the justification for giving this must be clear-cut. The actual mortality is difficult to assess; it has been estimated as 3 in 10 000 (Huestis 1983), but may be much less than this when albumin is the replacement fluid (*Lancet* Editorial 1982), and may differ between different patient groups. In the last few years, the results of two large series reporting the incidence of side-effects and mortality of plasma exchange, determined from national or regional registers, have been published. The French series covered 7538 plasma exchanges in 887 patients during a 3-year period (Bussel and Jais 1987). The overall incidence of side-effects was 16.8% of exchanges with termination of the procedure in 4%, but incidence varied amongst patients in different diagnostic categories. Transfusion reactions (7%) were mostly in those given FFP. Three deaths were considered to be plasma exchange-related; all had received FFP and two had thrombotic thrombocytopenia purpura.

A more recent multicentre Canadian study reported the incidence of side-effects in 627 patients who underwent 5235 plasma exchanges (Sutton *et al.* 1989). Thirty-nine per cent of exchanges were for neurological, 30% for haematological, 17% for connective tissue (including vasculitis) and 10% for renal conditions. Side-effects were classified as mild (transient with little or no clinical significance, e.g. fever, chills, urticaria, nausea and vomiting), moderate (considerable discomfort, but not requiring cessation of plasma exchange) or severe (requiring termination of exchange and vigorous resuscitation). Side-effects occurred in

12.5% of exchanges in 40% of patients — most commonly mild (9%) or moderate (3%). Twenty-eight severe episodes were reported (0.5%), including one cardiac and two respiratory arrests, but there were no deaths considered to be directly related to the procedure. Interestingly, the highest incidence of side-effects occurred in haematology patients (16%, of which two-thirds were for those with thrombotic thrombocytopenic purpura or haemolytic uraemic syndrome), and was lowest in the connective tissue disease and renal groups (5% and 7% respectively).

An increased incidence of infection during plasma exchange has been suggested, particularly since the patients are often immunosuppressed because of underlying disease or its treatment with steroids and cytotoxic drugs. A high level of life threatening infection in plasma exchanged patients with rapidly progressive glomerulonephritis has been reported (Wing *et al.* 1980), but this was a retrospective study without a control group. Cohen *et al.* (1982) did not find that plasma exchange significantly increased infection risk while the dose of steroids did. More recently a randomized controlled trial of plasma exchange in immunosuppressed lupus patients failed to demonstrate an increased risk of infection in the exchanged group (Pohl *et al.* 1991).

Large-volume therapeutic plasma exchange, removing 50 ml/kg or about 1–1.25 plasma volumes (around 4 litres for a 75 kg patient), requires replacement with a colloid solution to prevent a significant fall in plasma oncotic pressure. Synthetic plasma expanders have a short intravascular half-life, making them unsuitable as the major replacement fluid during intensive courses of exchange. Some gelatin-based solutions have been used as cheap partial replacement for patients receiving chronic intermittent plasma exchange. Pasteurized 5% albumin is most commonly used, with its very low risk of allergic reactions or disease transmission. Fresh frozen plasma is often given at the end of an exchange to replace clotting factors, particularly if there is a risk of haemorrhage or within 72 hours of a surgical procedure or biopsy.

Replacement of deficient plasma components has been suggested to play a beneficial role in plasma exchange when FFP is used as the major replacement fluid. Complement component replacement has possible theoretical advantages in diseases such as SLE, for instance by solubilizing immune complexes or enhancing their disposal by the RES. However, there is no good clinical evidence to support this notion. The benefit of replacement of other, undefined, factors (e.g. in the treatment of thrombotic thrombocytopenic purpura) has also been reported, but no convincing data exist.

Use of plasma exchange in specific diseases

There are now reports of the use of plasma exchange in a large number of immunological diseases. The following section reviews the data supporting (or otherwise) a role for plasma exchange in the major disorders in which it has been tried. Unfortunately adequately controlled trials are often lacking, and we can only comment on the small series or case reports published.

Anti-glomerular basement membrane disease

In anti-GBM disease, a single major antigen present in kidney and lung basement membrane has been shown to be the target of the autoimmune process (Pusey *et al.* 1987), and the pathogenicity of anti-GBM antibodies has been demonstrated experimentally (Lerner *et al.* 1967). Autoantibody removal would thus be expected to be an effective adjunct to the suppression of antibody synthesis by cytotoxic drugs, and this approach was justified by the rapid loss of renal function in untreated cases (Benoit *et al.* 1964; Proskey *et al.* 1970). Effective anti-GBM antibody removal is well documented (Pusey *et al.* 1983), although an intensive plasma exchange schedule is required to effectively lower antibody levels (daily 4-litre exchanges for around 14 days).

Clinical benefit was initially demonstrated by the dramatic improvement in treated patients compared with historical controls (Lockwood *et al.* 1975). Retrospective analysis of 29 patients treated with immunosuppression and plasma exchange revealed that 41% overall showed improved renal function, and 66% when oligoanuric patients were excluded (Savage *et al.* 1986). These results are much better than those previously reported for patients untreated or given drug treatment alone (Wilson and Dixon 1973). Similar favourable results have also been reported by other groups (Kincaid-Smith and d'Apice 1978; Erickson *et al.* 1979;

Walker *et al.* 1985). However, it is important to remember that most historical 'control' patients received neither plasma exchange nor what would now be considered adequate immunosuppression. The value of plasma exchange has thus generally been accepted, although clear-cut controlled data are not available. A controlled study (Johnson *et al.* 1985) found only equivocal benefit from plasma exchange, but the numbers in this study were small (17 patients) and a non-intensive plasma exchange regimen (1 × 4 litre exchange every 3 days) was used. Moreover their data revealed that only 1/9 control patients compared with 4/8 plasma-exchanged patients had improved renal function after treatment.

Early series suggested that oligoanuric patients and those on dialysis before treatment rarely improved, even with plasma exchange (Briggs *et al.* 1979; Simpson *et al.* 1982; Hind *et al.* 1983; Pusey *et al.* 1983). Treatment of such patients was therefore proposed only if lung haemorrhage was present (Savage *et al.* 1986). Subsequently, several groups have reported that occasional patients with advanced disease do respond — particularly if they are not anuric or the biopsy reveals a low crescent score and/or low proportion of sclerosed glomeruli (Walker *et al.* 1985). Our current short-term results, including all 59 patients treated since 1975, are shown in Table 48.1. Our current policy is to plasma-exchange all patients not dialysis-dependent on admission and those with pulmonary haemorrhage. Oliguric or dialysis-dependent patients without pulmonary haemorrhage are treated if the renal biopsy shows favourable features. An additional indication is to reduce anti-GBM antibody levels prior to renal transplantation if they do not spontaneously disappear (Flores *et al.* 1986). Recurrence of the disease is exceptional, so the long-term prognosis of successfully treated patients is good (see Chapter 99).

Focal necrotizing glomerulonephritis

The small-vessel vasculitides, including Wegener's granulomatosis (WG) and microscopic polyarteritis (MP), frequently cause a focal necrotizing glomerulonephritis (FNGN) with crescent formation (see Chapter 62). This is usually associated with the rapid development of renal failure, and the clinical description rapidly progressive glomerulonephritis (RPGN) is sometimes used. Focal necrotizing glomerulonephritis may also occur in the absence of evident extrarenal involvement, so-called 'idiopathic' RPGN, although this probably represents limited small-vessel vasculitis. Patients with WG, MP and idiopathic RPGN have recently been shown to have autoantibodies to cytoplasm of neutrophils and monocytes (anti-neutrophil cytoplasmic antibodies or ANCA) (Van der Woude *et al.* 1985; Savage *et al.* 1987). There is accumulating evidence that these antibodies are pathogenic (Falk *et al.* 1990), although associated antibodies which bind to glomerular endothelial cells may also be relevant (Abbot *et al.* 1989; Savage *et al.* 1991).

Plasma exchange was introduced because of the then current belief that immune complexes played a pathogenic role in RPGN, and in view of the successful treatment of anti-GBM disease. Initial, uncontrolled reports from several centres suggested benefit from plasma exchange (Lockwood *et al.* 1977). Furthermore, in contrast to results in anti-GBM disease, the majority of dialysis-dependent patients improved. Heaf *et al.* (1983), after reviewing the literature, concluded that advanced RPGN generally had a better outcome when treated with plasma exchange or pulse methylprednisolone in addition to immunosuppressive drugs. However, more than half of the patients reviewed had anti-GBM disease, infection-related or other secondary cause of

Table 48.1. Outcome at 2 months of 59 patients with anti-GBM disease treated with cytotoxic drugs, steroids and plasma exchange, stratified by renal function at presentation

Creatinine at presentation	No. of patients	Independent renal function	Dialysis	Died
Dialysis	30	4 (13%)	19	7
>600	8	4 (50%)	3	1
<600	21	18 (86%)	2	1
Total	59			

RPGN, and most of those treated with plasma exchange had anti-GBM disease. Despite the plethora of uncontrolled evidence suggesting that plasma exchange confers a benefit (Becker *et al.* 1977; d'Apice and Kincaid-Smith 1979; Russ and d'Apice 1981; Stevens *et al.* 1982; Stevens and Bone 1984; Thysell *et al.* 1982; Burran *et al.* 1986), it is clear that vasculitis generally responds well to immunosuppressive drug regimens including cyclophosphamide. Table 48.2 summarizes the outcome in 10 uncontrolled series of patients with RPGN (excluding, where possible, anti-GBM disease, SLE, Henoch–Schönlein purpura, infection-related and underlying glomerulonephritis) treated with plasma exchange. In interpreting these data, it must be realized that most patients also received immunosuppressive drugs (cyclophosphamide and/or azathioprine) and steroids in various regimens, including at least 24/111 non-Hammersmith patients who were given pulse methylprednisolone. Authors also had different (or unstated) criteria for improvement. However, improvement in renal function was reported to have occurred in 79% overall (range 60–100%), even in those patients on dialysis or with very high creatinines. The table also indicates that the initial improvement was often maintained medium- or long-term (Table 48.2). These results compare favourably with historical controls as recently assessed by Couser (1988), who reviewed published data on 78 patients with RPGN similar to those above. These patients received various combinations of cytotoxic drugs and steroids, but not plasma exchange or pulse methylprednisolone. Only 20% demonstrated significant clinical improvement and the remainder (including most dialysed or oliguric patients) developed end-stage renal failure. Our current short-term results for 78 patients with FNGN and a diagnosis of WG, MP or 'idiopathic' RPGN, and who received at least 3 plasma exchanges (average of 9, range 3–37) are shown in Table 48.3. All patients received cyclophosphamide and/or azathioprine and prednisolone as well as plasma exchange, but not pulse methylprednisolone. Three-quarters of the patients presenting on dialysis recovered independent renal function by 2 months, and most maintained function or improved further between 2 months and 1 year (Fig. 48.2), comparing favourably with published data on patients treated with cytotoxic drugs alone (Couser 1988).

The results of two controlled trials are available. Glockner *et al.* (1988) reported no statistically significant benefit from plasma exchange. They studied 26 patients, treated at 10 different centres, with a variety of diagnoses (including SLE, IgA disease and scleroderma), some of whom had received immunosuppressive drugs before entry into the trial. Immunosuppressive regimens varied depending on the underlying cause of RPGN, and the plasma exchange group had only three exchanges during the first week and two to three in each of the subsequent 3 weeks. At 4 weeks, 4/12 control and 7/14 plasma exchange patients showed a response (increase of > 20 ml/min above initial creatinine clearance or came off dialysis). By 6 months the results were 7/11 and 7/12 respectively, although by then three initial non-responders in the control group had improved after plasma exchange. These factors aside, their own statistical analysis predicted that many more patients would have been required to prove an effect of plasma exchange. Pusey *et al.* (1991) have reported a prospective, randomized, controlled trial of intensive plasma exchange in 48 patients with vasculitis-associated or idiopathic RNGN

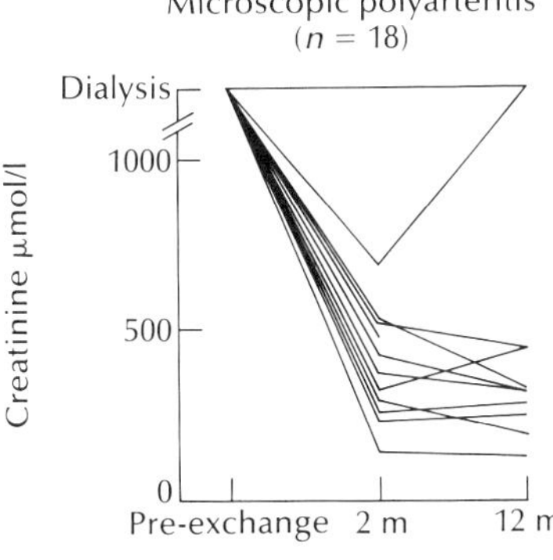

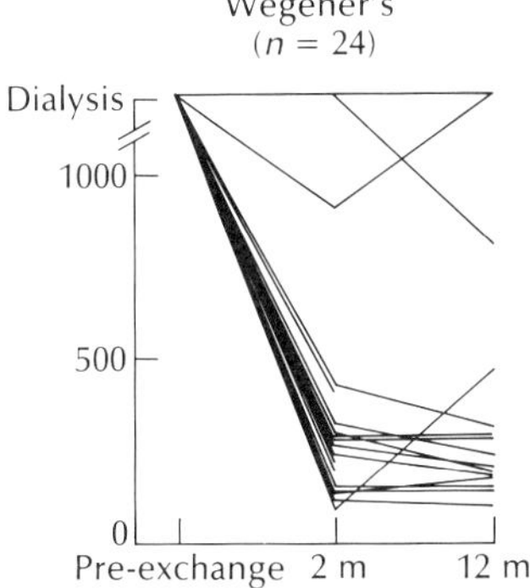

Fig. 48.2. Creatinines at 2 and 12 months of dialysis-dependent patients with focal necrotizing glomerulonephritis associated with Wegener's and microscopic polyarteritis following treatment with cytotoxic drugs, steroids and plasma exchange.

Table 48.2. Published series of the outcome of patients with RPGN (excluding where possible anti-GBM disease, SLE, Henoch–Schönlein purpura and underlying glomerulonephritis) treated by plasma exchange

Reference	No. of patients	Creatinine at presentation	No. of patients	Initial improvement	Maintained improvement	Comments
Becker *et al.* 1977	7	≥1000 or dialysis <1000	4 3	4/4 (100%) 1/3 (33%)	N/A N/A	Some patients had long periods of other therapy before PEx; 1 RPGN was in a transplant; 2 had background gouty and analgesic nephropathy
Thysell *et al.* 1982	22	≥1000 or dialysis <1000	11 11	8/11 (73%) 11/11 (100%)	6/8 (75%) 10/11 (91%)	Authors felt PEx was of definite benefit in 5 patients, probable in 8, doubtful in 4 and not at all in 5; 3 received pulse MP
Stratta *et al.* 1982	9	Unstratified	9	4/9 (44%)	3/4 (74%)	Few patient details given
D'Amico *et al.* 1982	4	≥1000 or dialysis <1000	2 2	1/2 (50%) 2/2 (100%)	1/1 (100%) 2/2 (100%)	Two patients also received pulse MP; a historical control group did worse
Stevens and Bone 1982, 1984	13	Unstratified	13	7/13 (54%)	6/7 (86%)	Included anti-GBM and HSP patients; 14 patients treated with pulse MP also described and this was concluded to be equally as effective as PEx, but superior to immunosuppressive drugs alone
Burran *et al.* 1986	8	≥1000 or dialysis <1000	7 1	6/7 (86%) 1/1 (100%)	3/6 (50%) 1/1 (100%)	All patients also received pulse MP
Glockner *et al.* 1988	14	≥1000 or dialysis <1000	9 5	6/9 (67%) 2/5 (60%)	6/6 (100%) 1/2 (50%)	Treated group from controlled study, included patients with SLE and scleroderma
Russ and d'Apice 1981	24	Unstratified	24	22/24 (92%)	14/22 (64%)	Included 5 patients with SLE; includes some patients reported by Becker *et al.* 1977
Keller *et al.* 1989	10	Unstratified	10	7/10 (70%)	5/7 (71%)	All patients also received pulse MP
Hammersmith unpublished	78	≥1000 or dialysis <1000	42 36	32/42 (76%) 24/36 (67%)	22/32 (69%) 22/24 (92%)	Includes 25 patients reported in a controlled trial by Pusey *et al.* 1991.
Overall total	189			138/189 (73%)	102/133 (77%)	

PEx = plasma exchange; MP = methylprednisolone; HSP = Henoch–Schönlein purpura.

Table 48.3. Outcome at 2 months of 78 patients with focal necrotizing glomerulonephritis (excluding anti-GBM disease, SLE, Henoch–Schönlein purpura and underlying glomerulonephritis) treated with cytotoxic drugs, steroids and plasma exchange, stratified by renal function at presentation

Creatinine at presentation	No. of patients	Independent renal function	Dialysis	Died
Dialysis	42	32 (76%)	6 (14%)	4 (10%)
>600	14	10 (71%)	1 (7%)	3 (22%)
<600	22	18 (82%)	1 (4%)	3 (13%)
Total	78			

(excluding anti-GBM disease, SLE, Henoch–Schönlein purpura and underlying glomerulonephritis). Patients were stratified into three groups on the basis of presenting creatinine; < 500 μmol/l (n = 17); > 500 μmol/l but not on dialysis (n = 12); or dialysis-dependent (n = 19). They were then randomized for treatment with prednisolone and cytotoxic drugs alone, or with the addition of plasma exchange. The only statistically significant difference was in the dialysis-dependent group, in which 10/11 plasma exchange and 3/8 control patients recovered renal function by 4 weeks ($p = 0.041$). Almost all patients not on dialysis, in both treatment groups, showed an improvement. Numbers were small, and several deaths between 1 month and 1 year in dialysis-dependent patients (four control and three plasma exchange) made longer-term analysis difficult. However, long-term survivors generally maintained independent renal function.

In conclusion, the evidence supporting a role for plasma exchange in FNGN is still not clear-cut, but it is likely that dialysis-dependent patients are the only group to benefit. We use plasma exchange in this situation, in the face of severe systemic disease unresponsive to drugs, or when cytotoxic treatment has to be withheld because of myelotoxicity in patients with uncontrolled disease.

Other renal diseases

Immunological mechanisms are implicated in most forms of glomerulonephritis (reviewed by Pusey *et al.* 1988; see Chapter 99), by the deposition of immunoglobulin and complement in renal biopsy material, and by analogy with experimental models of antibody-mediated or immune complex nephritis. However, apart from those disorders discussed elsewhere in this chapter, there is little substantive evidence that renal injury in man is caused by circulating autoantibodies or immune complexes which could be removed by plasma exchange. Since the clinical course of primary glomerulonephritis is often chronic, and may spontaneously improve, trials attempting to demonstrate benefit from plasma exchange need to include large numbers of patients and continue for long periods. Unfortunately, published data are limited to small uncontrolled series and case reports, and have usually described patients with rapidly declining renal function.

Plasma exchange and immunosuppressive drugs have been reported to be effective in mesangial IgA disease with crescents (Kauffmann and Houwert 1981; Nicholls *et al.* 1984), but a number of other studies have failed to support a long-term benefit from plasma exchange. These include a report of five patients with IgA nephropathy who showed early improvement in clinical state and immunological findings (IgA immune complex and complement C3 levels, and mononuclear cell and phagocyte function), of whom only two maintained long-term improvement (Coppo *et al.* 1985); and a report of two patients with rapidly progressing mesangial IgA disease, who showed initial but not long-term benefit of plasma exchange (Lai *et al.* 1987). A further uncontrolled study suggested that active mesangial IgA or Henoch–Schönlein nephritis may be more amenable to treatment than chronic progressive disease (Alcalay *et al.* 1987).

Plasma exchange has been claimed to be of value in uncontrolled studies of mesangiocapillary glomerulonephritis (Kincaid-Smith and Walker 1984; Roujeau *et al.* 1984b; McGinley *et al.* 1985), but also to be ineffective in acute (Espinel *et al.* 1984) and chronic (Kincaid-Smith and Walker 1984) mesangiocapillary glomerulonephritis. There are occasional reports of its use in focal segmental glomerulosclerosis, particularly for recurrent disease in renal transplantation (Munoz *et al.* 1985; Zimmerman 1985), and in membranous nephropathy, but these data are not persuasive of its benefit.

Renal transplantation

Plasma exchange has been used for three separate indications in renal transplantation: acute and chronic rejection; the highly sensitized recipient; and recurrent nephritis. First, it has been used to treat acute and chronic (especially 'vascular') rejection. Anti-HLA antibodies against mismatched antigens have been associated with vascular rejection, and anti-endothelial antibodies have been associated with accelerated vascular rejection unresponsive to high-dose steroids (Paul and Carpenter 1980). A non-randomized study demonstrated that plasma exchange and cyclophosphamide reduced anti-HLA antibody levels (undetectable after two to five exchanges) and that activity remained undetectable after stopping plasma exchange, but titres were unchanged by pulse methylprednisolone or cyclophosphamide alone (Vangelista *et al.* 1982). Removal of these antibodies was associated with improved renal function. A more recent uncontrolled study of plasma exchange claimed benefit, particularly for patients with acute endovasculitis (Franco *et al.* 1987). However, many reports have failed to find clinical benefit from plasma exchange (Allen *et al.* 1983; Soulillou *et al.* 1983). Gurland *et al.* (1983) reviewed 24 reports of the use of plasma exchange in renal transplantation published up until 1982. Response to plasma exchange was claimed by the authors in 59% of 214 episodes of acute rejection, and 19% of 26 episodes of chronic rejection, in patients who had failed to respond to other treatment. Controlled data have, however, been disappointing. The results of an early controlled trial with 24 patients treated with IV methylprednisolone or with eight plasma exchanges over 2 weeks suggested that the exchanged group actually did worse (although not statistically significant), but this group also received less steroids (Kirubakaran *et al.* 1981). In their review of the literature, Gurland *et al.* (1983) presented data from five controlled (but not all randomized or prospective) trials, including those already referred to. Overall, data on 157 patients were included and 53/87 (61%) of plasma exchange and 36/70 (51%) of control patients reportedly responded. More recently, Bonomini *et al.* (1985) reported a controlled trial of 44 patients, combining plasma exchange or methylprednisolone with cyclophosphamide, and found that plasma exchange reduced titres of cytotoxic antibodies and graft loss. However, this group of patients was unusual in that the treated rejection episodes occurred at a mean of more than 10 months after transplantation. Another controlled trial of 85 patients indicated benefit from additional plasma exchange compared with conventional anti-rejection therapy. However, there was no significant difference in graft survival when only those given pre-transplant blood transfusions were considered (Cardella *et al.* 1985). Overall, there is no convincing evidence to support a general role for plasma exchange in acute or chronic graft rejection, although selected patients with high titres of anti-HLA antibodies may respond. However, there are no studies comparing plasma exchange with other second-line rejection treatments, such as anti-lymphocyte globulin or monoclonal antibodies.

Secondly, plasma exchange has been used to treat highly sensitized potential recipients prior to transplantation. Patients with high panel reactivity often have antibodies directed against one or two HLA antigens in high titre, which cross-react with other HLA antigens resulting in a high incidence of positive cross-matches. Taube *et al.* (1984) reported five patients treated with intensive plasma exchange, cyclophosphamide and prednisolone, of whom four were successfully transplanted. Others have also reported similar success (Fauchald *et al.* 1987). The method has been refined, using protein A immunoadsorption of IgG from plasma and return of the depleted plasma to the patient (Palmer *et al.* 1989). In this study 7/8 transplanted patients had functioning allografts at 12–18 months, but larger numbers and longer-term follow-up is needed to confirm these promising results.

Finally, plasma exchange has been used to treat recurrent nephritis in allografts (especially focal segmental glomerulosclerosis), but with no clear evidence of benefit.

Systemic lupus erythematosus

Systemic lupus erythematosus is characterized by production of multiple autoantibodies, and it is suggested that these antibodies or related immune complexes are involved in pathogenesis (see Chapter 61). Although direct proof of pathogenicity in man is lacking, the strong circumstantial evidence for humoral immune involvement makes plasma exchange a logical therapeutic approach.

Since the use of plasma exchange in SLE was first reported in 1976 (Verrier-Jones *et al.* 1976), there have been many uncontrolled reports of benefit (Moran *et al.* 1977; Verrier-Jones *et al.* 1979; Lockwood *et al.* 1981; Lewis 1982; Moriconi *et al.* 1983; Leaker *et al.* 1986; Jordan *et al.* 1987), but disappointingly few controlled data. There is no doubt that plasma exchange reduces levels of autoantibodies and immune complexes (Wei *et al.* 1983; Haworth *et al.* 1985) and improves RES function with sustained falls in levels of circulating immune complexes (Lockwood *et al.* 1979; Walport *et al.* 1985), but it has been more difficult to demonstrate benefit. Part of the problem lies in the diversity of patterns and severity of disease, particularly renal involvement. Furthermore, SLE usually responds well to corticosteroids and immunosuppressive drugs. For these reasons, trials which are adequately controlled for pattern and severity of disease, including renal histology and function, require very large numbers to demonstrate conclusive benefit from plasma exchange. It is perhaps not surprising that the small controlled trials reported have not been informative. One controlled trial in 20 patients with lupus nephritis, using a non-intensive regimen of plasma exchange combined with low-dose steroids, failed to demonstrate benefit (Wei *et al.* 1983). However, these patients had only mild disease and received no concomitant cytotoxic drug therapy. Another controlled trial included patients treated with a variety of immunosuppressive regimes, or plasma exchange, and was too small to detect possible benefit (Derksen *et al.* 1988). Other small trials provided some support for the benefit of chronic plasma exchange in lupus glomerulonephritis, although there are difficulties in interpreting the results (Clark *et al.* 1983).

No appropriate prospective randomized trial, comparing the effect of adequate cytotoxic drug therapy with or without intensive plasma exchange has been fully reported, although the results of a large, prospective American trial (E.J. Lewis, pers. comm.) are awaited. Preliminary data on 86 patients in this trial have been published in abstract form only, and suggest that plasma exchange does not benefit clinical, renal or serological courses of patients with severe lupus nephritis (Herbert *et al.* 1987; Lewis *et al.* 1987), but it is necessary to know more about patient selection and treatment regimens. In the absence of definitive controlled data, it is reasonable to reserve plasma exchange for patients with life-threatening disease, for those who have not responded to cytotoxic drugs and steroids and for those in whom drugs have been temporarily withdrawn because of side-effects (Haworth *et al.* 1985). Table 48.4 summarizes the reasons for treatment and outcome in 30 consecutive lupus patients treated with plasma exchange at the Hammersmith Hospital. Many anecdotal reports and our own experience suggest that plasma exchange may be beneficial in cerebral lupus and those with lung haemorrhage or severe vasculitis, and it would be justifiable

Table 48.4. Outcome of 30 patients with lupus nephritis treated with plasma exchange, stratified by creatinine at presentation. Reasons for the use of plasma exchange are also given (from Haworth *et al.* 1985)

	No. of patients treated	Improved	No response	Died
Indications				
Drug failure	15	8	5	2
Severe disease	12	6	1	5
Drug toxicity	3	1	2	0
Creatinine at time of plasma exchange				
Dialysis	10	2	3	5
>500	6	2	3	1
<500	14	11	2	1
Total	30	15 (50%)	8 (27%)	7 (23%)

additional therapy in this group of patients with a severe morbidity and high mortality.

Myeloma

A proportion of patients with myeloma develop renal failure, for which there are many possible causes. The clinicopathological features of myeloma kidney or light chain nephropathy are thought to be directly related to the myeloma protein or the light chains. However a relationship between amount or type of Bence Jones proteinuria and serum creatinine has not been found. Recovery of renal function has been reported to occur following plasma exchange (Feest *et al.* 1976; Pozzi *et al.* 1987; Pasquali *et al.* 1990). Two controlled trials have been reported. The authors of the first, in 29 patients mostly on dialysis before treatment, concluded that at least five plasma exchanges on five consecutive days, in addition to chemotherapy, was more often associated with recovery of renal function (Zucchelli *et al.* 1988). However, 5/14 of the control group but only 1/15 of the plasma exchanged group died within 2 months, suggesting that they had worse disease. A more recent controlled trial in 21 patients failed to demonstrate benefit from plasma exchange (Johnston *et al.* 1990).

Cryoglobulinaemia

Type I cryoglobulinaemia consists of a monoclonal immunoglobulin of unknown specificity, and is often associated with myeloma or leukaemia (Grey and Kohler 1973). The condition may cause symptoms associated with hyperviscosity, or related to peripheral cryoprecipitation. The paraprotein is clearly pathogenic in these circumstances, and removal by plasma exchange has immediate benefit (Berkman and Orlin 1980). Maintenance of improvement generally requires the use of cytotoxic drugs to prevent or slow down resynthesis of the paraprotein. In type II cryoglobulinaemia, a monoclonal antibody (usually IgM) with rheumatoid factor activity appears in the circulation and forms complexes with autologous normal immunoglobulin. Although hyperviscosity is described (Gorevic *et al.* 1980), and cryoprecipitation may be a factor in peripheral and cutaneous features, most of the clinical manifestations, including glomerulonephritis, are associated with deposition of immune complexes. Whether these are formed *in situ* or are deposited from the circulation is unclear. Irrespective of the mechanism, because of their predominantly intravascular distribution, circulating complexes and the IgM monoclonal rheumatoid factor are efficiently removed by plasma exchange. However, the rate of recurrence of cryoglobulins (with or without other therapy) following plasma exchange is highly variable, and cryoglobulin levels do not always correlate with symptoms (Frankel *et al.* 1992). Reticuloendothelial system function has been demonstrated to improve following treatment (Walport *et al.* 1985) and this may be a factor in the clinical response. Type III cryoglobulinaemia consists of polyclonal mixed immunoglobulin, often associated with hyperglobulinaemia and present in a wide variety of infective, inflammatory and neoplastic conditions. It is often an epiphenomenon and usually does not cause symptoms separate from the underlying condition, but may do so. In these circumstances plasma exchange would seem a logical adjunct to therapy.

There have been many reports of the benefit of plasma exchange in MEC, using a variety of treatment regimens (reviewed by Valbonesi 1986), but there are no published controlled series. Plasma exchange has been used alone, or in combination with immunosuppressive drugs, for maintenance of chronic 'stable' disease and for acute therapy in cases with rapidly progressive renal failure. Our own and others' experience (Berkman and Orlin 1980; McLeod and Sassetti 1980) suggests that many clinical features, particularly Raynaud's phenomenon, skin lesions and arthralgia, are rapidly relieved following a small number of plasma exchanges. Patients vary considerably in the rate of resynthesis of cryoglobulins and recurrence of symptoms; in some, intermittent plasma exchange (for example, one or two treatments every month) may give symptomatic improvement, while in others, symptoms recur rapidly. Improvement in renal function, an important marker of prognosis, has been reported in some patients treated with plasma exchange and immunosuppressive drugs (D'Amico *et al.* 1985; Ferri *et al.* 1986; Frankel *et al.* 1992), although long-term benefit has not been convincingly demonstrated. In view of the lack of controlled data and variability of the disease, clear-cut guidelines for the use of plasma exchange are not possible. Our practice is to assess each patient individually, and tailor treatment accordingly. Patients are given an initial trial of five 4-litre plasma exchanges with steroids and, in patients with severe disease, cytotoxic drugs. Maintenance management, including the frequency of plasma exchange, then depends on the clinical response and rate of cyroglobulin resynthesis.

Rheumatoid arthritis

Trials of plasma exchange have been justified by the observation that rheumatoid factor-positive patients have a poorer prognosis than seronegative patients, and that there is an association between high levels of rheumatoid factor or circulating immune complexes and severe extra-articular disease, including vasculitis. There are numerous uncontrolled reports claiming improvement, some employing lymphoplasmaphaeresis (removal of lympocytes and plasma) rather than plasma exchange alone (Wallace *et al*. 1980; Karsh *et al*. 1981). The few controlled studies reported have been small and show conflicting results. An early controlled trial on 20 patients concluded that plasma exchange conferred no significant benefit (Rothwell *et al*. 1980), while a study of 14 patients with seropositive erosive rheumatoid arthritis, randomized to treatment with lymphoplasmaphaeresis or sham aphaeresis, found a modest improvement in subjective assessment and (at one time point) Ritchie score (Wallace *et al*. 1982). The authors of a further randomized study of 20 patients concluded that lymphoplasmaphaeresis had a minimal clinical effect, which was of short duration (Verdickt *et al*. 1983). Dwosh *et al*. (1983) conducted a well-controlled double-blind crossover trial on 26 patients with chronic rheumatoid arthritis who had failed to respond to, or tolerate, non-steroidal anti-inflammatory and second-line drugs (gold, penicillamine or chloroquine). No clinical benefit was demonstrated despite significant improvement in five laboratory parameters. In summary, there is no convincing evidence supporting benefit from plasma exchange in rheumatoid disease.

Its use in patients with rheumatoid vasculitis has been claimed to be effective (Goldman *et al*. 1979; Winkelstein *et al*. 1984).

Other rheumatological diseases

Plasma exchange has been claimed to be of value in scleroderma, particularly at an early stage in the disease (Dau *et al*. 1981; Ferri *et al*. 1987; Pourrat *et al*. 1987), but these uncontrolled data are unconvincing. Small series and case reports suggest benefit from plasma exchange in polymyositis (Dau 1981), dermatomyositis, (Cecere and Spiva 1982), Sjögren's syndrome and Behçet's disease (Raizman and Foster 1989).

Plasma exchange has been tried in Raynaud's phenomenon following the observation that sufferers have high blood viscosity (Goyle and Dormandy 1976). Several uncontrolled studies have suggested benefit (Taplos *et al*. 1978; Dodds *et al*. 1979), and in one small controlled trial none of the patients treated with placebo or intermittent heparinization improved, while five of eight patients plasma-exchanged showed amelioration of symptoms correlated with improved digital vessel patency (O'Reilly *et al*. 1979). It seems reasonable to try plasma exchange for the occasional patient with very severe disease (especially with digital ulcers) in whom other therapy has failed.

Myasthenia gravis

Antibodies to the acetylcholine receptor (AChR) are almost certainly pathogenic. Early reports of benefit in myasthenia gravis (Pinching *et al*. 1976; Dau *et al*. 1977) have been confirmed. There is an inverse relationship between clinical indices and AChR antibody titres, with a minimum lag phase of 2 days after exchange (Newsom-Davis *et al*. 1978), although electrophysiological improvement occurs earlier (Nielsen *et al*. 1982). Tindall and Rollins (1986) studied clearance of anti-AChR antibodies and found that exchange of six plasma volumes over 1 week reduced levels by 85%, but that rebound was seen in many patients, although this could be limited by concomitant administration of cytotoxic drugs. However, azathioprine alone results in clinical improvement with a decline in AChR antibody. Newsom-Davis *et al*. (1979) compared the long-term clinical response of patients to immunosuppressive therapy, with or without plasma exchange. Although the study was uncontrolled, no significant difference in rate of decline of anti-AChR antibody titres or overall clinical response was seen, apart from transient improvement after each exchange. There have been no trials examining the combined effects of plasma exchange and cyclophosphamide. In the absence of definitive randomized controlled trials, the data suggest that plasma exchange has no role in influencing the long-term outcome of myasthenia gravis. There is, however, a place for plasma exchange to relieve weakness which threatens respiration or swallowing while immunosuppressive therapy or thymectomy take effect.

Acute and chronic inflammatory demyelinating polyneuropathy

Certain patients with acute inflammatory demyelinating polyneuropathy, or Guillain–Barré syndrome, have been shown to benefit from plasma exchange. Trials were organized following anecdotal reports of response (Brettle *et al.* 1978), the detection of circulating serum factors capable of inducing demyelination in animals (Harrison *et al.* 1984), and the presence of antibodies to peripheral nerve myelin in many patients (reviewed by Cook and Dowling 1981; Koski *et al.* 1985). Several small trials reported conflicting results — both positive (Osterman *et al.* 1984) and negative (Greenwood *et al.* 1984). The situation has subsequently been clarified by two larger controlled studies. The Guillain–Barré Syndrome Study Group (1985) included 245 patients and demonstrated that short-term and 6-month improvement was significantly more likely in the plasma exchange group, in patients treated within 1 week of illness and in ventilator-dependent patients. The French co-operative randomized trial of plasma exchange (Raphael and Chastang 1984) included 183 patients and revealed similar findings. These studies have been criticized for the lack of a sham treated group, the exclusions and the statistical analysis. However, the consensus interpretation is that patients presenting within 1 week of symptoms, and those requiring ventilation, benefit from five 50 ml/kg exchanges in the first 7–14 days without steroids or other immunosuppressive therapy.

Chronic inflammatory demyelinating polyneuropathy has a slower time course than Guillain–Barré syndrome, and may be progressive or chronic and relapsing. Despite anecdotal reports of acute and continued benefit over several years, only one randomized controlled trial (which included sham treatment) has been published (Dyck *et al.* 1986). This study reported on 29 patients with 'severe' disease, randomized to twice-weekly plasma exchange (1–1.5 plasma volumes) for 3 weeks, with the sham treated group then proceeding to plasma exchange. Five of 15 treated patients responded transiently, and four of 14 control patients improved after they were plasma-exchanged. However, trials with larger numbers and longer follow-up, and perhaps with repeated courses of plasma exchange, are needed.

Multiple sclerosis

Although the aetiology of multiple sclerosis (MS) is unknown, there is accumulating evidence that it is immunologically mediated (see Chapter 109). However, there is little evidence to implicate circulating factors such as antibodies or immune complexes, although anti-myelin antibodies (Garcia-Merino *et al.* 1986) and non-antibody demyelinating factors (Bradbury *et al.* 1985) have been described. No treatment has been shown to modify the long-term outcome, and plasma exchange has been tried in both acute exacerbations and chronic MS. The many conflicting case reports and uncontrolled series are unhelpful. There are problems with conducting adequately controlled randomized studies in conditions like MS, which follow a relapsing–remitting clinical course over many years, with unknown pathogenesis and difficulties in quantifying disease activity. A prospective but unrandomized trial of azathioprine, with or without plasma exchange, in patients with chronic progressive disease, failed to demonstrate improvement in either group (Tindall *et al.* 1982). A randomized trial comparing adrenocorticotrophic hormone (ACTH), ACTH and cyclophosphamide, and ACTH with plasma exchange, in 58 patients with severe progressive MS, found that only the ACTH with cyclophosphamide arm showed any (albeit transient) improvement (Hauser *et al.* 1983). The authors of a double-blind controlled (but not randomized) study of patients with progressive chronic disease given cyclophosphamide and prednisolone, with or without plasma exchange, concluded that the plasma-exchanged group fared better than the sham control group (Khatri *et al.* 1985). However, the follow-up was relatively short (11 months) and at the end of this period the differences between control and treated group were less than at 5 months. There are a number of other criticisms of this trial (discussed by Weiner 1985), which make it unconvincing.

A large American, multicentre, double-blind randomized trial of plasma exchange in 116 patients with acute episodes of MS has recently been published (Weiner *et al.* 1989). Patients received intramuscular ACTH, oral cyclophosphamide, and 11 actual or sham plasma exchanges over 8 weeks. The results revealed that exchanged patients with relapsing–remitting disease ($n = 76$) had significantly greater and more rapid improvement at 4 weeks, although the effect was lost at 1 year. Indeed, disability scores were not significantly different at all time points from 2 to 24 months. In contrast to the studies reported by Khatri *et al.* (1985), patients with chronic progressive MS ($n = 40$) fared no better than controls at any stage (Weiner *et al.* 1989). Recently the randomized, placebo-controlled trial reported by the Canadian Co-operative multiple sclerosis study group (1991) failed to demonstrate benefit from plasma exchange or immunosuppression.

The balance of evidence thus cannot support a general role for plasma exchange in the management of MS. Possibly, in some patients with relapsing–remitting MS, with particularly severe acute attacks, the addition of plasma exchange to ACTH and cyclophosphamide may be useful.

Other neurological diseases

The Eaton–Lambert syndrome is probably due to autoantibodies to the presynaptic nerve terminal (see Chapter 106). Newsom-Davis and Murray (1984) assessed nine patients who received plasma exchange for 6 months to 2½ years together with steroids and azathioprine. It was concluded that plasma exchange was useful, and other reports have supported this view (Kranz *et al.* 1980; Dau and Denys 1982). However, clinical response generally takes longer than in myasthenia gravis, and randomized trials would be difficult in such a rare condition. Plasma exchange has also been tried in neuropathies due to paraproteinaemias and in motor neurone disease, but with no convincing evidence of benefit.

Pemphigus

Most patients with pemphigus (vulgaris and foliaceous) have antibodies which bind to stratified squamous epithelia, and which may have a pathogenic role (see Chapter 96). Before corticosteroids were used, pemphigus was a fatal disease. There have been many case reports and uncontrolled studies suggesting that plasma exchange allows lower doses of steroids to be used, or benefits corticosteroid-resistant patients (Ruocco *et al.* 1978; Roujeau *et al.* 1983), although rebound of antibody titres frequently occurs. Recently, a French multicentre study found that plasma exchange (10 × 60 ml/kg exchanges over 4 weeks) had no detectable effect on disease or steroid requirement; moreover, four of the plasma exchange group succumbed to sepsis, compared with none in the control group (Guillaume *et al.* 1988). It remains possible that plasma exchange may help in selected individuals with 'corticosteroid-resistant' severe pemphigus (Ruocco *et al.* 1984).

Bullous pemphigoid

Subepidermal bullae in pemphigoid are associated with deposition of IgG and C3 along the basement membrane, and circulating anti-basement membrane antibodies may be found (see Chapter 96). The condition generally responds to steroids, with or without cytotoxic drug therapy, and benefit from plasma exchange is reported. A medium-term but uncontrolled study claimed patients receiving three plasma exchanges per week for 3 months, followed by less frequent exchanges, had a lower relapse rate and needed less steroids than those taking steroids alone (Guillot *et al.* 1986). The only published controlled trial concluded that plasma exchange conferred a short-term steroid-sparing effect (Roujeau *et al.* 1984a), but no significant difference in recurrence rate was seen.

Other dermatological diseases

Many other skin disorders, often with evidence of circulating antibodies or immune complexes, have been treated with plasma exchange. These include: pyoderma gangrenosum, herpes gestationis, dermatitis herpetiformis, acquired bullous epidermolysis, psoriasis and atopic eczema. However, evidence for a beneficial role for plasma exchange in these disorders is restricted to a small number of anecdoctal reports, and has not been subjected to controlled trials (reviewed by Coffe 1986). There is also a subgroup of patients with severe drug-resistant cutaneous vasculitis who respond well to plasma exchange. Eight such cases have been treated at the Hammersmith Hospital, of whom five showed a good response, two a partial response and one no response. Four of these patients have been maintained on intermittent plasma exchange (4 litre every 2–4 weeks) for 5–12 years (Turner *et al.* 1990).

Immune thrombocytopenic purpura

In immune thrombocytopenic purpura (ITP) autoantibodies to platelets are believed to be responsible for the destruction of platelets by the RES, mainly in the spleen (see Chapter 95). Removal of antibody by plasma exchange is therefore logical, although most patients respond to steroids, splenectomy and/or immunosuppressive drugs. Many case reports, two uncontrolled series, but no controlled trials of plasma exchange in ITP have been published. Marder *et al.* (1981) described five patients with chronic ITP who failed to respond to steroids, splenectomy or plasma exchange, as compared with five of nine patients with acute ITP who had a limited response to exchange. In another study 6/9 refractory patients who showed a transient response when treated by immunoadsorption (Guthrie and Oral 1989). A more intensive plasma exchange regimen in an uncontrolled study, with FFP as replacement fluid, was claimed to result in responses in eight of ten cases, with the two failures (chronic ITP) responding to splenectomy (Blanchette *et al.* 1984). Plasma exchange has also been combined with intravenous IgG therapy, and one study reported responses in four of eight patients, although two treated with further courses failed to show a subsequent response (Bussel *et al.* 1988).

Thrombotic thrombocytopenic purpura

Plasma exchange is widely used in the treatment of thrombotic thrombocytopenic purpura (TTP) (Caggiano 1986). There have been many enthusiastic reports of plasma exchange, including a study of 17 patients, 14 of whom recovered (Blitzer *et al.* 1987). Other treatments, including plasma infusion alone, may produce a similar outcome and plasma exchange with FFP replacement has become a frequent part of the management of patients with TTP. Overall, the regimens used appear to be effective (Bell *et al.* 1991). We have treated isolated cases who appeared to respond to exchange for FFP, but not to exchange for albumin or infusion of FFP alone. Recently the results of a trial (in 102 patients) comparing plasma exchange (with FFP replacement) and FFP infusion alone have been published (Rock *et al.* 1991). The plasma exchange group did better when assessed on day 9 and at 6 months although they received three times as much plasma as the FFP alone group. The issue of whether efficacy is related to removal of pathogenic components or repletion of plasma factors is still an important unanswered question, but plasma exchange may allow more FFP to be given and appears to be the best therapy currently available (Moake 1991).

Other haematological diseases

Post-transfusion purpura, associated with allogeneic anti-phospholipase A_1 (PLA_1) antibodies, causes a self-limited but life-threatening thrombocytopenia lasting 4–6 weeks. The condition was first successfully treated with exchange transfusion in 1972 (Cimo and Aster 1972) and all reported cases have also responded to plasma exchange with a rapidly increasing platelet count. It is therefore regarded as the treatment of choice in this rare condition (reviewed by Rock 1986).

Haemophiliacs with anti-factor VIIIC antibodies, suffering life-threatening haemorrhage, have been treated with plasma exchange (Slocombe *et al.* 1981) or immunoadsorption with protein-A columns together with factor VIII infusion (Nilsson *et al.* 1981, 1984). Plasma exchange has been reported to be of value in the removal of AB blood group antibodies in preparation for ABO incompatible bone marrow transplants (Bensinger *et al.* 1981). There are a number of other rare conditions in which pathogenic autoantibodies are present which have been reported to respond to plasma exchange, including red cell aplasia (Messner *et al.* 1981), autoimmune haemolytic anaemia (Rosenfield and Jagathambal 1976), and prevention of rhesus haemolytic disease. However, all reports relating to these conditions are uncontrolled.

Graves' disease

Graves' ophthalmopathy is associated with an inflammatory myopathy of the extraocular muscles (see Chapter 102), and, although there is evidence for involvement of humoral and cell-mediated immunity, their relative contributions to pathogenesis are unknown. Plasma exchange was first reported to be successful in a single patient (Dandona *et al.* 1979). The same group reported success in four patients with acute, but not in three with chronic, ophthalmopathy (Dandona *et al.* 1980). Intensive plasma exchange with steroids and azathioprine has been reported to be beneficial in eight of nine patients (Glinoer *et al.* 1986), although another study using plasma exchange with or without azathioprine in 18 patients reported little success (Kelly *et al.* 1983).

Conclusions

It is disappointing that, although plasma exchange has been tried in a large number of immunologically mediated disorders over the past 15 years, there are few diseases in which it is of proved benefit. Adequate controlled studies are often lacking, although these are difficult to organize for rare and clinically variable conditions.

However, for certain diseases, there are either adequate controlled data, or convincing circumstantial evidence, to support a role for plasma exchange in primary management (Table 48.5). For other disorders, despite lack of clear-cut evidence from controlled trials, it seems likely that plasma exchange may prove useful (Table 48.6). It may be that only certain subgroups will benefit, for instance dialysis-dependent patients with systemic vasculitis, or steroid-resistant pemphigus. In these conditions, the use of plasma exchange looks promising, but larger numbers and longer follow-up are needed. Further, there will always be patients in whom there is a theoretical argument for the use of plasma exchange, and positive anecdotal reports, but little prospect of adequately controlled trials: for instance, the patients with rare antibody-mediated diseases such as post-transfusion purpura. Finally, there is a group of conditions (Table 48.7) in which there are only enthusiastic case reports and/or negative trial data. Obviously, in these disorders plasma exchange cannot at present be recommended.

In conclusion, it is clear that plasma exchange does have a role in certain defined clinical settings. The potential benefit must be balanced against the small, but definite, risk of the procedure, particularly if replacement with FFP is contemplated. However, plasma exchange is presently a rather crude treatment, and one hopes that, with increasing understanding of the immune mechanisms involved in disease pathogenesis, more specific forms of intervention will become available.

Table 48.5. Conditions for which plasma exchange has an established role with good supportive data

Condition	Comments
Guillain–Barré syndrome	Patients presenting within 1 week of symptoms or requiring ventilation; without steroids or immunosuppressive therapy
Myasthenia gravis	Alleviates weakness acutely; useful for myasthenic crises; no effect on long-term outcome
Anti-GBM disease	Indicated for pulmonary haemorrhage or non-oliguric nephritis; may be useful in oliguric/dialysis-dependent patients — see text; with immunosuppression
Haemophilia with antibodies	In patients unresponsive to factor VIII or IX with life-threatening haemorrhage
Post-transfusion purpura	If life-threatening haemorrhage occurs; only proved effective treatment
Hyperviscosity syndromes	With immediate relief of symptoms; other treatment may be necessary to prevent recurrence
Eaton–Lambert syndrome	Responds less quickly than myasthenia gravis; usually with immunosuppression
Mixed essential cryoglobulinaemia	Many patients symptomatically improved and may aid ulcer healing; little evidence for long-term disease modification; usually with immunosuppression

Table 48.6. Conditions for which plasma exchange may be useful

Condition	Comments
Rapidly progressive glomerulonephritis	Probably only in dialysis-dependent patients (with immunosuppression); reasonable additional therapy in severe systemic disease unresponsive to drugs
Systemic lupus erythematosus	Circumstantial evidence of benefit in severe lupus nephritis and cerebral lupus; reasonable additional therapy in severe systemic disease unresponsive to drugs
Pemphigus	Some evidence for a role in selected 'steroid-resistant' patients
Cutaneous vasculitis	Some patients seem to respond only to plasma exchange (± immunosuppression)
Renal transplantation	Possible role in occasional patients with vascular rejection (combined with cyclophosphamide); probable benefit for removal of anti-HLA antibodies in highly sensitized potential recipients (combined with immunosuppression)
ABO-incompatible bone marrow grafts	To remove anti-A or anti-B antibodies prior to bone marrow transplantation
Graves' ophthalmopathy	Uncontrolled series (± immunosuppression) with variable results
Raynaud's phenomenon	If severe (± ulcers) may be worth trying after failure of other therapy
Thrombotic thrombocytopenic purpura	Anecdotal reports of improvement with FFP as replacement fluid; prospective randomized trial comparing plasma exchange with plasma infusion in progress

Table 48.7. Conditions reported to respond to plasma exchange but with few convincing data or negative trials

Condition	Comments
Primary glomerulonephritides	Except anti-GBM nephritis
Rheumatoid arthritis	Possibly for patients with systemic vasculitis
Other rheumatological diseases	Including scleroderma, dermatomyositis, polymyositis, Sjögren's and Behçet's syndromes — uncontrolled reports combined with a variety of concomitant therapy
Multiple sclerosis	Several trials show no benefit, but one (which included immunosuppression) suggested temporary benefit
Pemphigoid	One controlled study suggested a steroid-sparing effect, but recurrence rate was the same as the control group
Other dermatological conditions	Including dermatitis herpetiformis, psoriasis and pyoderma gangrenosum
Chronic inflammatory polyradiculopathy	Great patient heterogeneity; adequate trials are needed
Immune thrombocytopenic purpura	Variable results reported but no controlled studies

References

Abbot, F., Jones, S., Lockwood, C.M. and Rees, A.J. (1988). Autoantibodies to glomerular antigens in patients with Wegener's granulomatosis. *Nephrol. Dial. Transplant.* **4**, 1.

Abel, J.J., Rowntree, L.G. and Turner, B.B. (1914). Plasma removal with return of corpuscles. *J. Pharmacol. Exp. Ther.* **5**, 625.

Alcalay, D., Deleplanque, P. and Alcalay, M. (1987). Plasma exchange in seven gastrointestinal and renal forms of Henoch–Schönlein purpura and primary IgA nephropathy. *Plasma Ther. Transfusion Technol.* **8**, 147.

Allen, N., Smith, J., Tate, D. *et al.* (1983). Intensive plasma exchange in acute renal allograft rejection — a controlled trial. *Transplant. Proc.* **15**, 1060.

Becker, G.J., d'Apice, A.J.F., Walker, R.G. and Kincaid-Smith, P. (1977). Plasmapheresis in the treatment of glomerulonephritis. *Med. J. Aust.* **2**, 693.

Bell, W.R., Braine, H.G., Ness, P.M. and Kickler, T.S. Improved survival in thrombotic thrombocytopenic purpura-hemolytic uremic syndrome-clinical experience in 108 patients. *N. Eng. J. Med.* **325**, 398.

Benoit, F.L., Rulon, D.B., Theil, G.B., Doolan, P.D. and Watten, R.H. (1964). Goodpasture's syndrome: a clinicopathologic entity. *Am. J. Med.* **37**, 424.

Bensinger, W.I., Baker, D.A., Buchner, C.D., Clift, R.A. and Thomas, E.D. (1981). Immunoadsorption for removal of A and B blood group antibodies. *N. Engl. J. Med.* **304**, 160.

Bensinger, W.I., Buckner, C.D. and Clift, R.A. (1985). Whole blood immunoadsorption of anti-A or anti-B antibodies. *Vox Sang.* **48**, 357.

Berkman, E.M. and Orlin, J.B. (1980). Use of plasmapheresis and partial plasma exchange in the management of patients with cryoglobulinaemia. *Transfusion* **20**, 171.

Blanchette, V.S., Hogan, V.A., McCombie, N.E. *et al.* (1984). Intensive plasma exhange therapy in ten patients with idiopathic thrombocytopenic purpura. *Transfusion* **24**, 388.

Blitzer, J.B., Granfortuna, J.M., Gottlieb, A.J. *et al.* (1987). Thrombotic thrombocytopenia purpura: treatment with plasmapheresis. *Am. J. Haematol.* **24**, 329.

Bonomini, V., Vangelista, A., Frasca, G.M., De Felice, A. and Liviano D'Arcangelo, G. (1985). Effects of plasmapheresis in renal transplant rejection: a controlled study. *Trans. Am. Soc. Artificial Intern. Organs* **31**, 698.

Bradbury, K., Aparicio, S.R., Sumner, D.W. *et al.* (1985). Comparison of *in vitro* demyelination and cytotoxicity of humoral factors in multiple sclerosis and other neurological diseases. *J. Neurol. Sci.* **70**, 167.

Brettle, R.P., Gross, M.L.P., Legg, N.J., Lockwood, C.M. and Pallis, C. (1978). Treatment of acute polyneuropathy by plasma exchange. *Lancet* **ii**, 1100.

Briggs, W.A., Johnson, J.P., Teichman, S., Yeager, H.C. and Wilson, C.B. (1979). Anti-GBM antibody mediated glomerulonephritis and Goodpasture's syndrome. *Medicine* **58**, 348.

Burran, W.P., Avasthi, P., Smith, K.J. and Simon, T.L. (1986). Efficacy of plasma exchange in severe idiopathic rapidly progressive glomerulonephritis: a report of ten cases. *Transfusion* **26**, 382.

Bussel, A. and Jais, J.P. (1987). Side effects and mortality associated with plasma exchange: a three year experience with a regional register. *Life Support Syst.* **5**, 353.

Bussel, J.B., Saal, S. and Gordon, B. (1988). Combined plasma exchange and intravenous gammaglobulin in the treatment of patients with refractory immune thrombocytopenic purpura. *Transfusion* **28**, 38.

Bygren, P., Freiburghaus, C., Lindholm, T., Simonsen, D., Thysell, H. and Wieslander, J. (1985). Goodpasture's syndrome with staphylococcal protein A immunoadsorption. *Lancet* **ii**, 1295.

Caggiano, V. (1986). Apheresis in the treatment of TTP. In *Therapeutic Hemapheresis*, ed. M. Valbonesi, A.A. Pineda and J.C. Biggs, p. 135, Wichtig Editore, Milan.

Canadian cooperative multiple sclerosis study group. (1991). The Canadian cooperative trial of cyclophosphamide and plasma exchange in progressive multiple sclerosis. *Lancet* **337**, 441.

Cardella, C.J., Sutton, D.M.C., Uldall, P.R., Cook, G.T. and de Veber, G.A. (1985). Factors influencing the effect of intensive plasma exchange on acute transplant rejection. *Transplant. Proc.* **17**, 2777.

Cecere, F.A. and Spiva, D.A. (1982). Combination plasmapheresis/leukocytapheresis for the treatment of dermatomyositis/polymyositis. *Plasma Ther. Transfusion Technol.* **3**, 401.

Cimo, P.L. and Aster, R.H. (1972). Post-transfusion purpura: successful treatment by exchange transfusion. *N. Engl. J. Med.* **287**, 290.

Clark, W.F. Cattran, D.C., Balfe, J.W., Williams, W., Lindsay, R.M. and Linton, A.L. (1983). Chronic plasma exchange in systemic lupus erythematosus nephritis. *Proc. Eur. Dialysis Transplant Assoc.* **20**, 629.

Coffe, C. (1986). Plasma exchange in dermatological disease. In *Therapeutic Hemapheresis*, ed. M. Valbonesa, A.A. Pineda and J.C. Biggs, p. 97, Wichtig Editore, Milan.

Cohen, J., Pinching, A.J., Rees, A.J. and Peters, D.K. (1982). Infection and immunosuppression. A study of the infective complications of 75 patients with immunologically-mediated disease. *Quart. J. Med.* **51**, 1.

Cook, S.D. and Dowling, P.C. (1981). The role of autoantibody and immune complexes in the pathogenesis of Guillain–Barré syndrome. *Ann. Neurol.* **9**, (suppl.), 70.

Coppo, R., Basolo, B., Roccatello, D. *et al.* (1985). Immunological monitoring of plasma exchange in primary IgA nephropathy. *Artificial Organs* **9**, 351.

Couser, W.G. (1988). Rapidly progressive glomerulonephritis: classification, pathogenetic mechanisms and therapy. *Am. J. Kidney Dis.* **11**, 449.

D'Amico, G., Ferrario, F., Colasanti, G. and Bucci, A. (1985). Glomerulonephritis in essential mixed cryoglobulinemia. In *Proceeding. 21st Congress of the European Dialysis and Transplant Association*, ed. P.J. Davison and P.J. Guillon, p. 527, Pitman, London.

Dandona, P., Marshall, N.J., Bidley, S.P., Nathan, A. and Havard, C.W.H. (1979). Successful treatment of exophthalmos and pretibial myxoedema with plasmapheresis. *Br. Med. J.* **i**, 374.

Dandona, P., Marshall, N.J., Bidley, S.P., Nathan, A. and Havard, C.W.H. (1980). Treatment of acute malignant exophthalmos with plasma exchange. In *Thyroid Research VIII*, ed. J.R. Stockigt and S. Nagataki, p. 583, Australian Academy of Science, Canberra.

d'Apice, A.J.F. and Kincaid-Smith, P. (1979). Plasma exchange in the treatment of glomerulonephritis. In *Progress in Glomerulonephritis*, ed. P. Kincaid-Smith, A. d'Apice and R. Atkins, p. 371, Wiley, New York.

Dau, P.C. (1981). Plasmapheresis in idiopathic inflammatory myopathy: experience with 35 patients. *Arch. Neurol.* **38**, 544.

Dau, P.C. and Denys, E.H. (1982). Plasmapheresis and immunosuppressive drug therapy in the Eaton–Lambert syndrome. *Ann. Neurol.* **11**, 570.

Dau, P.C., Lindstrom, J.M., Cassel, J.K., Denys, E.H., Shev, E.E. and Spitter, L.E. (1977). Plasmapheresis and immunosuppressive drug therapy in myasthenia gravis. *N. Engl. J. Med.* **297**, 1134.

Dau, P.C., Petajan, J.H., Johnson, K.P., Panitch, H.S. and Bornstein, M.B. (1980). Plasmapheresis in multiple sclerosis: preliminary findings. *Neurology* **30**, 1023.

Dau, P.C., Kahaleh, M.B. and Sagebiel, R.W. (1981). Plasmapheresis and immunosuppressive drug therapy in scleroderma. *Arthritis Rheum.* **24**, 1128.

Derksen, R.H.W.M., Hené, R.J., Kallenberg, C.G.M., Valentijn, R.M. and Kater, L. (1988). Prospective multicentre trial on the short-term effects of plasma exchange versus cytotoxic drugs in steroid-resistant lupus nephritis. *Neth. J. Med.* **33**, 168.

Derksen, R.H.W.M., Schuurman, H.J., Gmelig Meyling, F.H.J., Struyvenberg, A. and Kater, L. (1984). The efficiency of plasma exchange in the removal of plasma components. *J. Lab. Clin. Med.* **104**, 346.

Dodds, A.J., O'Reilly, M.J.G., Yates, C.J.P., Cotton, L.T., Flute, P.T. and Dormandy, J.A. (1979). Haemorrheological response to plasma exchange in Raynaud's syndrome. *Br. Med. J.* **2**, 1186.

Dwosh, I.L., Giles, A.R., Ford, P.M., Pater, J.L. and Anastassiades, T.P. (1983). Plasmapheresis therapy in rheumatoid arthritis: a controlled double-blind crossover trial. *N. Engl. J. Med.* **308**, 1124.

Dyck, P.J., Daube, J., O'Brien, P. *et al.* (1986). Plasma exchange in chronic inflammatory demyelinating polyradiculoneuropathy. *N. Engl. J. Med.* **314**, 461.

El-Habib, R., Laville, M. and Traeger, J. (1984). Specific adsorption of circulating antibodies by extracorporeal plasma perfusions over antigen coated collagen flat-membranes: applications to systemic lupus erythematosus. *J. Clin. Lab. Immunol.* **15**, 111.

Erickson, S.B., Kurtz, S.B., Donadio, J.V., Jr, Holley, K.E., Wilson, C.B. and Pineda, A.A. (1979). Use of combined plasmapheresis and immunosuppression in the treatment of Goodpasture's syndrome. *Mayo Clin. Proc.* **54**, 714.

Espinel, E., Vallés, M., Rodriguez, J.A., Rodriguez, A. and Piera, L. (1984). Crescentic mesangiocapillary glomerulonephritis and plasmapheresis. *Proc. IXth Int. Congress Nephrol.* 85A.

Falk, R.J., Terrell, R.S., Charles, L.A. and Jennette, J.C. (1990). Anti-neutrophil cytoplasmic autoantibodies induce neutrophils to degranulate and produce oxygen radicals *in vitro*. *Proc. Nat. Acad. Sci. (USA)* **87**, 4115.

Fauchald, P., Leivestad, T., Bratlie, A., Albrechtsen, D., Talseth, T. and Flatmark, A. (1987). Plasma exchange and immunosuppressive therapy before renal transplantation in allosensitized patients. *Transplant. Proc.* **14**, 3748.

Feest, T.G., Burge, P.S. and Cohen, S.L. (1976). Successful treatment of myeloma by diuresis and plasmapheresis. *Br. Med. J.* **i**, 503.

Ferri, C., Moriconi, L., Gremignai, G. *et al.* (1986). Treatment of the renal involvement in mixed cryoglobulinaemia with prolonged plasma exchange. *Nephron* **43**, 246.

Ferri, C., Bernini, L., Gremignai, G. *et al.* (1987). Plasma exchange in the treatment of progressive systemic sclerosis. *Plasma Ther. Transfusion Technol.* **8**, 169.

Flores, J.C., Taube, D., Savage, C.O. *et al.* (1986). Clinical and immunological evolution of oligoanuric anti-GBM nephritis treated by haemodialysis. *Lancet* **i**, 5.

Franco, A., Anaya, F., Niembro, E., Ahijado, F., Luno, J. and Valderrabano, F. (1987). Plasma exchange in the treatment of vascular rejection: relationship between histological changes and therapeutic response. *Transplant. Proc.* **14**, 3661.

Frank, M.M., Hamburger, M.I., Lawley, T.J., Kimberley, R.P. and Plotz, P.H. (1979). Defective reticuloendothelial system Fc receptor function in systemic lupus erythematosus. *N. Engl. J. Med.* **300**, 518.

Frankel, A.H., Singer, D.R.J., Winearls, C.G., Evans, D.J., Rees, A.J. and Pusey, C.D. (1992). Type II essential mixed cryoglobulinaemia: presentation, treatment and outcome in 13 patients. *Quart. J. Med.* (in press).

Garcia-Merino, A., Persson, M.A.A., Ernerudh, J. *et al.* (1986). Serum and cerebrospinal fluid antibodies against myelin basic protein and their IgG subclass distribution in multiple sclerosis. *J. Neurol. Neurosurg. Psychiatry* **49**, 1066.

Glinoer, D., Etienne-Decerf, J., Schrooyen, M. *et al.* (1986). Beneficial effects of intensive plasma exchange followed by immunosuppressive therapy in severe Graves' ophthalmopathy. *Acta Endocrinol.* **111**, 30.

Glockner, W.M., Sieberth, H.G., Wichmann, H.E. *et al.* (1988). Plasma exchange and immunosuppression in rapidly progressive nephritis: a controlled, multi-center study. *Clin. Nephrol.* **29**, 1.

Goldman, J.A., Casey, H.L., McIlwain, H., Kirby, J., Wilson, C.H. and Miller, S.B. (1979). Limited plasmapheresis in rheumatoid arthritis with vasculitis. *Arthritis Rheum.* **22**, 1146.

Gorevic, P.D., Kassab, H.J., Levo, Y. *et al.* (1980). Mixed cryoglobulinaemia: clinical aspects and long-term follow up of 40 patients. *Am. J. Med.* **69**, 287.

Goyle, K.B. and Dormandy, J.A. (1976). Abnormal blood viscosity in Raynaud's phenomenon. *Lancet* **i**, 1317.

Greenwood, R.J., Newson-Davis, J., Hughes, R.A.C. *et al.* (1984). Controlled trial of plasma exchange in acute inflammatory polyradiculoneuropathy. *Lancet* **i**, 877.

Grey, H.M. and Kohler, P.F. (1973). Cryoimmunoglobulins. *Semin. Hematol.* **10**, 87.

Guillain–Barré Syndrome Study Group (1985). Plasmapheresis and acute Guillain–Barré syndrome. *Neurology* **35**, 1096.

Guillaume, J.-C., Ronjeau, J.-C., Morel, P. *et al.* (1988). Controlled study of plasma exchange in pemphigus. *Arch. Dermatol.* **124**, 1659.

Guillot, B., Donadio, D., Guilhou, J.J. and Meynadier, J. (1986). Long-term plasma exchange therapy in bullous pemphigoid. *Acta Dermatol. Venereol.* **66**, 73.

Gurland, H.J., Blumenstein, M., Lysaght, M.J., Samtleben, W. and Stoffner, D. (1983). Plasmapheresis in renal transplantation. *Kidney Int.* **23** (suppl. 14), 82.

Gurland, H.J., Samtleben, W., Blumenstein, M., Randerson, D.H. and Schmidt, B. (1984). Comparative evaluation of filters used in membrane plasmapheresis. *Nephron* **36**, 173.

Guthrie, T.H. Jr, and Oral, A. (1989). Immune thrombocytopenia purpura: a pilot study of staphylococcal protein A immunomodulation in refractory patients. *Semin. Hematol.* **26**, (2 suppl. 1), 3.

Harrison, B.M., Hansen, L.A., Pollard, J.D. and McLeod, J.G. (1984). Demyelination induced by serum from patients with Guillain–Barré syndrome. *Ann. Neurol.* **15**, 163.

Hashimoto, H., Tsuda, H., Kanai, Y. *et al.* (1991). Selective removal of anti-DNA and anticardiolipin antibodies by adsorbent plasmapheresis using dextran sulfate columns in patients with systemic lupus erythematosus. *J. Rheumatol.* **18**, 545.

Hauser, S.L., Dawson, D.M., Lehrich, J.R. *et al.* (1983). Intensive immunosuppression in progressive multiple sclerosis: a randomised, three arm study of high-dose intravenous cyclophosphamide, plasma exchange and ACTH. *N. Engl. J. Med.* **308**, 173.

Haworth, S.J., Pusey, C.D. and Lockwood, C.M. (1985). Plasma exchange in lupus nephritis. *Proc. EDTA–ERA* **22**, 699.

Heaf, J.G., Jorgensen, F. and Nielsen, L.P. (1983). Treatment and prognosis of extracapillary glomerulonephritis. *Nephron* **35**, 217.

Herbert, L., Neilsen, E., Pohl, M., Lachin, J., Hunsicker, L. and Lewis, E. (1987). Clinical course of severe lupus nephritis during the controlled clinical trial of plasmapheresis therapy (PPT). *Kidney Int.* **31**, 201.

Hind, C.R.K., Paraskevakou, H., Lockwood, C.M., Evans, D.J., Peters, D.K. and Rees, A.J. (1983). Prognosis after immunosuppression of patients with crescentic nephritis. *Lancet* **i**, 263.

Huestis, D.W. (1983). Mortality in therapeutic haemapheresis. *Lancet* **i**, 1043.

Johnson, J.P., Moore, J., Austin, H.A., Balow, J.E., Antonovych T.T. and Wilson, C.B. (1985). Therapy of anti-glomerular basement membrane antibody disease: analysis of prognostic significance of clinical, pathologic and treatment factors. *Medicine* **64**, 219.

Jordan, S.C., Ho, W., Ettenger, R., Salusky, I.B. and Fine, R.N. (1987). Plasma exchange improves the glomerulonephritis of systemic lupus erythematosus in selected pediatric patients. *Pediatr. Nephrol.* **1**, 276.

Karsh, J., Klippel, J.H., Plotz, P.H., Decker, J.L., Wright, D.G. and Flye, M.W. (1981). Lymphapheresis in rheumatoid arthritis: a randomised trial. *Arthritis Rheum.* **24**, 867.

Kauffmann, R.H. and Houwert, D.A. (1981). Plasmapheresis in rapidly progressive Henoch Schönlein glomerulonephritis and the effect on circulating IgA immune complexes. *Clin. Nephrol.* **16**, 155.

Keller, F., Oehlenberg, B., Kunzendorf, U., Schwarz, A. and Offermann, G. (1989). Longterm treatment and prognosis of rapidly progressive glomerulonephritis. *Clin. Nephrol.* **31**, 190.

Kelly, W., Longson, D., Smithard, D. *et al.* (1983). An evaluation of plasma exchange for Graves' ophthalmopathy. *Clin. Endocrinol.* **18**, 485.

Khatri, B.O., McQuillen, M.P., Harrington, G.J., Schmoll, D. and Hoffmann, R.G. (1985). Chronic progressive multiple sclerosis: double-blind controlled study of plasmapheresis in patients taking immunosuppressive drugs. *Neurology* **35**, 312.

Khatri, B.O., McQuillen, M.P., Hoffmann, R.G., Harrington, G.J. and Schmoll, D. (1991). Plasma exchange in chronic progressive multiple sclerosis: A long-term study. *Neurology* **41**, 409.

Kincaid-Smith, P. and d'Apice, A.J.F. (1978). Plasmapheresis in rapidly progressive glomerulonephritis. *Am. J. Med.* **65**, 564.

Kincaid-Smith, P. and Walker, R.G. (1984). The case for plasmapheresis. In *Controversies in Nephrology and Hypertension*, ed. R.G. Nairns, p. 463, Churchill Livingstone, New York.

Kirubakaran, M.G., Disney, A.P.S., Norman, J., Pugsley, D.J. and Mathew, T.H. (1981). A controlled trial of plasmapheresis in the treatment of renal allograft rejection. *Transplantation* **32**, 164.

Koski, C.L., Humphrey, R. and Shin, M.L. (1985). Anti-peripheral myelin antibodies in patients with demyelinating neuropathy: quantitative and kinetic determination of serum antibodies by complement component and fixation. *Proc. Nat. Acad. Sci. (USA)* **82**, 905.

Kranz, H., Caddy, D.J., Williams, A.M. and Gay, W. (1980). Myasthenic syndrome: effect of choline, plasmapheresis and tests for circulating factor. *J. Neurol. Neurosurg. Psychiatry* **43**, 483.

Lai, K.N., Lai, F.M., Leung, A.C.T., Ho, C.P. and Vallance-Owen, J. (1987). Plasma exchange in patients with rapidly progressive idiopathic IgA nephropathy: a report of two cases and review of literature. *Am. J. Kidney Dis.* **10**, 66.

Lancet Editorial (1982). Hazards of apheresis. *Lancet* **ii**, 1025.

Law, A., Hotze, A., Krapf, F. *et al.* (1985). The non-specific clearance function of the reticuloendothelial system in patients with immune complex mediated diseases before and after plasmapheresis. *Rheumatol. Int.* **5**, 69.

Lazarus, H.M., Cohen, S.B., Clegg, D.O. *et al.* (1991). Selective *in vivo* removal of rheumatoid factor by an extracorporeal treatment device in rheumatoid arthritis patients. *Transfusion* **31**, 122.

Leaker, B.R., Becker, G.J., Dowling, J.P. and Kincaid-Smith, P. (1986). Rapid improvement in severe lupus glomerular lesions following intensive plasma exchange associated with immunosuppression. *Clin. Nephrol.* **25**, 236.

Lerner, R.A., Glassock, R.J. and Dixon, F.J. (1967). The role of anti-glomerular basement membrane antibody in the pathogenesis of human glomerulonephritis. *J. Exp. Med.* **126**, 989.

Lewis, E.J. (1982). Plasmapheresis for the treatment of severe lupus nephritis: uncontrolled observations. *Am. J. Kidney Dis.* **2**, (suppl. 1), 182.

Lewis, E., Lachin, J. and Lupus Nephritis Collaborative Study Group (LNCSG), (1987). Primary outcomes in the controlled trial of plasmapheresis therapy (PPT) in severe lupus nephritis. *Kidney Int.* **31**, 208.

Lockwood, C.M., Boulton-Jones, J.M., Lowenthal, R.M., Simpson, I.J., Peters, D.K. and Wilson, C.B. (1975). Recovery from Goodpasture's syndrome after immunosuppressive treatment and plasmapheresis. *Br. Med. J.* **ii**, 252.

Lockwood, C.M., Rees, A.J., Pinching, A.J. *et al.* (1977). Plasma exchange and immunosuppression in the treatment of fulminating immune-complex crescentic nephritis. *Lancet* **i**, 63.

Lockwood, C.M., Worlledge, S., Nicholas, A., Cotton, C. and Peters, D.K. (1979). Reversal of impaired splenic function in patients with nephritis of vasculitis (or both) by plasma exchange. *N. Engl. J. Med.* **300**, 524.

Lockwood, C.M., Pusey, C.D., Rees, A.J. and Peters, D.K.

(1981). Plasma exchange in the treatment of immune complex disease. *Clin. Immunol. Allergy* **1**, 433.

McGinley, E., Watkins, R., McLay, A. and Boulton-Jones, J.M. (1985). Plasma exchange in the treatment of mesangiocapillary glomerulonephritis. *Nephron* **40**, 385.

McLeod, B.C. and Sassetti, R.J. (1980). Plasmapheresis with return of cryoglobulin depleted autologous plasma (cryoglobulinpheresis) in cryoglobulinaemia. *Blood* **55**, 866.

Marder, V.J., Nusbacher, J. and Anderson, F.W. (1981). One year follow-up of plasma exchange therapy in 14 patients with idiopathic thrombocytopenic purpura. *Transfusion* **21**, 291.

Messner, H.A., Fauser, A.A., Curtis, J.E. and Dotten, D. (1981). Control of antibody mediated pure red cell aplasia by plasmapheresis. *N. Engl. J. Med.* **304**, 1334.

Moake, J.L. (1991). TTP-desperation, empiricism, progress. *N. Eng. J. Med.* **325**, 426.

Moran, C.J., Parry, H.F., Mowbray, J., Richards, J.D.M. and Goldstone, A.H. (1977). Plasmapheresis in systemic lupus erythematosus. *Br. Med. J.*, **1**, 1573.

Moriconi, L., Ferri, C., Fanara, G. *et al.* (1983). Plasma exchange in the treatment of lupus nephritis. *Int. J. Artificial Organs* **6**, 35.

Munoz, J., Sanchez, M., Perez-Garcia, R., Anaya, F. and Valderrabano, F. (1985). Recurrent focal glomerulosclerosis in renal transplants: proteinuria relapsing following plasma exchange. *Clin. Nephrol.* **24**, 213.

Newsom-Davis, J. and Murray, N. (1984). Plasma exchange and immunosuppressive drug treatment in the Lambert–Eaton myasthenic syndrome. *Neurology* **34**, 480.

Newsom-Davis, J., Pinching, A.J., Vincent, A. and Wilson, S.G. (1978). Function of circulating antibody to acetylcholine receptor in myasthenia gravis: investigation by plasma exchange. *Neurology* **28**, 266–72.

Newsom-Davis, J., Vincent, A., Wilson, S.G. and Ward, C.D. (1979). Long-term effects of repeated plasma exchange in myasthenia gravis. *Lancet* **i**, 464.

Nicholls, K., Walker, R.G., Kincaid-Smith, P. and Dowling, J. (1984). Malignant IgA nephropathy. *Am. J. Kidney Dis.* **5**, 42.

Nielsen, V.K., Paulson, O.B., Rosenkvist, J., Holsoe, E. and Lefvert, A.K. (1982). Rapid improvement of myasthenia gravis after plasma exchange. *Ann. Neurol.* **11**, 160.

Nilsson, I.M., Jonsson, S., Sundqvist, S.-B., Ahlberg, A. and Bergentz, S.E. (1981). A procedure for removing high titre antibodies by extracorporeal protein A sepharose adsorption in haemophilia: substitution therapy and surgery in a patient with hemophilia B and antibodies. *Blood* **58**, 38.

Nilsson, I.M., Freiburghaus, C., Sunqvist, S.-B. and Sandberg, H. (1984). Removal of specific antibodies from whole blood in a continuous extracorporeal system. *Plasma Ther. Transfusion Technol.* **5**, 127–34.

O'Reilly, M.J.G., Talpos, G., Roberts, V.C., White, J.M. and Cotton, L.T. (1979). Controlled trial of plasma exchange in treatment of Raynaud's syndrome. *Br. Med. J.* **i**, 1113.

Osterman, P.G., Lundemo, G., Pirskanen, R. *et al.* (1984). Beneficial effects of plasma exchange in acute inflammatory polyradiculopathy. *Lancet* **ii**, 1296.

Palmer, A., Taube, D., Welsh, K., Bewick, M., Gjorstrup, P. and Thick, M. (1989). Removal of anti-HLA antibodies by extracorporeal immunoadsorption to enable renal transplantation. *Lancet* **i**, 10.

Pasquali, S., Casanova, S., Zucchelli, A. and Zucchelli, P. (1990). Long-term survival patients with acute and severe renal failure due to multiple myeloma. *Clin. Nephrol.* **34**, 247.

Paul, L.C. and Carpenter, C.B. (1980). Antibodies against renal endothelial alloantigens. *Transplant. Proc.* **12** (suppl. 1), 43.

Pinching, A.J., Peters, D.K. and Newson-Davis, J. (1976). Remission of myasthenia gravis following plasma exchange. *Lancet* **ii**, 1373.

Pohl, M.A., Lan, S.-L., Berl, T. and the Lupus Nephritis Collaborative Study Group. (1991). Plasmapheresis does not increase the risk for infection in immunosuppressed patients with severe lupus nephritis. *Ann. Int. Med.* **114**, 924.

Pourrat, J.P., Begassi, F., Thierry, F.X., Dueymes, J.M., Vernier, I. and Conte, J.J. (1987). Plasma exchange therapy in progressive systemic sclerosis. *Plasma Ther. Transfusion Technol.* **8**, 113.

Pozzi, C., Pasquali, S., Donini, U. *et al.* (1987). Prognostic factors and effectiveness of treatment in acute renal failure due to multiple myeloma: a review of 50 cases. *Clin. Nephrol.* **28**, 1.

Proskey, A.J., Weatherbee, L., Easterling, R.E., Greene, J.A. and Weller, J.M. (1970). Goodpasture's syndrome: a report of 5 cases and review of the literature. *Am. J. Med.* **48**, 162.

Pusey, C.D., Lockwood, C.M. and Peters, D.K. (1983). Plasma exchange and immunosuppressive drugs in the treatment of glomerulonephritis due to antibodies to the glomerular basement membrane. *Int. J. Artificial Organs* **6**, 15.

Pusey, C.D., Ryan, C.J., Aslam, M., Lloveras, J.-J., Dileo, A.J. and Lockwood, C.M. (1985). Specific immunoadsorption in a rat model of Goodpasture's syndrome. *Proc. EDTA–ERA* **22**, 736.

Pusey, C.D., Dash, A., Kershaw, M.J. *et al.* (1987). A single autoantigen in Goodpasture's syndrome identified by a monoclonal antibody to human glomerular basement membrane. *Lab. Invest.* **56**, 23.

Pusey, C.D., Venning, M.C. and Peters, D.K. (1988). Immunopathology of glomerular and interstitial disease. In *Diseases of the Kidney*, ed. R.W. Schrier and C.W. Gottschalk, p. 1827, Little, Brown and Company, Boston.

Pusey, C.D., Rees, A.J., Evans, D.J., Peters, D.K. and Lockwood, C.M. (1991). Plasma exchange in focal necrotising glomerulonephritis without anti-GBM antibodies. *Kidney Int.* **40**, 757.

Raphael, J.C. and Chastang, C. (1984). Co-operative randomised trial of plasma exchange in Guillain–Barré syndrome: preliminary results. *Ann. Méd. Interne* **135**, 8.

Raizman, M.B. and Foster, C.S. (1989) Plasma exchange in the therapy of Behçet's disease. *Graeses Arch. Clin. Exp. Ophthalmol.* **227**, 360.

Rock, G. (1986). Apheresis in the treatment of immune mediated hematologic disease. In *Therapeutic hemapheresis*, ed. M. Valbonesi, A.A. Pineda and J.C. Biggs, p. 127, Wichtig Editore, Milan.

Rock, G.A., Shumak, K.H., Buskard, N.A. *et al.* (1991). Comparison of plasma exchange with plasma infusion in the treatment of thrombotic thrombocytopenic purpura. *N. Eng. J. Med.* **325**, 393.

Rosenfield, R.E. and Jagathambal (1976). Transfusion therapy for autoimmune haemolytic anaemia. *Semin. Hematol.* **13**, 311.

Rothwell, R.S., Davis, P., Gordon, P.A. *et al.* (1980). A controlled study of plasma exchange in the treatment of severe rheumatoid arthritis. *Arthritis Rheum.* **23**, 785.

Roujeau, J.-C., Andre, C., Fabre, M.J. *et al.* (1983). Plasma exchange in pemphigus; uncontrolled study of ten patients. *Arch. Dermatol.* **119**, 215.

Roujeau, J.-C., Guillaume, J.C., Morel, P.B. *et al.* (1984a). Plasma exchange in bullous pemphigoid. *Lancet* **ii**, 468.

Roujeau, J.-C., Quaranta, J.-F., Guillevin, L. *et al.* (1984b). Les échanges plasmatique thérapeutiques: indications et résultats. *Ann. Méd. Interne* **135**, 308.

Ruocco, V., Rossi, A., Argenziano, G. *et al.* (1978). Pathogenicity of the intercellular antibodies of pemphigus and their periodic removal from the circulation by plasmapheresis. *Br. J. Dermatol.* **98**, 237.

Ruocco, V., Astarita, C. and Pisani, M. (1984). Plasmapheresis as an alternative or adjunctive therapy in problem cases of pemphigus. *Dermatologica* **168**, 219.

Russ, G.R. and d'Apice, A.J.F. (1981). Plasma exchange and immunosuppression in crescentic glomerulonephritis. *Proc. VIIIth Int. Congress Nephrol.* 667.

Savage, C.O.S., Pusey, C.D., Bowman, C., Rees, A.J. and Lockwood, C.M. (1986). Antiglomerular basement membrane antibody mediated disease in the British Isles 1980–4. *Br. Med. J.* **i**, 301.

Savage, C.O.S., Winearls, C.G., Jones, S., Marshall, P.D. and Lockwood, C.M. (1987). Prospective study of radioimmunoassay for antibodies against neutrophil cytoplasm in diagnosis of systemic vasculitis. *Lancet* **i**, 1389.

Savage, C.O.S., Pottinger, B.E., Gaskin, G., Lockwood, C.M. and Pusey, C.D. (1991). Vascular damage in Wegener's granulomatosis and microscopic polyarteritis: presence of anti-endothelial cell antibodies and their relation to anti-neutrophil cytoplasm antibodies. *Clin. Exp. Immunol.* **85**, 14.

Schroeder, J.O., Euler, H.H. and Löffler, H. Synchronization of plasmapheresis and pulse cyclophosphamide in severe lupus erythematosus. *Ann. Intern. Med.* **107**, 344.

Simpson, I.J., Doak, P.B., Williams, L.C., Blacklock, H.A. and Hill, R.S. (1982). Plasma exchange in Goodpasture's syndrome. *Am. J. Nephrol.* **2**, 301.

Skoog, W.A. and Adams, W.S. (1959). Plasmapheresis in a case of Waldenström's macroglobulinaemia. *Clin. Res.* **7**, 96.

Slocombe, G.W., Newland, A.C., Colvin, M.P. and Colvin, B.T. (1981). The role of intensive plasma exchange in the prevention and management of haemorrhage in patients with inhibitors to factor VIII. *Br. J. Haematol.* **47**, 577.

Solomon, A. and Fahey, J.L. (1963). Plasmapheresis therapy in macroglobulinaemia. *Ann. Intern. Med.* **58**, 789.

Soulillou, J.P., Guyot, C., Guimbretiere, J. *et al.* (1983). Plasma exchange in early kidney graft rejection associated with anti-donor antibodies. *Nephron* **35**, 158.

Steven, M.M., Tanner, A.R., Holdstock, G.E. *et al.* (1981). The effect of plasma exchange on the *in vitro* monocyte function of patients with immune complex diseases. *Clin. Exp. Immunol.* **45**, 240.

Stevens, M.E. and Bone, J.M. (1984). Follow-up prednisolone dosage in rapidly progressive crescentic glomerulonephritis successfully treated with pulse methylprednisolone or plasma exchange. *Proc. EDTA–ERA* **21**, 594.

Stevens, M.E., McConnell, M. and Bone, J.M. (1982). Aggressive treatment with pulse methylprednisolone or plasma exchange is justified in rapidly progressive glomerulonephritis. *Proc. Eur. Dialysis Transplant Assoc.* **19**, 724.

Stratta, P. *et al.* (1982). Plasma exchange in immune complex glomerulonephritis: clinical and immunological correlations. *Int. J. Artif. Organs* **6**, 27.

Sturgill, B.C. and Worzniak, M.J. (1970). Stimulation of proliferation of 19S antibody-forming cells in the spleens of immunized guinea-pigs after exchange transfusion. *Nature* **228**, 1304.

Sutton, D.M.C., Nair, R.C., Rock, G. and the Canadian Apheresis study Group (1989). Complications of plasma exchange. *Transfusion* **29**, 124.

Taplos, G., Horrocks, M., Waite, J.M. and Cotton, L.T. (1978). Plasmapheresis in Raynaud's disease. *Lancet* **i**, 416.

Taube, D.H., Williams, D.G., Cameron, J.S. *et al.* (1984). Renal transplantation after removal and prevention of resynthesis of HLA antibodies. *Lancet* **i**, 824.

Theofilopoulos, A.N. and Dixon, F.J. (1979). The biology and detection of immune complexes. *Adv. Immunol.* **28**, 89.

Thysell, H., Bygren, P., Bengtsson, U. *et al.* (1982). Immunosuppression and the additive effect of plasma exchange in treatment of rapidly progressive glomerulonephritis. *Acta Med. Scand.* **212**, 107.

Tindall, R.S.A. and Rollins, J. (1986). Apheresis in the treatment of myasthenia gravis. In *Therapeutic Hemapheresis* ed. M. Valbonesi, A.A. Pineda and J.C. Biggs, p. 43, Wichtig Editore, Milan.

Tindall, R.S.A., Walker, J.E., Ehle, A.L., Near, L., Rollins, J. and Becker, D. (1982). Plasmapheresis in multiple sclerosis: prospective trial of pheresis and immunosuppression versus immunosuppression alone. *Neurology* **32**, 739.

Tsokos, G.L., Balow, J.E., Huston, D.P., Wei, N. and Decker, J.L. (1982). Effect of plasmapheresis on T and B lymphocyte functions in patients with systemic lupus erythematosus: a double blind study. *Clin. Exp. Immunol.* **48**, 449.

Turner, A.M., Whittaker, S., Banks, I., Russell Jones, R. and Pusey, C.D. (1990). Plasma exchange in refractory cutaneous vasculitis. *Br. J. Dermatol.* **122**, 411.

Valbonesi, M. (1986). Plasmapheresis in the management of cryoglobulinaemia. In *Therapeutic Hemapheresis*, ed. M. Valbonesi, A.A. Pineda and J.C. Biggs, p. 89, Wichtig Editore, Milan.

Van der Woude, F.J., Lobatto, S., Permin, H. *et al.* (1985). Autoantibodies against neutrophils and monocytes: tool for diagnosis and marker of disease activity in Wegener's granulomatosis. *Lancet* **i**, 425

Vangelista, A., Frasca, G.M., Nanni Costa, A., Stefoni, S. and Bonomini, V. (1982). Value of plasma exchange in renal transplant rejection induced by anti-HLA antibodies. *Trans. ASAIO* **28**, 599.

Verdickt, W., Dequeker, J., Ceuppens, J.L., Stevens, E., Gautama, K. and Vermylen, C. (1983). Effect of lymphoplasmapheresis on clinical indices and T cell subsets in rheumatoid arthritis: a double blind controlled study. *Arthritis Rheum.* **26**, 1419.

Verrier-Jones, J., Cumming, R.H., Bucknall, R.C. *et al.* (1976). Plasmapheresis in the management of acute systemic lupus erythematosus? *Lancet* **i**, 709.

Verrier-Jones, J., Cumming, R.H., Bacon, P.A. *et al.* (1979). Evidence for a therapeutic effect of plasmapheresis in patients with systemic lupus erythematosus. *Quart. J. Med.* **48**, 555.

Walker, R.G., Scheinkestel, C., Becker, G.J., Owen, J.E., Dowling, J.P. and Kincaid-Smith, P. (1985). Clinical and morphological aspects of the management of crescentic anti-glomerular basement membrane antibody (anti-GBM) nephritis/Goodpasture's syndrome. *Quart. J. Med.* **54**, 75.

Wallace, D.J., Goldfinger, D., Lowe, C. *et al.* (1982). A double blind, controlled study of lymphoplasmapheresis versus sham apheresis in rheumatoid arthritis. *N. Engl. J. Med.* **306**, 1406.

Wallace, D.J., Goldfinger, D., Thompson-Breton, R. *et al.* (1980). Advances in the use of therapeutic pheresis for the management of rheumatic diseases. *Semin. Arthritis. Rheum.* **10**, 81.

Walport, M.J., Peters, A.M., Elkon, K.B., Pusey, C.D., Lavender, J.P. and Hughes, G.R.V. (1985). The splenic extraction ratio of antibody-coated erythrocytes and its response to plasma exchange and pulse methyl prednisolone. *Clin. Exp. Immunol.* **60**, 465.

Wei, N., Klippel, J.H., Huston, D.P. *et al.* (1983). Randomised trial of plasma exchange in mild systemic lupus erythematosus. *Lancet* **i**, 17.

Weiner, H.L. (1985). An assessment of plasma exchange in progressive multiple sclerosis. *Neurology* **35**, 320.

Weiner, H.L., Dau, P.C., Khatri, B.O. *et al.* (1989). Double-blind study of true vs. sham plasma exchange in patients treated with immunosuppression for acute attacks of multiple sclerosis. *Neurology* **39**, 1143.

Wilson, C.B. and Dixon, F.J. (1973). Anti-glomerular basement membrane antibody-induced glomerulonephritis. *Kidney Int.* **3**, 74.

Wing, E.J., Bruns, F.J., Fraley, D.S., Segel, D.P. and Adler, S. (1980). Infectious complications with plasmapheresis in rapidly progressive glomerulonephritis. *JAMA* **244**, 2423.

Winkelstein, A., Starz, T.W. and Agarwal, A. (1984). Efficacy of combined therapy with plasmapheresis and immunosuppressants in rheumatoid vasculitis. *J. Rheumatol.* **11**, 162.

Zimmerman, S.W. (1985). Plasmapheresis and dipyrimadole for recurrent focal glomerular sclerosis. *Nephron* **40**, 241.

Zucchelli, P., Pasquali, S., Cagnoli, L. and Ferrari, G. (1988). Controlled plasma exchange trial in acute renal failure due to multiple myeloma. *Kid. Int.* **33**, 1175.

49: Immunoglobulin Therapy

R.J. Wedgwood

Introduction

Passive immunization with antiserum for the prevention and treatment of disease became part of medical therapy 100 years ago. By the turn of the century it was clear that serum sickness induced by the foreign serum proteins markedly limited the use of xenogeneic antisera. A decade later preliminary experiments showed the efficacy of convalescent human serum in the prevention of measles. Human sera obviated the risk of serum sickness. By the mid-1930s lyophilized pooled adult sera were being used and attempts were being made to purify and concentrate protective globulin fractions from both pooled human serum and placental extracts.

The need for plasma substitutes during World War II resulted in the development of the mass plasma fractionation techniques of E.J. Cohn (see historical review in Eibl and Wedgwood 1989). The technique evolved, which is the basis of most large-scale fractionation of human plasma used today, combines the use, in the cold, of reduction in ionic strength and pH in the presence of low concentrations of alcohol. The method provides a consistent stable source of purified (95%) immunoglobulin G (IgG) and is the basic source of most Ig products used today, whether for intramuscular or for intravenous use. By the end of World War II the intramuscular product had been shown effective for the prevention and mitigation of measles and for prophylaxis against poliomyelitis and hepatitis A.

Early clinical experience, however, showed that the standard intramuscular preparation was not safe for intravenous use. Intravenous infusion caused adverse reaction in 10% or more of normal persons; some reactions were potentially catastrophic. After the description of agammaglobulinaemia by O.C. Bruton in 1952 further attempts were made to give Ig intravenously; over 90% of immunodeficient patients had adverse reactions. The need for preparations safe for intravenous use increased as patients became older and required doses greater than those tolerable by the intramuscular route.

The reactions to intravenous infusion were primarily due to IgG aggregates. Proteolytic digestion prevented aggregation but diminished biological activity. In addition the resultant $F(ab')_2$ fragments were rapidly excreted (half-life 10 hours). Acidification of the Ig solution to pH 4.0 and the addition of amounts of pepsin too small to cause proteolysis (1 : 10 000) diminished aggregation, removed the anticomplementary activity and provided a stable preparation suitable for intravenous use

(Barandum and Isliker 1986). Over the next few years this and a variety of other processes, including the use of polyethylene glycol, chromatographic purification and treatment with minimal amounts of proteases or hydrolases that did not significantly cleave the IgG molecule, provided several safe, effective, 'intact' IgG preparations suitable for intravenous use.

Pharmacology

To ensure a consistent wide spectrum of antibodies a very large number of donors (generally more than 5000) is used to create the plasma pool for fractionation. If the donor pool is of sufficient size it can be assumed that antibody diversity and titres will reflect those found in the general population. While these are commonly thought to be sufficient for protection against most commonly encountered infectious agents, the actual levels achieved by administration cannot be assumed to be protective for any particular infection. For some special purposes (see intramuscular human immune serum globulin (HISG), below) smaller pools of convalescent or post-immunization donors are used to create hyper-immune preparations. Donors for both types of preparation are carefully screened to exclude persons with human immunodeficiency virus (HIV) or hepatitis. Additionally it has been shown that the fractionation techniques used both partition and inactivate many viruses, including HIV. No case of HIV has been shown to originate from any Ig preparation.

The currently available Ig preparations, having been prepared from human plasma, contain IgG subclasses in rough proportion to those found in normal human serum. One exception may be IgG-4, which can partition somewhat irregularly. While there are differences in the biological activity of IgG subclasses (see Chapter 9), differences in IgG subclass concentration in the preparations appear to have no clinical significance. The preparations contain primarily IgG-1 — the predominant serum IgG subclass. They contain only trace amounts of IgM and IgA. From the standpoint of therapy, the biological activity of the preparation is of far greater consequence than the concentrations of Ig isotypes and subclasses.

Following infusion into the bloodstream Ig preparations have a complex pattern of distribution, elimination and catabolism. Initially the IgG remains entirely in the intravascular space. Then, over 3–4 days aggregated and damaged molecules are removed and diffusion into the extravascular space occurs. About half of the infused dose remains in the vascular space itself. The catabolism of IgG thereafter is dependent both on IgG concentration and on availability of Fc receptors through which the IgG is removed for intracellular digestion. Although half-lives are often calculated, the fractional catabolic rates do not conform to the equilibrium states on which such calculations depend. For purposes of estimate it is safe to assume, on average, that the half-life of IgG approximates 17–25 days in normal persons, and 25–30 days in patients with humoral immunodeficiency. The half-life of IgG-1, IgG-2 and IgG-4 approximates that for total IgG; the half-life for IgG-3 is significantly shorter (Ochs *et al.* 1986). Catabolic rates in patients with protein loss through the skin (e.g. burns), kidneys or intestines can be very much faster, and dosage must be recalculated accordingly.

Current methods for the preparation of Ig for therapeutic use have eliminated most serious reactions. With intramuscular preparations, the major side-effect is pain at the site of injection. With large doses the pain can be severe. With very large doses (>5 ml per site) the inflammatory reaction can be sufficient to cause tissue damage and affect absorption; *in situ* proteolysis may occur. Preparations for intramuscular use commonly contain mercury-containing preservatives; with prolonged use at high doses accumulation of mercury, which is potentially toxic, can occur. With intravenous use, the reactions are generally mild and are most often associated with excessively rapid infusion. The symptoms are strikingly stereotyped. When they occur, they include tachycardia, a feeling of tightness in the anterior chest, back pain, and sometimes elevated blood pressure and low-grade fever. These side-effects almost always disappear on slowing the rate of, or discontinuing, the infusion. On very rare occasions severe reactions may be encountered; these may include anaphylaxis. The reasons for reactions are obscure. In patients who have active infection reactions may be due to the presence of circulating antigen and the *in vivo* formation of antigen–antibody complexes. *In vivo* complex formation has been demonstrated on some occasions. Immunoglobulin A-deficient individuals may have antibodies (especially IgE antibodies) to IgA and reactions have been reported from traces of IgA present in some IgG preparations.

There has been considerable concern about reports of isolated clusters of non-A non-B hepatitis in association with IgG use in immunodeficient patients. These have all been associated with single, presumably contaminated, lots and manufacturing processes. There have been literally thousands of doses of other lots of intravenous Ig (IVIG) prepared by identical processes given without any evidence of hepatitis. While it is advisable to monitor liver function tests on patients receiving IgG (or any other blood product), the current consensus is that Ig preparations produced commercially at this time do not transmit non-A non-B hepatitis.

Human immune serum globulin, for intramuscular use

As noted above, HISG is prepared from large pools of normal human plasma. There are two general types of preparation: (i) polyvalent HISG from normal adults, which is generally produced from pools of 5000 or more donors to ensure a consistent spectrum of antibody titres; and (ii) specific HISG from convalescent or hyperimmune immunized donors prepared for special restricted purposes.

Polyvalent human immune serum globulin

Polyvalent HISG generally comes as a 16.5% protein solution of which >95% is IgG. As noted above, it is safe only for intramuscular use. Because it is a concentrated protein solution administration is accompanied by local discomfort and often considerable pain. It must be administered deep in a large muscle mass. No more than 5 ml should be administered in any one site; the maximum tolerable dose in several sites at one time is probably 20 ml or 3300 mg of IgG.

It is a useful product. Very small doses (0.02–0.06 mg/kg) can prevent hepatitis A infections in exposed individuals if given within 14 days after exposure. It is also invaluable as pre-exposure prophylaxis for visitors to endemic areas, particularly in developing countries where exposure cannot be avoided. Specific HISG (hepatitis B immune globulin (HBIG), see below) should be used for hepatitis B. Studies are insufficient for recommendations in non-A non-B hepatitis.

With the advent of measles immunization prophylaxis with ISG for exposed non-immune persons is often forgotten: HISG in adequate dosage (0.25–0.5 mg/kg) given within 6 days after exposure will prevent or modify the disease. This should be followed by active immunization three months later (Committee on Infectious Diseases 1988).

Human immune serum globulin may be used for replacement therapy in antibody deficiency syndromes. The amount that can be given with comfort sharply limits its utility. The maximal dose for any one injection is probably 20 ml or 3300 mg given in 5 ml volumes in four sites. Weekly or even fortnightly injections of this amount are not well tolerated by even the most stoic individual. Since, as will be discussed below, the optimum dose for replacement therapy may approximate 400 mg/kg/month, intramuscular HISG is generally limited to individuals weighing less than 25 kg or younger than 8 years of age. Intravenous IgG is better tolerated and provides more assured blood levels.

Some centres have successfully circumvented these problems by the use of slow, prolonged, subcutaneous infusion of intramuscular HISG. This author does not consider this a satisfactory alternative because of the dangers of tissue damage, the possible introduction of infection and the potential cumulative toxicity from the mercury used in the preservatives.

Specific human immune serum globulin

There are now a variety of specific Ig preparations available for the prophylaxis and treatment of some major infectious diseases (Committee on Infectious Diseases 1988).

Varicella–zoster immune globulin (VZIG) is obtainable through the Red Cross or similar agencies and is indicated for prevention of varicella–zoster infections in persons at high risk for development of progressive varicella (e.g. persons on immunosuppressive therapy). The material is scarce. Patients should be screened for immunity to varicella before being placed on immunosuppressive therapy. Non-immune pregnant women and premature infants of non-immune mothers are also at risk for serious complications. Non-immune patients at risk should be given VZIG (15–25 units/kg), preferably within 48 hours (and not beyond 96 hours) of significant exposure. Concomitant treatment with vidarabine or acyclovir should be considered.

Hepatitis B immune globulin is commonly used for protection of non-immune persons immediately following significant exposure to hepatitis B. This includes accidental exposure to blood or blood products, wounds caused by contaminated needles or instruments, sexual and intimate household contacts and perinatal infections. For maximal effectiveness the HBIG (0.06 ml/kg) must be given within 24 hours of exposure and, because the incubation period of hepatitis B is long, the individual must either be immunized at the same time or be given a second dose of HBIG 1 month later. For this reason persons expected to be at long-term high risk for exposure should receive active immunization with hepatitis B vaccine. Newborn infants born to HBs antigen +ve mothers should be routinely given HBIG (0.5 ml) at birth, followed by active immunization.

Human tetanus immune globulin (HTIG) is now considered preferable to equine tetanus antitoxin. It is indicated for use (250–500 U) in persons who have serious, possibly contaminated, wounds who do not have a clear history of completed immunization. It is also indicated for persons who have developed the disease; the optimal therapeutic dose for treatment has not yet been established. Human tetanus immune globulin can only be administered intramuscularly and by local infiltration around the wounded area. Intrathecal or intravenous use is not recommended. Active immunization with tetanus toxoid should be initiated at the same time.

Persons with significant exposure to rabid animals who have not been previously fully immunized with a potent rabies vaccine should receive human rabies immune globulin (HRIG, 20 IU/kg) immediately; active immunization with human diploid cell vaccine should be initiated at the same time. Human rabies immune globulin is preferred to anti-rabies serum of equine or other xenogeneic origin because is not associated with hypersensitivity reactions.

The problem of maternal isosensitization to fetal erythrocytes is discussed in Chapter 95. The risk of initial sensitization in a rhesus (Rh) −ve mother can be reduced to less than 1% by the appropriate use of human anti-D immune globulin (HRhIG) given shortly after delivery or abortion of an Rh +ve infant or fetus. It can also be used during pregnancy to mitigate intrauterine fetomaternal transfer. The dose of HRhIG must be based on an estimate of the amount of fetal blood transferred: usually 1 vial for every 15 ml of Rh +ve blood to which the patient has been exposed.

Hyperimmune human serum globulin preparations have also been used for a variety of other infectious diseases; these have included prophylaxis of mumps, pertussis, diphtheria and *Haemophilus influenzae* b infections. There are not sufficient available data for recommendations. Undoubtedly additional human specific immune globulin preparations will be available in the future.

Intravenous immunoglobulin

The development during the last 20 years of gamma globulin preparations suitable for intravenous administration has resulted in a striking change in the use of HISG. Indications for use have expanded beyond prophylaxis of a limited number of viral diseases and replacement in agammaglobulinaemia to encompass treatment of several bacterial and viral diseases, replacement for a wide assortment of primary and secondary immunodeficiencies (including those associated with malignancies and transplantation) and the melioration, possibly through immunomodulation, of inflammatory diseases, including some due to autoimmunity and immune complex formation.

These uses require a preparation of Ig in which the tertiary structure of the molecule and the diverse biological activities of IgG remain intact (see Chapter 9). The biological activities of IgG — the optimal binding and activation of complement, the binding of IgG to Fc receptors on phagocytic and other cells, the interaction in idiotypic regulation — require that the molecular structure remain essentially unaltered. The IgG molecule can in some respects be considered as a molecular cascade mechanism; tertiary structure is vital. $F(ab')_2$ fragments can be used to neutralize toxins, but they cannot interact effectively with complement or Fc receptors. This requires not only an intact primary structure, but also a functional hinge region, apposition of domains and appropriate positioning of the carbohydrate moiety. It was learned quite early that any production method cleaving the molecule diminished biological activity. For example, beta propriolactone altered the molecule and reduced Fc-mediated function. In like manner both sulphonation and reduction and alkylation split the molecule and, although reassembly took place, Fc-mediated activity was reduced, limiting effectiveness in opsonization and protection against bacterial infections with organisms such as *Haemophilus influenzae* b. Modified IVIG preparations have therefore been replaced by intact, unmodified material (Eibl and Wedgwood 1989).

Several general approaches for the successful production of an intact IgG for intravenous use are employed. These include: (i) the use of minimal amounts of proteases or hydrolases which do not cleave the molecule but dissociate aggregates; the enzymes are then removed from the IgG; (ii) fractionation using polyethylene glycol and/or chromatographic purification with various supporting media, including sepharose and dextrans. Following purification the intact IgG solutions are stabilized by acidification with or without traces of pepsin, addition of sugars or amino acids, or addition of other serum proteins such as albumin.

In this manner preparations of intact IgG suitable for intravenous use with apparently full biological activity have been made widely available. It should be noted that these preparations lack significant amounts of IgA and IgM. They are not suitable for IgM or IgA replacement *per se*. Whether IgG replacement is sufficient for patients lacking IgM (and/or IgA) has not been well studied; a comparison of immunodeficient patients treated with IVIG or plasma infusions indicated that, with comparable amounts of IgG, the IVIG was preferable.

Immunodeficiency

The major use of IVIG is for replacement of IgG in patients with primary and secondary immunodeficiencies. These topics are discussed in detail in Chapters 66 and 69. Generally IgG replacement with IVIG should be considered for any patient with demonstrable antibody deficiency (Scientific Group on Immunodeficiency 1989).

PRIMARY IMMUNODEFICIENCY

Patients with X-linked agammaglobulinaemia, with the hyper-IgM syndrome, with common variable immunodeficiency, including certain patients with so-called subclass deficiency, and with severe combined immunodeficiency generally all require IgG replacement therapy. In the hyper-IgM syndrome IgG therapy may reduce serum IgM levels. Patients with ataxia telangiectasia and patients with the Wiscott–Aldrich syndrome can become severely antibody-deficient and will then require replacement. Patients with transient hypogammaglobulinaemia of infancy rarely require replacement; the condition corrects itself.

Immunoglobulin A deficiency, frequent in the normal Caucasian population (~ 1 : 800), is generally clinically unimportant unless associated with IgG deficiencies — most commonly deficiency of IgG-2 (and IgG-4). Replacement therapy for patients with selective IgG-2 deficiency (or other selective subclass defects) is controversial. Some authors suggest a cautious therapeutic trial of IVIG while monitoring infections.

Efficacy of IgG replacement in the primary immunodeficiencies was established with intramuscular HISG 30 years ago, but the optimal dose was never generally implemented because of 'discomfort and expense' (Medical Research Council 1969). Over the years with use of intramuscular HISG it became apparent that, while life was prolonged, bronchiectasis occurred with regularity and pulmonary function progressively decreased in most patients. Early death from pulmonary complications continued to occur. The development of IVIG obviated the problems of discomfort associated with intramuscular HISG and permitted much greater dosage than had been previously possible. Not only was IVIG as or more effective than intramuscular IgG at equivalent dose, but it became apparent that at higher doses (>400 mg/kg/month) pulmonary function consistently improved and the course of bronchiectasis was reversed. By adjusting dose and frequency of infusion, near normal serum IgG levels could be readily maintained. The hallmark of successful replacement therapy became maintenance or improvement of pulmonary function. These findings led to the recommendation (Scientific Group on Immunodeficiency 1989) that the 'trough' level of serum IgG be maintained at levels at least

200–400 mg/dl above those produced intrinsically by the patient. This in most instances requires an IVIG dose of 350–500 mg/kg/month or 150–250 mg/kg every 2 weeks. The latter may be preferable because levels are more consistently maintained and adverse reactions less frequent. The cost and inconvenience of the frequent infusions in some patients can be mitigated by self-infusion in the home. In all instances, replacement therapy should be initiated as soon as possible, to prevent recurrent infections and irreversible lung damage. This requires early and precise diagnosis.

SECONDARY IMMUNODEFICIENCIES

Striking deficiency of IgG can occur in the nephrotic syndrome as a result of urinary protein losses and a decreased IgG half-life. In most instances such patients do not have recurrent infections and IgG replacement is not needed. Protein-losing enteropathy can also be associated with large IgG losses (and lymphocytes in those patients with lymphangiectasia) even in the absence of diarrhoea. In burns significant IgG deficiency can occur from skin loss, immune suppression and hypercatabolism; generally the greater the burned surface, the shorter the IgG half-life. Replacement therapy in all instances is difficult because of the losses and hypercatabolism. Studies on the use of IVIG in burn patients have been inconclusive. The losses of Ig that occur with plasmaphaeresis can be successfully replaced with IVIG.

Secondary immunodeficiency also result from malignancies (e.g. chronic lymphocytic leukaemia — CLL) and as a consequence of the immunosuppressive treatment of such diseases. A well-controlled study of adjunctive treatment in CLL with IVIG (500 mg/kg every 3 weeks) showed a 50% reduction in the rate of bacterial infections, the greatest reduction being in infections of moderate rather than minor or severe degree. The reduction was surprisingly independent of serum IgG levels. Intravenous Ig has also been used successfully in patients with multiple myeloma and Waldenström's macroglobulinaemia. Such patients have elevated levels of Ig but poor antibody formation. Infection rates were also shown to be reduced with IVIG in the treatment of patients undergoing intensive induction therapy for small-cell carcinoma of the lung. The use of IVIG in transplantation is generally aimed at prevention or treatment of cytomegalovirus infections. Because of the large number of variables the several studies are difficult to interpret. Intravenous Ig appears to reduce Gram-negative and local infection and the risk of cytomegalovirus interstitial pneumonia. Intravenous Ig may also reduce the incidence of graft-versus-host disease. The two effects may be interrelated (Berkman *et al.* 1990).

Infections

The infections associated with surgery and severe trauma are perhaps at times due to secondary immunodeficiency. Studies on the effect of IVIG to date are inconclusive. One controlled study on poly-trauma showed a significant reduction in the number of patients developing pneumonia. Premature infants may also be considered secondarily immunodeficient since transplacental transfer of maternal antibody may be incomplete. The cumulative data from several studies suggest that premature infants (small neonates) may be protected from bacterial infections by IVIG (500 mg/kg/week for four doses). There is no apparent protection in full-term neonates.

There is little to suggest that IVIG will improve the course of an ongoing infection. In one otherwise normal male with long-standing pure red cell aplasia due to chronic parvovirus B19 infection, IVIG induced a rapid and apparently complete remission. Echovirus meningoencephalitis is a common complication in agammaglobulinaemia. These usually fatal infections have been successfully treated with high doses of IVIG. However, IVIG did not ameliorate one reported outbreak of echovirus 11 infections in a new-born nursery. Patients with acquired immune deficiency syndrome (AIDS) have impaired humoral immunity as well as T cell defects. There have been several studies on the use of IVIG in AIDS with reports of a reduction in the incidence of interstitial pneumonia, decreased bacterial infections and improved survival of infected neonates. Restoration of T cell functions has also been noted. The studies to date have unfortunately not been sufficient to provide conclusive answers. There have been reports of symptomatic improvement following the use of IVIG in chronic Epstein–Barr infection. Since the diagnosis of this syndrome is controversial and the studies were uncontrolled, the data are difficult to interpret. There have also been conflicting and inconclusive reports on IVIG in respiratory syncytial virus (RSV), adenovirus and para-influenza virus infections in infants and children. Double-blind controlled studies on the use of IVIG in RSV infections are reportedly under way (for more complete reviews and citations see Eibl and Wedgwood 1989; Berkman *et al.* 1990).

Autoimmune and inflammatory diseases

In a striking, serendipitous finding in the early 1960s it was noted that, while giving IVIG to three hypogammaglobulinaemic patients with concomitant haemolytic anaemia, the haemolytic anaemia abated. Subsequently a similar observation was made in two patients with idiopathic thrombocytopenic purpura (ITP) (Barandum and Isliker 1986). The observation has been confirmed by many others (Bussel and Pham 1987). The mechanism by which IVIG induces a prompt increase in platelet count is complex. Fc receptor blockade is one important factor. Intravenous Ig can block low-affinity Fc receptors pre-empting the uptake of antibody-coated platelets. Intravenous Ig can also down-regulate Fc receptors generally. But the long-lasting improvement seen in some patients cannot be explained in this manner. A longer-lasting immunomodulatory effect through an anti-idiotypic network (see below) may exist. Or, if ITP is the result of a prolonged viral infection, viral suppression may occur. Most cases of ITP in children are acute, are self-limited and require no therapy. Intravenous Ig is indicated (400 mg/kg/day for 5 consecutive days) in acute ITP when the platelet count is $<20\,000/mm^3$, particularly to prevent intracranial bleeding. In chronic ITP, IVIG may obviate the need for splenectomy. Intravenous Ig also appears to be of benefit in other autoimmune cytopenias.

In pregnant women IVIG crosses the placenta by Fc-mediated transport. In instances of maternal Rh sensitization or where the mother carries antinuclear antibodies (particularly anti-Ro), IVIG has been used to competitively inhibit the transport of these antibodies to the fetus.

A striking anti-inflammatory response is seen with IVIG treatment of Kawasaki's disease, a syndrome seen in young children, characterized by high fever, lymphadenopathy, rash, conjunctivitis and stomatitis. Approximately 25% of untreated affected children develop coronary artery aneurisms. In a randomized trial, administration of IVIG (400 mg/kg/day for 4 days) reduced the incidence of aneurysms more than fivefold. There was also a strikingly rapid clinical improvement within hours of the first infusion. In the blood CD8 +ve lymphocytes, which were initially decreased, rose rapidly to normal and the activated CD4 +ve and B lymphocytes found at onset decreased a thousandfold. In other studies similar results have been obtained. The rapid antiphlogistic effect of IVIG is unexplained. The cause of Kawasaki's disease is unknown. The rapidity of the response to IVIG is unlikely to be antiviral; immunomodulation through a cytokine network seems possible. Even though unexplained, the findings have given rise to studies in other inflammatory diseases, including asthma, juvenile rheumatoid arthritis, polymyositis, ulcerative colitis and intractable childhood epilepsy.

Pooled normal serum IgG naturally contains anti-antibodies, or anti-idiotypes. In autoimmune diseases anti-idiotypes could be expected to have two effects. Anti-idiotypes against the internal structure could, by molecular mimicry, block the activity of the autoantibody through competitive inhibition by occupation of the antigen binding site. Anti-idiotypes both to internal and to framework structure may also down-regulate antibody production through the anti-idiotypic network. If autoantibodies from different patients with the same disease share idiotypic determinants, IVIG from sufficiently large pools should contain anti-idiotypic antibodies to the common, shared determinants or cross-reactive idiotypes and should suppress the synthesis of allo- or autoantibody.

Anti-idiotypes against autoantibodies to factor VIII have been found in IVIG. Patients with autoimmune haemophilia may respond dramatically to IVIG with decreased autoantibody levels and increased factor VIII activity. Two patients studied with alloantibodies did not respond, and no anti-idiotypic antibodies to their alloantibodies were found (Kazatchkine *et al.* 1989). This striking clinical response in autoimmune haemophilia has been confirmed. Studies on patients with haemophilia A and haemophilia B who develop alloantibodies to factor VIII and factor IX respectively have suggested that tolerance can be reinduced by the combined use of IVIG, cyclophosphamide and the antigen.

The importance of anti-acetylcholine esterase receptor (AChR) antibodies in the pathogenesis of myasthenia gravis of both the adult and neonatal form is generally accepted. It appears probable that anti-idiotypic antibodies play a role in the regulation of this autoantibody formation. Administration of IVIG has been shown to result in striking improvement in some patients (Arsura *et al*. 1986). The improvement may be long-term and associated with a decrease in anti-AChR antibodies. The treatment appears to be effective also in some patients in whom the usual anti-AChR antibodies are not demonstrable. There is now supporting evidence that the Guillain–Barré syndrome, a neurological disease associated with autoantibodies to peripheral nerve myelin, may also respond favourably to IVIG; a controlled study is in progress.

Immune regulation through idiotypic–anti-idiotypic networks is neither widely understood nor uniformly accepted. It is, nevertheless, intriguing to speculate on this approach to the possible modulation of immunologically mediated diseases, as for example in anecdotal reports on the use of IVIG in early juvenile diabetes mellitus (see Eibl and Wedgwood 1989). There are clearly broader implications for the use of IVIG than protection against infections alone (Rosen and Wedgwood 1989).

References

Arsura, E.L., Bick, A., Brunner, N.G., Namba, T. and Grob, D. (1986). High-dose intravenous immunoglobulin in the management of myasthenia gravis. *Arch. Intern. Med.* **146**, 1365–8.

Barandum, S. and Isliker, H. (1986). Development of immunoglobulin in preparations for intravenous use. *Vox Sang.* **51**, 157–60.

Berkman, S.A., Lee, M.L. and Gale, R.P. (1990). Clinical uses of intravenous immunoglobulins. *Ann. Intern. Med.* **112**, 278–92.

Bussel, J.B. and Pham, L.C. (1987). Intravenous treatment with gammaglobulin in adults with immune thrombocytopenic purpura: review of the literature. *Vox Sang.* **52**, 1228–31.

Committee on Infectious Diseases (1988). *Report of the Committee on Infectious Diseases*, 21st edn. American Academy of Pediatrics, Elk Grove Village, Illinois 60009–0927.

Eibl M.M. and Wedgwood, R.J. (1989). Intravenous immunoglobulin: a review. *Immunodeficiency Rev.* **1** (suppl.), 1–42.

Kazatchkine, M.D., Rossi, F., Nydegger, V. and Sultan, Y. (1989). Anti-idiotypes against antoantibodies to procoagulant factor VIII (VIII.C) in intravenous immunoglobulins. *Int. Rev. Immunol.* **5**, 157–64.

Medical Research Council Working-Party (1969). Hypogammaglobulinaemia in the United Kingdom. *Lancet* **i**, 163–8.

Ochs, H.D., Morell, A., Skvaril, F., Fischer, S.H. and Wedgwood, R.J. (1986). Survival of IgG subclasses following administration of intravenous gammaglobulin in patients with primary immunodeficiency diseases. In *Clinical Use of Intravenous Immunoglobulins*, ed. A. Morell and U.E. Nydegger, pp. 77–85, Academic Press, London.

Rosen, F.S. and Wedgwood, R.J. (eds.) (1989). Immunomodulation: role of intravenous immunoglobulins. *Int. Rev. Immunol.* **5**, 97–202.

Scientific Group on Immunodeficiency (1989). Primary immunodeficiency diseases: report of a WHO sponsored meeting. *Immunodeficiency Rev.* **1**, 173–205.

50: Immunopotentiation

J.-F. Bach

Introduction

The discovery of the involvement of the immune system in the pathogenesis of an ever-increasing number of diseases has inevitably led to attempts to modify the course of these diseases, by manipulating the various elements of the immunological machinery. The first applications of this strategy dealt with autoimmune diseases and organ transplantation and, very logically, immunosuppressive agents were used in an attempt to abrogate undesirable immune responses. The successes and limitations of immunosuppression in terms of effectiveness or side-effects are presented in Chapter 51. Another approach of immunomanipulation has recently arisen from animal models, which consists of stimulating the immune system. This approach, for which there are several sets of potent agents available today, finds its best application in two major fields in medicine — cancer and infectious diseases. Paradoxically, it may also be applied to autoimmunity, a condition essentially treated thus far by immunosuppressive agents since studies on the pathogenesis of autoimmune diseases indicate that a selective deficiency of T cells is probably an important aetiological factor.

In these few pages, we shall review the principal classes of immunostimulating agents and discuss their main indications in the various clinical situations defined above.

Problems of definition

Adjuvants are commonly defined as agents that enhance immune responses against antigenic preparations into which they are incorporated. Immunostimulants are defined by their capacity to stimulate immune responses without simultaneous injection of the antigen (either at the same site or at the same time). This is an important difference. However, many adjuvants behave as immunostimulants (e.g. bacillus Calmette–Guérin (BCG), endotoxins). Similarly, the so-called polyspecific antibacterial vaccines may in fact elicit an immunostimulation that is not specific for the bacterial antigens present in the preparation given to patients. The potential effects of such vaccines, when they exist, will thus not be limited a priori to the bacteria initially used.

Immunopotentiating agents may be classified for the sake of simplicity into four classes as shown in Table 50.1.

Table 50.1. Immunopotentiating agents

Bacteria and bacterial products
Mycobacteria (BCG, MER, WSA, MDP)
Corynebacteria (*C. parvum*)
Endotoxins (lipid A)
Phospholipidic extract
Bordetella pertussis
Cytokines
Other physiologically relevant mediators
Thymic hormones (thymosins, thymopoietin, thymulin)
Transfer factor
Drugs
Levamisole
Isoprinosine
Polyribonucleotides
Tilorone
Pyran
Azimexon
Polyacrylic acids
Bestatin
Adjuvants
Complete Freund's adjuvant (CFA)
Incomplete Freund's adjuvant (IFA)
Alum

1 Bacterial products (e.g. BCG, *Corynebacterium parvum*, endotoxins, etc.).
2 Physiologically relevant mediators (e.g. thymic hormones, transfer factor and cytokines (e.g. interleukin 2 (IL-2), interferons (IFN), etc.)).
3 Chemicals (e.g. levamisole and polyribonucleotides).
4 True adjuvants.
This classification is imperfect, however, since all categories now include chemically well-defined agents (such as muramyl dipeptide (MDP) or some thymic hormones), and certain physiological mediators (e.g. transfer factor) have not been proved physiologically relevant and their physiological action is not necessarily the basis of their immunostimulating properties.

Main classes of immunopotentiating agents

Bacteria and bacterial products

The observation that animals infected by intracellular bacteria were resistant to non-antigenically related bacteria is not recent. It has led to a considerable number of experimental and clinical studies, dealing essentially with mycobacteria, corynebacteria and pertussis. We shall only consider here the products that are the most commonly used.

MYCOBACTERIA

Bacillus Calmette–Guérin

Bacillus Calmette–Guérin is a living non-virulent strain of mycobacteria (*Mycobacterium bovis*). Experimentally, it induces resistance to numerous bacteria. Its anti-infectious action probably operates through macrophage activation and stimulation of antibody production (Old *et al.* 1961). Its antitumour activities have been documented by extensive investigations (Bast *et al.* 1974; Mathé 1976). These immunostimulating properties may be modulated or even reversed in certain conditions of administration (particularly in high doses) by stimulation of suppressor cells (Asherson 1977). This suppression of immune responses has been reported for skin graft rejection (Zschiesche and Heinecke 1973) and tumour immunity (Glasèr 1978). Clinical use of BCG has been hampered by its local and general side-effects and by the variations of efficacy according to the source of mycobacteria.

Methanol extraction residue

Methanol extraction residue (MER) is an acetone–methanol extract of mycobacteria (Weiss *et al.* 1966). It includes various fragments of the bacterial membranes. It has been shown to protect animals from numerous infections, such as *Pasteurella* in the guinea-pig (Chedid *et al.* 1972; Weiss 1972). Like BCG, it also presents antitumour effects (Weiss *et al.* 1966). Its mechanism of action has not yet been perfectly determined but seems to involve stimulation of macrophages (Weiss *et al.* 1966) and T cells. B cell stimulation also occurs, but apparently secondarily to the action of a T cell factor (Maillard and Bloom 1972). Its clinical use has been limited by its toxicity in man (fever, spleen and liver reactions).

Muramyl dipeptide

Complete Freund's adjuvant (CFA) remains one of

the most potent known adjuvants. Several groups of investigators and notably Lederer in France have attempted to characterize chemically the active principle of CFA, which is located in the cell membrane (Lederer 1977). Soluble extracts were first prepared, such as the water-soluble adjuvant (WSA). More interesting is the characterization by Lederer and Petit of the minimal structure showing adjuvant properties, MDP. Muramyl dipeptide has been thoroughly studied by Chedid's group, who have shown that MDP has full adjuvant capacity without toxicity (Chedid *et al.* 1972, 1977). Its mechanism of action has not yet been determined but seems to involve, as a major action, stimulation of macrophages, which secondarily leads to an enhancement of B and T cell functions (Chedid *et al.* 1972, 1977; Sugimoto *et al.* 1978). Muramyl dipeptide can be considered as an immunostimulant since it keeps its potentiating activity when administered separately from the antigen, or even per os. It has not been clearly shown, however, that MDP had the antitumour effects of BCG. Muramyl dipeptide can be used in man (unlike CFA). Its potential clinical use, either in its original form or as one of the numerous analogues that have already been synthesized, is difficult to delineate: new vaccinations (unfeasible with present adjuvants, for example, against paludism), infectious diseases, etc.

Muramyl dipeptide has been used in many experimental and clinical settings in its original form and especially in the form of non-pyrogenic analogues. Promising, although not totally convincing, results have been obtained in vaccination against bacterial diseases (Parant and Chedid 1988). Perhaps more striking data have been obtained in anti gonadotrophin vaccination for contraception (Audibert *et al.* 1985).

CORYNEBACTERIUM PARVUM

A single injection of *C. parvum* induces a major lymphoid hyperplasia, activates macrophages and significantly enhances resistance against bacterial infections (Adlam 1972). This increased resistance is probably due to macrophage stimulation (Halpern *et al.* 1973). Unlike mycobacteria, T cells are not necessary for its action, and antibody responses to thymus-independent antigens are augmented as well as those to thymus-dependent antigens. In addition, *C. parvum* does not enhance delayed hypersensitivity reactions (Howard *et al.* 1973). Several clinical trials have been performed with *C. parvum*, with promising results (see later). However, like BCG, such clinical use is hampered by several side-effects (fever, hepatosplenomegaly) and by the variation in *C. parvum* strains. These difficulties might be alleviated by the use of purified fractions (Bizzini *et al.* 1978).

GRAM-POSITIVE BACTERIA

A number of Gram-positive bacteria extracts have been prepared (notably from *Klebsiella pneumoniae* and streptococci) and evaluated in upper respiratory infections. Although these trials have been essentially limited to France and Japan and have not always provided striking results, it seems fair to recognize that these extracts do show pharmacological activity and significantly reduce the rate of infections in chronically infected patients.

GRAM-NEGATIVE BACTERIA

Gram-negative bacteria and some of their products have been known as adjuvants for a long time. They have also been shown recently to possess potent systemic immunostimulant activity.

Endotoxins

Lipopolysaccharide (LPS) extracts of Gram-negative bacteria and specifically the lipidic part (lipid A) posses not only endotoxin activity but also strong immunoadjuvant and immunostimulant properties (Luderitz *et al.* 1973). This coincidence of toxic and immunostimulant activity has been an absolute obstacle so far, preventing clinical application of LPS. Attempts to detoxify LPS have failed since the detoxification eliminated the immunostimulating activity (Chedid *et al.* 1975). Lipopolysaccharide has multiple effects on the immune system. It is a B-cell-specific mitogen (Andersson *et al.* 1973) in the mouse, but this effect is not found in human peripheral blood lymphocytes. The selectivity of the action of LPS for B cells is assessed by its capacity to stimulate polyclonal antibody production. Such action on B cells appears to be independent of T cells and macrophages, although LPS also activates macrophages (Unanue *et al.* 1969). Interestingly, LPS also activates the alternative pathway of complement, which complicates the interpretation of its effects in immunopathological animal models.

Phospholipidic extract

Phospholipid fractions of numerous Gram-negative bacteria (salmonellae, *Escherichia coli*) and of other bacteria (*Vibrio cholerae*, *C. parvum*) enhance the immune defence against non-antigenically related infectious agents.

BORDETELLA PERTUSSIS

The important lymphocytosis observed in patients with whooping cough and in subjects vaccinated against this disease indicates that *Bordetella pertussis* significantly alters lymphocyte differentiation or migration. The bacterial component responsible for most of these effects has been characterized. The lymphocytosis-promoting factor (LPF) is a protein of MW 73 000, composed of four subunits (Morse and Morse 1976). Lymphocytosis-promoting factor is a T cell mitogen, and its immunostimulating activities appear to involve T cells, at least at low doses (Dresser 1972) *Bordetella pertussis* may also alter B cell and macrophage function by the intermediary of endotoxins and peptidoglycan moieties present in the bacteria.

Cytokines

Much interest has recently been shown in the use of various cytokines as immunopotentiating agents. The most thoroughly studied of these cytokines has been interleukin 2 (IL-2), which has been evaluated in several clinical settings, including anti-hepatitis (hepatitis B surface (HBs)) vaccination (Meuer *et al.* 1989) and especially cancer immunotherapy (Rosenberg *et al.* 1987; Lotze and Rosenberg 1989). In the latter model, it has been shown that IL-2 augmented the survival of patients with various forms of metastatic cancer. The effect, which needs to be confirmed in randomized trials in progress, was particularly dramatic when *in vivo* treatment was associated with *in vitro* treatment of patient's lymphoid cells with the lymphokine and reinfusion in the form of lymphokine-activated killer (LAK) cells. A serious problem related to the clinical use of IL-2 is its systemic side-effects. Other cytokines are being evaluated experimentally and clinically (in cancer patients), notably tumour necrosis factor (TNF) and IFN-γ. One should note, however, the difficulty met in the interpretation of the effect of these latter cytokines. It is always difficult to distinguish a true immunostimulatory effect from a direct antitumour or antiviral effect.

Other physiologically relevant mediators

THYMIC HORMONES

The hypothesis of the endocrine function of the thymus was put forward in the 1960s when the role of the thymus in immunity was discovered. Not until after 1970, however, were convincing reports published showing that it was possible to stimulate the immunological competence of thymus-deprived mice by injection of thymic extracts (Bach and Carnaud 1976).

Four groups of workers devoted important efforts to the isolation and the characterization of thymic factors. A.L. Goldstein and colleagues isolated a series of peptide 'thymosins' (one of which has been sequenced and synthesized, α_1 thymosin) (Goldstein *et al.* 1977). G. Goldstein characterized a 5500 MW polypeptide thymopoietin (Goldstein 1977). A pentapeptide was shown to possess most, if not all, activities of the whole molecule (Goldstein *et al.* 1979). Trainin and co-workers defined a 'thymic humoral factor' (THF) with an MW of approximately 3000, endowed with multiple biological properties, including stimulation of cyclic adenosine monophosphate (AMP) synthesis (Trainin *et al.* 1975). We ourselves, at the Necker Hospital in Paris, isolated a thymus-dependent factor from serum, thymulin, formerly called 'facteur thymique sérique' (FTS), which is capable of inducing T cell differentiation alloantigens in immature T cells. This factor was shown to be a non-apeptide and has been sequenced and synthesized (Bach *et al.* 1978). In addition to its capacity to induce most T cell markers *in vivo* or *in vitro*, thymulin is capable of enhancing a large number of T cell functions. It has been shown that thymulin is produced directly by the thymic epithelium and is bound on lymphoid cells by specific high-affinity receptors (Bach *et al.* 1979). It is not yet known whether these various factors are all distinct or if some of them are related (e.g. precursors or carriers) (Bach 1979).

Thymic peptides have been successfully used in

rheumatoid arthritis (Amor *et al.* 1987) and candidiasis (Bolla 1987).

TRANSFER FACTOR

In 1964, H.S. Lawrence reported that it was possible to transfer cutaneous delayed hypersensitivity in man by injecting dialysable leucocyte extracts (Lawrence 1969). The dialysable transfer factor has not yet been completely characterized, either immunologically or chemically. The preparations used by most workers seem to include two categories of molecules (Kirkpatrick 1975; Ascher *et al.* 1976; Khan *et al.* 1979): the first is antigen-specific; the second is non-antigen-specific and probably explains the increase in E-rosettes, the enhancement of lymphocyte responses to mitogens and, paradoxically, the transfer of skin reactivity to antigens against which the donor is apparently not sensitized. It is difficult to know to which of these activities the oligoribonucleotide and peptide components correspond. The possibility that the non-antigenic-specific activities are due to known biologically active materials, such as circulating thymic factors, which probably contaminate transfer factor preparations, cannot be excluded.

INTERFERONS

Interferons alpha and beta are glycoproteins produced by virus-infected cells. It has been shown to prevent or alleviate a number of viral diseases in various species (Cantell *et al.* 1974; Krim and Sanders 1977; Merigan *et al.* 1978). Immunological IFN (type II) is produced by mitogen- or antigen-stimulated lymphocytes. It also presents antiviral activity but is chemically distinct from viral interferon. In addition to their protective antiviral effect, IFNs have been shown to modulate the immune system, at the level of both membrane differentiation antigens and immune responses (De Maeyer-Guignard *et al.* 1975; Sonnenfeld *et al.* 1977). We shall see further that IFN chemical inducers, such as polyribonucleotides and tilorone, may have immunostimulating activities.

OTHER LYMPHOCYTE PRODUCTS

Lymphokines and immune ribonucleic acid (RNA) (extracted from immune spleen cells) (Coates and Pilch 1977) have been claimed to stimulate various immune responses. These data need confirmation and should be considered too preliminary for clinical application in the near future. One might also mention here the supernatants of concanavalin A (Con A)-activated lymphocytes (SIRS: soluble immune response suppressor), which have been shown to suppress immune response *in vitro* and *in vivo*, thus preventing the onset of autoimmune diseases in B/W mice (Krakauer *et al.* 1977).

Chemically defined compounds

We have already mentioned several immunopotentiating agents that are derived from biological preparations but that have been fully characterized chemically and are now available in synthetic form: MDP, α_1 thymosin, thymopoietin pentapeptide and thymulin. To these products one may add several chemicals that were not initially devised as immunostimulating agents — levamisole, isoprinosine, polyribonucleotides, tilorone, azimexon and bestatin.

LEVAMISOLE

Initially used as an antihelminthic agent in animals, levamisole was fortuitously shown by Renoux and Renoux (1971) to possess significant immunostimulant activities. Levamisole enhances immunity to numerous infectious agents, in particular to *Brucella abortus* (Renoux and Renoux 1971) and to Gram-positive bacteria (Fisher *et al.* 1974). It augments antibody production to thymus-dependent antigens and stimulates transplantation immunity and delayed-type hypersensitivity. It also stimulates phagocytosis. The mechanisms of these effects are not fully understood but probably involve macrophages and especially T cells (Renoux 1978). Levamisole has been reported to act in part through a serum factor. Its immunopotentiating effects are not as well demonstrated in man but are strongly suggested by the increase in E-rosettes and enhancement of skin delayed hypersensitivity (Levs *et al.* 1975; Renoux 1978). Its clinical use, however, is limited by the risk of induction of agranulocytosis in some patients.

IMUTHIOL

Sodium difluocarbonate (Imuthiol) has been reputed to exhibit immunostimulating activity and has been used successfully in patients with acquired immune deficiency syndrome (AIDS)-related complex (Lang *et al.* 1988).

ISOPRINOSINE (IONOSIPLEX)

Isoprinosine was first described as an antiviral agent (Gordon and Brown 1972). Its capacity to enhance lymphocyte proliferative responses to mitogens (Hadden *et al.* 1976) has prompted study of its immunostimulating properties and the possible use of the drug in viral infections presumably associated with immunodeficiencies, notably in subacute sclerosing panencephalitis. Promising results have been reported (Streletz 1977) but need confirmation.

Table 50.2. Clinical indications for immunostimulation

Malignancies
Leukaemia
Melanoma
Lung cancer
Head and neck cancer
Infectious diseases
Antibiotic-resistant bacterial infections
Lepromatous leprosy
Acute and severe viral infections (encephalitis, generalized herpes)
Infections in hosts with compromised immune system, congenital immunodeficiency, malignant haematological diseases, recipients of anticancer drugs or radiotherapy
Vaccination (in immunodeficient subjects)
Autoimmune diseases
Systemic lupus erythematosus
Rheumatoid arthritis

SYNTHETIC POLYNUCLEOTIDES

Complexes of synthetic ribonucleotides (poly A:U and to a lesser degree poly I:C) are potent immunostimulants. Poly A:U acts as a polyclonal T cell activator, at the level of both helper T cells and cytotoxic T cells (Cone and Johnson 1973; Bick and Moller 1977). This activation takes place in the absence of macrophages and may involve factors produced by T cells themselves (Bick and Johnson 1977).

OTHER DRUGS

A number of other chemicals have been shown to stimulate various aspects of immune responses. In particular the IFN inducers, tilorone (Bick and Johnson 1977), pyran (McCord *et al.* 1976; Morahan *et al.* 1977) and polyacrylic acids (De Clercq and De Somer 1973), represent interesting immunomodulators. Ubiquinone 8, initially characterized from *E. coli* extracts, protects mice against various bacterial infection (Block *et al.* 1978). Bestatin also shows various immunostimulating properties.

Adjuvants

Adjuvants have been used for many years for the stimulation of antibody production and delayed-type hypersensitivity reactions (Freund's adjuvant, alum, etc.). In this chapter, however, we will not review the numerous agents of this class, since they are essentially used for specific immunization, which, so far, represents a limited type of intervention in immunopathology. In addition, many of these adjuvants cannot be used in man because of toxicity, as is notably the case of Freund's adjuvants.

Indications for and effects of immunopotentiation in clinical medicine

Cancer

The involvement of the immune system in the control of cancer has been, and is still, a matter of considerable debate. According to the concept of immunosurveillance, the immune system eliminates malignant cells when they appear. The role of T cells, and more recently of macrophages, killer (K) cells and especially natural killer (NK) cells, has been emphasized but has not been proved. There exists, inconsistently, a depression of T cell number and functions in cancer patients but it is not known whether such depression is primary or secondary to the malignancy. In particular, it is important to note that nude mice, which totally lack T cells, do not show an abnormal incidence of spontaneous neoplasia. The antitumour response might also play an important role once the tumour is established. In any of these hypotheses, stimulating the immune system might be favourable for the host. In addition, even if the antitumour immune response does not normally play a major role in the control of tumour growth, it is likely that adequate immunostimulation could elicit an efficient immune response or render efficient an otherwise ineffective response. All these considerations have justified the use of immunostimulation in the treatment of cancer, as an auxiliary method to surgery, radiotherapy or chemotherapy.

Cancer immunotherapy still poses several major unresolved problems. The nature of the cells to be stimulated is open to question. The choice of the immunopotentiating agent is empirical since, in addition to the uncertainty of the relevant effector cell just mentioned, the cellular site of action of most available products is unknown. In fact, although considerable efforts have been devoted to experimental studies, much information still comes from the randomized clinical trials that are performed with products such as BCG, *C. parvum*, levamisole and thymic extracts.

Bacillus Calmette–Guérin is certainly the best documented of these agents. Positive clinical trials have been reported in acute lymphoid leukaemia, acute myeloid leukaemia, head and neck tumours and melanoma (Bast *et al*. 1974; Mathé 1976; Goodnight and Morton 1978). Bacillus Calmette–Guérin has also been used locally in intratumour injection, with apparently limited success. Negative trials have also been reported using systemic administration. It remains difficult to formulate definitive conclusions. The proponents of BCG argue that negative results may be explained by one or several of the following factors:

1 Use of inefficient BCG preparation.
2 Inadequate selection of patients (too heterogeneous).
3 Improper protocol of administration of BCG or of associated chemotherapy.

Clinical trials have been performed with other agents, such as MER (Mathé 1976; O'Connell *et al*. 1976), *C. parvum* (Israel 1975; Fischer *et al*. 1976), thymic extracts (Zaizov *et al*. 1977; Chretien *et al*. 1978) and levamisole (Ward 1974), notably in solid tumours (bronchus cancer, head and neck tumours), but the limited number of statistically interpretable trials prevents any hard conclusion. Note, however, the interesting report by Chretien and colleagues of a significant improvement in a randomized trial of survival of patients with oat-cell lung carcinoma after a 6-week treatment with thymic extracts (Chretien *et al*. 1978). It is fair to recognize that these results need confirmation. Let us also mention here again the very promising results discussed above for IL-2.

Infectious diseases

Immunology was born from bacteriology. Immunostimulating agents have been extensively studied in infectious disease in animal models. However, clinical trials of immunostimulants in human infectious diseases are still very scarce. One may predict that this situation will change and that several of the available immunostimulating agents mentioned in the preceding pages will be used in cases where conventional antibiotic, antiviral or antifungal therapy has failed.

The susceptibility toward infectious agents varies with individuals. In some epidemics a high percentage of the population is hit; in others only a minority will get the disease. Among these patients the severity of the infection varies considerably. The cellular, molecular and genetic bases of this individual variability are still imperfectly defined but should be recalled before discussing the potential indications for immunostimulating agents in infectious diseases. It is apparent that T cells play a major role in most viral and mycotic diseases, as well as in infections by intracellular bacteria, that antibody production is essential in defence against Gram-positive bacteria and that phagocytes (polymorphs, monocytes and macrophages) play an important role in most bacterial infections. The genetic control of anti-infectious defences is several-fold. One may distinguish immune response genes, controlling the response against well-defined antigens, and a polygenic control of the overall immune responses (particularly antibody-mediated), which seemingly operates at macrophage level. It is interesting, in that regard, that low antibody producers, having very active macrophages, are more resistant than high antibody producers against intracellular bacteria (Biozzi *et al*. 1979). Super-imposed on this genetic control there exists another level of susceptibility to infectious agents, which relates to the functional level of the various cellular subsets involved in the elimination of the pathogen. Immunodeficiencies may apply to part or the totality of immune responses. They may be congenital or acquired, particularly in the course of malignant haematological diseases. They may also be secondary to chemotherapy or irradiation.

Infected subjects presenting a recognized immunodeficiency, who often show infections with 'unusual' or 'opportunistic' microbes, should theoretically benefit from immunotherapy. It should be emphasized, however, that infections not obviously associated with immunodeficiency could also be improved by immunopotentiating agents, since enhancement of a physiological response might help to eliminate a particularly virulent agent that has overwhelmed normal responses. T-cell-stimulating agents, such as MDP, thymic extracts, levamisole or isoprinosine, should prove useful in cases of severe infections by viruses or of intracellular bacteria (e.g. herpes zoster, lepromatous leprosy, etc.). Promising data were reported for thymosin (Zaizov *et al.* 1977) and isoprinosine (Gordon and Brown 1972). Macrophage-stimulating agents (such as *C. parvum*) could be used in many bacterial infections. Particular attention should be given to the case of ageing subjects, who often respond poorly to a number of vaccines (e.g. influenza).

Autoimmune diseases

It may seem paradoxical to mention autoimmune diseases among possible indications for immunostimulation, since such diseases are defined by a high level of autoantibody. This is justified, however, by the present concepts of the aetiopathogenic mechanisms of autoimmune diseases. Indeed, arguments converge to indicate that a deficiency of suppressor T cells represents an important aetiological factor (Bach *et al.* 1977): neonatally thymectomized or nude mice present manifestations of autoimmunity; thymectomy aggravates spontaneous autoimmune diseases; spontaneously autoimmune NZB and B/W mice present a deficiency of suppressor T cells, an atrophy of the thymic epithelium and a premature decline in thymic hormone production. Data are less numerous in man but preliminary data obtained in systemic lupus erythematosus indicate that there is a deficiency of suppressor T cells. Such mechanisms have prompted several attempts to prevent or to cure autoimmunity in NZB and B/W mice (Bach and Droz 1980) by using thymocyte grafts (Gershwin and Steinberg 1976), supernatants of Con-A-activated lymphocytes, SIRS (Krakauer *et al.* 1977), thymic extracts or synthetic (M.A. Bach *et al.* 1978), prostaglandins (Zurier *et al.* 1977), or levamisole (Zulman *et al.* 1978): promising results have been reported with all these agents, but the extrapolation to human autoimmune diseases is hazardous. Only very limited data are available. The only trials performed in an interpretable fashion concern rheumatoid arthritis and levamisole, but the mode of action of levamisole in this situation is not yet clear. In any case, one should take into consideration the potential risks of immunostimulation of autoimmune patients. There is in fact no reason to believe that any of the agents mentioned above with selectively stimulate suppressor T cells and not helper T cells. Indeed, aggravation of autoimmunity has been reported for anti-deoxyribonucleic acid (DNA) antibodies with thymic hormones (M.A. Bach *et al.* 1978; Bach and Droz 1980): mice treated with FTS simultaneously showed improvement of haemolytic anaemia and Sjögren syndrome and aggravation of anti-DNA antibody production and glomerulonephritis. Similar phenomena could occur with other agents. This difficulty calls for great caution in selecting the indications for immunostimulants in autoimmune diseases but should not be considered as a cause of exclusion if the patients are carefully followed up.

One may hope that other approaches currently under experimental investigation will become applicable to human autoimmune diseases, notably anti-idiotypic sensitization, T cell vaccination and immunoregulatory cytokines: the case of TNF-α, which has been shown to inhibit the onset of murine lupus (Jacob and McDevitt 1988), is particularly intriguing.

Conclusion

Immunopotentiation is still at its beginning, at least in its clinical applications. Promising results have already been reported in the treatment of cancer but these results require confirmation. In any case they should be improved by the use of the well-defined products now available, and possibly by synthetic compounds. The indications should also be extended in particular to infectious and autoimmune diseases. The problem is complicated in the latter case, however, case by the risk of stimulating helper T cells and thus aggravating autoantibody production. This risk will probably decrease when the knowledge of the immunological mechanisms of autoimmune diseases and of the mode of action of immunostimulating agents on lymphocyte subsets has been improved.

References

Adlam, C., Broughton, E.S. and Scott, M.T. (1972). Enhanced resistance of mice to infection with bacteria following pretreatment with *C. parvum*. *Nature N. Biol.* **235**, 219.

Amor, B., Dougados, M., Mery, C., Dardenne, M. and Bach, J.F. (1987). Nonathymulin in rheumatoid arthritis: two double blind, placebo controlled trials. *Ann. Rheum. Dis.* **46**, 549.

Andersson, J.A., Melchers, F., Galanos, C. and Luderitz, O. (1973). The mitogenic effect of lipopolysaccharide on bone marrow derived mouse lymphocytes: lipid A as the mitogenic part of the molecule. *J. Exp. Med.* **137**, 943.

Ascher, M.S., Gottlieb, A.A. and Kirkpatrick, C.H. (eds) (1976). *Transfer Factor: Basic Properties and Clinical Applications.* Academic Press, New York.

Asherson, G.L. (1977). Depression of cell-mediated immunity by pretreatment with adjuvants. *Microbiology* **382**.

Audibert, F., Leclerc, C. and Chedid, L. (1985). Muramyl dipeptides as immunopharmacological response modifiers. In *Biologic Modifiers*, ed. P.F. Torrence, Academic Press, New York.

Bach, J.-F. (1979). Thymic hormones. *J. Immunopharmacol.* **1**, 277.

Bach, J.-F. and Carnaud, C. (1976). Thymic factors. *Prog. Allergy* **21**, 342.

Bach, J.-F., Bach, M.A., Carnaud, C., Dardenne, M. and Monier, J.C. (1977). Thymic hormones and autoimmunity. In *Autoimmunity*, ed. N. Talal, p. 207, Academic Press, New York.

Bach, J.-F., Bach, M.A., Blanot, D. *et al.* (1978). Thymic serum factor. *Bull. Inst. Pasteur* **76**, 325.

Bach, J.-F., Bach, M.A., Dardenne, M. *et al.* (1979). The serum thymic factor (FTS), a peptide lymphocyte differentiating hormone. In *Proc. Miles Symposium on Peptides*, Raven Press, New York.

Bach, M.A. and Droz, D. (1980). Experimental models in the search for new treatments of autoimmune renal diseases. *Adv. Nephrol.* **9**, 187.

Bach, M.A., Dardenne, M. and Droz, D. (1978). Effects of FTS on autoimmune disease in NZB and B/W mice. In *Pharmacology of Immunoregulation*, ed. G.H. Werner and F. Floc'h, p. 201, Academic Press, New York.

Bast, R.C., Zbar, B., Borsos, T. and Rapp, H.J. (1974). BCG and cancer (first of two parts). *N. Engl. J. Med.* **290**, 1413.

Bick, P.H. and Johnson, A.G. (1977). Poly A:U induced secretion of T lymphocyte helper factors. *Scand. J. Immunol.* **6**, 1133.

Bick, P.H. and Moller, G. (1977). Cytotoxic T-cell activation by polyribonucleotides: DNA synthesis is not required. *J. Exp. Med.* **146**, 844.

Biozzi, G., Mouton, D., Sant' Anna, O.A. *et al.* (1979). Genetics of immune responsiveness to natural antigens in the mouse. *Curr. Topics Microbiol. Immunol.* **85**, 31.

Bizzini, B., Maro, B. and Lallouette, P. (1978). Isolement et caractérisation d'une fraction dite P40 à partir de *Corynebacterium parvum*. *Méd. Malad. Infect.* **8**, 408.

Block, L.H., Georgopoulos, A., Mayer, P. and Drews, J. (1978). Non-specific resistance to bacterial infections: enhancement by Ubiquinone-8. *J. Exp. Med.* **148**, 1228.

Bolla, K. (1987). Therapeutic prophylactic effects of thymopentin with respect to its mechanism of action. In *Progress in Allergy and Clinical Immunology*, ed. N.J. Pichler, p. 537, Hogrefe and Huber, Toronto.

Cantell, K., Hirvonen, S. and Mogensen, K.E. (1974). Human leukocyte interferon: production, purification, stability and animals experiments. *In Vitro Monogr.* **3**, 35.

Chedid, L., Parant, M., Parant, F., Gustafson, R.H. and Berger, F.M. (1972). Biological study of a non-toxic water soluble immuno-adjuvant from mycobacterial cell walls. *Proc. Nat. Acad. Sci. (USA)* **69**, 855.

Chedid, L., Audibert, F., Bona, C., Damais, C., Parant, F. and Parant, M. (1975). Biological activities of endotoxins detoxified by alkylation. *Infect. Immun.* **12**, 714.

Chedid, L., Parant, M. and Le Francier, P. (1977). Enhancement of non specific immunity by a synthetic immunoadjuvant (*N*-acetyl muramyl-L-alanyl-D-isoglutamine) and several analogs. *Proc. Nat. Acad. Sci. (USA)* **74**, 2089.

Chretien, P.B., Lipson, S.D., Makuch, R., Kenady, D.E., Cohen, M.H. and Minna, J.D. (1978). Thymosin in cancer patients: *in vitro* effect and correlations with clinical response to thymosin immunotherapy. *Cancer Treatment Rep.* **62**, 1787.

Coates, M.R. and Pilch, Y.H. (1977). Conversion of normal human lymphocytes to tumor specific immuno-reactivity by xenogeneic immune RNA: blastogenic responses to soluble tumor antigens. *Cancer Immunol. Immunother.* **3**, 145.

Cone, R.E. & Johnson, A.G. (1973). Regulation of the immune system by synthetic polynucleotides. IV. Amplification of the proliferation of thymus-influenced lymphocytes. *Cell. Immunol.* **3**, 283.

De Clercq, E. and De Somer, P. (1973). Protection of rabbits against local vaccinia virus infection by *Brucella abortus* and polyacrylic acid in the absence of systemic interferon production. *Infect. Immun.* **8**, 669.

De Maeyer-Guignard, J., Cachard, A. and De Maeyer, E. (1975). Delayed type hypersensitivity to sheep red blood cells: inhibition of sensitization by interferon. *Science* **190**, 574.

Dresser, D.W. (1972). The role of T cells and adjuvant in the immune response of mice to foreign erythrocytes. *Eur. J. Immunol.* **2**, 50.

Fischer, B., Rubin, H., Sartiano, G., Ennis, L. and Wolmark, N. (1976). Observations following *Corynebacterium parvum* administration to patients with advanced malignancy: a phase 1 study. *Méd. Malad. Infect.* **8**, 408.

Fisher, G.W., Oi, V.T., Kelley, J.L. *et al.* (1974). Enhancement of host defense mechanisms against Gram-positive pyogenic infection with levotetramisole (levamisole) in neonatal rats. *Ann. Allergy* **33**, 193.

Gershwin, M.E. and Steinberg, A.D. (1976). Suppression of autoimmune hemolytic anemic in New Zealand (NZB) mice by syngeneic thymocytes. *Clin. Immunol. Immunopathol.* **4**, 38.

Glaser, M. (1978). Adjuvant-induced thymus-derived suppressive cells of cell-mediated tumour immunity. *Nature* **275**, 654.

Goldstein, A.L., Low, T.L.K., Mac Adoo, M. *et al.* (1977). Thymosin α_1: isolation and sequence analysis of an immunologically active thymic polypeptide. *Proc. Nat. Acad. Sci.*

(USA) **74**, 725.

Goldstein, G. (1977). What is a thymic hormone? In *Progress in Immunology III*, ed. T.E. Mandel, p. 390, North-Holland, Amsterdam.

Goldstein, G., Scheid, M.P., Boyse, E.A. and Van Wauwe, J. (1979). A synthetic pentapeptide with biological activity characteristic of the thymic hormone thymopoietin. *Science* **20**, 1309.

Goodnight, J.E. and Morton, D.L. (1978). Immunotherapy for malignant disease. *Ann. Rev. Med.* **29**, 231.

Gordon, P. and Brown, F.R. (1972). The antiviral activity of isoprinosine. *Can. J. Microbiol.* **18**, 1463.

Hadden, J.W., Hadden, E.M. and Coffey, R.G. (1976). Isoprinosine augmentation of phytohemagglutinin-induced lymphocyte proliferation. *Infect. Immun.* **13**, 382.

Halpern, B.N., Fray, A. and Crepin, V. (1973). *Corynebacterium parvum*, a potent immunostimulant in infections and in malignancies. In *Immunopotentiation*, vol. 18, p. 217, Ciba Foundation Symposium, Elsevier, Amsterdam.

Howard, J.D., Christie, G.H. and Scott, M.T. (1973). Biological effects of *Corynebacterium parvum*. IV. Adjuvant and inhibitory activities on B lymphocytes. *Cell. Immunol.* **7**, 290.

Israel, L. (1975). In Corynebacterium parvum: *Applications in Experimental and Clinical Oncology*, ed. B. Halpern, Plenum Press, New York.

Jacob, C.O. and McDevitt, H.O. (1988). TNF-α in murine autoimmune 'lupus' nephritis. *Nature* **331**, 356.

Khan, A., Kirkpatrick, C.H. and Hill, N.O. (eds) (1979). *Immune Regulators in Transfer Factor*. Academic Press, New York.

Kirkpatrick, C.H. (1975). Properties and activities of transfer factor. *Allergy Clin. Immunol.* **55**, 411.

Krakauer, R.S., Strober, W., Rippeon, D.L. and Waldmann, T.A. (1977). Prevention of autoimmunity in experimental lupus erythematosus by soluble immune response suppressor. *Science* **196**, 56.

Krim, M. and Sanders, F.K. (1977). In *Interferons and Their Actions*, ed. W.E. Stewart II, CRC Press, Chicago.

Lang, J.M., Touraine, J.L., Trepo, C. *et al.* (1988). Randomized, double blind placebo-controlled trial of ditiocarb sodium (Imuthiol) in human immunodeficiency virus infection. *Lancet* **ii**, 702.

Lawrence, H.S. (1969). Transfer factor. *Adv. Immunol.* **11**, 195.

Lederer, E. (1977). Natural and synthetic immunostimulants related to the mycobacterial cell wall. In *Proceedings of the 5th International Symposium on Medicinal Chemistry*, Elsevier, Amsterdam.

Levo, Y., Rotter, V. and Ramot, B. (1975). Restoration of cellular immune response by levamisole in patients with Hodgkin's disease. *Biomedicine* **23**, 198.

Lotze, M.T. and Rosenberg, (1989). The use of lymphokines in therapy. In *Progress in Allergy and Clinical Immunology*, ed. N.J. Pichler, p. 529, Hogrefe and Huber, Toronto.

Luderitz, O., Galanos, C., Lehmann, V. *et al.* (1973). Lipid A: chemical structure and biological activity. *J. Infect. Dis.* **128**, 17.

McCord, R.S., Breinig, M.K. and Morahan, P.S. (1976). Antiviral effects of pyran against systemic infection of mice with herpes virus simplex type 2. *Antimicrobial Agents Chemother.* **10**, 28.

Maillard, J. and Bloom, B.R. (1972). Immunological adjuvants and the mechanism of cell cooperation. *J. Exp. Med.* **136**, 185.

Mathé, G. (1976). Cancer active immunotherapy: immunoprophylaxis and immunorestoration: an introduction. In *Recent Results in Cancer Research*, Springer-Verlag, Berlin.

Merigan, T.C., Rand, K.H. and Pollard, R.B. (1978). Human leukocyte interferon for the treatment of herpes zoster in patients with cancer. *N. Engl. J. Med.* **198**, 981.

Meuer, S.C., Dumann, H., Meyer Zum Buschenfelde, K.H. and Kohler, H. (1989). Low dose interleukin 2 induces systemic immune responses against HBsAg in immunodeficient nonresponders to hepatitis B vaccination. *Lancet* **i**, 15.

Morahan, P.S., Kern, E.R. and Glasgow, L.A. (1977). Immunomodulator-induced resistance against herpes simplex virus. *Proc. Soc. Exp. Biol. Med.*, **154**, 615.

Morse, S.I. and Morse, J.M. (1976). Isolation and properties of the leukocytosis and lymphocytosis-promoting factor of *Bordetella pertussis*. *J. Exp. Med.* **143**, 1483.

O'Connell, M.J., Ritts, R.E. and Moertel, C.G. (1976). Immunological assessment of MER and placebo in advanced cancer, a double blind study. *Proc. Am. Assoc. Cancer Res.* **17**, 214.

Old, L.J., Benacerraf, B., Clarke, D.A., Carswell, E.A. and Stockert, E. (1961). The role of the reticuloendothelial system in the host-reaction to neoplasia. *Cancer Res.* **21**, 1281.

Parant, M. and Chedid, L. (1988). Muramyl dipeptides. In *The Pharmacology of Lymphocytes*, ed. M.A. Bray and J. Morley, p. 503. Springer-Verlag, Berlin.

Renoux, G. (1978). Modulation of immunity by levamisole. *Pharmacol. Ther.* **2**, 397.

Renoux, G. and Renoux, M. (1971). Effet immunostimulant d'un imidothiazole dans l'immunisation des souris contre l'infection par *Brucella abortus*. *C.R. Acad. Sci. (Paris) Sér. D* **272**, 349.

Rosenberg, S.A., Lotze, M.T., Muul, L.M. *et al.* (1987). A progress report on the treatment of 157 patients with advanced cancer using lymphokine-activated killer cells and interleukin 2 or high dose interleukin 2 alone. *N. Engl. J. Med.* **316**, 889.

Sonnenfeld, G., Mandel, A.D. and Merigan, T.C. (1977). The immunosuppressive effect of type II mouse interferon preparations on antibody production. *Cell. Immunol.* **34**, 193.

Streletz, L.J. and Cracco, J. (1977). The effect of isoprinosine in subacute sclerosing panencephalitis (SSPE). *Ann. Neurol.* **1**, 183–4.

Sugimoto, M., Germain, R.N., Chedid, L. and Benacerraf, B. (1978). Enhancement of carrier specific T cell functions by the synthetic adjuvant *N*-acetyl muramyl-L-alanyl-D-isoglutamine (MDP). *J. Immunol.* **120**, 980.

Trainin, N., Small, M., Zipori, D., Umiel, T., Kook, A.I. and Rotter, V. (1975). Characteristics of THF, a thymic hormone. In *The Biological Activity of Thymic Hormones*, ed. D.W. Van Bekkum, Kooyker Scientific Publications, Rotterdam.

Unanue, E.R., Askonas, B.A. and Allison, A.C. (1969). A role of macrophages in the regulation of immune response by adjuvants. *J. Immunol.* **103**, 71.

Ward, H.W.C. (1974). Levamisole in the treatment of cancer. *Lancet* **i**, 594.

Weiss, D.W. (1972). Non specific stimulation and modulation of the immune response and of state of resistance by the methanol extraction residue fraction of tubercle bacilli. *Nat. Cancer. Inst. Monogr.* **35**, 157.

Weiss, D.W., Bonhag, R.S. and Leslie, P. (1966). Studies on the heterologous immunogenicity of a methanol-insoluble fraction of attenuated tubercle bacilli (BCG). II. Protection against tumor isografts. *J. Exp. Med.* **124**, 1039.

Zaizov, R.R., Vogel, I., Cohen, I. *et al.* (1977). Thymic hormone (THF) therapy in immunosuppressed children with lymphoproliferative neoplasia and generalized varicella. *Biomedicine* **27**, 105.

Zschiesche, W.W. and Heinecke, H. (1973). Effects of variable bacillus Calmette-Guérin regiments on skin graft rejection. *Transplantation* **15**, 172.

Zulman, J., Michalski, J., McCombs, C., Greenspan, J. and Talal, N. (1978). Levamisole maintains cyclophosphamide induced remission in murine lupus erythematosus. *Clin. Exp. Immunol.* **31**, 321.

Zurier, R.B., Sayadoff, D.M., Torrey, S.B. and Rothfield, N.F. (1977). Prostaglandin E_1 treatment of NZB/NZW mice. I. Prolonged survival of female mice. *Arthritis Rheum.* **20**, 723.

51: Immunosuppressive Drugs in Clinical Practice

A.J. Rees and C.M. Lockwood

Introduction

The past decade has seen considerable advances in the understanding of how the immune system works and thus how it can be manipulated pharmacologically. There are many reasons for this, but four should be mentioned above all: first, the introduction of increasingly sophisticated molecular biological techniques to analyse gene expression and to produce reagents; second, the use of recombinant molecules and monoclonal antibodies to provide purified reagents and individual cell types for studying immune reactions, third, the demonstration that active mechanisms are involved in controlling immune responses and that these can be up-regulated or down-regulated therapeutically; and, fourth, a reappraisal of data derived from research in experimental models and cell cultures has clarified confusion which has hitherto attended their uncritical extrapolation of experimental results to man (see Table 51.1). In this chapter, information on the immunoregulatory effects of drugs will be presented in the context of their effects in man, and information from experimental animals has been included only where there are fundamentals relevant to any species.

Table 51.1. Constraints on interpretation of data from experimental studies with immunoregulatory drugs

1 Experimental studies *in vitro* and in animals have used high concentrations of drugs quite unobtainable pharmacologically in man.

2 Comparability of drug dosage between species has often been made on the basis of body-weight, not surface area. The rate of degradation and inactivation of a drug is proportional to metabolic rate, which in turn is proportional to surface area, not to body-weight. Thus, 1 mg/kg in an adult human is equivalent toxicologically to 13 mg/kg in a 20 mg mouse (Berenbaum 1975).

3 Species variation in drug metabolism. Rodents, for example, oxidize cyclophosphamide to its active metabolites far faster than does man.

4 Binding to plasma proteins may make it difficult to relate *in vitro* experiments to *in vivo* effects. Analogues of certain drugs may vary in this respect; for example, dexamethasone, now the most widely used steroid experimentally, shows little affinity for corticosteroid-binding globulin.

5 Certain drugs have a selective effect on lymphocyte populations. For example, cyclophosphamide depletes certain T cell subpopulations and glucocorticoids redirect lymphocyte traffic. Studies on circulating cells after *in vivo* treatment with these agents necessarily examine only the residual populations.

Steroids

Biochemistry and metabolism

Glucocorticoids are the most effective steroids used for immunotherapy (Dougherty *et al.* 1964; Rosenberg and Lysz 1980); the most commonly used are cortisone, hyrocortisone (cortisol), prednisone and prednisolone (molecular weights 358–362). Their solubility in water depends on the preparation; for example, hydrocortisone succinate is highly soluble whereas hydrocortisone acetate is much less so. They are metabolized to water-soluble glucocorticoids, which are excreted in the urine. This is predominantly by the hepatic microsomes, which can be induced by steroids themselves. Extensive methyl group substitution of the molecule, as in dexamethasone and methylprednisolone, can slow the rate of metabolism and extend the half-life. Thus the plasma half-life of glucocorticoids varies from 30–60 minutes for hydrocortisone and presnisone to 180–200 minutes for dexamethasone and methylprednisolone (Baxter and Forsham 1972; Berenbaum 1975).

Transport

Eight per cent of native cortisol exists free in plasma, and this provides the hormonal effect. The remainder is transported by a specific corticosteroid-binding globulin (CBG) (77%) or loosely bound to albumin (15%) (Ballard 1979). Although CBG has a high affinity for cortisol, it has a low binding capacity and, at concentrations of 10^{-6} M or greater, most of the cortisol exists free because albumin has low binding affinity (Ballard 1979). Synthetic glucocorticoids, with the exception of prednisolone, have a low affinity for CBG, and they exist in plasma as two-thirds loosely bound to albumin and one-third free. Since it is the free steroid which is active, increasing doses of synthetic glucocorticoids will bring about comparatively greater increases in effect than similar increases in cortisol (or prednisolone).

Pharmacokinetics

The concentrations of glucocorticoid achievable physiologically and pharmacologically in man are shown in Table 51.2. Generally it is useful to consider concentrations of 10^{-7} M or less as physiological and those greater than 10^{-6} M as being pharmacological. Concentrations of 10^{-5} M can be attained transiently after a single intravenous dose, but this is rarely indicated clinically.

Clinically the most commonly used glucocorticoid is prednisone, which is metabolized to prednisolone by liver enzymes. The metabolism is rapid and not rate-limiting except in severe liver failure. Both prednisone and prednisolone are poorly soluble in water and cannot be used for intravenous preparations. Comparison of peak steroid concentrations after administration shows that concentrations achieved by intravenous prednisolone phosphate are up to 10-fold higher than after the same dose of oral prednisone or intravenous prednisolone phthalate (Frey *et al.* 1984). The difference is matched by a corresponding difference in biological activity (inhibition of the mixed lymphocyte reaction (MLR) or inter-

Table 51.2. Glucocorticoid levels under physiological and pharmacological conditions

Physiological		Pharmacological[a]	
Diurnal variation[b]	1–5 × 10^{-7} M	Prednisolone 10 mg oral[g]	0.4–1 × 10^{-6} M
Pregnancy[c]	up to 7.4 × 10^{-7} M	Hydrocortisone 100 mg iv[h]	3.6–1.5 × 10^{-6} M
Stress (surgery)[d,e,f]	11–19 × 10^{-7} M	Prednisone 60 mg oral[i]	1.7–3.4 × 10^{-6} M
		Hydrocortisone 400 mg iv[h]	7–2 × 10^{-6} M
		Methylprednisolone 1 g iv[j,k]	2.7–4.0 × 10^{-5} M

Peak drug concentration usually achieved between 30 and 120 minutes, dependent on route of administration and individual variation. Enteric-coated preparations achieved similar levels but with a lag time of 30–60 minutes compared with non-coated preparations.

a Studies have shown that there is considerable variability in pharmacokinetic measurement between individuals at any single glucocorticoid dose (Wilson *et al.* 1975), although separate studies in the same individuals are reproducible (Tanner *et al.* 1979). **b** de Lacardi *et al.* 1973. **c** Rosenthal *et al.* 1969. **d** Mukundraike *et al.* 1968. **e** Plumpton *et al.* 1969. **f** Carter and James 1970. **g** Morrison *et al.* 1977. **h** Fauci and Dale 1974. **i** Colburn and Buller 1973. **j** Webel *et al.* 1974. **k** Coburg *et al.* 1970.

leukin 2 (IL-2) production), emphasizing the importance of the differences in pharmacokinetics of substances having a complex and variable metabolism.

Receptors

The effect of steroids is mediated through binding to specific receptors located in the cytoplasm of cells. These translocate to the nucleus when coupled with steroids and interact with chromatin to modulate gene expression (Baxter and Funder 1979). It is not known how the steroids enter the cell, although passive diffusion and specific uptake mechanisms have both been suggested. The effects of glucocorticoids on lymphoid cells were thought to be mainly inhibitory (Claman 1972), but they induce synthesis of specific proteins in many types of cells (Saltonick *et al.* 1983), and it is now known that the inhibitory effects on cells of the immune system are mediated by such proteins (Shephard *et al.* 1985; Strickland *et al.* 1986). Receptors for other steroid hormones have comparable effects, which may explain why they can also be immunoregulatory (Hall and Goldstein 1984; Grossman 1985).

Glucocorticoid receptors are found on all mammalian cells, in numbers varying from 3000 to 100 000 per cell. In the immune system, they have been characterized on rat thymocytes (Turnell *et al.* 1974), human lymphocytes (Smith *et al.* 1977), mouse peritoneal macrophages and human monocytes (Werb 1978). However, it has not been possible to relate overall receptor numbers to steroid sensitivity (Lippman and Barr 1977), and variations in receptor numbers during the cell cycle may be important (Crabtree *et al.* 1980; Distelhorst *et al.* 1984).

Mechanisms of action

The immune system is regulated by at least three different fundamental mechanisms, hormonal (as exemplified by glucocorticoids), the cytokine system (including interleukins and interferons) and network connectivity (through idiotypic–anti-idiotypic responses). Glucocorticoids have extensive effects on the immune system and these are so diverse that their study is not straightforward (Claman 1972; Cupps and Fauci 1982). For example, it is difficult to equate the results of *in vitro* experiments that examine the behaviour of a particular cell type with the effects of glucocorticoids *in vivo*. Species differences present a further problem, man and guinea-pigs being relatively resistant to the immunoregulatory effects of glucocorticoids, whilst rats and mice are susceptible (Claman 1972).

Species differences at a cellular level have also been reported; for example, murine CD4 +ve cells are steroid-sensitive (Vann 1974; Lee *et al.* 1975; Markham *et al.* 1978), whereas the function of the CD8 +ve T cell is inhibited in man (Gupta and Good 1977). Differences do not correlate with expression of steroid receptors (Fauci *et al.* 1980). More recently some of the species differences have been reconciled by careful phenotypical definition of cells involved, and the allowance for the presence or absence of exogenous growth factors (Claesson and Ropke 1983). Nevertheless, differences do exist, and so we shall concentrate on the human immune response wherever possible, and will draw on studies in experimental animals only to provide greater details when necessary. We will concentrate on three effects of glucocorticoids, which are believed to be important for their immunoregulatory effect, namely on cytokine production, immune cell function and immune cell traffic.

Glucocorticoids and cytokine synthesis

In the last 10 years there has been a considerable increase in knowledge about the cytokines, which are important for cell proliferation and activation pathways during the development of an immune response. Studies *in vitro* have shown repeatedly that physiological and pharmacological concentrations of glucocorticoids inhibit synthesis of cytokines, but have little effect on their function (see Table 51.3).

A detailed discussion of the effects of cytokines on the immune response would be inappropriate here and so a few examples will suffice: IL-1 is a co-factor released by antigen-presenting cells which stimulates T cells and B cells, and possesses powerful pro-inflammatory properties on neutrophils and endothelial cells; stimulation of T cell receptor initiates synthesis of IL-2, which acts as an autocrine growth factor for T cells; stimulated T cells also synthesize interferon gamma (IFN-γ), which activates macrophages and primes polymorphonuclear leucocytes; IL-6 stimulates B cell growth, whilst IL-4 promotes B cell differentiation. Microbial products stimulate macrophages to produce tumour necrosis factor (TNF), which has important major pro-inflammatory actions similar to IL-1. Table 51.3 shows that many of these responses can be influenced by glucocorticoids, which gives these agents a powerful role in the control of the immune response. This was first suggested by Balow and Rosenthal (1973), who described suppression of macrophage migration inhibition factor by corticosteroids, and has since been described in other systems (Wahl *et al.* 1975; Waage and Bakko 1988). It is uncertain how glucocorticoids achieve this but it involves interference with arachidonic acid metabolism in the case of IL-2 (Goodwin *et al.* 1986). Steroids inhibit translation of IL-1 (Kern *et al.* 1988) and TNF (Beutler *et al.* 1986) but have no direct effect on transcription. The activity of physiological concentrations of glucocorticoids on cytokine release has encouraged the hypothesis that they have a major homoeostatic role to play in the immune response in normal individuals (Guyre *et al.* 1988).

Cell function

LYMPHOCYTES

Glucocorticoids at physiological and pharmacological concentrations have no effect on proliferative responses by human T lymphocytes, although suprapharmacological concentrations have been reported to be inhibitory (see Table 51.4). However, glucocorticoids in physiological concentrations affect monocytes and inhibit their accessory cell function in the autologous MLR. Hydrocortisone appears to render T cells unresponsive to IL-1 and thus unable to synthesize IL-2 (Palacios and Sugawara 1982). This has led to speculation that the physiological rise in steroid levels after injury might be to inhibit T cell response to self antigens (Craddock 1978; Hahn *et al.* 1980).

Table 51.3. Effect of steroids on cytokines production

Stimulus	Cell stimulated	Cytokine	Inhibit
LPS	Human monocyte	TNF[a]	Dex 10^{-8}–10^{-6} M Cort 10^{-7}–10^{-6} M
LPS	Human monocyte	IL-1[b]	Dex 10^{-6}–5×10^{-6} M
	Human lymphocytes	IFN[b,c]	Dex 10^{-7} M
	Human lymphocytes	IL-2[c,d]	Dex 10^{-7} M
	MLC	IL-3[e]	Dex 10^{-7} M

LPS = lipopolysaccharide; MLC = mixed lymphocyte culture; TNF = tumour necrosis factor; IL = interleukin; IFN = interferon; Dex = dexamethasone; Cort = cortisone.

a Waage and Backko 1988. **b** Kern *et al.* 1988. **c** Guyre *et al.* 1988. **d** Orson and Auzenne 1988. **e** Schreiber *et al.* 1989.

Table 51.4. Steroids and T cell function

Response	Inhibition dose
Proliferation	
Lymphocyte proliferation (antigens or mitogens)	*In vitro* >2.8×10^{-5} M[a,b]
	In vivo 80 mg methylprednisolone[c] 400 mg hydrocortisone[d]
Lymphocyte proliferation	>4×10^{-7} M[e,f]
Allogeneic cells	*In vitro* >3×10^{-8} M[e,f]
Autologous cells	*In vivo* >40 mg prednisolone[g]
Cytotoxicity	
Direct cytotoxicity (lymphocytes)	*In vitro* >2.8×10^{-5} M[f,h,i]
K cell function	*In vitro* >10^{-4} M[j]
	In vivo >40 mg prednisolone[k]
NK cell activity	>10^{-4} M[l,m]
In vitro	>10^{-6} M (2 hours preincubation)[n,o]
In vivo	>12 mg dexamethasone
	>400 mg hydrocortisone IV[l]
	Cortisol (infusion equivalent to stress levels)[q]
Colony formation	
CD4	>10^{-4} M[r]
CD8	>10^{-6} M[r]

K = killer; NK = natural killer.
a Kissling *et al.* 1972. **b** Ruhl *et al.* 1974. **c** Webel *et al.* 1974. **d** Fauci *et al.* 1976. **e** Ilfeld *et al.* 1977. **f** Balow *et al.* 1977. **g** Katz and Fauci 1979. **h** Lundgren 1970. **i** Thong *et al.* 1975. **j** Parillo and Fauci 1978a. **k** Clark *et al.* 1977. **l** Parillo and Fauci 1978b. **m** Bray *et al.* 1983. **n** Gatting *et al.* 1987. **o** Nair and Schwartz 1984. **p** Katz *et al.* 1984. **q** Tonnesen *et al.* 1987. **r** Claesson and Ropke 1983.

In vitro synthesis of immunoglobulin by B cells is enhanced by the addition of glucocorticoids to the culture system, first, through inhibition of T-mediated suppression (Gupta and Good 1977; Lipsky *et al.* 1978; Haynes and Fauci 1978; Knapp *et al.* 1982) and, second, by influencing B cell interactions with monocytes (Cooper *et al.* 1981; Jeang *et al.* 1986; Orson and Auzenne 1988). It is likely that the latter process is the more important. Regulation of B cells by monocytes demonstrates the central role of the accessory cell in governing the immune response and the potential influence of steroids, since many of the accessory cell functions are readily moderated by fluctuations of steroid concentrations within the physiological range.

The influence of steroids on B cell maturation has also been examined *in vitro*, including effects on activation, proliferation and differentiation (Cupps *et al.* 1984, 1985). Steroids inhibit the earliest stage of B cell activation by blocking of macrophage generation of IL-1, and consequently T cell production of IL-2. B cell proliferation is initiated by one of two pathways, one dependent on monocytes and the other independent of them. Both are steroid-sensitive; however, the later stages of B cell differentiation are resistant to steroids, and indeed steroids can enhance immunoglobulin production. Recently, this has been shown in mice to be due to stimulating effect of steroids on production of B cell differentiation factors (IL-4, IL-5 and IL-6) (Jeang *et al.* 1986; Orson and Auzenne 1988). Intriguingly, a mechanism for focusing this steroid-enhanced effect has been defined: cell–cell contact between monocyte and B cell is required before steroid and IL-5 can increase immunoglobulin production (Orson and Auzenne 1988). It should be pointed out, however, that IL-5 is not a growth factor for human B cells.

The complex pathways by which steroids influence B cell function *in vitro* probably explain the variable action they are reported to have *in vivo*. Thus methyl prednisolone 96 mg daily for up to 5 days produced a small decrease in total immunoglobulin concentrations due to reduced synthesis and increased catabolism (Butler and Rossen 1973). Specific antibody responses were not affected (Butler *et al.* 1974) and under some conditions were even enhanced (Tuchinda *et al.* 1972).. The *in vivo* counterpart of steroid abrogation of T-cell-mediated suppression of immunoglobulin production has been shown in patients with common variable hypogammaglobulinaemia. Immunoglobulin synthesis can be restored by exposure of patients' cells to corticosteroids *in vitro* or *in vivo*; it can also be restored by T depletion of peripheral blood lymphocyte cultures from patients with the disease (Waldmann *et al.* 1976; Soothill 1975).

MONONUCLEAR PHAGOCYTES

Two major functions of monocytes are the elaboration of cytokines and the disposal of foreign particles with subsequent presentation of antigenic material to instigate the immune response. Steroids inhibit the production of monokines such as IL-1 and TNF (see above), but do not block the effect of other cytokines on monocyte function; indeed, they can even promote them. Thus the binding IFN-γ and subsequent expression of human leucocyte antigen HLA-DR molecules and Fc receptors are increased by relatively low doses of dexamethasone (2×10^{-7} M) (Girard *et al.* 1984; Shen *et al.* 1986). This is most probably due to a steroid-mediated increase in monocyte receptors for IFN-γ (Strickland *et al.* 1986). In contrast, immune activation (Ia) antigen expression in the mouse is inhibited by hydrocortisone (Warren and Vogel 1985), another example of differences between man and mouse.

In vitro exposure of monocytes to 10^{-8} M prednisone markedly inhibits monocyte chemotaxis, and the effect is maximal at 10^{-7} M (Tanner *et al.* 1980). However, cells harvested from individuals being treated with steroids had normal chemotaxis *in vitro*, irrespective of whether they derived from patients receiving long-term steroids (Tanner *et al.* 1980) or were from normal individuals given 50 mg prednisolone twice daily for 3 days (Rinehart *et al.* 1975). Both immune-mediated (antibody-dependent) and non-immune-mediated phagocytosis by monocytes is resistant to steroids *in vitro* except when concentrations greater than 10^{-4} M are used. Similar concentrations are needed to inhibit phagocytosis of cryptococci and of *Candida* (Rinehart *et al.* 1974), latex particles or immunoglobulin G (IgG)-coated erythrocytes (Schreiber *et al.* 1975). However, there was marked impairment of Fc receptor function in humans *in vivo* when tested 4 hours after 32 mg methylprednisolone had been taken orally.

Concentrations of steroid of 4×10^{-5} M are needed to inhibit monocyte bactericidal activity *in vitro*. Prolonged high-dose steroid therapy *in vivo* (prednisolone 50 mg twice daily for 3 days) markedly reduces both bactericidal and fungicidal activity, which remains impaired for up to 48 hours (Rinehart *et al.* 1974, 1975).

The function of polymorphonuclear leucocytes is resistant to levels of steroid achievable pharmacologically, as judged by tests of chemotaxis (Rinehart *et al.* 1974), phagocytosis (Dale and Petersdorf 1973) and antibody-dependent cytotoxicity (Parillo and Fauci 1978a, b).

Cell traffic

Administration of steroids causes striking changes in circulating leucocyte numbers, even when small doses are used. One gram of prednisolone IV (Coburg *et al.* 1970), 100 mg or 400 mg of hydrocortisone IV (Fauci and Dale 1974), 30 or 60 mg of prednisolone orally (Yu *et al.* 1974a) or even the administration of steroids in quantities to produce physiological concentrations in previously adrenalectomized patients (Thomson *et al.* 1984) causes lymphocytopenia, which is maximal at 4–6 hours and returns to normal by 24 hours. T cells are affected more than B cells (Yu *et al.* 1974a; Haynes and Fauci 1978), and within T cell subsets the numbers of CD4+ve cells fall to a much greater extent than those expressing CD8 (Haynes and Fauci 1978; Bast *et al.* 1983; Slade and Hepburn 1983). A similar phenomenon has been observed in guinea-pigs and shown to be due to redistribution of cells to the bone marrow and spleen (Fauci 1975). Circulating lymphocyte counts and endogenous cortisol concentrations both show diural variation, but careful analysis has failed to show any significant link (Levi *et al.* 1988). Interestingly, numbers of circulating natural killer (NK) cells remain constant throughout the 24 hours (Tonnesen *et al.* 1987).

Monocyte numbers in normal individuals decrease profoundly 2–6 hours after a single dose of steroids (hydrocortisone 100 mg IV) but recover by 24 hours (Fauci and Dale 1974), even if glucocorticoids are continued (prednisolone 50 mg twice daily) (Rinehart *et al.* 1975). However, alternate-day administration of steroids causes repeated cycles of monocytopenia (Dale *et al.* 1974; Fauci and Dale 1975b).

Modest doses of steroids produce neutrophilia, which is maximal at 4 hours and returns to baseline at 24 hours (Dale *et al.* 1975). This is due partly to release of mature neutrophils from bone marrow (Dale *et al.* 1975) and partly to reduction in the number of cells leaving the circulation, the latter being demonstrated using Roebuck skin windows to show that neutrophil influx into inflammatory exudates is reduced in normal individuals being treated with corticosteroids. A marked and prolonged (up to 72 hours) fall in circulating eosinophils and basophils has been documented after steroid treatment in normals (Zweiman *et al.* 1976; Dunsley *et al.* 1979), and this contrasts markedly with the neutrophilia observed at the same time.

Summary of the effects of glucocorticoids

At present it is thought that the major effect of steroids on the immune response is by regulation of production of cytokines. This may be an important aspect of the physiological control of the immune response in normal and diseased individuals. Such mechanisms could explain the effects of steroids in controlling inflammation (for example, by limiting TNF and IL-1 synthesis), as well as their effects on augmenting antibody responses, perhaps mediated by IL-4 and IL-6. Whether they also explain the striking effects of glucocorticoids on cell traffic is less certain.

Thiopurines

Purine analogues with immunosuppressive activity have been synthesized since the early 1950s, but only the thiopurines, 6-mercaptopurine and azathioprine, have been used extensively for this purpose in clinical medicine. Mercaptopurine is related to hypoxanthine but has a thiol group at the 6-hydroxyl position (Fig. 51.1). Azathioprine is a further modification and has an imidazole group added to the sulphur atom; it was originally conceived as a slow-release preparation but is converted to 6-mercaptopurine very rapidly *in vivo*. This conversion takes place non-enzymatically in whole blood but not in plasma, and can be accelerated by the addition of glutathione, which is normally found in erythrocytes. Azathioprine can also be metabolized through other pathways (Chalmers *et al.* 1967) but neither the products of these reactions nor the imidazole group released by conversion to 6-mercaptopurine have important immunosuppressive effects (Chalmers *et al.* 1969; Speafico *et al.* 1973).

Metabolism and biological effects

The metabolism and biological effects of azathioprine and 6-mercaptopurine are similar in experimental animals and man (Fig. 51.2). Neither parent drug is active, and both are metabolized intracellularly to active compounds, principally thio-inosinic acid. This reaction is catalysed by hypoxanthine–guanine phosphoribosyl transferase (HGPRT) — the enzyme that is absent in the Lesch–Nyhan syndrome. Azathioprine and 6-mercaptopurine are simultaneously catabolized to

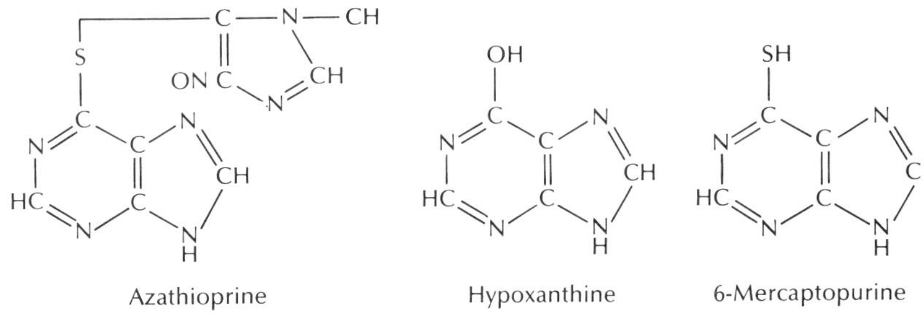

Azathioprine Hypoxanthine 6-Mercaptopurine

Fig. 51.1. Chemical formulae of azathioprine, hypoxanthine and 6-mercaptopurine.

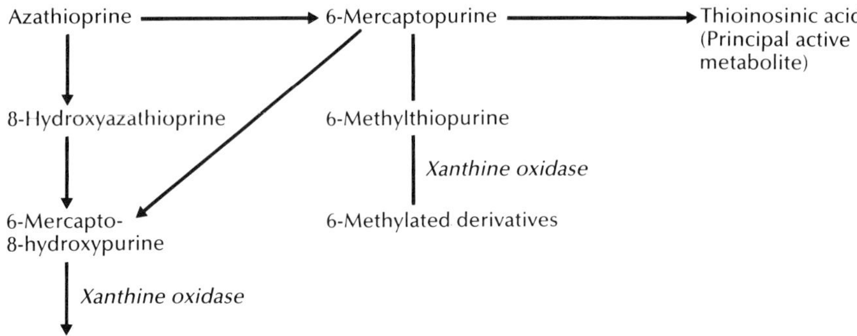

Fig. 51.2. Metabolism of azathioprine and 6-mercaptopurine.

inactive metabolites by xanthine oxidase, and the balance between these two pathways determines the immunosuppressive effect. Allopurinol, which inhibits xanthine oxidase activity, increases the effective dose of azathioprine and 6-mercaptopurine four- to sixfold.

Thio-inosinic acid inhibits synthesis of deoxyribonucleic acid (DNA), ribonucleic acid (RNA) and protein by interference with a number of steps in purine metabolism. These include competitive inhibition of enzymes which convert inosinic acid to xanthylic acid and adenylosuccinic acid, and feedback inhibition of enzymes necessary for conversion of phosphoribosylpyrophosphate to inosinic acid, perhaps by incorporation of fraudulent purine bases into DNA (Fig. 51.3). As the main effects are on DNA synthesis, thiopurines are only active against dividing cells. These reactions and the metabolism of thiopurines have been extensively reviewed (Elion and Hitchings 1975; Bach and Strom 1985).

Pharmacology

There are considerable difficulties in interpreting the pharmacokinetics of azathioprine because of its rapid metabolism to mixtures of compounds, only some of which are immunosuppressive. These difficulties are compounded by the fact that the immunosuppressive metabolites are produced intracellularly, close to their presumed site of action. The original pharmacokinetic studies used ^{35}sulphur- and ^{14}carbon-labelled azathioprine and 6-mercaptopurine (Bach and Dardenne 1972a; Elion 1972), and the problems were identified when results of these studies were compared with plasma drug activity (Bach and Dardenne 1972a). Some of these difficulties have been circumvented more recently by using high-performance liquid chromatography to measure parent drug and individual metabolites specifically (Maddocks and Davidson 1975; Lavi and Hoecenberg 1985; Lennard 1985). The sensitivity of these assays is about 0.5 ng/ml.

The combined use of these approaches shows that azathioprine and 6-mercaptopurine are both well absorbed after an oral dose and that peak plasma concentrations of 1–2 μg/ml are reached after 2 hours; it had previously been shown that concentrations as high as 20–25 μg/ml are attained for a few hours after high (13 mg/kg) intravenous doses (Loo *et al.* 1968; Coffey *et al.* 1972). The half-life of unchanged azathioprine and 6-mercaptopurine varies between 30 minutes and 4 hours, and is

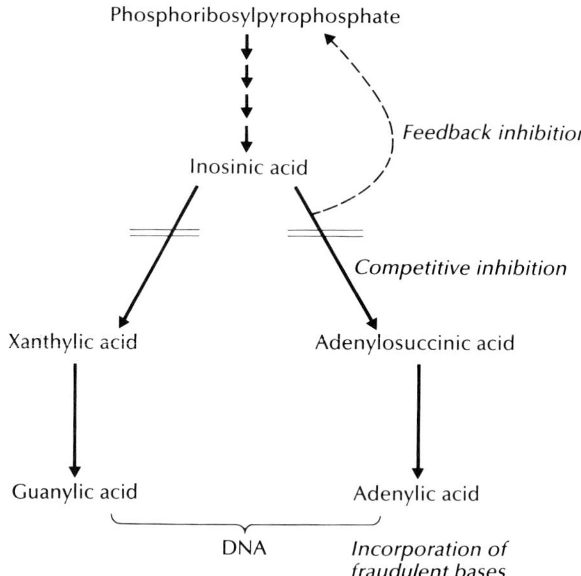

Fig. 51.3. Sites of inhibition of purine metabolism by thiopurines.

much shorter than the apparent half-lives assessed by ^{35}S-labelled drug or of the plasma immunosuppressive activity, both of which are about 4 hours. Protein binding of 6-mercaptopurine is less than 30% and urinary excretion is more than 50%, mostly in the form of inactive metabolites; 10–25% of an oral dose appears in the stools (Bach and Strom 1985).

In experimental animals, maximum tolerated chronic oral doses of azathioprine are 20 mg/kg/day in mice and rats and 10 mg/kg/day in rabbit (Elion and Hitchings 1975). In man, the usual dose of azathioprine long-term treatment is 1–3 mg/kg/day and 6-mercaptopurine is given in equivalent molar doses (0.5–1.5 mg/kg/day). Bone marrow toxicity is the limiting factor. Exceptional patients are exquisitely sensitive to azathioprine, which, in some cases, is due to delayed catabolism of immunosuppressive metabolites (Bach and Strom 1985).

Dosage does not need to be modified in patients with renal failure (Bach and Dardenne 1972) but, as much of the conversion of azathioprine to 6-mercaptopurine takes place in the liver, severe hepatic failure may limit its therapeutic effect (Mitchell *et al.* 1970; Bach and Dardenne 1972a; Elion 1972). Neither azathioprine nor 6-mercaptopurine is effective in patients with the Lesch–Nyhan syndrome (see above), and allopurinol should be avoided whenever possible in patients receiving thiopurines because inhibition of xanthine oxidase prevents their inactivation. If allopurinol is essential, the dose of thiopurine should be reduced to 25%.

The pharmacology of the thiopurines has been reviewed by Elion and Hitchings (1974).

In vitro effects of thiopurines

In short-term cultures, neither azathioprine nor 6-mercaptopurine is directly cytotoxic at concentrations attainable *in vivo* (Bach and Strom 1985), nor do these concentrations depress protein synthesis. However, they can be toxic to long-term cultures; for example, 5-day cultures of human lymphocytes are inhibited by 50 μg/ml of azathioprine, and concentrations as low as 0.5–1 μg/ml reduce the mitosis of bone marrow cultures (Boll *et al.* 1971).

Mixed lymphocyte reactivity in mice and in men is completely suppressed by 10 μg/ml azathioprine *in vitro*, but only if added within the first 48 hours of culture (Bach and Bach 1972); there is partial suppression with 0.1–1 μg/ml (see Bach and Strom 1985). Generation of cytotoxic T cells in mice can also be suppressed by these concentrations of azathioprine, although, once generated, the T cells function normally (Rollinghoff *et al.* 1973). Antigen-specific proliferation in response to keyhole limpet haemocyanin is similarly affected (Swanson and Schwartz 1967; Denman *et al.* 1970; Dimitriu and Fauci 1978) but phytohaemagglutinin (PHA) responses are much more resilient.

In vitro murine antibody responses to thymus-dependent antigens are suppressed by azathioprine 1–2 μg/ml in the culture medium, but again only when added within the first 48 hours (Galanaud *et al.* 1975). Responses to thymus-independent antigens are also suppressed, provided that they do not activate B cells polyclonally (Rollinghoff *et al.* 1973; Galanaud *et al.* 1976).

In vitro, azathioprine has no effect on monocyte chemotaxis, phagocytosis or microbial killing when concentrations attainable *in vivo* are used (Ward 1971; Losito *et al.* 1978).

In vivo effects of thiopurines in rodents

Most studies in experimental animals have used single high-dose or very short courses of thiopurines, and so the results have limited relevance to the chronic administration of azathioprine used clinically. Consequently only a brief description will be given here; fuller accounts may be found in Bach and Strom (1985) and Winkelstein (1979).

CELL NUMBERS

Short courses of high-dose azathioprine reduce thymic cellularity in mice, rats and guinea-pigs (Poulter *et al.* 1974; Berenbaum 1975). The greatest effect is on cortisone-sensitive thymocytes in the cortex. Cellularity of lymph nodes is unaffected (Miller and Cole 1967), as are circulating T and B cell numbers (Winkelstein 1977). Killer (K) cell activity of mice is strikingly depressed by a short course of very low-dose azathioprine (Purves 1975; Purves and Berenbaum 1975) and NK cell activity is also suppressed by low doses (Mantovani *et al.* 1978).

Peripheral blood monocyte counts are exquisitely sensitive to azathioprine in mice: azathioprine 3 mg/kg for 9 days depresses the monocyte count by 50%, due to inhibition of the mitotic rate of promonocytes (Van Furth *et al.* 1975). Reduction in the number of peritoneal macrophages needs higher doses and more prolonged courses (Gassman and Van Furth 1975).

IMMUNE RESPONSE *IN VIVO*

The effects of immune response *in vivo* have been studied repeatedly in mice, rats, guinea-pigs and rabbits, and have been related to the timing of antigen challenge (see Bach and Strom (1985) and Winkelstein (1979) for comprehensive reviews).

Primary antibody responses to a wide range of antigens are suppressed by a single high dose of azathioprine or 6-mercaptopurine in all the species tested, and the effect is maximal when the drug is given within 4 days of antigenic challenge. Secondary responses can also be suppressed but are more resilient; in both cases the IgG response is more severely affected than that of IgM. Large doses of antigen given simultaneously with the thiopurine sometimes induce prolonged specific unresponsiveness (Sela *et al.* 1963; Bach and Strom 1985). However, azathioprine and 6-mercaptopurine given for a brief period before immunization can result in enhanced antibody responses. This phenomenon was originally demonstrated by Chanmougan and Schwartz (1966) and has been confirmed repeatedly by others (for example Kipilman and Smith 1979; Drössler *et al.* 1981).

Suppression of delayed hypersensitivity and contact hypersensitivity has been variously reported in mice, rats, guinea-pigs and rabbits (Bach and Strom 1985). Single high doses given with antigen inhibit induction of specific cytotoxic T cells. However, there are also powerful anti-inflammatory effects when the drug is given continuously after sensitization (Phillips and Zweiman 1973). Again, single doses of azathioprine given before immunization can enhance the subsequent delayed hypersensitivity responses (Smith *et al.* 1981).

Thiopurines suppress inflammation non-specifically in mice (Gassman and Van Furth 1975) and rabbits (Page *et al.* 1962). The degree of suppression correlates with reduction in circulating monocyte counts. Neither 6-mercaptopurine nor azathioprine has any effect on clearance of particles from the circulation by the reticulophagocytic system (Schwartz and Andre 1960; Kaufman and McIntosh 1971).

In vivo effects of thiopurines in man

Interpretation of the effect of thiopurines on lymphocyte numbers in man has to be guarded, as most studies are of patients concurrently taking small doses of corticosteroids.

CELL NUMBERS

Lymphocyte counts are reduced by prolonged courses of 2–3 mg/kg/day azathioprine (Campbell *et al.* 1974, 1976; Yu *et al.* 1974b; Clements and Levy 1977; Thomas *et al.* 1977), without a change in the proportions of T and B cells (Ellis *et al.* 1981; Chatenoud *et al.* 1983). Striking reductions in K cell activity have been reported in patients with Crohn's disease after 6 months' treatment with azathioprine (Campbell *et al.* 1976; Shih *et al.* 1982), but the effect wears off 2–3 weeks after stopping the drug. Similar observations have been made in patients after renal transplantation (Thomas *et al.* 1977), but only in those also taking small doses of prednisolone (Descamps *et al.* 1977). Natural killer cell activity has been reported to be even more sensitive to azathioprine (Shih *et al.* 1982), as has the NK activity generated in response to interferon (Lipinsky *et al.* 1980). Peripheral blood monocyte counts are also reduced by azathioprine or 6-mercaptopurine (Page *et al.* 1962; Hersh *et al.* 1966).

IMMUNE RESPONSE *IN VIVO* (Table 51.5)

Short courses of high-dose azathioprine or 6-mercaptopurine suppress antibody responses when given with antigen but not if given before (Hersh *et al.* 1966; Santos and Owens 1966); as in rodents, IgG responses are affected to a greater extent than IgM (Swanson and Schwartz 1967; Rowley *et al.* 1969), and occasionally prolonged specific unresponsiveness may result (Levin *et al.* 1964). These regimens carry a high risk of toxicity and are not used for immunosuppression clinically, and there is little convincing evidence that chronic administration of either drug in conventional dosage inhibits humoral immunity. Delayed hypersensitivity is not convincingly depressed by conventional doses of thiopurines (Epstein and

Table 51.5. Effect of azathioprine on immune responsiveness in man

Daily dose (po) (mg/kg)	Duration before immunization	Concomitant therapy	Study group	Control groups	Effect on immune response: Delayed hypersensitivity	Primary antibody response	Second antibody response	Others	Toxicity	Authors
3	Day of immunization	None	Various	Healthy	Suppressed	Suppressed	Suppressed	—	Moderate	Swanson and Schwartz 1967
3	>3 months	None	Renal transplant	Healthy	—	—	—	K cell activity not suppressed	Slight	Descamps *et al.* 1977
2.5	>3 months	Prednisolone approx. 11 mg od	RA/Stills	(a) Patients (b) Healthy	No effect	No effect	No effect	—	Moderate	Denman *et al.* 1970
2.5	1 year	None	Ulcerative colitis	(a) Patients (b) Healthy	—	—	—	K cell activity suppressed	Slight	Campbell *et al.* 1976
2.4	1 year	Prednisolone approx. 28 mg od	Renal transplant	Healthy	—	Attenuated	—	—	Slight	Rowley *et al.* 1969
2	3–12 months	Prednisolone approx. 13 mg od	Various	(a) Patients (b) Healthy	—	No effect	—	—	Slight	Mackay *et al.* 1973
2	>3 months	None	Crohn's disease	(a) Patients (b) Healthy	No effect	—	—	—	None	Gyte and Willoughby 1977
1.4–2.8		Prednisolone approx. 13 mg od	Various	(a) Patients (b) Healthy	—	No effect	—	—	Slight	Lee *et al.* 1975
1.4	6 weeks	None	Healthy	Healthy	No effect	Attenuated	—	Booster response suppressed	None	Epstein and Maibach 1965
1.4	6 weeks	None	Healthy	Healthy	—	Attenuated	—	Booster response suppressed	None	Maibach and Epstein 1965

RA = rheumatoid arthritis

Maibach 1965; Swanson and Schwartz 1967; Gyte and Willoughby 1977). Mitogenic responses to pokeweed mitogen (PWM) of lymphocytes from patients taking azathioprine are suppressed (Abdou *et al.* 1973) but response to PHA is not (Denman *et al.* 1970).

The most striking immunosuppressive effect of these doses of azathioprine or mercaptopurine is the depression of K cell and NK cell activity (Campbell *et al.* 1976; Lipinsky *et al.* 1980; Shih *et al.* 1982). Non-specific inflammation is suppressed after 3–4 weeks' treatment with 6-mercaptopurine 1.5 mg/kg (Page *et al.* 1962; Hersh *et al.* 1966), and suppression correlates with a fall in circulating monocyte counts (Hurd and Ziff 1968).

Effect of thiopurines on experimental diseases

Neither azathioprine nor 6-mercaptopurine prevents the development of autoimmune disease in New Zealand B/W (NZB/W) mice, even when given for prolonged periods at the maximum tolerated dose (Casey 1968b; Gelfand and Steinberg 1972). In rabbits (Hoyer *et al.* 1962), guinea-pigs (Field 1961) and rats (Vogel and Calabresi 1969), 6-mercaptopurine will suppress experimental allergic encephalomyelitis. It also prevents the development of experimental uvetis (Wirotsko and Halbert 1962), allergic experimental thyroiditis (Speigelberg and Meischer 1963) and experimental autoimmune myasthenia in rabbits (Abramsky *et al.* 1976; Tarrab-Hazdai *et al.* 1977).

Azathioprine has been shown to prolong renal allograft survival in rats (Tinbergen 1968) and more particularly in dogs (Calne 1960; Calne *et al.* 1962; Simonian and Murray 1971). Modest prolongation of skin grafts had also been reported (Elion and Hitchings 1975).

Specific toxicity of thiopurines

As with other cytotoxic drugs, myelosuppression is the commonest toxic reaction to azathioprine in both experimental animals and man. Granulocytes and platelets are particularly susceptible and leucopenia often persists for more than a week after stopping the drug. In man the erythroid series is also affected by the prolonged administration of azathioprine, and macrocytosis (MCV 95–105) is common. Occasional patients develop pure red cell aplasia (McGrath *et al.* 1975; Old *et al.* 1978; Williams *et al.* 1978). Intrahepatic cholestasis (Sparberg *et al.* 1969) and acute pancreatitis (Nogueira and Freedman 1972) have also been ascribed to azathioprine in man, but interstitial pneumonitis and bladder cancers are exceptional.

Alkylating agents

General comments

Alkylating agents are compounds that attach alkyl groups covalently to other compounds. Their cytotoxic effect has been known since the end of the nineteenth century but they were not extensively developed for use in medicine until the 1940s, when the toxicity for lymphoid tissue and other rapidly dividing cells suggested their use as anticancer agents. Since then, numerous alkylating agents have been synthesized but only chlorambucil and cyclophosphamide (Fig. 51.4) have been used extensively for immunosuppression.

Metabolism and biological effects

The action of an alkylating agent depends on its ability to interfere with DNA reduplication. Alkylation of purine bases in DNA weakens the DNA strand and may interfere with recognition of the nucleotides. Attempts to repair the damage further

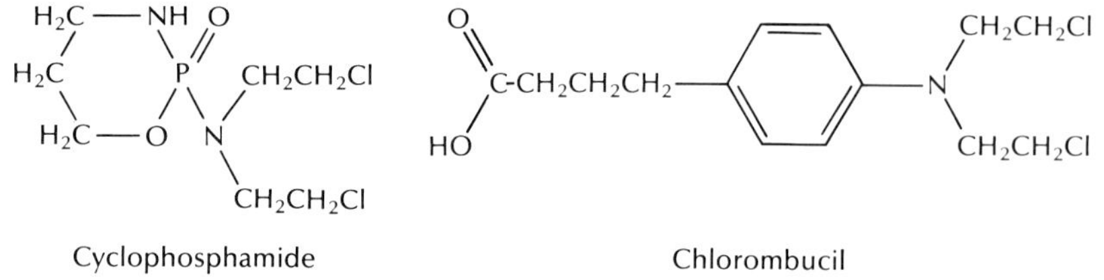

Cyclophosphamide

Chlorombucil

Fig. 51.4. Chemical formulae of cyclophosphamide and chlorambucil.

weaken the DNA, and its tendency to break during mitosis before repair is complete is lethal to the cell. The overall effect is to reduce the functional activity of DNA; for instance, methylated DNA *in vivo* has about 3% of the transforming activity of the native DNA molecule (Strauss *et al.* 1969). Some alkylating agents, including the active metabolites of cyclophosphamide, have two active groups and so have the additional property of covalently cross-linking strands of DNA and preventing their separation during reproduction (Roberts *et al.* 1971). Cells of different tissue vary in their capacity to repair DNA after alkylation. This, together with differing rates of cell division, determines the sensitivity of individual tissue to the toxic effects of alkylating agents.

Cyclophosphamide itself has no alkylating activity and is not cytotoxic, but many of its metabolites are (Fig. 51.5). Initially, it is oxidized by hepatic microsomes and to a lesser extent by mitrochondria (Brock and Hohorst 1963), utilizing metabolic pathways that are similar in rodents and man (Brock *et al.* 1971). The initial oxidation product is 4-hydrocyclophosphamide, which is in equilibrium with aldophosphoramide. These are the principal alkylating and immunosuppressive metabolites. Aldophosphoramide then decays to phosphoramide mustard (Connors *et al.* 1974; Jardine *et al.* 1978) and further metabolism yields nornitrogen mustard, which has some activity, and 4-ketocyclophosphamide and carboxyphosphoramide, which have none (Shand and Howard 1979).

Pharmacology

The pharmacology of cyclophosphamide has been extensively reviewed by Mellet (1971), Hill (1975) and Balis *et al.* (1983). In man, it has been studied after injection of radiolabelled drugs (Mellet 1971; Bagley *et al.* 1973), and more recently using simple reliable assays for cyclophosphamide (Jarman *et al.* 1975; Faccinetti *et al.* 1978; Juma *et al.* 1978) and its metabolites (Connors *et al.* 1974). Cyclophosphamide is rapidly, though incompletely, absorbed. Maximal serum concentrations of 1–2 mg/ml are reached 2 hours after an oral dose of 2–3 μg/kg, and plasma concentrations as high as 40–50 μg/ml are found after large intravenous injections (25 mg/kg). Cyclophosphamide is not bound to plasma proteins and its volume of distribution is about 60 litres (Bagley *et al.* 1973). Only 3–5% is excreted unchanged in the urine, even after massive intravenous doses (Jarman *et al.* 1975; Juma *et al.* 1978). Impaired renal function has no effect on the plasma half-time of cyclophosphamide but does prolong the alkylating activity detectable in plasma (Bramwell *et al.* 1979); both drug and metabolites are cleared by dialysis.

The half disappearance time after intravenous cyclophosphamide is about 6 hours (range 2–12 hours) and perhaps faster (1–6 hours) after ingestion (Juma *et al.* 1978), whilst that of alkylating activity is 5–6 hours (Bramwell *et al.* 1979). The conversion of cyclophosphamide to active metabolites can be increased by drugs that induce hepatic microsomal enzymes; this has been shown for phenobarbitone (Mellet 1971), prednisolone (Faber *et al.* 1974) and even cyclophosphamide itself (D'Incalci *et al.* 1979), all of which increase the concentration of active metabolites by about 25%.

In man, dosage of cyclophosphamide is usually limited by marrow toxicity to 2–3 mg/kg/day for prolonged courses, or single intravenous doses of 500–750 mg/m^2 body surface area, which may be repeated at 3-weekly to monthly intervals.

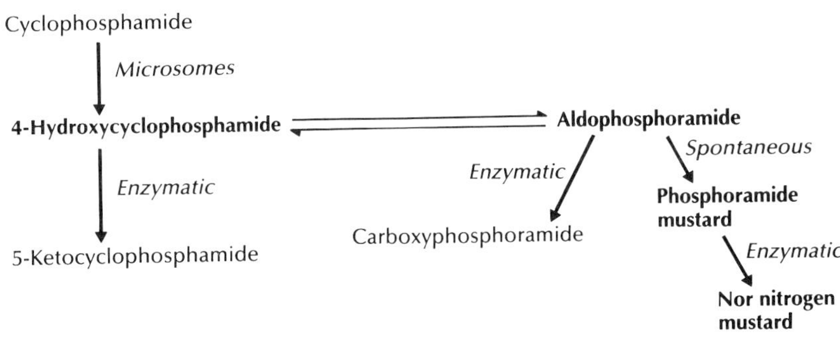

Fig. 51.5. Metabolism of cyclophosphamide. Compounds that are underlined having alkylating and immunosuppressive activity.

In vitro effects of cyclophosphamide in rodents

Cyclophosphamide itself is not cytotoxic to lymphocytes or other cells, even at high concentrations, but must be activated by hepatic microsomes; this can be accomplished *in vitro* (Connors *et al.* 1970). Purified metabolites with alkylating activity are also cytotoxic and immunosuppressive at concentrations equivalent to those attained *in vivo*. T cell functions are abrogated by *in vitro* treatment with activated cylophosphamide or purified metabolites; suppressor functions are more sensitive than those of helper T cells (Diamentsen *et al.* 1979). Proliferation induced by concanavalin A is suppressed by cyclophosphamide *in vitro*, apparently under the influence of adherent cells (Ikezawa 1981). The MLR is also inhibited (Smith *et al.* 1981). The effects need not all be due to the cytotoxic effects as cyclophosphamide has been shown to have more subtle influences on certain cells. Murine B cells incubated with activated cyclophosphamide lose their ability to re-express surface-bound immunoglobulin after capping with anti-immunoglobulin sera, and are unable to mount antibody responses when used in cell transfer experiments *in vivo* (Shand and Howard 1979). Neither activated cyclophosphamide (Hunninghake and Fauci 1976) nor chlorambucil affects chemotaxis, phagocytosis or killing by inflammatory cells (Losito *et al.* 1978).

In vivo effects in rodents

CELL NUMBERS

In mice, rats and guinea-pigs, cyclophosphamide destroys B cells and T cells (Bach and Dardenne 1972b). Single small doses of cyclophosphamide cause a marked reduction in cellularity of the thymus, as well as thymic areas of spleen and lymph nodes (Turk and Poulter 1972; Stockman *et al.* 1973; Neta *et al.* 1977). Chronic courses of cyclophosphamide in guinea-pigs cause wasting of T-independent areas as well (Winkelstein 1977), but there are no comparable data for man. Single high doses of cyclophosphamide induce a profound lymphopenia of B and T cells, which is maximal after 3 days (Poulter and Turk 1972; Turk and Poulter 1972; Winkelstein 1977). Chronic low dosage induces a proportionately greater fall in B cells (Winkelstein 1977; Hunninghake and Fauci 1976) in guinea-pigs and also decreases the number of resident peritoneal macrophages (Buhles and Shifrine 1977).

IMMUNE RESPONSES *IN VIVO*

Cyclophosphamide is a powerful inhibitor of humoral immune responses for a wide range of antigens in mouse, rat and guinea-pig (reviewed by Bach and Strom 1985). Both 19S and 7S antibodies are affected (Santos and Owens 1966) in a dose-dependent fashion. Single high doses and continued low doses are both effective and the timing, though important, is less critical than with the thiopurines. The effect is maximal when cyclophosphamide is given with the antigen or in the succeeding 4 days (Berenbaum 1975). Recovery after stopping cyclophosphamide is complete by 7 days in the absence of repeated antigenic challenge. If animals are rechallenged with antigen, a state of prolonged specific unresponsiveness can be obtained (Aisenberg and Davies 1968), which has been attributed to development of specific suppressor T cells (Aisenberg and Murray 1973). This is unlikely to be the only mechanism as cyclophosphamide can induce tolerance to T-independent antigens (Shand and Howard 1979), which may be related to its ability to inhibit re-expression of surface membrane immunoglobulin on B cells.

Cyclophosphamide does not always depress antibody responses. Increased antibody titres have been described when low doses are given 3–4 days before antigen challenge (Duclos *et al.* 1977; Noble *et al.* 1977), possibly because of abrogation of suppressor T cells in a manner similar to that more regularly described for cell-mediated immunity. Cyclophosphamide can also reverse genetically controlled unresponsiveness to synthetic antigens (Debre *et al.* 1976) and IgE responsiveness (Taniguchi and Tada 1971; Chiorazzi *et al.* 1976).

Cyclophosphamide suppresses delayed hypersensitivity and contact sensitivity in dose-dependent fashion when given with the antigen or in the days following (reviewed by Bach and Strom 1985). However, if given 4 days before the antigen, both contact sensitivity and delayed hypersensitivity are usually enhanced, even when the concurrent antibody response is suppressed (Maguire and Ettore 1967; Turk *et al.* 1972; Langrange *et al.* 1974; Turk and Parker 1979). At first it was thought that release from the depressive effects of antibody liberated the enhanced response, but subsequent experiments have shown that enhancement is not dependent on a change in antibody titre (Askenase *et al.* 1975). Later interpretations suggested that suppressor T cell activity was abrogated (Rollinghoff *et al.* 1977). It should, however, be remembered that suppressor T cells are not a homogeneous population and not all are sensitive to cyclophosphamide (Zembala and Ascherson 1976; Shand 1979).

Cyclophosphamide has direct anti-inflammatory effects in rodents (Stevens and Willoughby 1969; Curry 1971) but these are probably less potent than those of the thiopurines. Hunninghake and Fauci (1976) showed that antibody-dependent cytotoxicity by guinea-pig alveolar macrophages was suppressed by five daily doses of 20 mg cyclophosphamide, but not when the same total dose is given as a single injection.

Thus the effects of cyclophosphamide in rodents can be summarized as follows: (i) it suppresses humoral and cell-mediated immunity when given after the antigen; (ii) under certain circumstances it can promote tolerance to T-dependent and T-independent antigens; and (iii) cell-mediated responses, and to a lesser extent humoral responses, are enhanced when cyclophosphamide is given before antigen challenge.

In vivo effects of cyclophosphamide in humans

CELL NUMBERS

Chronic treatment with cyclophosphamide (1–3 mg/kg/day) in man results in a modest reduction of total lymphocyte count (Winkelstein *et al.* 1972; Clements *et al.* 1974; Fauci *et al.* 1974; Horwitz 1974; Clements and Levy 1977), with B cells being affected rather more than T cells (Horwitz 1974; Cupps *et al.* 1982; Zhu *et al.* 1987).

Immune responses *in vivo*

A short course of high-dose cyclophosphamide, such as 7 mg/kg/day for 5 days, completely suppresses an antibody response provided it starts at the time of antigenic challenge (Santos *et al.* 1969). Single doses of 125 mg/kg are less effective. Chronic administration at very low dose (0.5–1 mg/kg/day) does not depress the antibody response (Curtis *et al.* 1973; Winkelstein 1974), but higher doses (2–3 mg/kg/day) are effective (Townes *et al.* 1972; MacKay *et al.* 1973) (Table 51.6).

Cyclophosphamide 3 mg/kg/day suppressed delayed hypersensitivity to mumps, purified protein derivative (PPD) and candidin (Alepa *et al.* 1970; Santos *et al.* 1971; MacKay *et al.* 1973). Cyclophosphamide has little effect on inflammation in humans.

Effects on experimental disease

Cyclophosphamide significantly delays or even suppresses the autoimmune disease in NZB/W mice (Casey 1968a; Gelfand and Steinberg 1972; Walker and Bole 1975). Experimental allergic encephalomyelitis can also be prevented by cyclophosphamide (Paterson *et al.* 1966), as can experimental allergic thyroiditis in rats (Paterson *et al.* 1971) and immune complex disease in aleutian minks (Cheema *et al.* 1972).

Cyclophosphamide has been used much less extensively than thiopurines to prolong allograft survival in experimental animals. In general, prolonged survival has been reported for rat renal allografts (Husberg 1972; Kawabe *et al.* 1972), whereas results in dogs are unimpressive (Reams 1963; Zukoski *et al.* 1963). Modest survival of skin grafts in mice (Sutton *et al.* 1963), rats and rabbits (Brody *et al.* 1965) have been reported, but again there is no effect in dogs (Reams 1963; Zukoski *et al.* 1963).

Toxicity of cyclophosphamide

Prolonged azoospermia occurs regularly in adults given courses of cyclophosphamide lasting more than 1 year (Fairley *et al.* 1972; Kumar *et al.* 1972); occasionally this improves after considerable delay (Buchanan *et al.* 1975). Children are similarly affected but the prepubertal testis appears less susceptible, particularly when the total dose is less than 200 mg/kg (Penso *et al.* 1974; Parra *et al.* 1978). However, Trompeter *et al.* (1980) have reported significantly reduced sperm counts in young adults given cyclophosphamide 2 mg/kg for 8 weeks (168 mg/kg total) 7 years previously.

Haemorrhagic cystitis complicates treatment with cyclophosphamide in rats, dogs and man, and it is thought to be due to acrolein, one of the

Table 51.6. Effect of cyclophosphamide on immune response in man

Daily dose	Duration before challenge	Concomitant therapy	Study group	Control group	Effect on immune response				Toxicity	Authors
					Delayed hypersensitivity	Primary antibody response	Secondary antibody response	Other		
>7 mg/kg IV × 7	None	None	Cancer	None	—	Suppressed	—	—	Severe	See Berenbaum 1975
3.5 mg/kg IV × 7	None	None	Cancer	None	—	Suppressed	—	—	Moderate	See Berenbaum 1975
2.5 mg/kg po	3 months	Prednisolone approx. 13 mg	Various	(a) Patients (b) Healthy	—	Suppressed	—	—	Mild	Mackay *et al.* 1973
2 mg/kg po	Not stated	Salicylates	RA	Patients	Suppressed	No effect	—	—	Moderate	Townes *et al.* 1972
0.5–1.5 mg/kg po	>3 months	Prednisolone 5–7 g od	RA	Patients	—	—	No effect	—	None	Winkelstein *et al.* 1974
0.7–1 mg/kg po	8 weeks	Salicylates	RA	Patients	No effect	No effect	—	—	None	Curtis *et al.* 1973

RA = rheumatoid arthritis

alkylating metabolites in urine (Cox 1979; Brock *et al.* 1979). The occurrence does not correlate directly with the dose, and in some patients the cystitis is complicated by bladder carcinoma. High fluid intake should be given to all patients on cyclophosphamide. The dangers can be eliminated, in patients being treated with pulses of intravenous cyclophosphamide, by co-administration of mesna, which reacts specifically with acrolein.

Cyclophosphamide occasionally causes interstitial pneumonitis and pulmonary fibrosis (reviewed by Sostman *et al.* 1977). Usually it follows massive intravenous doses of cyclophosphamide, but it has been reported after chronic low dosage (Mark *et al.* 1978).

Cyclosporin and related drugs

The immunosuppressive properties of cyclosporin were first identified by Borel and his colleagues (1976), who also showed that it had a novel mode of action. Subsequently two other drugs, FK506 (Kino *et al.* 1987) and rapamycin (Morris 1991), have been shown to have broadly similar properties and analogous mechanisms of action. Thus, they join cyclosporin in a new class of immunosuppressive drugs (Fig. 51.6). However, it should be emphasized that rapamycin differs from the other two in important respects. Cyclosporin has been used extensively in patients after transplantation and is being assessed increasingly in patients with autoimmune and immunoinflammatory diseases. FK506 has been used clinically in transplantation but not yet for autoimmune disease (Starzl *et al.* 1989), and rapamycin has yet to pass beyond the experimental stage (Morris 1991).

Cyclosporin is a cyclical peptide containing 11 amino acids, 10 of which are aliphatic and one of which is unique. It has a molecular weight of 1200 and is soluble in lipids and other organic solvents. It is a natural product of the fungus *Tolypocladeium inflatium* (Gams), and has now been synthesized, together with a number of analogues (Wenger 1984). FK506 is a macrolide lactone with a molecular weight of 822. It is derived from the fungus *Streptomyces tsukubaensis*. Rapamycin is also a macrolide lactone, and the two molecules share structural similarities (Schreiber 1991). All three drugs are united by their capacity to bind to a class of cytoplasmic proteins with peptidyl–prolyl isomerase (rotamase) activity; these have been named the immunophilins and are believed to play a crucial role in transducing signals from the cell surface to the nucleus (Schreiber 1991) (Table 51.7). Studies to correlate the immunosuppressive properties of analogues of these three drugs implicate drug–immunophilin complexes in the mechanism of action of these drugs.

Pharmacology

Cyclosporin is available as an intravenous preparation and as solutions and capsules for oral use. Both oral preparations have similar absorption characteristics and, weight for weight, are equivalent to roughly one-third of the intravenous dose. After absorption, cyclosporin is rapidly metabolized by enzymes of the cytochrome P_{450} system to at least 13 metabolites (Maurer and Lemaire 1986), two or more of which are strongly immunosuppressive (Rosano *et al.* 1986; Freed *et al.* 1987). There is considerable difficulty in assessing the appropriate dose of cyclosporin from drug concentrations, as metabolism and absorption profiles vary considerably from patient to patient (and

Table 51.7. Immunophilins and their binding proteins

Drug	Binding protein	M_r(kD)	Activity
Cyclosporin A	Cyclophilin	17.7	Rotamase
	Cyclosporin A-binding phosphoprotein	45	
FK506	FK-binding protein	11.8	Rotamase
	FK-binding phosphoprotein	60	
	FK-binding phosphoprotein	40	
Rapamycin	FK-binding protein	11.8	Rotamase

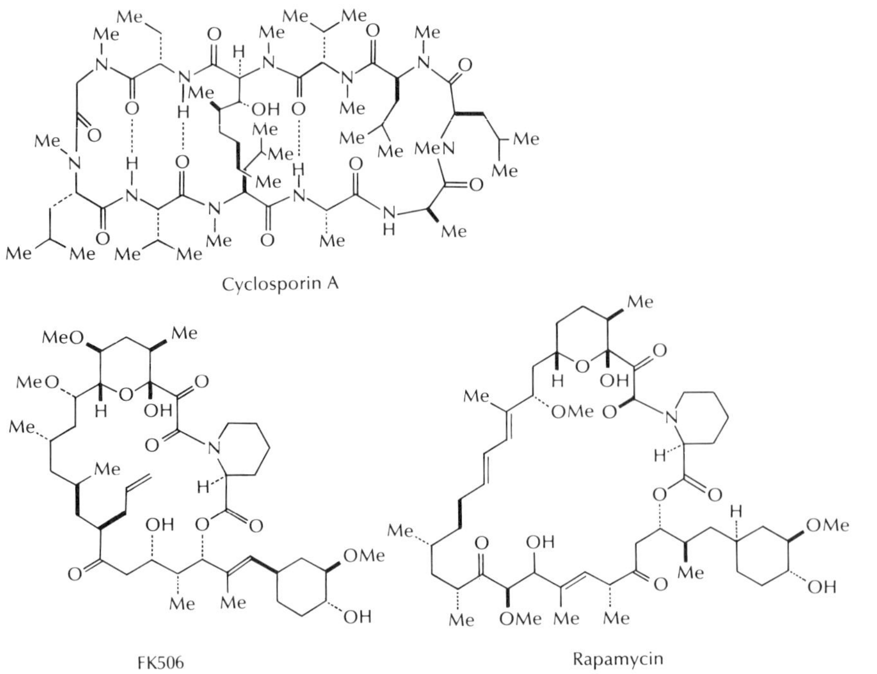

Cyclosporin A

FK506

Rapamycin

Fig. 51.6. Chemical formulae of cyclosporin A, FK506 and rapamycin.

even within the same patient) (Holt *et al.* 1986). Specific assays have been developed to improve the monitoring of cyclosporin concentrations in blood, with the use of either high-performance liquid chromatography (Christians *et al.* 1988) or capture radio-immunoassays, some of which are specific for the parent drug, such as the 'Sandimmune kit' (Quesniaux *et al.* 1987a), whilst others are not.

Detailed comparisons between assays have been made (Rosano *et al.* 1988). Disappearance time in plasma is biphasic, with half-times of 1.2 hours and 27 hours respectively (Quesniaux 1989). Recommended dose schedules are much lower now than where advocated when cyclosporin was introduced initially, and currently doses of up to 10 mg/kg/day orally are used for renal transplants and, more usually, 5 mg/kg/day for autoimmune disease (Dontasch and Ryffel 1986). Approaches to optimizing the dose of drugs have been reviewed (Keown 1988; Quesniaux 1989).

Table 51.8. Comparison of some functions of immunophilins

	Cyclosporin A	FK506	Rapamycin
Binding to NFAT	+	+	–
Lymphokine secretion (IL-2, IL-3, IL-4, IL-6 GM-CSF, IFN-γ)	↓	↓	– or ↑
IL-2 receptor expression	↓	↓	–
Inhibition of response to IL-2	–	–	+
Induction of apoptosis	+	+	–
Inhibition of proliferation	+	+	+
Autoreactive MLR	+	+	+
TcR ligation	+	+	+
Mitogens			

GM–CSF = granulocyte macrophage–colony stimulating factor; TcR = T cell receptor.

Effects of cyclosporin on cells of the immune system

Cyclosporin is not cytotoxic but has powerful inhibitory effects on certain populations of lymphocytes, and possibly on some antigen-presenting cells and on basophils (reviewed by Shevach 1985; Di Padova 1989) (Table 51.8). The original observation of Leoni *et al.* (1978) and Gordon and Singer (1979) showed that cyclosporin bound to murine and human lymphocytes; however, it is now known that cellular uptake of cyclosporin is much more widespread (LeGrue *et al.* 1983). Cyclosporin powerfully inhibits T cell proliferation in MLR, autologous MLR and the responses to the T cell mitogens concanavalin A and PHA. Early studies established that cyclosporin needed to be present within the first 24 hours of culture (Leoni 1978; Borel *et al.* 1977; White *et al.* 1979; Hess and Tutschka 1980). More recently, attempts have been made to define the cyclosporin-sensitive pathway of T cell activation more accurately (reviewed by Ryffel 1989). Lymphocyte activation that depends on calcium influx, for example exposure to concanavalin A or calcium ionophone A23187, is very sensitive to cyclosporin (Kay *et al.* 1983), even though cyclosporin does not affect the calcium influx itself (Metcalf 1984). In contrast, stimulation of T cell proliferation by phorbol ester plus IL-2, which is not dependent on calcium influx, is resistant to cyclosporin A (Sugawara and Ishizaka 1983). This approach has been further refined by studying the responses of allospecific T cell clones, which show that cyclosporin appears to inhibit antigen-specific T helper cell function (assessed by IL-2 generation) and cytotoxic T cell precursor proliferation, but not the expression of IL-2 receptors or the proliferative response to IL-2 (Orosz *et al.* 1982, 1983). These and later studies showing that cyclosporin inhibits IL-2 messenger RNA (mRNA) and protein synthesis (Kronke *et al.* 1984) raised the question whether the products of T helper cells that promote B cell and macrophage development might be similarly affected. This has proved to be the case; mRNA for IL-3, IL-4, IFN-γ, TNF-α, and granulocyte–macrophage colony-stimulating factor (GM-CSF) are inhibited by cyclosporin (Elliot *et al.* 1984; Granelli-Piperino *et al.* 1984, 1986; Espevik *et al.* 1987; Zipfel 1989). Cyclosporin also has direct effects on cytotoxic T cells by inhibiting exocytosis (Lancki *et al.* 1989; Trenn *et al.* 1989).

Cyclosporin affects B cells under certain circumstances, as first demonstrated by Kunkl and Klaus (1980). The proliferative response of B cells to anti-immunoglobulin is very susceptible to cyclosporin (Dongworth and Klaus 1982; Klaus 1988), whereas the response to lipopolysaccharide (LPS) is unaffected (Borel *et al.* 1977; Dongworth and Klaus 1982). Similarly, the response of human B cells stimulated with anti-heavy-chain antibodies is also sensitive to cyclosporin (Muraguchi *et al.* 1983), but proliferative responses induced by *Staphylococcus cowan* and Epstein–Barr virus are relatively resistant (Tosato *et al.* 1982). The effects of IL-5 on murine B cell proliferation are also inhibited by cyclosporin (O'Garra *et al.* 1986); but it should be noted that human B cells are unresponsive to IL-5.

Cyclosporin may inhibit antigen presentation by monocytes (Palay *et al.* 1986; Snyder *et al.* 1987; Esa *et al.* 1987) and by Langhans' cells (Furue and Katz 1988). There are also tentative reports that cyclosporin reduces receptor-mediated exocytosis by basophils (Trenn *et al.* 1989; Hultsh *et al.* 1990), that is decreases surface expression of Class II major histocompatibility complex (MHC) molecules of monocytes (Groenewegen *et al.* 1985) and that it increases synthesis of prostaglandin E_2 (Whistler *et al.* 1985). Thus it is clear that cyclosporin has rather broader immunoregulatory effects than were originally supposed. Certainly, it cannot be regarded as a drug that affects T cells exclusively.

Molecular mechanisms of action

Cyclosporin probably binds to cells non-specifically, because it is lipophilic and is concentrated in the cytoplasm by binding to immunophilins. Cyclosporin binds to cyclophilin (Handschumacher *et al.* 1984; Handschumacher and Harding 1989), whereas FK506 and rapamycin both bind to FK-binding protein (FKBP) (Harding *et al.* 1989; Siekierka *et al.* 1989; reviewed by Schreiber 1991). Cyclosporin binding to cyclophilin is probably dependent on its unique amino acid (Quesniaux *et al.* 1987b; Durrette *et al.* 1988), whilst FK506 and rapamycin probably have a common binding domain characterized by the ketone carbonyl adjacent to the homopropyl bond (Rosen *et al.* 1990). The immunophilin drug complex probably mediates many of the immunosuppressive properties of these drugs, although not in a straightforward way. It now appears that the cyclosporin/cyclophilin complex binds to calcineurin, a calcium/calmodulin-dependent phosphatase B, and that this is responsible for its effects (McKeon 1991). Cyclosporin/cyclophilin complex inhibits expression of 'early genes' activated by T cell receptor ligation, including those encoding the interleukins and the proto-oncogene c-Myc. The effects are mediated by inhibition of the nuclear *trans*-activity factors, which increase cytokine gene expression (Crabtree 1989). Emmel *et al.* (1989) have shown that cyclosporin inhibits one such factor, NFAT-1, in human T cells, and Randak *et al.* (1990) have produced data implicating purine boxes (homologues of NFAT-1) in mice.

FK506 probably has the same effects as cyclosporin, albeit acting with a different immunophilin. However, the effects of rapamycin are distinct, even though it binds to FKBP. Rapamycin does not inhibit the expression of early genes by activated T cells, and may even augment them (Morris 1991). In contrast, it inhibits the effects of IL-2 binding to its receptors, a process unaffected by cyclosporin and FK506.

In summary, cyclosporin and the other drugs in this group interfere with essential steps in the transduction of signals from receptors on the surface of T cells, B cells and probably a limited range of other cell types. These steps certainly involve immunophilins and possibly other pathways as well. Additional complexity comes from the different effects of FK506 and rapamycin bound to FKBP, which suggests that the immunophilins have multiple discrete functions. It also suggests the possibility of synergy between different immunophilin-binding drugs.

Effects on immune responses *in vivo*

The effect of cyclosporin *in vivo* was originally studied by Borel and his colleagues (1977) and has recently been reviewed by Borel (1989). Early reports showed that primary antibody responses were suppressed in rodents, results subsequently confirmed by others (Homan *et al.* 1980a, b; Lindsey *et al.* 1980). Cyclosporin has less consistent effects on secondary antibody responses. Both Borel *et al.* (1977) and Homan *et al.* (1980a) reported significant suppression in rats, using plaque-forming assays and serology respectively, whereas Lindsey *et al.* (1980) found cyclosporin to have no effect on the secondary antibody response to bovine serum albumin in rabbits. It is impossible to judge from these studies whether the differences in results are due to the protocols used or to species differences.

Primary and secondary contact sensitivity and delayed hypersensitivity in rodents and guinea-pigs are suppressed by cyclosporin (Borel *et al.* 1977). These reactions have been investigated in detail by Thomson *et al.* (1983a, b), who found that the delayed hypersensitivity response to dinitrophenol (DNP) in guinea-pigs was suppressed not only when cyclosporin was given daily from immunization to skin testing 14 days later, but also when guinea-pigs were first treated just prior to rechallenge. There are striking parallels with results of experiments with cytotoxic drugs, because cyclosporin given for the 4 days after immunization also caused an augmented response to skin testing on day 14 (Thomson *et al.* 1983a, b). Taken together, these results are consistent with inhibition of lymphokine synthesis by cyclosporin when the animals were skin-tested, and possibly with some type of inactivation of regulatory mechanisms at the time of immunization. They also presage the apparently contradictory findings when cyclosporin is used to treat experimental autoimmune disease.

In man, cyclosporin in doses of 10 mg/kg/day has been reported to inhibit delayed hypersensitivity responses, whilst leaving antibody responses intact (Palastine *et al.* 1985).

Cyclosporin A and experimental autoimmunity

Cyclosporin A has been used extensively to treat experimental autoimmune disease (reviewed by Borel 1989). Unsurprisingly, cyclosporin given before antigen challenge can prevent the development of a variety of organ-specific autoimmune diseases, including experimental allergic encephalomyelitis in mice (Schuller-Levis *et al.* 1986) and rats (Borel *et al.* 1987), autoimmune uveitis in rats (Nussenblatt *et al.* 1981; Chan *et al.* 1985; Caspi *et al.* 1988), collagen-induced arthritis (Kaibara *et al.* 1984, 1985; Hom *et al.* 1988), experimental allergic glomerulonephritis (Reynolds *et al.* 1991), Heymann nephritis (a model of membranous nephropathy) (de Heer *et al.* 1985; Cattran 1988) and tubulo-interstitial nephritis (Gimenez *et al.* 1987; Shih *et al.* 1988). Cyclosporin has also been shown to suppress the development of mercuric chloride-induced autoimmune disease in Brown Norway rats (Baran *et al.* 1986; Aten *et al.* 1988) and the spontaneous development of diabetes in Bio Breeding (BB) rats (Laupacis *et al.* 1983; Like *et al.* 1984) and non-obese diabetic (NOD) mice (Mori *et al.* 1986; Formby *et al.* 1988) and of lupus syndrome in NZB/W mice (Israel-Biet *et al.* 1983; Berden *et al.* 1986). Cyclosporin has to be continuously present to be effective in each of these diseases.

Cyclosporin has also been used to treat established disease in some of these models, and the results are variable. Late treatment is effective in autoimmune encephalomyelitis (Borel *et al.* 1987), uveitis, glomerulonephritis (Aten *et al.* 1988; Reynolds *et al.* 1991) and tubulo-interstitial nephritis (Shih *et al.* 1988), but has no effect on rats with Heymann nephritis that have already developed proteinuria (Cattran 1988). These differences may reflect the continued involvement of T cells in injury in the former conditions, and that of antibody and complement in the latter. Collagen-induced arthritis has been reported to be aggravated by later treatment with cyclosporin (Kaibara *et al.* 1984), as have some models of nephritis (Wood *et al.* 1988). It is speculative whether these seemingly paradoxical responses are caused by interference with immunoregulatory circuits, effects on cytokine release, or whether they are a direct result of cyclosporin toxicity.

Toxicity of cyclosporin A

Cyclosporin A has little or no bone marrow toxicity, which remains one of its chief attractions as an immunosuppressive drug. There are, however, other worrisome toxic effects (reviewed by Kahan 1989; Mason 1989). Many patients complain of slight nausea or a bloated feelings after taking the drug; light-headedness, facial flushing and a sensation of hotness are also common. Hypertension occurs in at least 50% of patients on long-term cyclosporin (Bencini *et al.* 1986; Kahan *et al.* 1987) and is particularly troublesome in Indian Caucasoids. A high proportion of patients develop gingival hyperplasia, which can be severe enough to necessitate gingivectomy (Wysocki *et al.* 1983). Hepatotoxicity is potentially more serious and is usually signalled by an increase in hepatic enzymes. Liver biopsies show centrolobular fatty change and necrosis of hepatocytes. Prolonged use of cyclosporin is associated with increased incidence of gallstones. Nephrotoxicity is common and can be evident within the first week of treatment with cyclosporin. Early changes reflect the effect of cyclosporin on renal blood flow and are probably due to effects on glomerular filtration of cyclosporin-induced constriction of the afferent arteriole. Prolonged use of cyclosporin is associated with structural damage, with tubular interstitial fibrosis (Mihatsch *et al.* 1988). Other less common side-effects are venous thrombosis, haemolytic uraemic syndrome (Van Buren *et al.* 1985) and epileptic fits.

Effects of immunosuppressive drugs on disease

General comments

The development of concepts of autoimmune and inflammatory disease has led to the increasingly frequent use of steroids and immunosuppressive drugs, often to treat disease of uncertain aetiology and variable course. It has proved extremely difficult, using conventional controlled clinical trials, to get clear-cut answers to questions of whether steroids and, more particularly, cytotoxic drugs are beneficial in a particular disease and, if so, how to define the optimal regimen.

The ideal conditions for controlled clinical trials are: first, that a disease is not life-threatening, has a homogeneous population of patients and presents in suitable numbers; and, secondly, that it should be a disease in which easily defined endpoints develop rapidly. These conditions are almost completely satisfied in the case of frequently relapsing steroid-responsive nephrotic syndrome and, not surprisingly, controlled trials have been used to great effect in this disease.

It has proved much more difficult to document the effect of immunosuppressive drugs in other conditions by controlled trials. Some diseases, such as various types of chronic nephritis, are very slowly progressive and would necessitate trials continuing for many years before an answer was reached. Some present as life-threatening illnesses demanding immediated treatment and others, such as Crohn's disease and ulcerative colitis, run a variable course without clear-cut indices of disease activity. Many are very heterogeneous, which precludes proper matching of patients.

Another problem is the gradual onset of the therapeutic effect of some immunosuppressive drugs. For instance, the anti-inflammatory effect of azathioprine takes 3–4 weeks to develop and occurs through effects on dividing cells. On *a priori* grounds, it follows that, when azathioprine is used to treat chronic inflammatory lesions, which themselves may contain long-lived cells, study periods of at least 6 months should be used before the effects of treatment are assessed.

Difficulties also arise when applying controlled trials to clinical practice. The results of trials cannot be extrapolated beyond the protocol used. Many trials of immunosuppressive drugs have studied only a subgroup of patients with a particular disease in order to get uniform samples, and there is inevitable uncertainty about generalizing these results to the disease as a whole. Similarly, negative results from a short course of immunosuppressive drugs cannot be regarded as definitive.

Finally, even when a definite early benefit has been established, the problem of what place immunosuppressive drugs have in the treatment still arises because of their potential dangers. Marrow suppression from cytotoxic drugs should be avoidable by meticulous monitoring of dosage, but there are risks of infection, particularly from pharmacological doses of corticosteroids and the long-term usage of cytotoxic drugs. The most important of these is the increased risk of development of malignancy. The increased use of cytotoxic drugs for prolonged periods makes this danger increasingly apparent (see Boitard and Bach 1989).

Gastrointestinal disease

AUTOIMMUNE CHRONIC ACTIVE HEPATITIS

Autoimmune chronic active hepatitis is characterized by the presence of autoantibodies (for example, antinuclear, anti-smooth muscle) and hyperglobulinaemia in a patient with typical hepatitis on liver biopsy. Attempts to halt the progression of chronic active hepatitis by steroids and immunosuppressive drugs have been made for nearly 20 years (Mackay and Wood 1963), and early positive results have been confirmed by controlled trials (Cook *et al.* 1971; Soloway *et al.* 1972; Murray-Lyon *et al.* 1973; Summerskill *et al.* 1975). From these, one can conclude, first, that prednisolone significantly improves mortality in this disease and, secondly, that it can induce complete clinical and histological remissions in some patients (Baggenstoss *et al.* 1972). The optimum duration of therapy has not been defined, but is likely to be a very long time in most patients. However, a substantial proportion of patients in complete clinical and biochemical remission do not relapse in the first 6 months after stopping prednisolone (Czaja *et al.* 1980; Hegarty *et al.* 1983). Nevertheless, most patients are maintained on low-dose prednisolone, which is often combined with azathioprine as a steroid-sparing agent (Soloway *et al.* 1972; Summerskill *et al.* 1975). Azathioprine has even been used alone to control hepatitis, apparently with success (Johnson *et al.* 1988). An uncontrolled study suggested that cyclophosphamide may confer additional benefit (Naccarato *et al.* 1974).

PRIMARY BILIARY CIRRHOSIS

There appears to be little, if any, place for immunosuppressive drugs in the treatment of primary biliary cirrhosis; steroids and contra-indicated because of the osteomalacia that may complicate this condition, and two controlled trials of azathioprine 2 mg/kg over 6 years showed no benefit (Heathcote *et al.* 1976; Christiansen 1985). A controlled trial of chlorambucil showed apparent benefit (Hoofnagel *et al.* 1984), but the potential dangers of prolonged treatment with alkylating agents needs to be considered carefully.

CROHN'S DISEASE

Crohn's disease is a chronic inflammatory disease of uncertain aetiology that affects both small and large intestines. Treatment with corticosteroids was introduced in the 1960s, with enthusiastic reports of their use in acute exacerbations. A substantial placebo-controlled trial (Summers *et al.* 1979) confirmed significant improvement in symptoms during acute exacerbations when a 4-month course of prednisolone 0.25–0.75 mg/kg (depending on the severity of the disease) was compared with placebo control or with azathioprine 2.5 mg/kg. Prednisolone, however, had little or no advantage over placebo in preventing relapses when continued for a further 4 months. Similarly negative conclusions were reached by Smith *et al.* (1978) and Bergman and Krause (1976) in studies to assess the capacity of prednisolone to prevent relapse. Despite negative results from a large international controlled trial (Summers *et al.* 1979), the long-term use of azathioprine is probably beneficial in preventing relapses. There are now a large number of placebo-controlled trials to contradict this result (Rhodes *et al.* 1971; Willoughby *et al.* 1971; Klein *et al.* 1974; Watson and Bukousky 1974; Rosenberg *et al.* 1975; Present *et al.* 1980), both for acute exacerbations and for maintenance therapy (O'Donaghue *et al.* 1978; Nyman *et al.* 1985). In each of the trials lasting longer than 6 months, using 1.5 mg/kg azathioprine or an equivalent dose of 6-mercaptopurine produced a positive result, and there is now little doubt of their efficacy.

ULCERATIVE COLITIS

Oral corticosteroids were introduced as treatment for ulcerative colitis in 1950 and their efficacy was validated by controlled clinical trials (Truelove and Witts 1955) for hydrocortisone and, subsequently, for prednisolone (Lennard-Jones *et al.* 1960). An attempt by Barron *et al.* (1962) to define optimal dose schedules showed that prednisolone 40 or 60 mg/day was more effective than 20 mg. There is no difference in effect between once- and four-times-daily doses (Powell-Tuck *et al.* 1978). Whether to persist with high doses in patients with particularly severe disease before proceeding to early surgery is controversial (Kristensen *et al.* 1974).

Local treatment with steroid enemas is also effective but it is not known how much this is due to local actions and to what extent the results of absorbed drug; trials to distinguish between the possibilities have been inconclusive (Truelove 1960; Lennard-Jones *et al.* 1960). An effective treatment to prevent relapse would be a great advantage but, unfortunately, neither steroids nor azathioprine has been shown to do this (Lennard-Jones *et al.* 1965; Jewell and Truelove 1964; Caprilli *et al.* 1975; Rosenberg *et al.* 1975), although azathioprine may have a steroid-sparing effect (Rosenberg *et al.* 1975b; Kirk and Lennard-Jones 1982).

Renal disease

MINIMAL-CHANGE NEPHROTIC SYNDROME

Minimal-change nephropathy is the commonest cause of nephrotic syndrome in childhood. Minor histological changes may be seen by light microscopy and podocyte spreading by electron microscopy. The effectiveness of corticosteroids in minimal-change nephrotic syndrome was established many years ago (see Cameron 1979a), as was the effectiveness of an 8-week course of cyclophosphamide for frequently relapsing patients (Barratt and Soothill 1970). More recently, cyclosporin has also been shown to be effective treatment for both children and adults (Meyrier 1989). At present, the usual approach to minimal-change nephrotic syndrome in children is to start treatment with prednisolone 80 mg/m^2 (to a maximum of 80 mg daily) per day as a single morning dose for 4 weeks, followed by the same dose on alternate days; roughly 90% of children go into remission by 4 weeks on this regimen. Those not in remission may benefit from boluses of methylprednisolone (1 g/1.73 m^2). Relapses, which occur in about two-thirds of patients, can either be treated in the same manner as the initial attack (prednisolone 60 mg/m^2 daily for 4 weeks) or, preferably, by using lower doses for shorter periods. Cyclophosphamide is now reserved for those in whom very frequent relapses result in the patient receiving unacceptably high doses of corticosteroids. Controlled trials have established that doses of 3 mg/kg/day for 6 to 8 weeks are more effective than the same dose for 2 weeks (International Study of Kidney Disease in Children 1974). More recently, a trial of a 12-week course of cyclophosphamide 2 mg/kg/day showed it to be significantly more effective than an 8-week one (Arbeitsgemeinschaft für pädiatrische Nephrologie 1987). More prolonged treatment does not appear to improve the results further. Nor are there grounds for believing that other alkylating agents such as chlorambucil are more effective when used in equivalent dosage. Similar results with cyclophosphamide have been obtained in adults with minimal-change nephrotic syndrome and have recently been reviewed critically by Meyrier and Simon (1988). Again, it is usual to give doses of 2–3 mg/kg/day for 8–12 weeks.

Treatment with cyclosporin has emerged as

another approach to the patient needing unacceptably high doses of corticosteroids to maintain remission. Its effectiveness was first reported by Hoyer *et al*. (1986) and subsequently confirmed by others, both in children (for example, Niaudet *et al*. 1988; Tejani *et al*. 1988) and in adults (Meyrier *et al*. 1989; Favre *et al*. 1989). From these results it is clear that cyclosporin induces remission in the majority of patients with responsive nephrotic syndrome. Remissions are maintained for as long as the drug is continued, albeit at the risk of irreversible nephrotoxicity.

MEMBRANOUS NEPHROPATHY

Membranous nephropathy is the commonest cause of nephrotic syndrome in adults living in developed countries. It is associated with deposition of immunoglobulin on the subepithelial side of the glomerular basement membrane (GBM). If untreated, about 50% of patients go into spontaneous remission and 50% progress to end-stage renal failure over 15 years (Cameron 1979a; Noel *et al*. 1979). There is a lot of anecdotal evidence that corticosteroids and immunosuppressive drugs can induce remission in patients with membranous nephropathy (Hopper 1973; Lagrue *et al*. 1975; Row *et al*. 1975). Azathioprine appears ineffective (Western Canadian Glomerulonephritis Study Group 1976). Controlled trials designed to examine the value of prednisolone and of chlorambucil combined with prednisolone have now been reported.

There have been three substantial trials to examine the effects of corticosteroids alone (Collaborative Study of the Adult Nephrotic Syndrome 1979; Cameron *et al*. 1990; Cattran *et al*. 1989). Only the Collaborative Study (1979) reported that steroids were effective for treatment, and most would now regard them as being of uncertain benefit. The case for the combined use of prednisolone and chlorambucil appears to be more secure. Ponticelli *et al*. (1984; 1989) have reported highly significant and sustained benefit from a 6-month course of prednisolone (for months 1, 3 and 5) and chlorambucil (0.2 mg/kg/day) for months 2, 4 and 6. This regimen induced sustained remission in all of patients in the trial. The regimen is also effective in a proportion of patients with more severe disease (Mathieson *et al*. 1988). The case for using immunosuppressive drugs for treating membranous nephropathy has been reviewed by Mathieson and Rees (1991).

RAPIDLY PROGRESSIVE GLOMERULONEPHRITIS

Rapidly progressive glomerulonephritis is a severe renal disorder which progresses to end-stage renal failure within weeks or months if left untreated. It is characterized by a focal necrotizing glomerulonephritis and may be caused by a number of distinct diseases (discussed fully in Chapter 99). The two commonest causes are: autoimmunity to GBM (Goodpasture's syndrome); and small-vessel vasculitis associated with anti-neutrophil cytoplasmic antibodies (ANCA), even though this may appear to be confined to the kidney. Other less common causes are systemic lupus erythematosus and post-infective glomerulonephritis.

There is general agreement that high-dose steroids alone or in combination with cytotoxic drugs do nothing to alter the course of the most severely affected patients with Goodpasture's syndrome (Bierne *et al*. 1977; Briggs *et al*. 1979; reviewed by Turner and Rees 1991). However, the regimen originally described by Lockwood *et al*. (1976) provides the best approach. It combines the use of high-dose prednisolone and oral cyclophosphamide with daily whole-volume plasma exchange to remove circulating anti-GBM antibodies (see Chapter 99). The regimen has now been used with apparent benefit by a number of groups (Peters *et al*. 1982; Walker *et al*. 1985). Johnson *et al*. (1985) attempted to evaluate the use of less intensive plasma exchange in Goodpasture's syndrome in a controlled prospective trial. Unfortunately, the study was ineffective because of the small number of patients and differences between the control and plasma exchange groups. Thus the current approach to Goodpasture's syndrome should combine plasma exchange with immunosuppression for all but the least severely affected patients.

Patients with ANCA-associated rapidly progressive glomerulonephritis respond to immunosuppressive drugs in the same way as do those with clear evidence of systemic vasculitis (see below).

SYSTEMIC VASCULITIS

The considerable developments in understanding of the pathogenesis of systemic vasculitis are discussed fully in Chapter 62. It is now apparent that both Wegener's granulomatosis and microscopic polyarteritis are associated with ANCA and that both respond to steroids and cytotoxic drugs in a similar manner. Today there is a trend to treat both in a similar fashion. The use of corticosteroids was established during the 1950s for both the microscopic and the macroscopic variants of polyarteritis (Rose and Spencer 1957; Medical Research Council 1960; Frohnert and Sheps 1967), as well as for acute exacerbations of Wegener's granulomatosis (Walton 1958; Hollander and Manning 1967). Cyclophosphamide was introduced for both diseases during the 1960s and shown to be more effective, particularly as part of long term regimens to treat chronic disease (Fauci and Wolff 1973; Reza *et al.* 1975; Israel *et al.* 1977; Fauci *et al.* 1979; Lieb *et al.* 1979; Raitt 1971). The use of cyclophosphamide in these diseases has not been subjected to controlled trial, but there is abundant clinical evidence of its effectiveness; thiopurines, such as azathioprine, have a similar but less potent effect (Fauci *et al.* 1983; Savage *et al.* 1985; Ten Berge *et al.* 1985; Coward *et al.* 1986; Fuiano *et al.* 1988). The most severely affected patients are frequently treated with pulses of methylprednisolone in addition to oral corticosteroids (Bolton and Couser 1979; Oredugba *et al.* 1980; Stevens *et al.* 1983; Fuiano *et al.* 1988; Bolton and Sturgill 1989). Although uncontrolled, these reports suggest that these are additional to the patients with severe renal failure. Plasma exchange has also been used in this group of patients (Lockwood *et al.* 1977; Glockner *et al.* 1988) and shown to be beneficial to patients who are already in renal failure when treatment was started (Pusey *et al.* 1991).

Modern immunosuppressive regimens control disease acutely in most patients with ANCA-associated vasculitis. The real challenge now is long-term control of the disease with minimal toxic effects. It is clear that the traditional approach of long-term oral cyclophosphamide (1–2 mg per day) is associated with considerable toxicity, including gonadal dysfunction in men and women (Fauci *et al.* 1983), and, even more worrying, with myelodysplasia, haematological malignancies (Ten Berge *et al.* 1985; Ohyashiki *et al.* 1986) and lymphomas (Colburn *et al.* 1985; Ambrus and Fauci 1984). Various strategies have been adopted in attempts to minimize this risk. We substitute azathioprine for cyclophosphamide once disease has been controlled in the acute phase (Peters *et al.* 1982; Gaskin *et al.* 1991). Gross and his colleagues have given intravenous pulses of cyclophosphamide instead of an oral preparation (Steppat and Gross 1989; Hoffman *et al.* 1990) and Cohen Tervaert *et al.* (1990) have made use of the observation that relapses can be correlated with the ANCA titre to individualize immunosuppressive regimens in particular patients.

LUPUS NEPHRITIS

Because of the dramatic palliative effect of corticosteroids in the treatment of extrarenal manifestations of lupus, few physicians have been willing to withhold steroid therapy in patients with renal involvement. As a result, there are few data concerning the course of untreated renal lupus and, in addition, the value of steroid therapy has never been tested.

Low doses of prednisolone (0.2–0.5 mg/kg/day) control symptoms in many patients, but it is more usual in the severely affected to start prednisolone in a dose of 1 mg/kg/day. Pollak *et al.* (1964) were the first to demonstrate the effectiveness of this regimen and to demonstrate its superiority to lower doses. However, there are a considerable number of adverse effects with the prolonged use of high-dose steroids in this regimen, especially those of infection (Cohen *et al.* 1982; Rubin *et al.* 1985) and nowadays the dose is tapered rapidly to 20 mg daily by 4 weeks. Alternatively, pulses of methylprednisolone can be given at the outset in an attempt to induce a remission (Kimberley *et al.* 1983).

The use of cytotoxic drugs or adjunctive therapy is thought to be the reason why patients' disease can now be controlled with lower doses of steroids, although this has been very difficult to prove. Early trials of azathioprine (Sztejnbok *et al.* 1971; Donadio *et al.* 1972, 1974, 1978; Cade *et al.* 1973; Decker *et al.* 1975; Ginzler *et al.* 1976) and of cyclophosphamide (Steinberg *et al.* 1971; Decker *et al.* 1975; Ginzler *et al.* 1976; Donadio *et al.* 1978) failed to show any benefit from treatment, but it is clear that many of these studies were flawed in design, usually because far too few patients were treated and the types of patients studied were too heterogeneous. Even so, there was clear evidence that withdrawal of azathioprine was associated with relapse of disease activity (Sharon *et al*. 1973). Felson and Anderson (1984) undertook a meta-analysis of 8 trials of cytotoxic drugs and concluded that the use of either azathioprine or cyclophosphamide was associated with significantly less deterioration of renal function than steroids alone. This conclusion has been sustained by a very careful long-term follow-up study by Balow and his colleagues at the National Institute of Health, Bethesda (Austin *et al*. 1986). This trial shows a clear benefit of the addition of immunosuppressive drugs to steroids in the treatment of severe lupus nephritis. They compared 4 different immunosupressive regimens with steroids, namely: oral azathioprine 4 mg/kg/day; oral cyclophosphamide up to 4 mg/kg/day; combined azathioprine and cyclophosphamide, each in doses of 1 mg/kg/day; and intravenous infusions of cyclophosphamide, initially 0.75 g/m^2 body surface area. All the groups being treated with immunosuppressive drugs did better than those given prednisolone, but the difference was greatest for the group given intravenous pulses of cyclophosphamide. The effectiveness of intravenous cyclophosphamide has been confirmed by others (McCune *et al*. 1988) and its use has been reviewed by McCune and Fox (1989). What makes these results all the more impressive is that the side-effects of pulse cyclophosphamide are less than those of oral cyclophosphamide. Nevertheless, the dangers of long-term cyclophosphamide are appreciable and there is considerable uncertainty about how long the treatment should be continued, especially as excellent long-term results have been reported in patients converted from oral cyclophosphamide to azathioprine for maintenance therapy (Cameron 1979b; Ponticelli *et al*. 1987).

Our present policy is to use oral cyclophosphamide (2.3 mg/kg/day), together with high-dose prednisolone (1 mg/kg/day) for induction therapy, to reduce the dose of prednisolone to 20 mg od by 4 weeks and to convert the cyclophosphamide to azathioprine (2–3 mg/kg/day) after 2–3 months. Intravenous cyclophosphamide is reserved for patients who cannot be controlled on this regimen. Pulse methylprednisolone and plasma exchange are reserved for those with fulminant disease. Cyclosporin has not been used extensively to treat patients with systemic lupus, despite efficacy in lupus strains of mice (Israel-Biet *et al*. 1983; Berden *et al*. 1986). It has been reported to be effective occasionally (Miescher *et al*. 1987; Feutren *et al*. 1987).

Rheumatoid arthritis

Despite the fact that nearly 40 years have elapsed since corticosteroids were introduced for treatment of rheumatoid arthritis, controlled trials demonstrating the efficacy of these are not available. Thus, although it is widely recognized that the dose of prednisolone should not exceed 10 mg/day, the morbidity and the mortality of this regimen are not known.

Most physicians recognize that a small proportion of patients with rheumatoid arthritis (5–10%) develop a fulminating form characterized by aggressive vasculitis, for which immunosuppressive treatment is essential. This and the attempt to use lower doses of prednisolone in maintenance therapy have prompted investigation of cytotoxic drugs as suitable therapeutic agents.

A number of controlled trials have demonstrated the beneficial effect of azathioprine (Mason *et al*. 1969; Harris *et al*. 1971; Curry *et al*. 1974; DeSilva and Hazleman 1981; Woodland *et al*. 1981; Thompson *et al*. 1985), cyclophosphamide (Cooperative Clinics Committee of the American Rheumatism Association 1970; Urowitz *et al*. 1973; Curry *et al*. 1974; Townes *et al*. 1976; Williams *et al*. 1980) for symptomatic relief, but their role in management remains the subject of debate. More recently, methotrexate has also been shown to be beneficial in short-term double-blind controlled studies (Thomson *et al*. 1984; Anderson *et al*. 1985; Weinblatt *et al*. 1985; Williams *et al*. 1985), but the results of long-term treatment are less impressive (Kremer and Lee 1986, 1988; Weinblatt *et al*. 1988). The dilemma with each of these treatment is to weigh benefits against potential long-term risks, especially those of long-term malignancy. This is especially obvious in rheumatoid arthritis, in which a controlled study has demonstrated a four-fold excess of solid tumours and a 16-fold excess of lymphoreticular malignancies in those treated with alkylating agents (Kinlen 1985).

Constraints upon therapy

There are two important dangers to the use of long-term immunosuppression: infection and malignancy (reviewed by Boitard and Bach 1989). The risk from infection consequent upon the prolonged use of immunosuppressive agents, both in renal transplant recipients (Anderson *et al.* 1973; Rubin and Tolkoff-Rubin 1988) and in other non-neoplastic conditions (Dale and Petersdorf 1973; Cohen *et al.* 1982), has received much attention but inadequate experimental study. Basic homoeostatic mechanisms are important in host defence and are compromised by immunosuppressive agents, as discussed above, but detailed studies in experimental animals are lacking.

The other area which has received attention is the potential danger of malignancy. It is theorized that interference with the surveillance function of the immune system permits malignancy. Studies of immunosuppressed patients showed that the incidence of malignant disease was raised 100-fold over that expected in the general population (Kinlen *et al.* 1983; Penn 1987). In these and other studies (Kinlen *et al.* 1979), the frequency of lymphoma (of the non-Hodgkin's variety) was found to be disproportionately increased. More recently, the risks of bone marrow dysplasia and the development of leukaemia have become increasingly apparent (Cameron 1977; Grunwald and Rosner 1979; Sabouraud *et al.* 1983; Lhermitte *et al.* 1984; Patapanian *et al.* 1988).

The constraints to prolonged use of immunosuppressive agents have highlighted the need for careful tailoring of treatment to disease activity and reduction of dosage wherever possible. In the case of steroids, the possibility of early transfer to alternate-day regimens has received widespread support. It has been clearly demonstrated that numerous harmful side-effects can be avoided using alternate-day steroids (Harter *et al.* 1963). A further problem when treating disease affecting the immune system, however, is the difficulty attendant upon reducing drug therapy, since most of these are indolent and long-lasting processes.

References

Abdou, N.I., Zweiman, B. and Casella, S.R. (1973). Effects of azathioprine therapy on bone marrow dependent and thymus dependent cells in man. *Clin. Exp. Immunol.* **13**, 55.

Abramsky, O., Tarrab-Hazdai, R., Aharonov, A. and Fuchs, S. (1976). Immunosuppression of experimental autoimmune myasthenia gravis by hydrocortisone and azathioprine. *J. Immunol.* **117**, 225.

Aisenberg, A.C. and Davis, C. (1968). The thymus and recovery from cyclophosphamide induced tolerance to sheep erythrocytes. *J. Exp. Med.* **128**, 35.

Aisenberg, A.C. and Murray, C. (1973). Cell transfer studies in cyclophosphamide induced tolerance. *Cell. Immunol.* **7**, 143.

Alepa, F.B., Zcaifler, N.J. and Sliwinski, A.J. (1970). Immunologic effects of cyclophosphamide treatment in rheumatoid arthritis. *Arthritis Rheum.* **13**, 754.

Ambrus, J.L., Jr and Fauci, A.S. (1984). Diffuse histocytic lymphoma in a patient treated with cyclophosphamide for Wegener's granulomatosis. *Am. J. Med.* **76**, 745.

Anderson, P.A., West, S.A., O'Dell, J.R., Via, C.S., Claypool, R.G., and Kotzin, B.L. (1985). Weekly pulse methotrexate in rheumatoid arthritis. *Ann. Intern. Med.* **103**, 489.

Anderson, R.J., Shafer, L.A., Olin, D.B. and Eickhoff, T.C. (1973). Infectious risk factors in the immunosuppressed host. *Am. J. Med.* **54**, 453.

Arbeitsgemeinschaft für pädiatrische Nephrologie (1981). Alternate-day prednisone is more effective than intermittent prednisone in frequently relapsing nephrotic syndrome. *Eur. J. Pediatr.* **135**, 229.

Askenase, P.W., Hayslen, B.J. and Gershon, R.K. (1975). Augmentation of delayed type hypersensitivity by doses of cyclophosphamide which do not effect antibody responses. *J. Exp. Med.* **141**, 697.

Aten, J., Bosman, C.B., De Heer, E., Heodemaeker, P.J. and Weening, J.J. (1988). Cyclosporin A induces long term unresponsiveness in mercuric chloride-induced autoimmune glomerulonephritis. *Clin. Exp. Immunol.* **73**, 307.

Austin, H.A., Kippel, J.H., Balow, J.E. *et al.* (1986). Therapy of lupus nephritis: controlled trial of prednisone and cytotoxic drugs. *N. Engl. J. Med.* **314**, 614.

Bach, M.A. and Bach, J.-F. (1972). Activities of immunosuppressive agents *in vitro* II. Different timing of azothioprine and methotrexate inhibition and stimulation of mixed lymphocyte reaction. *Clin. Exp. Immunol.* **11**, 89.

Bach, J.-F. and Dardenne, M. (1972a). Serum immunosuppressive activity of azathioprine in normal subjects and patients with liver disease. *Proc Roy. Soc. Med.* **65**, 260.

Bach, J.-F. and Dardenne, M. (1972b). Antigen recognition by T lymphocytes. I. Thymus and bone marrow dependence of spontaneous rosette forming cells in normal and neonatally thymectomised mice. *Cell. Immunol.* **3**, 1.

Bach, J.-F. and Strom, T. (1985). *The Mode of Action of Immunosuppressive Agents*, 2nd edn. North-Holland, Amsterdam.

Baggenstoss, A.H., Soloway, R.D. and Summerskill, W.H.J. (1972). Chronic active liver disease: the range of histological lesions, their response to treatment and evaluation. *Hum. Pathol.* **3**, 183.

Bagley, C.M., Bostick, F.W. and De Vita, V.T. (1973). Clinical pharmacology of cyclophosphamide. *Cancer Res.* **33**, 226.

Balis, F.M., Holcenberg, J.S. and Bleyer, M.A. (1983). Clinical pharmacokinetics of commonly used anti-cancer drugs. *Clin. Pharmacokinetics* **8**, 202.

Ballard, P.L. (1979). Delivery and transport of glucocorticoids to target cells. In: *Glucocorticoid Hormone Action*, ed. J.D. Baxter and G.G. Rousseau, p. 25, Springer-Verlag, New York.

Balow, J.E. and Rosenthal, A.S. (1973). Glucocorticoid suppression of macrophage migration inhibition factor. *J. Exp. Med.* **137**, 1031.

Balow, J.E., Hunninghake, G. and Fauci, A.S. (1977). Corticosteroids in human lymphocyte mediated cytotoxic reactions. *Transplantation* **23**, 322.

Baran, D., Vendeville, B., Vial, M.C. *et al.* (1986). Effect of cyclosporin A on mercury-induced autoimmune glomerulonephritis in the Brown Norway rat. *Clin. Nephrol.* **25**, 175.

Baron, J.H., Connell, A.M., Kanaghinis, T.G., Lennard-Jones, J.E. and Jones, F.A. (1962). Outpatient treatment of ulcerative colitis: comparison between 3 doses of oral prednisolone. *Br. Med. J.* **2**, 441.

Barratt, T.M. and Soothill, J.F. (1970). Controlled trial of cyclophosphamide in steroid sensitive nephrotic syndrome of childhood. *Lancet* **ii**, 479.

Barratt, T.M., Cameron, J.S., Chantler, C., Ogg, C.S. and Soothill, J.F. (1974). Comparative trial of 2 weeks and 8 weeks cyclophosphamide in steroid sensitive relapsing nephrotic syndrome of childhood. *Arch. Dis. Child.* **48**, 286.

Bast, R.C., Reinherz, E.L., Maver, C., Lavin, P. and Schlossman, S.F. (1983). Contrasting effects of cyclophosphamide and prednisolone on the phenotype of human peripheral blood leucocytes. *Clin. Immunol. Immunopathol.* **28**, 101.

Baxter, J.D. and Forsham, P.H. (1972). Tissue effect of glucocorticoids. *Am. J. Med.* **53**, 573.

Baxter, J.D. and Funder J.W. (1979). Hormone receptors. *N. Engl. J. Med.* **301**, 1149.

Bencini, P.L., Montagnino, G., Sala, F., De Vecchi, A., Crosti, C. and Tarrantino, A. (1986). Cutaneous lesions in 67 cyclosporin-treated renal transplant recipients. *Dermatologica* **172**, 30.

Berden, J.H.M., Faaber, P., Assmann, K.J.H. and Rijke, T.P.M. (1986). Effects of cyclosporin A on autoimmune disease in MRL/lpr and BXSB mice. *Scand. J. Immunol.* **24**, 405.

Berenbaum, M.C. (1975). The clinical pharmacology of immunosuppressive agents. In: *Clinical Aspects of Immunology*, ed. P.G.J. Gell, R.R.A. Coombs and P.J. Lachmann, p. 689, Blackwell Scientific Publications, Oxford.

Bergman, L. and Krause, G. (1976). Postoperative treatment with corticosteroids and salazosulphapridine (salazopyrin) after radical resection for Crohn's disease. *Scand. J. Gastroenterol.* **11**, 651.

Beutler, B., Krochin, N., Milsark, I., Luedke, C. and Cerami A. (1986). Control of cachectin (tumour necrosis factor) synthesis: mechanisms of endotoxin resistance. *Science* **232**, 977.

Bierne, G.J., Wagnild, J.P., Zimmerman, S.W., Macken, P.D. and Burkholder, P.M. (1977). Idiopathic crescentic nephritis. *Medicine (Baltimore)* **56**, 349.

Boitard, C. and Bach, J.-F. (1989). Long-term complications of conventional immunosuppressive treatment. *Adv. Nephrol.* **18**, 335.

Boll, I., Klimas, J. and Willigeroot, B. (1971). Die Wirkung von 6-Mercaptopurin und Azathioprin auf menschlichen Knochenmark *in vitro*. *Arzneimittelforschung* **21**, 502.

Bolton, W.K. and Couser, W.G. (1979). Intravenous pulse methyl prednisolone therapy of acute crescentic rapidly progressive glomerulonephritis. *Am. J. Med.* **66**, 495.

Bolton, W.K. and Sturgill, B.C. (1989). Methylprednisolone therapy for acute crescentic rapidly progressive glomerulonephritis. *Am. J. Nephrol.* **9**, 368.

Borel, J.F. (1989). Pharmacology of cyclosporine (Sandimmune): pharmacological properties *in vivo*. *Pharmacol. Rev.* **41**, 259.

Borel, J.F. and Weisinger, D. (1977). Effects of cyclosporin A in murine lymphoid cells. In *Regulatory Mechanisms in Lymphocyte Activation: Proceedings of the 11th Leucocyte Culture Conference*, p. 716, Academic Press, New York.

Borel, J.F., Feurer, C., Gubler, M.U. and Stahelin, H. (1976). Biological effects of cyclosporine A: a new antilymphocyte agent. *Agents Actions* **6**, 468.

Borel, J.F., Feurer, C., Magnee, C. and Stahelin, H. (1977). Effects of the new antilymphocyte peptide cyclosporin A in animals. *Immunology* **32**, 1017.

Borel, J.F., Weisinger, D. and Gubler, H.U. (1987). Effects of the antilymphocytic agent cyclosporin A in chronic inflammation. *Eur. J. Rheumatol. Inflamm.* **1**, 237.

Bramwell, V., Calvert, R.T., Edwards, G., Scarffe, H. and Crowther, D. (1979). Disposition of cyclophosphamide in a group of myeloma patients. *Cancer Chemother. Pharmacol.* **3**, 253.

Bray, R., Abrams, S. and Brahmi, Z. (1983). Studies of the mechanism of human natural killer cell-mediated cytolysis. *Cell. Immunol.* **78**, 100.

Briggs, W.A., Johnson, J.P., Teichman, S., Yeager, H.C. and Wilson, C.B. (1979). Antiglomerular basement membrane antibody-mediated glomerulonephritis and Goodpasture's syndrome. *Medicine (Baltimore)* **58**, 348.

Brock, N. and Hohorst, H.J. (1963). Uber di Activierung von Cyclophosphamid *in vivo* und *in vitro*. *Arzneimittelforschung* **13**, 1021.

Brock, N., Gross, R., Hohorst, H.J., Klein, H.D. and Schneider, B. (1971). Activation of cyclophosphamide in man and animals. *Cancer* **27**, 1512.

Brock, N., Stekar, J., Pohe, J., Niemeyer, U. and Scheffer, G. (1979). Acrolein, the causative factor of urotoxic side effects of cyclophosphamide. *Arzneimittelforschung* **29**, 659.

Brody, G.L., Jones, J.W. and Haines, R.F. (1965). Influence of cyclophosphamide on homograft rejection. *JAMA* **191**, 297.

Brown, T.G., Ahmed, A., Filo, R.S., Knudsen, R.C. and Sell, K.W. (1976). The immunosuppression mechanism of azathioprine. *Transplantation* **21**, 27.

Buchanan, J.D., Fainley, K.F. and Barrie, J.U. (1975). Return of spermatogenesis after stopping cyclophosphamide therapy. *Lancet* **ii**, 156.

Buhles, W.C. and Shifrine, M. (1977). Effects of cyclophosphamide on macrophage numbers, functions and progenitor cells. *J. Reticuloendothelial Soc.* **21**, 285.

Butler, W.T. and Rossen, R.D. (1973). Effects of corticosteroids on immunity in man. I. Decreased serum IgG concentration caused by 3 or 5 days of high dose methyl prednisolone. *J. Clin. Invest.* **52**, 2629.

Butler, W.T., Couch, R.B., Rossen, R.D. and Hersh, E.M. (1974). Methyl prednisolone fails to inhibit primary and secondary antibody responses but causes marked suppression of ongoing antibody formation in man. *J. Clin. Invest.* **53**, 14A.

Cade, R., Spooner, G., Schlein, E. *et al.* (1973). Comparison of azathioprine, prednisone and heparin alone or combined in treating lupus nephritis. *Nephron* **10**, 37.

Calne, R.Y. (1960). The rejection of renal homografts: inhibition in dogs by 6 mercaptopurine. *Lancet* **i**, 417.

Calne, R.Y., Alexandre, G.P.J. and Murray, J.E. (1962). A study of the effects of drugs in prolonging survival of homologous renal transplants in dogs. *Ann. NY Acad. Sci.* **99**, 743.

Cameron, J.S. (1977). Chlorambucil and leukemia. *N. Engl. J. Med.* **296**, 1065.

Cameron, J.S. (1979a). The natural history of glomerulonephritis. In *Renal Disease*, ed. D.A.J. Black and N.F. Jones, p. 329, Blackwell Scientific Publications, Oxford.

Cameron, J.S. (1979b). Systemic lupus with nephritis: a long-term study. *Quart. J. Med.* **48**, 1.

Cameron, J.S., Healy, M.J.R. and Adu, D. (1990). The Medical Research Council trial of short-term high dose alternate day prednisolone in idiopathic membranous nephropathy with nephrotic syndrome in adults. *Quart. J. Med.* **274**, 133.

Campbell, A.C., Skinner, J.M., Hensey, P., Roberts-Thomson, P., MacLennan, I.C.M. and Truelove, S.C. (1974). Immunosuppression in the treatment of inflammatory bowel disease. I. Changes in lymphoid sub-populations in the blood and rectal mucosa following cessation of treatment with azathioprine. *Clin. Exp. Immunol.* **16**, 521.

Campbell, A.C., Skinner, J.M., MacLennan, I.C.M. *et al.* (1976). Immunosuppression in the treatment of inflammatory bowel disease. II. The effects of azathioprine on lymphoid cell populations in a double blind trial in ulcerative colitis. *Clin. Exp. Immunol.* **24**, 249.

Caprilli, R., Carrata, R. and Babbini, M.A. (1975). A double blind comparison of the effectiveness of azathioprine and sulphasalazine in idiopathic proctocolitis. *Am. J. Dig. Dis.* **20**, 115.

Carter, M.E. and James, V.H.T. (1970). Pituitary-adrenal response to surgical stress in patients receiving corticotrophin treatment. *Lancet* **i**, 328.

Casey, T.P. (1968a). Immunosuppression by cyclophosphamide in NZB.MZW mice with lupus nephritis. *Blood* **32**, 436.

Casey, T.P. (1968b). Azathioprine (imuran) administration and the development of lymphomas in NXB mice. *Clin. Exp. Immunol.* **3**, 305.

Caspi, R.R., McAllister, C.G., Gery, I. and Nussenblatt, R.B. (1988). Differential effects of cyclosporin A and G on functional activation of a T-helper-lymphocyte line mediating experimental autoimmune uveoretinitis. *Cell. Immunol.* **113**, 350.

Cattran, D.C. (1988). Effects of cyclosporin on active Heymann nephritis. *Nephron* **48**, 142.

Cattran, D.C., Delmore, T., Roscoe, J. *et al.* (1989). A randomized controlled trial of prednisone in patients with idiopathic membranous nephropathy. *N. Engl. J. Med.* **320**, 210.

Chalmers, A.M., Knight, P.R. and Atkinson, M.R. (1967). Conversion of azathioprine into mercaptopurine and mercaptomidazole derivatives *in vitro* during immunosuppressive therapy. *Aust. J. Exp. Biol. Med. Sci.* **45**, 681.

Chalmers, A.M., Knight, P.R. and Atkinson, M.R. (1969). 6 thiopurines as substrates and inhibitors of purine oxidase: a pathway for conversion of azathioprine into 6-thiouric acid without release of 6 mercaptopurine. *Aust. J. Exp. Biol. Med. Sci.* **47**, 263.

Chan, C.C., Mochizuki, M., Palestine, A., Benezra, D., Gergy, I. and Nussenblatt, R.B. (1985). Kinetics of T-lymphocyte subsets in the eyes of Lewis rats with experimental autoimmune uveitis. *Cell. Immunol.* **96**, 430.

Chanmougan, D. and Schwartz, R.S. (1966). Enhancement of antibody synthesis by 6 mercaptopurine. *J. Exp. Med.* **124**, 363.

Chatenoud, L., Chkofpl, N., Kreis, H. and Bach, J.-F. (1983). Interest in and limitations of monoclonal anti-T cell antibodies for follow up of renal transplant patients. *Transplantation* **36**, 45.

Cheema, A., Henson, J.B. and Gorham, J.R. (1972). Aleutian disease of mink: prevention of lesions by immunosuppression. *Am. J. Pathol.* **66**, 543.

Chiorazzi, N., Fox, D.A. and Katz, D.H. (1976). Hapten specific IgE antibody production by low doses of X-irradiation and by cyclophosphamide. *J. Immunol.* **117**, 1624.

Christians, U., Zimmer, K.O., Wonigeit, K., Maurer, G. and Sewing, K.F. (1988). Liquid-chromatographic measurement of cyclosporin A and its metabolites in blood, bile and urine. *Clin. Chem.* **34**, 34.

Christiansen, E., Neuberger, E., Crowe, J. *et al.* (1985). Beneficial effects of azathioprine and prediction and prognosis in primary biliary cirrhosis. *Gastroenterology* **89**, 1084.

Claesson, M.H. and Ropke, C. (1983). Colony formation by subpopulations of T lymphocytes IV inhibitory effect of hydrocortisone on human and murine T cell subsets. *Clin. Exp. Immunol.* **54**, 554–60.

Claman, H.N. (1972). Corticosteroid and lymphoid cells. *N. Engl. J. Med.* **287**, 388.

Clarke, J.R., Gagnon, R.F., Gotch, F.M. *et al.* (1977). The effect of prednisolone on leucocyte function in man. *Clin. Exp. Immunol.* **28**, 292.

Clements, P.J. and Levy, J. (1977). Relative cell size of lymphocyte populations: the effect of immunosuppressive therapy. *Clin. Immunol. Immunopathol.* **7**, 69.

Clements, P.J., Yu, D.T.Y., Levy, J., Paulus, H.E. and Barnett, E.V. (1974). Effects of cyclophosphamide on B and T lymphocytes in rheumatoid arthritis *Arthritis Rheum.* **17**, 347.

Coburg, A.J., Gray, S.J., Katz, F.H., Penn, L., Halgrimson, C. and Starzl, T.E. (1970). Disappearance rates and immunosuppression of intermittent intravenously administered prednisolone in rabbits and human beings. *Surg. Gynecol. Obstet.* **131**, 933.

Coffey, J.J., White, C.A., Lesk, A.B., Rogers, W.I. and Serpick, A.A. (1972). Effect of allopurinol on the pharmacokinetics of 6 mercaptopurine (NSC-755) in cancer patients. *Cancer Res.* **32**, 1283.

Cohen, J., Pinching, A.J., Rees, A.J. and Peters, D.K. (1982). Infection and immunosuppression: a study of the infective complications in 75 patients with immunologically mediated disease. *Quart. J. Med.* **51**, 1.

Cohen Tervaert, J.W. *et al.* (1990). Autoantibodies against myeloid lysosomal enzymes in crescentic glomerulonephritis. *Kidney Int.* **37**, 799.

Colburn, W.A. and Buller, R.H. (1973). Radioimmunoassay for prednisolone. *Steroids* **21**, 833.

Colburn, K.K., Cao, K.D., Krick, E.H., Mortensen, S.E. and Wong, L.G. (1985). Hodgkins lymphoma in a patient treated for Wegeners granulomatosis with cyclophosphamide and azathioprine. *J. Rheumatol.* **12**, 599.

Collaborative Study of the Adult Nephrotic Syndrome (1979). A controlled study of short term prednisone treatment in adults with membranous nephropathy. *N. Engl. J. Med.* **301**, 1301.

Connors, T.A., Grover, P.L. and McLoughlin, A.M. (1970). Microsomal activation of cyclophosphamide *in vivo*. *Biochem. Pharmacol* **19**, 1533.

Connors, T.A., Cox, P.J., Farmer, P.B., Foster, A.B. and Jarman, M. (1974). Some studies of active intermediates formed in the microsomal metabolism of cyclophosphamide and isophosphamide. *Biochem. Pharmacol.* **23**, 115.

Cook, G.C., Mulligan, R. and Sherlock, S. (1971). Controlled prospective trial of corticosteroid therapy inactive chronic hepatitis. *Quart. J. Med.* **40**, 159.

Cooper, D.A., Duckett, M., Hansen, P., Petts, V. and Rennie, R.

(1981). Glucocorticoid enhancement of immunoglobulin synthesis by pokeweed nitrogen-stimulated human lymphocytes. *Clin. Exp. Immunol.* **44**, 129.

Cooperative Clinics Committee of the American Rheumatism Association (1970). A controlled trial of cyclophosphamide in rheumatoid arthritis. *N. Engl. J. Med.* **283**, 883.

Coward, R.A., Hamdy, N.A.T., Shortland, J.S. and Brown, C.B. (1986). Renal micropolyarteritis: a treatable condition. *Nephrol. Dialysis Transplant.* **1**, 31.

Cox, P.J. (1979). Cyclophosphamide cystitis: Identification of acrolein as the causative agent. *Biochem. Pharmacol* **28**, 2045.

Crabtree, G.R. (1989). Contigent genetic regulatory events in T-lymphocyte activation. *Science* **243**, 355.

Crabtree, G.R., Munck, A. and Smith, K.A. (1980). Glucocorticoids and lymphocytes, II. Cell cycle dependent changes in glucocorticoid receptor content. *J. Immunol.* **125**, 13.

Craddock, C.G. (1978). Corticosteroid induced lymphopenia, immunosuppression and body defence. *Ann. Intern. Med.* **88**, 564.

Cupps, T.R. and Fauci, A.S. (1982). Corticosteroid-mediated immunoregulation in man. *Immunol. Rev.* **65**, 133.

Cupps, T.R., Edgar, L.C. and Fauci, A.S. (1982). Suppression of human B-lymphocyte activation by cyclophosphamide. *J. Immunol.* **128**, 2453.

Cupps, T.R., Edgar, L.C., Thomas, C.A. and Fauci, A.S. (1984). Multiple mechanisms of B cell immunoregulation in man after administration of *in vivo* corticosteroids. *J. Immunol.* **132**, 170.

Cupps, T.R., Gerrard, T.L., Falkoff, R.J.M., Whalen, G. and Fauci, A.S. (1985). Effects of *in vitro* corticosteroids on B cell activation, proliferation and differentiation. *J. Clin. Invest.* **75**, 754.

Curry, H.L.F. (1971). A comparison of immunosuppressive and anti-inflammatory agents in the rat. *Clin. Exp. Immunol.* **9**, 879.

Curry, H.L.F., Harris, J., Mason, R.M. *et al.* (1974). Comparison of azathioprine cyclophosphamide and gold in treatment of rheumatoid arthritis. *Br. Med. J.* **iii**, 763.

Curtis, J.E., Sharp, J.Y., Lidsky, M.D. and Hersch, E.M. (1973). Immune response of patients with rheumatoid arthritis during cyclophosphamide treatment. *Arthritis Rheum.* **16**, 34.

Czaja, A.J., Ammonh, V. and Summerskill, W.H.J. (1980). Clinical features and prognosis of severe chronic active liver disease (CALD) after corticosteroid induced remission. *Gastroenterology* **78**, 518.

Dale, D.C. and Petersdorf, R.G. (1973). Corticosteroids and infectious diseases. *Med. Clin. North Am.* **57**, 1277.

Dale, D.C., Fauci, A.S. and Wolff, S.M. (1974). Alternate day prednisone: leucocyte kinetics and susceptibility to infection. *N. Engl. J. Med.* **291**, 1154.

Dale, D.C., Fauci, A.S., Guerry, D. and Wolff, S.M. (1975). Comparison of agents producing a neutrophil leucocytosis in man: hydrocortisone, prednisone, endotoxin and etiocholanolone. *J. Clin. Invest.* **56**, 808.

Debre, P., Waltenbaugh, C., Dorf, M.E. and Benacerraf, B. (1976). Genetic control of specific immune suppression. IV. Responsiveness to the random copolymers L glutamic acid^{50}–L tyrosine^{50}. *J. Exp. Med.* **144**, 277.

Decker, J.L., Klippel, J.H., Plotz, P.H. and Steinberg, A.D. (1975). Cyclophosphamide or azathioprine in lupus glomerulonephritis: a controlled trial: results at 28 months. *Ann. Intern. Med.* **83**, 606.

de Heer, E., Daha, M.R., and Van Es, L.A. (1985). The autoimmune response in active Heymann's nephritis in Lewis rats in regulated by T-lymphocyte subsets. *Cell. Immunol.* **92**, 254.

de Lacerda, L. Kowarski, A. and Migeon, C.J. (1973). Integrated concentration and diurnal variation of plasma cortisol. *J. Clin. Endocrinol. Metab.* **36**, 227.

Denman, E.J., Denman, A.M., Greenwood, B.M., Gall, D. and Heath, R.B. (1970). Failure of cytotoxic drugs to suppress immune reponse of patients with rheumatoid arthritis. *Ann. Rheum. Dis.* **29**, 220.

Descamps, B., Gagnon, R., Van der Gaag, R., Meyer, O. and Cronei, J. (1977). Influence of azathioprine and prednisolone *in vivo* treatment on lymphocyte dependent antibody mediated cytotoxicity (LDAC) in 57 renal allograft recipients. *Transplant. Proc.* **9**, 981.

DeSilva, M. and Hazleman, B.L. (1981). Long term azathioprine in rheumatoid arthritis: a double blind study. *Ann. Rheum. Dis.* **40**, 560.

Diamentsen, T., Willinger, E. and Reimann, J. (1979). T suppressor cells sensitive to cyclophosphamide and its *in vitro* active derivatives 4-hydrophenoxy-cyclophosphamide control the mitogenic response of immune B splenic B cells to dextran sulphate: a direct proof of different sensitivities of lymphocyte subsets to cyclophosphamide. *J. Exp. Med.* **150**, 1571.

Dimitriu, A. and Fauci, A.S. (1978). Activation of human B lymphocytes. XI. Differential effects of azathioprine on B lymphocytes and lymphocyte subpopulations regulating B cell function. *J. Immunol.* **121**, 2335.

D'Incalci, M., Bolis, G., Facchinetti, T. *et al.* (1979). Decreased half life of cyclophosphamide in patients under control treatment. *Eur. J. Cancer* **15**, 7.

di Padova, F.E. (1989). Pharmacology of cyclosporine (Sandimmune): pharmacological effects on immune function: *in vitro* studies. *Pharmacol. Rev.* **41**, 373.

Distelhorst, C.W., Benutto, B.M. and Berganini, R.A. (1984). Effect of cell cycle position as dexamethasone binding by mouse and human lymphoid cell lines: correlation between an increase in dexamethasone binding during S phase and dexamethasone sensitivity. *Blood* **63**, 105.

Donadio, J.V., Holley, K.E., Wagoner, R.D., Ferguson, R.H. and McDuffie, F.C. (1972). Treatment of lupus nephritis with prednisolone and combined prednisolone and azathioprine. *Ann. Intern. Med.* **77**, 829.

Donadio, J.V., Holley, K.E., Wagoner, R.D., Ferguson, R.H. and McDuffie, F.C. (1974). Further observations on the treatment of lupus nephritis with prednisolone and combined prednisolone and azathioprine. *Arthritis Rheum.* **17**, 573.

Donadio, J.V., Holley, K.E., Ferguson, R.H. and Ilstrup, D.M. (1978). Treatment of diffuse proliferative lupus nephritis with prednisolone and combined prednisolone and cyclophosphamide. *N. Engl. J. Med.* **299**, 1151.

Dongworth, D.W. and Klaus, G.G.B. (1982). Effects of cyclosporin A on the immune system of the mouse. I. Evidence for a direct selective effect of cyclosporin A on B cells responding to anti-immunoglobulin antibodies. *Eur. J. Immunol.* **12**, 1018.

Dontasch, P. and Ryffel, B. (1986). Pharmacokinetics of cyclosporine in toxical studies. *Transplant. Proc.* **18**, 71.

Dougherty, T.F., Berliner, M.L., Schneebeli, G.L. and Berliner, D.L. (1964). Hormonal control of lymphatic structure and function. *Ann. NY Acad. Sci.* **113**, 825.

Drössler, K., Klima, F. and Ambrosius, H. (1981). Influence of cyclophosphamide and 6-mercaptopurine on Ig1 and Ig2 immune responses in guinea-pigs. *Immunology* **44**, 61.

Duclos, H., Galandaud, P., Devinsky, O., Maillot, M.-C. and Dormonst, J. (1977). Enhancing effect of low dose cyclophosphamide treatment on the *in vitro* antibody response. *Eur. J. Immunol.* **7**, 679.

Dunsley, E.H., Zweiman, B., Fischler, E. and Levy, D.A. (1979). Early effects of corticosteroids on basophils, leucocyte histamine and tissue histamine. *J. Allergy Clin. Immunol.* **63**, 426.

Durette, P.L., Boger, J., Dumont, F. *et al.* (1988). A study of the correlation between cyclophilin binding and *in vitro* immunosuppressant activity of cyclosporin A and analogous. *Transplant. Proc.* **20** (suppl. 2). 51.

Elion, G.B. (1972). Significance of azathioprine metabolites. *Proc. Roy. Soc. Med.* **65**, 257.

Elion, G.B. and Hitchings, G.H. (1975). Azathioprine Ch 48 in antineoplastic and immunosuppressive agents. In *Handbook of Experimental Pharmacology (N.S.)*, vol. 38, pt 2, ed. A.C. Sartorelli and D.G. Johns, Springer-Verlag, Berlin.

Elliot, J.F., Lin, Y., Mizel, S.B., Bleackley, R.C., Harnish, D.G. and Paetkau, V. (1984). Induction of interleukin 2 messenger RNA inhibited by cyclosporin A. *Science* **226**, 1439.

Ellis, T.H., Lee, H.M. and Mohanakumar, T. (1981). Alterations in human regulatory T lymphocyte sub-populations after renal allografting. *J. Immunol.* **127**, 2199.

Emmel, E.A., Verweij, C.L., Durand, D.B., Higgins, K.M., Lacy, E. and Crabtree, G.R. (1989). Cyclosporin A specifically inhibits functions of nuclear proteins involved in T cell activation. *Science* **246**, 1617.

Epstein, W.L. and Maibach, H.I. (1965). Immunologic competence of patients with psoriasis recieving cytotoxic drug therapy. *Arch. Dermatol.* **91**, 599.

Esa, A.H., Converse, P.J. and Hess, A.D. (1987). Cyclosporine inhibits soluble antigen and alloantigen presentation by human monocytes *in vitro*. *Int. J. Immunopharmacol.* **9**, 893.

Espevik, T., Figari, I.S., Refaat Shalaby, R. *et al.* (1987). Inhibition of cytokines production by cylosporin A and transforming growth factors β *J. Exp. Med.* **166**, 571.

Faber, O.K., Mouridsen, H.T. and Skovsted, L. (1974). The biotransformation of cyclophosphamide in man: influence of prednisone. *Acta Pharmacol. Toxicol.* **35**, 195.

Faccinetti, T., D'Incalci, M., Martelli, G., Cantoni, L., Belveldere, G. and Salmona, M. (1978). Simple and sensitive method of the determination of cyclophosphamide by means of a nitrogen–phosphorus selective detector. *J. Chromatog.* **145**, 315.

Fairley, K.F., Barrie, J.A. and Johnson, W. (1972). Sterility and testicular atrophy related to cyclophosphamide therapy. *Lancet* **i**, 568.

Fauci, A.S. (1975). Mechanisms of corticosteroid on lymphocyte subpopulation. I. Redistribution of circulating T and B lymphocytes to the bone marrow. *Immunology* **28**, 669.

Fauci, A.S. and Dale, D.C. (1974). The effect of *in vitro* hydrocortisone on subpopulations of human lymphocytes. *J. Clin. Invest.* **53**, 240.

Fauci, A.S. and Dale, D.C. (1975a). The effect of hydrocortisone on the kinetics of normal human lymphocytes. *Blood* **46**, 235.

Fauci, A.S. and Dale, D.C. (1975b). Alternate day prednisone therapy and human lymphocyte subpopulations. *J. Clin. Invest.* **55**, 22.

Fauci, A.S. and Wolf, S.M. (1973). Wegener's granulomatosis: studies in eighteen patients and a review of the literature. *Medicine (Baltimore)* **52**, 535.

Fauci, A.S., Dale, D.C. and Wolf, S.M. (1974). Cyclophosphamide and lymphocyte subpopulations in Wegener's granulomatosis. *Arthritis Rheum.* **17**, 355.

Fauci, A.S., Dale, D.C. and Balow, J.E. (1976). Corticosteroid therapy: mechanism of action and clinical considerations. *Ann. Int. Med.* **84**, 304.

Fauci, A.S., Katz, P., Haynes, B.F. and Wolf, S.M. (1979). Cyclophosphamide therapy for severe necrotising vasculitis. *N. Engl. J. Med.* **301**, 235.

Fauci, A.S., Murukami, T., Brandon, D.D., Loriaux, D.L. and Lipsett, M.B. (1980). Mechanism of corticosteroid action on lymphocyte subpopulations. VI. Lack of correlation between glucocorticosteroid receptors and the differential effects of glucocorticosteroids on T-cell subpopulations. *Cell. Immunol.* **49**, 43.

Fauci, A.S., Haynes, B.F., Katz, P. and Wolff, S.M. (1983). Wegener's granulomatosis: prospective clinical and therapeutic experience with 85 patients for 21 years. *Ann. Intern. Med.* **98**, 76.

Favre, H., Meischer, P., Huang, Y.P., Chaternat, F. and Mihatsch, M.-H. (1989). Cyclosporin in the treatment of the nephrotic syndrome. *Am. J. Nephrol.* **9** (suppl. 1), 57.

Felson, D.T. and Anderson, J. (1984). Evidence for the superiority of immunosuppressive drugs and prednisone over prednisone alone in lupus nephritis. *N. Engl. J. Med.* **311**, 1528.

Feutren, G., Querin, S., Noël, L.H. *et al.* (1987). Effects of cyclosporine in severe systemic lupus erythematosus. *J. Pediatr.* **111**, 1063.

Field, E.J. (1961). Experimental allergic encephalomyelitis. *Proc. Roy. Soc. Med.* **54**, 15.

Formby, B., Miller, N. and Peterson, C.M. (1988). Adoptive immunotherapy of diabetes in autologous nonobese diabetic mice with lymphoid cells *in vivo* exposed to cyclosporin plus interleukin 2. *Diabetes* **37**, 1305.

Freed, B.M., Rosano, T.G. and Lempert, N. (1987). *In vitro* immunosuppressive properties of cyclosporine metabolites. *Transplantation* **42**, 123.

Frey, B.M., Walker, C., Frey, F.J. and de Weck, A.L. (1984). Pharmacokinetics and pharmacodynamics of three different prednisolone: effect on circulating lymphocyte subtests and function. *J. Immunol.* **133**, 2479.

Frohnert, P.P. and Sheps, S.G. (1967). Long term follow up study of periarteritis nodosa. *Am. J. Med.* **43**, 8.

Fuiano, G., Cameron, J.S., Raftery, M., Hartley, B.H., Williams, D.G. and Ogg, C.S. (1988). Improved prognosis of renal microscopic polyarteritis in recent years. *Nephrol. Dialysis Transplant.* **3**, 383.

Furue, M. and Katz, S.I. (1988). Cyclosporin A inhibits accessory cell and antigen-presenting functions of epidermal Langhans cells. *Transplant. Proc.* **20** (suppl. 2), 87.

Galanaud, P., Crevon, M.-C. and Dormont, J. (1975). Effect of azathioprine on *in vitro* antibody response. *Clin. Exp. Immunol.* **22**, 139.

Galanaud, P., Crevon, M.-C., Errard, D., Wallon, C. and

Dormont, J. (1976). Two processes for B-cell triggering by T-independent antigens as evidenced by the effect of azathioprine. *Cell. Immunol.* **22**, 83.

Gaskin, G., Savage, C.O.S., Ryan, J.J. *et al.* (1991). Anti-neutrophil cytoplasmic antibodies and disease activity during follow-up of 70 patients with systemic vasculitis. *Nephrol. Dialysis Transplant.* **6**, 689.

Gassman, A.E. and Van Furth, R. (1975). The effect of azathioprine (in man) on the kinetics of monocyte and macrophage during the normal steady state and on acute inflammatory reaction. *Blood* **46**, 51.

Gatting, G., Cavalla, R., Sartori, M.L. *et al.* (1987). Inhibition by cortisol of human natural killer (MK) cell activity. *J. Steroid Biochem.* **26**, 49.

Gelfand, M.C. and Steinberg, A.D. (1972). Therapeutic studies in NZB/W mice. II. Relative efficiency of azathioprine, cyclophosphamide and methylprednisolone. *Arthritis Rheum.* **15**, 247.

Gimenez, A., Leyva-Cobian, F., Fierro, C., Rio, M., Bricio, T. and Mampaso, F. (1987). Effects of cyclosporin A on autoimmune tubulointerstitial nephritis in the Brown Norway rat. *Clin. Exp. Immunol.* **69**, 550.

Ginzler, E., Biamond, H., Guttadauria, M. and Kaplan, D. (1976). Prednisolone and azathioprine compared to prednisone plus low-dose azathioprine and cyclophosphamide in the treatment of diffuse lupus nephritis. *Arthritis Rheum.* **19**, 693.

Girard, M.T., Guyre, P., Fejes-Toth, A. and Munck, A. (1984). Glucocorticoids enhance the immuno-interferon-induced increase in monocyte IgG Fc receptors. *Fed. Proc.* **43**, 1434.

Glockner, W.M. *et al.* (1988). Plasma exchange and immunosupression in rapidly progressive glomerulonephritis: a controlled, multi-center study. *Clin. Nephrol.* **29**, 1.

Goodwin, J.S., Durgaprasadarao, A., Sierakowski, S. and Lianos, E.A. (1986). Mechanism of action of glucocorticoids: inhibition of T cell proliferation and interleukin-2 production is reversed by leucotriene B4. *J. Clin. Invest.* **77**, 1244.

Gordon, M.Y. and Singer, J.W. (1979). Selective effects of cyclosporin A on colony-forming lymphoid and myeloid cells in man. *Nature* **297**, 433.

Granelli-Piperino, A., Inaba, K. and Steinman, R.M. (1984). Stimulation of lymphokine release from T lymphoblasts: requirement for mRNA synthesis and inhibition by cyclosporin A. *J. Exp. Med.* **160**, 1792.

Granelli-Piperino, A., Andrus, L. and Steinman, R.M. (1986). Lymphokine and nonlymphokine mRNA levels in stimulated human T cells: kinetics, mitogen requirements, and effects of cyclosporin A. *J. Exp. Med.* **163**, 992.

Groenewegen, G., Buurman, W.A., Jeunhomme, G.M.A.A. and van der Linden (1985). Effect of cyclosporin on MHC class II antigen expression on arterial and venous endothelium *in vitro*. *Transplantation* **40**, 21.

Grossman, S. (1985). Interactions between gonadal steroids and the immune system. *Science* **227**, 257.

Grunwald, H.W. and Rosner, F. (1979). Acute leukaemia and immunosuppressive drug use: a review of patients undergoing immunosuppressive therapy for non-neoplastic disease. *Arch. Intern. Med.* **139**, 461.

Gupta, S. and Good, R.A. (1977). Subpopulations of human T lymphocytes. II. Effect of thymopoietin, corticosteroids and irradiation. *Cell. Immunol.* **34**, 10.

Guyre, P.M., Girard, M.T., Morganelli, P.M. and Manganiello, P.D. (1988). Glucocorticoid effects in the production and action of immune cytokines. *J. Steroid Biochem.* **30**, 89.

Gyte, G.M.L. and Willoughby, J.M.T. (1977). The effect of azathioprine on cell mediated immunity (CMI) to *Candida albicans* in Crohn's disease. *Clin. Exp. Immunol.* **30**, 242.

Hahn, B.H., MacDermott, R.P., Burkholder, S., Pletcher, L.S. and Beale, M.G. (1980). Immunosuppressive effect of low doses of glucocorticoids: effects on autologous and allogeneic mixed leucocyte reactions. *J. Immunol.* **124**, 2812.

Hall, N.R. and Goldstein, A.L. (1984). Endocrine regulation of host immunity: the role of steroids and thymosin. In *Immune Modulation, Agents and their Mechanisms*, ed. R.L. Fenichel and M.A. Chirigos, p. 533, *Immunology Series 25*, Marcel Dekker, New York.

Handschumacher, R.E. and Harding, M.W. (1989). Cyclophilin, a primary molecular target for cyclosporin. *Transplantation* **46**, 295.

Handschumacher, R.E., Harding, M.W., Riace, J. and Drugge, R. (1984). Cyclophilin: a specific cytosolic binding protein for cyclosporin A. *Science* **226**, 544.

Harding, M.W., Galat, A., Ueling, D.E. and Schreiber, S.L. (1989). A receptor for the immunosuppressant FK-506 is a *cis–trans* peptidyl–polyl isomerase. *Nature* **341**, 758.

Harris, J., Jessop, J.D. and Chaput de Saintonge, D.M. (1971). Further experience with azathioprine in rheumatoid arthritis. *Br. Med. J.* **iv**, 463.

Hapter, J.G., Reddy, W.J. and Thorn, G.W. (1963). Studies of intermittent corticosteroid dosage regimen. *New Engl. J. Med.* **269**, 591.

Haynes, B. and Fauci, A.S. (1978). The differential effect of *in vivo* hydrocortisone on the kinetics of subpopulations of human peripheral blood thymus derived lymphocytes. *J. Clin. Invest.* **61**, 703.

Heathcote, J., Ross, A. and Sherlock, S. (1976). A prospective controlled trial of azathioprine in primary biliary cirrhosis. *Gastroenterology* **70**, 656.

Hegarty, J.E., Nouria-Aria, K.T.N., Portmann, B., Eddleston, A.L.W.F. and Williams, R. (1983). Relapse following treatment withdrawal in patients with autoimmune chronic active hepatitis. *Hepatology* **3**, 685.

Hersh, E.M., Wong, V.G. and Freireich E.J. (1966). Inhibition of the local inflammatory response in man by antimetabolites. *Blood* **27**, 38.

Hess, A.D. and Tutschka, P.J. (1980). Effects of cyclopsorin A on human lymphocyte responsed *in vitro*. *J. Immunol.* **124**, 2601.

Hill, D.L. (1975). *A Review of Cyclophosphamide*. Charles G. Thomas, Springfield.

Hoffman, G.S., Leavitt, R.Y., Fleischer, T.A., Minor, J.R. and Fauci, A.S. (1990). Treatment of Wegener's granulomatosis with intermittent high-dose intravenous cyclophosphamide. *Am. J. Med.* **89**, 403.

Hollander, D. and Manning, R.T. (1967). The use of aklylating agents in the treatment of Wegener's granulomatosis. *Ann. Intern. Med.* **67**, 393.

Holt, D.W., Marsden, J.T. and Johnston, A. (1986). Measurement of cyclosporine: methodological problems. *Transplant. Proc.* **18**, 101.

Hom, J.T., Butler, I.D., Riedl and Bendele, A.M. (1988). The progression of the inflammation in established collagen-induced arthritis can be altered by treatments with immunological or pharmacological agents which inhibit T cell activities. *Eur. J. Immunol.* **18**, 881.

Homan, W.P., Fabre, J.W., Millard, P.R. and Morris, P.J. (1980a). Interaction of cyclosporin A with antilymphocyte serum and with enhancing serum for suppression of renal allograft rejection in the rat. *Transplantation* **29**, 219.

Homan, W.P., Fabre, J.W., Millard, P.R. and Morris, P.J. (1980b). Effect of cyclosporin A upon second-set rejection of rat renal allograft. *Transplantation* **30**, 354.

Hoofnagel, J.H., Davis, G.L., Schafer, D.F. *et al.* (1984). Randomized trial of chlorambucil for primary biliary cirrhosis. *Hepatology* **4**, 1062.

Hopper, J. (1973). Membranous glomerulonephritis. *Ann. Intern. Med.* **79**, 285.

Horwitz, D.A. (1974). Selective depletion of Ig bearing lymphocytes by cyclophosphamide in rheumatoid arthritis and systemic lupus erythematosis. *Arthritis Rheum.* **17**, 363.

Hoyer, L.W., Good, R.A. and Vondie, R.M. (1962). Experimental encephalomyelitis: the effect of 6 mercaptopurine. *J. Exp. Med.* **116**, 311.

Hoyer, P.E., Krull, F. and Brodehl, J. (1986). Cyclosporin in frequently relapsing minimal-change nephrotic syndrome. *Lancet* **ii**, 335.

Hultsh, T., Rodriguez, J.L., Kaliner, M.A. and Hohman, R.J. (1990). Cyclosporin A inhibits rat basophilic leukaemia cells and human basophils. *J. Immunol.* **144**, 2659.

Hunninghake, G.W. and Fauci, A.S. (1976). Divergent effects of cyclophosphamide administration on mononuclear killer cells: quantitative depletion of cell numbers versus qualitative suppression of functional capabilities. *J. Immunol.* **117**, 337.

Hurd, E.R. and Ziff, M. (1968). Studies in the anti-inflammatory activity of 6-mercaptopurine. *J. Exp. Med.* **128**, 785.

Husberg, B.S. (1972). Influence of cyclophosphamide on the rejection of allogeneic rat kidney transplants: an *in vitro* study of cell bound and antibody mediated immunity. *Clin. Exp. Immunol.* **10**, 697.

Ikezawa, Z. (1981). Regulation of the *in vitro* concanavalin A response of lymphocytes by cyclophosphamide sensitive cells — a possible role for cyclophosphamide sensitive regulatory cells. *J. Exp. Med.* **50**, 225.

Ilfeld, D.N., Krakauer, R.S. and Blaese, R.M. (1977). Suppression of the human autologous mixed lymphocyte reaction by physiologic concentrations of hydrocortisone. *J. Immunol.* **119**, 428.

International Study of Kidney Disease in Children (1974). Prospective controlled trial of cyclophosphamide therapy in children with the nephrotic syndrome. *Lancet* **ii**, 423.

Israel, H.L., Patchevsky, A.S. and Saldana, M.J. (1977). Wegener's granulomatosis, lymphomatoid granulomatosis and benign lymphocyte angiitis and granulomatosis of lung. *Ann. Intern. Med.* **87**, 691.

Israel-Biet, D., Noel, L.H., Bach, M.A., Dardenne, M. and Bach, J.-F. (1983). Marked reduction of DNA antibody production and glomerulopathy in thymulin (FTS-Zn) or cyclosporin A treated (NZB × NZW) F_1 mice. *Clin. Exp. Immunol.* **54**, 359.

Jardine, I., Fenselau, C., Appler, M., Kan, M.-N., Brundrett, R.B. and Colvin, M. (1978). Quantitation by gas chromatography–chemical ionisation mass spectrometry: cyclophosphamide, phosphanamide mustard, and nor-nitrogen mustard in plasma and urine of patients receiving cyclophosphamide therapy. *Cancer Res.* **38**, 408.

Jarman, N., Gilby, E.D., Foster, A.B. and Bondy, P.K. (1975). The quantitation of cyclophosphamide in human blood and urine by mass spectrometry — stable isotope dilution. *Clin. Chim. Acta.* **58**, 61.

Jeang, G., Nakoinz, I. and Ralph, P. (1986). Independent regulation of B cell inducing factor and IL-2 production by T lymphocytes, and direct and indirect promotion of immunoglobulin secretion by glucocorticoids. *Cell. Immunol.* **103**, 199.

Jewell, D.P. and Truelove, S.C. (1964). Azathioprine in ulcerative colitis: final report on a controlled therapeutic trial. *Br. Med. J.* **iv**, 627.

Johnson, J.P., Moore, J., Jr, Austin, H.A., Balow, J.E., Antonovych, T.T. and Wilson, C.D. (1985). Therapy of anti-glomerular basement membrane antibody disease: analysis of prognostic significance of clinical, pathological and treatment factors. *Medicine (Baltimore)* **64**, 219.

Johnson, J.P., McFarlane, I.G. and Williams, R. (1988). Long term follow up of patients with chronic active hepatitis maintained in remission by azathioprine alone. *Gut* **29**, 726.

Juma, F.D., Rogers, H.J., Trounce, J.R. and Bradbrook, I.D. (1978). Pharmacokinetics of intravenous cyclophosphamide in man, estimated by gas–liquid chromatography. *Cancer Chemother. Pharmacol.* **1**, 229.

Kahan, B.D. (1989). Cyclosporine. *N. Engl. J. Med.* **321**, 1725.

Kahan, B.D., Flechner, S.M., Lorber, M.I., Golden, D., Conley, S. and Van Buren, C.T. (1987). Complications of cyclosporin — prednisone immunosuppression in 402 renal allograft recipients exclusively followed at a single center from one to five years. *Transplantation* **43**, 197.

Kaibara, N., Hotokebuchi, T., Takagishi, K. *et al.* (1984). Pathogenetic differences between collagen arthritis and adjuvant arthritis. *J. Exp. Med.* **158**, 1388.

Kaibara, N., Morinaga, M., Arita, C., Hotokebuchi, T. and Takagishi, K. (1985). Serum transfer of collagen arthritis to cyclosporin-treated type, type II collagen-tolerant rats. *Clin. Immunol. Immunopathol.* **35**, 252.

Katz, P. and Fauci, A.S. (1979). Autologous and allogeneic intercellular interactions: Modulation by adherent cells irradiation and *in vitro* and *in vivo* corticosteroids. *J. Immunol.* **123**, 2270.

Katz, P., Zaytoun, A.M. and Lee, J.H. (1984). The effects of *in vivo* hydrocortisone on lymphocyte-mediated cytotoxicity *Arthritis Rheum.* **27**, 72.

Kaufman, D.B. and McIntosh, R.M. (1971). The effects of azathioprine on reticuloendothelial clearance. *Clin. Res.* **19**, 221.

Kawabe, S., Guttman, R.D., Levin, B., Merrill, J.P. and Lindquist, R.P. (1972). Renal transplantation in the inbred rat. XVII. Effect of cyclophosphamide on acute rejection and long survival of recipients. *Transplantation* **13**, 21.

Kay, J.E., Benzie, C.R. and Borghetti, A.F. (1983). Effect of cyclosporin A on lymphocyte activation by the calcium ionophore A23187. *Immunology* **50**, 441.

Keown, P.A. (1988). Optimizing cyclosporine therapy: dose, levels and monitoring. *Transplant. Proc.* **20** (suppl. 2), 382.

Kern, J.A., Lamb, R.J., Reed, J.C., Daniele, R.P. and Nowell, P.C. (1988). Dexamethasone inhibition of interleukin 1 beta production by human monocytes. *J. Clin. Invest.* **81**, 237.

Kimberly, R.P., Lockshin, M.D., Sherman, R.L., Mouradian, J.

and Saal, S. (1983). Reversible 'end-stage' lupus nephritis. *Am. J. Med.* **74**, 361.

Kinlen, L.J. (1985). Incidence of cancer in rheumatoid arthritis and other disorders after immunosuppressive treatment. *Am. J. Med.* **78** (suppl. 1A), 44.

Kinlen, L.J., Sheil, A.G.R., Peto, J. and Doll, R. (1979). Collaborative United Kingdom–Australasian study of cancer in patients treated with immunosuppressive drugs. *Br. Med. J.* **ii**, 1461.

Kinlen, L.J., Doll, R. and Peto, J. (1983). The incidence of tumours in renal transplants. *Transplant. Proc.* **15**, 1039.

Kino, T., Hatanaa, H., Miyata, S. *et al.* (1987). FK506, a novel immunosuppressant isolated from a streptomyces. II. Immunosuppressive effects of FK-506 *in vitro*. *J. Antibiotics* **40**, 1256.

Kipilman, C.T. and Smith, Y. (1979). Comparative effects of azathioprine, cyclophosphamide, and frentizole on humoral immunity in mice. *J. Immunopharmacol.* **1**, 455.

Kirk, A.P. and Lennard-Jones, J.E. (1982). Controlled trial of azathioprine in chronic ulcerative colitis. *Br. Med. J.* **284**, 1291.

Kissling, M., Speck, B. and Goselink, H. (1972). Effect of hydrocortisone on lymphocytes stimulated by phytohaemagglutinin and pokeweed mitogen. *Vox Sang.* **23**, 344.

Klaus, G.G.B. (1988). Cyclosporine-sensitive and cyclosporine-insensitive modes of B cell stimulation. *Transplantation* **46**, 11.

Klein, M., Binder, H.J., Mitchell, M., Aaronso, R. and Spiro, H. (1974). Treatment of Crohn's disease with azathioprine: a controlled evaluation. *Gastroenterology* **66**, 916.

Knapp, W., Berger, R. and Posch, B. (1982). Regulation of pokeweed mitogen-induced human B cell differentiation: effects of hydrocortisone. *Immunopharmacology* **5**, 1.

Kremer, J.M. and Lee, J.K. (1986). The safety and efficacy of the use of methotrexate in rheumatoid arthritis. *Arthritis Rheum.* **29**, 822.

Kremer, J.M. and Lee, J.L. (1988). A long term prospective study of the use of methotrexate in rheumatoid arthritis: update after a mean of 53 months. *Arthritis Rheum.* **31**, 577.

Kristensen, M., Koudahl, G., Fischerman, K. and Jarnum, S. (1974). High dose prednisolone treatment in severe ulcerative colitis. *Scand. J. Gastroenterol.* **9**, 177.

Kronke, M., Leonard, W.J., Depper, J.M. *et al.* (1984). Cyclosporin A inhibits T cell growth factor gene expression at the level of mRNA transcription. *Proc. Nat. Acad. Sci. (USA)* **81**, 5214.

Kumar, R., Biggard, J.D., McEvory, J. and McGeon, M.G. (1972). Cyclophosphamide and reproductive function. *Lancet* **i**, 1212.

Kunkl, A. and Klaus, G.G.B. (1980). Selective effects of cyclosporin A on functional B cell subsets in the mouse. *J. Immunol.* **125**, 2526.

Lancki, D.W., Kaper, B.P. and Firch, F.W. (1989). The requirements for triggering of lysis by cytolytic T lymphocyte clones. *J. Immunol.* **142**, 416.

Langrange, P.H., Mackaness, G.B. and Miller, T.E. (1974). Potentiation of T cell mediated immunity by selective suppression of antibody formation with cyclophosphamide. *J. Exp. Med.* **139**, 1529.

Laupacis, A., Stiller, C.R., Gardell, C. *et al.* (1983). Cyclosporin prevents diabetes in BB Wistar rats. *Lancet* **i**, 10.

Lavi, L.E. and Hoecenberg, J.S. (1985). A rapid and sensitive HPLC assay for 6-mercaptopurine metabolites in red blood cells. *Ann. Biochem.* **144**, 514.

Lee, K.C., Langman, R.E., Paetkan, V.H. and Diener, E. (1975). The cellular basis of cortisone induced immunosuppression of the antibody response studied by its reversal *in vitro*. *Cell Immunol.* **17**, 405.

Legrue, G., Bernard, D., Bariety, J., Druet, P. and Guenel, J. (1975). Controlled trial of chlorambucil and azathioprine in idiopathic chronic glomerulonephritis. *Kidney Int.* **8**, 274.

LeGrue, S., Friedmann, A. and Kahan, B. (1983). Binding of cyclosporine by human lymphocytes and phospholipid vesicles. *J. Immunol.* **131**, 712.

Lennard, L. (1985). Assay for 6-mercaptopurine in human plasma. *J. Chromatog.* **345**, 441.

Lennard-Jones, J.E., Longmore, A.J., Newell, A.C., Wilson, C.W.E. and Jones, F.A. (1960). Assessment of prednisolone, Salazopyrin and topical hydrocortisone hemisuccinate used on outpatient treatment for ulcerative colitis. *Gut* **1**, 217.

Lennard-Jones, J.E., Misiewicz, J.J., Connell, A.M., Baron, J.H. and Jones, A.F. (1965). Prednisone as a maintenance treatment for ulcerative colitis in remission. *Lancet* **i**, 188.

Leoni, P., Garcia, R.C. and Allison, A.C. (1978). Effects of cyclosporin A on human lymphocytes in culture. *J. Clin. Lab. Immunol.* **1**, 67.

Levi, F.A., Canon, C., Touiton, Y. *et al.* (1988). Circadian rhythms in circulating T lymphocyte subtypes and plasma testosterone, total and free cortisol in five healthy men. *Clin. Exp. Immunol.* **71**, 329.

Levin, R.J., Landy, M. and Frei, E. (1964). The effect of 6-mercaptopurine on the immune response in man. *N. Engl. J. Med.* **271**, 16.

Lhermitte, F., Marteau, R. and Roullet, E. (1984). Not so benign long-term immunosuppression in multiple sclerosis. *Lancet* **i**, 276.

Lieb, E.S., Restivo, C. and Paulus, H.E. (1979). Immunosuppressive and corticosteroid therapy of polyarteritis nodosa. *Am. J. Med.* **67**, 941.

Like, A.A., Dirodi, V., Thomas, S., Guberski, D.L. and Rossini, A.A. (1984). Prevention of diabetes mellitus in the BB/W rat with cyclosporin A. *Am. J. Pathol.* **117**, 92.

Lindsey, N.J., Harris, K.R., Norman, H.B., Smith, J.E., Lee, H.A. and Slapak, M. (1980). The effect of cyclosporin A on the primary and secondary immune responses in the rabbit. *Transplant. Proc.* **12**, 252.

Lipinsky, M., Tursz, T., Kreis, H., Finall, Y. and Amiel, J.L. (1980). Dissociation of natural killer cell activity and antibody-dependent cell-mediated cytotoxicity in kidney allograft recipients receiving high dose immunosuppressive therapy. *Transplantation* **29**, 214.

Lippman, M. and Barr, R. (1977). Glucocorticoid receptors in purified subpopulations of human peripheral blood lymphocytes. *J. Immunol.* **118**, 1977.

Lipsky, P.E., Ginsberg, W.W., Fnikelman, F.D. and Ziff, M. (1978). Control of human and lymphocyte responsiveness: enhanced suppressor T cell activity after *in vitro* incubation. *J. Immunol.* **120**, 902.

Lockwood, C.M., Rees, A.J., Pearson, R.A., Evans, D.B., Peters, D.K. and Wilson, C.B. (1976). Immunosuppression and plasma exchange in the treatment of Goodpasture's syndrome. *Lancet* **i**, 711.

Lockwood, C.M., Rees, A.J., Pinching, A.J. *et al.* (1977). Plasma exchange and immunosuppression in the treatment of fulminating immune complex nephritis. *Lancet* **i**, 63.

Loo, T.L., Luce, J.K., Sullivan, M.L. and Frei, E. (1968). Clinical pharmacologic observation on 6 mercaptopurine and 6-methylthiopurine ribonucleoside. *Clin. Pharmacol. Ther.* **9**, 180.

Losito, A., Williams, D.G., Cooke, G. and Harris, L. (1978). The effects on polymorphonuclear leucocyte function of prednisolone and azathioprine *in vivo* and prednisolone, azathioprine and 6 mercaptopurine *in vitro*. *Clin. Exp. Immunol.* **32**, 423.

Lundgren, G. (1970). *In vitro* cytotoxicity by human lymphocytes from individuals immunised against histocompatibility antigens. *Clin. Exp. Immunol.* **6**, 661.

McCune, W.J. and Fox, D.A. (1989). Intravenous cyclophosphamide therapy for severe SLE. *Rheum. Dis. Clin. North Am.* **15**, 455.

McCune, W.J., Golbus, J., Zeldes, W., Bohlke, P., Dunne, R. and Fox, D.A. (1988). Clinical and immunologic effects of monthly administration of intravenous cyclophosphamide in severe systemic lupus erythematosus. *N. Engl. J. Med.* **318**, 1423.

McGrath, B.P., Ibels, L.S., Raik E., Hargrave, M., Mahony, J.F. and Stewart, J.M. (1975). Erythroid toxicity of azathioprine *Quart. J. Med.* **44**, 57.

Mackay, I.R. and Wood, I.J. (1963). The cause and treatment of chronic active hepatitis. *Gastroenterology* **45**, 4.

Mackay, I.R., Dwyer, J.M. and Rowley, M.J. (1973). Differing effects of azathioprine and cyclophosphamide on immune responses to flagellin in man. *Arthritis Rheum.* **16**, 455.

McKeon, F. (1991). When worlds collide: Immunosuppressants meet protein phosphatases. *Cell* **66**, 823.

MacLeod, A.M. and Thomson, A.W. (1991). FK-506: an immunosuppressant for the 1990s? *Lancet* **337**, 25.

Maddocks, J.L. and Davidson, J.L. (1975). Separation and detection of picomole quantities of azathioprine metabolites. *Br. J. Clin. Pharmacol.* **2**, 359.

Maguire, H.C. and Ettore, V.L. (1967). Enhancement of dinitrochlorobenzene (DNCB) contact sensitisation by cyclophosphamide in guinea-pigs. *J. Invest. Dermatol.* **48**, 39.

Maibach, H.I. and Epstein, W.L. (1965). Immunologic responses of healthy volunteers receiving azathioprine (in man). *Int. Arch. Allergy* **27**, 102.

Manca, F., Kunkl, A. and Celada, F. (1985). Inhibition of the accessory function of immune macrophages *in vitro* by cyclosporin. *Transplantation* **39**, 644.

Mantovani, A., Luini, W., Pesi, G., Vecchi, A,. and Spreafico, F. (1978). Effect of chemotherapeutic agents on natural cell-mediated cytotoxicity in mice. *J. Nat. Cancer Inst.* **61**, 1255.

Mark, G.J., Lehimger-Zadeh, A. and Ragsdale, B.D. (1978). Cyclophosphamide pneumonitis. *Thorax* **33**, 89.

Markham, R.B., Stashak, P.W., Prescott, B., Amsbaugh, D.F. and Baker, P.J. (1978). Selective sensitivity to hydrocortisone of regulatory functions that determine the magnitude of the antibody response to type III pneumococcal polysaccharide. *J. Immunol.* **121**, 829.

Mason, J. (1989). Pharmacology of cyclosporine (Sandimmune): pathophysiology and toxicity of cyclosporine in humans and animals. *Pharmacol. Rev.* **41**, 423.

Mason, M., Curry, H.L.F., Barnes, C.G., Dunne, J.F., Hazelman, B.L. and Strickland, I.D. (1969). Azathioprine in rheumatoid arthritis. *Br. Med. J.* **i**, 420.

Mathieson, P.W. and Rees, A.J. (1991). A critical review of treatment for membranous nephropathy. *Adv. Nephrol.* **20**, 151.

Mathieson, P.W., Turner, A.N., Maidment, C.G.H., Evans, D.J. and Rees, A.J. (1988). Prednisolone and chlorambucil treatment in idiopathic membranous nephropathy with deteriorating renal function. *Lancet* **ii**, 869.

Maurer, G. and Lemaire, M. (1986). Biotransformation and distribution in blood of cyclosporine and its metabolites. *Transplant. Proc.* **18**, 25.

Medical Research Council (1960). Treatment of polyarteritis nodosa with cortisone: results after three years. *Br. Med. J.* **i**, 1399.

Mellet, L.B. (1971). Chemistry and metabolism of cyclophosphamide. In: *Workshop on the Immunosuppressive Properties of Cyclophosphamide*, ed. M.E. Vancil, p. 6, Mead Johnson Research Centre, Indianapolis.

Metcalf, S. (1984). Cyclosporin does not prevent cytoplasmic Ca^{2+} changes with lymphocyte activation. *Transplantation* **38**, 161.

Meyrier, A. (1989). Treatment of glomerular disease with cyclosporin A. *Nephrol. Dialysis Transplant.* **4**, 923.

Meyrier, A. and Simon P. (1988). Treatment of corticoresistant idiopathic nephrotic syndrome in the adult: minimal-change disease and focal-segmental glomerulosclerosis. *Adv. Nephrol.* **17**, 127.

Meyrier, A., Collaborating Group of the Société de Nephrologie (1989). Cyclosporin in the treatment of nephrosis — minimal-change disease and focal segmental glomerulosclerosis. *Am. J. Nephrol.* **9** (suppl. 1), 65.

Miescher, P.A., Favre, H., Chatelanat, F. and Mihatsch, M.J. (1987). Combined steroid–cyclosporin treatment of chronic autoimmune disease. *Klin. Wochenschr.* **65**, 727.

Mihatsch, M.J., Thiel, G. and Ryeffel, B. (1988). Histopathology of cyclosporine nephrotoxicity. *Transplant. Proc.* **20**, 759.

Miller, J.J. and Cole, L.J. (1967). Resistance of long lived lymphocytes and plasma cells in rat lymph nodes to treatment with prednisone, cyclophosphamide, 6 merceptopurine and actinomycin D. *J. Exp. Med.* **126**, 109.

Mitchell, C.G., Eddleston, A.L.W.F., Smith, M.G.M. and Williams, R. (1970). Serum immunosuppressive activity due to azathioprine and its relation to hepatic function after liver transplantation. *Lancet* **i**, 1196.

Mori, Y., Suko, M., Okudaira, H. *et al.* (1986). Preventive effects of cyclosporin on diabetes in NOD mice. *Diabetologia* **29**, 244.

Morris, R.E. (1991). Rapamycin: FK-506's fraternal twin or distant cousin? *Immunol. Today* **12**, 137.

Morrison, P.J., Bradbrook, I.D. and Rogers, H.J. (1977). Plasma prednisolone levels from enteric and non enteric coated tablets estimated by an original technique. *Br. J. Pharmacol.* **4**, 597.

Mukundraik, J., Freeman, P.A., Boyle, J.A., Reid, A.M., Diver, M.J. and Buchanan, W.W. (1968). Studies of the rise in plasma 11-hydroxycorticosteroids (11-OHCS) in corticosteroid-treated patients with rheumatoid arthritis during surgery: correlations with the functional integrity of the hypothalamo-pituitary-adrenal axis. *Quart. J. Med.* **147**, 407.

Muraguchi, A., Butler, J.L., Kehrl, J.H., Falkoff, R.J.M. and Fauci, A.S. (1983). Selective suppression of an early step in human B cell activation by cyclosporin A. *J. Exp. Med.* **158**, 690.

Murray-Lyon, I.M., Stern, R.B. and Williams, R. (1973). Controlled trial of prednisone and azathioprine in active chronic hepatitis. *Lancet* **i**, 735.

Naccarato, R., Farini, R., Chiaramonte, M., Fagiolo, U. and Sturniogl. (1974). Treatment of active chronic hepatitis with cyclophosphamide. *Postgrad. Med. J.* **50**, 16.

Nair, M.P.N. and Schwartz, S.A. (1984). 'Immunomodulatory effects of corticosteroids on natural killer and antibody dependent cellular cytotoxic activities of human lymphocytes. *J. Immunol.* **132**, 2876.

Neta, R., Winkelstein, A., Salvin, S.B. and Turk, J.L. (1977). The effect of cyclophosphamide on suppressor cells in guinea pigs. *Cell. Immunol.* **33**, 402.

Niaudet, P., Tete, M.J., Broyer, M. and Habib, R. (1988). Cyclosporin and childhood idiopathic nephrosis. *Transplant. Proc.* **20**, 265.

Noble, B., Parker, D., Scheper, R.J. and Turk, J.L. (1977). The relation between B-cell stimulation and delayed hypersensitivity: the effect of cyclophosphamide pretreatment on antibody production. *Immunology* **32**, 885.

Noel, L.H., Zanetti, M., Droz, D. and Barbanel, C. (1979). Long term prognosis idiopathic membranous glomerulonephritis: study of 116 untreated patients. *Am. J. Med.* **66**, 82.

Nogueira, J.R. and Freedman, M.A. (1972). Acute pancreatitis as a complication of immune therapy in regional enteritis. *Gastroenterology* **62**, 1040.

Nussenblatt, R.B., Rodrigues, M.M., Wacker, W.B., Cevario, S.J. and Salinas-Carmona, M.C. (1981). Cyclosporin A: inhibition of experimental autoimmune uveitis in Lewis rats. *J. Clin. Invest.* **67**, 1228.

Nyman, M., Hassan, I. and Eriksson, S. (1985). Long term immunosuppressive treatment in Crohns disease. *Scand. J. Gastroenterol.* **20**, 1197.

O'Donaghue, D.P., Dawson, A.M., Powell-Tuck, J., Brown, R.L. and Lennard-Jones, J.E. (1978). Double blind withdrawal trial of azathioprines as maintenance treatment for Crohn's disease. *Lancet* **ii**, 955.

O'Garra, A., Warren, D.J., Holman, M., Popham, A.M., Sanderson, C.J. and Klaus, G.G.B. (1986). The effects of cyclosporin on responses of murine B cells to T cell derived lymphokines. *J. Immunol.* **137**, 2220.

Ohyashiki, K., Kocova, M., Ryan, D.H., Rowe, J.M. and Sandberg, A.A. (1986). Secondary acute myeloblastic leukaemia with a Ph translocation in a treated Wegener's granulomatosis. *Cancer Genet. Cytogenet.* **19**, 331.

Old, C.W., Flannery, E.P., Grogan, T.M., Stone, W.H. and San Antonio, R.P. (1978). Azathioprine-induced pure red cell aplasia. *JAMA* **240**, 552.

Oredugba, O., Mazumdar, D.C., Meyer, J.S. and Lubowitz, H. (1980). Pulse methylprednisolone therapy in idiopathic rapidly progressive glomerulonephritis. *Ann. Intern. Med.* **92**, 504.

Orosz, C.G., Fidelus, R.K., Roopenian, D.C., Widmer, M.B., Ferguson, R.M. and Bach, F.H. (1982). Analysis of cloned T cell function. I. Dissection of cloned T cell proliferative responses using cyclosporin A. *J. Immunol.* **129**, 1865.

Orosz, C.G., Roopenian, D.C., Widmer, M.B. and Bach, F.H. (1983). Analysis of cloned T cell function. II. Differential blockade of various cloned T cell functions by cyclosporin. *Transplantation* **36**, 706.

Orson, F.M. and Auzenne, C.A. (1988). Glucocorticosteroid-induced immunoglobulin production requires intimate contact between B cells and monocytes. *Cell. Immunol.* **112**, 147.

Page, A.R., Condie, R.M. and Good, R.A. (1962). Effect of 6 mercaptopurine on inflammation. *Am. J. Pathol.* **40**, 519.

Palacios, R. and Sugawara, I. (1982). Hydrocortisone abrogates proliferations of T cells in autologous mixed lymphocyte reactions by rendering the interleukin-2 producer T cells unresponsive to interleukin-1 and unable to synthesise the T-cell growth factor. *Scand. J. Immunol.* **15**, 25.

Palastine, A.G., Roberge, F., Charous, B.L., Lane, H.C., Fauci, A.S. and Nussenblatt, R.B. (1985). The effect of cyclosporine on immunization with tetanus and keyhole limpet hemocyanin (KLH) in humans. *J. Clin. Immunol.* **5**, 115.

Palay, D.A., Cluff, C.W., Wentworth, P.A. and Zeigler, H.K. (1986). Cyclosporin inhibits macrophage-mediated antigen presentation. *J. Immunol.* **136**, 4348.

Parillo, J.E. and Fauci, A.S. (1978a). Mechanisms of corticosteroid action on lymphocyte subpopulations. III. Differential effects of dexamethasone administration on subpopulations of effector cells mediating cellular cytotoxicity in man. *Clin. Exp. Immunol.* **31**, 116.

Parillo, J.E. and Fauci, A.S. (1978b). Comparison on the effector cells in human spontaneous cell mediated and antibody dependent cytotoxicity: differential sensitivity of effector cells to *in vivo* and *in vitro* corticosteroids. *Scand. J. Immunol.* **8**, 99.

Parra, A., Santos, D., Cervantes, C., Sojo, I., Carranco, A. and Cortes-Gollegas, V. (1978). Plasma gonadotrophins and gonadal steroids in children treated by cyclophosphamide. *J. Pediatr.* **92**, 117.

Patapanian, H., Graham, S., Sambrook, P.N. (1988). The oncogenicity of chlorambucil in rheumatoid arthritis. *Br. J. Rheumatol.* **27**, 44.

Paterson, P.Y., Gerner, E.W., Steele, F.M. and Hanson, M.A. (1966). Cyclophosphamide inhibition of an autoimmune disease, allergic encephalomyelitis. *J. Clin. Invest.* **45**, 1055.

Paterson, P.Y., Drobish, D.G. and Biddick, A.S. (1971). Cyclophosphamide inhibition of experimental allergic thyroiditis and thyroid antibody production in rats. *J. Immunol.* **106**, 570.

Penn, I. (1987). Cancers following cyclosporin therapy. *Transplant. Proc.* **19**, 2211.

Penso, J., Lippe, B., Ehrlich, R. and Smith, F.G. (1974). Testicular function in prepubertal and pubertal male patients treated with cyclophosphamide for nephrotic syndrome. *J. Pediatr.* **84**, 831.

Peters, D.K., Rees, A.J., Lockwood, C.M. and Pusey, C.D. (1982). Treatment and prognosis in antibasement membrane antibody-mediated nephritis. *Transplant. Proc.* **14**, 513.

Phillips, S.M. and Zweiman, B. (1973). Mechanisms in the suppression of delayed hypersensitivity in the guinea-pig by 6 mercaptopurine. *J. Exp. Med.* **137**, 1494.

Plumpton, F.S., Besser, G.M. & Cole, P.V. (1969) Corticosteroid treatment and surgery. *Anaesthesia* **24**, 3.

Pollak, V.E., Pirani, C.L. and Schwartz, F.D. (1964). The natural history of the renal manifestations of systemic lupus erythematosus. *J. Lab. Clin. Med.* **63**, 537.

Ponticelli, C., Zucchelli, P., Imbasciati, E. *et al.* (1984). Controlled trial of methyl prednisolone and chlorambucil in idiopathic membranous nephropathy. *N. Eng. J. Med.* **310**, 946.

Ponticelli, C., Zucchelli, P., Moroni, G., Cagnoli, L., Banfi, G.

and Pasquali, S. (1987). Long-term prognosis of diffuse lupus nephritis. *Clin. Nephrol.* **28**, 263.

Ponticelli, C., Zucchelli, P., Passerini, P. *et al.* (1989). A randomized trial of methyl prednisolone and chlorambucil in idiopathic membranous nephropathy. *N. Engl. J. Med.* **320**, 8.

Poulter, L.W. and Turk, J.L. (1972). Proportional increase in the theta carrying lymphocytes in peripheral lymphoid tissue following treatment with cyclophosphamide. *Nature N. Biol.* **238**, 17.

Poulter, L.W., Bradley, N.J. and Turk, J.L. (1974). Differential effect of azathioprine on θ-antigenicity of mouse lymphocytes. *Immunology* **26**, 777.

Powell-Tuck, J., Brown, R.L. and Lennard-Jones, J.E. (1978). A comparison of oral prednisolone given as single or multiple daily doses for active protocolitis. *Scand. J. Gastroenterol.* **13**, 833.

Present, D.H., Korelitz, B.I., Wisch, N., Glass, J.L., Sochan, D.B. and Pasternack, B.S. (1980). Treatment of Crohn's disease with 6 mercaptopurine: a long term, randomised, double blind study. *N. Engl. J. Med.* **302**, 981.

Purves, E.C. (1975). Mechanisms of specific and non-specific tumour immunity after azathioprine treatment of mice. *Clin. Exp. Immunol.* **22**, 348.

Purves, E.C. and Berenbaum, M.C. (1975). Selective suppression of murine antibody-dependent cell mediated cytotoxicity by azathioprine. *Transplantation* **19**, 274.

Pusey, C.D., Rees, A.J., Evans, D.J., Peters, D.K. and Lockwood, C.M. (1991). A randomised controlled trial of plasma exchange in rapidly progressive glomerulonephritis without anti-G&M antibodies. *Kidney International* **40**, 757.

Quesniaux, V.F.J. (1989). Pharmacology of cyclosporine (Sandimmune): immunochemistry and monitoring. *Pharmacol. Rev.* **41**, 449.

Quesniaux, V.F.J., Tees, R., Schreier, M.H., Maurer, G. and Van Regenmortel, M.H.V. (1987a). Potential of monoclonal antibodies to improve therapeutic monitoring of cyclosporine. *Clin. Chem.* **33**, 32.

Quesniaux, V.F.J., Schreier, M.N., Wenger, R.M., Hiestand, P.C., Harding, M.W. and Van Regenmortel, M.H.V. (1987b). Cyclophilin binds the region of cyclosporine involved in its immunosuppressive activity. *Eur. J. Immunol.* **17**, 1359.

Raitt, J.W. (1971). Wegener's granulomatosis: treatment with cytotoxic agents and adrenocorticoids. *Ann. Intern. Med.* **74**, 344.

Randak, C., Brabletz, T., Hergenrother, M., Sobotta, I. and Serfling, E. (1990). Cyclosporin A suppresses the expression of the interleukin 2 gene by inhibiting the binding of lymphocyte-specific factors to the IL-2 enhancer. *EMBO J.* **9**, 2529.

Reams, G.B. (1963). Use of cyclophosphamide in an attempt to modify the canine renal homograft response. *Nature* **197**, 713.

Reynolds, J., Cashman, S.J., Evans, D.J. and Pusey, C.D. (1991). Cyclosporin A in the prevention and treatment of experimental autoimmune glomerulonephritis in the Brown Norway rat. *Clin. Exp. Immunol.* **85**, 28.

Reza, M.J., Dornfield, L., Goldberg, L.S., Bluestone, R. and Pearson, C.M. (1975). Wegener's granulomatosis: long term follow-up of patients treated with cyclophosphamide. *Arthritis Rheum* **18**, 501.

Rhodes, J., Beck, P., Bainton, D. and Campbell, H. (1971). Controlled trial of azathioprine in Crohn's disease. *Lancet* **ii**, 1273.

Rinehart, J.J., Balcerzak, S.P., Sagone, A.L. and Lobuglio, A.F. (1974). Effect of corticosteroids on human monocyte function. *J. Clin. Invest.* **54**, 1337.

Rinehart, J.J., Sagone, A.L., Balcerzak, S.P., Ackerman, G.A. and Lobuglio, A.F. (1975). Effect of corticosteroid on human monocyte function. *N. Engl. J. Med.* **22**, 236.

Roberts, J.J., Brent, T.P. and Crathorn, A.R. (1971). Evidence for inactivation and repair of the mammalian DNA template after aklylation by mustard gas and half mustard gas. *Eur. J. Cancer* **7**, 515.

Rollinghoff, M., Schrader, J. and Wagner, H. (1973). Effect of azathioprine and cytosine arabinodine on humoral and cellular immunity *in vitro*. *Clin. Exp. Immunol.* **15**, 261.

Rollinghoff, M., Starzinski-Powitz, A., Pfizenmaier, K. and Wagner, H. (1977). Cyclophosphamide sensitive T cells suppress the *in vivo* generation of antigen specific cytotoxic T lymphocytes. *J. Exp. Med.* **145**, 455.

Rosano, T.G., Freed, B.M., Cerilli, J. and Lempert, N. (1986). Immunosuppressive metabolites of cyclosporine in the blood of renal allograft recipients. *Transplantation* **42**, 262.

Rosano, T.G., Fell, M.A. Freed, B.M., Dybas, M.T. and Lempert, N. (1988). Cyclosporine and metabolites in blood from renal allograft recipients with nephrotoxicity, rejection or good renal function: comparative high performance liquid chromatography and monoclonal radioimmunoassay studies. *Transplant. Proc.* **20** (suppl, 2), 330.

Rose, G.A. and Spencer, M. (1957). Polyarteritis nodosa. *Quart. J. Med.* **26**, 43.

Rosen, M.K., Standaert, R.F., Galat, A., Nakatsuka, M. and Schreiber, S.L. (1990). Inhibition of FKBP rotamase activity by immunosuppressant FK-506. *Science* **248**, 863.

Rosenberg, J.C. and Lysz, K. (1980). Suppression of the immune response by steroids: comparative potency of hydrocortisone, methyl prednisolone and dexamethasone. *Transplantation* **29**, 425.

Rosenberg, J.L., Levin, B., Wall, A.J. and Kirstner, J.B. (1975a). A controlled trial of azathioprine in Crohn's disease. *Dig. Dis.* **20**, 721.

Rosenberg, J.L., Wall, A.J., Levin, B., Binder, H.J. and Kirstner, J.B. (1975b). A controlled trial of azathioprine in the management of chronic ulcerative colitis. *Gastroenterology* **69**, 96.

Row, P.G., Cameron, J.S., Turner, D.R., Evans, D.J., White, R.H.R., Ogg, C.S., Chantler, C. and Brown, C.B. (1975). Membranous nephropathy: long term follow up and association with neoplasia. *Quart. J. Med.* **44**, 207.

Rowley, M.J., Mackay, I.R. and McKenzie, I.F.C. (1969). Antibody production in immunosuppressed recipients of renal allografts. *Lancet* **ii**, 708.

Rubin, L.A., Urowitz, M.B. and Gladman, D.D. (1985). Mortality in systemic lupus erythematosus: the bimodal pattern revisited. *Quart. J. Med.* **216**, 87.

Rubin, R.H. and Tolkoff-Rubin, N.E. (1988). Opportunist infections in renal transplant recipients. *Transplant Proc.* **20** (suppl. 8), 12.

Rühl, H., Vogt, W., Bochert, G., Schmidt, S., Moelle, R. and Schaoua, H. (1974). Effect of L-asparaginase and hydrocortisone on human lymphocyte transformation and production of a mononuclear leucocyte chemotactic factor *in vitro*. *Immunology* **26**, 989.

Ryffel, B. (1989). Pharmacology of cyclosporine (Sandimmune): cellular activation: regulation of intracellular events by cyclosporine. *Pharmacol. Rev.* **41**, 407.

Sabouraud, O., Auger, J., Darcel, F. *et al.* (1972). Immunosuppression au long cours dans le sclérose en plaque: évaluation des traitements commencés avant. *Ren. Neurol. (Paris)* **140**, 125.

Saltonick, A.I., Krupp, M.N. and Amatruda, J.M. (1983). Dexamethasone stimulates insulin receptor synthesis in cultured rat hepatocytes. *J. Biol. Chem.* **258**, 1413.

Santos, G.W. and Owens, A.H. (1966). 19S and 7S antibody production in cyclophosphamide or methotrexate treated rats. *Nature* **209**, 622.

Santos, G.W., Burke, P.J., Sensenbrenner, L.L. and Owens, A.H. (1969). Rationale for the use of cyclophosphamide as an immunosuppressant for marrow transplants in man. In *Pharmacological Treatment in Organ and Tissue Transplantation*, p. 24, Excerpta Medica International Congress Series No. 196, Amsterdam.

Santos, G.W., Sensenbrenner, L.L., Burke, P.J., Colvin, M. and Owens, A.H. (1971). Marrow transplantation in man following cyclophosphamide. *Transplant. Proc.* **3**, 400.

Savage, C.O.S., Winnearls, C.G., Evans, D.J., Rees, A.J. and Lockwood, C.M. (1985). Microscopic polyarteritis: presentation, pathology prognosis. *Quart. J. Med.* **56**, 467.

Schreiber, A.D., Parsons, J., MacDermot, P. and Cigar, R.A. (1975). Effect of corticosteroids on the human monocyte IgG and complement receptors. *J. Clin. Invest.* **56**, 1189.

Schreiber, R.P., Derse, C.P., Friedman, B., Gillis, S., Plant, M., Lichtenstein, L.M. and MacGlashan, D.W. (1989). Regulation of human basophil mediator release by cytokines. *J. Immunol.* **143**, 1310.

Schreiber, S.L. (1991). Chemistry and biology of the immunophilins and their immunosuppressive ligands. *Science* **251**, 283.

Schuller-Levis, G.B., Kozlowski, P.B. and Wisniewski, H.M. (1986). Cyclosporin A treatment of an induced attack in a chronic relapsing model of experimental allergic encephalomyelitis. *Clin. Immunol. Immunopathol.* **40**, 244.

Schwartz, R.S. and Andre, J. (1960). Clearance of protein from blood of normal and 6 mercaptopurine-treated rabbits. *Proc. Soc. Exp. Biol.* **104**, 228.

Sela, M., Fuchs, S. and Feldman, M. (1963). Specific immunologic unresponsiveness to synthetic polypeptide antigens. *Science* **139**, 342.

Shand, F.L. (1979). The immunopharmacology of cyclophosphamide. *Int. J. Immunopharmacol.* **1**, 165.

Shand, F.L. and Howard, J.G. (1979). Induction *in vitro* of reversible immunosuppression and inhibition of B cell receptor regeneration by defined metabolites of cyclophosphamide. *Eur. J. Immunol.* **9**, 17.

Sharon, E., Kaplan, D. and Diamond, H.S. (1973). Exacerbation of systemic lupus erythematosus after withdrawal of azathioprine therapy. *N. Engl. J. Med.* **288**, 122.

Shen, L., Guyre, P.M., Ball, E.D. and Fanger, M.W. (1986). Glucocorticoid enhances gamma interferon effects on human monocyte antigen expression and ADCC. *Clin. Exp. Immunol.* **65**, 387.

Shephard, V.L., Konish, M.G. and Stahl, P. (1985). Dexamethasone increases expression of mannose receptors and decreases extracellular lysosomal enzyme accumulation in macrophages. *J. Biol. Chem.* **260**, 160.

Shevach, E.M. (1985). The effects of cyclosporin A on the immune system. *Ann. Rev. Immunol.* **3**, 397.

Shih, W.W.H., Ellison, G.W., Myers, L.W., Durkos-Smith, D. and Fahey, J.L. (1982). Locus of selective depression of human natural killer cells by azathioprine. *Clin. Immunol. Immunopathol.* **23**, 672.

Shih, W.W.H., Hines, W.H. and Neilson, E.G. (1988). Effects of cyclosporin A on the development of immune-mediated interstitial nephritis. *Kidney Int.* **33**, 1113.

Siekierka, J.J., Hung, S.H.Y., Poe, M., Lln, C.S. and Sigal, N.H. (1989). A cytosolic binding protein for the immunosuppressant FK-506 has peptidyl–prolyl isomerase activity but is distinct from cyclophilin. *Nature* **341**, 755.

Simonian, S.J. and Murray, J.E. (1971). Further analysis of the mechanism of prolonged survival of canine renal allografts. *Transplant. Proc.* **3**, 470.

Slade, J.D. and Hepburn, B. (1983). Prednisone-induced alterations of circulating human lymphocyte subsets. *J. Lab. Clin. Med.* **101**, 479.

Smith, K.A., Crabtree, G.R., Kennedy, S.R. and Munck, A.U. (1977). Glucocorteroid receptors and glucocorticoid sensitivity of mitogen stimulated and unstimulated lymphocytes. *Nature* **267**, 523.

Smith, R.C., Rhodes, J., Heatley, R.V. *et al.* (1978). Low dose steroid and clinical relapse in Crohn's disease: a controlled trial. *Gut* **19**, 606.

Smith, S.R., Termmellie, C., Kipilman, C.T. and Smith, Y. (1981). Comparative effects of azathioprine, cyclophosphamide and frentizole on cellular immunity in mice. *J. Immunopharmacol.* **3**, 133.

Snyder, D.S., Wright, C.L. and Ting, C. (1987). Inhibition of human monocyte antigen presentation, but not HLA-DR expression, by cyclosporine. *Transplantation* **44**, 407.

Soloway, R.D., Summerskill, W.H.J., Baggenstoss, A.H. *et al.* (1972). Clinical, biochemical and histological remission of severe chronic active liver disease: a controlled study of treatment and early prognosis. *Gastroenterology* **63**, 820.

Soothill, J. (1975). In *Immunodeficiency in Man and Animals*. ed. D. Bergsma, R.A. Good and J. Finstad, p. 50, Sinauer Assoc. Inc., Sunderland, Massachusetts.

Sostman, H.D., Matthay, R.A. and Putman, C.E. (1977). Cytotoxic drug-induced lung disease. *Am. J. Med.* **62**, 608.

Sparberg, M., Simon, N. and Greco, F. (1969). Intrahepatic cholestosis due to azathioprine. *Gastroenterology* **57**, 439.

Speigelberg, H.L. and Meischer P.A. (1963). Effects of 6-MP on experimental autoimmune thyroiditis in guinea pigs. *Fed. Proc.* **22**, 501.

Spreafico, F., Donelli, M.G., Bossi, A., Vecchi, A., Standen, S. and Garattinin, S. (1973). Immunodepressant activity and 6 mercaptopurine levels after administration of 6 mercaptopurine and azathioprine. *Transplantation* **16**, 269.

Starzl, T.E., Todo, S., Fung, J. Demetris, A.J., Venkataramman, R. and Jain, A. (1989). FK-506 for liver, kidney, and pancreas transplantation. *Lancet* **ii**: 1000.

Steinberg, A.D., Kaltreider, H.B., Staples, P.J., Goetzl, E.J., Talal, N. and Decker, J.L. (1971). Cyclophosphamide in lupus nephritis: a controlled trial. *Ann. Intern. Med.* **75**, 165.

Steppat, J.D. and Gross, W.L. (1989). Stage adapted treatment of

Wegener's granulomatosis. *Klin. Wochenschr.* **67**, 666.

Stevens, L.E. and Willoughby, R.S. (1969). The anti-inflammatory effects of some immunosuppressive agents. *J. Pathol.* **97**, 367.

Stevens, M.E., McConnell, M. and Bone, J.M. (1983). Aggressive treatment with pulse methyl prednisolone or plasma exchange is justified in rapidly progressive glomerulonephritis. *Proc. Eur. Dialysis Transplant. Assoc. Eur. Renal Assoc.* **19**, 724.

Stockman, G.D., Heim, L.R., Smith, M.A. and Trentin, J.J. (1973). Differential effects of cyclophosphamide on the B and T cells compartments of adult mice. *J. Immunol.* **110**, 277.

Strauss, B., Coyle, M. and Robbins, M. (1969). Consequences of alkylating for the behaviour of DNA. *Ann. NY Acad. Sci. (USA)* **163**, 765.

Strickland, R.W., Wahl, L.M. and Firbloom, D.S. (1986). Corticosteroids enhance the binding of recombinant interferon to cultured human monocytes. *J. Immunol.* **137**, 1577.

Sugawara, I. and Ishizaka, S. (1983). The degree of monocyte participation in human B- and T-cell activation by phorbol myristate acetate. *Clin. Immunol. Immunopathol.* **26**, 299.

Summers, R.W., Switz, D.M., Sessions, J.T. *et al.* (1979). National cooperative Crohn's disease study: results of drug treatment. *Gastroenterology* **77**, 847.

Summerskill, W.H.J., Korman, M.G., Ammon, H.G. and Baggenstoss, A.M. (1975). Prednisolone for chronic active liver disease: dose titration, standard dose and combination with azathioprine compared. *Gut* **16**, 876.

Sutton, W.T., Van Hagen, F., Griffith, B.H. and Preston, F.W. (1963). Drug effects on survival of homografts of skin. *Arch. Surg.* **87**, 840.

Swanson, M.A. and Schwartz, R.S. (1967). Immunosuppressive therapy: the relation between clinical response and immunologic competences. *N. Engl. J. Med.* **277**, 163.

Sztejnbok, M., Stewart, A., Diamond, H. and Kaplan, D. (1971). Azathioprine in the treatment of systemic lupus erythematosus. *Arthritis Rheum.* **14**, 639.

Taniguchi, M. and Tada, T. (1971). Regulation of homocytotropic antibody formation in the rat. IV. Effects of various immunosuppressive drugs. *J. Immunol.* **107**, 579.

Tanner, A.R., Halliday, J.W. and Pavell, L.W. (1980). Effect of long term corticosteroid therapy on monocyte chemotaxis in man. *Scand. J. Immunol.* **11**, 335.

Tarrab-Hazdai, R., Abramsky, O. and Fuchs, S. (1977). Immunosuppression of experimental autoimmune myasthenia gravis by azathioprine. II. Evaluation of immunological mechanisms. *J. Immunol.* **119**, 702.

Tejani, A., Butt, K., Trachtman, H., Suthantiran, M., Rosenthal, C. and Khawar, M. (1988). Cyclosporin A-induced remission of relapsing nephrotic syndrome in children. *Kidney Int.* **33**, 729.

Ten Berge, I.J.M. *et al.* (1985). Clinical and immunological follow-up of patients with severe renal disease in Wegener's granulomatosis. *Am. J. Nephrol.* **5**, 21.

Thomas, F., Thomas, J., Mendez, G., Lower, R. and Lee, H.M. (1977). Differential effects of immunosuppressive drugs on human T, B and K lymphocytes. *Transplantation* **24**, 435.

Thomson, A.W., Moon, D.K., Inoue, Y., Geczy, C.L. and Nelson, D.S. (1983a). Modification of delayed-type hypersensitivity reactions to ovalbumin in cyclosporin A treated guinea pigs. *Immunology* **48**, 301.

Thomson, A.W., Moon, D.K. and Nelson, D.S. (1983b). Suppression of delayed type hypersensitivity reactions and lymphokine production by cyclosporin A in the mouse. *Immunology* **52**, 599.

Thomson, R.N., Watts, C., Edelman, J., Esdaile, J. and Russell, A.S. (1984). A controlled two centre trial of parenteral methotrexate therapy for refractory rheumatoid arthritis. *J. Rheumatol.* **11**, 760.

Thomspson, P.W., Kirwan, J.R. and Barnes, C.G. (1985). Practical results of treatment with disease-modifying anti-rheumatoid drugs. *Br. J. Rheumatol.* **24**, 167.

Thong, Y.H., Henson, S.A., Vincent, M.M., Rola-Pleszczynski, M., Walser, J.B. and Bellanti, J.A. (1975). Effect of hydrocortisone on *in vitro* cellular immunity to viruses in man. *Clin. Immunol. Immunopathol.* **3**, 363.

Tinbergen, W.J. (1968). The effects of some immunosuppressive agents on kidney graft survival in rats. *Transplantation* **6**, 203.

Tonnesen, E., Christiensen, N.J. and Brinklow, M.M. (1987). Natural killer cell activity during cortisol and adrenalin infusion in healthy volunteers. *Eur. J. Clin. Invest.* **17**, 497.

Tosato, G., Pike, S.E., Koski, I.R. and Blaese, R.M. (1982). Selective inhibition of immunoregulatory cell functions by cyclosporin A. *J. Immunol.* **128**, 1986.

Townes, A.S., Sowa, J.M. and Shulman, L.E. (1972). Controlled trial of cyclophosphamide in rheumatoid arthritis: an 18 month double-blind crossover study. *Arthritis Rheum.* **15**, 129.

Townes, A.S., Sowa, J.M. and Shulman, L.E. (1976). Controlled trial of cyclophosphamide in rheumatoid arthritis. *Arthritis Rheum.* **19**, 563.

Trenn, G., Taffs, R., Hohman, R., Kincaid, R. and Shevach, R.M. (1989). Biochemical characterisation of the inhibitory effects of CsA on cytolytic T lymphocytes effector function. *J. Immunol.* **142**, 3792.

Trompeter, R.S., Evans, P.R. and Barratt, T.M. (1980). Gonadal function in males treated with limited cyclophosphamide for steroid sensitive nephrotic syndrome. *Pediatr. Res.* **14**, 1007.

Truelove, S.C. (1960). Systematic and local corticosteroid therapy in ulcerative colitis. *Br. Med. J.* **i**, 464.

Truelove, S.C. and Witts S.J. (1955). Cortisone in ulcerative colitis: final report on a therapeutic trial. *Br. Med. J.* **ii**, 1041.

Tuchinda, M., Newcombe, R.W. and De Vald, B.L. (1972). Effect of prednisone treatment on the human immune response to keyhole limpet neurocyamin. *Int. Arch. Allergy* **42**, 533.

Turk, J.L. and Parker, D. (1979). The effect of cyclophosphamide on the immune response. *J. Immunopharmacol.* **1**, 127.

Turk, J.L. and Poulter, L.W. (1972). Selective depletion of lymphoid tissue by cyclophosphamide. *Clin. Exp. Immunol.* **10**, 285.

Turk, J.L., Parker, D. and Poulter, L.W. (1972). Functional aspects of selective depletion of lymphoid tissue by cyclophosphamide. *Immunology* **23**, 493.

Turnell, R.W., Kaiser, N., Milholland, R.J. and Rosen, F. (1974). Glucocorticoid receptors in rat thyrocytes. *J. Biol. Chem.* **249**, 1133.

Turner, A.N. and Rees, A.J. (1992). Antiglomerular basement membrane disease. In *Oxford Textbook of Clinical Nephrology*, ed. J.S. Cameron, A.M. Davison, J.-P. Grunfeld, D.N.S. Kerr and E. Ritz. ch. 3.10, p. 438, Oxford University Press, Oxford.

Urowitz, M.B., Gorden, D.A., Smuthe, H.A., Pruzanski, W. and Orgryzlo, M.A. (1973). Azathioprine in rheumatoid arthritis: a double-blind crossover study. *Arthritis Rheum.* **16**, 411.

Van Buren, D., Van Buren, C.T., Flechner, S.M., Maddox, A.M., Verani, R. and Kahan, B.D. (1985). *De novo* hemolytic uremic syndrome in real transplant recipients immunosuppressed with cyclosporine. *Surgery* **98**, 54.

Van Furth, R., Gassman, A.E. and Diessehoff-Den Dulk, M.M.C. (1975). The effect of azathioprine (imuran) on cell cycle of promonocytes and the production of monocytes in the bone marrow. *J. Exp. Med.* **141**, 531.

Vann, D.C. (1974). Restoration of the *in vivo* responses of corticosteroid treated spleen cells by T cells or soluble factors. *Cell. Immunol.* **11**, 11.

Vogel, C.L. and Calabresi, P. (1969). Enhanced suppression of experimental allergic encephalomyelitis by combination therapy with diazomycin-A and 6-mercaptopurine. *Proc. Soc. Exp. Biol. (NY)* **131**, 251.

Waage, A. and Bakko, O. (1988). Glucocorticoids suppress the production of tumour necrosis factor by lipopolysaccharide-stimulated human monocytes. *Immunology* **63**, 299.

Wahl, S.M., Altman, L.C. and Rosenstreich, D.L. (1975). Inhibition of *in vitro* lymphokine synthesis by steroids. *J. Immunol.* **115**, 476.

Waldmann, T.A., Broder, S., Krakauer, R. *et al.* (1976). The role of suppressor cells in the pathogenesis of common variable hypogammaglobulinaemia and the immune deficiency associated with myeloma. *Fed. Proc.* **35**, 2067.

Walker, R.G., D'Apice, A.J.F. and Kincaid-Smith, P. (1977). Plasmapheresis in Goodpasture's syndrome with renal failure. *Med. J. Aust.* **1**, 875.

Walker, R.G., Scheinkestel, C., Becker, G.J., Owen, J.E., Dowling, J.P. and Kincaid Smith, P. (1985). Clinical and morphological aspects of the management of crescentic anti-glomerular basement membrane antibody (anti-GBM) nephritis/Goodpasture's syndrome. *Quart. J. Med.* **54**, 75.

Walker, S.E. and Bole, G.G. (1975). Selective suppression of autoantibody responses in NZB/NZW mice treated with long term cyclophosphamide. *Arthritis Rheum.* **18**, 265.

Walton, E.W. (1958). Giant-cell granuloma of the respiratory tract (Wegener's granulomatosis). *Br. Med. J.* **ii**, 265.

Ward, P.A. (1971). Leucotoxic factors in health and disease. *Am. J. Pathol.* **64**, 521.

Warren, M.K. and Vogel, S.N. (1985). Opposing effects of glucocorticoids on interferon induced murine macrophage Fc receptor and Ig antigen expression. *J. Immunol.* **134**, 2462.

Watson, W.C. and Bukowsky, M. (1974). Azathioprine in management of Crohn's disease: a randomised crossover study. *Gastroenterology* **66**, 796.

Webel, M.L., Ritts, R.E., Taswell, H.E., Donadio, J.V. and Woods, J.E. (1974). Cellular immunity after intravenous administration of methyl prednisolone. *J. Lab. Clin. Med.* **83**, 383.

Weinblatt, M.E., Colbyn, J.S., Fox, D.A. *et al.* (1985). Efficacy of low dose methotrexate in rheumatoid arthritis. *N. Engl. J. Med.* **312**, 818.

Weinblatt, M.E., Trentham, D.E., Fraser, P.A., Holdsworth, D.E., Ialchuk, K.R., Weissman, B. and Coblyn, J.S. (1988). Long term prospective trial of low dose methotrexate in rheumatoid arthritis. *Arthritis Rheum.* **31**, 167.

Wenger, R.M. (1988). Cyclosporin: conformation and analogues for studying its mechanism of action. *Transplant Proc.* **29** (suppl. 2), 313.

Werb, Z. (1978). Biochemical actions of glucocorticoids on macrophages in culture: specific inhibition of elastase, collagenase and plasminogen activator secretion and effects on other metabolic functions. *J. Exp. Med.* **147**, 1695.

Western Canadian Glomerulonephritis Study Group (1976). Controlled trial of azathioprine in the nephrotic syndrome secondary to idiopathic membranous glomerulonephritis. *Can. Med. Assoc. J.* **115**, 1209.

Whistler, R.L., Lindsey, J.A., Proctor, K.V.W., Marisaki, N. and Cornwell, D.G. (1984). Characteristics of cyclosporin induction of increased prostaglandin levels from human peripheral blood monocytes. *Transplantation* **38**, 377.

White, D.J.G., Plumb, A.M., Pawelec, G. and Brons, G. (1979). Cyclosporin A: an immunosuppressive agent preferentially active against proliferating T cells. *Transplantation* **27**, 55.

Williams, D., Wickramasinghe, S.N. and Hulme, B. (1978). Effects of azathioprine therapy on MCV in patients with renal grafts. *Scand. J. Haematol.* **20**, 258.

Williams, H.J., Reading, J.C., Ward, J.R. and O'Brien, W.M. (1980). Comparison of high and low dose cyclophosphamide therapy in rheumatoid arthritis. *Arthritis Rheum.* **23**, 521.

Williams, H.J., Wilkens, R.F., Samuelson, C.O. *et al.* (1985). Comparison of low dose oral pulse methotrexate and placebo in treatment of rheumatoid arthritis: a controlled clinical trial. *Arthritis Rheum.* **28**, 721.

Willoughby, J.M.T. and Kumar, P.J., Beckett, J. and Dawson, A.M. (1971). Controlled trial of azathioprine in Crohn's disease. *Lancet* **ii**, 944.

Wilson, C.G., Ssendagire, R., May, C.S. and Paterson, J.W. (1975). Measurement of plasma prednisolone in man. *Br. J. Clin. Pharmacol.* **2**, 321.

Winkelstein, A. (1977). Effect of immunosuppressive drugs on T and B lymphocytes in guinea pigs. *Blood* **50**, 81.

Winkelstein, A. (1979). The effects of azathioprine on immunity. *J. Immunopharmacol.* **1**, 429.

Winkelstein, A., Mikulla, J.M., Nankin, H.R., Pollock, B.H. and Stolzer, B.L. (1972). Mechanisms of immunosuppression: effects of cyclophosphamide on lymphocytes. *J. Lab. Clin. Med.* **80**, 506.

Winkelstein, A., Rubin, F.L., Tolchin, S.F. and Pollock, B.H. (1974). Mechanisms of immunosuppression: effect of cyclophosphamide on responses to influenza immunisation. *J. Lab. Clin. Med.* **83**, 504.

Wirotsko, E. and Halbert, S.P. (1962). Suppression of allergic uveitis by 6-mercaptopurine. *J. Exp. Med.* **116**, 653.

Wood, A., Adu, D., Birtwistle, R.J., Brewer, D.B. and Michael, J. (1988). Cyclosporin A and anti-glomerular basement membrane antibody glomerulonephritis in rats. *Br. J. Exp. Pathol.* **69**, 189.

Woodland, J., Sharman, V.L. and Currey, H.L.F. (1981). Azathioprine in rheumatoid arthritis: a double blind study of full versus half dose versus placebo. *Ann. Rheum. Dis.* **40**, 355.

Wysocki, G.P., Gretzinger, H.A., Laupacis, A., Ulan, R.A. and Stiller, C.R. (1983). Fibrous hyperplasia of the gingiva: a side effect of cyclosporin A therapy. *Oral Surg. Oral Med. Oral Pathol.* **55**, 274.

Yu, D.T., Clements, P.J., Panlus, H.E., Peters, J.B., Levy, J. and

Barnett, E.V. (1974a). Human lymphocyte subpopulations: effects of corticosteroids. *J. Clin. Invest.* **53**, 565.

Yu, D.T., Clements, P.J., Peters, J.B., Levy, J., Panlus, H.E. and Barnett, E.V. (1974b). Lymphocyte characteristics in rheumatic patients and the effect of azathioprine. *Arthritis Rheum.* **17**, 37.

Zembala, M. and Ascherson, G.L. (1976). The effect of cyclophosphamide and irradiation on cells which suppress contact sensitivity in the mouse. *Clin. Exp. Immunol.* **23**, 445.

Zhu, L., Cupps, T.R., Whalen, G. and Fauci, A.S. (1987). Selective effects of cyclophosphamide therapy on activation, proliferation and differentiation of human B cells. *Lab. Invest.* **7**, 1082.

Zipfel, P.F., Irving, S.G., Kelly, K. and Siebenlist, U. (1989). Complexity of the primary genetic response to mitogenic activation of human T cells. *Mol. Cell. Biol.* **9**, 1041.

Zukoski, C.F., Callaway, J.M. and Rhea, W.G. (1963). Prolongation of canine renal homograft survival by antimetabolites. *Transplantation* **1**, 293.

Zweiman, B., Scott, R.J. and Atkins, P.C. (1976). Histologic study of human skin test response to ragweed and compared 48/80. III. Effects of alternate day steroid therapy. *J. Allergy. Clin. Immunol.* **58**, 657.

Section 6
Allergy

52: The Immunobiology of Immunoglobulin E: Immediate or Type I Hypersensitivity

T.A.E. Platts-Mills

Historical introduction: hypersensitivity and immunoglobulin E

The word 'allergy', which is so delightfully abused in normal usage today, derives from the Greek words 'allos ergos', meaning altered reactivity. Originally the term was meant to define any altered state that resulted from prior exposure to an antigen, and thus included all forms of immunity (Silverstein 1989). At that time there was confusion about the role of immunity in human anaphylaxis and hay fever, because, although the patients clearly gave altered responses, there was no evidence of serum antibodies which could be measured using the available techniques (i.e. precipitin tests or complement fixation). This led to the confused concept of allergens that gave rise to 'no production of antibodies but to supersensitivity' (Von Pirquet 1906). In 1921 Küstner, who was allergic to fish, injected his serum into Prausnitz's skin and demonstrated that immediate or weal-and-flare skin responses could be passively transferred (the P–K test) (Prausnitz and Küstner 1921). The substance responsible for this transfer was called reagin (or active substance), but it was still not generally recognized as antibody, although there was good evidence that P–K transfer was immunologically specific. The scientific study of allergy had actually started much earlier, when Blackley demonstrated in 1873 that grass pollen was the cause of 'cattarhus aestivus' (or spring hay fever) and that sensitive individuals could be identified by skin testing. When Robert Cooke was made head of the division of immunology at Cornell (in 1919), many substances had already been shown to give positive weal-and-flare skin tests, including pollens, animal dander, foods, fungal spores and house dust. The common feature of these substances was that they were otherwise harmless. Coca, who founded the *Journal of Immunology*, introduced the term atopy to describe the tendency of some individuals to develop this immediate hypersensitivity to common environmental substances that were otherwise harmless (Coca and Cooke 1923). These substances were called atopic allergens (or atopens) but came to be called allergens. From that time on, the word 'allergy' has developed its modern meaning, i.e. referring to those forms of immunity that cause hypersensitivity against otherwise harmless antigens.

As early as 1931 Taliafero and Taliafero reported from Puerto Rico that patients with schistosomiasis gave positive immediate skin responses to extracts of schistosomules and that this skin response could be passively transferred with serum. Immediate sensitivity to schistosomules is presumed to cause 'swimmers' itch' as these larvae burrow through the skin. The severe itching that occurs when chiggers or scabies mites burrow in the skin almost certainly involves immediate hypersensitivity and may well help in dislodging these parasites from the skin (Mellanby 1943; Arlian *et al.* 1988). It is now clear that specific immunoglobulin E (IgE) antibodies, raised total IgE and systemic and local eosinophilia are common features of the immune response to helminth invasion or allergen exposure. This pattern of immunity is not a feature of virus infections, protozoal infections or the great majority of bacterial infections. Similarly, most forms of therapeutic immunization (e.g. smallpox, diphtheria, tetanus, polio, pertussis) do not give rise to persistent immediate hypersensitivity.

For many years it was assumed that the substances that gave rise to immediate hypersensitivity were different from the antigens that gave rise to other forms of immunity. Much early work on purifying and characterizing allergens aimed to identify these special properties (see Marsh 1975). It has been shown that helminths produce factors (other than the antigens) that non-specifically boost IgE production. Some similar non-specific effects have been reported with allergen extracts (Berrens 1974). However, most purified allergens do not activate complement, do not boost IgE production non-specifically in animal experiments and are not irritant to the skin of non-allergic individuals. Purification of an increasing number of allergens has not revealed any common properties. Indeed, allergens are remarkably diverse, e.g. digestive enzymes of mites, recognition proteins from pollens, a skin protein from cats and a urinary protein from rodents. Further, it was obvious from early experiments on pollen allergens that *Amb a* I from ragweed was a very labile protein easily denatured by heat, pH or reduction (King and Norman 1962). By contrast, the major allergen from grass pollen was so stable to heating that initially it seemed unlikely that it was a protein (Johnson and Marsh 1965; Marsh 1975).

By 1965 it seemed certain that the reagins that could passively transfer immediate skin sensitivity were a special kind of antibody. However, there was still no convincing way of measuring these antibodies *in vitro* and no clear understanding of how they might lead to the release of mediators in the skin. In 1967 Ishizaka established that reaginic activity was carried by an antigenically distinct form of immunoglobulin, which he named IgE (Ishizaka *et al.* 1967; see Ishizaka and Ishizaka 1975). Shortly afterwards, Johansson and Bennich demonstrated that a previously uncharacterized myeloma (ND, the patient's initials) was antigenically IgE and would block P–K tests (Stanworth *et al.* 1968; Bennich and Johansson 1971). The discovery of IgE was followed rapidly by the formal proof that this isotype alone has the ability to bind to a high-affinity Fc receptor which is present on basophils and mast cells (Ishizaka *et al.* 1972). These cells, which are the only important source of histamine in humans, will release mediators if their surface receptors ($Fc_{\varepsilon}RI$) are cross-linked by antigen, anti-IgE or antibodies to the receptors themselves (Ishizaka and Ishizaka 1975). These findings explained how IgE antibodies could mediate weal-and-flare skin responses, and, indeed, for a great variety of antigens there was found to be an excellent correlation between immediate skin reactivity and serum IgE antibodies (Johansson *et al.* 1971, 1972). It is important to realize that these results did not establish that IgE antibodies are responsible for the immunopathology of allergic diseases. Indeed, it was clear that, although virtually all patients with hay fever caused by pollen (or asthma caused by cats) have IgE antibodies to the relevant allergen, the quantitative correlation between disease and IgE antibodies is generally poor.

The ability to measure IgE antibodies led to a great increase in interest in the factors controlling IgE antibody production in man and animals. There is no doubt that a wide range of factors are involved, including several T-cell-derived interleukins. It is also clear that there are specific potentiating pathways for IgE production in mice which may play an important role in enhancing an IgE response (Ishizaka 1985). The recent demonstration that interleukin 4 (IL-4) has a central role in mouse IgE responses and that it is produced by a subtype of helper T cells has led to enthusiastic efforts to identify similar subtypes of CD4+ve cells in man (Snapper *et al.* 1988; Umetsu *et al.* 1988). However, in many ways the most useful result obtained from mouse experiments remains the simple observation that immunizing dose and adjuvant are more important than the nature of the protein (Levine and Vaz 1970). Repeated immunization with antigen in alum starting with ≤0.001 μg and using progressively higher doses will give rise to persistent IgE antibody responses (Jarrett and Stewart 1974; Prouvost-Danon *et al.* 1977). By contrast, in rabbits and most strains of mice 'high'-dose immunization with >1 μg or immunization using complete Freund's adjuvant will produce IgG antibody responses without IgE antibody. These 'high'-dose immunization regimes prime T cells that will not help and often appear to suppress IgE antibody production (Kishimoto and Ishizaka 1973). For most inhalant allergens, natural exposure represents a very low-dose immunization 'regime'. Exposure to pollen allergens has been estimated as ~1 μg/season or 10 ng/day (Marsh 1975). Similarly, studies on airborne house dust suggest that average daily exposure to group I mite allergens is unlikely to be greater than 20 ng (Tovey *et al.* 1981b).

Taking the mouse experiments together with the observations on natural exposure led to the conclusion that atopic patients are those individuals who can make an immune response to very low-dose immunization (see Marsh 1975; Platts-Mills 1982). From the results on mice it is also clear that, when mice make IgE antibody responses to low-dose immunization, they are always accompanied by IgG responses. Similarly, human IgE antibody responses to inhalants are accompanied by IgG antibody. Indeed, for immune responses to pollen and dust mite allergens, there is a reasonable quantitative correlation between serum IgE and IgG antibodies (Platts-Mills 1979). In keeping with this, studies that have used radiolabelled purified allergens to assay IgG antibodies find that most non-allergic individuals do not have detectable IgG antibodies to pollen or mite antigens (Ishizaka *et al.* 1967; Tse *et al.* 1973; Platts-Mills 1979; Chapman *et al.* 1980; Marsh *et al.* 1982). The situation is clearly different for those allergens where natural exposure is higher in dose, e.g. egg (or milk) proteins, rat urinary allergen or bee venom. Many individuals who are exposed but who are not allergic to these antigens are found to have serum IgG antibodies (Kemeny *et al.* 1982, 1983; Platts-Mills *et al.* 1987b; Van der Zee and Aalberse 1987).

The preceding paragraph implies that most allergic individuals are immunologically 'high responders' who respond to inhaled allergens under conditions where most non-allergic individuals make no response. It has been extensively reported that the tendency to become allergic and, specifically, the disease hay fever are inherited, which implies that there are genetic differences between allergic and non-allergic individuals (Cooke and Van Der Veer 1916; Marsh 1975). In order to study the genetic control of any immune response, it is essential that all the individuals being studied have been equally exposed. Thus, it is no surprise that most studies on the genetics of allergy have been carried out using patients with pollen hay fever. The most convincing studies have come from Baltimore, where both grass pollen in the spring and ragweed in the late summer cause epidemic disease. The results show multiple associations between human leucocyte antigen (HLA) typing and IgE antibody responses. In particular, there are close associations between DR type and the IgE response to certain low-molecular-weight antigens (Marsh *et al.* 1982). It is assumed that these associations are clearest in response to low-molecular-weight antigens because they have a restricted number of B cell or T cell epitopes and therefore they can only be recognized in a limited number of ways. There are also general genetic controls over total IgE which probably affect the ability to respond to antigens in general; however, these are not directly related to HLA type (Gerrard *et al.* 1974; Marsh *et al.* 1974). The studies by Marsh and his colleagues (1982) on the association between allergy to *Amb a* V and Dw2 concluded that this genetic linkage was as close with IgG antibody responses as it was with IgE antibody responses. Recently it has been reported that there is a linkage between IgE antibody responses and chromosome 11q. However, the relationship between this observation and other genetic studies is not yet clear (Cookson *et al.* 1989).

Having briefly considered the background to present understanding of allergic disease, this chapter will outline some further aspects of immediate hypersensitivity before discussing the possible significance of the system. The issues to be considered are the nature of allergens, the immune response to allergens and the mechanisms giving rise to the different diseases associated with immediate hypersensitivity. In addition, the immunological basis for two other 'allergic' diseases (contact sensitivity and extrinsic allergic alveolitis) will be discussed briefly in order to put IgE responses into perspective. The hypothesis is that immune (or allergic) responses to otherwise harmless proteins in our environment are a consequence of maintaining a sensitive immune system. The response to allergens is special in that it is dominated by IgE antibodies; none the less, the response is complex, involving both regulator and effector roles for T cells and also a role for IgG antibodies. As we will discuss, there are many parallels between the immune response to allergens and that to parasites. However, it is likely that different elements of the immediate hypersensitivity responses are important in immune defences against many different pathogens.

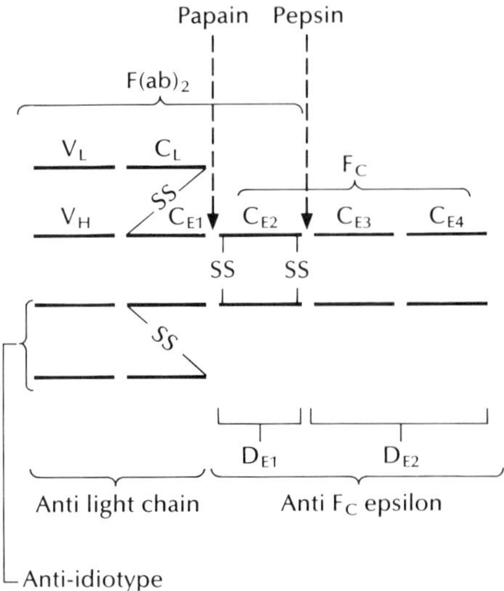

Fig. 52.1. Immunoglobulin E, showing only interchain disulphide bonds. The light chain consists of a variable (V_L) and constant (C_L) domain, while the heavy chain consists of one variable (V_H) and four constant (C_{E1-4}) domains. The molecule can be fractionated by using papain, which yields Fab and Fc fragments or with pepsin which yields $F(ab)_2$ fragments. When rabbits are immunized with purified IgE myeloma protein, they produce antibodies against the epsilon (ε) heavy chain, against the light chains and also against the idiotype on the variable domains. The epsilon-specific antibodies can be separated into those directed against antigens on the $F(ab)_2$ fragment (D_{E1}) and those on the remainder of the heavy chain (D_{E2}). Structures in the Fc portion are responsible for binding to the IgE receptor and are very susceptible to heat and reduction.

Immunoglobulin E

Immunoglobulin E is present in the circulation as monomers of molecular weight 190 000 daltons, composed of two heavy and two light chains (Bennich and Johansson 1971) (Fig. 52.1). The main isotype-specific antigens, referred to as DE1 and DE2, are on the Fc portion of the molecule. The ability to bind to IgE receptors is associated with an extra domain in the constant region CE_4. The light chains can be either kappa or lambda, and the Fab fragment includes the antigen-binding site. Heating at 56°C for 30 minutes will damage the Fc portion sufficiently to prevent skin sensitization. Mild reduction with dithiothreitol will also destroy skin-sensitizing activity without damaging antigen-binding activity. Although it has been reported that a short peptide from IgE can block binding of IgE to the skin, this has not been confirmed and seems most unlikely from the results of previous experiments (Bennich *et al.* 1977). The affinity of IgE for $Fc_{\varepsilon}RI$ is approximately 1×10^9 l/M. This binding is reversible slowly at pH 7 and rapidly at pH 4. *In vivo* IgE bound to skin mast cells stays *in situ* for weeks. It is likely that IgE released from mast cells rapidly rebinds to the same cell. In addition, it has been suggested that enzymes in the tissues destroy IgE released from mast cells (Bach *et al.* 1978). Using radiolabelled IgE or infusions of high-IgE plasma, it is clear that IgE is removed from the serum with a half-life of <2 days (Waldmann *et al.* 1976). There is still no clear explanation of how the serum half-life can be <2 days while the skin half-life is closer to 10 days.

The high-affinity receptor for IgE has now been sequenced and defined in great detail (Metzger 1988). It is composed of four amino acid chains, each of which contains one or more transmembrane segments. The alpha subunit has the largest extracellular segment and by itself is capable of binding IgE. The first evidence that histamine release required cross-linking came from studies with dimers and monomers of pencilloyl determinants (Levine and Redmond 1968). This tended to imply that cross-linking normally involved two IgE antibodies of the same specificity. However, it is now clear from the known sequences of allergens that they do not in general have repeat determinants. Thus, most cross-linking by allergens is likely to involve IgE antibodies against at least two different epitopes on the same molecule. However, detailed studies with monoclonal antibodies to allergens have suggested that there are only a few 'IgE'-binding epitopes on most major allergens (Esch and Klapper 1989; Platts-Mills and Chapman 1987). Following cross-linking of IgE on receptors, the histamine-containing granules rapidly come in contact with the outside wall of the cell. The two membranes, which are apparently identical, fuse and a direct channel to the exterior is created. In basophils, the granule contents rapidly dissolve, causing the granule to expand and then discharge to the exterior (Hastie 1971). In mast cells, the granule contents are often released without dissolving. Neither mast cells nor basophils are damaged by degranulation; indeed, it seems likely that regranulation usually occurs within 24 hours. The sequence of mediators released from these cells is discussed in Chapter 29.

Allergens: the antigens that induce immunoglobulin E antibody responses in man

Over the last few years allergen immunochemistry has advanced, not only because of the continued purification and characterization of different allergens but also from a series of new developments:

1 The establishment of International Standards (IS) and a new nomenclature system.

2 The advent of monoclonal antibodies to allergens.

3 Cloning and/or sequencing of some important allergens.

World Health Organization International Standards and the new nomenclature

Since the early part of this century there have been repeated attempts to establish standard preparations of allergens. Until recently these have failed because there was no *in vitro* technique for measuring the potency of allergen extracts. At least as far as the World Health Organization (WHO) is concerned, the corner-stone of establishing an IS is to demonstrate that laboratories in different countries can measure the activity or potency of the extract *in vitro*. The RAST inhibition technique, despite its many problems, has provided such an assay. In addition, for many allergen extracts it is now possible to measure the content of a representative major allergen using immunochemical techniques, e.g. immunodiffusion, RIA or enzyme-linked immunosorbent assay (ELISA).

Since 1981 a vigorous campaign, headed by de Weck, Norman and Lowenstein, has succeeded in establishing five WHO ISs. In each case the collaborative data accepted by WHO have been RAST inhibition and major allergen content (Ford *et al.* 1985; Norman 1986). It appears likely that future standards will be based on major allergen content, because the measurements can be made in absolute units and are more easily validated. The use of these standards to monitor clinical extracts has not expanded rapidly, because they are not easily used with the techniques currently recommended, e.g. biological units in Scandinavia, allergy units in the USA. The IS will become progressively more important with the introduction of more and simpler assays for major allergens.

The increasing recognition of specific allergens led to a wide proliferation of different abbreviations and also, in several cases, the multiple names for the same or similar allergens. In 1986 the International Union of Immunological Societies formally adopted a new nomenclature system (Marsh *et al.* 1986). Very briefly, the system adopts the first three letters of the genus name and the first letter of the species followed by a roman numeral. Major allergens are numbered in the order in which they were first purified (see Table 52.1). Allergens can only be adopted into the system once they have been purified and characterized. Thus, allergens identified only as IgE-binding bands on crossed radio-immunoelectrophoresis (CRIE) or on Western blotting after sodium

Table 52.1. Properties of some major purified allergens

Allergen source	Nomenclature for purified allergen	MW	Monoclonal antibodies	Sequence data
Pollens				
Grass				
Perennial rye	*Lol p* I	29 000	Esch and Klapper 1989	Yes[a]
	Lol p II	11 000		Yes
Kentucky blue	*Poa p* I		Ekramoddoullah *et al.* 1986	Yes
Ragweed				
Short ragweed	*Amb a* I	35 000	Olson and Klapper 1986	Yes
	Amb a III	11 000		—
	Amb a V	5 000		Yes[b]
Parietaria judaica	*Par j* I	47 000	Corbi *et al.* 1985	—
House dust allergens				
Cat				
Felis domesticus	*Fel d* I	34 000	Chapman *et al.* 1987	Yes
	Cat albumin	68 000	—	Yes
Cockroach				
Blatella germanica	*Bla g* I	25 000	Pollart *et al.* 1991	—
Dust mites				
Dermatophagoides				
Group I	*Der p* I	24 000	Chapman *et al.* 1984	Yes[c]
	Der f I	24 000	Heymann *et al.* 1986 Lind *et al.* 1988	Yes
Group II	*Der p* II	15 000		Yes
	Der f II	15 000	Heymann *et al.* 1989	Yes

a For analysis of the grass pollen allergens, see Ansari *et al.* 1987. Sequence data for all three rye grass pollen allergens have now been reported by this group.
b The first full sequence of an inhalant allergen was reported for *Amb a* V by Mole *et al.* 1975.
c The full sequence for *Der p* I was reported by Chua *et al.* 1988.

dodecyl sulphate polyacrylamide gel electrophoresis (SDS-PAGE) separation (immunoblotting) cannot be allotted new nomenclature.

Monoclonal antibodies to allergens

Developing monoclonal antibodies to allergens generally requires initial purification of an allergen. The procedure for establishing hybridomas has become routine; however, the selection of cell lines producing useful monoclonal antibodies is not simple. For most purposes, it is essential to obtain a monoclonal antibody with high affinity, and at present that means mouse monoclonal antibody of the IgG isotype. The advantages of monoclonal antibodies are that their specificity remains constant as long as the cell line is maintained and that they can be produced in much larger quantities than conventional antibodies. The main roles for monoclonal antibodies in allergy are purification, analysis and measurement of allergens (see Fig. 52.2). Many studies have used monoclonal antibodies to identify B cell epitopes on allergens and to inhibit the binding of IgE antibodies (Lind *et al.* 1988; Esch and Klapper 1989). Although inhibition of human IgE by mouse monoclonal antibody (or a combination of monoclonal antibodies) has been demonstrated, many of these antibodies appear to be directed against epitopes that are not important in the human IgE response (Chapman *et al.* 1984). These results have suggested that the immunizing conditions that are normally used for priming mice prior to producing hybridomas (i.e. high dose in complete Freund's adjuvant) may produce antibodies against different epitopes. Indeed, it is now clear that immunization of mice with repeated low-dose antigen in alum will produce antibodies against different, pre-

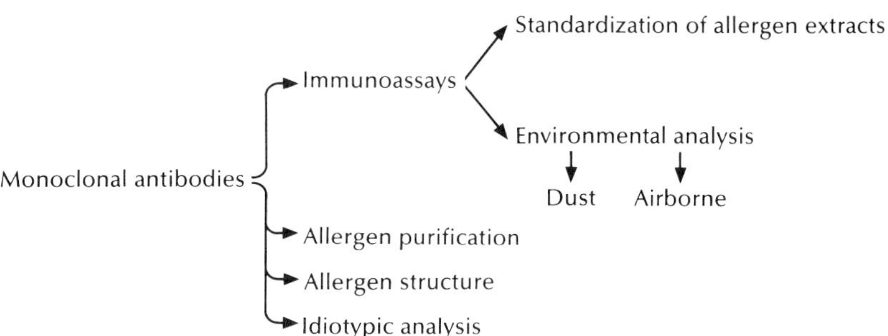

Fig. 52.2. Uses of monoclonal antibodies in allergy. Reproduced by permission of Dr Martin Chapman.

dominantly cross-reacting, antigens on dust mite group I allergens. By contrast, the monoclonal antibodies produced against group I allergens are predominantly against species-specific epitopes (Platts-Mills and Chapman 1987). Cross-reactivity between different allergens is an important feature of human allergy. For example, there is extensive cross-reactivity between proteins derived from different species of grasses, trees and mites. This cross-reactivity has often been found to be less obvious when the proteins are compared using antisera raised in animals or murine monoclonal antibodies. At present, this observation would best be explained if low-dose chronic natural exposure to airborne allergens favoured a special form of antigen processing.

Monoclonal antibodies have practical uses in purification, identification and measurement of allergens (Fig. 52.1). Affinity purification of *Fel d* I from cat extract has made it possible to purify this allergen directly from house dust, with yields of up to 5 mg of purified protein (Chapman *et al.* 1988). This purification made it possible to determine the N-terminal 35 amino acids of *Fel d* I and to clone the molecule (Morganstern *et al.* 1991). Monoclonal antibodies have also been used to develop two-site immunometric assays, using either radio- or enzyme labelling techniques (Chapman *et al.* 1987; Luczynska *et al.* 1989a). A two-site assay of this kind is not only an excellent way of measuring the protein but also a very effective way of defining the molecule. These assays are now the simplest approach to measuring natural exposure. The approach of measuring specific allergens has particular advantages in relation to indoor exposure, because the results (in absolute units) can be standardized and the results for different allergens can be directly compared, e.g. comparing airborne cat allergen with airborne mite allergen. Perhaps most important, the advent of monoclonal antibodies means that these assays are sufficiently simple to be used in epidemiological surveys and to consider their use in routine clinical practice.

Cloning and sequencing allergens

The first allergen sequenced was a low-molecular-weight protein from ragweed pollen *Amb a* V (Mole *et al.* 1975). The results yielded little insight into either the nature of the protein or the reasons why it was an allergen. Indeed, some cynics (including the author) felt that sequencing of allergens would not yield useful results. Now that the sequence of several allergens is known, it seems increasingly unlikely that analysing protein structure will identify a common property that makes some proteins allergens. On the other hand, there are many reasons for wanting to understand the primary and tertiary structure of the major allergens. Perhaps the most obvious objective is to identify those parts of the molecule or epitopes that react with antibodies or T cells. It is hoped that repeated injections of small fragments, i.e. <20 amino acids, could be used to modify the immune response in allergic individuals. These T-cell-reactive fragments might be used either alone or in combination with univalent B cell epitopes. The development of human T cell clones reactive with allergens provides an important tool for identifying these T cell epitopes (O'Hehir *et al.* 1988). Attempts have been made to predict the sites on a molecule that are likely to be recognized by T cells. However, these programmes are based largely on mouse data and it is possible that natural, i.e. repeated low-dose, immunization with allergens leads to the recognition of different T cell epitopes.

Sequencing proteins has already produced benefits in terms of understanding the function of these molecules. The dust mite allergen *Der p* I was known to be present in the gut lining and faeces of mites (Tovey *et al.* 1981a). In keeping with this, the molecule shows significant homology with papain and other proteolytic enzymes (Chua *et al.* 1988). This finding has renewed interest in older views that the enzymic activity of allergens might be important for their immunogenicity (Berrens 1974). On the other hand, the group II allergens of dust mites (*Der p* II and *Der f* II) show no sequence homology with known enzymes and they have no enzymic activity *in vitro*. Recently Stewart has reported that the N-terminal sequence of *Der f* III (MW 29 000) (see Heymann *et al.* 1989; Stewart *et al.* 1989) has sequence homology with chymotrypsin. The results with group I and group II allergens of mites do not support the view that any one type of molecule is more likely to become an allergen. The two groups of proteins are almost equally important as allergens but are strikingly different. Group I proteins are highly labile to heat, pH and reduction, as well as having potent protease activity. By contrast, the group II allergens are remarkably stable to heat, pH and reduction and do not apparently have enzymic activity. There are still several important allergens, e.g. α-2u-globulins in rodent urine and *Fel d* I in cat skin, where the primary function of the protein is not known.

Conclusions regarding allergens

Until recently, maintaining the definition of a specific allergen required repeated purification and the production of monospecific antisera. The definition of *Amb a* I from ragweed pollen and *Lol p* I from rye-grass pollen has been maintained in this way for over 20 years. For non-pollen antigens, where source material is available in grams rather than kilograms, the task of maintaining specific reagents has been more difficult. Recent developments with monoclonal antibodies and sequencing have made it much simpler to identify, measure and, in some cases, purify specific allergens. In addition, the International Standards have allowed for better definition of the measurements being made in different laboratories. Standardization is of great importance both for defining the quantities of extracts used for diagnosis and treatment and for measurements of natural exposure. The recent proposal of levels of mite allergen that represent a risk factor for asthma was only possible because measurements of mite allergens in house dust in different countries were being standardized relative to the *Dermatophagoides pteronyssinus* WHO IS (82/518) (Platts-Mills and de Weck 1989).

The progressive structural analyses of allergens has not demonstrated any particular biochemical structure or property that could explain why some proteins become allergens. Indeed, the sequence results tend to confirm that important allergens have physical (but not biochemical) properties in common. The major inhalant allergens are freely soluble glycoproteins with MW between 10 000 and 50 000. In general, the important allergens represent a significant and sometimes large proportion of the soluble protein in a source (Chapman and Platts-Mills 1980). Furthermore, for most of the important inhalant allergens (e.g. grass pollen, dust mite, cat, ragweed, cockroach, parietaria, birch pollen, etc.), the proteins derived from that allergen can become the dominant foreign protein that is being inhaled. Thus, grass pollen in England is the most prevalent pollen, the commonest cause of IgE antibody production and the main cause of hay fever (Blackley 1873). Similarly, in a dry (i.e. few mites or fungi) house with cats, *Fel d* I becomes an important and probably the dominant foreign protein in house dust. In some carpet or bedding dust samples, mite faecal pellets have been estimated at 500 000 per gram, which makes them the commonest protein-carrying particle in the house (Tovey *et al.* 1981b; Dowse *et al.* 1985; Smith *et al.* 1985; Platts-Mills *et al.* 1986).

An apparent discrepancy occurs with airborne fungal spores. Airborne fungal spores may reach very large numbers in the outside air, often exceeding the number of pollen grains. Despite this, 'epidemic' allergic disease caused by fungal spores has only been documented in a few areas, e.g. *Alternaria* in the Midwest of the United States (O'Holleran *et al.* 1988). Furthermore, in most studies on asthmatics the prevalence of fungal sensitivity is not as high as that to pollens or dust mites (Green *et al.* 1986). There are two factors that may reduce the significance of fungal spores. First, many fungal spores are smaller than other particles and thus cannot carry as much protein. Spores of 5 μm or 2 μm diameter have respectively only 1/64 or 1/100 the volume of a pollen grain or mite faecal particles of 20 μm diameter. Second, and perhaps equally important, many fungal spores appear not to release proteins rapidly without physical disruption. Finally, estimates of the prevalence of sensitization assume that the diagnostic skin test reagents or *in vitro* assays have equivalent sensitivity. At present we do not know whether fungal extracts are equivalent in allergen content to pollen extracts. Rapid solubility of proteins carried on airborne particles is essential for the delivery of proteins to nasal lymphoid tissue. This is because particles landing on the mucus blanket of the nose are passed posteriorly by ciliary action and will be swallowed within 10–15 minutes. The acidity of the stomach contents will denature most allergens rapidly. For this reason it may be that mycelial elements of fungi with permeable or semi-permeable walls are more important than spores as sources of airborne allergens (Burge *et al.* 1987).

There are still many unanswered questions about the events that lead to IgE antibody responses. However, it remains true that the common allergens are those soluble proteins (or sources or proteins) which humans inhale repeatedly (i.e. over weeks or months) in the largest quantities. Although the quantities that become airborne are limited, it appears to be those proteins that are delivered to the nasal lymphoid tissue in the largest quantities for the longest period of time that give rise to persistent IgE antibody responses.

The immune response to inhalant allergens

The discovery of IgE and demonstration of its special ability to trigger mediator release from mast cells and basophils explained a large part of immediate hypersensitivity. Since it was also known that the serum of patients with atopic diseases did not contain precipitins and that their skin did not produce delayed hypersensitivity (DH) skin responses, it was easy to reach the conclusion that IgE antibodies explained allergic disease. However, a more realistic interpretation of the data suggests that IgE antibodies are necessary but not sufficient for the development of allergic disease. This conclusion is reached because some individuals have IgE antibodies but do not have symptoms, and the quantitative correlation between serum IgE antibodies and severity of disease is generally poor. A quantitative correlation has been reported between skin reactivity to *Amb a* I (from ragweed pollen) and severity of ragweed hay fever, but for other diseases this correlation is less clear (Norman *et al.* 1973). Thus, further understanding of the immune response to inhalants is essential in order to understand the relationship of IgE antibodies to disease.

Isotype-specific antibodies: systemic and local production

The first evidence for antibodies to allergens other than reagins came with the demonstration that serum from patients who had received immunotherapy would 'block' *in vitro* histamine release (Cooke *et al.* 1935). Following the recognition of IgG and IgA as separate isotypes, it became possible to identify IgG and IgA antibodies to allergens (Ishizaka *et al.* 1967; Tse *et al.* 1973). Using radiolabelled purified allergens to measure antibodies (either by radio-immunoelectrophoresis (RIEP) or with fluid-phase binding assays), the data have consistently shown that allergic individuals have IgG antibodies as well as IgE antibodies. These studies have also reported that IgG antibodies were at low levels or absent in the serum of non-allergic individuals. There have been several confusing reports that IgG antibodies to allergen are present in the serum of individuals without IgE antibodies (e.g. Soliman and Rosenstreich 1986). Most of these studies have used solid-phase techniques, i.e. RAST or ELISA, to measure IgG. The problem with these studies is to exclude non-specific binding of IgG to the solid phase. It is important to remember that IgG levels in serum are ~10 mg/ml, while total IgE levels are generally ≤1 μg/ml. Thus, even a very low percentage level of non-specific binding for IgG may make it difficult to interpret IgG antibody assays.

Since pollen grains are inhaled and deposited predominantly on the nasal mucosa, it is logical to consider in what sense the immune response is local to the nose. In considering the response to immunotherapy, it is also relevant to ask whether changes occur in local antibodies. Some early studies suggested that non-allergic individuals had nasal antibodies or nasal blocking activity (Turk *et al.* 1970; Stokes *et al.* 1974; Taylor 1974). These observations formed part of the argument that led to the now generally discarded view that allergy was in some sense a form of immune deficiency (Soothill 1976; see Platts-Mills 1982 for further discussion). Similarly, the view that delayed maturation of IgA in infancy predisposed to allergy has not been supported by studies on local antibody or by subsequent studies of serum IgA (Kaufman and Hobbs 1970; Kaufmann and Frick 1976; Cogswell *et al.* 1982). With all assays for antibodies, it is important to confirm the results. None of the reports of IgA or IgG antibodies in non-allergic individuals have been confirmed by alternative techniques, and at present it seems most likely that these results can be attributed to non-specific binding of either IgG or IgA to solid-phase immunosorbents.

The quantities of antibodies present in the nasal secretion of allergic individuals are not large and have generally required the use of radiolabelled antigens to detect them. However, the results have been confirmed by RIEP, by antigen-binding immunoprecipitation and by isotype-specific blocking of *in vitro* histamine release (Tse *et al.* 1973; Platts-Mills *et al.* 1976; Platts-Mills 1979) (Fig. 52.3). The presence of IgG and IgA antibodies in nasal secretions has been demonstrated convincingly, using *Amb a* I, *Lol p* I or *Der p* I as radiolabelled antigens. The simple presence of antibodies in nasal secretions does not define in what sense the response is local. Certainly, similar antibodies are present in the circulation. Most allergic individuals are sensitized in all relevant tissues, i.e. nose, conjunctiva, lungs and skin (Bruce *et al.* 1974; Cavanaugh *et al.* 1977). A detailed study relating nasal antibody and serum antibody concluded that the IgG and IgA antibodies in nasal secretions must be locally produced (Platts-Mills 1979). That study also found that antibodies to grass pollen were not present in saliva. This is interesting because it implies that the local response requires continuing exposure of tissues to allergen. It seems likely that antigens are transported from the nasal mucosa to the local lymph nodes and that B cells primed there return to mucosal surfaces. However, it appears that these B cells do not produce antibodies locally unless they are re-exposed to allergen. This is in contrast to B cells primed in the gut to bacterial antigens, which will produce antibodies locally in the breast in the absence of re-exposure to antigen. Analysing the changes in IgG antibodies to allergens that occur following immunotherapy shows a sharp increase ($\geq$10-fold) in serum antibodies with only modest ($\sim$ twofold) increases in local IgG (or IgA) antibody. This has two implications: first that the immune response to immunotherapy is probably in the central lymphoid tissue and second that the

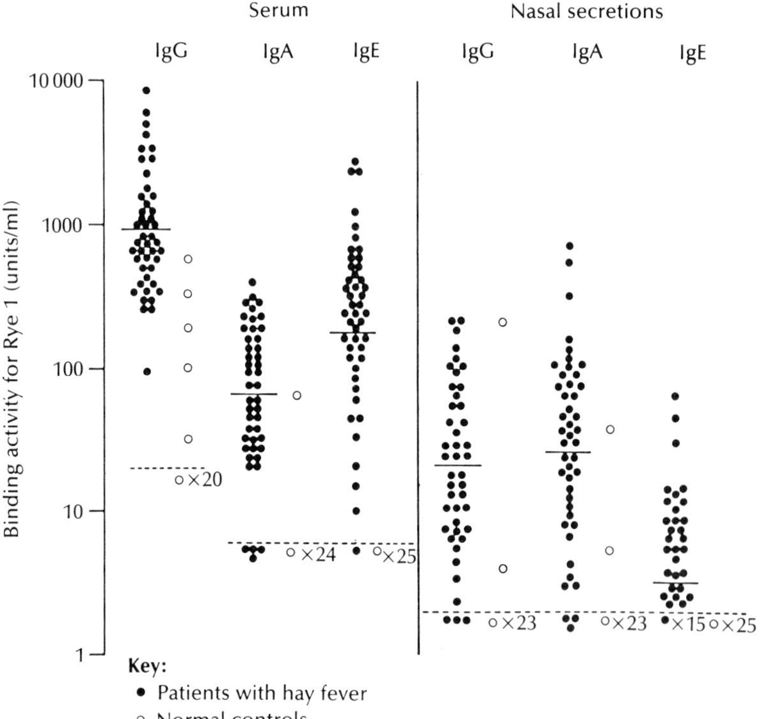

Fig. 52.3. Class-specific antibodies to a major grass pollen allergen (Rye I = *Lol p* I) in patients with hay fever and normal controls. Antibodies were measured by antigen-binding radioimmunoassay and are expressed in units of binding activity/ml of serum or concentrated nasal secretions. (Platts-Mills 1979.)

therapeutic effect of immunotherapy cannot be explained by increased blocking activity in nasal secretions.

Isotype-specific antibodies to allergens: immunoglobulin G subclasses

Analysis of the role of IgG subclasses in allergic disease was hampered for many years by confusion over the specificity of the reagents. With increasing availability of monoclonal antibodies to subclasses and WHO workshop agreement about the reagents, several conclusions are now becoming clear. Initially it was suggested that (as in mice) some subclass of human IgG might play a role in mediator release; both IgG-2 and IgG-4 were suggested. These views generally ignored the clear evidence that purified IgG (or IgA) antibodies were inactive in passive transfer (P–K) experiments. Several studies found that anti-IgG-4 could release mediators from mast cells or basophils. However, experiments using specifically purified IgG-4 antibodies to sensitize basophils for allergen-induced histamine release were consistently negative. In addition, individuals who make IgG-4 antibodies to such antigens as castor bean dust or common foods do not get either symptoms or positive skin tests unless they also have IgE antibodies. Thus, it is no longer considered likely that either IgG-4 or IgG-2 antibodies play a significant role in triggering mediator release from basophils or mast cells (see Van der Zee and Aalberse 1987 for detailed discussion).

Allergic individuals do have higher total serum IgG-4 than non-allergic individuals. In addition, IgG responses to allergens include a disproportionate quantity of IgG-4 antibodies (Aalberse *et al.* 1983). Interestingly, a similar relative increase in this subclass is found in the IgG response to parasites (Iskander *et al.* 1981; Ottessen *et al.* 1985). Aalberse and his colleagues in Amsterdam have made major contributions to this area and his work has also shown that IgG-4 antibodies (which were known not to fix complement) not only do not produce precipitin lines in gel but actually inhibit precipitation by IgG-1 antibodies. This appears to reflect the fact that they are functionally monovalent. The importance of this observation is that production of IgG-4 may represent a form of protection. The possibility is that an initial response that includes IgG-1 antibodies (precipitating and complement fixing) is beneficial in terms of neutralizing and clearing some antigens. On the other hand, an IgG-1 response that continues with a persistent exposure such as a parasite worm load or a commonly eaten food would have the potential for severe 'immune complex' disease. Thus, a progressive change to IgG-4 antibodies (non-precipitating and non-complement fixing) might reduce the likelihood of harmful effects from continued exposure. This kind of change in subclass could well be important in the mechanism by which non-IgE-mediated 'inflammatory' diseases related to food exposure (e.g. milk gastroenteropathy or pulmonary haemosiderosis) spontaneously improve as the children reach 2–3 years of age. Using an antigen-binding technique with radiolabelled antigens and monoclonal anti-IgG-4, we studied IgG-4 antibodies to several different allergens (Rowntree *et al.* 1987). The level of IgG-4 antibodies were raised relative to overall IgG antibodies, and this proportion further increased with desensitization treatment. For milk proteins, we observed changes in IgG-4, as a percentage of IgG antibodies, from 11% at 3 months of age to 50% at 5 years (Fig. 52.4).

In conclusion, there is excellent evidence that

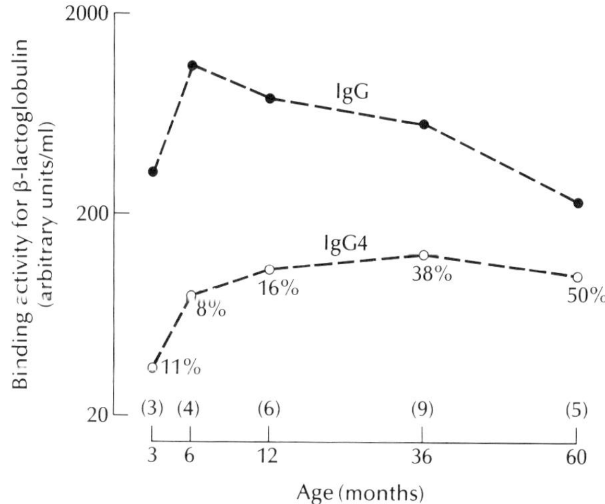

Fig. 52.4. Changes in IgG-4 antibodies relative to total IgG antibodies to β-lactoglobulin during the first 5 years of life. Total IgG antibody was measured using polyclonal goat anti-human IgG to precipitate IgG and radiolabelled β-lactoglobulin. IgG-4 antibodies were measured by using a monoclonal anti-IgG-4 antibody and a polyclonal rabbit anti-mouse IgG. The values under the IgG-4 data indicate IgG-4 antibody as a percentage of total IgG binding (see Rowntree *et al.* 1987).

the IgG response to inhalant, food and injected allergens includes a high proportion of IgG-4, and that this proportion can increase with persistent exposure. There is very little evidence that IgG-4 or any other subclass of IgG plays a role in mediator release *in vivo*. It is assumed that IgG-4 is not especially effective as a blocking antibody, since the *in vitro* evidence suggests that it is functionally monovalent. However, it is possible that the shift in IgG responses to IgG-4 which occurs with persistent exposure reduces the risk of immune complex or other inflammatory effects mediated by IgG-1 antibodies.

T cell responses to allergens

From the earliest work on hay fever, it was clear that the common inhalant allergens (i.e. pollens, animal dander, house dust) did not give rise to DH skin responses. This was true both for allergic and non-allergic individuals. Thus, in a clinic where intradermal skin testing is routinely performed (if prick tests are negative), the only antigens that commonly produce an indurated response at 24 and 48 hours are *Trichophyton* and *Candida*. The inhalants often give a 'late' reaction maximum at 6–8 hours but these generally follow large immediate reactions and are usually reduced or negative at 24–48 hours. On the other hand, it is now clear that IgE antibody responses in animals are absolutely T-cell-dependent. Thus, it seems reasonable to assume that allergic individuals make T cell responses but that these T cells in general do not give rise to DH skin responses. It is possible that the lack of delayed responses in allergic individuals occurs because the weal response 'washes out' or neutralizes antigen at the local site (Brostoff and Roitt 1969). Indeed, it was suggested shortly after the discovery of IgE that its primary role was as a 'gatekeeper' triggering the mobilization of serum (with antibodies) and effector cells to the local site (Steinberg *et al.* 1974). However, one would expect to see typical DH responses in some patients or non-allergic individuals if T cells of this kind were primed to inhalants. In 1963 Slavin and his colleagues showed that lymphocytes from patients with hay fever would not transfer DH unless the donor had received desensitization treatment. Until very recently, the only approach used to evaluate T cell sensitivity *in vitro* was to culture cells with antigen and demonstrate a specific proliferative response (Girard *et al.* 1967; Ishizaka *et al.* 1974; Rocklin *et al.* 1974; Black and Marsh 1980). Using cell separation experiments, surface marker studies and T cell cloning, it is clear that the responding cells are T cells predominantly of the helper phenotype (Lanzavecchia *et al.* 1983; Rawle *et al.* 1984; O'Hehir *et al.* 1988).

Recently analysis of the role of T cells in allergic disease has focussed on the development of T-cell clones. In particular clones specific for mite allergens have been developed by several groups (O'Hehir *et al.* 1991, Wierenga *et al.* 1990, Yssel *et al.* 1990, Parronichi *et al.* 1991). All groups have reported the production of T cell clones from allergic individuals and increasingly it is clear that these CD4 +ve clones produce IL-4 and will help IgE production *in vitro*. Similar clones can also be cloned from lesional skin of patients with atopic dermatitis (van der Heijden *et al.* 1991). Although lymphocytes from non-allergic individuals generally make very poor proliferative responses *in vitro*, several groups have reported the development of mite-specific T-cell clones. Clones from nonallergic individuals are also CD4 + ve but have properties more like Th-I cells in mice (Cherwinski *et al.* 1987, Snapper *et al.* 1988, Umetsu *et al.* 1988). Indeed the results on allergen specific T-cell clones represent some of the best evidence for a human analogy of ThI and Th2 cells.

T cell control of diseases associated with immediate hypersensitivity

In addition to playing a dominant role in the control of specific antibody responses, T cells may play other roles in the inflammation of allergic diseases. The ability of human T cells to produce local inflammatory responses in obvious. Contact sensitivity reactions caused by chemicals such as nickel (or the oils in poison ivy) are considered to be T-cell-mediated. Furthermore, positive patch responses to these chemicals include an eosinophil and basophil infiltrate and are histologically very similar to cutaneous basophil hypersensitivity reactions in guinea-pigs (Dvorak *et al.* 1974; Askenase 1979). The effector role of T cells in the inflammation associated with immediate hypersensitivity is less obvious but may be equally important. It is important to recognize that T cells may play several different roles, including: stimulating bone marrow production of granulocytes; recruitment of cells to local sites; and influencing the function of both granulocytes and mast cells in local tissues.

For many years, it was generally held that the number of mast cells in the nose of allergic individuals was the same as in normals. However, this view was based on nasal biopsies, in which the epithelium was disrupted and the mucus was not visible (see Mygind 1979). On the other hand, it was well known that nasal 'reactivity' to allergens could change. McLean *et al.* (1977) reported that nasal non-specific reactivity increased during the pollen season and then fell again. Since 1977, there have been several reports clearly establishing that both basophils in the mucus and mast cells in the nasal epithelium increase during the pollen season (Okuda and Otsuka 1977; Hastie *et al.* 1979; Mitchell and Askenase 1983; Denburg *et al.* 1985; Otsuka *et al.* 1986; Bochner *et al.* 1988). It has not been formally established that localization of these metachromatic cells to the nose is mediated by T cells in the human. However, there is good evidence that mast cell or basophil localization in animals is T-cell-dependent and that human T cells can release basophil chemotactic factors.

The possible role of T cells in atopic dermatitis (AD) is suggested both by the presence of T cells in the natural skin lesions and by the parallels between skin responses to a patch test with contact sensitizers on the one hand or allergens on the other. The skin lesions of naturally occurring atopic dermatitis include a lymphocyte infiltrate, and Geha and his colleagues (Leung *et al.* 1983, 1987) have demonstrated that these T cells are CD4 +ve. Recently Frew and Kay (1988) have shown that injection of sufficient antigen into the skin of allergic individuals will routinely lead to a local accumulation of CD4 +ve cells. Injection of allergen into the dermis is not an effective way of producing a patch of atopic dermatitis; however, application of allergen (e.g. *Der p* I) as a patch test for 48 hours will produce an eczematous response (Mitchell *et al.* 1982; Adinoff *et al.* 1988; Bruijnzeel-Koomen *et al.* 1988). Microscopically these patches of eczema induced in patients with AD include basophils, eosinophils and lymphocytes. In order to ask how much of this 'eczematous' response was mediated by IgE on mast cells, we carried out local passive transfer experiments (Mitchell *et al.* 1984). The skin response to a patch of *Der p* I after passive transfer of IgE antibody is erythematous (rather than eczematous) and includes eosinophils (but not basophils). However, the simple view that the presence of basophils demonstrates a local role for T cells was weakened by finding that the local transfer of whole serum from patients with AD to a normal recipient would transfer the ability to recruit both basophils and eosinophils (Mitchell *et al.* 1984). The local response to allergen has a marked eosinophil infiltrate, which is not obvious in naturally occurring lesions of AD. It is assumed that eosinophils degranulate locally, since the skin of AD patients is heavily infiltrated with eosinophil major basic protein (MBP) (Leiferman *et al.* 1985); and continued application of allergen to a patch test site (for 8 days) leads to a sharp fall in the eosinophil infiltrate (Mitchell *et al.* 1986). Adinoff and his colleagues (1988) have reported that eczematous patch responses to allergens are poor or absent in allergic patients who have asthma but not AD. This implies that the patch response may actually be a model for the way in which this allergic response is localized to the skin. At present, the mechanisms controlling the localization of allergic inflammation to the skin (or lungs or nose) are very poorly understood.

Either dust mite allergens or poison ivy extract applied to the skin of appropriately sensitive individuals can produce an eczematous response which is, histologically, cutaneous basophil hypersensitivity (Dvorak *et al.* 1974; Mitchell *et al.* 1982). If the sensitized T cells found in patients with AD play a major role in the skin inflammation, an obvious question to ask is how these T cells relate to the T cells produced against contact sensitizing agents. There is a wealth of animal work on contact sensitization (Asherson *et al.* 1980; Van Loveren and Askenase 1984; Askenase 1992). However, very little is known about the T cells that give rise to contact dermatitis in man. It is likely that T cell sensitization in the skin requires Langerhans' cells, since ultraviolet (UV) treatment can block sensitization (Stingl *et al.* 1981; Bergstressor and Streilein 1983). The use of UV light and psoralens may have a similar effect in man.

It is now 20 years since it was first suggested that the ease with which basophils released histamine on exposure to allergen was an important factor influencing the severity of allergic disease (Sadan *et al.* 1969; Lichtenstein and Levy 1972; May and Williams 1973). Initially it was assumed that this releasability was a property of the individual's basophils or mast cells. However, it proved difficult to establish a clear relationship between releasability and severity of disease. In 1984 Lett-Brown and his colleagues reported that human lymphocytes could produce a factor which increased the 'releasability' of basophils. Initially these histamine-releasing factors (HRF) were greeted with considerable scepticism. However, the work has been confirmed in several laboratories and the properties of T-cell-derived HRF are increasingly well defined (Sedgwick *et al.* 1981; Kaplan *et al.* 1985; Alam *et al.* 1988; Lichtenstein 1988). A major area of interest is in understanding why basophils from some individuals respond to HRF and in particular whether this reflects differences in the IgE (MacDonald *et al.* 1987). Since the amino acid sequence of HRF has not been established, it remains possible that HRF is related to one of the already defined interleukins. Interleukin 3 has activity in stimulating growth of basophils and mast cells but does not appear to explain HRF activity (Ihle *et al.* 1982; Alam *et al.* 1988). Whatever the exact nature of HRF, the demonstration that a product of T cells can influence the ease with which mediators are released from basophils is clearly of great importance in understanding the symptoms of allergic disease. Similar T cell products could play a role in contact sensitivity, mediating both the initial recruitment of T cells and the wealing and severe pruritus so common in poison ivy skin lesions. Indeed, the interesting question is whether human T cells produce antigen-specific products which can sensitize skin mast cells (as well as basophils), comparable to those demonstrated in mice (Van Loveren and Askenase 1984). Such antigen-specific T-cell-derived molecules could play a central role in atopic dermatitis but have not yet been demonstrated in humans.

Eosinophilia, both of purified blood and of local tissues, is a striking feature of allergic disease. It is well established that eosinophilia and eosinophil bone marrow production in animals is T-cell-dependent (Sanderson *et al.* 1985). In man it is assumed that T cells stimulate the production of eosinophils from the bone marrow, presumably by release of IL-5 or a similar lymphokine. Local recruitment of eosinophils may be primarily mediated by mast cell products, such as leucotriene B-4 or platelet-activating factor (PAF), but T cells are also capable of recruiting eosinophils to local tissues. An important implication is that, since T cells are most likely to be driven by a foreign antigen, the presence of eosinophilia may be taken to imply that there is persistent stimulation by a foreign antigen. Recently, it has been shown that circulating basophil precursors, presumably bone marrow-derived, increase during exacerbations of allergic diseases, particularly asthma (Denburg *et al.* 1985). It is assumed that bone marrow production of basophils and their precursors is also T-cell-dependent.

In conclusion, there are now a series of ways in which T cells could influence the severity of allergic disease (Table 52.2). While it seems inevitable that T cells play some role in symptoms, the relative importance of these different roles will be difficult to sort out *in vivo*. However, with the availability of T cell clones, fragments of allergens that selectively stimulate T cells and accurate assays for interleukins, answering these questions becomes a possibility. While most of the possible roles of T cells act to enhance IgE-mediated responses, there are ways in which T cells could contribute to 'inflammation' unrelated to IgE. Data available at present suggest that the common inhalant allergens only produce significant symptoms in patients who have produced IgE antibodies. This implies either that T cells alone are not sufficient to produce symptoms under conditions of natural exposure or that T cell responses of this kind 'only' occur in parallel with IgE antibody responses. Contact sensitizing agents can induce a T cell

Table 52.2. The role of T cells in 'allergic' disease

Helper cells for IgE production
Production of interleukins that control bone marrow production of eosinophils (IL-5) and basophils (TCGF) (IL-3)
Recruitment of basophils and mast cells to local sites. Local increases of these cells have been demonstrated in hay fever and atopic dermatitis
Recruitment of eosinophils to local sites:[a] Probably a dominant role for T cells in contact sensitivity Potentially an inflammatory role for T cells in other 'allergic' diseases which is independent of IgE
Production of factors that influence the releasability of mast cells and basophils — histamine — releasing factors (HRF)

a T cells may also play a role in eosinophil degranulation.
TCGF = T-cell growth factor.

response which produces local 'inflammation' without a role for IgE antibody. Presumably, responses of this kind cannot be (or are not) induced by antigens absorbed through the nasal mucosa. Understanding the details of the way(s) in which T cells influence the severity of allergic disease will inevitably increase our understanding of the way these responses could act in the immune response to parasites. In addition, these experiments may well make it possible to understand how injections of allergens (acting on T cells?) could alter the symptoms of allergic disease.

Asthma as a disease of chronic bronchial inflammation

The complex nature of allergic disease is well illustrated by asthma. Developing immediate hypersensitivity to common inhalant allergens is a major risk factor for asthma. This is true for chronic disease in children, for bronchial reactivity in school populations and for acute asthma in adults (Smith *et al.* 1969; Pollart *et al.* 1988, 1989; Peat *et al.* 1989; Sporik *et al.* 1990). However, the disease is not explained by immediate hypersensitivity and many (if not most) allergic individuals do not develop asthma. Furthermore, it is now clear that the response of the lung to allergen exposure includes chronic changes. These may persist for weeks after a single exposure, and may take months to resolve when patients are removed from chronic exposure (Kerrebijn 1970; Cartier *et al.* 1982; Platts-Mills *et al.* 1982). The mechanism of these prolonged effects is not fully understood, but it is likely that a secondary infiltration with eosinophils plays an important role in producing inflammation and epithelial damage (Gleich *et al.* 1988). Over the last few years the use of bronchial biopsy and broncho-alveolar lavage has provided better understanding of the pathological changes in mild asthma and following allergen challenges (Metzger *et al.* 1987; Beasley *et al.* 1989). However, although it seems inevitable that T cells play a role in inflammation of the bronchi either directly or by recruiting granulocytes to the lung, it is still difficult to provide an estimate of the importance of these events (Corrigan *et al.* 1991). Thus, as with other allergic diseases, IgE antibodies are necessary but not sufficient and T cells may be very important in controlling the severity of the disease. Since the inflammatory response is not immediate in onset and is persistent, it is not surprising that patients are often unaware of the factors that lead to progressive increases in bronchial reactivity (Fig. 52.5). By contrast, patients clearly understand the many non-specific triggers that can make their already irritable lungs go into bronchospasm. Most of the common triggers are not causes of asthma, e.g. cold air, exercise, tobacco smoke, diurnal variation and emotion.

The impact of allergens on the lung must depend on the local concentration of allergen and thus on the characteristics of the particles carrying allergen. It is very striking that the major form in which dust mite allergen becomes airborne is as faecal pellets with a mean diameter of >10 μm (Tovey *et al.* 1981a, b) (Fig. 52.6). Natural exposure to a few (i.e. <200) faecal particles or pollen grains per day may be the ideal way to produce increased bronchial reactivity without noticeable acute episodes of bronchospasm at the time of exposure. By contrast, the cat allergen *Fel d* I is airborne on small

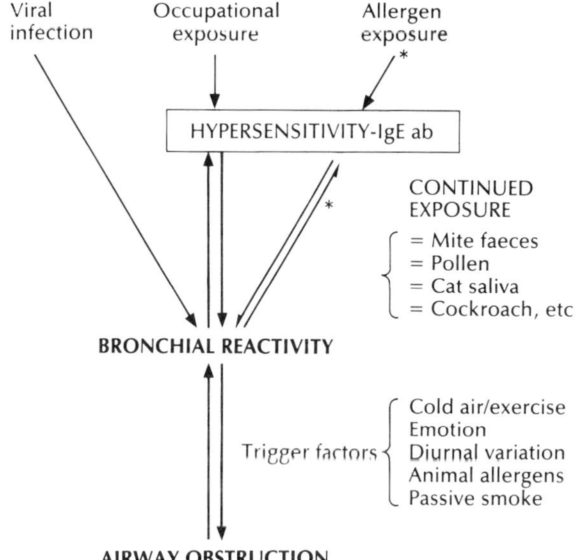

Fig. 52.5. Causes of asthma. The initial role of allergens is to provoke immediate-hypersensitivity immune responses. The patients who develop IgE are at increased risk of bronchial reactivity and symptomatic asthma if they have continued exposure. The development of bronchial reactivity is shown as a reversible phenomenon, but it may, at least in part, be irreversible. Patients are generally aware of the 'trigger factors' that precipitate acute attacks, but are generally unaware of the underlying exposure that gives rise to bronchial reactivity.

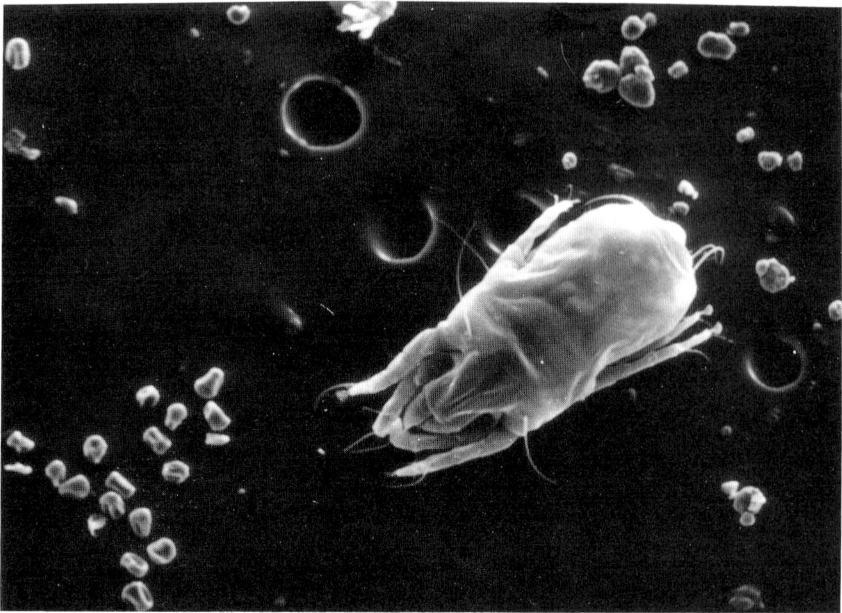

Fig. 52.6. Female *Dermatophagoides pteronyssinus* under scanning electron microscopy (approx. real size 300 μm long). In the bottom left are a group of biconcave rye grass pollen grains; at the upper left are mite faecal particles (see Tovey *et al.* 1981a).

particles which remain airborne and are inhaled in much larger numbers (Findlay *et al.* 1983; Swanson *et al.* 1985; Luczynska *et al.* 1989b). The size and number of particles carrying cat allergen explains why cat-allergic patients often develop acute symptoms, including bronchospasm, on entering a house with a cat. The importance of particles to lung disease is strongly supported by the contrasts between asthma and extrinsic allergic alveolitis (EAA). The antigens that give rise to EAA are often airborne as 10^9 particles of ≤ 2 μm diameter/m^3 (Pepys 1971; Belin 1980, 1982; Fink 1986) (see Chapter 98). The immune response includes precipitating antibodies and a T cell response which in animals can transfer the disease (Bice *et al.* 1976; Belin 1980; Strickler *et al.* 1986). Furthermore, the T cells found in the lungs of patients with EAA are predominantly CD8 +ve (Leatherman *et al.* 1984). Thus, the disease of EAA is completely different from asthma, the form of exposure is strikingly different, and the immune response of these patients is distinct from immediate hypersensitivity responses. Furthermore, there is very little 'crossover' between EAA and asthma. The allergens that give rise to asthma are not recognized as causes of EAA and neither mouldy hay (actinomycete spores), bagasse nor mould on lumber in Scandinavia has been recognized as a cause of asthma.

Understanding the role of allergens in bronchial inflammation becomes more complicated when it comes to non-inhaled antigens, such as foods or dermatophytes. Recent evidence has confirmed that some patients who would otherwise be classified as cases of intrinsic asthma are specifically sensitive to antigens derived from the athletes' foot fungus, *Trichophyton* (Platts-Mills *et al.* 1987a; Ward *et al.* 1989). Here the exposure is continuous and presumably is blood-borne. In contrast to the inhaled allergens, many 'normal', i.e. non-allergic, individuals have profound delayed hypersensitivity to *Trichophyton*. Thus, *Trichophyton* represents an example of a different dichotomy, where infected individuals can develop either DH or IgE antibody responses. Several previous studies have suggested that the nature of the immune response to *Trichophyton* influences the progression of the skin disease (Hay and Shennan 1984; Honbo *et al.* 1984). At present, asthma and rhinitis have only been associated with those individuals who develop IgE antibodies and have persistent infection of their feet and toe-nails (Ward *et al.* 1989). Again, it is presumably the nature of the initial T cell response that dictates the difference between an IgE response and a DH response. It is increasingly likely that the primary role of allergens in asthma is to maintain chronic inflammation of the bronchi. This inflammation is dominated by eosinophils but also includes metachromatic cells and in some way leads to increased bronchial reactivity. Although IgE is a remarkably consistent feature of the immune responses associated with asthma, the reaction to antigens is chronic and delayed rather than immediate.

Immunobiology of immediate hypersensitivity

By definition allergy is an immune response that causes harmful or annoying symptoms on exposure to an otherwise harmless environmental antigen. If so, there cannot be a beneficial effect of allergy itself. No convincing argument has been presented that hay fever, anaphylaxis or asthma is beneficial to the sufferer. The question is, what is or was the biological significance of this form of immunity? As we have discussed, the response is complex and it is not likely that the significance is restricted to a single situation. The obvious parallels are with the system for defence against helminths (Butterworth *et al.* 1975; Chapter 83). Helminths induce IgE antibodies and eosinophilia; they can also lead to localization of mast cells and basophils. It is very likely that mast cell triggering at the site of entry of a larva, with subsequent arrival of both IgG antibodies and eosinophils, represents an important mechanism for controlling excessive worm load.

In the following section, the possible roles for some of the different elements that make up the immune response to allergens will be discussed:

1 Isotype-specific antibody responses.
2 Mast cells and basophils.
3 T cells as effector cells.
4 Antigen-presenting cells and T cells as helper cells for isotype-specific responses.

Isotype-specific antibody responses

The dominant view of IgE is as a specific trigger for mediator release from those cells bearing a high-affinity receptor for IgE ($Fc_\varepsilon RI$). It is important not to underestimate the effectiveness of this system. With many purified proteins, *in vitro* histamine release or *in vivo* skin tests can be achieved with as little as 0.05 ml of 10^{-7} μg/ml. For a protein with a molecular weight of 24 000 (e.g. *Der p* I), this represents $\leq 10^{-13}$ M. In addition, the response is very rapid. Weal formation can often be seen within 2 minutes, sneezing can occur in 30 seconds and *in vitro* histamine release can occur within 2 minutes (Hastie *et al.* 1979). Thus, IgE-mediated histamine release represents an extremely sensitive and rapid mechanism for detecting the arrival of a foreign protein into the skin or respiratory tract. That similar mechanisms can occur in the gut is obvious from animal studies on helminths, but our understanding of local allergic reactions in human intestines is still limited (Lessof *et al.* 1988; see Chapter 56). Given that many larvae entering the body rapidly develop systems to avoid the host's immune response, it is obvious that a system that is both sensitive and rapid may be very important.

Whether IgE has any other role is an interesting question. It is most unlikely to have any role other than those dependent on its homocytropic properties. This is because the quantities of IgE are small, and IgE is rarely, if ever, produced in the absence of an IgG antibody response. It has been suggested that IgE antibodies play a role in triggering eosinophils. This area has become confused with the whole issue of low-affinity IgE receptors ($Fc_\varepsilon RII$). There is no doubt that many cells, including lymphocytes, bear low-affinity receptors for IgE. However, there is some doubt about whether IgE does bind to these receptors *in vivo* and whether binding IgE is the biological function of these receptors (Delespesse *et al.* 1988, 1989). The situation with regard to eosinophils is further confused because some studies have difficulty demonstrating low-affinity IgE receptors on these cells, while other groups have consistently reported IgE-mediated triggering of eosinophils (Joault *et al.* 1988). A recent study on eosinophil triggering found no evidence for a role of IgE but surprisingly found that both IgG and IgA antibodies could cause mediator release (Abu-Ghazaleh *et al.* 1989). Eosinophils are well known to have a high-affinity receptor for Fc_γ which can trigger mediator release. This presence of a specificity control over eosinophil triggering may be important biologically, because eosinophils carry extremely toxic substances, e.g. MBP, eosinophil cationic protein (ECP) and neurotoxins. At present, the clear evidence is that IgE plays a primary role in controlling mediator release from basophils and mast cells but has no other established role. By contrast, IgG (and IgA), which binds poorly if at all to mast cells and basophils, is an important trigger for eosinophils.

Mobilization of mast cells and basophils

The simple view that mast cells were fixed in the tissues while basophils were circulating cells is no longer tenable. Our understanding of basophil localization was limited for many years because most common fixation techniques (e.g. formalin) left basophils microscopically indistinguishable from neutrophils. It is now clear that mobilization of basophils to a local site is a significant element of many immune responses in animals, as well as of allergic responses in man. While it is obvious that basophils moving into the mucus of the respiratory tract could increase the speed and sensitivity of mediator release, it is likely that basophils have other roles. The clearest example is the tick model described by Bagnall (1975) in Australia. On primary exposure, ticks feed for several days on guinea-pigs and finally fall off satiated. On repeated exposure of these animals, the ticks fall off within a day and die. Examination of the gut of the dead ticks reveals large numbers of guinea-pig-derived basophils. While it is probable that the toxicity of these basophils is related to their mediators, it is unlikely that this release is dependent on IgE antibodies. The normal mechanisms for basophil and mast cell recruitment are dependent on T cells. Askenase and associates have made a very strong case that these T cells can also specifically sensitive mast cells and basophils (Meade *et al.* 1988). Certainly, the intense itching and wealing of contact sensitivity reactions would best be understood if T cells not only recruited these cells but also sensitized them to react to the antigen locally. As Michael Jagger so clearly explained, one of the true advantages of the United States is a proper appreciation for the morbidity that can be caused by contact sensitivity to a common plant.

The important conclusion in terms of biological role is that mast cells and basophils have a role independent of IgE antibodies. Indeed, cells of this kind probably had a role in immunity prior to the evolution of antibody isotypes. The next question is whether these cells have or have had a biological role other than defence. Histamine and other vasoactive mediators (e.g. serotonin) released in small quantities could play an important role in homoeostasis of local tissue pressure, blood supply, etc. Several mechanisms for non-anaphylactic release of mediators from mast cells have been proposed; however, it is very difficult to assess whether these systems play a role *in vivo* (Galli and Dvorak 1979). An interesting new light has been shed on the whole area by the demonstration that most tissue mast cells are directly innervated by autonomic nerves (Bienenstock 1988). With increasing appreciation of the biological activity of neuropeptides, it now seems likely that these nerves have the capability of controlling local mast cell release of histamine and other mediators. Indeed, many of the clinical patterns of angio-oedema would be very difficult to explain if the nervous system did not play a role: for example, patients who always have one-sided angio-oedema of the face or body, or individuals whose hives are triggered at a precise time each day.

Thus, both mast cells and basophils should be seen as cells that:

1 Can be recruited to local areas of 'inflammation'.
2 Can probably be specifically sensitized by T cell products as well as IgE antibodies.
3 Have mediators which may be released gradually as well as anaphylactically.
4 May well be controlled or modulated by the autonomic system.

T cells as effector cells

If the primary role of T cells in human immunity were as helper cells for antibody production, then one would expect that the acquired immune deficiency syndrome (AIDS) could be managed with injections of immunoglobulin. In fact, patients with AIDS develop a series of rather specific diseases which are otherwise relatively uncommon. The disease can present with yeast infection of the oropharynx and gastrointestinal (GI) tract; *Pneumocystis* infection of the lungs; atypical tuberculosis (TB); Kaposi's sarcoma; or cryptococcal meningitis. Many physicians have never seen these diseases except in patients with AIDS. The patients progressively lose CD4 +ve cells, DH skin responses and *in vitro* proliferative responses to phytohaemagglutinin (PHA). Prior to the onset of AIDS, near complete loss of *in vitro* proliferative responses to PHA was very rare, even in an immune deficiency referral centre (Asherson and Webster 1980). At present, it is not clear why a viral infection that is cytotoxic to CD4 +ve T cells should produce this particular group of diseases (Fauci 1988). However, the likely answer is that they are all conditions where normal immunity depends on the effector role of these T cells.

In animal models, mucosal immunity to yeasts is T-cell-dependent, while the primary defence against fungal or yeast invasion of the bloodstream is provided by neutrophils. Very little is known about the normal immune mechanisms for preventing *Pneumocystis* infection (which must be very effective). In thinking about the reasons why deficiency of CD4 +ve cells leads to these diseases, it may be important to think of T cells both as effectors of local inflammation and in the role of controlling bone marrow production of eosinophils and basophils. Patients with AIDS commonly have short episodes of eosinophilia related to atypical TB or *Pneumocystis* infection but generally do not have persistent eosinophilia. Terminally, many AIDS patients become eosinophil-'deficient', with few or no eosinophils detectable in the peripheral blood. This is a pattern that is rare otherwise, but has been seen in patients with primary immune deficiency associated with thymoma and a decreased percentage of CD4 +ve cells (Mitchell *et al.* 1982). It is likely that the loss of eosinophils reflects failure of bone marrow production secondary to lack of IL-5, which is normally produced by CD4 +ve cells. The interesting question is whether eosinophil responses are quantitatively or functionally deficient from an early stage of the disease. In turn, it is possible that much of clinical AIDS could reflect subsequent failure of the effector role of T cells in recruiting granulocytes to local tissues.

In the progression of AIDS, many patients initially have difficulty with 'allergy', but in the later stages, as expected, they get progressively less reaction to environmental allergens. Interestingly, total serum IgA levels, but not IgE levels, rise with progression of AIDS (Fling *et al.* 1988). This phenomenon has also been observed in patients with hypogammaglobulinaemia associated with thymoma and a low CD4 : CD8 ratio (Platts-Mills *et al.* 1981; Mitchell *et al.* 1983). Overall, the devastation wrought by AIDS leaves no doubt that these T cells play a very important and probably constant role in defence that is not restricted to tropical parasites.

Antigen-presenting cells and T cells as 'helpers' for antibody production

What is the real difference between allergic (or atopic) individuals and non-allergic individuals? Although it has been proposed that there are differences in mast cells/basophils; or that their IgE is different; or that they have deficient T cell function, the evidence is not compelling for any of these differences. It has also been proposed that allergic individuals would be more effective at clearing helminths; however, there is little or no evidence for this. It appears that everyone is capable of making an IgE response to schistosomes, hookworm or scabies and that subtle differences between atopic and non-atopic individuals are not critical. Mast cell deficiency in humans is extremely rare, if it exists, and is certainly not the basis for a difference between allergic and non-allergic individuals. The real difference is that atopic individuals recognize and respond to the very low concentrations of airborne foreign proteins while non-allergic individuals do not. We assume that the immune response occurs in the draining lymph nodes, since IgE-producing plasma cells are found in these nodes (Tada and Ishizaka 1970; Mayerhoffer *et al.* 1976). It is not clear how inhaled proteins actually move from the nasal mucosa to the lymph nodes. Physical constraints would suggest that proteins of molecular weight less than 60 000 could penetrate the basement membrane, while molecules less than 5000 would pass straight into the circulation. Thus, molecules the size of most important allergens (i.e. $<60\,000$ and >5000) might be expected to end up in lymphatics. On the other hand, there are Ia +ve cells in the epithelial lining of the respiratory tract (Holt *et al.* 1985; Holt and Sedgwick 1987). These cells are thought to be capable of accumulating antigen and carrying it to the local lymph nodes. Thus, the difference between atopic and non-atopic individuals may well be in the function of these antigen-presenting cells of the upper respiratory tract.

Why do almost one-third of all humans maintain a recognition system that is so sensitive that it responds to otherwise irrelevant environmental proteins? At present, there are two probable answers.

1 Under natural circumstances of poor hygiene, no immunization, helminth load, poor diet, etc., humans normally do not make these responses. Alternatively, under these conditions allergic disease never reaches a level where the morbidity is significant. Certainly asthma is in general a more severe problem in developed countries, which may reflect different housing conditions but may also reflect a protective effect of primitive conditions. However, a recent severe epidemic of asthma in natives of Papua New Guinea suggests that, given adequate exposure to dust mites, almost any group can develop IgE responses and asthma (Dowse *et al.* 1985).

2 The second explanation is that individuals who have an increased ability to recognize foreign antigens have a survival advantage. In order to identify this advantage, we would need to search for negative associations between atopy and other diseases (Platts-Mills 1982). It is certainly possible that 'atopic' individuals had a significant survival advantage in one of the major epidemics of the past, e.g. influenza, tuberculosis, plague or smallpox. Under current circumstances in the Western world, it would be very difficult to identify such an advantage. However, a minor survival advantage in any of these epidemics could well explain why this 'genetic' trait should persist at such a high frequency in the population.

Conclusion

When humans are exposed to otherwise harmless environmental antigens, they can make a variety of different immune responses. Low-molecular-weight chemicals applied to the skin produce a T cell response which is capable of producing a dermatitis which is, histologically, cutaneous basophil hypersensitivity. Inhaling very large numbers of small fungal or actinomycete spores (≤ 2 μm diameter) can give rise to precipitating IgG antibodies and an associated T cell response. Further exposure of these individuals produces a characteristic inflammation focused on the peripheral lung — EAA. Repeated exposure of the nose to particles carrying soluble proteins, e.g. pollen grains, mite faecal pellets or cat 'dander', can produce an immune response, including IgE antibodies and CD4 +ve T cells. Repeated exposure of these individuals can produce anaphylaxis, hay fever, asthma or AD. Increasingly, it appears that T cells play a critical role in the inflammation induced by common allergens and that these effector T cells have much in common with the T cells that produce contact sensitivity. Overall, it is clear that 'allergic' disease involves many different forms of immune response, and it would be wrong to interpret the biological significance of immediate hypersensitivity simply as the role of IgE.

The close parallels between allergy and the immune response to helminths are obvious. Indeed, it seems reasonable to describe much of allergic disease as a mistaken attempt to kill, cough out or scratch out invading helminth larvae. The simple sequence is rapid release of mediators from mast cells sensitized with specific IgE antibodies, which leads to an influx of serum and granulocytes. Following this, IgG and possibly IgE antibodies bind to the 'invader' and trigger eosinophils through Fc receptors. The role of T cells in this process is not immediately obvious. However, it is likely that T cells can sensitize local tissues specifically, recruit granulocytes and stimulate eosinophil production from the bone marrow. Finally, although these immune mechanisms all represent important aspects of protective immunity, they do not appear to be the difference between allergic and non-allergic individuals. Non-allergic individuals are equally able to make IgE responses to helminths, to localize basophils, mast cells or eosinophils and to make T cell responses to contact sensitizing agents. The real difference appears to be that allergic individuals are able to recognize and respond to levels of antigen in the environment that are 'ignored' by non-allergic individuals. Inhalant allergy is the price we pay for maintaining an immune system capable of killing helminth larvae, and also an antigen recognition system sufficiently sensitive to respond to 1 μg pollen antigen inhaled over a 100-day season, i.e. 10 ng soluble protein/day. Although the exact biological role of such a sensitive system is not clear, it may well have been relevant to survival during one of the major pandemics of the past. It is also possible that these recognition systems are essential for monitoring the body for the development of abnormal or malignant changes in surface antigens. The fact that symptomatic allergic disease persists in up to 25% of the population suggests strongly that these diseases represent the consequence of a system that has or has had a significant survival advantage.

Acknowledgements

I am grateful to my many colleagues in Virginia for discussion and help with this chapter. I am particularly grateful to Nancy Malone for preparing the manuscript. This work was supported by NIH Grant No. AI-20565.

References

Aalberse, R.C., van de Gaag, R. and van Leeuven, J (1983). Serologic aspects of IgG4 antibodies. 1. Prolonged immunization results in an IgG4-restricted response. *J. Immunol.* **130**, 722.

Abu-Ghazaleh, R.I., Fujisawa, T., Mestecky, J., Kyle, R.A. and Gleich, G.J. (1989). IgA induced eosinophil degranulation. *J. Immunol.* **142**, 2393.

Adinoff, A.D., Teller, P. and Clark, R.A.F. (1988). Atopic dermatitis and aeroallergen contact sensitivity. *J. Allergy Clin. Immunol.* **81**, 736.

Alam, R., Grant, J.A. and Lett-Brown, M.A. (1988). Identification of a histamine release inhibitory factor produced by human mononuclear cells *in vitro*. *J. Am. Soc. Clin. Invest.* **82**, 2056.

Ansari, A.A., Kihara, T.K. and Marsh, D.G. (1987). Immunochemical studies of *Lolium perenne* (rye grass) pollen allergens, *Lol p* I, II and III. *J. Immunol.* **139**, 4034.

Arlian, L.G., Vyszenski-Moher, D.L. and Gilmore, A.M. (1988). Cross-antigenicity between *Sarcoptes scabiei* and the house dust mite, *Dermatophagoides farinae* (Acari: Sarcoptidae and Pyroglyphidae). *J. Med. Entomol.* **25**, 240.

Asherson, G.L. and Webster, A.D.B. (1980). *Diagnosis and Treatment of Immunodeficiency Diseases*. Blackwell Scientific Publications, Oxford.

Asherson, G.L., Zembala, M., Thomas, W.R. and Perera, M.A. (1980). Suppressor cells and the handling of antigen. *Immunol. Rev.* **50**, 3.

Askenase, P.W. (1979). Basophil arrival and function in tissue hypersensitivity reactions. *J. Allergy Clin. Immunol.* **64**, 79.

Askenase, P.W. (1992). Delayed-type hypersensitivity (DTH) recruitment of T cell subsets via antigen-specific non IgE factors or IgE antibodies. In *Progress in Chemical Immunology*. ed. R. Coffman Karger, Basel.

Bach, M.K., Bach, S., Brashler, J.R., Ishizaka, T. and Ishizaka, K. (1978). On the nature of the presumed receptor for IgE on mast cells. V. Enhanced binding of ^{125}I labelled IgE to cell-free particulate fractions in the presence of protease inhibitors. *Int. Arch. Allergy Appl. Immunol.* **56**, 1.

Bagnall, B.G. (1975). Cutaneous immunity to the tick *Ixodes halacyclus*. Thesis, University of Sydney.

Beasley, R., Roche, W.R., Roberts, J.A. and Holgate, S.T. (1989). Cellular events in the bronchi in mild asthma and after bronchial provocation. *Am. Rev. Respir. Dis.* **139**, 806–817.

Belin, L. (1980). Clinical and immunological data on 'Wood trimmer's disease' in Sweden. *Eur. J. Respir. Dis.* **61**, 169.

Belin, L. (1982). Experimental and clinical aspects of allergic alveolitis. In *Theoretical and Clinical Aspects of Allergic Disease*, ed. H. Bostrom and N. Ljungstedt, p. 77, Almqvist and Wiksell International, Stockholm.

Bennich, H. and Johansson, S.G.O. (1971). Structure and function of human immunoglobulin E. *Adv. Immunol.* **13**, 1.

Bennich, H., Ragnarsson, U., Johansson, S.G.O. *et al.* (1977). Failure of the putative IgE pentapeptide to compete with IgE for receptors on basophils and mast cells. *Int. Arch. Allergy Appl. Immunol.* **53**, 459.

Berrens, L. (1974). Inhalant allergens in human atopic disease: their chemistry and mode of action. *Ann. NY Acad. Sci.* **221**, 183.

Bergstressor, P.R. and Streilein, J.W. (1983). Ultraviolet radiation produces selective immune incompetence. *J. Invest. Dermatol.* **81**, 85.

Bice, D.E., Salvaggio, J.E. and Hofmann, E. (1976). Passive transfer of experimental hypersensitivity pneumonitis with lymphoid cells in the rabbit. *J. Allergy Clin. Immunol.* **58**, 250.

Bienenstock, J. (1988). An update on mast cell heterogeneity including comments on mast cell/nerve relationships. *J. Allergy Clin. Immunol.* **81**, 763.

Black, P.L. and Marsh, D.G. (1980). Correlation between lymphocyte responses and immediate hypersensitivity to purified allergens. *J. Allergy Clin. Immunol.* **66**, 394.

Blackley, C.H. (1873). *Experiments and Researches on the Causes and Nature of Catarrhus Aestivus*. Baillière, London.

Bochner, B.S., Schleimer, R.P., Charlesworth, E.N., Lamas, A.M. and Lichtenstein, L.M. (1988). Basophil activation and recruitment in allergic disease. In *Progress in Allergy and Clinical Immunology: Proceedings of the 13th International Congress on Allergology and Clinical Immunology*, ed. W.J. Pichler, B.M. Stadler, C. Dahinden *et al.*, p. 12, Hogrefe and Huber, Toronto.

Brostoff, J. & Roitt, I.M. (1969). Cell mediated (delayed) hypersensitivity in patients with summer hay fever. *Lancet*, **ii**, 269.

Bruce, C.A., Rosenthal, R.R., Lichtenstein, L.M. and Norman, P.S. (1974). Diagnostic tests in ragweed-allergic asthma: a comparison of direct skin tests, leukocyte histamine release and quantitative bronchial challenge. *J. Allergy Clin. Immunol.* **53**, 230.

Bruijnzeel-Koomen, C.A.F.M., van Wichen, D.F., Spry, C.J.F., Venge, P. and Bruijnzeel, P.L.B. (1988). Active participation of eosinophils in patch test reactions to inhalant allergens in patients with atopic dermatitis. *Br. J. Dermatol.* **118**, 229.

Burge, H.A. *et al.* (1987). Guidelines for the assessment and sampling of saprophytic bioaerosols in the indoor environment. *Appl. Indust. Hyg.* **2**, R10.

Butterworth, A.E., Sturrock, R.F., Houba, V., Mahmoud, A.A.F., Sher, A. and Rees, P.H. (1975). Eosinophils as mediators of antibody-dependent damage to schistosomula. *Nature* **256**, 727.

Cartier, A., Thomson, N.C., Frith, P.A., Roberts, M. and Hargreave, F.E. (1982). Allergen-induced increase in bronchial responsiveness to histamine: relationship to the late asthmatic response and change in airway caliber. *J. Allergy Clin. Immunol.* **70**, 170.

Cavanaugh, M.J., Bronsky, E.A. and Buckley, J.M. (1977). Clinical value of bronchial provocation testing in childhood asthma. *J. Allergy Clin. Immunol.* **59**. 41.

Chapman, M.D. and Platts-Mills, T.A.E. (1980). Purification and characterization of the major allergen from *Dermato-*

phagoides pteronyssinus-antigen P_1. *J. Immunol.* **125**, 587.

Chapman, M.D., Platts-Mills, T.A.E., Gabriel, M. *et al.* (1980). Antibody response following prolonged hyposensitization with *Dermatophagoides pteronyssinus* extract. *Int. Arch. Allergy Appl. Immunol.* **61**, 431.

Chapman, M.D., Sutherland, W.M. and Platts-Mills, T.A.E. (1984). Recognition of two *Dermatophagoides pteronyssinus*-specific epitopes on antigen P_1 using monoclonal antibodies: binding to each epitope can be inhibited by sera from dust mite-allergic patients. *J. Immunol.* **133**, 2488.

Chapman, M.D., Heymann, P.W., Wilkins, S.R., Brown, M.B. and Platts-Mills, T.A.E. (1987). Monoclonal immunoassays for the major dust mite (*Dermatophagoides*) allergens, *Der p* I and *Der f* I, and quantitative analysis of the allergen content of mite and house dust extracts. *J. Allergy Clin. Immunol.* **80**, 184.

Chapman, M.D., Aalberse, R.C., Brown, M.J. and Platts-Mills, T.A.E. (1988). Monoclonal antibodies to the major feline allergen *Fel d* I. II. Single step affinity purification of *Fel d* I, N-terminal sequence analysis, and development of a sensitive two-site immunoassay to assess *Fel d* I exposure. *J. Immunol.* **140**, 812.

Cherwinski, H.M., Schumacher, J.H., Brown, K.D. and Mosmann, T.R. (1987). Two types of mouse helper T cell clone. III. Further differences in lymphokine synthesis between Th1 and Th2 clones revealed by RNA hybridization, functionally monospecific bioassays and monoclonal antibodies. *J. Exp. Med.* **166**, 1229.

Chua, K.Y., Stewart, G.A., Thomas, W.R. *et al.* (1988). Sequence analysis of cDNA coding for a major house dust mite allergen, *Der p* I: homology with cysteine proteases. *J. Exp. Med.* **167**, 175.

Coca, A.F. and Cooke, R.A. (1923). On the classification of the phenomena of hypersensitiveness. *J. Immunol.* **8**, 163.

Cogswell, J.J., Halliday, D.F. and Alexander, J.R. (1982). Respiratory infections in the first year of life in children at risk of developing atopy. *Br. Med. J.* **284**, 1011.

Cooke, R.A. and Van Der Veer, A. (1916). Human sensitization. *J. Immunol.* **1**, 201.

Cooke, R.A., Barnard, J., Hebald, S. and Stull, A. (1935). Serological evidence on immunity with co-existing sensitization in a type of human allergy, hay fever. *J. Exp. Med.* **62**, 733.

Cookson, W.O.C.M., Faux, J.A., Sharp, P.A. and Hopkin, J.M. (1989). Linkage between immunoglobulin E responses underlying asthma and rhinitis and chromosome. 11q. *Lancet*, **i**, 1292.

Corbi, A.L., Ley, V., Sanchez-Madrid, F. and Carreira, J. (1985). Isolation of the major IgE binding protein from *Parietaria judaica* pollen using monoclonal antibodies. *Mol. Immunol.* **22**, 1081.

Corrigan, C.G., Brown, P.H., Barnes, N.C. *et al.* (1991). Glucocorticoid resistance in chronic asthma. *Am. Rev. Respir. Dis.* **144**, 1016.

Delespesse, G. Sarfati, M., Hofstetter, H., Letellier, M. and Peleman, R. (1988). Human IgE-binding factors. In *Progress in Allergy and Clinical Immunology: Proceedings of the 13th International Congress on Allergology and Clinical Immunology*, ed. W.J. Pichler, B.M. Stadler, C. Dahinden, p. 133, Hogrefe and Huber, Toronto.

Delespesse, G., Sarfati, M. and Peleman, R. (1989). Influence of recombinant interleukin 4, interferon alpha and interferon gamma on the production of human IgE-binding factors. *J. Immunol.* **142**, 134.

Denburg, T.A., Otsuka, H., Telizyn, S. *et al.* (1985). Peripheral blood basophils, basophil progenitors and nasal metachromatic cells in allergic rhinitis. *J. Allergy Clin. Immunol.* **75**, 153.

Dowse, G.K., Turner, K.J., Stewart, G.A., Alpers, M.P. and Woolcock, A.J. (1985). The association between *Dermatophagoides* mites and the increasing prevalence of asthma in village communities within the Papua New Guinea Highlands. *J. Allergy Clin. Immunol.* **75**, 75.

Dvorak, H.F., Mihm, M.C., Dvorak, A.M. *et al.* (1974). Morphology of delayed type hypersensitivity reactions in man. I Quantitative description of the inflammatory response. *Lab. Invest.* **31**, 111.

Ekramoddoullah, A.K.M., Kisil, F.T. and Sehon, A.H. (1986). Isolation of a Kentucky bluegrass pollen allergen using a murine monoclonal antibody immunosorbent. *Int. Arch. Allergy Appl. Immunol.* **80**, 100.

Esch, R.E. and Klapper, D.G. (1989). Identification and localization of allergenic determinants on grass Group I antigens using monoclonal antibodies. *J. Immunol.* **142**, 179.

Fauci, A.S. (1988). The human immunodeficiency virus: infectivity and mechanisms of pathogenesis. *Science* **239**, 617.

Findlay, S.R., Stotsky, E., Leitermann, K., Hemady, Z. and Ohman, J.L., Jr (1983). Allergens detected in association with airborne particles capable of penetrating into the peripheral lung. *Am. Rev. Respir. Dis.* **128**, 1008.

Fink, J.N. (1986). Hypersensitivity pneumonitis. In *Allergy*, ed. A.P. Kaplan, p. 525, Churchill Livingstone, New York.

Fling, J.A., Fischer, J.R., Boswell, R.N. and Reid, M.J. (1988). The relationship of serum IgA concentration to human immunodeficiency virus (HIV) infection: a cross-sectional study of HIV-seropositive individuals detected by screening in the United States Air Force. *J. Allergy Clin. Immunol.* **82**, 965.

Ford, A.W., Rawle, F.C., Lind, P., Spieksma, F.T.M., Lowenstein, H. and Platts-Mills, T.A.E. (1985). Standardization of *Dermatophagoides pteronyssinus*: assessment of potency and allergen content in ten coded extracts. *Int. Arch. Allergy Appl. Immunol.* **76**, 58.

Frew, A.J. and Kay, A.B. (1988). The relationship between infiltrating CD4+ lymphocytes, activated eosinophils, and the magnitude of the allergen-induced late phase cutaneous reaction in man. *J. Immunol.* **141**, 4158.

Galli, S.J. and Dvorak, H.F. (1979). Basophils and mast cells: structure, function and role in hypersensitivity. In *Comprehensive Immunology. 6. Cellular, Molecular, and Clinical Aspects of Allergic Disorders*, ed. S. Gupta and R.A. Good, p. 1, Plenum, New York and London.

Gerrard, J.W., Horne, S., Vickers, P. *et al.* Serum IgE levels in parents and children. *J. Pediatr.* **85**, 660.

Girard, J.P., Rose, N.R., Kunz, M., Kobayashi, S. and Arbesman, C.E. (1967). *In vitro* lymphocyte transformation in atopic patients: induced by antigens. *J. Allergy* **39**, 65.

Gleich, G.J., Flavahan, A., Fujisawa, T. and Vanhoutte, P.M. (1988). The eosinophil as a mediator of damage to respiratory epithelium: a model for bronchial hyperreactivity. *J. Allergy Clin. Immunol.* **81**, 776.

Green, W.F., Wookcock, A.J., Stuckey, M., Sedgwick, C. and

Leeder, S.R. (1986). House dust mites and skin tests in different Australian localities. *Aust. NZ J. Med.* **16**, 639.

Hastie, R. (1971). The antigen-induced degranulation of basophil leucocytes from atopic subjects, studied by phase contrast microscopy. *Clin Exp. Immunol.* **8**, 45.

Hastie, R., Heroy, J.H. and Levy, D.A. (1979). Basophil leukocytes and mast cells in human nasal secretions and scrapings studied by light microscopy. *Lab. Invest.* **40**, 554.

Hay, R.J. and Shennan, G. (1984). Antibody responses in tinea imbricata: the role of immunoglobulin E. *Trans Roy. Soc. Trop. Med. Hyg.* **78**, 653.

Heymann, P.W., Chapman, M.D. and Platts-Mills, T.A.E. (1986). Antigen *Der f* I from the dust mite *Dermatophagoides farinae*: structural comparison with *Der p* I from *Dermatophagoides pteronyssinus* and epitope specificity of murine IgG and human IgE antibodies. *J. Immunol.* **137**, 2841.

Heymann, P.W., Chapman, M.D., Fox, J., Aalberse, R.C. and Platts-Mills, T.A.E. (1989). Antigenic and structural analysis of Group II allergens (*Der p* II and *Der f* II) from house dust mites (*Dermatophagoides* spp.). *J. Allergy Clin. Immunol.* **83**, 1055.

Holt, P.G. and Sedgwick, J.D. (1987). Suppression of IgE responses following antigen inhalation: a natural homeostatic mechanism which limits sensitization to aeroallergens. *Immunol. Today* **8**, 14.

Holt, P.G., Degebrodt, A. and O'Leary, L. (1985). Extraction of immune and inflammatory cells from human lung parenchyma: evaluation of an enzymatic digestion procedure. *Clin. Exp. Immunol.* **66**, 188.

Honbo, S., Jones, H.E. and Artis, W.M. (1984). Chronic/dermatophyte infection: evaluation of the class specific antibody response reactive with polysacharide and peptide antigens derived from *Trichophyton mentagraphytes*. *J. Invest. Dermatol.* **82**, 287.

Ihle, J.N., Keller, J., Oroszlan, S., *et al.* (1982). Biologic properties of homogenous interleukin 3. 1. Demonstration of WEHI-3 growth factor activity, mast cell growth factor activity, P cell stimulating factor activity, colony stimulating factor activity, and histamine producing cell stimulating activity. *J. Immunol.* **131**, 282.

Ishizaka, K. (1985). Twenty years with IgE: from the identification of IgE to regulatory factors for the IgE response. *J. Immunol.* **135**, 1.

Ishizaka, K. and Ishizaka, T. (1975). Biology of immunoglobulin E: molecular basis of reaginic hypersensitivity. *Prog. Allergy* **19**, 60.

Ishizaka, K., Ishizaka, T. and Hornbrook, M.M. (1967). Allergen binding activity of γE, γG and γA, antibodies in sera from atopic patients: *in vitro* measurements of reaginic antibody. *J. Immunol.* **98**, 490.

Ishizaka, K., Kishimoto, T., Delespesse, G. and King, T.P. (1974). Immunogenic properties of modified antigen E. I. Presence of specific determinants for T-cells on urea denatured antigen E and polypeptide chains. *J. Immunol.* **113**, 70.

Ishizaka, T., De Bernardo, R., Tomioka, H., Lichtenstein, L.M. and Ishizaka, K. (1972). Identification of basophil granulocytes as a site of allergic histamine release. *J. Immunol.* **108**, 848.

Iskander, R., Das, P.K. and Aalberse, R.C. (1981). IgG antibodies in Egyptian patients with schistosomiasis. *Int. Arch. Allergy Appl. Immunol.* **66**, 200.

Jarrett, E.E.E. and Stewart, D.C. (1974). Rat IgE production: effect of dose of antigen on primary and secondary reaginic antibody responses. *Immunology* **27**, 365.

Johansson, S.G.O., Bennich, M. and Berg, T. (1971). *In vitro* diagnosis of atopic allergy. III. Quantitative estimation of circulating IgE antibodies by the radioallergosorbent test. *Int. Arch. Allergy Appl. Immunol.* **41**, 443.

Johansson, S.G.O., Bennich, M. and Berg, T. (1972). The clinical significance of IgE. In *Progress in Clinical Immunology*, ed. R.S. Schwartz, vol. I, p. 157, Grune and Stratton, New York.

Johnson, P. and Marsh, D.G. (1965). 'Iso allergens' from rye grass pollen. *Nature (London)* **206**, 935.

Joualt, T., Capron, M., Balloul, J.M., Ameisen, J.C. and Capron, A. (1988). Quantitative and qualitative analysis of the Fc receptor for IgE (Fc_εRII) on human eosinophils. *Eur. J. Immunol.* **18**, 237.

Kaplan, A.P., Haak-Frendscho, M., Fauci, A., Dinarello, C. and Halbert, E. (1985). A histamine releasing factor from activated human mononuclear cells. *J. Immunol.* **135**, 2027.

Kaufman, H.S. and Frick, O.L. (1976). Immunological development in infants of allergic parents. *Clin Allergy* **6**, 321.

Kaufman, H.S. and Hobbs, J.R. (1970). Immunoglobulin deficiencies in an atopic population. *Lancet* **ii**, 1061.

Kemeny, D.M., Miyachi, S., Platts-Mills, T.A.E., Wilkins, S. and Lessof, M.H. (1982). The immune response to bee venom: comparison of the antibody response to phospholipase A_2 with the response to inhalant antigens. *Int. Arch. Allergy Appl. Immunol.* **68**, 268.

Kemeny, D.M., MacKenzie-Mills, M., Harries, M.G., Youlten, L.J.F. and Lessof, M.H. (1983). Antibodies to purified bee venom proteins and peptides. II. A detailed study of changes in IgE and IgG antibodies to individual bee venom antigens. *J. Allergy Clin. Immunol.* **72**, 376.

Kerrebijn, K.F. (1970). Endogenous factors in childhood CNSLD: methodological aspects in population studies. In *Bronchitis*, ed. N.G.M. Orie and R. van der Lende, vol. III, p. 38, Royal Vangorcum Assen, The Netherlands.

King, T.P. and Norman, P.S. (1962). Isolation studies of allergens from ragweed pollen. *Biochemistry* **1**, 709.

Kishimoto, T. and Ishizaka, K. (1973). Regulation of antibody response *in vitro*. VI. Carrier-specific helper cells for IgE and IgG antibody response. *J. Immunol.* **111**, 720.

Lanzavecchia, A., Santini, P., Maggi, E. *et al.* (1983). *In vitro* selective expansion of allergen specific T cells from atopic patients. *Clin. Exp. Immunol.* **52**, 21.

Leatherman, J.W., Michael, A.F., Schwartz, B.A. and Hoidal, J.R. (1984). Lung T cells in hypersensitivity pneumonitis. *Ann. Intern. Med.* **100**, 390.

Leiferman, K., Ackerman, S., Sampson, M., Haugen, M., Venencie, P. and Gleich, G. (1985). Dermal deposition of eosinophil granule major basic protein in atopic dermatitis. *N. Engl. J. Med.* **313**, 282.

Lessof, M.H., Murdoch, R.D., Pollock, I. and Young, E. (1988). Intolerance to food and food additives. In *Progress in Allergy and Clinical Immunology: Proceedings of the 13th International Congress of Allergology and Clinical Immunology*, ed. W.J. Pichler, B.M. Stadler, C. Dahinden *et al.*, p. 353, Hogrefe and

Huber, Toronto.

Lett-Brown, M.A., Thueson, D.O., Plank, D.E., Langford, M.P. and Grant, J.A. (1984). Histamine-releasing activity. IV. Molecular heterogeneity of the activity from stimulated human thoracic duct lymphocytes. *Cell. Immunol.* **87**, 434.

Leung, D.Y.M., Bhan, A.K., Schneeberger, E.E. and Geha, R.S. (1983). Characterization of the mononuclear cell infiltrate in atopic dermatitis using monoclonal antibodies. *J. Allergy Clin. Immunol.* **71**, 47.

Leung, D.Y.M., Schneeberger, E.E., Siraganian, R.P., Geha, R.S. and Bhan, A.K. (1987). The presence of IgE on macrophages and dendritic cells infiltrating into the skin lesion of atopic dermatitis. *Clin. Immunol. Immunopathol.*, **42**, 328.

Levine, B.B. and Redmond, A.P. (1968). The nature of the antigen antibody complexes initiating the specific wheal-and-flare reaction in sensitized man. *J. Clin. Invest.* **47**, 556.

Levine, B.B. and Vaz, N.M. (1970). Effect of combinations of inbred strain, antigen and antigen dose on immune responsiveness and reagin production in the mouse: a potential mouse model for immune aspects of human atopic allergy. *Int. Arch. Allergy Appl. Immunol.* **39**, 156.

Lichtenstein, L.M. (1988). Histamine releasing factors and IgE heterogeneity. *J. Allergy Clin. Immunol.* **81**, 814.

Lichtenstein, L.M. and Levy, D.A. (1972). Is 'desensitization' for ragweed hayfever immunologically specific? *Int. Arch. Allergy Appl. Immunol.* **42**, 615.

Lind, P.O., Hansen, C. and Horn, N. (1988). The binding of mouse hybridoma and human IgE antibodies to the major fecal allergen, *Der p* I, of *Dermatophagoides pteronyssinus*. *J. Immunol.* **140**, 4256.

Luczynska, C.M., Arruda, L.K., Platts-Mills, T.A.E., Miller, J.D., Lopez, M. and Chapman, M.D. (1989a). A two-site monoclonal antibody ELISA for the quantitation of the major *Dermatophagoides* spp. allergens, *Der p.* I and *Der f* I. *J. Immunol. Methods* **118**, 227.

Luczynska, C.M., Li, Y., Chapman, M.D. and Platts-Mills, T.A.E. (1990). Airborne concentrations and particle size distribution of allergen derived from domestic cats (*Felis domesticus*): measurements using cascade impactor, liquid impinger and a two site monoclonal antibody assay for *Fel d* I. *Am. Rev. Respir. Dis.* **141**, 361.

MacDonald, S.M., Lichtenstein, L.M., Proud, D. *et al.* (1987). Studies of IgE-dependent histamine releasing factors: heterogeneity of IgE. *J. Immunol.* **139**, 506.

McLean, J.A., Mathews, K.P., Solomon, W.R., Brayton, D. and Ciarkowski, A.A. (1977). Effect of histamine and methacholine on nasal airway resistance in atopic and nonatopic subjects. *J. Allergy Clin. Immunol.* **59**, 165.

Marsh, D.G. (1975). Allergens and the genetics of allergy. In *The Antigens*, ed. M. Sela, vol. III, p. 271, Academic Press, New York.

Marsh, D.G., Bias, W.B. and Ishizaka, K. (1974). Genetic control of basal serum immunoglobulin E level and its effect on specific reaginic sensitivity. *Proc. Nat. Acad. Sci. (USA)* **71**, 3588.

Marsh, D.G., Meyers, D.A., Freidhoff, L.R. *et al.* (1982). HLA-Dw2: a genetic marker for human immune response to short ragweed pollen allergen Ra5. II. Response after ragweed immunotherapy. *J. Exp. Med.* **155**, 1452.

Marsh, D.G., Goodfriend, L., King, T.P., Lowenstein, M. and Platts-Mills, T.A.E. (1986). Allergen nomenclature. *Bull. World Health Org.* **64**, 767.

May, C.D. and Williams, C.S. (1973). Further studies of concordant fluctuation in sensitivity of peripheral leukocytes to unrelated allergens and the meaning of nonspecific 'desensitization'. *Clin Allergy* **3**, 319.

Mayerhoffer, G., Bazin, H. and Gowans, J.L. (1976). Nature of cells binding anti-IgE in rats immunized with *Nipostrongylus brasiliensis*: IgE synthesis in regional nodes and concentration in mucosal mast cells. *Eur. J. Immunol.* **6**, 537.

Meade, R., Van Loveren, H., Parmentier, H., Iverson, G.M. and Askenase, P.W. (1988). The antigen-binding T cell factor PC1-F sensitizes mast cells for *in vitro* release of serotonin: comparison with monoclonal IgE antibody. *J. Immunol.* **141**, 2704.

Mellanby, K. (1943). *Scabies*. Oxford University Press, Oxford.

Metzger, H. (1988). Molecular aspects of receptors and binding factors for IgE. *Adv. Immunol.* **43**, 277.

Metzger, W.J., Zavaia, D., Richerson, H.B. *et al.* (1987). Local allergen challenge and bronchoalveolar lavage of allergic asthmatic lungs: description of the model and local airway inflammation. *Am. Rev. Respir. Dis.* **135**, 433.

Mitchell, E.B. and Askenase, P.W. (1983). Basophils in human disease. *Clin. Rev. Allergy* **1**, 427.

Mitchell, E.B., Crow, J., Chapman, M.D., Jouhal, S.S., Pope, F.M. and Platts-Mills, T.A.E. (1982). Basophils in allergen-inhaled patch tests in atopic dermatitis. *Lancet* **i**, 127.

Mitchell, E.B., Platts-Mills, T.A.E., Pereira, R.S., Malkovska, V. and Webster, A.D. (1983). Acquired basophil and eosinophil deficiency in a patient with hypogammaglobulinaemia associated with thymoma. *Clin. Lab. Haematol.* **5**, 253.

Mitchell, E.B., Crow, J., Rowntree, S., Webster, D.B. and Platts-Mills, T.A.E. (1984). Cutaneous basophil hypersensitivity to inhalant allergens: local transfer of basophil accumulation with immune serum but not IgE antibody. *J. Invest. Dermatol.* **83**, 290.

Mitchell, E.B., Crow, J., Williams, G. and Platts-Mills, T.A.E. (1986). Increase in skin mast cells following chronic house dust mite exposure. *Br. J. Dermatol.* **114**, 65.

Mole, L.E., Goodfriend, L., Lapkoff, C.B., Kehoe, J.M. and Capra, J.D. (1975). The amino acid sequence of ragweed pollen allergen Ra5. *Biochemistry* **14**, 1216.

Morganstern, J., Griffith, I., Bauer, A. *et al.* (1991). Determination of the amino acid sequence of *Fel d* I, the major allergen of the domestic cat: protein sequence analysis and CDNA cloning. *Proc. Nat. Acad. Sci.* **88**, 9690.

Mygind, N. (1979). *Nasal Allergy*, 2nd edn. Blackwell Scientific Publications, Oxford.

Norman, P.S. (1986). Why standardized extracts? *J. Allergy Clin. Immunol.* **77**, 405.

Norman, P.S., Lichtenstein, L.M. and Ishizaka, K. (1973). Diagnostic tests in ragweed hay fever. *J. Allergy Clin. Immunol.* **52**, 210.

O'Hollaren, M.T., Sachs, M.I., O'Connell, E.J. and Yunginger, J. (1988). Allergen exposure as a possible precipitating factor for respiratory arrest in young adults with asthma. *J. Allergy Clin. Immunol.* **81**, 246.

O'Hehir, R.E., Eckels, D.D., Frew, A.J., Kay, A.B. and Lamb, J.R. (1988). MHC class II restriction specificity of cloned human T lymphocytes reactive with *Dermatophagoides farinae* (house dust mite). *Immunology* **64**, 627.

O'Hehir, R.E., Garman, R.D., Greenstein, J.L. and Lamb, J.R. (1991). The specificity and regulation of T-cell responsiveness to allergens. *Ann. Rev. Immunol.* **9**, 67.

Okuda, M. and Otsuka, H. (1977). Basophilic cells in allergic nasal secretions. *Arch. Oto-Rhino-Laryngol.* **214**, 283.

Olson, J.R. and Klapper, D.G. (1986). Two major human allergenic sites on ragweed pollen allergen antigen E identified by using monoclonal antibodies. *J. Immunol.* **136**, 2109.

Otsuka, H., Dolovitch, J., Befus, D., Bienenstock, J. and Denburg, J. (1986). Peripheral blood basophils, basophil progenitors, and nasal metachromatic cells in allergic rhinitis. *Am. Rev. Respir. Dis.* **133**, 757.

Ottesen, E.A., Skvaril, F., Tropathy, S.P., Poindexter, R.W. and Hussain, R. (1985). Prominence of IgG4 in the IgG antibody response to human filariasis. *J. Immunol.* **134**, 2707.

Parronchi, P., Macchia, D., Piccinni, M.P. *et al.* (1991). Allergen and bacterial antigen specific T cell clones established from atopic donors show a different pattern of cytokine production. *Proc. Nat. Acad. Sci. USA* **88**, 4538.

Peat, J.K., Salome, C.M., Sedgwick, C.J., Kerrebijn, J. and Woolcock, A.J. (1989). A prospective study of bronchial hyperresponsiveness and respiratory symptoms in a population of Australian schoolchildren. *Clin. Exp. Allergy* **19**, 299.

Pepys, J. (1971). Pulmonary aspergillosis, farmers lung and related diseases. In *Immunological Diseases*, ed. M. Samter, p. 693, Little, Brown, Boston.

Platts-Mills, T.A.E. (1979). Local production of IgG, IgA, and IgE antibodies in grass pollen hayfever. *J. Immunol.* **122**, 2218.

Platts-Mills, T.A.E. (1982). Type I or immediate hypersensitivity. In *Clinical Aspects of Immunology*, 4th edn, ed. P.J. Lachmann and D.K. Peters, p. 579, Blackwell Scientific Publications, Oxford.

Platts-Mills, T.A.E. and Chapman, M.D. (1987). Dust mites: immunology, allergic disease and environmental control. *J. Allergy Clin. Immunol.* **80**, 755.

Platts-Mills, T.A.E. and de Weck, A.L. (1989). Dust mite allergens and asthma — a world wide problem. *Bull. WHO* **66**, 6; and *J. Allergy Clin. Immunol.* **83**, 416.

Platts-Mills, T.A.E., von Maur, R.K., Ishizaka, K., Norman, P.S. and Lichtenstein, L.M. (1976). IgA and IgG anti-ragweed antibodies in nasal secretions: quantitative measurements of antibodies and correlation with inhibition of histamine release. *J. Clin. Invest.* **57**, 1041.

Platts-Mills, T.A.E., de Gast, G.C., Webster, A.D.B., Asherson, G.L. and Wilkins, S.R. (1981). Two immunologically distinct forms of late-onset hypogammaglobulinaemia. *Clin. Exp. Immunol.* **44**, 383.

Platts-Mills, T.A.E., Tovey, E.R., Mitchell, E.B., Moszoro, H., Nock, P. and Wilkins, S.R. (1982). Reduction of bronchial hyperreactivity during prolonged allergen avoidance. *Lancet* **ii**, 675.

Platts-Mills, T.A.E., Hayden, M.L., Chapman, M.D. and Wilkins, S.R. (1986). Seasonal variation in dust mite and grass pollen allergens in dust from the houses of patients with asthma. *J. Allergy Clin. Immunol.* **79**, 781.

Platts-Mills, T.A.E., Fiocco, G., Hayden, M.L., Guerrant, J.L., Pollart, S.M. and Wilkins, S.R. (1987a). Serum IgE antibodies to *Trichophyton* in patients with urticaria, angioedema, asthma and rhinitis: development of a radioallergosorbent test. *J. Allergy Clin. Immunol.* **79**, 40.

Platts-Mills, T.A.E., Longbottom, J., Edwards, J., Cockroft, A. and Wilkins, S.R. (1987b). Occupational asthma and rhinitis related to laboratory rats: serum IgG and IgE antibodies to the rat urinary allergen. *J. Allergy Clin. Immunol.* **79**, 505.

Pollart, S.M., Reid, M., Brown, M. *et al.* (1988). Epidemiology of emergency room asthma in northern California: association with IgE antibody to rye grass pollen. *J. Allergy Clin. Immunol.* **82**, 224.

Pollart, S.M., Chapman, M.D., Fiocco, G.P., Rose, G. and Platts-Mills, T.A.E. (1989). Epidemiology of acute asthma: IgE antibodies to common inhalant allergens as a risk factor for emergency room visits. *J. Allergy Clin. Immunol.* **83**, 875.

Pollart, S.M., Platts-Mills, T.A.E., Vailes, L., Sutherland, W. and Chapman, M.D. (1991). Purification of a major allergen from the German cockroach. *J. Allergy Clin. Immunol.* **87**, 505.

Prausnitz, C. and Küstner, H. (1921). Studien veber die verbering Findlichkeit. *Zentralbl. Bakteriol. Parasitenk. Infectionskr. Hyg.* Abt. 1, Orig 86, 160.

Prouvost-Danon, A., Mouton, D., Abadie, A., Mevel, J.C. and Biozzi, G. (1977). Genetic regulation of IgE and agglutinating antibody synthesis in lives of mice selected for high and low immune responsiveness. *Eur. J. Immunol.* **7**, 342.

Rawle, F.C., Mitchell, E.B. and Platts-Mills, T.A.E. (1984). T cell responses to the major allergen from the house dust mite *Dermatophagoides pteronyssinus* antigen P_1: comparison of patients with asthma, atopic dermatitis, and perennial rhinitis. *J. Immunol.* **133**, 195.

Rocklin, R.E., Sheffer, A.L., Greineder, D.K. and Melmon, K.L. (1980). Generation of antigen specific suppressor cells during allergy desensitization. *N. Engl. J. Med.* **302**, 1213.

Rowntree, S., Platts-Mills, T.A.E., Cogswell, J.J. and Mitchell, E.B. (1987). A subclass IgG_4 specific antigen binding radioimmunoassay (RIA): comparison between IgG and IgG_4 antibodies to food and inhaled antigens, in adult atopic dermatitis, after desensitization treatment and during development of antibody responses in children. *J. Allergy Clin. Immunol.* **80**, 622.

Sadan, N., Rhyne, M.B., Mellitis, E.A., Levy, D.A. and Lichtenstein, L.M. (1969). Immunotherapy of pollinosis in children: investigation of its immunological basis of clinical improvement. *N. Engl. J. Med.* **280**, 623.

Sanderson, C.J., Warren, D.J. and Strath, M. (1985). Identification of a lymphokine that stimulates eosinophil differentiation *in vitro*: its relationship to IL3, and functional properties of eosinophils produced in cultures. *J. Exp. Med.* **162**, 60.

Sedgwick, J.D., Holt, P.G. and Turner, K.J. (1981). Production of a histamine-releasing lymphokine by antigen- or mitogen-stimulated human peripheral T cells. *Clin. Exp. Immunol.* **45**, 409.

Silverstein, A.M. (1989). *A History of Immunology*. Academic Press, Inc., New York.

Slavin, R.G., Tennenbaum, J.I., Becker, R.J., Feinburg, A.R. and Feinberg, S.M. (1963). Cell transfer of delayed hypersensitivity to ragweed from atopic subjects treated with emulsified ragweed extracts. *J. Allergy* **34**, 368.

Smith, J.M., Disney, M.E., Williams, J.P. and Goels, Z.A. (1969). Clinical significance of skin reactions to mite extracts in children with asthma. *Br. Med. J.* **2**, 723.

Smith, T.F., Kelly, L.B., Heymann, P.W., Wilkins, S.R. and Platts-Mills, T.A.E. (1985). Natural exposure and serum antibodies to house dust mite of mite-allergic children with asthma in Atlanta. *J. Allergy Clin. Immunol.* **76**, 782.

Snapper, C.M., Finkelman, F.D. and Paul, W.E. (1988). Differential regulation of IgG1 and IgE synthesis by interleukin-4. *J. Exp. Med.* **167**, 183.

Soliman, M.Y. and Rosenstreich, D.L. (1986). Natural immunity to dust mites in adults with chronic asthma. I. Mite-specific serum IgG and IgE. *Am. Rev. Respir. Dis.* **134**, 962.

Soothill, J.F. (1976). Some intrinsic and extrinsic factors predisposing to allergy. *Proc. Roy. Soc. Med.* **69**, 439.

Sporik, R., Holgate, S.T., Platts-Mills, T.A.E. and Cogswell, J. (1990). Exposure to house dust mite allergen (*Der p* I) and the development of asthma in childhood: A prospective study. *New Eng. J. Med.* **323**, 502.

Stanworth, D.R., Humphrey, J.H., Bennich, H. and Johansson, S.G.O. (1968). Inhibition of Prausnitz–Küstner reaction by proteolytic cleavage fragments of a human myeloma protein of immunoglobulin class E. *Lancet* **ii**, 17.

Steinberg, P., Ishizaka, K. and Norman, P.S. (1974). Possible role of IgE-mediated reaction in immunity. *J. Allergy Clin. Immunol.* **54**, 359.

Stewart, G.A., Thompson, P.J. and Simpson, R.J. (1989). Protease antigens from house dust mite. *Lancet* **ii**, 154 (NB See also erratum published subsequently).

Stingl, G., Gazze-Stingl, L.A., Aberer, W. and Wolff, K. (1981). Antigen presentation by murine epidermal Langerhans cells and its alteration by ultra-violet B light. *J. Immunol.* **127**, 1707.

Stokes, C.R., Taylor, B. and Turner, M.W. (1974). Association of house dust and grass pollen allergies with specific IgA antibody deficiency. *Lancet* **ii**, 485.

Strickler, J., Layton, J.E., Homburger, H.A. *et al.* (1986). Immunologic response to aerosols of affinity-purified antigen in hypersensitivity pneumonitis. *J. Allergy Clin. Immunol.* **78**, 411.

Swanson, M.C., Agarwal, M.K. and Reed, C.E. (1985). An immunochemical approach to indoor aeroallergen quantitation with a new volumetric air sampler: studies with mite, roach, cat, mouse, and guinea pig antigens. *J. Allergy Clin. Immunol.* **76**, 724.

Tada, T. and Ishizaka, K. (1970). Distribution of gamma E forming cells in lymphoid tissues of the human and monkey. *J. Immunol.* **104**, 377.

Taliafero, W.H. and Taliafero, L.G. (1931). Skin reaction in persons infected with *Schistosoma mansoni*. *Puerto Rico J. Publ. Health Trop. Med.* **7**, 23.

Taylor, G. (1974). The nose as a model for the study of respiratory tract allergic disease. *Ann. NY Acad. Sci.* **211**, 117.

Tovey, E.R., Chapman, M.D. and Platts-Mills, T.A.E. (1981a). Mite faeces are a major source of house dust allergens. *Nature* **289**, 592.

Tovey, E.R., Chapman, M.D., Wells, C.W. and Platts-Mills, T.A.E. (1981b). The distribution of dust mite allergen in the houses of patients with asthma. *Am. Rev. Respir. Dis.* **124**, 630.

Tse, K.S., Wicher, K. and Arbesman, C.E. (1973). Effect of immunotherapy on the appearance of antibodies to ragweed in external secretions. *J. Allergy Clin. Immunol.* **51**, 208.

Turk, A., Lichtenstein, L.M. and Norman, P.S. (1970). Nasal secretory antibody to inhalant allergens in allergic and non-allergic individuals. *Immunology* **19**, 85.

Umetsu, D.T., Jabara, H.H., DeKruyff, R.H., Abbas, A.K., Abrams, J.S. and Geha, R.S. (1988). Functional heterogeneity among human inducer T cell clones. *J. Immunol.* **140**, 4211.

Van der Heijden, F.L., Wierenga, E.A., Bos, J.D. and Kapsenberg, M.L. (1991). High frequency of IL-4-producing CD4+ allergen specific T lymphocytes in atopic dermatitis lesional skin. *J. Invest. Dermatol.* **97**, 389.

Van der Zee, J.S. and Aalberse, R.C. (1987). The role of IgG. In *Allergy: an International Textbook*, ed. M. Lessoff, M. Kemeny and T. Lee, pp. 49–67, Wiley, Chichester.

Van Loveren, H. and Askenase, P.W. (1984). Delayed-type hypersensitivity is mediated by a sequence of two T cell activities. *J. Immunol.* **133**, 2397.

Von Pirquet, C. (1906). Allergy. In *Clinical Aspects of Immunology*, 3rd edn, ed. P.G.H. Gell *et al.* Blackwell Scientific Publications, Oxford.

Waldmann, T.A., Ito, A., Ogawa, M., McIntyre, O.R. and Strober, W. (1976). The metabolism of IgE: studies in normal individuals and in a patient with IgE myeloma. *J. Immunol.* **117**, 1139.

Ward, G.W., Karlsson, G., Rose, G. and Platts-Mills, T.A.E. (1989). *Trichophyton* asthma: specific sensitization of the bronchi and upper airways to a dermatophyte antigen. *Lancet* **i**, 259.

Wierenga, E.A., Snoek, M., De Groot, C., Bos, C.I., Jansen, H.M. and Kapsenberg, M.L. (1990). Evidence for compartmentalization of functional subsets of CD4+ lymphocytes in atopic patients. *J. Immunol.* **144**, 4651.

Yssel, H., Hsu, G., Schneider, P.V. *et al.* (1990). Mapping of the minimal T cell inducing epitopes on the *Der p* I allergen. *Clin. Exp. Allergy* **20**, S46.

53: General Anaphylaxis

J.R.W. Wilkinson and T.H. Lee

History

Although fatal allergic reactions have been described for at least 4000 years (Feinberg *et al.* 1956), since the hieroglyphic recording of the death of King Menes of Egypt from an insect sting, it was not until the studies of Portier and Richet in the early years of the twentieth century that the biological mechanisms began to be unravelled (Fig. 53.1). Portier and Richet (1902) demonstrated that injection of extract of sea anemone into a dog was well tolerated on the first occasion but induced a rapidly fatal reaction when reinjected in the same amount several weeks later. They coined the term 'anaphylaxis', distinguishing it from the protective prophylaxis commonly induced by injection of biological substances. It was soon realized (Arthus 1921) that the effect was not necessarily due to a toxin but that any injected foreign protein could induce anaphylaxis in a suitably sensitized individual.

The increasing use of hyperimmune horse serum, as a source of antitoxins against tetanus and diphtheria toxins and antisera to such organisms as *Pneumonococcus*, *Meningococcus* and tubercle bacillus led to a substantial number of reports of fatalities caused by anaphylaxis (Lamson 1924, 1929). A review of the literature by Vaughan and Pipes in 1936 attributed half of 68 cases of fatal anaphylaxis to serum therapy and the remainder to other, mainly proteinaceous, foreign materials. The advent of penicillin treatment in the 1940s provided another source of anaphylactic reactions. The first case of fatal anaphylaxis to penicillin was reported by Waldbloot in 1949. The incidence increased with more widespread use and by the 1960s the mortality was estimated at between 100 and 500 per year in the USA (Parker 1963, 1972). By the 1970s penicillin was estimated to account for approximately 75% of all cases of severe anaphylaxis (Delage and Irey 1972; Parker 1972), and this

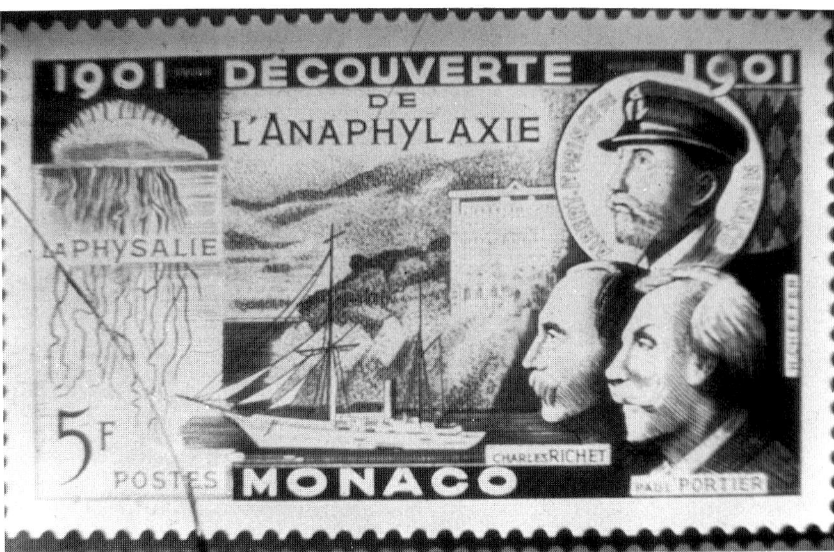

Fig. 53.1. Stamp commemorating the discovery of anaphylaxis by Portier and Richet in 1902. (Kindly donated to Tak Lee by Dr K.F. Austen.)

is probably unchanged at present. Despite the increasing number of pharmaceutical agents capable of causing anaphylaxis, the most important cause of anaphylaxis after penicillin remains, to this day, the venom of Hymenoptera. Serious reactions to insect stings have been estimated to occur in 0.4% of the population (Sobotka *et al.* 1974) and account for 60 to 80 deaths per year in the USA (Patterson and Valentine 1982).

Epidemiology of anaphylaxis

There is no evidence that race, sex, occupation, geographical or seasonal factors affect the risk of anaphylactic reactions, except that such factors may influence the availability of, and exposure of individuals to, the offending agents. A large proportion of anaphylactic reactions is due to either drugs or insect stings. Figures for the incidence of reactions to different drugs are often difficult to obtain but the prevalence of reactions to drugs has been estimated at between 15 and 40 per 100 000 patients (Boston Collaborative Drug Surveillance Program 1973; Giansiracus and Upchurch 1985), whereas fatal reactions to penicillin — the most common agent — occur in 0.002%, or one fatality for every 7.5 million injections (Idsoe *et al.* 1968). Radiological contrast media provoke anaphylactic reactions in 1 : 600 patients (Lasser *et al.* 1987) and anaesthetic drugs in 1 : 20 000 (Fisher and Baldo 1984). At the other extreme, horse anti-human lymphocyte globulin, used in the suppression of allograft rejection, induced anaphylaxis in 2% (Ring *et al.* 1974) to 21% (Kashiwagi *et al.* 1968) of patients. Serious reactions to Hymenoptera stings occur in 0.4–0.8% of the population (Settipane *et al.* 1972; Sobotka *et al.* 1974). Mortality has been estimated by Parrish (1965) at 1 in 6.5×10^6 stings.

Age may affect the severity of anaphylactic reactions. Parrish (1965) found that 93% of fatal reactions occurred after 19 years of age and, in general, most severe reactions tend to occur above this age. However, anaphylactic deaths can and do occur in infancy (Delage and Irey 1972) and those resulting from ingested proteins occur predominantly in this age-group (Despres *et al.* 1971). Evidence concerning the relationship between anaphylaxis and atopy has been conflicting. Early observations (Lamson 1929; Kern and Wimberley 1953; Welch *et al.* 1953) suggested a considerably higher incidence of severe anaphylaxis in patients with a previous history of atopic disease. Studies in the 1970s found 25% of patients with systemic reactions to Hymenoptera stings had other atopic diseases and a further 8% had positive scratch tests to common inhaled allergens but were asymptomatic (Schwartz and Kahn 1970; Settipane *et al.* 1972; Settipane and Chaffe 1979). More recent studies have shown no evidence of correlation between the propensity to develop severe anaphylaxis due to penicillin (Green and Rosenblum 1971; Horowitz 1975) and other agents such as suxamethonium (Adkinson 1984; Charpin *et al.* 1988) or bee stings (Settipane *et al.* 1978) and personal or family history of atopy, skin testing or radioallergosorbent tests (RAST) for common allergens.

Definition and aetiology

The term anaphylaxis is used in two ways. First, it denotes a specific immunoglobulin E (IgE)-mediated antigen-induced reaction by mast cells and basophils: the type 1 immediate hypersensitivity of Coombs and Gell. Second, it is used in clinical practice to describe the clinical syndrome resulting from the release of a variety of mast cell-derived mediators and affecting the respiratory, cardiovascular and other organ systems. In this latter context, the initiating event may be mediated by specific antibodies, either IgE or, more rarely, IgG, or by non-immunological mechanisms. Such non-immunologically mediated reactions are often termed anaphylactoid reactions in that, although the initiating event may not be a true type 1 reaction, the subsequent mediator release is similar and the clinical manifestation is identical.

Aetiological agents

Some of the more common aetiological agents causing anaphylactic or anaphylactoid reactions are listed in Table 53.1. Precipitating agents may be broadly classified into those causing IgE-mediated (anaphylactic) and those causing non-IgE-mediated (anaphylactoid) reactions.

IMMUNOGLOBULIN E-MEDIATED ANAPHYLAXIS

Characteristically, the antigens that trigger anaphylactic reactions are large molecules (>10 000 daltons) and include both proteins and polysaccharides. Low-molecular-weight drugs, such as antibiotics, are classically not considered antigenic in their own right and require carrier proteins before they are capable of inducing an immune response. Such molecules are called haptens. The higher the affinity of the hapten to its carrier protein, the more likely it is to induce an allergic reaction. More recent work (Baldo and Fisher 1983) has suggested that some small molecules are able to stimulate IgE responses without the necessity of binding the carrier proteins.

Antibiotics

By far the most frequently implicated agent in systemic anaphylaxis is penicillin, which accounts for 75% of all anaphylactic reactions. These occur most frequently in the 40 to 49 years age-group and are more common and more severe with parenterally administered drugs. Although almost all patients treated with penicillin mount an immunological response (de Weck and Blum 1965; Levine 1966), only a small proportion develop adverse reactions. Specific IgE is directed either against the major metabolic product, the penicilloyl group (called the major determinant), or against minor determinants, which include crystalline penicillin, sodium penicilloate and sodium benzylpenicilloylamine. The presence of IgG-blocking antibody specific for the major determinant prevents the major determinant from triggering sensitized mast cells. The minor determinants, unlike the major determinant, do not induce specific IgG antibodies and the presence of the specific IgE directed against these minor determinants appears to be responsible for penicillin anaphylaxis (Levine and Redmond 1969). As all penicillin derivatives possess the same 6-amino-penicillamic acid nucleus, there is a high degree of cross-reactivity between them. Any patient with a history of a severe reaction to one penicillin should be considered at risk of similar reactions to any other penicillin (Stewart 1962; Green 1970).

Cephalosporins share the beta-lactam ring structure and similar metabolic pathways with penicillins and consequently cross-react immunologically (Batchelor *et al.* 1966). Early estimates of clinical cross-reactivity were as high as 30% but subsequent reviews (Petz 1978) lowered this figure to approximately 8% of patients with a history of penicillin allergy reacting to cephalosporins. Positive skin tests for the major determinant (in the form of penicilloyl polylysine) or a mixture of minor determinants, in addition to a clinical history of penicillin hypersensitivity, indicate a high risk of further anaphylaxis to penicillin, and approximately 50% risk of a reaction to cephalosporins.

Although virtually all antibiotic and antimicrobial agents have been recorded as causing anaphylaxis by a variety of routes of administration, the major antigenic determinants, apart

Table 53.1. Agents producing anaphylaxis

IgE-mediated	Non-IgE-mediated
Proteins	*Haptens*
Antisera	Antibiotics
Tetanus	Penicillins
Diphtheria	Cephalosporins
Venoms	Tetracycline
Antilymphocyte	Chlortetracycline
Hormones	Demethylchlortetracycline
Insulin	Sulphonamides
Relaxin	Neomycin
Corticotrophin	Streptomycin
Parathormone	Polymixin B
Enzymes	Amphotericin B
Chymotrypsin	Vitamins
Trypsin	Thiamine
Penicillinase	Folic acid
Chymopapain	Miscellaneous
Venoms	Procaine
Hymenoptera	Ethylene oxide
Fire ants	Suxamethonium
Snake	
Allergen extracts	*Complement-mediated*
Ragweed	Cuprammonium cellulose
Food	Radiocontrast media
Egg white	
Milk	*Immune complexes*
Crustacea (shrimp, lobster)	IgA deficiency
Nuts (Brazil, cashew)	
Legumes (soya bean, peanut)	*Direct mast cell activation*
Fish (cod, halibut, salmon)	Opiates
Grains (rice, buckwheat)	Muscle relaxants
Potato	Dextran
Chocolate	Radiocontrast media
Citrus fruit (orange, tangerine)	
Mango	*Arachidonic acid metabolism*
Strawberry	Aspirin
Seminal plasma	NSAIDs
Polysaccharides	
Dextran	
Iron–Dextran	
Acacia	

from those of the beta-lactam antibiotics, have not yet been completely elucidated. The most commonly involved drug classes after penicillins are sulphonamides, followed by tetracyclines and macrolides.

Proteins used in therapy

Hormones, enzymes and therapeutic allergen extracts, are all well-recognized causes of anaphylaxis. A few specific examples are worthy of comment because of a particularly high incidence of reactions. Animal-derived sera, initially the most commonly recognized cause of anaphylaxis, are still used for prophylaxis against snake venoms, botulinum toxin and gas gangrene and for anti-lymphocyte immunosuppression. Anti-lymphocyte globulin therapy has a particularly high rate of anaphylaxis, varying from 2 to 20% (Kashiwagi *et al*. 1968; Ring *et al*. 1974).

Chymopapain is a plant protease used for the enzymatic digestion of herniated intervertebral discs. It cross-reacts with papain, used as a meat tenderizer and in fruit juices, beers, toothpaste, cosmetics and contact lens cleaning fluid. There is a significant incidence of anaphylaxis in chemonucleosis procedures, with a prevalence of 0.8% (Simmons *et al.* 1984). Interestingly, there is a higher incidence in women (1.5%) than in men (0.5%) (Levy *et al.* 1986), which may reflect differences in exposure to cross-reacting substances. The majority of reactions are IgE-mediated (McCullough *et al.* 1985) but, in rare instances, anaphylaxis occurs in patients with a negative skin test and no *in vitro* evidence of specific IgE (Bernstein and Bernstein 1986). These reactions have been attributed, with little evidence, to a direct non-immunological effect on mast cells causing mediator release.

Hymenoptera venom

Following antibiotics, hymenoptera stings are the most common cause of anaphylaxis. The order Hymenoptera contains two families: Apidae (bees) and Vespidae (wasps, hornets and yellow-jackets). The genus *Apis* contains only the honey-bee (*A. mellifera*), the genus *Vespula* contains hornets and yellow-jackets, and *Polistes* contains the wasps. Various subspecies occur with different frequencies around the world. The major allergens in both bees and wasps are different types of phospholipase A. In addition to this protein, bee venom contains a number of mediators, including dopamine, noradrenaline, a neurotoxin apamin, melittin (which causes haemolysis) and peptide 401 (which causes mast cell degranulation), and a variety of enzymes, including hyaluronidase and acid phosphatase. Wasp venoms contain similar but not identical toxins and a different phospholipase A (Habermann 1972). Whilst a single bee sting may be fatal for a sensitized individual, multiple stings are normally well tolerated, with patients surviving over 500 stings despite severe toxic effects (Murray 1964). Venom allergy is not predictable. Although skin tests in children can confirm sensitivity, Schuberth *et al.* (1983a, b) found, on follow-up of such children, that it did not accurately predict their response to further stings. Clayton *et al.* (1985) found that 2% of patients with anaphylactic reactions had both negative skin tests to venom and negative RAST for venom-specific IgE. In addition, patients with a history of anaphylactic sting reactions may have no reaction to subsequent stings (Schuberth *et al.* 1983a, b).

Foods

The huge variety of foods which have been shown to be capable of inducing anaphylaxis includes almost everything eaten by humans. The most commonly implicated foods are milk and milk-derived products, eggs, *Crustacea*, nuts and legumes. Rather less commonly involved foods include fruits, grains and chocolate.

NON-IMMUNOGLOBULIN-MEDIATED ANAPHYLAXIS (ANAPHYLACTOID REACTIONS)

The mechanisms of anaphylactoid reactions are not well understood. There are a number of possible pathways whereby substances may bypass the antibody/antigen reaction and directly or indirectly stimulate mast cells. Some anaphylactoid reactions may be mediated by other inflammatory mechanisms which are independent of mast cells. Examples of possible mechanisms include: (i) activation of coagulation or fibrinolysis, with resultant generation of kinins, such as bradykinin, and the anaphylatoxins C3a and C5a; (ii) activation of the complement cascade to generate anaphylatoxins; and (iii) modulation of arachidonic acid metabolism in favour of the generation of pro-inflammatory mediators.

Immune complexes

Anaphylaxis may occur during infusion of blood, plasma, γ-globulin (Ellis and Henney 1969) or serum products, such as cryoprecipitate (Burman *et al.* 1973). Such reactions are thought to be associated with immune complex formation and subsequent complement activation via the alternative pathway. The clinical and physiological signs of anaphylaxis are closely mimicked by acute complement activation *in vitro* with the release of vasoactive amines, oxygen radicals, mast cell degranulation and increased arachidonic acid and leucotriene metabolism (Bolt and Herman 1983), and altered vascular permeability. Immune complexes, especially those containing IgA, are known to activate the alternative complement pathway, and IgG aggregates are able to mimic clinical anaphylaxis (Christian 1960).

Patients who lack IgA (1 in 700 of the population) form IgG antibodies against IgA in about 50% of individuals. Such antibodies may also occur in patients lacking only a subclass of IgA and in patients who have been repeatedly transfused (Vyas *et al*. 1975). If such patients are transfused blood containing IgA, or therapeutic preparations of IgG, which may also be contaminated with IgA (Wells *et al*. 1977), immune complexes of recipient IgG and donor IgA form and are demonstrable in these individuals in association with anaphylactic reactions (Wells *et al*. 1977; Vyas *et al*. 1968, 1969).

Complement activation

As mentioned above, the alternative pathway of complement may be activated by IgA-containing immune complexes. Complement may also be activated directly by contact with cuprammonium cellulose, a material commonly used for haemodialysis membranes, with generation of C3a and C5a, and mast cell degranulation (Craddock *et al*. 1977; Wauters and Lambert 1977; Hakim *et al*. 1984). Dialysis membranes may also cause anaphylaxis by an IgE-dependent mechanism, due to production of specific IgE to ethylene oxide, used to sterilize membranes. Radiocontrast media are also known to activate the complement cascade, both *in vivo* and *in vitro* (Aroyave and Tan 1977; Lieberman and Siegle 1979), with consequent generation of anaphylatoxins (Till *et al*. 1978; Westaby *et al*. 1985). This is a short-lived phenomenon, with demonstrable loss of complement components occurring immediately after administration and with complement levels returning to normal within 30 minutes (Freyria *et al*. 1982). Unlike the activation produced by immune complexes, that induced by radiocontrast media does not progress in an orderly sequential manner and is independent of calcium and magnesium. Several components may be cleared simultaneously and there is evidence for the secondary generation of plasmin-like activity (Lieberman *et al*. 1987). Strongly ionic contrast media appear to act partly by altering the conformation of C3 and C4 through disruption of their thiol–ester bonds to result in conformations similar to C3b and C4b, with a similar ability to activate further components. Non-ionic agents may act in different ways. Metrizamide interferes with the normal inhibition of the complement pathway and also acts directly on C2 (von Zabern *et al*. 1984).

Complement activation is also seen in other clinical syndromes that share some features with anaphylaxis. Hereditary angio-oedema is inherited as an autosomal dominant trait. A deficiency in the activity of C1 esterase inhibitor, either due to absence or to a functionally inactive inhibitor (Rosen *et al*. 1971), results in unpredictable acute episodes of angio-oedema, which may result in asphyxia and death due to laryngeal oedema in up to 30% of patients (Donaldson and Evans 1963; Frank *et al*. 1976).

Activation of coagulation

Activation of Hageman factor by complex insoluble materials, such as collagen (Wilner *et al*. 1968) and endotoxin (Morrison and Cochrane 1974), has been described. Such activation results in the generation of kinins, including bradykinin, which is a potent vasodilator, and the activation of the complement cascade, generating C3a and C5a. This mechanism of mediator release has been demonstrated to occur with radiological contrast media (Lieberman *et al*. 1987), and has been postulated as a cause of some anaphylactoid mechanisms.

Direct action on mast cells

A variety of agents have been shown to cause histamine release from mast cells and basophils by pharmacological mechanisms. Both hypo- and hyperosmotic stimuli induce histamine release (Lasser *et al*. 1987). Hyperosmolar solutions, such as mannitol, 50% dextrose and radiocontrast media (Rice *et al*. 1983), have also been shown *in vitro* to cause histamine release. The risk of anaphylaxis may be reduced by decreasing the infusion rate of hypertonic solutions. Other agents recorded as causing histamine release directly include opiates (Schoenfeld 1960), muscle relaxants (Fisher 1975) and dextran (Hedin *et al*. 1976).

Modulation of arachidonic acid metabolism

The ability of aspirin and related non-steroidal anti-inflammatory drugs (NSAIDs) to induce bronchospasm and anaphylactic reactions has been recognized for some time, and has been estimated to occur in approximately 1% of individuals (Chafee and Settipane 1974). There may be cross-reactivity amongst different NSAIDs and also with azo dyes such as tartrazine (Chafee and Settipane 1967) and benzoate preservatives (Samter and Beers 1968). The ability of NSAIDs to induce anaphylaxis appears related to their potency as inhibitors of the enzyme cyclo-oxygenase (see section on mediators) (Flower *et al.* 1972; Szczeklik *et al.* 1975) rather than to similarities of structure. This may affect the balance of pro-inflammatory mediators in two ways: (i) by preferential metabolism of arachidonic acid by the lipoxygenase pathway to form leucotrienes, which are potent pro-inflammatory mediators, causing bronchoconstriction and increased vascular permeability; and (ii) by decreasing production of prostaglandin E_2 (PGE_2), which acts as a bronchodilator. Although Ferreri *et al.* (1988) demonstrated changes in leucotriene generation, with increased leucotriene C-4 (LTC-4) generation in aspirin-sensitive subjects after challenge with aspirin, a corresponding decrease in PGE_2 release was seen in both sensitive and normal control subjects.

Multiple mechanisms

Some agents causing anaphylaxis may work via more than one mechanism. For example, radiocontrast media may cause mast cell activation by a combination of direct osmotic effects, complement activation and activation of the coagulation and fibrinolytic systems via the Hageman factor, or possibly by immunological mechanisms (McClennan *et al.* 1976; Sweeney and Klotz 1983). Any of these mechanisms may contribute to the final common pathway of mast cell degranulation and mediator release.

Anaphylaxis of unknown mechanism

Exercise-induced anaphylaxis

This has been recognized only relatively recently (Sheffer and Austen 1980) and is distinct from the other exercise-induced phenomena of asthma and cholinergic urticaria. In affected individuals, exercise provokes the classical symptoms and signs of anaphylaxis, often culminating in circulatory collapse if continued. Attacks are more likely in hot, humid weather and may be precipitated by exercise ranging in severity from tennis warm-ups and jogging to sprinting in track events. About 50% of individuals are atopic and some familial occurrences have been reported (Soter *et al.* 1982). Approximately a third of subjects develop symptoms following ingestion of aspirin prior to exercise (Sheffer and Austen 1980), but not following aspirin alone. Some subjects experience symptoms only if they exercise shortly after ingestion of foods such as shellfish or celery (Maulitz *et al.* 1979; Kidd *et al.* 1982). The frequency of attacks varies from a single isolated episode to weekly attacks occurring over many years. Symptoms are reproducible on challenge under controlled conditions, and Sheffer *et al.* (1985) demonstrated that these were accompanied by increased levels of circulating histamine and histological and ultrastructural evidence of mast cell degranulation, similar to that seen in mast cells challenged with IgE (Caulfield *et al.* 1980). In these studies, no abnormality of mast cells or circulating histamine was found before exercise, or in normal subjects before or after exercise.

Idiopathic anaphylaxis

Idiopathic anaphylaxis is essentially a diagnosis of exclusion (Sale *et al.* 1981; Sonin *et al.* 1983). Care must be taken to rule out uncommon antigens (Stricker *et al.* 1986) and factitious self-administration of antigens. However, even after exhaustive investigation, there remains a group of individuals with recurrent attacks of anaphylaxis, in whom no agent or mechanism can be identified.

Pathogenesis

The essential common factor in anaphylaxis, whether initiated by immunological mechanisms or by others previously outlined, is the activation of mast cells and circulating basophils, with the release of preformed mediators by degranulation and the generation and release of newly formed mediators. The mast cell is capable of releasing a wide variety of inflammatory mediators, with effects on vascular and bronchial smooth muscle, and vascular permeability. Many of these mediators are also able to recruit other inflammatory cells, such as eosinophils, which are prominent in anaphylactic reactions. Once recruited, these cells are, in turn, able to amplify the inflammatory response by secondary generation of mediators (Fig. 53.2)

Preformed mediators of mast cells

Preformed mediators are stored in cytoplasmic granules and are rapidly released in response to a variety of stimuli, including the cross-linking by antigen of two or more IgE molecules bound to surface receptors (Ishizaka and Ishizaka 1984), the anaphylatoxins C3a and C5a (Dvorak *et al.* 1981) and osmotic stimuli (Findlay *et al.* 1981). Granule-associated factors thought to be implicated in the genesis of anaphylaxis include histamine, eosinophil and neutrophil chemotactic factors, heparin, tryptase and kininogenase.

HISTAMINE

The first mast cell mediator to be recognized, histamine has been identified in the venous blood of individuals in conjunction with anaphylaxis (Sheffer *et al.* 1983). Subcutaneous injection of histamine increases vascular permeability in post-capillary venules (Majno and Palade 1961). Infusions of histamine have been shown to mimic the signs and symptoms of anaphylaxis, including urticaria, angio-oedema, hypotension, bronchospasm and coronary vasoconstriction (Levi 1972), and their intensity correlates with histamine levels (Lorenz *et al.* 1982).

CHEMOTACTIC FACTORS

While not implicated in the acute anaphylactic response, neutrophil and eosinophil chemotactic factors are released by immunological stimuli (Goetzl and Austen 1975; Czarnetzki *et al.* 1976). They may account for the accumulation of eosinophils seen in anaphylactic reactions. In addition, these mediators may be involved in the severe late-phase reactions, which occur in up to 20% of patients (Stark and Sullivan 1986), and in the persistent sequelae of anaphylactic reactions.

ENZYMES

Neutral proteases such as tryptase account for up to 25% of total mast cell mass (Schwartz *et al.* 1981). Although the role of tryptase in anaphylactic

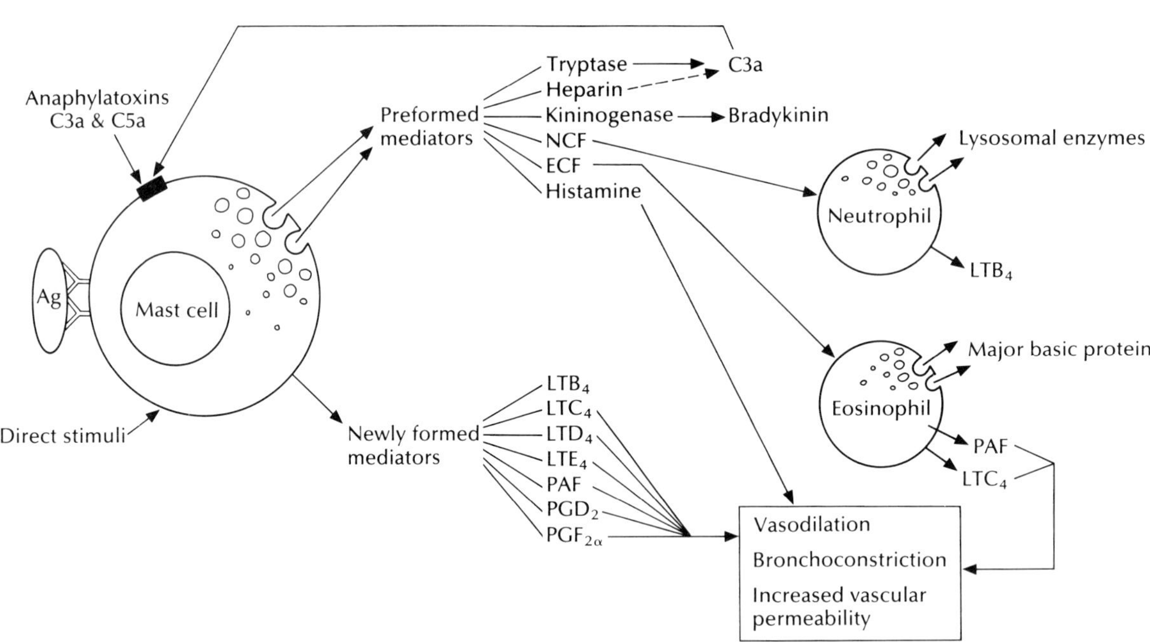

Fig. 53.2. Mediators which may participate in anaphylactic reactions. Ag = antigen, NCF = neutrophil chemotactic factors, ECF = eosinophil chemotactic factors, LT = leukotriene, PAF = platelet-activating factor, PG = prostaglandin.

reactions remains to be fully clarified, it has been shown to cleave C3 to generate C3a and C3b *in vitro* (Schwartz *et al.* 1983). This effect is potentiated by the presence of heparin, another granule-derived mast cell product. Such an effect, if occurring *in vivo*, provides an additional amplifying mechanism.

Basophils and mast cells both produce kininogenases, which cause increased generation of bradykinin *in vitro* (Newball *et al.* 1979). Bradykinin, which is a vasodilator, also increases vascular permeability. It has been detected in venous blood following antigen challenge in sensitized subjects (Proud *et al.* 1983) but not, as yet, in systemic anaphylaxis.

Newly generated mediators of mast cells

Newly generated mediators are all derived from the mobilization of membrane lipids by the action of phospholipase A_2. They are not present in stored form but are rapidly generated following cell activation. This group of mediators comprises the prostaglandins, thromboxanes, leukotrienes and platelet-activating factor (PAF).

PROSTAGLANDINS

Prostaglandins are formed from arachidonic acid by the cyclo-oxygenase pathway. Immunoglobulin E-mediated stimulation of human lung mast cells causes generation and release of PGD_2, thromboxane A_2 (TXA_2) (Peters *et al.* 1984), which is rapidly metabolized to TXB_2, and possibly PGF_2 (Lichtenstein *et al.* 1984). These are all potent pro-inflammatory mediators, which cause smooth-muscle contraction, bronchoconstriction and mucus secretion, and activation of human basophils to enhance mediator release.

LEUKOTRIENES

The sulphidopeptide leukotrienes, LTC-4, LTD-4 and LTE-4, constitute the activity previously termed slow-reacting substance of anaphylaxis (SRS-A). They are formed by the activity of the 5-lipoxygenase pathway and are produced by a number of types of inflammatory cells, including mast cells and eosinophils (Lichtenstein *et al.* 1984). Leukotriene C-4, LTD-4 and LTE-4 increase vascular permeability and contract non-vascular smooth muscle (Drazen *et al.* 1980), causing bronchoconstriction. Leukotriene B-4, also generated by mast cells, neutrophils and monocytes, is a potent neutrophil and eosinophil chemotactic agent (Nagy *et al.* 1982).

PLATELET-ACTIVATING FACTOR

Platelet-activating factor was first discovered in the supernatants of antigen-challenged rabbit basophils. It has potent bronchoconstrictor (Rubin *et al.* 1987) and coronary vasoconstrictor (Levi *et al.* 1984) actions and has been shown to cause both vasoconstriction and vasodilation in the pulmonary circulation (Barnes *et al.* 1988). It is approximately 1000 times more active than histamine in inducing vascular permeability (Evans *et al.* 1987). Platelet-activating factor activates a wide variety of inflammatory cells, including platelets, eosinophils and neutrophils, and is a potent eosinophil chemotactic agent. In animal models, infusion of PAF has been shown to mimic most of the features of anaphylaxis (Halonen *et al.* 1980). In addition, specific PAF antagonists, such as BN52021, inhibit the haemodynamic changes of shock induced by injection of IgG aggregates (Sanches-Crespo *et al.* 1985) in dogs and rats, and bronchoconstriction induced by antigen challenge in sensitized guinea-pigs (Lagente *et al.* 1987). The role of PAF in human anaphylaxis is less certain. Although human mast cells generate PAF following stimulation with IgE, they do not release it under such conditions (Lichtenstein *et al.* 1984).

Clinical manifestations

Anaphylaxis is the most serious emergency in allergic disease. Although individuals may vary greatly in the onset, clinical manifestations and time course, the hallmark of the anaphylactic reaction is the onset of symptoms within seconds or minutes of exposure to the precipitating agent. The initial signs and symptoms are often sensations of warmth, pruritis and tingling, especially of the hands, feet, groins and axillae, accompanied by a generalized flush. Subjects commonly feel an ovewhelming sense of impending doom and may complain of abdominal cramps and a feeling of faintness.

Cutaneous effects are not life-threatening and may progress from a flush through to generalized urticaria or to angio-oedema over several hours. Such effects are transient and resolve within 24 hours. Gastrointestinal disturbance may progress from the initial cramping pains and nausea to diarrhoea, which may be bloodstained, and profuse vomiting.

The most serious manifestations of acute anaphylaxis are those affecting the respiratory tract and cardiovascular system. Together with the initial flush and angio-oedema, these form the most common manifestations of anaphylaxis, with one series of 276 patients studied by Fisher and Baldo (1988) finding cardiovascular collapse in 92%, erythema in 48%, bronchospasm in 29% and angio-oedema in 24%. In another series, Delage and Irey (1972) found that 70% of fatalities were due to respiratory complications and 24% due to cardiovascular collapse.

Respiratory tract involvement may take the form of upper airways obstruction due to laryngeal oedema, or lower airways obstruction due to bronchospasm and oedema. Initial symptoms and signs suggesting upper airways obstruction include hoarseness, dysphagia, a sense of fullness or constriction of the throat and the development of respiratory stridor. Lower respiratory tract manifestations include wheezing, coughing, chest tightness and increasing shortness of breath. Both may progress to asphyxia.

Cardiovascular collapse is often rapid in onset, with a feeling of faintness and retrosternal pain, followed by syncope, due either to a combination of vasodilation and suppressed cardiac function, or to asphyxia or cardiac arrhythmia. Myocardial infarction has been reported in acute anaphylaxis (Levine 1976).

Up to 20% of patients treated for an initial episode of anaphylaxis may have a further life-threatening episode up to 8 hours after the apparent remission of symptoms. This phenomenon has been termed biphasic anaphylaxis (Popa and Lerner 1984; Stark and Sullivan 1986) and may reflect release of secondary mediators by recruited inflammatory cells, a situation analogous to the late-phase asthmatic response seen after antigen bronchial challenge in sensitized subjects. Death from anaphylaxis may occur within minutes of exposure (James and Austen 1964) but may occur up to several weeks after the initial event, secondary to organ damage incurred in the acute reaction (Barnard 1973).

Laboratory investigations

Few laboratory tests are ever carried out during acute anaphylactic episodes, due to the unpredictable onset, the rapid course and the urgency of treatment. Chest X-ray may show evidence of hyperinflation caused by bronchospasm, and areas of atelectasis due to oedema and mucus plugging of the smaller airways (Edde and Burtis 1973). Electrocardiogram (ECG) recordings may show signs of ischaemia or infarction, conduction disturbances, including bundle branch block, and various supraventricular arrhythmias (Booth and Patterson 1970). Blood count may reveal haemoconcentration if the patient is in shock due to the increased vascular permeability. Biochemical tests may reveal raised concentrations of creatine phosphokinase and glutamo-oxaloacetic transferase in the days following the acute episode. Acute abnormalities of the coagulation and complement systems have been reported in connection with anaphylaxis (Tannenbaum *et al.* 1975; Smith, P.L. *et al.* 1980), as have elevations of serum histamine levels (Smith, P.L. *et al.* 1980). The presence of a positive RAST to a known allergen may confirm the diagnosis and may be used *post mortem*.

Pathological abnormalities

Post-mortem investigation in fatal episodes of anaphylaxis in humans reveals acute pulmonary hyperinflation in up to 50% of cases, and laryngeal and upper respiratory tract oedema in up to two-thirds. There is submucosal oedema and an eosinophilic infiltrate in the bronchial walls (James and Austen 1964) and the peribronchial vessels are dilated and congested. There are increased quantities of mucus and oedema fluid in the airway lumen and alveolar spaces. Investigation of other organs reveals similar vascular changes in the abdominal viscera, including the liver and spleen. As many as 80% of cases may show evidence of myocardial damage (Delage *et al.* 1973).

Differential diagnosis

The combination of symptoms and signs leaves the diagnosis rarely in doubt in the acute situation. However, in some cases the first manifestation may be loss of consciousness and, in these cases, the possibility of cardiac arrhythmia or infarction, pulmonary embolism or acute respiratory obstruction due to inhalation must be considered. Vasovagal attacks may look superficially similar, but are not accompanied by urticaria or any evidence of respiratory obstruction, such as stridor or wheeze. In addition, there is pallor rather than evidence of vasodilation, the pulse is slow rather than fast and symptoms are rapidly relieved by lying flat. Laryngeal oedema may occur in the syndrome of hereditary angioneurotic oedema but there is no associated hypotension or urticaria and the onset is generally somewhat slower. In angioneurotic oedema a family history may be elicited and the diagnosis may be confirmed by testing for C1 esterase inhibitor activity.

Cold urticaria may simulate the other features of anaphylaxis, although there is usually a history of cold exposure and this may be confirmed by challenge testing. A combination of careful history-taking and skin or RAST testing for suspected allergens results in diagnosis for a large number of IgE-mediated reactions.

Treatment

The early recognition and initiation of treatment in acute general anaphylaxis is of paramount importance. Death may occur within minutes and is more likely the greater the delay in treatment (Barnard 1973). As death is ultimately due to hypoxia, as in all forms of shock, the initial treatment should be aimed at protecting respiratory and cardiovascular function and tissue oxygenation. The treatment of choice is adrenaline in a dose of 10 μg/kg up to 1 mg (1.0 ml of a 1:1000 solution) given subcutaneously. Adrenaline blocks the end-organ effects of histamine, causing bronchodilation via β_2-adrenergic receptors and vasoconstriction via α-receptors, and is positively inotropic. It also inhibits release of histamine and leucotrienes by mast cells. As the effect is short-lived, repeat injections of adrenaline may be necessary at frequent intervals until the reaction subsides.

If the site of injection of allergen is peripheral, as in an insect sting, absorption may be delayed by the application of a tourniquet proximal to the site and removal of the sting if still embedded. Some authors recommend local subcutaneous injection at the site of the sting of a further 0.15 ml of 1:1000 adrenaline to slow absorption (Soto-Aguillar *et al.* 1987). If a tourniquet is applied, it should be loosened for 1 minute every 3 minutes. If severe systemic symptoms of anaphylaxis appear, other measures should be taken. These can be conveniently divided into those preserving airway function and those preserving cardiovascular function.

Respiratory tract obstruction

Oxygen should be administered in the highest concentration available. In the absence of hypotension, nebulized β agonists such as salbutamol may be effective. If not, slow intravenous infusion of aminophylline 5 mg/kg over 10–20 minutes, followed by infusion at 0.9 mg/kg/hour, is frequently used. Alternatively, intravenous infusions of a specific β_2 agonist or adrenaline may be used to control bronchospasm. If adequate airway patency is not maintained, early intubation and assisted ventilation may be required. Occasionally, bronchospasm in anaphylaxis may respond to administration of anaesthetic agents such as ether, halothane, ketamine and endotracheal instillation of procaine (Fisher and Baldo 1988).

Cardiovascular collapse

Hypotension is usually due to a combination of vasodilation and fluid loss into the extracellular space, resulting in a hypovolaemic state. Fluid replacement should be aggressive and primarily with colloid solutions, such as Haemaccel, dextran or plasma protein solution. Although these compounds themselves can cause anaphylactoid reactions, this rarely occurs in anaphylactic shock states. Central venous pressure (CVP) and, if possible, pulmonary capillary wedge pressure (PCWP) should be monitored and infusions continued if PCWP is less than 6 mmHg or CVP is less than 5 cm H_2O and the patient remains hypotensive. If CVP or PCWP are elevated (CVP >15 cm H_2O, PCWP >18 mmHg) inotropic agents should be used. Dopamine at doses above 5 μg/kg/minute has the advantage of combining a positive inotropic effect and a vasoconstrictor adrenergic effect. Some patients fail to respond to any sympathomimetic other than noradrenaline.

Bradycardia may require injections of atropine to maintain cardiac rate. In any severe anaphylactic reaction, particularly if it involves an element of angio-oedema, it is recommended practice to administer H_1 antagonists, such as chlorpheniramine 20 mg intravenously. There are also some grounds for adding H_2 antagonists, as the combination has been shown to suppress late-phase cutaneous responses (Smith, J.A. *et al.* 1980) and also the clinical manifestations of chemically induced anaphylaxis in dogs (Schoning *et al.* 1982). However, there is little direct evidence that histamine antagonists offer any therapeutic value in the treatment of anaphylactic reactions, although they may be of use in premedication to prevent or ameliorate anaphylaxis. Likewise, corticosteroids, in the form of intravenous hydrocortisone or methylprednisolone, and oral prednisolone are recommended for suppression of late-phase and persistent reactions. However, Stark and Sullivan (1986) found that 10/12 patients with persistent or biphasic anaphylaxis had been given oral or parenteral corticosteroids during the treatment of the initial reaction, and yet still had severe prolonged or recurrent symptoms within 12 hours. In view of the risk of severe late reactions, patients with severe anaphylactic reactions should be monitored closely for 24 hours.

Prevention

Many cases of anaphylaxis may be avoided by taking a careful, detailed medical history, avoiding agents known to have caused, or suspected of causing, previous reactions, and giving drugs orally rather than parenterally when possible. Once a substance is suspected, sensitivity may be determined by RAST or by skin testing, although these are not completely reliable. Skin testing itself carries a risk of anaphylaxis and should be performed with caution, with resuscitation equipment available.

Patient education plays an important part in avoiding exposure to relevant antigens and, in addition, patients may be taught to carry and self-administer preloaded adrenaline-containing syringes, in cases of recurrent anaphylaxis. If a known anaphylactic agent is required in treatment, or if exposure is unavoidable for other reasons, there is a place for desensitization, although this is dangerous in itself (Warner and Kerr 1987) and should only be carried out in experienced hands and with appropriate facilities. An alternative sometimes adopted for the use of radiocontrast media is to pretreat patients for 24 hours with corticosteroids (Lasser *et al.* 1987), either alone or in combination with H_1 and H_2 antagonists.

Prognosis

Recovery from acute anaphylaxis is usually rapid and complete and occurs within a few hours, although in a minority it may persist or recur within 12–24 hours. Long-term sequelae are rare unless cardiac or neurological damage is incurred in the initial episode. In general, further anaphylactic attacks become more severe with each successive episode.

References

Adkinson, N.F. (1984). Risk factors for drug allergy. *J. Allergy Clin. Immunol.* **74**, 567–72.

Aroyave, C.M. and Tan, E.M. (1977). Mechanism of complement activation by radiographic contrast media. *Clin Exp. Immunol.* 89–94.

Arthus, M. (1921). *De l'anaphylaxie à l'immunité*. Masson, Paris.

Baldo, B.A. and Fisher, M.M. (1983). Anaphylaxis to muscle relaxant drugs: cross-reactivity and molecular basis of binding of IgE antibodies detected by radioimmunoassay. *Mol. Immunol.* **20**, 1393–400.

Barnard, J.H. (1973). Studies of 400 Hymenoptera stings in the United States. *J. Allergy Clin. Immunol.* **52**, 259–64.

Barnes, P.J., Chung, K.F. and Page, C.P. (1988). Platelet activating factor as a mediator of allergic disease. *J. Allergy Clin. Immunol.* **81**, 919–34.

Batchelor, F.R., Dewdney, J.M., Weston, R.D. and Wheeler, A.W. (1966). The immunogenicity of cephalosporin derivatives and their cross reaction with penicillin. *Immunology* **10**, 21–33.

Bernstein, D.I. and Bernstein, I.L. (1986). Chymopapain induced allergic reactions. *Clin Rev. Allergy* **4**, 201–13.

Bolt, H. and Herman, A.G. (1983). Inflammatory mediators released by complement-derived peptides. *Agents Actions* **13**, 405–14.

Booth, P.H. and Patterson, R. (1970). Electrocardiographic changes during human anaphylaxis. *JAMA* **211**, 627–31.

Boston Collaborative Drug Surveillance Program (1973). Drug induced anaphylaxis. *JAMA* **224**, 613–15.

Burman, D., Hodson, A.K., Wood, C.B.S. and Brueton, F.W. (1973). Acute anaphylaxis, pulmonary oedema and intravascular hemolysis due to cryoprecipitate. *Arch. Dis. Child.* **48**, 483–5.

Caulfield, J.P., Lewis, R.A., Hein, A. and Austen, K.F. (1980). Secretion in dissociated human pulmonary mast cells: evidence for solubilisation of granule contents before discharge. *J. Cell Biol.* **85**, 299–312.

Chafee, F.H. and Settipane, G.A. (1967). Asthma caused by FDC approved dyes. *J. Allergy* **40**, 65–72.

Chafee, F.H. and Settipane, G.A. (1974). Aspirin intolerance. I.

Frequency in an allergic population. *J. Allergy Clin. Immunol.* **53**, 193–9.

Charpin, D., Benzarti, M., Hemon, Y., *et al.* (1988). Atopy and anaphylactic reactions to suxamethonium. *J. Allergy Clin. Immunol.* **82**, 356–60.

Christian, C.L. (1960). Studies of aggregated γ-globulin. II. Effect *in vivo*. *J. Immunol.* **84**, 117–21.

Clayton, W.F., Georgitis, J.W. and Reisman, P.E. (1985). Insect sting anaphylaxis in patients without detectable serum venom specific IgE. *Clin. Allergy* **15**, 329–33.

Craddock, P.R., Fehr, J., Brigham, K.L., Kronenberg, R.S. and Jacob, H.A. (1977). Complement and leukocyte-mediated pulmonary dysfunction in hemodialysis. *N. Engl. J. Med.* **296**, 769–74.

Czarnetzki, B.M., Konig, W. and Lichtenstein, L.M.G. (1976). Antigen induced eosinophil chemotactic factor (ECF) release by human leukocytes. *Inflammation* **201**, 215–18.

Delage, C. and Irey, N.S. (1972). Anaphylactic deaths: a clinicopathologic study of 43 cases. *J. Forensic Sci.* **17**, 525.

Delage, C., Mullick, F.G. and Irey, N.S. (1973). Myocardial lesions in anaphylaxis: a histochemical study. *Arch. Pathol. Lab. Med.* **95**, 185–9.

Despres, P., Plainfosse, B., Papiernic, T. *et al.* (1971). Les intolérances digestives aux protéines du lait de vache chez l'enfant. *Ann. Paediatr.* **18**, 464–82.

de Weck, A.L. and Blum, G. (1965). Recent clinical and immunological aspects of penicillin allergy. *Int. Arch. Allergy* **27**, 221–56.

Donaldson, V.H. and Evans, R.R. (1963). A biochemical abnormality in hereditary angioneurotic oedema: absence of serum inhibitor of C1 estarase. *Am. J. Med.* **35**, 37–44.

Drazen, J.M., Austen, K.F., Lewis, R.A. *et al.* (1980). Comparative airway and vascular activities of leukotrienes C1 and D *in vivo* and *in vitro*. *Proc. Nat. Acad. Sci. (USA)* **77**, 4354–8.

Dvorak, A.M., Lett-Brown, M., Thueson, D. and Grant, J.A. (1981). Complement-induced degranulation of human basophils. *J. Immunol.* **126**(2), 523–8.

Edde, R.R. and Burtis, B.B. (1973). Lung injury in anaphylactic shock. *Chest* **63**, 636–8.

Ellis, E.F. and Henney, C.S. (1969). Adverse reactions following administration of human gamma globulin. *J. Allergy* **13**, 45–54.

Evans, T.W., Chung, K.F., Rogers, D.F. and Barnes, P.J. (1987). Effect of platelet-activating factor on airway vascular permeability: possible mechanisms. *J. Appl. Physiol.* **63**, 479–84.

Feinberg, A.R., Feinberg, S.M. and Bernarm-Pinto, C. (1956). Asthma and rhinitis from insect allergens: clinical importance. *J. Allergy* **27**, 437–44.

Ferreri, N.R., Howland, W.C., Stevenson, D.D. and Spiegelberg, H.L. (1988). Release of leukotrienes, prostaglandins and histamine into nasal secretions of aspirin-sensitive asthmatics during reaction to aspirin. *Am. Rev. Respir. Dis.* **137**, 847–54.

Findlay, S.R., Dvorack, A.M., Kagey-Sobotka, A. and Lichtenstein, L.M. (1981). Hyperosmolar triggering of histamine release from human basophils. *J. Clin. Invest.* **67**, 1604–13.

Fisher, M.M. (1975). Severe histamine mediated reactions to intravenous drugs used in anaesthesia. *Anaesthesia Intensive Care* **3**, 180–97.

Fisher, M.M. and Baldo, B.A. (1984). Anaphylactoid reactions during anaesthesia. In *Adverse Reactions*, ed. M.M. Fisher, vol. 3, pp. 677–92, W.B. Saunders, London.

Fisher, M.M. and Baldo B.A. (1988). Acute anaphylactic reactions. *Med. J. Aust.* **149**, 34–8.

Flower, R.J., Gryglewski, R., Herbaczynska-Cerdro, K. and Vane, J.R. (1972). Effects of anti-inflammatory drugs on prostaglandin biosynthesis. *Nature* **238**, 104–6.

Frank, M.M., Gelfaud, J.A. and Atkinson, J.P. (1976). Hereditary angioedema: the clinical syndrome and its management. *Ann. Intern. Med.* **84**, 580–93.

Freyria, A.M., Belleville, J., Eloy, R. and Trager, J. (1982). Effects of five different contrast agents on serum complement and calcium levels after excretory urography. *J. Allergy Clin. Immunol.* **69**, 397–403.

Giansiracus, D.F. and Upchurch, K.S. (1985). Anaphylactic and anaphylactoid reactions. In *Intensive Care Medicine*, ed. J.M. Rippe and M. Caste, pp. 1102–12, Little Brown & Co., Boston.

Goetzl, E.J. and Austen, K.F. (1975). Purification and synthesis of eosinophilotactic tetrapeptides of human lung tissue: identification as eosinophil chemotactic factor of anaphylaxis. *Proc. Nat. Acad. Sci. (USA)* **72**, 4123–7.

Grammer, L.C., Schafer, M., Bernstein, D. *et al.* (1987). Prevention of chymopapain anaphylaxis by screening chemonucleosis candidates with cutaneous chymopapain testing: a preliminary report. *Clin. Orthopaedics* **221**, 202–6.

Green, G.R. (1970). Antibiotic therapy in patients with a history of penicillin allergy. In *Penicillin Allergy: Clinical and Immunological Aspects*, ed. G.T. Stewart and J.P. McGovern, pp. 162–75, Charles C. Thomas, Springfield.

Green, G.R. and Rosenblum, A. (1971). Report of the Penicillin Study Group — American Academy of Allergy. *J. Allergy Clin. Immunol.* **48**, 331–43.

Habermann, E. (1972) Bee and wasp venoms. *Science* **177**, 314–22.

Hakim, R.M., Breillat, J., Lazarus, J.M. and Port, F.K. (1984). Complement activation and hypersensivity reactions to dialysis membranes. *N. Engl. J. Med.* **311** (14), 878–82.

Halonen, M., Palmer, J.D., Lohman, I.C., McManus, L.M. and Pinckard, R.N. (1980). Respiratory and circulatory alterations induced by acetyl-glyceryl ether phosphorylcholine, a mediator of IgE anaphylaxis in the rabbit. *Am. Rev. Respir. Dis.* **122**, 915–24.

Hedin, H., Richter, W. and Ring, J. (1976). Dextran-induced anaphylactoid reactions in man. *Int. Arch. Allergy Appl. Immunol.* **52**, 145–59.

Horowitz, L. (1975). Atopy as a factor in penicillin reactions. *N. Engl. J. Med.* **292**, 1243–4.

Idsoe, O., Gruthe, T., Willcox, R.R. and de Weck, A.L. (1968). Nature and extent of penicillin side-reactions with particular reference to fatalities from anaphylactic shock. *Bull. WHO* **38**, 159–68.

Ishizaka, T. and Ishizaka, K. (1984). Activation of mast cells for receptor release through IgE receptors. *Prog. Allergy* **34**, 188–235.

James, L.P. and Austen, K.F. (1964). Fatal systemic anaphylaxis in man. *N. Engl. J. Med.* **270**, 597–603.

Kashiwagi, N., Brantigan, C.O., Brettschneider, L., Groth, C.G. and Starzl, T.E. (1968). Clinical reactions and serologic changes after the administration of heterologous antilymphocyte globulin to human recipients of renal homografts. *Ann. Intern. Med.* **68**, 275–86.

Kern, R.A. and Wimberley, N.A., Jr (1953). Penicillin reactions: their nature, growing importance, recognition, management and prevention. *Am. J. Med. Sci.* **226**, 357–75.

Kidd, J.M., Cohen, S.H., Sosman, A.J. and Fink, J.N. (1982). Food dependent exercise-induced anaphylaxis. *J. Allergy Clin. Immunol.* **71**, 407–11.

Lagente, V., Touvay, C., Randon, J. *et al.* (1987). Interference of the PAF-acether antagonist BN52021 with passive anaphylaxis in the guinea pig. *Prostaglandins* **33**, 265–74.

Lamson, R.W. (1924). Fatal anaphylaxis and sudden death associated with the injection of foreign substances. *JAMA* **82**, 1091–4.

Lamson, R.W. (1929). So-called fatal anaphylaxis in man with especial reference to diagnosis and treatment of clinical allergies. *JAMA* **93**, 1775–8.

Lasser, E.C., Berry, C.C., Talner, L.B. *et al.* (1987). Pretreatment with corticosteroids to alleviate reactions to intravenous contrast material. *N. Engl. J. Med.* **317**, 845–9.

Levi, R. (1972). Effects of exogenous and immunologically released histamine on the isolated heart: a quantitative comparison. *J. Pharmacol. Exp. Ther.* **182**, 227–38.

Levi, R., Burke, J.A., Guo, Z.G., *et al.* (1984). Acetyl glyceryl ether phosphorylcholine (AGEPC): a putative mediator of cardiac anaphylaxis in the guinea pig. *Circ. Res.* **54**, 117–24.

Levine, B.B. (1966). Immunologic mechanisms of penicillin allergy: a haptenic model system for the study of allergic diseases of man. *N. Engl. J. Med.* **275**, 1115–25.

Levine, B.B. (1973). Antigenicity and cross-reactivity of penicillins and cephalosporins. *J. Infect. Dis.* **128**, S364–S366.

Levine, B.B. and Redmond, A.P. (1969). Minor haptenic determinant-specific reagins of penicillin hypersensitivity in man. *Int. Arch. Allergy Appl. Immunol.* **35**, 445–55.

Levine, H.D. (1976). Acute myocardial infarction following wasp sting: report of two cases and critical survey of the literature. *Am. Heart J.* **91**, 365–74.

Levy, J.H., Roizen, M.F. and Morris, J. (1986). Anaphylactic and anaphylactoid reactions: a review. *Spine* **11** (3), 282–91.

Lichtenstein, L.M., Schleimer, R.P., MacGlashan, D.W. Jr, *et al.* (1984). *In vitro* and *in vivo* studies of Mediator release from human mast cells. In *Asthma: Physiology, Immunopharmacology and Treatment*, ed. A.B. Kay, R.F. Austen and L.M. Lichtenstein, pp. 1–19. Academic Press, London.

Lieberman, P. and Siegle, R.L. (1979). Complement activation following intravenous contrast material administration. *J. Allergy Clin. Immunol.* **64**, 13–17.

Lieberman, P., Siegle, R.L. and Treadwell, G. (1987). Radiocontrast reactions. In *Clinical Reviews in Allergy*, ed. L.L. Lieberman, Elsevier Science, Amsterdam.

Lorenz, W., Doenicke, A., Schoning, B., Ohmann, C., Grote, B. and Neugebaver, E. (1982). Definition and classification of the histamine release response to drugs in anaesthesia and surgery: studies in the conscious human subject. *Klin. Wochenschr.* **60**, 896–913.

McClennan, B.L., Periman, P.O. and Rockoff, S.D. (1976). Positive immunological response to contrast media. *Invest. Radiol.* **11**, 240.

McCullough, J., Canham, W. and Dolovich, J. (1985). Skin testing for chymopapain allergy — a preliminary report. *Ann Allergy* **55**, 609–11.

Majno, G. and Palade, G.E. (1961). Studies on inflammation. I. The effect of histamine and seratonin on vascular permeability: an electron microscope study. *J. Biophys. Biochem. Cytol.* **11**, 571–605.

Maulitz, R.M., Pratt, D.S. and Schochet, A.L. (1979). Exercise-induced anaphylactic reaction to shellfish. *J. Allergy Clin. Immunol.* **63**, 433–4.

Morrison, D.C. and Cochrane, C.G. (1974). Direct evidence for Hageman factor (Factor XII) activation by bacterial lipopolysaccharides (endotoxins). *J. Exp. Med.* **140**, 797–811.

Murray, J.A. (1964). Case of multiple bee stings. *Central Afr. J. Med.* **10**, 249–51.

Nagy, L., Lee, T.H., Goetzl, E.J., Pickett, W.C. and Kay, A.B. (1982). Complement receptor enhancement and chemotaxis of human neutrophils and eosinophils by leukotrienes and other lipoxygenase products. *Clin Exp. Immunol.* **47**, 541–7.

Newball, H.H., Berninger, R.W., Talamo, R.C. and Lichtenstein, L.M. (1979). Anaphylactic release of basophil kallikrein-like activity. I. Purification and characterisation. *J. Clin. Invest.* **64**, 457–65.

Parker, C.W. (1963). Penicillin allergy. *Am. J. Med.* **34**, 747–52.

Parker, C.W. (1972). Allergic drug responses — mechanisms and unsolved problems. *CRC Crit. Rev. Toxicol.* **1**, 261–5.

Parrish, H.M. (1965). Analysis of 460 fatalities from venomous animals in the United States. *Am. J. Med. Sci.* **245**, 129–41.

Patterson, R. and Valentine, M. (1982). Anaphylaxis and related allergic emergencies including reactions to insect stings. *JAMA* **248**, 2632–6.

Peters, S.P., MacGlashan, D.W., Jr, Schulman, E.S. *et al.* (1984). Arachidonic acid metabolism in purified human lung mast cells. *J. Immunol.* **132**, 1972–9.

Petz, L.D. (1978). Immunologic cross reactivity between penicillins and cephalosporins: a review. *J. Infect. Dis.* **137S**, 74–9.

Popa, V.T. and Lerner, S.A. (1984). Biphasic systemic anaphylactic reaction: three illustrative cases. *Ann. Allergy* **53**, 151–5.

Portier, P. and Richet, C. (1902). De l'action anaphylactique de certains venins. *C.R. Soc. Biol. (Paris)* **54**, 170.

Proud, D., Togias, A., Naclerio, R.M. *et al.* (1983). Kinins are generated *in vivo* following nasal airway challenge of allergic individuals with allergen. *J. Clin. Invest.* **72**, 1678–85.

Reisman, R.E., Rose, N.R. and Witebsky, E. (1962). Penicillin allergy and desensitisation. *J. Allergy* **33**, 178–87.

Rice, M.C., Leiberman, P., Siegle, R.L. and Mason, J. (1983). *In vitro* histamine release induced by radio-contrast media and various chemical analogues in reactor and control subjects. *J. Allergy Clin. Immunol.* **72**, 180–6.

Ring, J., Seifert, J., Lob, G., Hopf, U., Land, W. and Brendel, W. (1974). Allergic reactions to horse globulin therapy and their prevention by induction of immunological tolerance. *Allergol. Immunopathol.* **2**, 93–8.

Rosen, F.S., Alper, C.A., Pensky, J., Klemperer, M.R. and Donaldson, V.H. (1971). Genetic heterogeneity of the C1 esterase inhibitor in patients with hereditary angioneurotic oedema. *J. Clin. Invest.* **50**, 2143–9.

Rubin, A.E., Smith, L.J. and Patterson, R. (1987). The bronchoconstricting properties of platelet-activating factor in humans. *Am. Rev. Respir. Dis.* **136**, 1145–51.

Sale, S., Greenberger, P.A. and Patterson, R. (1981). Idiopathic anaphylactoid reactions. *JAMA* **246**, 2336–9.

Samter, M. and Beers, R.F. (1968). Intolerance to aspirin: clinical studies and consideration of its pathogenesis. *Ann. Intern. Med.* **68**, 975–83.

Sanches-Crespo, M., Fernandes-Gallardo, S., Nieto, M.L., Baranes, J. and Braquet, P. (1985). Inhibition of the vascular actions of IgG aggregates by BN52021, a highly-specific antagonist of paf-acether. *Immunopharmacology* **10**, 69–75.

Schoenfeld, M.R. (1960). Acute allergic reactions to morphine, codeine, meperidine hydrochloride and opium alkaloids. *NY State J. Med.* **60**, 2591–3.

Schoning, B., Lorenz, W. and Doenicke, A. (1982). Prophylaxis of anaphylactoid reactions to a polypeptidal plasma substitute by H1–plus H2– receptor antagonists: synopsis of three randomised controlled trials. *Klin. Wochenschr.* **60**, 1048–55.

Schuberth, K.C., Golden, D.B.K., Kagey-Sobotka, A., Valentine, M.D. and Lichtenstein, L.M. (1983a). Allergie aux venins d'hyménoptères chez l'enfant. *Rev. Fr. Allergol.* **23**, 73–8.

Schuberth, K.C., Lichtenstein, L.M., Kagey-Sobotka, A., Szklo, M., Kwiterovich, K.A. and Valentine, M.D. (1983b). Epidemiologic study of insect allergy in children. II. Effect of accidental stings in allergic children. *J. Pediatr.* **102**, 361–5.

Schwartz, H.J. and Kahn, B. (1970). Hymenoptera sensitivity. II. The role of atopy in the development of clinical hypersensitivity. *J. Allergy* **45**, 87–91.

Schwartz, L.B., Lewis, R.A., Seldin, D. and Austen, K.F. (1981). Acid hydrolases and tryptase from secretory granules of dispersed human lung mast cells. *J. Immunol.* **126**, 1290–4.

Schwartz, L.B., Kawahara, M.S., Hugli, T.E., Vik, D., Fearon, D.T. and Austen, K.F. (1983). Generation of C3a anaphylatoxin from human C3 by human mast cell tryptase. *J. Immunol.* **130**, 1891–5.

Settipane, G.A. and Chaffe, F.H. (1979). Natural history of allergy to hymenoptera. *Clin Allergy* **9**, 385–90.

Settipane, G.A., Newstead, G.J. and Boyd, G.K. (1972). Frequency of hymenoptera allergy in an atopic and normal population. *J. Allergy* **50**, 146–50.

Settipane, G.A., Klein, D.E. and Boyd, G.K. (1978). Relationship of atopy and anaphylactic sensitisation: a bee sting allergy model. *Clin. Allergy* **8**, 259–65.

Sheffer, A.L. and Austen, K.F. (1980). Exercise-induced anaphylaxis. *J. Allergy Clin. Immunol.* **66**, 106–11.

Sheffer, A.L., Soter, N.A., McFadden, E.R. and Austen, K.F. (1983). Exercise-induced anaphylaxis: a distinct form of physical allergy. *J. Allergy Clin. Immunol.* **71**, 311–16.

Sheffer, A.L., Tong, A.K.F., Murphy, G.F., Lewis, R.A., McFadden, E.R. and Austen, K.F. (1985). Exercise-induced anaphylaxis: a serious form of physical allergy associated with mast cell degranulation. *J. Allergy Clin. Immunol.* **75**, 479–84.

Simmons, J.W., Stavinoha, W.B. and Knodel, L.S. (1984). Update and review of chemonucleolysis. *Clin. Orthopaedics* **183**, 51–60.

Smith, J.A., Mansfield, L.E., de Shazo, R.D. and Nelson, H.S. (1980). An evaluation of the pharmacologic inhibition of the immediate and late cutaneous reaction to allergen. *J. Allergy Clin. Immunol.* **65**, 118–21.

Smith, P.L., Kagey-Sobotka, A., Bleecker, E.R. *et al.* (1980). Physiologic manifestations of human anaphylaxis. *J. Clin. Invest.* **66**, 1072–80.

Sobotka, A.K., Valentine, M.D., Benton, A.W. and Lichtenstein, L.M. (1974). Allergy to insect stings. I. Diagnosis of IgE-mediated hymenoptera sensitivity by venom-induced histamine release. *J. Allergy Clin. Immunol.* **53**, 170–84.

Sonin, L., Grammer, L.C., Greenberger, P.A. and Patterson, R. (1983). Idiopathic anaphylaxis: a clinical summary. *Ann. Intern. Med.* **99** (S), 634–5.

Soter, N.A., Sheffer, A.L., McFadden, E.R., Jr and Austen, K.F. (1982). Exercise-related physical allergy. *J. Allergy Clin Immunol.* **69**, 103.

Soto-Aguillar, M.C., de Shazo, R.D. and Waring, N.P. (1987). Anaphylaxis: why it happens and what to do about it. *Postgrad. Med.* **82**, 154–70.

Stark, B.J. and Sullivan, T.J. (1986). Biphasic and protracted anaphylaxis. *J. Allergy Clin. Immunol.* **78**, 76–83.

Steward, G.T. (1962). Cross-allergenicity of penicillin G and related substances. *Lancet* **i**, 509–10.

Stricker, W.E., Anorve-Lopez, E. and Reed, C.E. (1986). Food skin testing in patients with idiopathic anaphylaxis. *J. Allergy Clin. Immunol.* **77** (3), 516–19.

Sweeney, M.J. and Klotz, S.D. (1983). Frequency of IgE mediated radiocontrast dye reactions. *J. Allergy Clin. Immunol.* **71**, 147.

Szczeklik, A., Gryglewski, R.J. and Czerniawska-Mysik, G. (1975). Relationship of inhibition of prostaglandin biosynthesis by analgesis to asthma attacks in aspirin-sensitive patients. *Br. Med. J.* **1**, 67–9.

Tannenbaum, H., Ruddy, S. and Schur, P.H. (1975). Acute anaphylaxis associated with serum complement depletion. *J. Allergy Clin. Immunol.* **56**, 226–34.

Till, G., Rother, U. and Gemsa, D. (1978). Activation of complement by radiographic contrast media: generation of chemotactic and anaphylatoxin activities. *Int. Arch. Allergy Appl. Immunol.* **56**, 543–50.

Vaughan, W.T. and Pipes, D.M. (1936). On the probable frequency of allergic shock. *Am. J. Dig. Dis.* **3**, 558–64.

von Zabern, I., Pryzyklenk, H., Nolte, R. and Vogt, W. (1984). Effect of metrizamide, a non-ionic radiographic contrast agent, on human serum complement: comparison with ionic contrast media. *Int. Arch. Allergy Appl. Immunol.* **73**, 321–9.

Vyas, G.N., Perkins, H.A. and Fudenberg, H.H. (1968). Anaphylactoid transfusion reactions associated with anti-IgA. *Lancet* **ii**, 312–15.

Vyas, G.N., Homdahl, L., Perkins, H.A. and Fudenberg, H.H. (1969). Serologic specificity of human anti-IgA and its significance in transfusion. *Blood* **34**, 573–81.

Vyas, G.N., Perkins, H.A., Yang, Y.M. and Fudenberg, H.H. (1975). Healthy blood donors with selective absence of immunoglobulin A: prevention of anaphylactic transfusion reactions caused by antibodies to IgA. *J. Lab. Clin. Med.* **85**, 838–42.

Waldbott, G.L. (1949). Anaphylactic death from penicillin. *JAMA* **139**, 526–7.

Warner, J.O. and Kerr, J.W. (1987). Hyposensitisation. *Br. Med. J.* **294**, 1179–80.

Wauters, J.P. and Lambert, P.H. (1977). Haemodialysis-induced leukopenia: role of cellophane membrane and complement activation. *Kidney Int.* **12** (1), 77.

Welch, H., Lewis, L.N., Kerlan, L. and Putnam, L.E. (1953). Acute anaphylactoid reactions attributable to penicillin. *Antibiotic Chemother.* **3**, 891.

Wells, J.V., Buckley, R.H., Schanfield, M.S. and Fundenberg,

H.H. (1977). Anaphylactic reactions to plasma infusions in patients with hypogammaglobulinaemia and anti-IgA antibodies. *Clin. Immunol. Immunopathol.* **5**, 265–71.

Westaby, S., Dawson, P., Turner, M.W. and Pridie, R.B. (1985). Angiography and complement activation: evidence for generation of C3a anaphylotoxin by intravascular contrast agents. *Cardiovasc. Res.* **19**, 85–8.

Wilner, G.D., Nossel, H.L. and Le Roy, E.C. (1968). Activation of Hageman factor by collagen. *J. Clin Invest.* **47**, 2608–15.

54: The Immunopharmacology of Asthma

Q.A. Summers and S.T. Holgate

Introduction

Asthma is a common disease, with a high prevalence in the developed world and a rising death-rate (Burney 1987), the cause of which is not understood. In the last two decades, there have been great advances in the treatment of asthma and in our understanding of the inflammatory basis of the disease, as well as in our understanding of inflammation in general. In this review, we shall concentrate on the evidence for the inflammatory basis of asthma, and specifically examine the role of cells and mediators released and derived from cells in the pathogenesis of this condition.

The definition of asthma

Despite the recent advances in our understanding of allergic disease and asthma, there remains great difficulty in reaching an acceptable definition of the disorder. The most recent description includes clinical, physiological and pathological features (American Thoracic Society 1987). Asthma is a clinical syndrome characterized by increased responsiveness of the tracheobronchial tree to a variety of stimuli, the primary physiological disturbance being reversible airflow limitation, which may be spontaneous or drug-related, and the pathological hallmark being inflammation of the airways (Lopez-Vidrierio and Reid 1983; Beasley *et al.* 1989a). Clinically, it is useful to subdivide asthma into extrinsic and intrinsic variants. Extrinsic asthma has an identifiable precipitant, and can be thought of as being atopic, occupational and drug-induced. Atopic asthma is associated with positive skin tests to common aeroallergens and/or atopic symptoms, and it can be divided further into seasonal and perennial forms according to the seasonal timing of symptoms. Occupational asthma may be related to the development of specific immunoglobulin E (IgE) to a protein hapten such as acid anhydrides in plastic workers and plicatic acid in some western red cedar-induced asthma, or to non-IgE related mechanisms, such as that seen in toluene di-isocyanate-induced asthma (O'Neil and Salvaggio 1988). Drug-induced asthma can be seen after the exhibition of aspirin or other non-steroidal anti-inflammatory drugs, most often in a certain subset of patients who may display other features such as nasal polyposis and sinusitis. Intrinsic or cryptogenic asthma is reported to develop after upper respiratory tract infections, but can arise *de novo* in middle-aged or older people, in whom it is more difficult to treat than extrinsic asthma. Thus, asthma should not be considered as a single disease entity, but rather is the result of a final common pathway of reaction of the airways to a variety of injurious agents in predisposed persons.

Bronchial hyper-responsiveness and airway inflammation

Reversible airflow limitation is manifest by symptoms of dyspnoea, wheeze and cough of varying severity, which are related to the underlying hyper-responsiveness of the airways. Hyper-responsiveness may be defined as the exaggerated bronchoconstrictor response of the airways to a wide variety of specific and non-specific stimuli (Boushey *et al.* 1980). It is commonly expressed as the amount of an inhaled substance (for example, histamine or methacholine) required to produce a predetermined fall in a physiological measurement, such as the volume of air exhaled in the first second of a forced expiration (FEV_1) (Fig. 54.1), or specific airways conductance (sGAW). The term is also used to describe the propensity toward bronchoconstriction on exposure to environmental stimuli such as cold air or irritant substances (Mortagy *et al.* 1986). Hyper-responsiveness relates to the exaggerated diurnal rhythm of airway calibre that is a characteristic of asthma, and which manifests as nocturnal asthma and prominent early morning symptoms of dyspnoea and wheeze (Ryan *et al.* 1982).

Bronchial hyper-responsiveness is present in all forms of asthma, regardless of the type, and in susceptible individuals it may arise after a single exposure to a sensitizing agent (Hargreave *et al.* 1981). Hyper-responsiveness is not found solely in asthmatic patients, as individuals with atopy and even some normal individuals can react to the provocative substances used to measure this phenomenon, although these latter two groups require greater doses to produce the required effect (Cockcroft *et al.* 1977). The level of bronchial hyper-responsiveness is variable over time (Josephs *et al.* 1987) and, although it may change markedly without a concomitant change in symptoms or pulmonary function, it is considered a good reflection of disease severity and need for medication (Juniper *et al.* 1981).

Bronchial hyper-responsiveness and airway inflammation are related directly. The more hyper-

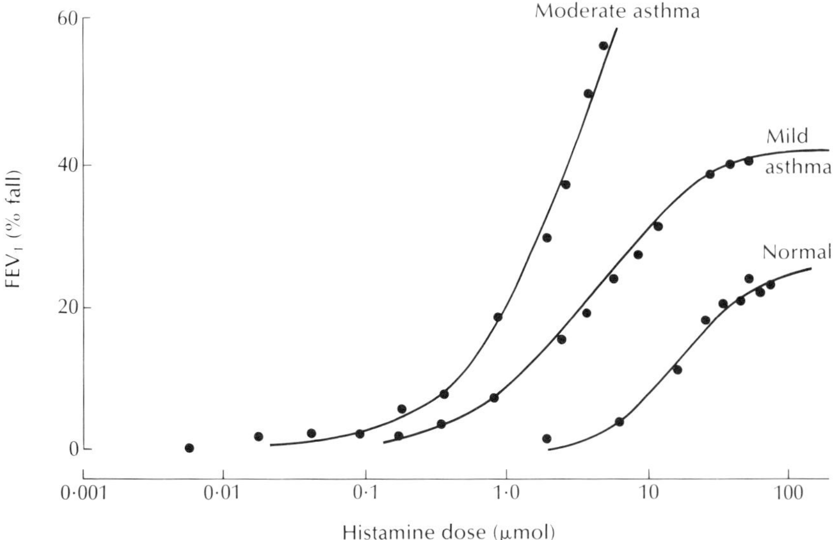

Fig. 54.1. Typical dose–response curves to inhaled histamine in normal subjects, and in mild and moderate asthmatics. The greater sensitivity of the asthmatic subjects to histamine-induced bronchoconstriction as compared with the normal subject is shown and also the 'plateau' achieved in normal subjects but not in asthmatics to increasing doses of inhaled histamine.

responsive the individual (i.e. lower provocative concentration required to produce a 20% fall in FEV_1, designated the PC_{20}), the greater the evidence for inflammation reflected in the cellular and mediator content of bronchoalveolar lavage (BAL) fluid. In this respect the prominent markers of inflammation are the eosinophil, lymphocyte and mast cell and the presence of histamine and eosinophil-derived major basic protein (MBP) in the fluid phase of BAL (Kelly *et al.* 1988; Wardlaw *et al.* 1988). Airway inflammation is a constant feature of both acute and chronic asthma. Patients who have died during an acute attack of asthma have marked inflammatory cell infiltration of their airways with especially eosinophils and prominent damage to the pseudostratified epithelium (Dunnill 1960) (Fig. 54.2). These and other features of inflammation have also been found in bronchial biopsies taken from patients with chronic asthma (Glynn and Michaels 1960; Laitinen *et al.* 1985; Beasley *et al.* 1989a). In comparison with 'normal airways', these changes include mucus and protein plugging, hypertrophy of airways smooth muscle, and the demonstration of sub-basement membrane

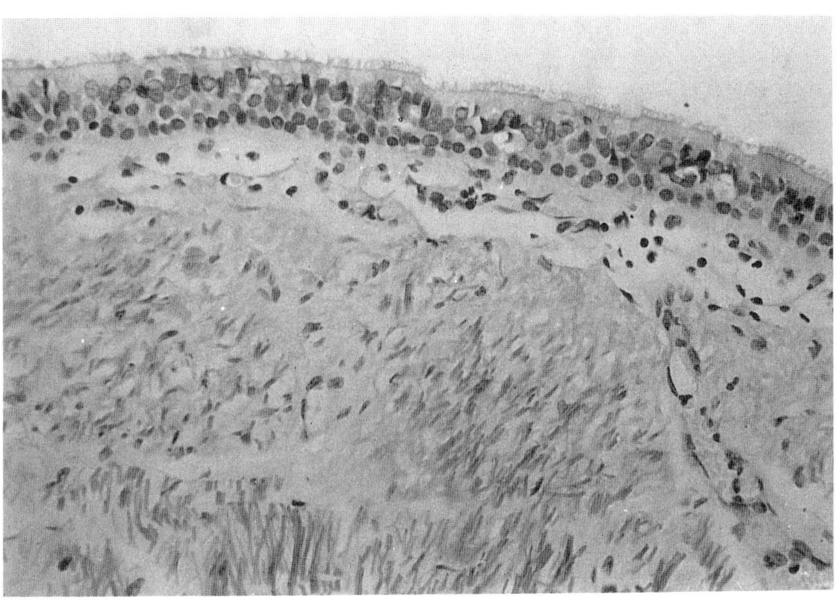

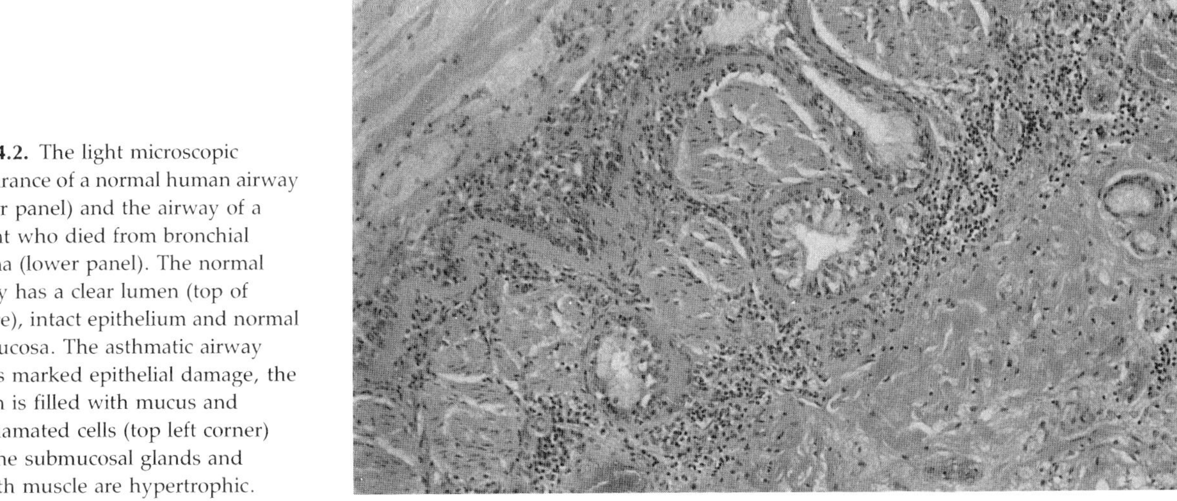

Fig. 54.2. The light microscopic appearance of a normal human airway (upper panel) and the airway of a patient who died from bronchial asthma (lower panel). The normal airway has a clear lumen (top of picture), intact epithelium and normal submucosa. The asthmatic airway shows marked epithelial damage, the lumen is filled with mucus and desquamated cells (top left corner) and the submucosal glands and smooth muscle are hypertrophic.

type 3 and 5 collagen deposition (Beasley *et al.* 1989a). It is possible that this collagen deposition may be related to the development of irreversible airflow limitation seen in some long-standing asthmatics (Brown *et al.* 1984; Connolly, C.K. *et al.* 1988). Inflammation of the airways following exposure to ozone and di-isocyanates also leads to bronchial hyper-responsiveness, but in this case the inflammatory infiltrate is principally of neutrophils (Seltzer *et al.* 1986; Fabbri *et al.* 1987). Further evidence of the link between bronchial hyper-responsiveness and airway inflammation is the similar time course of cellular infiltration into the airway and the development of hyper-responsiveness after allergen inhalation (de Monchy *et al.* 1985; Cockcroft and Murdock 1987).

The early and late asthmatic reaction: a model of asthma

Following allergen inhalation, there is a well-defined pattern of airways response which has provided a useful and reliable model to investigate mechanisms in asthma. Some 15 minutes after exposure to allergen or sensitizing agent, there is a fall in pulmonary function (usually measured as FEV_1) which recovers spontaneously within 1–2 hours (Robertson *et al.* 1974). This is referred to as the early asthmatic response, or the rapid spasmogenic phase. In up to 60% of asthmatics, the early asthmatic response is followed 4–6 hours later by a further fall in pulmonary function, the late asthmatic response, which may last for up to 6 hours before resolving, and may be followed by recurring episodes of airflow limitation for days or even weeks (Booij-Noord *et al.* 1972). The late asthmatic response is preceded by the development of bronchial hyper-responsiveness (Thorpe *et al.* 1986; Cockcroft & Murdock 1985), which may persist for days or weeks depending on the sensitizing agents (Hargreave *et al.* 1981). The early reaction is mediated by the release of preformed and newly generated inflammatory mediators, predominantly from mast cells, following cross-linkage of cell-bound IgE by allergen and bridging of high-affinity Fc_ε receptors (IgE $Fc_\varepsilon RI$).

By contrast, the late asthmatic response occurs through the recruitment of inflammatory leucocytes, particularly neutrophils and eosinophils, and may also involve the effects of cellular activation through antigen-specific T cells (Corrigan *et al.* 1988). The association of the late asthmatic response with the development of bronchial hyper-responsiveness, and the ability of sodium cromoglycate (SCG) and corticosteroids to inhibit the late asthmatic response (Booij-Nord *et al.* 1971) and allergen-acquired hyper-responsiveness (Cockcroft and Murdock 1987) suggest that the late asthmatic response may be a valid model of asthma mechanisms. Furthermore, both of these drugs have been shown to reduce bronchial hyper-responsiveness after long-term therapy (Löwhagen and Rak 1985; Woolcock *et al.* 1988), whilst β-2-adrenoceptor agonists such as salbutamol have been shown to have no effect either on the magnitude of the late asthmatic response or on the associated acquisition of increased bronchial responsiveness (Cockcroft and Murdock 1987).

Salbutamol and other β-2-agonists are potent 'mast cell stabilizing agents' *in vitro* (Church and Hiroi 1987). On the other hand, SCG, while being inhibitory to mast cell mediator release, is approximately 1000 times less potent in molar terms (Church *et al.* 1983). Sodium cromoglycate has also been found to inhibit the activation of neutrophils following allergen challenge of the airways (Moqbel *et al.* 1986a) and the eosinophilia seen in BAL after continuous treatment for 4 weeks (Diaz *et al.* 1984). Both SCG and the more recently developed drug, nedocromil sodium (Cairns and Orr 1988), have been shown to inhibit the activation of neutrophils and eosinophils *in vitro* (Kay *et al.* 1987; Moqbel *et al.* 1988), and the former drug also inhibits neutrophil chemotaxis and the mobilization of intracellular calcium in relation to stimulus–secretion coupling (Skedinger *et al.* 1987). These agents should therefore be regarded as anti-inflammatory drugs, and their clinical effects in asthma may relate more to this property than to 'stabilization' of mast cells.

The pharmacological evidence casts some doubt over the assumption that the late asthmatic response is a mast cell-dependent event, and suggests that other cells are important in its pathogenesis. This view is supported by the finding that the late, but not the early, asthmatic response is accompanied by an influx of neutrophils and activated eosinophils into the tissues (de Monchy *et al.* 1985; Metzger *et al.* 1986) and a similar accumulation of cells is seen in skin (Fowler and Louvel 1966).

The mast cell

The most prominent effector cell involved in the pathogenesis of bronchoconstriction during the early asthmatic response is the mast cell (Holgate *et al.* 1987a). Mast cells are distributed widely throughout the lung, especially within the airways where they are situated adjacent to the airway lumen, within airway epithelium and between the bronchial epithelium and basement membrane (Pearce 1988). Mast cells situated superficially are those most likely to be involved in the early asthmatic response, although mediators released from these cells can increase epithelial permeability, allowing subsequent penetration of allergen to submucosal mast cells. Mast cells located superficially are those most likely to be recovered by BAL (Lewis and Austen 1981).

In non-asthmatic subjects, mast cells comprise 0.25–0.5% of the differential nucleated cell count in BAL, macrophages being by far the most abundant cells (Flint *et al.* 1985a). Several studies have reported an increase in the BAL mast cell population from patients with asthma (Flint *et al.* 1985b; Kelly *et al.* 1988; Wardlaw *et al.* 1988), with the increase correlating with indices of baseline airway calibre and bronchial hyper-responsiveness (Flint *et al.* 1985a; Kelly *et al.* 1988). Mast cells from the lung may also be recovered following enzymatic dispersion of lung tissue, where they constitute 3–5% of total nucleated cells. Both BAL and enzymatically dispersed mast cells have similar staining characteristics: (i) they are sensitive to formalin fixation; (ii) they stain orthochromatically with alcian blue; (iii) they stain metachromatically with toluidine blue; and (iv) their granules do not counter-stain with safranin (Pearce 1988). The secretory granules of human mast cells contain amongst their preformed mediators neutral proteases, particularly tryptase, chymase and carboxypeptidase B (Schwartz 1988). There is evidence for mast cell heterogeneity in pulmonary tissue. Between 77% and 93% of lung mast cells are of the tryptase-only type (T mast cells), the remaining cells containing both tryptase and chymase (TC mast cells), which is the predominant mast cell found in skin. The TC mast cell also contains carboxypeptidase B which is not found in the T mast cell (Schwartz 1988). This level of mast cell heterogeneity has its counterpart in rodents of the mucosal (similar to human T mast cells) and connective tissue mast cells (similar to human TC mast cells) containing rat mast cell protease II (RMCP II) and RMCP I (chymase) respectively (Lai and Holgate 1988). There are also functional differences between the mast cells obtained from different sites. For example, compound 48/80, which elicits histamine release from skin mast cells, has no effect on mast cells from the lung (Church *et al.* 1982; Benyon *et al.* 1987). Furthermore, in contrast to lung mast cells the skin mast cells are refractory to the inhibitory action of SCG (Church and Hiroi 1987). Sodium cromoglycate is a more effective inhibitor of mediator release from BAL mast cells than from mast cells derived from enzymatic dispersion of lung tissue, and, different from dispersed lung mast cells, those recovered by BAL do not display tachyphylaxis to the drug (Flint *et al.* 1985b).

Transmission electron microscopy shows that BAL and tissue mast cells have a similar ultrastructure (Holgate *et al.* 1986), both being 5–15 μm in diameter, and containing lysosomal secretory granules with crystalline scroll, lattice and grating ultrastructures. The presence of scrolls parallels the distribution of tryptase alone and is the structural counterpart of the T mast cell whereas a grating and lattice appearance of the granule matrix identifies the TC mast cell (Craig *et al.* 1988). In addition to tryptase and chymase, mast cell granules contain a variety of other preformed mediators, including histamine, exoglycosidases, chemotactic factors for eosinophils and neutrophils, superoxide dismutase and heparin (Kaliner 1989). The array and functions of the preformed mediators of human lung mast cells are displayed in Table 54.1.

Mast cells can also synthesize *de novo* a number of lipid-derived inflammatory mediators, including prostaglandin D_2 (PGD_2), a component of slow-reacting substance of anaphylaxis (leucotriene C_4 (LTC_4)), LTB_4 and platelet-activating factor (PAF, 1-*O*-alkyl-2-acetyl-*sn*-glyceryl/3-phosphorylcholine). These newly generated products have potent chemotactic and broncho- and vasoactive properties pertinent to the pathogenesis of asthma (Freeland *et al.* 1988; Pearce 1988). The physicochemical properties of these products are displayed in Table 54.1, and will be considered in further detail.

Table 54.1. Preformed and newly generated mediators of human lung mast cells

Classification	Name	Physiochemical Characteristics	Function	
Amines	Histamine	Imidazole	Bronchoconstrictor, vasoactive, chemotactic, nerve stimulant, mucus secretagogue	
Exoglycosidases	β-glucuronidase	Tetrameric glycoprotein	Hydrolysis of tissue ground substance containing glycoproteins and proteoglycans	
	β-hexosaminidase	Tetrameric glycoprotein		
	β-galactosidase	Tetrameric glycoprotein		
	Aryl-sulphatase	Glycoprotein		
Neutral proteases	Tryptase	Tetrameric protein	Activates C3, fibrinolytic proteolytic	Hydrolysis of tissue ground substance in concert with exoglycosidases
	Chymase	Monomeric protein	General proteolysis	
	Carboxypeptidase B	Monomeric protein	Proteolytic	
	Kininogenase	Monomeric protein	Generates bradykinin	
Prostaglandin generating factor	PGF-A	Oligopeptide	Stimulates PGF_2 and TXA_2 formation	
Chemotactic factors	ECF-A	Oligopeptide	Eosinophil chemotaxis and priming	
	HMW NCF	Glycoprotein	Neutrophil chemotaxis and priming	
Proteoglycan	Heparin	Oligopeptide, glycosaminoglycan complex	Anticoagulant, anticomplementary	
Active radicals	Superoxide	O_2	Lipid peroxidation and cytolysis	
	Superoxide dismutase	Monomeric protein	Conversion of superoxide to H_2O_2	
Purines	Adenosine	Purine nucleoside	Bronchoconstrictor, vasodilator, augmentation of mast cell mediator release, suppression of T-lymphocytes	
Prostanoids	PGD_2	Prostaglandin	Bronchoconstrictor, vasodilator, antiplatelet chemokinetic	
	TXA_2	Thromboxane	Bronchoconstrictor, vasoconstrictor, proplatelet	
Leukotrienes	LTC_4 (SRS-A)	Sulphidopeptide lipid	Bronchoconstrictor, vasoconstrictor, mucus secretagogue, nerve stimulant	

ECF-A = eosinophil chemotactic factor of anaphylaxis; HMW NCF = high molecular weight neutrophil chemotactic factor; PGF-A = prostaglandin generating factor of anaphylaxis.

Mast cell activation

Following allergen inhalation, the sequence of events leading to cellular activation is initiated by cross-linkage of cell-bound IgE, and the subsequent calcium- and energy-dependent release of preformed and newly generated mediators of inflammation (Benyon 1988). The cellular receptors for IgE can be divided into two categories, high- and low-affinity, designated $Fc_{\varepsilon}RI$ and $Fc_{\varepsilon}RII$ respectively (Conrad 1988). High-affinity receptors are found on mast cells and basophils, whilst low-affinity receptors, probably equivalent to the CD23 antigen, can be found on macrophages, monocytes, eosinophils, platelets and subpopulations of T lymphocytes. A summary of the biochemical events thought to be involved in mast cell activation–secretion coupling is depicted in Fig. 54.3. The bridging of IgE receptors initiates the activity of membrane-associated serine protease, with subsequent activation of a series of enzymes involved in the catalytic cleavage and synthesis of phospholipids and the stimulation of adenylate cyclase (Ishizaka *et al.* 1987). These events are calcium-dependent, and lead to the turnover of membrane-bound phosphatidylinositol (PI), the accumulation of 1,2-diacylglycerol (DAG) within the cell membrane and release of inositol tri-

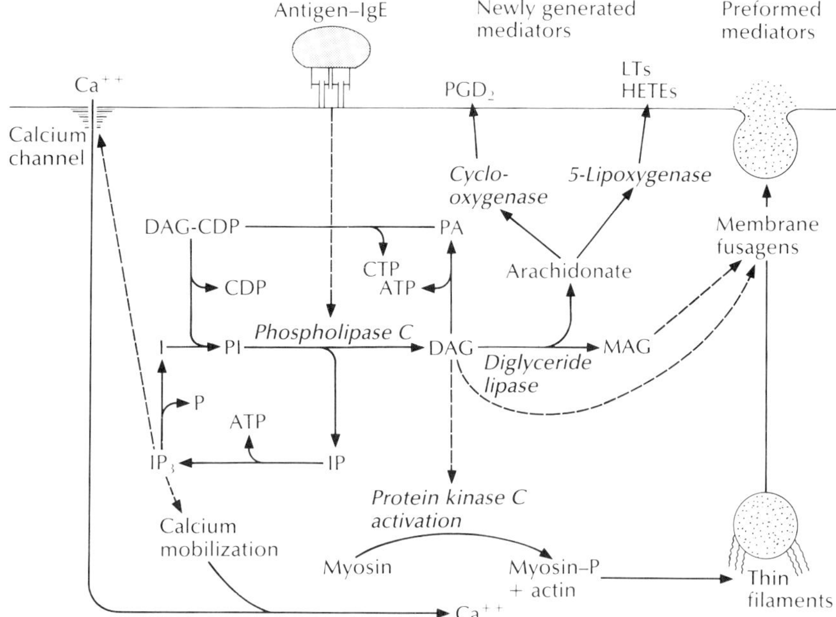

Fig. 54.3. Schematic representation of the biochemical steps involved in mast cell activation-secretion coupling. PI, phosphatidylinositol; IP_3, inositol triphosphate; PA, phosphatidic acid; CDP, cytidyl-5′-diphosphate.

phosphate (IP_3) into the cell cytosol. Inositol triphosphate is considered to trigger the release of calcium from cytoplasmic stores while DAG activates protein kinase C. As part of the PI cycle, DAG-lipase is activated to generate arachidonic acid and monoacylglycerol (MAG). Another source of arachidonic acid is the calcium-dependent stimulus of phospholipase A_2, which probably occurs sequential to the enhanced metabolism of PI. The arachidonate generated by these processes provides the necessary substrate for the generation of an array of eicosanoids. There appears to be an intimate association in mast cells of those mechanisms which are linked to the energy-dependent secretion of lysosomal granules and the enzyme pathways responsible for the generation of eicosanoids. The presence of PGD_2 synthetase and 5-lipoxygenase together with γ-glutamyl transferase provides further evidence that the major eicosanoids from human lung mast cells are PGD_2 and LTC_4.

Mast cells obtained by BAL from patients with asthma and normal controls release histamine and PGD_2 spontaneously, with those cells from asthmatics releasing more histamine than those from controls. Mast cells derived from dispersed lung tissue also spontaneously release histamine, although less than from BAL mast cells (Pearce *et al.* 1987). Similarly, mast cells derived by BAL from asthmatics show an enhanced response towards IgE-induced histamine release when compared with those derived from normal controls (Flint *et al.* 1985a). In accordance with the biochemical scheme shown in Fig. 54.3 these cells also generate appreciable amounts of PGD_2 and LTC_4 in addition to releasing a wide array of other preformed mediators (Table 54.1).

Allergen challenge in atopic asthmatics is rapidly followed by an increase in the concentration of histamine in peripheral venous plasma (Howarth *et al.* 1987) and BAL fluid (Casale *et al.* 1987a), and mast cells recovered by BAL from asthmatic airways shortly after allergen challenge exhibit the ultrastructural features of degranulation (Metzger *et al.* 1986). The increase in BAL histamine observed after provoking the airways with allergen is also accompanied by an increase in its τ-methyl metabolite in the urine (de Monchy *et al.* 1986). After local challenge of the airways with allergen, increased levels of BAL tryptase have been reported (Wenzel *et al.* 1988), together with increased concentrations of PGD_2 and its metabolite, 9α,11β-PGF_2 (Dworski *et al.* 1988). The features of mast cell degranulation have been observed in the airways of asthmatic children (Cutz *et al.* 1978) and in endobronchial biopsies obtained from adults with mild atopic asthma (Beasley *et al.* 1989a), where mucosal mast cells showed widespread loss of the crystalline granule structure and dissolution of the granular contents. Both inhaled salbutamol and SCG inhibit the early asthmatic response and the rise in plasma histamine and neutrophil chemotactic activity seen after allergen challenge (Howarth *et al.* 1985), which provides pharmacological evidence for the participation of mast cells in the response (Church and Hiroi 1987). Further evidence of the mast cell's role in the early asthmatic response comes from the ability of the potent and selective histamine antagonist terfenadine to inhibit this response by approximately 50% following allergen inhalation (Holgate *et al.* 1987b). This effect occurs within the first 15 minutes after challenge, which coincides with the time when most of the histamine is released from the airway mast cells (Church and Hiroi 1987). The role of mast cell-derived PGD_2 in the early asthmatic response has been examined in two ways: the orally active prostaglandin antagonist, GR32191, has been reported to inhibit the allergen-induced early asthmatic response by approximately 25% (Beasley *et al.* 1989b), and the use of a potent cyclo-oxygenase inhibitor, flurbiprofen, was found to inhibit allergen-induced bronchoconstriction by a similar amount (Curzen *et al.* 1987).

The role of the mast cell in the maintenance of the asthmatic state is suggested by studies that have shown a correlation between airway responsiveness to histamine and the percentage of BAL mast cells (Flint *et al.* 1985a; Kirby *et al.* 1987). Furthermore, Flint and co-workers (1985a) found an inverse correlation between the baseline FEV_1 and the BAL content of airway mast cells, and only those asthmatics with increased bronchial responsiveness to histamine have increased spontaneous release of histamine by their mast cells (Wardlaw *et al.* 1988). The direct relationship between the level of histamine in the cell-free supernatant of BAL fluid and the degree of bronchial responsiveness to histamine further extends these observations (Casale *et al.* 1987b). A group of histamine-releasing factors have been described (Thueson *et al.* 1979) that are generated by a variety of cells, including neutrophils (White and Kaliner 1987) and peripheral blood lymphocytes (Alam *et al.* 1987), and which are able to induce the release of histamine from human lung mast cells (MacDonald *et al.* 1987) and basophils. For one of these factors, the magnitude of its spontaneous production by mononuclear cells has been shown to correlate with the level of bronchial hyper-responsiveness in asthmatic patients (Alam *et al.* 1987).

Mast cell activation is not only a feature of allergen-induced early asthmatic responses. Exercise-induced asthma (EIA) is also thought to be related in part to the activation of mast cells, as histamine and neutrophil chemotactic factor are released during EIA (Lee, T.H. *et al.* 1984), and both inhaled salbutamol and SCG are highly effective in the prevention of EIA (Anderson 1988). During exercise, or hyperventilation, water is lost from the airway lining fluid in order to condition the inspired air to body temperature and full humidity. The resultant increase in the osmolarity of the lining fluid is thought to lead to mast cell activation (Eggleston *et al.* 1987; Anderson 1988; Silber *et al.* 1988). Histamine release by mast cells from BAL and dispersed lung can be enhanced in a dose-dependent manner by incubation in a hyperosmolar medium (Pearce *et al.* 1987). Further evidence of mast cell involvement in this process is the ability of the potent H_1-receptor blocker, terfenadine, in inhibiting bronchoconstriction following hypertonic saline inhalation (Wilmot *et al.* 1988). Exercise-induced asthma may also result from other mechanisms including stimulation of neural reflexes, both central and local, and possibly rebound vasodilatation following recovery from hypothermic vasoconstriction (McFadden and Ingram 1979) (Fig. 54.4).

Macrophages and monocytes

The majority of cells recovered from BAL fluid both in normal and asthmatic subjects are macrophages. These cells express low-affinity receptors for IgE ($Fc_{\varepsilon}RII$), and the BAL recovered from atopic asthmatic subjects has more of these cells than does that from normal subjects (Joseph *et al.* 1983; Capron *et al.* 1986). Furthermore, peripheral blood monocytes bearing these receptors are found in increased numbers in allergic individuals (Melewicz *et al.* 1981). Following local challenge of the airways with allergen, there occurs an increase in the number of macrophages recovered by BAL (Metzger *et al.* 1987), and it is thought that these cells are responsible for the increased levels of free β-glucuronidase identified in BAL fluid (Tonnel *et al.* 1983).

Fuller and co-workers (1986) have shown that stimulation of the IgE receptor on macrophages leads to the production of inflammatory mediators such as LTB_4, $PGF_{2\alpha}$ and thromboxane

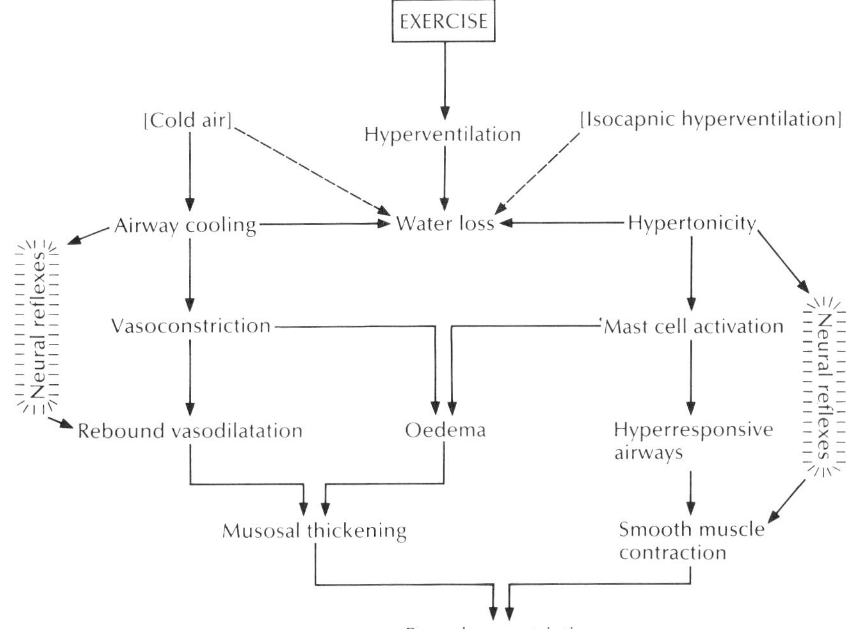

Fig. 54.4. Events leading to exercise-induced asthma. Water loss is provoked by hyperventilation and inspiring cold air, leading respectively to mast cell activation and stimulation of neural reflexes. These are considered to have a combined effect in reducing airway calibre by direct effects on smooth muscle and by vascular engorgement of the submucosa.

(TX) B_2. When macrophages from atopic subjects are stimulated *in vitro* by zymosan or allergen, PAF, its derivative and precursor lyso-PAF, and β-glucuronidase are all released. In contrast, the same stimuli do not cause the release of these phospholipids from the alveolar macrophages of non-atopic individuals or from those of atopic subjects treated with theophylline and/or corticosteroids (Arnoux *et al*. 1987). Finally, macrophages recovered from the airways are capable of releasing chemoattractants for neutrophils and eosinophils after IgE-dependant stimulation (Gosset *et al*. 1984). This chemotactic activity is thought, in part, to be due to LTB_4. Peripheral blood monocytes and other leucocytes have been shown to be activated after provoking allergen-induced asthma (Durham *et al*. 1984). The inhibition of leucocyte activation by SCG may therefore explain some or all of the ability of this agent to inhibit the late asthmatic response, and lends some support for the role of the macrophage in the pathogenesis of asthma.

Further evidence that implicates macrophages and monocytes in the pathogenesis of asthma is the ability of corticosteroids to inhibit the increased expression of complement (complement receptor 1 (CR1)) and IgG Fc receptors on peripheral blood monocytes isolated from asthmatic patients (Gin and Kay 1985). Furthermore, the improvement in airways function seen after the exhibition of corticosteroids was shown to correlate with the inhibition of leucocyte activation (Gin *et al*. 1985), and patients who were resistant to corticosteroids were shown to have defective inhibition of phytohaemagglutinin-stimulated monocyte growth following incubation with prednisolone (Poznansky *et al*. 1984). The possession of the $Fc_{\varepsilon}II$ receptor indicates that this cell has the potential to respond to the presence of inhaled antigen. The demonstration that it can release many different inflammatory mediators and chemoattractants implies a role in the development or maintenance of the asthmatic diathesis. The cell may also have a role in determining the response of inflammation to suppression by corticosteroids.

Eosinophils

Eosinophils have long been known to be associated with asthma. In 1975, Horn and colleagues found that there was an inverse relationship between the severity of asthma in non-atopic subjects, as measured by the FEV_1, and the level of circulating eosinophils in the peripheral blood. In atopic subjects, Durham and Kay (1985) found that blood eosinophilia accompanied the late but not the early asthmatic response, and that the degree of eosinophilia correlated inversely with the measured level of non-specific bronchial responsiveness. These findings were confirmed in a study by Taylor and Luksza (1987), who found a relationship between eosinophil count and bronchial responsiveness in both atopic and non-atopic asthmatic subjects.

Bronchoalveolar lavage fluid obtained during and after the allergen-induced late asthmatic response contains increased numbers of eosinophils and eosinophil products (de Monchy *et al.* 1985), and others have found that the eosinophils recovered from the airway after inhalation of allergen have the features of cell activation (Metzger *et al.* 1986). The BAL fluid of asthmatics with hyper-responsive airways also contains increased numbers of eosinophils and eosinophil products such as myelin basic protein (MBP), which correlate inversely with the level of non-specific bronchial hyper-responsiveness (Wardlaw *et al.* 1988). These features were absent in the BAL fluid of stable asthmatics (as defined by the absence of symptoms or hyper-responsiveness), although other studies have reported the presence of eosinophils in the airway lumen regardless of the presence or absence of symptoms (Godard *et al.* 1982; Flint *et al.* 1985b; Kirby *et al.* 1987). Sodium cromoglycate, which is known to inhibit the activation of eosinophils (Moqbel *et al.* 1988), has been shown to prevent the eosinophilia in BAL fluid, which, in turn, is related to clinical improvement (Diaz *et al.* 1984).

Eosinophils are produced in the bone marrow and distributed to the tissues via the blood stream. Eosinophils contain distinctive cytoplasmic granules which, because of the basic substances they contain, produce the characteristic staining pattern with acidic dyes such as eosin. The bulk of each granule is comprised of four cationic proteins: MBP, eosinophil cationic protein (ECP), eosinophil peroxidase (EPO) and eosinophil-derived neurotoxin (EDN) (Fig. 54.5). Major basic protein is localized to the core of the granule, and is responsible for the central crystalloid structures found in the granules, whilst the other three proteins are found in the granule matrix (Dahl *et al.* 1988). Both MBP and ECP are cytotoxic to the respiratory epithelium (Gleich *et al.* 1979), causing desquamation, and they are also able to induce histamine release from basophils and rodent mast cells (Bergstrand *et al.* 1985). Eosinophil cationic protein and EPO are able to inhibit the response of T lymphocytes to phytohaemagglutinin (Venge

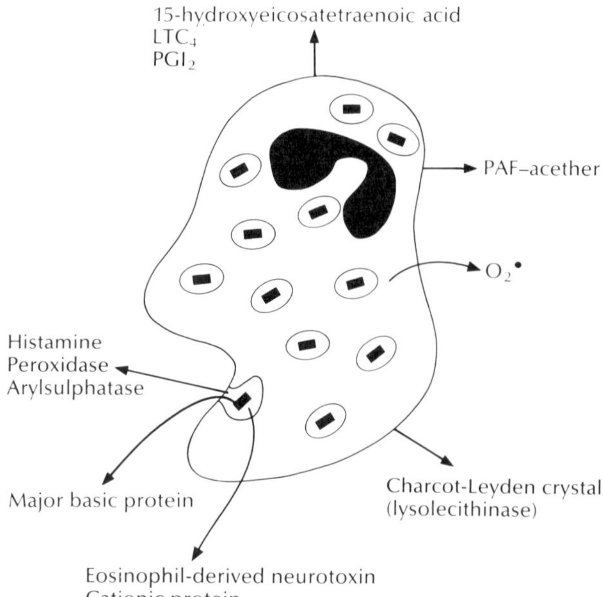

Fig. 54.5. Inflammatory mediators released from the human eosinophil which may be relevant to the pathogenesis of asthma.

1985), and EPO is able to inactivate inflammatory mediators such as LTD_4 and LTB_4 (Henderson *et al.* 1982). In the presence of eosinophil-generated H_2O_2 and halide, EPO is able to kill a variety of micro-organisms (Slifman *et al.* 1988).

The level of MBP in the BAL fluid of symptomatic asthmatics correlates inversely with the level of non-specific bronchial hyper-responsiveness (Wardlaw *et al.* 1988). Studies in guinea-pig trachea have shown that MBP is capable of inducing hyper-reactivity of smooth muscle to acetylcholine and histamine only in the presence of an intact epithelium (Flavahan *et al.* 1988). This may imply that MBP is interfering with epithelial cell function, perhaps by affecting the release, diffusion or action of the putative epithelium-derived relaxant factor (Vanhoutte 1988).

Charcot–Leyden crystals (CLC) were initially described in the last century in a patient with leukaemia and then in the sputa of asthmatic patients. The CLC protein is derived from the cell membranes of eosinophils, but is not entirely specific to this type of cell as it is also associated with basophils (Ackerman *et al.* 1982). The CLC protein has lysophospholipase activity, and its function may be to inactivate toxic products of phospholipase A_2 activity (Dahl *et al.* 1988).

Once activated, eosinophils are able to synthesize LTC_4 and LTD_4, 15-hydroxyeicosatetraenoic acid (15-HETE) and PAF (Lee, T.C. *et al.* 1984; Shaw *et al.* 1985), and they appear to have a capacity for self-modulation, as LTC_4 synthesis is increased when the EPO−halide−H_2O_2 system is inhibited (Henderson *et al.* 1982). The synthesis of PAF by the eosinophil involves the enzyme 1-alkyl-2-lyso-*sn*-glycero-3-phosphocholine:acetyl-CoA acetyltransferase, and its secretion from the cell can be stimulated by a variety of naturally occurring chemotactic factors for eosinophils, such as eosinophil chemotactic factor of anaphylaxis (ECF-A) and C5a (Lee, T.C. *et al.* 1984). Platelet-activating factor itself is a potent chemotactic factor for eosinophils (Wardlaw *et al.* 1986), and it may also enhance, or induce, the zymosan-induced production of LTC_4 by these cells (Bruynzeel *et al.* 1986). Eosinophils can be primed for activation by other mediators, including LTB_4 and interleukin 5 (IL-5) (Kay 1988), and in turn, at higher concentrations, these mediators may influence the function of eosinophils in other ways, such as the stimulation of chemotaxis by LTB_4 (Lewis *et al.* 1981). Interleukin 5 is able to promote the growth and subsequent differentiation of eosinophil, precursor cells in the bone marrow, resulting in enhanced functional activity (Harriman and Strober 1989), and can also act in concert with IL-1 and IL-3 in eosinophil differentiation (Warren and Moore 1988).

Eosinophils express receptors for IgE and IgG, and surface IgE has been demonstrated on eosinophils from patients with increased serum IgE levels (Capron *et al.* 1985). There are two populations of eosinophils, and, although both types are able to bind IgE on their surface, only the hypodense and not the normodense eosinophil population is able to degranulate in response to an IgE-directed stimulus (Khalife *et al.* 1986). Immunoglobulin E- but not IgG-dependent stimulation can cause the release of both MBP and EPO, whilst the exocytosis of ECP appears to depend on IgG stimulation (Capron 1989). Furthermore, PAF is produced only in response to IgE-dependent stimulation. The clinical relevance of this differential mediator release is not yet known.

Neutrophils

Neutrophils are polymorphonuclear leucocytes characterized by a multilobed nucleus and by cytoplasm which contains specific and azurophil granules. The azurophil granules contain acid hydrolases such as cathepsin B and β-glucuronidase, the serine proteases elastase and cathepsin G, and the antibacterial enzyme myeloperoxidase. The specific granules contain alkaline phosphatase and collagenase. Neutrophils are also able to synthesize arachidonic acid-derived mediators of inflammation such as LTB_4 and TXA_2, as well as superoxide anions (Ford-Hutchinson 1988).

Neutrophils are known to play an important role in the acute inflammatory response (Marchesi 1985), and there is established evidence of neutrophil involvement in the pathogenesis of asthma. A neutrophilia is present in BAL fluid before, during and after late asthmatic responses induced by allergen (Diaz *et al.* 1986; Metzger *et al.* 1987), toluene di-isocyanate (TDI) and plicatic acid (Fabbri *et al.* 1987; Lam *et al.* 1987), and after exposure to ozone (Seltzer *et al.* 1986), and an increase in neutrophil counts accompanies the increase in eosinophils seen in these studies. However, a neutrophilia was not found in the BAL fluid of mild, stable asthmatics (Wardlaw *et al.* 1988; Beasley *et al.* 1989a). The increase in BAL neutrophils and airway hyper-responsiveness following TDI challenge can be inhibited by oral corticosteroids, suggesting that in at least this form of asthma they may be causally linked to the disease (Boschetto *et al.* 1987). Peripheral blood neutrophils also become activated as evidenced by enhanced expression of complement and IgG Fc receptors with exercise- and allergen-provoked asthma (Carroll *et al.* 1985; Moqbel *et al.* 1986b), and both SCG and corticosteroids inhibit late-phase responses and neutrophil activation (Gin and Kay 1985; Kay *et al.* 1987).

Following either allergen- or exercise-induced bronchoconstriction, a high-molecular-weight neutrophil chemotactic activity (NCA) has been found in the peripheral blood (Lee *et al.* 1982; Nagy *et al.* 1982). This activity, which at one time was thought to be derived from mast cells, has also been demonstrated to be present in the serum of individuals with acute severe asthma (Buchanan *et al.* 1987a), and its level falls with treatment. The same study demonstrated only very low levels of NCA in subjects with mild stable asthma (i.e. patients not taking corticosteroids or SCG), and

NCA activity has been found in the supernatant of cultured mononuclear cells from patients with acute severe asthma (Buchanan *et al.* 1987b). The more recent data suggest that an array of NCAs are secreted, possibly from activated lymphocytes and monocytes, following stimulation. The significance of the presence of NCA is not yet understood, but it is possible that it is acting to attract and subsequently immobilize neutrophils once recruited into the airways.

Neutrophils are capable of producing LTB_4 (Ford-Hutchinson *et al.* 1980), itself a powerful chemotactic factor for neutrophils and to a lesser extent eosinophils, and therefore cellular activation may lead to a cycle of cell attraction and activation. The fact that neutrophils have been reported in the bronchial epithelium of asthmatic airways (Laitinen *et al.* 1985), and that they are able to release lipid mediators which can increase airways responsiveness, at least in animals (Irvin *et al.* 1986), provides some circumstantial evidence of their possible involvement in the pathogenesis of asthma.

Because of the difficulties inherent in studying the events that take place during asthma in human airways, animal models of the disease process have been developed. One of the most useful of these is the guinea-pig model as it allows airway sensitization and challenge by the administration of aerosols to the conscious animal (Hutson *et al.* 1988a). After sensitization of the guinea-pig airways with inhaled ovalbumin, the effects of allergen challenge can be studied, both physiologically and by examining BAL fluid and airway histopathology. Thus, following aerosol challenge of sensitized animals with allergen there occurred an early asthmatic response, which resolved within 2 hours, followed by two late responses, maximal at 17 and 72 hours after challenge (Fig. 54.6). Bronchoalveolar lavage studies showed that these falls were associated with increases in eosinophil and neutrophil counts at 17 and 72 hours, with the eosinophils showing features of cell activation. These findings were mirrored by an infiltration of both cell types in the guinea-pig airways (Hutson *et al.* 1988a). In a further study, salbutamol inhalation prior to challenge was able to inhibit the allergen-induced early asthmatic response, but neither of the late responses, whereas SCG inhibited the early and the 17 hour responses, but not the 72 hour response. When cromoglycate was given 6 hours after challenge, both late asthmatic responses were inhibited. The rise in neutrophils, but not eosinophils, at 17 hours was also inhibited by cromoglycate inhaled before challenge, but the cellular changes at 72 hours were unaffected. When cromoglycate was given at 6 hours after challenge, the sole effect was inhibition of the 72 hour

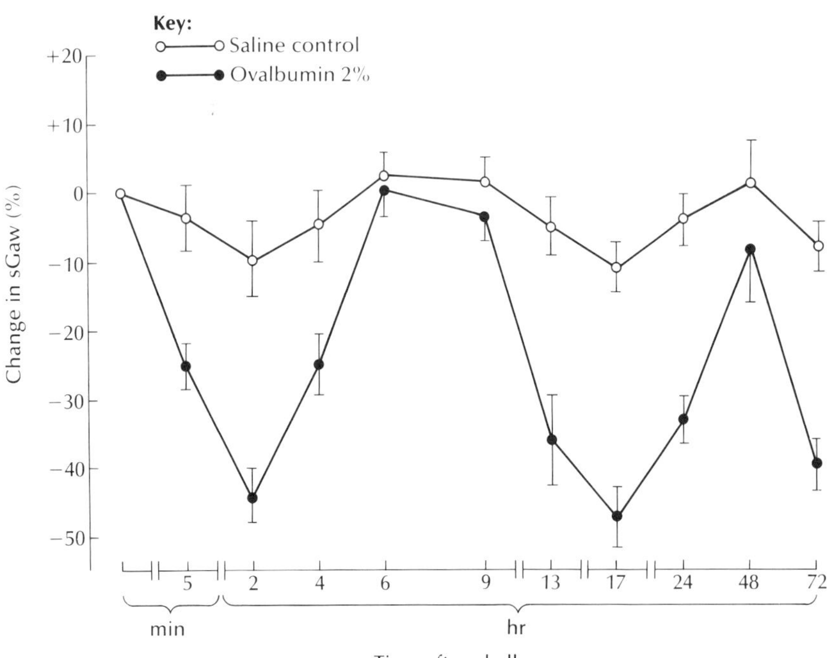

Fig. 54.6. Changes in specific airway conductance (sGaw) after ovalbumin challenge of sensitized guinea-pigs. The early, late and very late asthmatic responses can be clearly seen at 2, 17 and 72 hours after allergen but not after saline.

eosinophilia. Inhalation of salbutamol inhibited only the early asthmatic response when given before challenge, and both the early and late asthmatic responses when given before and 6 hours after challenge. Salbutamol inhalation was able to inhibit the rise in neutrophils during the late asthmatic response if given before challenge, and, if given before and 6 hours after, it inhibited the rise in neutrophils at 17 hours and the eosinophil rise at 72 hours (Hutson *et al.* 1988b). In a further study, nedocromil sodium given before challenge was able to inhibit the early and late asthmatic responses and the associated neutrophilia, although the eosinophilia was unaffected, whilst when nedocromil was given 6 hours after challenge, both the 17 and 72 hour late asthmatic responses were inhibited, but not the neutrophilia, suggesting that the influx of neutrophils is somehow dependent on the presence of an intact early asthmatic response, whilst the late asthmatic response is not related to the neutrophilia (Hutson *et al.* 1988c).

The utility of this guinea-pig model is shown by the similarity between these findings and those of Cockcroft and Murdock (1987), who gave salbutamol, beclomethasone dipropionate (BDP) and SCG by inhalation to a group of atopic asthmatic subjects in order to assess their effect on the development of early and late asthmatic responses and bronchial hyper-responsiveness after allergen inhalation. Both salbutamol and SCG inhibited the early asthmatic responses by >50%, whereas BDP had little or no effect. In contrast, the late asthmatic response and the development of bronchial hyper-activity were attenuated by SCG and BDP, but not by salbutamol. These authors suggested that the inhibition of the late asthmatic response by SCG and BDP may have been due to the ability of these drugs to stabilize inflammatory cells other than mast cells, particularly eosinophils and neutrophils.

Platelets

A role for the platelet as an effector cell in the pathogenesis of the asthmatic inflammatory response has been suggested because platelet depletion can inhibit PAF-induced airway hyperreactivity in guinea-pigs (Mazzoni *et al.* 1985). Platelet activation and accumulation within the pulmonary circulation have been reported to be associated with bronchoconstriction or anaphylaxis (Vargaftig *et al.* 1980; Morley *et al.* 1984). Following allergen inhalation, platelets have been found in BAL fluid (Metzger *et al.* 1985) and are in an activated state in the peripheral blood (Knauer *et al.* 1981). Platelet activation occurs through at least two mechanisms, IgG- and IgE-dependent. Immunoglobulin G stimulation leads to platelet aggregation and serotonin release, whilst stimulation of the low-affinity IgE receptor (Joseph *et al.* 1987) induces the release of cytocidal factors and oxygen metabolites (Capron *et al.* 1987). Although this evidence is scanty, it does suggest that the platelet can be activated by exposure to antigen, and it may be that this property has a specific role in the pathogenesis of aspirin-induced asthma (Ameisen *et al.* 1985).

Lymphocytes

The T lymphocyte is known to be intimately involved in the regulation of IgE production, and thus may be responsible for some of the manifestations of the atopic state (Leung and Geha 1987). There has been a great deal of recent interest in the role of this cell type in the pathogenesis of asthma. T lymphocyte activation has been described as occurring with acute severe asthma (Corrigan *et al.* 1988); activated CD4 (T helper) cells were found in the peripheral blood of asthmatic patients admitted to hospital with acute exacerbations, and the percentage of activated cells (as defined by the presence of markers for the expression of Class II major histocompatibility complex antigens, the receptor for IL-2 and the very late activation antigen, VLA) was found to decrease with treatment and corresponding clinical improvement, although there was no change in the relative distribution of T cell subtypes in either the patient or the control groups. Further evidence of the involvement of these cells is the demonstration of raised serum levels of interferon-γ and soluble IL-2 receptor, which are both markers of T lymphocyte activation, in the blood of patients with acute severe asthma (Corrigan and Kay 1988). These workers found a linear correlation between levels of these markers and the admission peak expiratory flow, and the levels decreased with treatment. Those patients with chronic asthma who are relatively unresponsive to corticosteroid therapy have been found to have a reduction in the numbers of circulating CD8 (T suppressor) cells as well as an abnormality of IL-2-stimulated T cell growth (Poznansky *et al.* 1984, 1985).

A study examining the variation in cellular content of BAL fluid between patients with single early responses and those with dual or late asthmatic responses to allergen inhalation has shown that the early responders have reduced CD4, increased CD8 and a decreased CD4 : CD8 ratio in BAL fluid with the inverse being shown in the peripheral blood, whilst the late-phase responders had an increase in both CD4 and CD8 in BAL fluid (Gonzalez *et al.* 1987). It appears that there may be a preferential recruitment of CD8 lymphocytes into the airways following allergen challenge, and that this may be one factor that protects the airways against the development of the late asthmatic response. CD4 cells have been found in BAL fluid 48 hours after segmental bronchial challenge via the bronchoscope in subjects who developed a late asthmatic response (Metzger *et al.* 1987), and after allergen inhalation a decrease in CD4 cells in the peripheral blood has been reported in asthmatics (Gerblich *et al.* 1984), implying that there is a selective pulmonary recruitment and retention of these cells during the late asthmatic response.

A study of bronchial biopsies from symptomatic asthmatic patients has shown a prominent infiltrate of lymphocytes and macrophages throughout the lamina propria and in clusters just below the epithelium. The cell clusters were predominantly composed of T lymphocytes, generally with equal numbers of CD4 and CD8 cells (Poulter *et al.* 1988). These findings were interpreted as being evidence of an ongoing cell-mediated reaction in the bronchial wall of asthmatics. A study of the late-phase response in human skin, which is thought to mirror the late asthmatic response in the airways, has shown that this phenomenon is accompanied by an influx of activated eosinophils and a perivascular accumulation of CD4 lymphocytes, and that the numbers of cells correlate directly with the size of the late-phase response (Frew and Kay 1988).

There is increasing evidence of the involvement of T lymphocytes in the pathogenesis of asthma, and since these cells have the capacity to secrete an array of cytokines pertinent to the inflammatory response of asthma, e.g. IL-2, IL-3, IL-4 and IL-5, they may play a role as central effectors of the asthmatic response. Interleukin-2 is a growth factor for activated T cells and can stimulate the synthesis of other interleukins; IL-3 (multi-colony-stimulating factor-(CSF)) promotes the growth of precursor cells in the bone marrow; IL-4 is a growth factor for resting T cells and enhances the activity of cytotoxic T cells; and IL-5 has been discussed above (Dinarello and Mier 1987). Furthermore, T lymphocytes are able to produce an eosinophil CSF (Raghavachar *et al.* 1987) which influences eosinophil differentiation, a lymphokine which stimulates neutrophil chemotaxis (Maestrelli *et al.* 1987) and a leukotriene release-enhancing factor which increases LTB_4 generation by neutrophils (Tsai *et al.* 1987). The ability to study BAL cells and tissue from the airways of patients with asthma will undoubtedly provide an invaluable new approach for dissecting the contribution of various cytokines in the induction of airway inflammation.

The inflammatory mediators

Histamine

Histamine was first shown to be a potent bronchoconstrictor agonist in guinea-pigs by Dale and Laidlaw (1911), since which time its role in the pathogenesis of asthma has been studied extensively, particularly since highly selective H_1 and H_2 receptor antagonists are now available. Histamine is formed by decarboxylation of L-histidine by L-histidine decarboxylase (Fig. 54.7), and is stored in cytoplasmic granules of mast cells and basophils in close association with the proteoglycans (predominantly heparin) that form the granule matrix. Once released, histamine is found in the peripheral blood within minutes, and is then metabolized by two major pathways with only 2–3% being excreted in the urine unchanged (White and Kaliner 1988). *N*-methyltransferases metabolize histamine to τ-methylhistamine, with some histamine undergoing further degradation by monoamine oxidase to τ-methylimidazole-acetic acid. Diamine oxidase metabolizes the remaining 30% to imidazole-acetic acid.

Histamine acts through two distinct receptors, H_1 and H_2 (Table 54.2). H_1 receptors mediate smooth muscle contraction, increased vascular permeability, prostaglandin generation and activation of airway vagal afferent nerves. They are stimulated by 2-methylhistamine and inhibited by selective antagonists such as terfenadine and

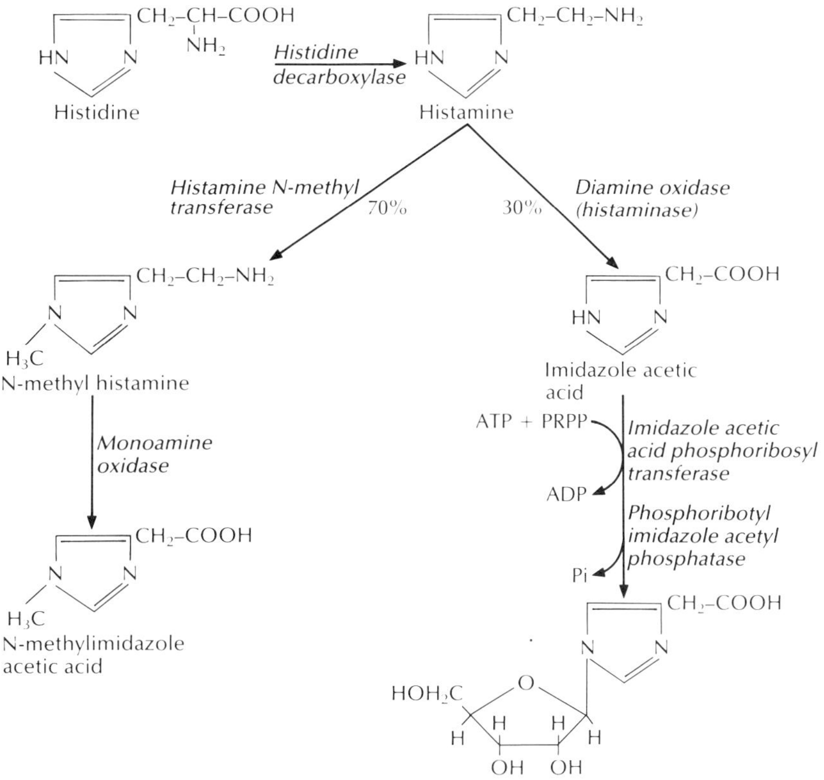

Fig. 54.7. Histamine metabolic pathway. The two major routes of histamine degradation in humans are shown, with the final products being excreted in the urine.

astemizole. H_2 receptors mediate gastric acid secretion, airway mucus secretion, the inhibition of basophil histamine release and stimulation of CD8 (suppressor) T lymphocytes. They are stimulated by 4-methylhistamine, and inhibited by cimetidine and ranitidine (White and Kaliner 1988).

The involvement of histamine in asthma is suggested by the finding of higher levels of plasma histamine in perennial asthmatics when compared with non-asthmatic controls (Barnes *et al.* 1982), and also by the release of histamine into the peripheral circulation following allergen- or exercise-induced bronchoconstriction (Lee, T.H. *et al.* 1984; Howarth *et al.* 1985). After the inhalation of histamine, airflow limitation is due to airway smooth muscle contraction and to mucosal oedema consequent on increased vascular permeability, both mechanisms being H_1 receptor-mediated. Many investigators have shown that the airways in asthma are exquisitely sensitive to inhaled histamine, being up to 1000 times more reactive than normal subjects, whereas non-asthmatic atopic subjects and those with chronic bronchitis and emphysema are intermediate in their responsiveness to this mediator (Townley *et al.* 1979; Woolcock *et al.* 1984).

The potent H_1 receptor antagonists, astemizole and terfenadine, are both able to attenuate histamine-induced bronchoconstriction (Howarth and Holgate 1985; Rafferty and Holgate 1987), and are free of the side-effects experienced with the older antihistamines. Astemizole has a long onset and prolonged duration of action (over a period of 15 to 30 days), and is able to inhibit bronchoconstriction induced by histamine, antigen and exercise one week after it has been ceased (Holgate *et al.* 1985). Terfenadine has a more rapid onset of action and a half-life of 12 hours, and is also able to inhibit exercise-induced asthma (O'Hickey *et al.* 1988). Because histamine is only one of many mediators that are likely to contribute to bronchoconstriction, it is most unlikely that H_1 antagonists alone will offer much benefit as therapeutic agents in asthma. Although terfenadine does have a bronchodilator action in man (Cookson 1987; Rafferty and Holgate 1987), in doses of 120 mg twice daily it has been shown to have only a small

Table 54.2. Biological role of histamine

Target organ and cells	Physiological and pharmacological action	Receptor subtype
Monocytes	Inhibits secretion of complement proteins	H_2
Neutrophils	Inhibits lysosomal enzyme release	H_2
	Inhibits superoxide and peroxide production	H_2
	Modulates chemotactic response	H_2
Platelets	Inhibits platelet aggregation	
Nervous system		
1 Central	Neuroregulatory role	H_1, H_2
2 Peripheral	Stimulates afferent cutaneous nerves, flare of the triple response, stimulates cough receptors directly and indirectly	H_1
Nose	Increases nasal secretion	H_1
	Oedema: vasodilation and increased vascular permeability	H_1
Mucus secreting cells — glands	Increases glycoprotein secretion	H_2
Whole lung	Increases cyclic AMP	H_2
	Increases cyclic GMP	H_1
	Modulates prostanoid release	H_1, H_2
Smooth muscle		
1 Vascular —		
Large arteries & veins	Constrict	
Small arteries & veins	Dilate	H_2
2 Bronchial	Constrict (reflex and direct actions)	H_1
Endothelial cells (vascular)	Increases permeability	H_1 and H_2
	Releases PGI_2	H_1
Epithelial cells	Short lived increased permeability	H_2
Immune system		
Basophils	Negative feedback on histamine release at the antigen dependent stage	H_2
	Inhibits chemotactic responses	
	Increases uptake of histidine	H_1
Eosinophils	Modulates chemotactic responsiveness	H_1/H_2
	Chemotactic	H_1 and H_2
	Elevates cyclic AMP	H_2
	Receptor enhancement	H_1
Lymphocytes	Reduces cytolytic ability	H_2
	Reduces lymphokine production	H_2
	Inhibits lymphocyte proliferation	H_2
	Activates suppressor cells (monocyte factor dependent)	H_2
	Inhibits immunoglobulin production	
	Influences receptor expression regulation	
	Produces histamine induced suppressor factor (HSF_1 SRS)	

effect on the symptoms of allergic asthma (Taytard *et al.* 1987). Clearly, further studies are needed to define the place, if any, of this new generation of antihistamines in the treatment of asthma. The selective H_2 antagonists have not been shown to have any detectable effect upon clinical or provoked asthma, suggesting that this receptor subtype plays a relatively small role in asthma mechanisms.

Mast cell activation and histamine release is also a feature of the bronchial response to inhaled adenosine and adenosine monophosphate (AMP). Both atopic and non-atopic asthmatics react to inhaled AMP, and the resultant bronchoconstriction can be almost totally inhibited by H_1 antagonists (Phillips *et al.* 1987; Rafferty *et al.* 1987), and also by inhaled theophylline, a histamine purinoceptor antagonist (Cushley *et al.* 1984). The findings of the latter study strongly suggest that the mechanism of action of adenosine is via cell surface purinoceptors, as the concentration of inhaled theophylline was lower than that needed to inhibit phosphodiesterase. Adenosine monophoshate-induced bronchoconstriction can also be inhibited by nedocromil sodium and SCG. (Phillips *et al.* 1988a). Further evidence for involvement of the mast cell and release of histamine is the lack of a late-phase response or the development of bronchial hyper-responsiveness after AMP inhalation (Phillips and Holgate 1989). Adenosine is released following allergen challenge, both rising in concert with the initial bronchoconstriction followed by a later peak, and this sequence of events is also seen after methacholine provocation (Mann *et al.* 1986). The role of adenosine in the pathogenesis of asthma is not certain, but it appears to be a secondary mediator in causing release of histamine and other mediators via purinoceptor activation of mast cells. As it can be released following certain bronchoconstrictor stimuli, it may be a mediator that can augment a bronchoconstrictor response rather than being primarily causative.

Proteoglycans and proteases

Proteoglycans are large molecules comprising repeating disaccharide units (glycosaminoglycans) attached to a peptide core. They are the constituents of the mast cell and basophil granules that are responsible for the metachromatic staining characteristics of these cells (Schwartz 1988). Heparin is the principal proteoglycan of the human lung mast cell, although its functions in allergic disease processes have not been clearly established. It is likely that heparin is responsible for regulating the stability and activity of mast cell enzymes, and may facilitate the uptake and packaging of contents of the secretory granules. Heparin has been found to regulate the activity of tryptase, which may be important for the full expression of this and other mast cell enzymes (Schwartz and Bradford 1986). Known extracellular functions of heparin include binding of antithrombin III and inhibition of complement activation.

The two predominant neutral proteases in the human lung mast cell are chymase and tryptase. They form 20–50% of the protein content of mast cells, and are specific markers for these cells as basophils contain very small quantities (Castells *et al.* 1987). The biological role of tryptase is not clear, although it is thought to generate the anaphylotoxin C3a from C3, which may cause smooth muscle contraction and increased vascular permeability (Schwartz 1988). Chymase is present in the TC mast cells but is lacking from T mast cells. Chymase converts angiotensin I to angiotensin II, although it is not known whether angiotensin II is released during activation of TC mast cells (Reilly *et al.* 1982). Other neutral proteases that have been identified within the human lung mast cell include elastase, carboxypeptidase B and dipeptidase.

The eicosanoids

All of the cells discussed earlier are able to synthesize a variety of inflammatory mediators from the products of membrane-derived arachidonic acid breakdown, once cell activation has taken place. As a group, these substances are the eicosanoids, and can be subdivided into agents derived from cyclo-oxygenation (the prostanoids — prostaglandins and thromboxanes) or from lipoxygenation (the sulphidopeptide leucotrienes and the lipoxins).

THE PROSTANOIDS

Cyclo-oxygenase acts on arachidonic acid to produce an endoperoxide, PGG_2, which in turn is converted by a C-15 peroxidase to PGH_2

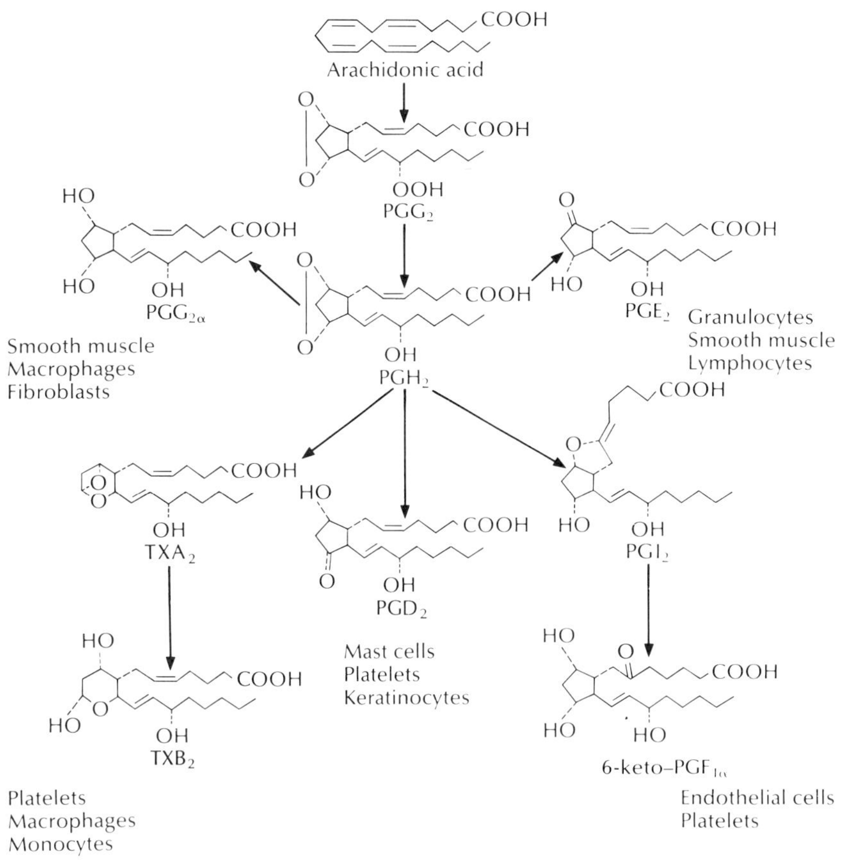

Fig. 54.8. Metabolism of arachidonic acid by the cyclo-oxygenase pathway to prostanoids.

(Fig. 54.8). This is an unstable cyclic endoperoxide, and is rapidly converted into the bronchoconstrictor PGs, PGD_2 and $PGF_{2\alpha}$, and a bronchodilator, PGE_2. Prostacyclin (PGI_2) and TXA_2 are also derived from the endoperoxides. The most abundant of the cyclo-oxygenase products synthesized and released by stimulated lung cells is PGD_2, along with smaller quantities of TXA_2, PGI_2 and the other prostaglandins (Holgate *et al*. 1984). The release of PGD_2 paralleled the release of histamine, although the amount of histamine released was up to 20-fold greater than PGD_2, depending on the stimulus to activation. This study showed that the majority of the PGD_2 originated from mast cells, while TXA_2 and prostacyclin were released from macrophages, monocytes and lymphocytes. These cells are known to carry IgE $Fc_{\varepsilon}RII$ receptors (Conrad 1988), through which cell activation by allergen for mediator release may occur. Alternatively, these cells may be activated by the mediators released by the mast cell (Robinson and Holgate 1986a).

Prostaglandin D_2 is released into the BAL fluid of atopic asthmatics following allergen challenge (Murray *et al*. 1986). When inhaled by asthmatic and normal subjects, PGD_2 is a potent bronchoconstrictor in the asthmatic group, and a less potent constrictor in normals (Hardy *et al*. 1984). It is approximately 30 times more potent than histamine in molar terms. Some of its constrictor activity is due to its metabolite, $9\alpha,11\beta$-PGF_2 (Beasley *et al*. 1987a) (Fig. 54.9), which is of equivalent potency to PGD_2, and is formed by the stereospecific reduction of the 11-ketone group of PGD_2. Both PGD_2 and its metabolite produce their effects upon the airway by a combination of direct and cholinergic-mediated mechanisms (Beasley *et al*. 1987b). Histamine and PGD_2 are released in parallel by stimulated mast cells with 30–100 times as much histamine being released as PGD_2 (Agius *et al*. 1986), and, since PGD_2 and its metabolite are 30–40 times more potent than histamine as a bronchoconstrictor, the constrictor activity of the two mediators when released into the airways during the early asthmatic response is likely to be similar. Indeed, Hardy *et al*. (1986a) have shown that, when both agents are inhaled in the molar ratios in which they are released from mast cells,

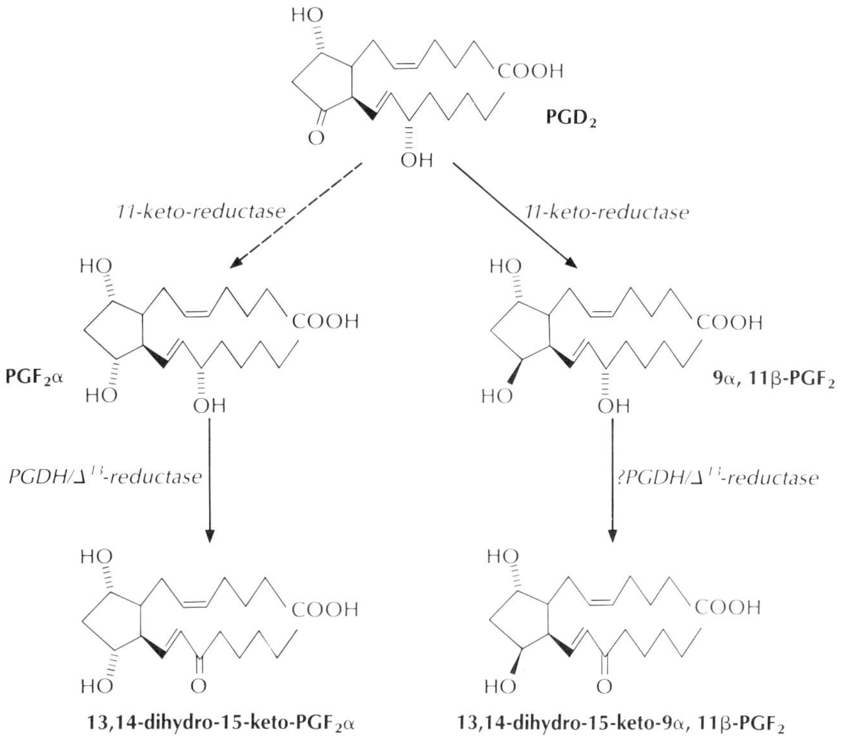

Fig. 54.9. Metabolism of the predominant cyclo-oxygenase product from mast cells, PGD_2, to $9\alpha,11\beta\text{-}PGF_2$.

the same degree of bronchoconstriction is produced. Further supportive evidence of the role of PGD_2 and its metabolite derives from the work using the potent cyclo-oxygenase inhibitor, flurbiprofen. This agent has been found to inhibit the allergen-induced early asthmatic response by about one-third in atopic non-asthmatic subjects (Curzen *et al.* 1987) and more recently in asthmatic patients. However, this activity is unrelated to the opposite response of bronchoconstriction produced by non-steroidal anti-inflammatory drugs in up to 5% of asthma patients.

Prostaglandin is another bronchoconstrictor prostanoid derived from arachidonate that is less potent than PGD_2, but 3.5 times as potent as histamine (Hardy *et al.* 1984). Following inhalation it is rapidly metabolized to the inactive product 13,14-dihydro-15-keto-$PGF_{2\alpha}$ (Hardy *et al.* 1986b). It has variable effects on the airways in asthmatic subjects, and can produce complex biphasic and triphasic bronchoconstriction which is not inhibited by anticholinergic medication (Beasley *et al.* 1987b). Like PGD_2, it produces cough and tachycardia in volunteers after inhalation.

Thromboxane A_2 is released from lung fragments during anaphylaxis (Schulman *et al.* 1981) and is a potent bronchoconstrictor (Svensson *et al.* 1977). It is released into the plasma (measured as its metabolite, TXB_2) during allergen-induced bronchoconstriction (Shephard *et al.* 1985), and oral administration of a thromboxane synthetase inhibitor has been shown to reduce bronchial responsiveness to acetylcholine (Fujimura *et al.* 1986), implicating this mediator in this aspect of disordered airway function.

Prostaglandin E_2 is a bronchodilator in asthmatic patients, but it also produces cough and, occasionally, paradoxical bronchoconstriction that limits its usefulness (Smith and Cuthbert 1972; Roberts *et al.* 1985). It is also an inhibitory agent in that it can prevent the bronchoconstriction produced by inhaled $PGF_{2\alpha}$, and it has been shown to reduce bronchial hyper-responsiveness (Walters *et al.* 1982). It has been postulated that cyclo-oxygenase inhibition by drugs such as aspirin may be responsible for asthma induced by these agents, as they may selectively inhibit the synthesis of PGE_2, rather than by shifting arachidonate metabolism towards the over-production of lipoxygenase products (Barnes and Thompson 1988). Release of PGE_2 may also be responsible for the refractory period seen after exercise-provoked asthma (O'Byrne and Jones 1986).

LEUKOTRIENES AND LIPOXYGENASE PRODUCTS

The enzyme 5-lipoxygenase acts on arachidonate to produce the important intermediary compound, 5-hydroperoxy-6,8,11,14-eicosatetraenoic acid (5-HPETE). This unstable product gives rise to 5-HETE via the glutathione peroxidase system, or to the leukotrienes, a group of compounds characterized by their conjugated triene structure (Henderson 1987). Leukotriene A_4 is an unstable derivative of 5-HPETE, and from this compound LTB_4 and the sulphidopeptide leukotrienes (LTC_4, LTD_4 and LTE_4) are derived (Fig. 54.10). The sulphidopeptide LTs comprise the activity previously recognized as slow-reacting substance of anaphylaxis which in addition to contracting airways smooth muscle also increases vascular permeability and mucus secretion (Samuelsson 1983). Both LTD_4 and LTE_4 are enzymatically derived from the peptide chain shortening of LTC_4, and retain the original biological activities.

There is abundant evidence from *in vitro* studies that these compounds might be involved in the pathogenesis of asthma. Their production by human lung or by isolated cells is selective and requires the activation of 5-lipoxygenase. This can be brought about by allergen challenge, exposure to PAF, to the chemotactic peptide *N*-formyl-L-methionyl-L-leucyl-phenylalanine (FMLP) or to C5a, an anaphylatoxin derived from the complement cascade (Drazen and Austin 1987), and can be inhibited by drugs acting on the 5-lipoxygenase enzyme system both in enzymatically dispersed lung tissue and from non-dispersed lung fragments (Dahlén *et al.* 1983; Robinson and Holgate 1986b). Eosinophils and mast cells are able to synthesize only LTC_4, with eosinophils from asthmatics producing three times as much LTC_4 as cells isolated from normal controls (McGlashan *et al.* 1982; Weller *et al.* 1983; Shaw *et al.* 1984). In contrast, human neutrophils produce only LTB_4, with the production of this mediator also being enhanced in asthmatic subjects (Mita *et al.* 1985).

The sulphidopeptide LTs are potent bronchoconstrictor agents when given by inhalation in both normal subjects and those with asthma (Bisgaard *et al.* 1985). When administered to human bronchi *in vitro*, they are some 100–1000 times more potent than histamine on a molar basis. They are also able to increase microvascular permeability by an effect on post-capillary venules, and stimulate mucus production in human airways (Dahlén *et al.* 1987a). They are thus able to produce many of the observed abnormalities known to occur in clinical asthma. Most of these effects occur by direct mechanisms involving the activation of specific cell surface LT receptors. However, LTE_4 is a less potent constrictor than the other two agents (Davidson *et al.* 1987), and it can also enhance bronchial reactivity to histamine in asthmatic subjects (Arm *et al.* 1987). A synergistic interaction between the airway effects of inhaled histamine and LTC_4 (possibly after metabolism to LTE_4), and between inhaled PGD_2 and LTC_4, has been shown, which suggests a role for mediator interaction in the pathogenesis of airflow limitation (Phillips and Holgate 1989).

Leukotriene B_4 is also a bronchospastic agent but is considerably less potent in this regard than the sulphidopeptide LTs. It can also increase microvascular permeability by a different mechanism than the sulphidopeptide LTs. The plasma leakage induced by LTB_4 is slow in onset and correlates with the wave of leucocyte diapedesis that is a characteristic of the inflammatory response. The primary activity of LTB_4 is to stimulate neutrophil and eosinophil chemotaxis and chemokinesis (Dahlén 1988), and to prime these cells via mobilization of intracellular calcium. Neutrophils possess specific high-affinity receptors for LTB_4 that mediate chemotaxis and increased adherence, and low-affinity receptors that mediate the production of superoxide and the release of lysosomal enzymes (Burrell *et al.* 1988).

There have been a number of studies examining the effect of leukotriene inhibitors in asthma. Fujimura and co-workers (1986) administered a 5-lipoxygenase inhibitor by mouth for 4 days prior to acetylcholine challenge in asthmatic volunteers. The compound, AA-861, has been shown to inhibit the generation of LTC_4 by stimulated human peripheral blood leucocytes, but had no activity against acetylcholine-induced bronchoconstriction. The putative LT inhibitor (U-60257, piriprost) was found to be inactive when given by inhalation against exercise- and allergen-induced bronchoconstrictor early and late responses, and it had no effect on the fall in peak expiratory flow measured on the morning after allergen challenge (Mann *et al.* 1986). The effects of an oral LTD_4 antagonist

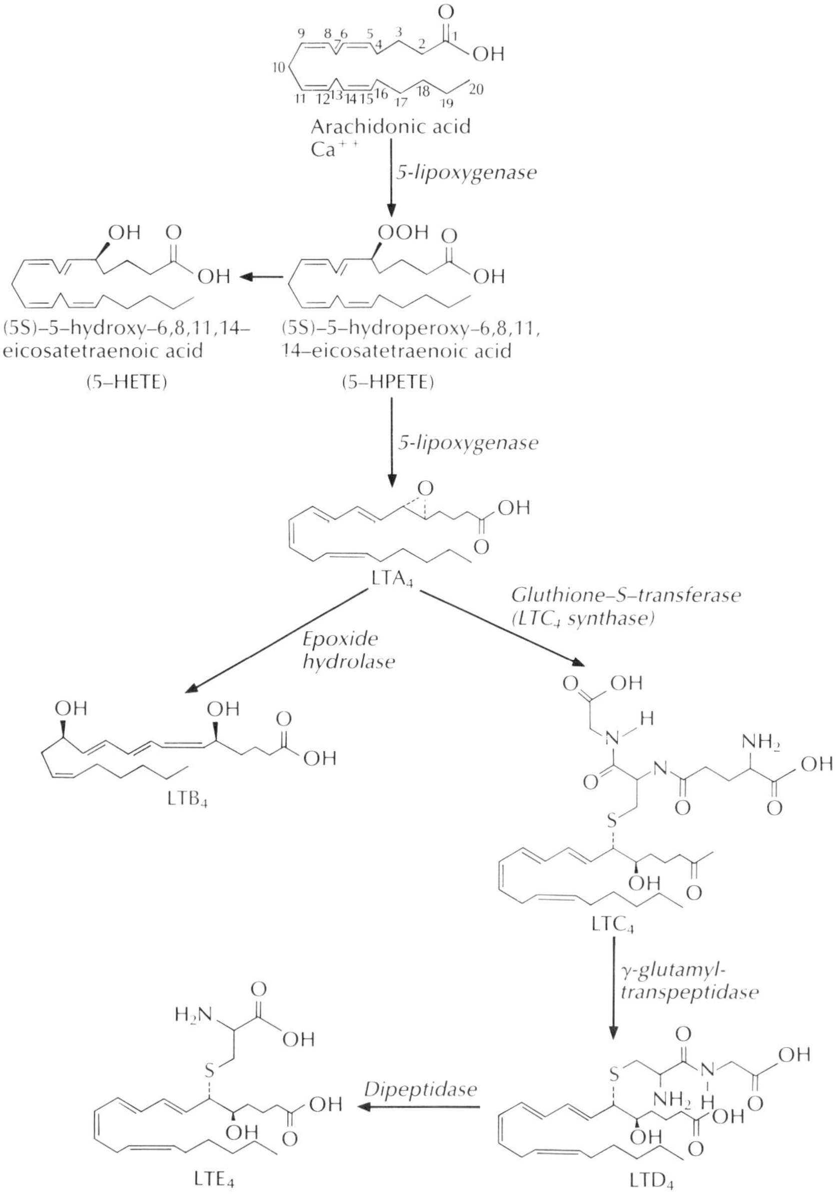

Fig. 54.10. Metabolism of arachidonic acid by the lipoxygenase pathway. The major products of this pathway relevant to the mast cell are the sulphidopeptide LTs (LTC_4 and LTD_4) and LTB_4.

(Jones *et al.* 1986) have also been examined in asthma. Britton and colleagues (1987) gave the compound to hyper-reactive asthmatics 2 hours prior to allergen challenge, and followed the subjects for 9 hours. They found only minor protection, and most subjects experienced adverse side-effects of acute abdominal discomfort or profuse watery diarrhoea soon after ingestion. Barnes and colleagues (1987) examined the effect of the same dose of the drug against histamine- and leukotriene-induced bronchoconstriction in normal men, and found that it inhibited the response to LTD_4 but not to histamine. These subjects also experienced similar side-effects. The most recent published study examined the effects of another LTD_4 antagonist, LY-171883, on LTD_4-induced bronchoconstriction (Phillips *et al.* 1988b). The drug was given by mouth 2 hours before challenge in non-asthmatic subjects, and was found to produce a dose-dependent inhibition of bronchoconstriction. No adverse effects were noted. Clearly, further work is required to assess the place of the LT synthesis inhibitors and antagonists as potential treatment modalities in asthma, especially with drugs of greater potency and selectivity, such as ICI 198,615, a highly potent LT receptor antagonist in the guinea-pig (Krell *et al.* 1987), and the acetohydroxamic acid group of 5-lipoxygenase inhibitors, which have been reported to partially inhibit the bronchospastic response to inhaled antigen in the guinea-pig (Payne *et al.* 1988).

PRODUCTS DERIVED FROM THE 15-LIPOXYGENASE PATHWAY

The enzyme 15-lipoxygenase is able to convert arachidonic acid into a variety of mono- and di-HETEs, in addition to a group of newly recognized lipid mediators, the lipoxins, which require an interaction between 5- and 15-lipoxygenase for their biosynthesis (Serhan *et al.* 1984). The major product of this pathway that has been implicated as a mediator of asthma is 15-HETE, which is produced by both normal and asthmatic lung homogenates in the presence of arachidonate (Hamberg *et al.* 1980). When lung tissue is subjected *in vitro* to allergen challenge, 15-s-HETE is released in molar amounts approximately 100 times greater than that of LTC_4 (Dahlén *et al.* 1983). When atopic asthmatic subjects were challenged with an extract of house dust mite instilled into a segmental bronchus, the amount of 15-HETE recovered from BAL fluid was observed to increase by up to 30-fold, along with a 40-fold increase of PGD_2 (Murray *et al.* 1986). The most likely cellular sources of the mediator are airway epithelial cells and eosinophils. When suspensions of purified human tracheal epithelial cells were incubated with arachidonic acid (Hunter *et al.* 1985), they were found to generate 10 times the amount of 15-HETE as that synthesized by eosinophils when studied under the same conditions (Turk *et al.* 1982). Both cell lines produced smaller quantities of other 15-lipoxygenase metabolites, although the significance of these findings is not yet clear.

In vitro, 15-HETE is reported to be a potent stimulator of mucus glycoprotein secretion from cultured human airway explants (Marom *et al.* 1981). It is a weak contractile agonist of human bronchial muscle, being 10 times less potent than histamine (Copas *et al.* 1982). It can either activate (Goetzl *et al.* 1983) or inhibit (Vanderhoek *et al.* 1980; Camp and Fincham 1985) the 5-lipoxygenase pathway and may therefore be an important modulator of LT production. In the dog airway, it is able to induce neutrophil and mast cell chemotaxis, cause interalveolar oedema and induce mucus secretion (Johnson *et al.* 1985). Lipoxin A_4 is an activator of protein kinase C (Hansson *et al.* 1986), and is able to cause contraction of airway smooth muscle and vasodilatation (Dahlén *et al.* 1987b), although it remains to be seen what role these substances will have in the pathogenesis of the type of inflammation characteristic of asthma.

To our knowledge, only one study has been undertaken observing the effects of inhaled 15-HETE in normal and asthmatic subjects (Lai *et al.* 1989). The effect of inhaled 15-HETE on bronchial responsiveness to methacholine and histamine was studied. 15-Hydroxyeicosatetraenoic acid produced no changes in either FEV_1 or an index of small airway function (maximum expiratory flow rate at 70% baseline vital capacity below total lung capacity) in either group of subjects. Moreover, 15-HETE had the effect of reducing the sensitivity of airways to both methacholine and histamine, for up to 24 hours after inhalation. The mechanism of this effect is not known, but it may have some biological importance in the modulation of the airway inflammatory response to injurious stimuli. The place of these substances in the production or maintenance of the asthmatic process is not yet clear, although at the time of writing there seems to be little to implicate a pro-inflammatory role.

Platelet-activating factor

Platelet-activating factor is a unique ether-linked phospholipid mediator of inflammation, which has the same molecule as its precursor and immediate metabolite, lyso-PAF (Fig. 54.11). It can be synthesized and released from a number of cells, including eosinophils (Lee, T.C. *et al.* 1984), neutrophils (Clay *et al.* 1984), macrophages (Arnoux *et al.* 1987), basophils (Benveniste *et al.* 1972), endothelial cells (Camussi *et al.* 1983a) and platelets (Chignard *et al.* 1980). Eosinophils and macrophages derived from asthmatic subjects produce more PAF than those from non-asthmatic subjects (Godard *et al.* 1982; Lee, T.C. *et al.* 1984). Platelets, neutrophils, macrophages and lung tissue have all been found to have high-affinity binding sites for PAF that may reside within cell membranes. Following the binding of PAF to its receptor, there is internalization of the PAF receptor complex (Kloprogge and Akkerman 1984), followed by a series of cellular biochemical events

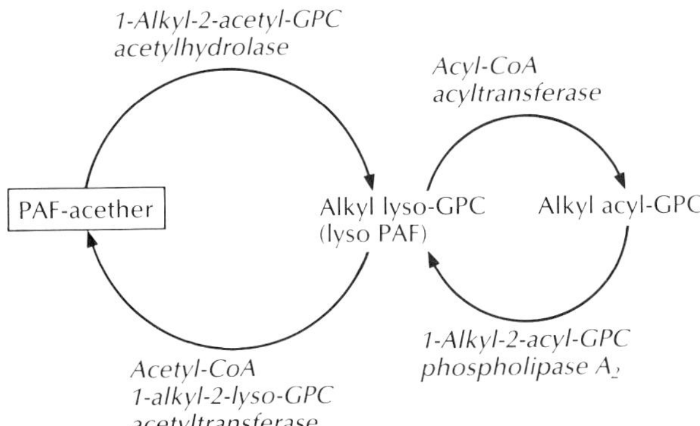

Fig. 54.11. The synthesis and catabolism of platelet-activating factor (PAF).

which transduce the signal to cellular activation (Page 1988).

Platelet-activating factor has a variety of actions that are relevant to asthma (Barnes 1988a). These include bronchoconstriction both in normal subjects and in asthmatic volunteers (Chung *et al.* 1987a; Rubin *et al.* 1987), the induction of long-standing bronchial hyper-responsiveness in animals (Robertson *et al.* 1988) and non-asthmatic humans (Cuss *et al.* 1986; Rubin *et al.* 1987), increase in capillary permeability (Evans *et al.* 1987), and a reduction in the rate of mucociliary transport (Aursudkij *et al.* 1987). It is also a potent chemotactic and activating agent for eosinophils (Wardlaw *et al.* 1986), neutrophils (Archer *et al.* 1985), macrophages (Camussi *et al.* 1983b) and platelets (Lellouch-Tubiana *et al.* 1985).

The significance of those studies that report a rapid onset of bronchoconstriction followed by increased bronchial responsiveness after inhaling increasing concentrations of PAF is unclear as tachyphylaxis occurs in this setting (Cuss *et al.* 1986). Furthermore, both the studies of Rubin *et al.* (1987) and Cuss *et al.* (1986) demonstrated that the increased bronchial responsiveness to methacholine was of the order of one doubling concentration less than that required to produce a response prior to PAF inhalation, and it is known that the repeatability of the methacholine inhalation test varies from half to twice the initial dose or concentration that produces the required result (Connolly, M.J. *et al.* 1988). The mechanism of PAF-induced bronchial hyper-responsiveness is unclear, although it is partially inhibited by β adrenoceptor agonists (Chung *et al.* 1987b), and it is not affected by ketotifen, an agent with potent antihistamine activity (Chung *et al.* 1988). At least one study has failed to confirm the ability of PAF when administered as a single dose to enhance airways responsiveness in healthy subjects (Jenkins *et al.* 1989), and in two studies asthmatic subjects given PAF by inhalation did not develop bronchial hyper-responsiveness to methacholine (Rubin *et al.* 1987; Chung and Barnes 1989).

The recent development of specific PAF antagonists may help elucidate the role of this substance in the pathophysiology of asthma. One such compound, BN52063, is a mixture of three naturally occurring gingkolides (A, B, C) derived from the leaves of a chinese tree, *Gingko biloba* (Braquet *et al.* 1985). When given by mouth, it produces a dose-dependent inhibition of PAF-induced wheal and flare in the skin, and an *ex vivo* inhibition of PAF-induced platelet aggregation (Chung *et al.* 1987c). Furthermore, it can inhibit the late, but not the early, cutaneous response to antigen challenge (Roberts *et al.* 1988a), while the same dose affords only partial protection against PAF-induced bronchoconstriction in normal subjects (Roberts *et al.* 1988b). Although PAF seems likely to be an important mediator in the pathogenesis of asthma, further clinical work with more potent and selective antagonists such as WEB 2086 are needed to fully elucidate its role.

Bradykinin and airway peptides

Bradykinin is a nonapeptide, one of a family of three peptides that is formed from a plasma precursor during inflammation. Bradykinin is one of several kinins that are generated from kininogens (α-2-globulins) by the action of kininogenases, the other kinins being kallidin (lys-bradykinin) and met-lys-bradykinin. Bradykinin has been implicated in the development of inflammatory reactions (Regoli and Barabe 1980), as it can be released by inflammatory cells or tissues in which an inflammatory response has been provoked (Newball *et al.* 1979; Proud *et al.* 1985) and it is found in nasal washings of allergic individuals following nasal challenge with antigen (Proud *et al.* 1983). It is a potent constrictor of isolated guinea-pig tracheal rings, an effect that can be inhibited by cyclo-oxygenase inhibitors (Fuller and Barnes 1988), and of isolated human lung (Regoli and Barabe 1980). Bradykinin causes the release of prostaglandins and thromboxane from isolated guinea-pig lungs (Bakhle *et al.* 1985), and release is enhanced by the prior administration of an angiotensin-converting enzyme inhibitor such as captopril, supporting the view that these agents inhibit bradykinin degradation (Greenberg *et al.* 1979).

Bradykinin can induce extravasation of plasma (Williams and Peck 1977), and by stimulation of afferent C fibres causes bronchoconstriction and mucous gland secretion in the dog airways (Kaufman *et al.* 1980; Davis *et al.* 1982). Fuller and co-workers (1987) administered bradykinin by inhalation to normal and asthmatic subjects, and found that it produced a dose-dependent bronchoconstriction in the asthmatics but not in the normal subjects; it was more potent than histamine or methacholine, and its effects were inhibited by the prior administration of ipratropium bromide and by SCG, but not by aspirin. It seems likely that its effects are partially mediated via cholinergic nerves with a contribution made by local peptide-containing nerves, and it can be considered as a secondary inflammatory mediator as it does not produce a late asthmatic response or an increase in bronchial hyper-responsiveness.

Recently, another group of peptides have been identified in the human respiratory tract, known as the sensory neuropeptides or the tachykinins. These peptides were first found in the human gastrointestinal tract, where they are involved in the regulation of gut motility, sphincter control and secretion, and where they appear to act as neurotransmitters or neuromodulators. As the human respiratory tract has a similar embryological origin to the foregut, much attention has been focused on this group of peptides, which comprise vasoactive intestinal peptide (VIP), substance P (SP), neurokinin A (NKA), neurokinin B (NKB) and calcitonin gene-related peptide (CGRP).

When these agents were given intravenously to rats, it was found that they were potent bronchoconstrictors (NKA>SP>NKB), and were accompanied by prominent cardiovascular changes, including hypotension and the development of a metabolic acidosis (Joos *et al.* 1986). In healthy non-asthmatic subjects, inhalation of SP and NKA produces no detectable change in sGAW while in asthmatics inhaled SP has no effect, but NKA produces a concentration-dependent reduction in sGAW. No correlation has been found between bronchial responsiveness to methacholine and that to NKA (Joos *et al.* 1987). Nedocromil sodium was found to significantly protect against NKA-induced bronchoconstriction (Joos *et al.* 1988a), whilst the synthetic antimuscarinic anticholinergic agent, oxitropium bromide, failed to provide any protection (Joos *et al.* 1988b). Neurokinin A probably causes bronchoconstriction through an indirect mechanism (Joos 1989), possibly due to an increase in the number or affinity of tachykinin receptors in the airways. Enkephalinase is a membrane-bound metallo-endopeptidase found in specific airway cells, particularly in sensory nerve endings, tracheal epithelium, airways smooth muscle and submucosal glands. It can modulate tachykinin-induced secretion and constriction in ferret trachea preparations (Nadel and Borson 1988), and, because it is present at sites where tachykinins are released (sensory nerves) and where they have their effects (smooth muscle, submucosal glands and epithelium) (Sekizawa *et al.* 1987), it is likely that it exerts some local control over the responses to SP and other tachykinins.

Calcitonin gene-related peptide is also localized to afferent nerves in the airways. It is a potent vasodilator and inducer of microvascular leakage, and *in vitro* is a more potent constrictor of human airways than SP (Barnes 1988b). Vasoactive intestinal peptide is a potent dilator of airway smooth muscle preparations, although it has no activity when inhaled by humans, and only a very small protective effect against histamine-induced bronchoconstriction (Barnes and Dixon 1984). The role of these and other peptides in the development of airway disease has yet to be established but it is highly likely that they contribute to the magnitude and distribution of inflammation within the airways (Barnes 1986).

Conclusion

Much of the evidence concerning the involvement of inflammatory cells and chemical mediators in the pathogenesis of asthma has been discussed in this review. How do these abnormalities become translated into the development of clinical asthma and bronchial hyper-responsiveness? Many pathological and clinical features of asthma can be caused or reproduced by the cells and mediators discussed above, and complex intercellular and inter-mediator interactions must take place in the

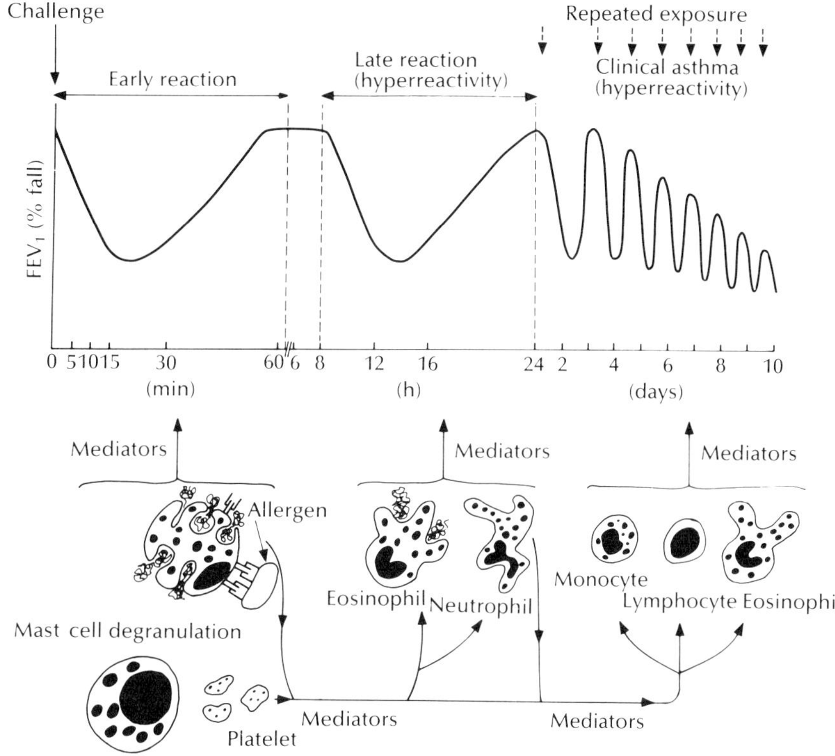

Fig. 54.12. Schematic representation of the inflammatory events underlying the development and maintainance of asthma. The early asthmatic response is associated with mediator release from mast cells and possibly from macrophages and platelets. The mediators attract eosinophils and neutrophils to the airway, which also release mediators and toxic substances, provoking the late asthmatic response. Repeated allergen exposure is associated with clinical asthma and airway hyperreactivity, and is associated with airway infiltration by cells such as lymphocytes and eosinophils.

airways of asthmatic patients to produce the final 'product' of airway smooth muscle shortening and hypertrophy, mucosal oedema, epithelial damage and increased mucus production (Fig. 54.12). Snashall and colleagues (1988) have proposed that a variety of factors operate to heighten the individual's response to inhaled allergen or other irritant substances which combine to produce bronchial hyper-responsiveness; the link between these factors is almost certainly inflammation. Further research, in particular with agents that inhibit these inflammatory responses, may yet enhance our understanding of this increasingly common condition.

Acknowledgements

Dr Summers is supported by a grant from The Lillian Roxon Memorial Asthma Research Travel Grant.

References

Ackerman, S.J., Weil, G.J. and Gleich, G.J. (1982). Formation of the Charcot–Leyden crystals by human basophils. *J. Exp. Med.* **155**, 1597–609.

Agius, R.M., Godfrey, R.C. and Holgate, S.T. (1986). Mast cell and histamine content of human bronchoalveolar lavage fluid. *Thorax* **40**, 760–7.

Alam, R., Kuna, P., Rozniecki, J. and Kuzminska, B. (1987). The magnitude of the spontaneous production of histamine-releasing factor (HRF) by lymphocytes *in vitro* correlates with the state of bronchial hyperreactivity in patients with asthma. *J. Allergy Clin. Immunol.* **79**, 103–8.

Ameisen, J.C., Capron, A., Joseph, M. *et al.* (1985). Aspirin-sensitive asthma: abnormal and physiopathological implications. *Int. Arch. Allergy Appl. Immunol.* **78**, 438–48.

American Thoracic Society (1987). Standards for the diagnosis and care of patients with chronic obstructive pulmonary disease (COPD) and asthma. *Am. Rev. Respir. Dis.* **136**, 225–44.

Anderson, S.D. (1988). Exercise-induced asthma. In *Asthma: Basic Mechanisms and Clinical Management*, ed. P.J. Barnes, I.W. Rodger and N.C. Thompson, pp. 503–22, Academic Press, London.

Archer, C.B., MacDonald, D.M., Morley, J., Page, C.P., Paul, W. and Sanjar, S. (1985). Effects of serum albumin, indomethacin and histamine H_1-antagonists on paf-acether-induced inflammatory responses in the skin of experimental animals and man. *Br. J. Pharmacol.* **85**, 109–13.

Arm, J.P., Spar, B.W. and Lee, T.H. (1987). Leukotriene E_4 (LTE_4) enhances airway histamine responsiveness in asthmatic subjects. *Thorax* **42**, 220 (abstract).

Arnoux, B., Joseph, M., Simoes, M.H. *et al.* (1987). Antigenic release of PAF-Acether and β-glucuronidase from alveolar macrophages of asthmatics. *Clin. Respir. Physiol.* **23**, 119–24.

Aursudkij, B., Rogers, D.F., Evans, T.W., Alton, E.W.F.W., Chung, K.F. and Barnes, P.J. (1987). Reduced tracheal mucus velocity in guinea-pig *in vivo* by platelet-activating factor. *Am. Rev. Respir. Dis.* **135**, A160.

Bakhle, Y.S., Moncada, S., de Nucci, G. and Salmon, J.A. (1985). Differential release of eicosanoids by bradykinin, arachidonic acid and calcium ionophore A23187 in guinea-pig isolated perfused lung. *Br. J. Pharmacol.* **86**, 55–62.

Barnes, N., Piper, P.J. and Costello, J. (1987). The effect of an oral leukotriene antagonist L-649,923 on histamine and leukotriene D_4-induced bronchoconstriction in normal men. *J. Allergy Clin. Immunol.* **79**, 816–21.

Barnes, P.J. (1986). Asthma as an axon reflex. *Lancet* **i**, 242–5.

Barnes, P.J. (1988a). Platelet-activating factor. In Asthma — what are the important experiments? ed. A.J. Woolcock. *Am. Rev. Respir. Dis.* **138**, 730–44.

Barnes, P.J. (1988b). Airway neuropeptides. In *Asthma: Basic Mechanisms and Clinical Management*, ed. P.J. Barnes, I.W. Rodger and N.C. Thompson, pp. 395–413, Academic Press, London.

Barnes, P.J. and Dixon, C.M.S. (1984). The effect of inhaled vasoactive intestinal peptide on bronchial hyperreactivity in man. *Am. Rev. Respir. Dis.* **130**, 162–6.

Barnes, P.J. and Thompson, N.C. (1988). Drug-induced asthma. In *Asthma: Basic Mechanisms and Clinical Management*, ed. P.J. Barnes, I.W. Rodger and N.C. Thompson, pp. 533–49, Academic Press, London.

Barnes, P.J., Ind, P.W. and Brown, M.J. (1982). Plasma histamine and catecholamines in stable asthmatic subjects. *Clin. Sci.* **62**, 661–5.

Beasley, C.R.W., Robinson, C., Featherstone, R.L. *et al.* (1987a). $9\alpha,11\beta$-prostaglandin F_2, a novel metabolite of prostaglandin D_2 is a potent contractile agonist of human and guinea pig airways. *J. Clin. Invest.* **79**, 978–83.

Beasley, C.R.W., Varley, J., Robinson, C., Holgate, S.T. (1987b). Cholinergic-mediated bronchoconstriction induced by prostaglandin D_2, its initial metabolite $9\alpha,11\beta$-PGF_2, and $PGF_{2\alpha}$ in asthma. *Am. Rev. Respir. Dis.* **136**, 1140–4.

Beasley, C.R.W., Roche, W.R., Roberts, J.A. and Holgate, S.T. (1989a). Cellular events in the bronchi in mild asthma and after bronchial provocation. *Am. Rev. Respir. Dis.* **139**, 806–17.

Beasley, C.R.W., Featherstone, R.L., Church, M.K. *et al.* (1989b). Receptor antagonism of bronchoconstrictor prostanoids *in vitro* and *in vivo* by GR 32191: implications for the contribution of these mediators to immediate allergen-induced bronchoconstriction in asthma. *J. Appl. Physiol.* **66**, 1685–93.

Benveniste, J., Henson, P.M. and Cochrane, C.G. (1972). Leukocyte-dependant histamine release from rabbit platelets: the role of IgE, basophils and a platelet-activating factor. *J. Exp. Med.* **136**, 1356–77.

Benyon, R.C. (1988). Stimulus-secretion coupling in mast cells and basophils. In *Mast Cells, Mediators and Disease*, ed. S.T. Holgate, pp. 195–226, Kluwer Academic, Dordrecht.

Benyon, R.C., Lowman, M.A. and Church, M.K. (1987). Human skin mast cells: their dispersion, purification and secretory characterisation. *J. Immunol.* **138**, 861–7.

Bergstrand, H., Lundquist, B., Petersson, B.-Å., Petersson, C. and Venge, P. (1985). Eosinophil derived cationic proteins and human leukocyte histamine release. In *Inflammation: Basic Mechanisms, Tissue Injuring Principles and Clinical Models*, ed. P. Venge and A. Lindbom, pp. 361–6, Almqvist & Wiksell International, Stockholm.

Bisgaard, H., Groth, S. and Flemming, M. (1985). Bronchial hyperreactivity to leukotriene D_4 and histamine in exogenous asthma. *Br. Med. J.* **290**, 1468–71.

Booij-Noord, H., Orie, N.G.M. and de Vries, K. (1971). Immediate and late bronchial obstructive reactions to house dust mite and protective effects of disodium cromoglycate and prednisolone. *J. Allergy Clin. Immunol.* **48**, 344–54.

Booij-Noord, H., de Vries, K., Sluiter, H.J. and Orie, N.G.M. (1972). Late bronchial obstructive reaction to experimental inhalation of house dust extract. *Clin. Allergy* **2**, 43–61.

Boschetto, P., Fabbri, L.M., Zocca, E. *et al.* (1987). Prednisone inibits late asthmatic reactions and airway inflammation induced by toluence diisocyanate in sensitized subjects. *J. Allergy Clin. Immunol.* **80**, 261–7.

Boushey, H.A., Holtzman, M.J., Sheller, J.R. and Nadel, J.A. (1980). Bronchial hyperreactivity. *Am. Rev. Respir. Dis.* **121**, 389–413.

Braquet, P., Spinnewyn, B., Braquet, M. *et al.* (1985). BN52021 and related compounds: a new series of highly specific PAF-receptor antagonists isolated from *Gingka biloba. Blood Vessels* **16**, 559–72.

Britton, J.R., Hanley, S.P. and Tattersfield, A.E. (1987). The effect of an oral leukotriene antagonist L-649,923 on the response to inhaled antigen in asthma. *J. Allergy Clin. Immunol.* **79**, 811–16.

Brown, P.J., Greville, H.W. and Finucane, K.E. (1984). Asthma and irreversible airflow obstruction. *Thorax* **39**, 131–6.

Bruynzeel, P.L.B., Koenderman, L., Kok, P.T.M., Hameling, M.L. and Verhagen, J. (1986). Platelet-activating factor (PAF-acether) induced leukotriene C_4 formation and luminol dependant chemiluminescence by human eosinophils. *Pharmacol. Res. Commun.* **18** (suppl.), 61–9.

Buchanan, D.R., Cromwell, O. and Kay, A.B. (1987a). Neutrophil chemotactic activity in acute severe asthma ('status asthmaticus'). *Am. Rev. Respir. Dis.* **136**, 1397–402.

Buchanan, D.R., Fitzharris, P., Cromwell, O. and Kay, A.B. (1987b). Neutrophil chemotactic activity from cultured blood mononuclear cells in acute severe asthma. *Thorax* **42**, 749 (abstract).

Burney, P.G.J. (1987). Asthma mortality: England and Wales. *J. Allergy Clin. Immunol.* **80** (2), 379–82.

Burrell, B.A., Payan, D.G. and Goetzl, E.J. (1988). Arachidonic acid-derived mediators of hypersensitivity and inflammation. In *Allergy: Principles and Practice*, ed. E. Middleton, Jr, C.E. Reed, E.F. Ellis, N.F. Adkinson and J.W. Yunginger, pp. 164–78, C.V. Mosby, Washington.

Cairns, H. and Orr, T.S.C. (1988). The development of a new agent for the treatment of inflammatory/allergic conditions. *Int. Arch. Allergy Appl. Immunol.* **82**, 513–17.

Camp, R.D.R. and Fincham, N.J. (1985). Inhibition of ionophore-stimulated leukotriene B_4 production in human leukocytes by monohydroxy fatty acids. *Br. J. Pharmacol.* **85**, 837–41.

Camussi, G., Anglietta, M., Malavasi, F. *et al.* (1983a). The release of platelet-activating factor from human endothelial cells in culture. *J. Immunol.* **131**, 2397–403.

Camussi, G., Pawlowski, I., Tetla, C. *et al.* (1983b). Acute lung inflammation induced in the rabbit by local instillation of

1-*O*-octadecyl-2-acetyl-*sn*-glyceryl-*s*-phosphorylcholine or of native platelet-activating factor. *Am. J. Pathol.* **112**, 75–88.

Capron, A., Ameisen, J.C., Joseph, M. and Tonnel, A.B. (1987). Platelets as effectors of hypersensitivity reactions. In *Allergy and Inflammation*, ed. A.B. Kay, pp. 125–38, Academic Press, London.

Capron, M. (1989). Eosinophils: receptors and mediators in hypersensitivity. *Clin. Allergy* **19** (suppl. 1), 3–8.

Capron, M., Kusnierz, J.P., Prin, L. *et al.* (1985). Cytophilic IgE on human blood and tissue eosinophils: detection by flow microfluorometry. *J. Immunol.* **134**, 3013–18.

Capron, M., Jouault, T., Prin, C. *et al.* (1986). Functional study of a monoclonal antibody to IgE Fc receptor of eosinophils, platelets and macrophages ($Fc_\epsilon R2$). *J. Exp. Med.* **164**, 72–89.

Carroll, M.P., Durham, S.R., Walsh, G.M. and Kay, A.B. (1985). Activation of neutrophils and monocytes after allergen- and histamine-induced bronchoconstriction. *J. Allergy Clin. Immunol.* **75**, 290–6.

Casale, T.B., Wood, D.S., Richerson, H.B., Zehr, B., Zavala, D. and Hunninghake, G.W. (1987a). Direct evidence of a role for mast cells in the pathogenesis of antigen-induced bronchoconstriction. *J. Clin. Invest.* **80**, 1507–11.

Casale, T.B., Wood, D.S., Richerson, H.B. *et al.* (1987b). Elevated bronchoalveolar lavage fluid histamine levels in allergic asthmatics are associated with methacholine bronchial responsiveness. *J. Clin. Invest.* **79**, 1197–203.

Castells, M., Irani, A.A. and Schwartz, L.B. (1987). Evaluation of human peripheral blood leukocytes for mast cell tryptase. *J. Immunol.* **138**, 2184–9.

Chignard, M., LeCouedic, J.P., Vargaftig, B.B. and Benveniste, I. (1980). Platelet-activating factor (PAF-acether) secretion from platelets effect of aggregating agents. *Br. J. Haematol.* **46**, 455–64.

Chung, K.F. and Barnes, P.J. (1989). Effects of platelet activating factor on airway calibre, airway responsiveness, and circulating cells in asthmatic subjects. *Thorax* **44**, 108–15.

Chung, K.F., Dixon, C.M.S. and Barnes, P.J. (1987a). Plàtelet-activating factor (PAF) and asthmatic airways: effects on calibre, responsiveness and circulating cells. *Am. Rev. Respir. Dis.* **135**, A159.

Chung, K.F., Dent, G., McCusker, M. and Barnes, P.J. (1987b). Effect of a β_2-adrenergic agonist on bronchoconstriction, airway hyper-responsiveness, neutropenia and neutrophil activation after platelet-activating factor in man. *Am. Rev. Respir. Dis.* **135**, A181.

Chung, K.F., McCusker, M., Page, C.P., Dent, G., Guinot, P. and Barnes, P.J. (1987c). Effect of a gingkolide mixture (BN52063) in antagonising skin and platelet responses to platelet activating factor in man. *Lancet* **i**, 248–51.

Chung, K.F., Minette, P., McCusker, M. and Barnes, P.J. (1988). Ketotifen inhibits the cutaneous but not the airway responses to platelet-activating factor in man. *J. Allergy Clin. Immunol.* **81**, 1192–8.

Church, M.K. and Hiroi, J. (1987). Inhibition of IgE-dependent histamine release from human dispersed lung mast cells by anti-allergic drugs and salbutamol. *Br. J. Pharmacol.* **90**, 421–9.

Church, M.K., Pao, G.J.-K. and Holgate, S.T. (1982). Characterisation of histamine secretion from dispersed human lung mast cells: effects of anti-IgE, calcium ionophore A23187, compound 48/80, and basic polypeptides. *J. Immunol.* **129**, 2116–21.

Church, M.K., Holgate, S.T. and Pao, G.J.-K. (1983). Histamine release from mechanically and enzymatically dispersed human lung mast cells: inhibition by salbutamol and cromoglycate (abstract). *Br. J. Pharmacol.* **79** (suppl.), 374.

Clay, K.L., Murphy, R.C., Andres, J.L., Lynch, J. and Henson, P.M. (1984). Structure elucidation of platelet-activating factor derived from human neutrophils. *Biochem. Biophys. Res. Commun.* **121**, 815–25.

Cockcroft, D.W. and Murdock, K.Y. (1985). Bronchial responsiveness to inhaled histamine is increased 7 and 30 hours but not 2 hours after allergen inhalation in subjects with dual asthmatic response. *Clin. Invest. Med.* **8**, A44.

Cockcroft, D.W. and Murdock, K.Y. (1987). Comparative effects of inhaled salbutamol, sodium cromoglycate and beclomethasone dipropionate on allergen-induced early asthmatic responses, late asthmatic responses and increased bronchial responsiveness. *J. Allergy and Clin. Immunol.* **79**, 734–40.

Cockcroft, D.W., Killian, D.N., Mellon, J.J.A. and Hargreave, F.E. (1977). Bronchial reactivity to inhaled histamine: a method and clinical survey. *Clin. Allergy* **7**, 235–43.

Connolly, C.K., Chan, N.S. and Prescott, R.J. (1988). The relationship between age and duration of asthma and the presence of persistent obstruction in asthma. *Postgrad. Med. J.* **64**, 422–5.

Connolly, M.J., Avery, A.J., Walters, E.H. and Hendrick, D.J. (1988). The relationship between bronchial responsiveness to methacholine and bronchial responsiveness to histamine in asthmatic subjects. *Pulmonary Pharmacol.* **1**, 53–8.

Conrad, D.H. (1988). The receptor for immunoglobulin E. In *Mast Cells, Mediators and Disease*, ed. S.T. Holgate, pp. 99–127, Kluwer Academic, Dordrecht.

Cookson, W.O.C.M. (1987). Bronchodilator action of the antihistaminic terfenadine. *Br. J. Clin. Pharmacol.* **24**, 120–1.

Copas, J.L., Borgeat, P. and Gardiner, P.J. (1982). The actions of 5-, 12- and 15-HETE on tracheobronchial smooth muscle. *Prostaglandins Med.* **8**, 105–14.

Corrigan, C.J. and Kay, A.B. (1988). T lymphocyte activation in acute severe asthma is accompanied by a rise in serum concentrations of interferon and the soluble interleukin-2 receptor. *Thorax* **43**, 814P.

Corrigan, C.J., Hartnell, A. and Kay, A.B. (1988). T lymphocyte activation in acute severe asthma. *Lancet* **i**, 1129–32.

Craig, S.S., Schechter, N.M. and Schwartz, L.B. (1988). Ultrastructural analysis of human T and TC mast cells identified by immunoelectron microscopy. *Lab. Invest.* **58**, 682–91.

Curzen, N., Rafferty, P. and Holgate, S.T. (1987). Effects of a cyclooxygenase inhibitor, flurbiprofen, and an H_1 histamine receptor antagonist, terfenadine, alone and in combination on allergen induced immediate bronchoconstriction in man. *Thorax* **42**, 946–52.

Cushley, M.J., Tattersfield, A.E. and Holgate, S.T. (1984). Adenosine induced bronchoconstriction in asthma: antagonism by inhaled theophylline *Am. Rev. Respir. Dis.* **129**, 380–4.

Cuss, F.M., Dixon, C.M.S. and Barnes, P.J. (1986). Effects of inhaled platelet-activating factor on pulmonary function and bronchial responsiveness in man. *Lancet* **ii**, 189–92.

Cutz, E., Levison, H. and Cooper, D.M. (1978). Ultrastructure of airways in children with asthma. *Histopathology* **2**, 407–21.

Dahl, R., Venge, P. and Fredens, K. (1988). Eosinophils. In *Asthma: Basic Mechanisms and Clinical Management*, ed. P.J. Barnes, I.W. Rodger and N.C. Thompson; pp. 115–29. Academic Press, London.

Dahlén, S.-E. (1988). Leukotrienes and related lipoxygenase products. In *Asthma: Basic Mechanisms and Clinical Management*, ed. P.J. Barnes, I.W. Rodger and N.C. Thompson, pp. 213–30, Academic Press, London.

Dahlén, S.-E., Hansson, G., Hedqvist, P., Bjork, T., Granstrom, E. and Dahlén, B. (1983). Allergen challenge of lung tissue from asthmatics elicits bronchial contraction that correlates with the release of leukotrienes C_4, D_4 and E_4. *Proc. Nat. Acad. Sci. (USA)* **80**, 1712–18.

Dahlén, S.-E., Kumlin, A., Bjorck, T., Raud, J. and Hedqvist, P. (1987a). Leukotrienes and related eicosanoids. *Am. Rev. Respir. Dis.* **136**, S24–S28.

Dahlén, S.-E., Raud, J., Serhan, C.N., Bjork, J. and Samuelsson, B. (1987b). Biological activities of lipoxin A include lung strip contraction and dilation of arterioles *in vivo*. *Acta Physiol. Scand.* **130**, 643–8.

Dale, H.H. and Laidlaw, P.P. (1911). The physiologic action of β-imidazolylethylamine. *J. Physiol.* **41**, 318–44.

Davidson, A.E., Lee, T.H., Scanlon, P.D. *et al.* (1987). Bronchoconstrictor effects of leukotriene E_4 in normal and asthmatic subjects. *Am. Rev. Respir. Dis.* **135**, 333–7.

Davis, B., Roberts, A.M., Coleridge, H.M. and Coleridge, J.C.G. (1982). Reflex tracheal gland secretion evoked by stimulation of bronchial C-fibres in dogs. *J. Appl. Physiol.* **53**, 985–91.

de Monchy, J.G.R., Kauffman, H.F., Venge, P. *et al.* (1985). Bronchoalveolar eosinophilia during allergen-induced late asthmatic reactions. *Am. Rev. Respir. Dis.* **131**, 373–6.

de Monchy, J.G., Keyzer, J.J. and Kauffman, H.F. (1986). Histamine in late asthmatic reactions following house dust mite inhalation. *Agents Actions* **16**, 252–5.

Diaz, P., Galleguillos, F.R., Gonzalez, M.C., Pantin, C.F.A. and Kay, A.B. (1984). Bronchoalveolar lavage in asthma: the effect of disodium cromoglycate (cromolyn) on leukocyte counts, immunoglobulins and complement. *J. Allergy Clin. Immunol.* **74**, 41–8.

Diaz, P., Gonzalez, M.C., Galleguillos, F.R., Ancic, P. and Kay, A.B. (1986). Eosinophils and macrophages in bronchial mucus and bronchoalveolar lavage during allergen-induced late-phase reactions. *J. Allergy Clin. Immunol.* **77**, 244 (abstract).

Dinarello, C.A. and Mier, J.W. (1987). Lymphokines. *N. Engl. J. Med.* **317**, 940–5.

Drazen, J.M. and Austen, K.F. (1987). Leukotrienes and airway responses. *Am. Rev. Respir. Dis.* **136**, 985–98.

Dunnill, M.S. (1960). The pathology of asthma with special reference to changes in the bronchial mucosa. *J. Clin. Pathol.* **13**, 27–33.

Durham, S.R. and Kay, A.B. (1985). Eosinophils, bronchial hyperreactivity and late-phase asthmatic reactions. *Clin. Allergy* **15**, 411–18.

Durham, S.R., Carroll, M., Walsh, G.M. and Kay, A.B. (1984). Leukocyte activation in allergen-induced late phase reactions. *N. Engl. J. Med.* **311**, 1398–402.

Dworski, R., Fitzgerald, G.A., Roberts, L.J., Oates, J.A., Schwartz, L.B. and Sheller, J.R. (1988). Eicosanoid formation in atopic human lung: effect of indomethacin. *Am. Rev. Respir. Dis.* **137**, 375a.

Eggleston, P.A., Kagey-Sobotka, A. and Lichtenstein, L.M. (1987). A comparison of the osmotic activation of basophils and human lung mast cells. *Am. Rev. Respir. Dis.* **135**, 1043–8.

Evans, T.W., Chung, K.F., Rogers, D.F. and Barnes, P.J. (1987). Effect of platelet-activating factor on airway vascular permeability: possible mechanisms. *J. Appl. Physiol.* **63**, 479–84.

Fabbri, L.M., Boschetto, P., Zocca, E. *et al.* (1987). Bronchoalveolar neutrophilia during late asthmatic reactions induced by toluene diisocyanate. *Am. Rev. Respir. Dis.* **136**, 36–42.

Flavahan, N.A., Slifman, N.R., Gleich, G.J. and Vanhoutte, P.M. (1988). Human eosinophil major basic protein causes hyperreactivity of respiratory smooth muscle. *Am. Rev. Respir. Dis.* **138**, 685–8.

Flint, K.C., Leung, K.B.P., Hudspith, B.N., Brostoff, J., Pearce, F.L. and Johnson, N.McI. (1985a). Bronchoalveolar mast cells in extrinsic asthma: a mechanism for the initiation of antigen specific bronchoconstriction. *Br. Med. J.* **291**, 923–6.

Flint, K.C., Leung, K.B.P., Pearce, F.L., Hudspith, B.N., Brostoff, J. and Johnson, N.McI. (1985b). Human mast cells recovered by bronchoalveolar lavage: their morphology, histamine release and effects of sodium cromoglycate. *Clin. Sci.* **68**, 427–32.

Ford-Hutchinson, A.W. (1988). The neutrophil and lymphocytes. In *Asthma: Basic Mechanisms and Clinical Management*, ed. P.J. Barnes, I.W. Rodger and N.C. Thompson, pp. 131–42, Academic Press, London.

Ford-Hutchinson, A.W., Bray, M.A., Doig, M.V., Shipley, M.E. and Smith, M.J.H. (1980). Leukotriene B, a potent chemokinetic and aggregating substance released from polymorphonuclear leukocytes. *Nature* **286**, 264–5.

Fowler, II, J.W. and Louvel, F.C. (1966). The accumulation of eosinophils as an allergic response to allergen applied to the denuded skin surface. *J. Allergy Clin. Immunol.* **37**, 19–28.

Freeland, H.S., Schleimer, R.P., Schulman, E.S., Lichtenstein, L.M. and Peters, S.P. (1988). Generation of leukotriene B_4 by human lung fragments and purified human lung mast cells. *Am. Rev. Respir. Dis.* **138**, 389–94.

Frew, A.J. and Kay, A.B. (1988). Relation between T lymphocytes, activated eosinophils and human late phase skin reactions. *Thorax* **43**, 810P.

Fujimura, M., Sasaki, F., Nakatsumi, Y. *et al.* (1986). Effects of a thromboxane synthetase inhibitor (OKY-046) and a lipoxygenase inhibitor (AA-861) on bronchial responsiveness to acetylcholine in asthmatic subjects. *Thorax* **41**, 955–9.

Fuller, R.W. and Barnes, P.J. (1988). Kinins. In *Asthma: Basic Mechanisms and Clinical Management*, ed. P.J. Barnes, I.W. Rodger and N.C. Thompson, pp. 259–72, Academic Press, London.

Fuller, R.W., Morris, P.K., Richmond, R. *et al.* (1986). Immunoglobulin E-dependent stimulation of human alveolar macrophages: significance in type I hypersensitivity. *Clin. Exp. Immunol.* **65**, 416–26.

Fuller, R.W., Dixon, C.M.S., Cuss, F.M.C. and Barnes, P.J. (1987). Bradykinin-induce bronchoconstriction in humans. *Am. Rev. Respir. Dis.* **135**, 176–80.

Gerblich, A.A., Campbell, A. and Schuyler, M. (1984). Changes in T lymphocyte subpopulations after antigenic bronchial provocation in asthmatics. *N. Engl. J. Med.* **310**, 1349–52.

Gin, W. and Kay, A.B. (1985). Effect of corticosteroids on

monocyte and neutrophil activation in bronchial asthma. *J. Allergy Clin. Immunol.* **76**, 675–82.

Gin, W., Shaw, R.J. and Kay, A.B. (1985). Airways reversibility following prednisolone therapy in chronic asthma in associated with changes in leukocyte function. *Am. Rev. Respir. Dis.* **132**, 1199–203.

Gleich, G.J., Frigas, E., Loegering, D.A., Wassom, D.L. and Steinmuller, D. (1979). Cytotoxic properties of the eosinophil major basic protein. *J. Immunol.* **123**, 2925–7.

Glynn, A.A. and Michaels, L. (1960). Bronchial biopsy in chronic bronchitis and asthma. *Thorax* **15**, 142–53.

Godard, P., Chaintreuil, J., Damon, M. *et al.* (1982). Functional assessment of alveolar macrophages: comparison of cells from asthmatics and normal subjects. *J. Allergy Clin. Immunol.* **70**, 88–95.

Goetzl, E.J., Phillips, M.J. and Gold, W.M. (1983). Stimulus specificity of the generation of leukotrienes by dog mastocytoma cells. *J. Exp. Med.* **158**, 731–7.

Gonzalez, C., Diaz, P., Galleguillos, F., Ancic, P., Cromwell, O. and Kay, A.B. (1987). Allergen-induced recruitment of bronchoalveolar helper (OKT4) and suppressor (OKT8) cells in asthma: relative increases in OKT8 cells in single early responders compared with those in late-phase responders. *Am. Rev. Respir. Dis.* **136**, 600–4.

Gosset, P., Tonnel, A.B., Joseph, M. *et al.* (1984). Secretion of a chemotactic factor for neutrophils and eosinophils by alveolar macrophages from asthmatic patients. *J. Allergy Clin. Immunol.* **74**, 827–34.

Greenberg, R., Osman, G.H., O'Keefe, E.H. and Antonaccio, M.J. (1979). The effects of captopril (SQ 14,225) on bradykinin-induced bronchoconstriction in the anaesthetised guinea-pig. *Eur. J. Pharmacol.* **57**, 287–94.

Hamberg, M., Hedqvist, P. and Radegran, K. (1980). Identification of 15-hydroxy-5,8,11,13-eicosatetraenoic acid (15-HETE) as the major metabolite of arachidonic acid in the lung. *Acta Physiol. Scand.* **110**, 219–21.

Hansson, A., Serhan, C.N., Haeggström, J., Ingelman-Sundberg, M. and Samuelsson, B. (1986). Activation of protein kinase C lipoxin and other eicosandoids. *Biochem. Biophys. Res. Commun.* **134**, 1215–22.

Hardy, C.C., Robinson, C., Tattersfield, A.E. and Holgate, S.T. (1984). The bronchoconstrictor effect of inhaled prostaglandin D_2 in normal and asthmatic men. *N. Engl. J. Med.* **311**, 209–213.

Hardy, C.C., Bradding, P., Robinson, C. and Holgate, S.T. (1986a). The combined effect of two pairs of mediators, adenosine with methacholine and prostaglandin D_2 with histamine, on airway calibre in asthma. *Clin. Sci.* **71**, 385–92.

Hardy, C.C., Holgate, S.T. and Robinson, C. (1986b). Evidence against the formation of 13,14-dihydro-15-keto-prostaglandin $F_{2\alpha}$ following inhalation of prostaglandin D_2 in man. *Br. J. Pharmacol.* **87**, 563–8.

Hargreave, F.E., Ryan, G., Thomson, N.C. *et al.* (1981). Bronchial responsiveness to histamine or methacholine in asthma: measurement and clinical significance. *J. Allergy Clin. Immunol.* **68**, 347–55.

Harriman, G.R. and Strober, W. (1989). The immunobiology of interleukin-5. In *The Year in Immunology 1988: Immunoregulatory Cytokines and Cell Growth*, ed. J.M. Cruse and R.E. Lewis, Jr, pp. 160–77, Karger, Basel.

Henderson, W.R. (1987). Eicosanoids and lung inflammation. *Am. Rev. Respir. Dis.* **135**, 1176–85.

Henderson, W.R., Jorg, A. and Klebenoff, S.J. (1982). Eosinophil peroxidase-mediated inactivation of leukotrienes B_4, C_4 and D_4. *J. Immunol.* **128**, 2609–13.

Holgate, S.T., Burns, G.B., Robinson, C. and Church, M.K. (1984). Anaphylactic- and calcium-dependent generation of prostaglandin D_2 (PGD_2), thromboxane B_2, and other cyclo-oxygenase products of arachidonic acid by dispersed human lung cells and relationship to histamine release. *J. Immunol.* **133**, 2138–44.

Holgate, S.T., Emanuel, M.B. and Howarth, P.H. (1985). Astemizole and other H_1-antihistaminic drug treatment of asthma. *J. Allergy Clin. Immunol.* **76**, 375–80.

Holgate, S.T., Hardy, C., Robinson, C., Agius, R.M. and Howarth, P.H. (1986). The mast cell as a primary effector cell in the pathogenesis of asthma. *J. Allergy Clin. Immunol.* **77**, 275–82.

Holgate, S.T., Twentyman, O.P., Rafferty, P. *et al.* (1987a). Primary and secondary effector cells in the pathogenesis of bronchial asthma. *Int. Arch. Allergy Appl. Immunol.* **82**, 498–506.

Holgate, S.T., Mann, J.S., Church, M.K. and Cushley, M.J. (1987b). Mechanisms and significance of adenosine-induced bronchoconstriction in asthma. *Allergy* **42**, 727–30.

Horn, B.R., Robin, E.D., Theodore, J. and Van Kessel, A. (1975). Total eosinophil counts in the management of bronchial asthma. *N. Engl. J. Med.* **292**, 1152–5.

Howarth, P.H. and Holgate, S.T. (1985). Astemizole, an H_1 antagonist in allergic asthma. *J. Allergy Clin. Immunol.* **75**, 166.

Howarth, P.H., Durham, S.R., Lee, T.H., Kay, A.B., Church, M.K. and Holgate, S.T. (1985). Influence of albuterol, cromolyn sodium and ipratropium bromide on the airway and circulating mediator responses to allergen bronchial challenge in asthma. *Am. Rev. Respir. Dis.* **132**, 986–92.

Howarth, P.H., Durham, S.R., Kay, A.B. and Holgate, S.T. (1987). The relationship between mediator release and bronchial reactivity in allergic asthma. *J. Allergy Clin. Immunol.* **80**, 703–11.

Hunter, J.A., Finkbeiner, W.E., Nadel, J.A., Goetzl, E.J. and Holtzman, M.J. (1985). Predominant generation of 15-lipoxygenase metabolites of arachidonic acid by epithelial cells from human trachea. *Proc. Nat. Acad. Sci. (USA)* **82**, 4633–7.

Hutson, P.A., Church, M.K., Clay, T.P., Miller, P. and Holgate, S.T. (1988a). Early and late phase bronchoconstriction after allergen challenge of nonanaesthetised guinea-pigs. *Am. Rev. Respir. Med.* **137**, 548–57.

Hutson, P.A., Holgate, S.T. and Church, M.K. (1988b). The effect of cromolyn sodium and albuterol on early and late phase bronchoconstriction and airway leukocyte infiltration after allergen challenge of nonanaesthetised guinea-pigs. *Am. Rev. Respir. Med.* **138**, 1157–63.

Hutson, P.A., Holgate, S.T. and Church, M.K. (1988c). Inhibition by nedocromil sodium of early and late phase bronchoconstriction and airway cellular infiltration provoked by ovalbumin inhalation in conscious guinea-pigs. *Br. J. Pharmacol.* **94**, 6–8.

Irvin, C.G., Baltopoulos, G., Honour, J., Seccombe, J.F. and Henson, P.M. (1986). Lipid mediators released by activated human neutrophils which increase airways reactivity. *Am. Rev. Respir. Dis.* **133**, A175 (abstract).

Ishizaka, T., White, J.R. and Saito, H. (1987). Activation of basophils and mast cells for mediator release. *Int. Arch. Allergy Appl. Immunol.* **82**, 327–32.

Jenkins, J.R., Lai, C.K.W. and Holgate, S.T. (1989). Effect of increasing doses of platelet activating factor on normal human airways. *J. Allergy Clin. Immunol.* **83**, 282.

Johnson, H.G., McNee, M.L. and Sun, F.F. (1985). 15-Hydroxyeicosatetraenoic acid is a potent inflammatory mediator and agonist of canine tracheal mucus secretion. *Am. Rev. Respir. Dis.* **131**, 917–22.

Jones, T.R., Young, R., Champion, E. *et al.* (1986). L-649,923, sodium (βS*, gamma R*)-4-(3-(4-acetyl-3-hydroxy-2-propylphenoxy)-propylthio)-gamma-hydroxy-beta-methylbenzene butanoate, a selective, orally active leukotriene receptor antagonist. *Can. J. Physiol. Pharmacol.* **64**, 1068–75.

Joos, G. (1989). The role of sensory neuropeptides in the pathogenesis of bronchial asthma. *Clin. Allergy* **19** (Suppl. 1), 9–13.

Joos, G., Kips, J., Pauwels, R. and Van Der Straeten, M. (1986). The effect of tachykinins on the conducting airways of the rat. *Arch. Int. Pharmacodynamics* **180** (suppl.), 176–90.

Joos, G., Pauwels, R. and Van Der Straeten, M. (1987). The effect of inhaled substance P and neurokinin A on the airways of normal and asthmatic subjects. *Thorax* **42**, 779–83.

Joos, G., Pauwels, R. and Van Der Straeten, M. (1988a). The effect of nedocromil sodium on the bronchoconstrictor effect on neurokinin A in asthmatics. *J. Allergy Clin. Immunol.* **81**, A433.

Joos, G., Pauwels, R. and Van Der Straeten, M. (1988b). The effect of oxitropium bromide on neurokinin A-induced bronchoconstriction in asthmatic subjects. *Pulmonary Pharmacol.* **1**, 41–5.

Joseph, M., Tonnel, A.B., Torpier, G., Capron, A., Arnoux, B. and Benveniste, J. (1983). Involvement of IgE in the secretory processes of alveolar macrophages from asthmatic patients. *J. Clin. Invest.* **71**, 221–30.

Joseph, M., Capron, A., Ameisen, J.C. *et al.* (1987). The receptor for IgE on blood platelets. *Eur. J. Immunol.* **16**, 306–12.

Josephs, L.K., Gregg, I., Bain, D.J.G. and Holgate, S.T. (1987). A longitudinal study of non-specific bronchial responsiveness in asthma. *Thorax* **42**, 711 (abstract).

Juniper, E.F., Frith, P.A. and Hargreave, F.E. (1981). Airway hyper-responsiveness to histamine and methacholine: relationship to minimum treatment to control symptoms of asthma. *Thorax* **38**, 575–9.

Kaliner, M. (1989). Asthma and mast cell activation. *J. Allergy Clin. Immunol.* **83**, 510–20.

Kaufman, M.P., Coleridge, H.M., Coleridge, J.C.G. and Baker, D.G. (1980). Bradykinin stimulates afferent vagal C-fibres in intrapulmonary airways of dogs. *J. Appl. Physiol.* **48**, 511–17.

Kay, A.B. (1988). Inflammatory cells in allergic disease. In *Mast Cells, Mediators and Disease*, ed. S.T. Holgate, pp. 227–39, Kluwer Academic, London.

Kay, A.B., Walsh, G.M., Moqbel, R. *et al.* (1987). Disodium cromoglycate inhibits activation of human inflammatory cells *in vitro*. *J. Allergy Clin. Immunol.* **80**, 1–8.

Kelly, C., Ward, C., Stenton, C.S., Bird, G., Hendrick, D.J. and Walters, E.H. (1988). Number and activity of inflammatory cells in bronchoalveolar lavage fluid in asthma and their relation to airway hyper-responsiveness. *Thorax* **43**, 684–92.

Khalife, J., Capron, M., Cesbron, J.Y. *et al.* (1986). Role of specific IgE antibodies in peroxidase (EPO) release from human eosinophils. *J. Immunol.* **137**, 1659–64.

Kirby, J.G., Hargreave, F.E., Gliech, G.J. and O'Byrne, P.M. (1987). Bronchoalveolar cell profiles of asthmatic and nonasthmatic subjects. *Am. Rev. Respir. Dis.* **136**, 379–83.

Kloprogge, E. and Akkerman, J.W.N. (1984). Binding kinetics of PAF-acether (1-*O*-alkyl-2-acetyl-*sn*-glycero-3-phosphorylcholine) to intact human platelets. *Biochem. J.* **223**, 901–9.

Knauer, K.A., Lichtenstein, L.M., Franklin Adkinson, Jr, N. and Fish, J.E. (1981). Platelet activation during antigen-induced airway reactions in asthmatic subjects. *N. Engl. J. Med.* **304**, 1404–7.

Krell, R.D., Giles, R.E., Yee, Y.K. and Snyder, D.W. (1987). *In vivo* pharmacology of ICI 198,615: a novel, potent and selective leukotriene antagonist. *J. Pharmacol. Exp. Ther.* **243**, 557–64.

Lai, C.K.W. and Holgate, S.T. (1988). The mast cell and asthma. In *Clinical Immunology and Allergy: the Allergic Basis of Asthma*, ed. A.B. Kay, vol. II, no. 1, pp. 37–66, Baillière, Tindall, London.

Lai, C.K.W., Phillips, G.D., Jenkins, J.R. and Holgate, S.T. (1989). The effect of inhaled 15-(s)-hydroxyeicostatetraenoic acid on normal airways. *Am. Rev. Respir. Dis.* **139**, A499.

Laitinen, L.A., Heino, M., Laitinen, A., Kava, T. and Haahtela, T. (1985). Damage of the airway epithelium and bronchial reactivity in patients with asthma. *Am. Rev. Respir. Dis.* **131**, 599–606.

Lam, S., LeRiche, J., Phillips, D. and Chan-Yeung, M. (1987). Cellular and protein changes in bronchial lavage fluid after late asthmatic reactions in patients with red cedar asthma. *J. Allergy Clin. Immunol.* **80**, 44–50.

Lee, T.C., Lenihan, D.J., Malone, B., Ruddy, L.L. and Wasserman, S.I. (1984). Increased biosynthesis of platelet activating factor in activated human eosinophils. *J. Biol. Chem.* **259**, 5526–30.

Lee, T.H., Nagy, L., Nagakura, T., Walport, M.J. and Kay, A.B. (1982). Identification and partial characterisation of an exercise-induced neutrophil chemotactic factor in bronchial asthma. *J. Clin. Invest.* **69**, 889–99.

Lee, T.H., Nagakura, T., Papageogiou, N., Cromwell, O., Ikura, Y. and Kay, A.B. (1984). Mediators in exercise-induced asthma. *J. Allergy Clin. Immunol.* **73**, 634–9.

Lellouch-Tubiana, A., Lefort, J., Pirotzky, E., Vargaftig, B.B. and Pfister, A. (1985). Ultrastructural evidence for extravascular platelet recruitment in the lung upon intravenous injection of platelet-activating factor (paf-acether) to guinea-pigs. *Br. J. Exp. Pathol.* **66**, 345–55.

Leung, D.Y.M. and Geha, R.S. (1987). Regulation of the human IgE antibody response. *Int. Rev. Immunol.* **2**, 75–91.

Lewis, R.A. and Austen, K.F. (1981). Mediators of local homeostatic and inflammation of leukotrienes and the other mast cell-dependant compounds. *Nature* **293**, 103–8.

Lewis, R.A., Goetzl, E.J., Drazen, J.M., Soter, N.A., Austen, K.F. and Corey, E.J. (1981). Functional characterization of synthetic leukotriene B_4 and its stereochemical isomers. *J. Exp. Med.* **154**, 1243–8.

Lopez-Vidriero, M. and Reid, L. (1983). Pathological changes in asthma. In *Asthma*, ed. T.J.H. Clark and S. Godfrey, pp. 73–98, Chapman and Hall, London.

Löwhagen, O. and Rak, S. (1985). Modification of bronchial hyperreactivity after treatment with sodium cromoglycate during pollen season. *J. Allergy Clin. Immunol.* **75**, 460–7.

MacDonald, S.M., Lichtenstein, L.M., Proud, D. *et al.* (1987). Studies of IgE-dependent histamine releasing factors: heterogeneity of IgE. *J. Immunol.* **139**, 506–12.

McFadden, E.R. Jr and Ingram, R.H. Jr (1979). Exercise-induced asthma. *N. Engl. J. Med.* **301**, 763–9.

McGlashan, D.W. Jr, Schleimer, R.P., Peters, S.P. *et al.* (1982). Generation of leukotrienes by purified human lung mast cells. *J. Clin. Invest.* **70**, 747–51.

Maestrelli, P., Tsai, J.J. and Kay, A.B. (1987). Human lymphocyte derived neutrophil chemotactic activities. *J. Allergy Clin. Immunol.* **79**, 160.

Mann, J.S., Robinson, C., Sheridan, A.Q., Clement, P., Bach, M.K. and Holgate, S.T. (1986). Effect of inhaled piriprost (U-60,257) a novel leukotriene inhibitor, on allergen and exercise induced bronchoconstriction in asthma. *Thorax* **41**, 746–52.

Marchesi, V.T. (1985). Inflammation and healing. In *Anderson's Pathology*, ed. J.M. Kissure and W.A.D. Anderson, pp. 22–60, C.V. Mosby, St. Louis.

Marom, Z., Shelhamer, J.H. and Kailner, M. (1981). The effects of arachidonic acid, monohydroxyeicosatetraenoic acid, and prostaglandins on the release of mucous glycoproteins from human airways *in vitro*. *J. Clin. Invest.* **67**, 1695–703.

Mazzoni, L., Morley, J., Page, C.P. and Sanjar, S. (1985). Induction of airway hyperreactivity by platelet activating factor in the guinea-pig. *J. Physiol.* **365**, 107.

Melewicz, F.M., Zeiger, R.S., Mellon, M.N., O'Connor, R.D. and Spiegelberg, H.L. (1981). Increased IgE-dependent cytotoxicity by blood mononuclear cells of allergic patients. *Clin. Exp. Immunol.* **49**, 364–70.

Metzger, W.J., Hunninghake, G.W. and Richerson, H.B. (1985). Late asthmatic responses: inquiry into mechanisms and significance. *Clin. Rev. Allergy* **3**, 145–65.

Metzger, W.J., Richerson, H.B., Warden, K., Monick, M. and Hunninghake, G.W. (1986). Bronchoalveolar lavage of allergic asthmatic patients following allergen provocation. *Chest* **89**, 477–83.

Metzger, W.J., Zavala, D., Richerson, H.B. *et al.* (1987). Local allergen challenge and bronchoalveolar lavage of allergic asthmatic lungs: description of the model and local airway inflammation. *Am. Rev. Respir. Dis.* **135**, 433–40.

Mita, H., Yui, Y., Taniguchi, N., Yasyeda, H. and Shida, T. (1985). Increased activity of 5-lipoxygenase in polymorphonuclear leukocytes in asthmatic patients. *Life Sci.* **37**, 907–14.

Moqbel, R., Walsh, G.M., Macdonald, A.J. and Kay, A.B. (1986a). Effect of disodium cromoglycate on activation of human eosinophils and human neutrophils following reversed (anti-IgE) anaphylaxis. *Clin. Allergy* **16**, 73–84.

Moqbel, R., Durham, S.R, Shaw, R.J., Walsh, G.M., Macdonald, A.J., Mackay, J.A., Carroll, M.P. and Kay, A.B. (1986b). Enhancement of leukocyte cytotoxicity after exercise-induced asthma. *Am. Rev. Respir. Dis.* **133**, 609–13.

Moqbel, R., Cromwell, O., Walsh, G.M., Wardlaw, A.J., Kurlak, L. and Kay, A.B. (1988). Effects of nedocromil sodium (Tilade®) on the activation of human eosinophils and neutrophils and the release of histamine from mast cells. *Allergy* **43**, 268–76.

Morley, J., Sanjar, S. and Page, C.P. (1984). The platelet in asthma. *Lancet* **ii**, 1142–4.

Mortagy, A.K., Howell, J.B.L. and Waters, W.E. (1986). Respiratory symptoms and bronchial reactivity: identification of a syndrome and its relation to asthma. *Br. Med. J.* **293**, 525–9.

Murray, J.J., Tonnel, A.B., Brash, A.R. *et al.* (1986). Release of prostaglandin D_2 into human airways during acute antigen challenge. *N. Engl. J. Med.* **315**, 800–4.

Nadel, J.A. and Borson, D.B. (1988). Modulation of tachykinins and bradykinin by enkephalinase. In *Mechanisms in Asthma: Pharmacology, Physiology, and Management*, ed. C.L. Armour and J.L. Black, pp. 123–30, Alan R. Liss, New York.

Nagy, L., Lee, T.H. and Kay, A.B. (1982). Neutrophil chemotactic activity in antigen-induced late asthmatic reactions. *N. Engl. J. Med.* **306**, 497–501.

Newball, H.H., Berninger, R.W., Talamo, R.C. and Lichtenstein, L.M. (1979). Anaphylactic release of a basophil kallidrein-like activity. I. Purification and characterisation. *J. Clin. Invest* **64**, 457–65.

O'Byrne, P.M. and Jones, G.L. (1986). The effect of indomethacin on exercise-induced bronchoconstriction and refractoriness after exercise. *Am. Rev. Respir. Dis.* **134**, 69–72.

O'Hickey, S.P., Belcher, N., Rees, P.J. and Lee, T.H. (1988). Effect of terfenadine on the bronchoconstrictor response to hypertonic saline and exercise in asthmatic subjects. *Thorax* **43**, 865P (abstract).

O'Neil, C.E. and Salvaggio, J.E. (1988). The pathogenesis of occupational asthma. In *The Allergic Basis of Asthma Series: Clinical Immunology and Allergy — International Practice and Research*, ed. A.B. Kay, pp. 143–75, Baillière, Tindall, London.

Page, C.P. (1988). The role of platelet-activating factor in asthma. *J. Allergy Clin. Immunol.* **81**, 144–52.

Payne, A.N., Garland, L.G., Lees, I.W. and Salmon, J.A. (1988). Selective inhibition of arachidonate 5-lipoxygenase by novel acetohydroxamic acids: effects on bronchial anaphylaxis in anaesthetized guinea-pigs. *Br. J. Pharmacol.* **94**, 540–6.

Pearce, F.L. (1988). Mast cell heterogeneity. In *Mast Cells, Mediators and Disease*, ed. S.T. Holgate, pp. 175–93, Kluwer Academic, Dordrecht.

Pearce, F.L., Flint, K.C., Leung, K.B.P. *et al.* (1987). Some studies on human pulmonary mast cells obtained by bronchoalveolar lavage and by enzymic dissociation of whole lung tissue. *Int. Arch. Allergy Appl. Immunol.* **82**, 507–12.

Phillips, G.D. and Holgate, S.T. (1989). The interaction of inhaled leukotriene C_4 with histamine and prostaglandin D_2 on airway calibre in asthma. *J. Appl. Physiol.* **66**, 304–12.

Phillips, G.D., Rafferty, P., Beasley, R. and Holgate, S.T. (1987). Effect of oral terfenadine on the bronchoconstrictor response to inhaled histamine and adenosine 5′-monophosphate. *Thorax* **42**, 939–45.

Phillips, G.D., Richards, R., Scott, V.L. and Holgate, S.T. (1988a). Sodium cromoglycate and nedocromil sodium inhibit bronchoconstriction provoked by adenosine 5′-monophosphate in atopic and non-atopic asthma. *Am. Rev. Respir. Dis.* **137**, 87 (abstract).

Phillips, G.D., Rafferty, P., Robinson, C. and Holgate, S.T. (1988b). Dose-related antagonism of leukotriene D_4-induced bronchoconstriction by p.o. administration of LY-171883 in nonasthmatic subjects. *J. Pharmacol. Exp. Ther.* **246**, 732–8.

Poulter, L.W., Burke, C., Gallagher, E. and Kidney, J. (1988). Does a cell mediated reaction contribute to asthma? *Thorax* **43**, 813P (abstract).

Poznansky, M.C., Gordon, A.C.H., Douglas, J.G., Krajewski, A.S., Wyllie, A.H. and Grant, I.W.B. (1984). Resistance to methylprednisolone in cultures of blood mononuclear cells from glucocorticoid-resistant asthmatic patients. *Clin. Sci.* **67**, 639–45.

Poznansky, M.C., Gordon, A.C.H., Grant, I.W.B. and Wyllie, A.H. (1985). A cellular abnormality in glucocorticoid resistant asthma. *Clin. Exp. Immunol.* **61**, 135–42.

Proud, D., Togias, A., Naclerio, R.M., Crush, S.A., Norman, P.S. and Lichtenstein, L.M. (1983). Kinins are generated *in vivo* following nasal airway challenge of allergic individuals with allergen. *J. Clin. Invest.* **72**, 1678–85.

Proud, D., Maglashan, D.W., Newball, H.H., Schulmans, A. and Lichtenstein, L.M. (1985). Immunoglobulin E-mediated release of a kininogenase from purified human lung mast cells. *Am. Rev. Respir. Dis.* **132**, 405–6.

Rafferty, P. and Holgate, S.T. (1987). Terfenadine (Seldane®) is a potent and selective histamine H_1 receptor antagonist in asthmatic airways. *Am. Rev. Respir. Dis.* **135**, 181–4.

Rafferty, P., Beasley, R. and Holgate, S.T. (1987). The contribution of histamine to immediate bronchoconstriction provoked by inhaled allergen and adenosine 5′ monophosphate in atopic asthma. *Am. Rev. Respir. Dis.* **136**, 369–73.

Raghavachar, A., Fleischer, S., Frickhofen, N., Heimpel, H. and Fleischer, B. (1987). T lymphocyte control of human eosinophilic granulopoiesis: clonal analysis of an idiopathic hypereosinophilic syndrome. *J. Immunol.* **139**, 3753–8.

Regoli, D. and Barabe, J. (1980). Pharmacology of bradykinin and related peptides. *Pharmacol. Rev.* **32**, 1–46.

Reilly, C.F., Tewksbury, D.A., Schechter, N.M. and Travis, J. (1982). Rapid conversion of angiotensin I to angiotensin II by neutrophil and mast cell proteinases. *J. Biol. Chem.* **257**, 8619–22.

Roberts, A.M., Schultz, H.D., Green, J.F. *et al.* (1985). Reflex tracheal contraction evoked in dogs by bronchodilator prostaglandins E_2 and Iy_2. *J. Appl. Physiol.* **58**, 1823–41.

Roberts, N.M., Page, C.P., Chung, K.F., Barnes, P.J. (1988a). Effect of a PAF antagonist, BN52063, on antigen-induced acute and late-onset cutaneous response in atopic subjects. *J. Allergy Clin. Immunol.* **82**, 236–41.

Roberts, N.M., McCusker, M., Chung, K.F. and Barnes, P.J. (1988b). Effects of a PAF antagonist, BN52063, on PAF-induced bronchoconstriction in normal subjects. *Br. J. Clin. Pharmacol.* **26**, 65–72.

Robertson, D.G., Kerigan, A.T., Hargreave, F.E., Chalmers, R. and Dolovich, J. (1974). Late asthmatic responses induced by ragweed pollen allergen. *J. Allergy Clin. Immunol.* **54**, 244–54.

Robertson, D.N., Coyle, A.J., Rhoden, K.J., Grandordy, B., Page, C.P. and Barnes, P.J. (1988). The effect of platelet-activating factor on histamine and muscarinic receptor function in guinea-pig airways. *Am. Rev. Respir. Dis.* **137**, 1317–22.

Robinson, C. and Holgate, S.T. (1986a). Prostaglandins in the lung. In *Asthma: Clinical Pharmacology and Therapeutic Progress*, ed. A.B. Kay, pp. 213–25, Blackwell Scientific Publications, Oxford.

Robinson, C. and Holgate, S.T. (1986b). Ionophore-dependent generation of eicosanoids in human dispersed lung cells. Modulation by 6,9-deepoxy-6,9-(phenylimino)-$\Delta^{6,8}$-prostaglandin I_1 (U-60,257). *Biochem. Pharmacol.* **35**, 1903–8.

Rubin, A.E., Smith, L.J. and Patterson, R. (1987). The bronchoconstricting properties of platelet-activating factor in humans. *Am. Rev. Respir. Dis.* **136**, 1145–51.

Ryan, G., Latimer, K.M., Dolovitch, J. and Hargreave, F.E. (1982). Bronchial responsiveness to histamine: relationship to diurnal rhythm in peak flow rate, improvement after bronchodilator usage and airway calibre. *Thorax* **37**, 423–9.

Samuelsson, B. (1983). Leukotrienes: mediators of immediate hypersensitivity reactions and inflammation. *Nature* **220**, 568–75.

Schulman, E.S., Newball, H.H., Demers, L.M., Fitzpatrick, F.A. and Adkinson, N.F. (1981). Anaphylactic release of thromboxane A_2, prostaglandin D_2 and prostacycline from human lung parenchyma. *Am. Rev. Respir. Dis.* **124**, 402–6.

Schwartz, L.B. (1988). Preformed mediators of human mast cells and basophils. In *Mast Cells, Mediators and Disease*, ed. S.T. Holgate, pp. 129–47, Kluwer Academic, Dordrecht.

Schwartz, L.B. and Bradford, T.M. (1986). Regulation of tryptase from human lung mast cells by heparin: stabilization of the active tetramer. *J. Biol. Chem.* **261**, 7372–9.

Sekizawa, K., Tamaoki, J., Graf, P.D., Basbaum, C.B., Borson, D.B. and Nadel, J.A. (1987). Enkephalinase inhibitor potentiates mammalian tachykinin-induced contraction in ferret trachea. *J. Pharmacol. Exp. Ther.* **243**, 1211–17.

Seltzer, J., Bigby, B.G., Stulbarg, M. *et al.* (1986). Ozone-induced change in bronchial reactivity to methacholine and airway inflammation in human subjects. *J. Appl. Physiol.* **60**, 1321–6.

Serhan, C.N., Hamberg, M. and Samuelsson, B. (1984). Lipoxins: a novel series of compounds formed from arachidonic acid in human leukocytes. *Proc. Nat. Acad. Sci. (USA)* **81**, 5335–9.

Shaw, R.J., Cromwell, O. and Kay, A.B. (1984). Preferential generation of leukotriene C_4 by human eosinophils. *Clin. Exp. Immunol.* **56**, 716–22.

Shaw, R.J., Walsh, G.M., Cromwell, O., Moqbel, R., Spry, C.J.F. and Kay, A.B. (1985). Activated human eosinophils generate SRS-A leukotrienes following physiological (IgG-dependent) stimulation. *Nature* **316**, 150–2.

Shephard, E.G., Malan, L., Macfarlane, C.M., Mouton, W. and Joubert, J.R. (1985). Lung functional and plasma levels of thromboxane B_2, 6-ketoprostaglandin $F_{1\alpha}$ and β-thromboglobulin in antigen-induced asthma before and after indomethacin pretreatment. *Br. J. Clin. Pharmacol.* **19**, 459–70.

Silber, G., Proud, D., Warner, J. *et al.* (1988). *In vivo* release of inflammatory mediators by hyperosmolar solutions. *Am. Rev. Respir. Dis.* **137**, 606–12.

Skedinger, M.C., Augustine, N.H., Morris, E.Z., Nielson, D.W., Zimmerman, G.A. and Hill, H.R. (1987). Effect of disodium cromoglycate on neutrophil movement and intracellular calcium mobilization. *J. Allergy Clin. Immunol.* **80**, 573–7.

Slifman, N.R., Adolphson, C.R. and Gleich, G.R. (1988). Eosinophils: biochemical and cellular aspects. In *Allergy: Principles and Practice*, ed. E. Middleton, Jr, C.E. Reed, E.F. Ellis, N.F. Adkinson and J.W. Yunginger, pp. 179–205, C.V. Mosby, Washington.

Smith, A.P. and Cuthbert, M.F. (1972). Antagonist action of

aerosols of prostaglandins $F_{2\alpha}$ and E_2 on bronchial muscle tone in man. *Br. Med. J.* **3**, 212–13.

Snashall, P.D., Gillett, M.K. and Chung, K.F. (1988). Factors contributing to bronchial hyper-responsiveness in asthma. *Clin. Sci.* **74**, 113–18.

Svensson, J., Strandberg, K., Tuvemo, T. and Hamberg, M. (1977). Thromboxane A_2: effects on airway and vascular smooth muscle. *Prostaglandins* **14**, 425–36.

Taylor, K.J. and Luksza, A.R. (1987). Peripheral blood eosinophil counts and bronchial responsiveness. *Thorax* **42**, 452–6.

Taytard, A., Beaumont, D., Pujet, J.C., Sapene, M. and Lewis, P.J. (1987). Treatment of bronchial asthma with terfenadine; a randomised controlled trial. *Br. J. Clin. Pharmacol.* **24**, 743–6.

Thorpe, J., Steinberg, D., Bernstein, D., Bernstein, I.L. and Murlas, C. (1986). Bronchial hyper-reactivity occurs soon after the immediate asthmatic response in dual responders. *Am. Rev. Respir. Dis.* **133**, A33 (abstract).

Thueson, D.O., Speck, L.S., Lett-Brown, M.A. and Grant, J.A. (1979). Histamine releasing activity (HRA). I. Production by mitogen- or antigen-stimulated human mononuclear cells. *J. Immunol.* **123**, 626–32.

Tonnel, A.B., Gosset, P., Joseph, M., Fournier, E. and Capron, A. (1983). Stimulation of alveolar macrophages in asthmatic patients after local provocation test. *Lancet* **i**, 1406–8.

Townley, R.G., Bewtra, A.K., Nair, N.M., Brodkey, F.D., Watt, G.D. and Burke, K.M. (1979). Methacholine challenge studies. *J. Allergy Clin. Immunol.* **64**, 569–73.

Tsai, J.J., Maestrelli, P., Fitzharris, P., Parish, N., Knight, R.A. and Kay, A.B. (1987). A lymphocyte derived activity which enhances IgG-dependant release of leukotriene B_4 from human neutrophils. *J. Allergy Clin. Immunol.* **79**, 167.

Turk, J., Maas, R.L., Brash, A.R., Roberts, L.J. II and Oates, J.A. (1982). Arachidonic acid 15-lipoxygenase products from human eosinophils. *J. Biol. Chem.* **257**, 7068–76.

Vanderhoek, J.Y., Bryant, R.W. and Bailey, J.M. (1980). 15-Hydroxy-5,8,11,13-eicosatetraenoic acid: a potent and selective inhibitor of platelet lipoxygenase. *J. Biol. Chem.* **255**, 5996–8.

Vanhoutte, P.M. (1988). Epithelium derived relaxing factor: myth or reality? *Thorax* **43**, 665–8.

Vargaftig, B.B., Lefort, J., Chignard, M. and Benveniste, J. (1980). Platelet-activating factor induces a platelet-dependent bronchoconstriction unrelated to the formation of prostaglandin derivatives. *Eur. J. Pharmacol.* **65**, 185–92.

Venge, P. (1985). The eosinophil in inflammation. In *Inflammation: Basic mechanisms, Tissue Injuring Principles and Clinical Models*, ed. P. Venge and A. Lindbom, pp. 85–103, Almqvist & Wiksell International, Stockholm.

Walters, E.H., Bevan, C., Parrish, R.W., Davies, B.H. and Smith, A.P. (1982). Time-dependant effect of prostaglandin E_2 inhalation on airway responses to bronchoconstrictor agents in normal subjects. *Thorax* **37**, 438–42.

Wardlaw, A.J., Moqbel, R., Cromwell, O. and Kay, A.B. (1986). Platelet-activating factor. A potent chemotactic and chemokinetic factor for human eosinophils. *J. Clin. Invest.* **78**, 1701–6.

Wardlaw, A.J., Dunnette, S., Gleich, G.J., Collins, J.V. and Kay, A.B. (1988). Eosinophils and mast cells in bronchoalveolar lavage in subjets with mild asthma. *Am. Rev. Respir. Dis.* **137**, 62–9.

Warren, D.J. and Moore, M.A.S. (1988). Synergism among interleukin, 1, interleukin 3, and interleukin 5 in the production of eosinophils from primitive hemopoietic stem cells. *J. Immunol.* **140**, 94–9.

Weller, P.F., Lee, C.W., Foster, D.W., Corey, E.J., Austen, K.F. and Lewis, R.A. (1983). Generation and metabolism of 5-lipoxygenase pathway leukotrienes by human eosinophils: predominant production of leukotriene C_4. *Proc. Nat. Acad. Sci. (USA)* **80**, 7626–30.

Wenzel, S.E., Fowler, A.A. and Schwartz, L.B. (1988). Activation of pulmonary mast cells by bronchoalveolar allergen challenge: *in vivo* release of histamine and tryptase in atopic subjects with and without asthma. *Am. Rev. Respir. Dis.* **137**, 1002–8.

White, M.V. and Kaliner, M.A. (1987). Neutrophils and mast cells. I. Human neutrophil-derived histamine releasing activity. *J. Immunol.* **139**, 1624–30.

White, M.V. and Kaliner, M.A. (1988). Histamine. In *Asthma: Basic Mechanisms and Clinical Management*, ed. P.J. Barnes, I.W. Rodger and N.C. Thompson, pp. 231–57, Academic Press, London.

Williams, T.J. and Peck, M.J. (1977). Role of prostaglandin-mediated vasodilatation in inflammation. *Nature* **270**, 530–2.

Wilmot, C., Finnerty, J.P. and Holgate, S.T. (1988). Role of histamine and prostaglandins in the bronchial response to inhaled hypertonic saline. *Thorax* **43**, 865P (abstract).

Woolcock, A.J., Salome, C.M. and Yan, K. (1984). The shape of the dose–response curve to histamine in asthmatic and normal subjects. *Am. Rev. Respir. Dis.* **130**, 71–5.

Woolcock, A.J., Yan, K. and Salome, C.M. (1988). Effect of therapy on bronchial hyper-responsiveness in the long-term management of asthma. *Clin. Allergy* **18**, 165–76.

55: Allergic Rhinitis

P.W. Ewan

Allergic rhinitis is common. It is an important cause of morbidity, but much underdiagnosed. Treatment is highly effective and recognition of the allergic basis and identification of causative allergens can contribute to better management of the disorder. There is now considerable understanding of the pathophysiology. The first requirement for the development of this disorder is the generation of specific immunoglobulin E (IgE) antibodies; these become bound to specific receptors ($Fc_{\varepsilon}RI$) on mast cells in a variety of sites, including the nasal mucosa. Interaction of allergen and cell-bound specific IgE leads to activation of the mast cell, with release of preformed and newly generated mediators, which are responsible for the clinical manifestations.

Hay fever — seasonal allergic rhinitis — is due to pollen allergy. While grass pollens are the major cause in the UK, symptoms can also be provoked by tree, flower, shrub and weed pollens. The dominant pollens differ in different parts of the world: ragweed and birch pollens are the main causes of seasonal allergy in the United States and Scandinavia respectively while olive trees cause problems in Southern Europe. The moulds, *Alternaria* and *Cladosporium*, which are well known for causing isolated seasonal asthma (July–August), may also cause rhinoconjunctivitis.

The major cause of perennial rhinitis is house dust mite allergy, but allergy to animal dander, particularly cats and dogs, is also common.

Estimates of prevalence and incidence vary (WHO report 1986) but at least 10% of the population suffer from allergic rhinitis. Studies from the United States suggest a prevalence of childhood allergic rhinitis, both seasonal and perennial, of between 3.1 and 9% (WHO report 1986), whereas in adults a prevalence of 18% was estimated from health interview surveys (Meltzer *et al.* 1983), which means that about 40 million Americans were affected. In a London general practice, 2.2% of the patients were found to have hay fever (Blair 1974), but the accumulative frequency (those who have or have had hay fever) is probably 10% or more. A prevalence of 15% was found in Danish medical students (Johnsen and Mygind 1978) and 8% in a study involving 77 000 children and 18-year-olds (Aberg 1989).

The variation in figures for prevalence and incidence may, in part, be due to underdiagnosis and to the use of different criteria for identification of disease in different studies. That underdiagnosis or misdiagnosis of rhinitis is common is suggested from a study of about 3000 patients in a London general practice. Although patients with seasonal symptoms were twice as likely as those with perennial symptoms to be labelled as rhinitic, more than 25% of the subjects who actually had hay fever were still not diagnosed (Sibbald and Rink 1991). There has been a steep rise in consultation rates for rhinitis in recent years: between 1970 and 1981 the number of consultations for hay fever in general practice doubled from about 10 to 20 per 1000 population (Fleming and Crombie 1987). It does seem that there has been a real rise in the prevalence of allergic rhinitis in recent decades; the reasons for this are not clear, but changes in the environment, including increased exposure to air pollutants and allergens such as house dust mite, may be important.

Factors influencing the development of allergy

Atopy is defined as the presence of specific IgE antibodies to one or more of the common inhalant allergens (usually demonstrated by a positive skin prick test). In the UK, atopy can be determined by testing for IgE to house dust mite, grass pollen and animal (cat or dog) dander. About one-third of the population is atopic; yet only a proportion of these (about one-third) will ever develop allergic symptoms. Although the pathophysiology of the IgE–antigen interaction is well understood, the mechanisms which determine an individual's propensity to develop IgE antibodies are not clear. It is also not clear why only a proportion of subjects with IgE to inhalant allergens develop allergic disease.

A number of factors seem important for the development of atopic disease. Genetic factors determine the general propensity: the familial occurrence of both atopy and allergic disorders is well known. When there are no atopic family members, 5–15% of the children are likely to be atopic. This figure rises to 20–40% when one parent is atopic, and 40–75% when both parents are atopic (Kjellman 1988). Genetic factors also determine the type of allergic disease and the age at which symptoms begin. Work is in progress to identify the gene(s) for atopy. Although genetic factors are important, it is the interaction of both genetic and environmental influences that seems to determine atopy.

Raised total IgE levels at birth appear to have predictive value for the development of allergies in children (Kjellman 1976). Smoking during pregnancy has been shown to increase cord blood IgE levels.

Neonatal exposure to allergen can be important. Long-term studies in Sweden have shown that the risk of developing allergy appears to be related to the month of birth; for example, children born just before the birch pollen season and exposed to birch pollen in their early months are more likely to develop this sensitivity (Björksten and Suoniemi 1976; Björksten *et al.* 1980). The importance of the month of birth and consequent neonatal sensitization has been confirmed in studies in the UK, for house dust mite and grass pollen, and in the USA, for ragweed. Early exposure to house dust mites and cats may also result in a higher incidence of sensitization and clinical allergy. The relation between early exposure to inhalant allergens and allergic disease seems to be limited to children with a genetic predisposition to allergy.

Exposure to airborne pollutants in industrial areas and to cigarette smoke in the home also influence the development of allergic symptoms in babies and young children (Rantakallio 1978; Cogswell *et al.* 1987; Andrae *et al.* 1988). Virus infection may have a role; clinically, it is often noted that the onset of allergic disease coincides with or follows a viral upper respiratory infection (Frick *et al.* 1979). The mechanism is unclear, but certain viral infections, including respiratory syncytial virus, are associated with generation of virus-specific IgE antibody (Welliver *et al.* 1981); virus products such as interferon cause increased histamine release from basophils; and subtle but predictable and consistent increases in airway reactivity occur after viral infections, even in non-asthmatics. It is also possible that virus-induced damage to the respiratory epithelium may allow greater access of inhaled allergens to the IgE-producing plasma cells.

These environmental factors seem to be particularly important in the genetically predisposed (at-risk) individual. Thus it is the interaction of genetic susceptibility, exposure to allergen (possibly at a critical time) and other environmental factors which determines outcome.

Allergic disorders are more likely to occur in individuals whose ability to modulate their IgE response has been impaired by some form of immunodeficiency, possibly affecting T cell function. This has been suspected because of the association of some congenital immune deficiencies (the Wiskott–Aldrich syndrome) with allergy (Asherson and Webster 1980), and has been apparent in some patients with the acquired immune deficiency syndrome (AIDS) (Parkin *et al.* 1987). Allergic manifestations in two AIDS patients improved, in parallel with *in vitro* tests of cellular immunity, during treatment with interferon, and recurred when treatment was stopped. Other studies support this view. A high incidence of atopic eczema is reported in infants with AIDS, and atopic eczema in haemophiliacs became worse when they developed infection with human immunodeficiency virus, as shown by a positive antibody test (Ball and Harper 1987).

Pathogenesis of allergic rhinitis

Mediators

The interaction of allergen with the Fab portion of specific IgE antibodies bound to mast cells or basophils leads to activation of the cell and release of mediators, which are either stored in granules in the mast cell or newly synthesized by the cell. The preformed mediators include histamine and neutrophil and eosinophil chemotactic factors; platelet-activating factor (PAF) and the prostaglandins and leukotrienes are newly synthesized on cell activation.

The pattern of mediator release has been extensively studied following nasal challenge with allergen. More recently mediators have also been measured following natural allergen exposure.

The clinical response to nasal challenge, e.g. with grass pollen in a hay fever patient, includes sneezing, a rapid increase in nasal secretions and the development of congestion or obstruction, which can be demonstrated as increased nasal airway resistance. The immediate reaction (early phase) occurs minutes after allergen challenge. After a quiescent period of about 6 hours, a late-phase reaction occurs in up to 50% of patients with a recurrence of symptoms and further mediator release. If patients are rechallenged 12–24 hours after the immediate reaction, many show an enhanced reactivity and increased mediator release (rechallenge response). The development of nasal lavage models for the recovery of secretions has allowed identification of a post-challenge increase in a number of mediators *in vivo* in man.

IMMEDIATE REACTION

During the immediate reaction, which occurs within minutes and is short-lived, an increase in histamine levels in nasal secretions can be demonstrated (Naclerio *et al.* 1983a). Prostaglandin D_2 (PGD_2) (Naclerio *et al.* 1983a) and leukotrienes B_4, C_4 and D_4 (LTB_4, LTC_4 and LTD_4) (Shaw *et al.* 1985; Miadonna *et al.* 1987; Freeland *et al.* 1989) are also generated. There is also a rise in kinin levels and in tosyl-L-arginine methyl esterase (TAME) activity, a non-specific marker of inflammation of plasma origin (Naclerio *et al.* 1983a). Of these, TAME is the marker that best reflects the symptoms obtained at challenge (Naclerio *et al.* 1983b). This suggests plasma leakage may be important in the pathogenesis of symptoms of nasal allergy. Plasma-derived mediators, such as kinins and complement factors, could augment the inflammatory response.

LATE REACTION

The pattern of mediator release has also been studied in the late reaction, which occurs in up to 50% of patients (Dvoracek *et al.* 1984). Similar late reactions occur in the skin after intradermal skin tests and in the lung after bronchial challenge. It has been suggested, from studies on the skin, that, if large enough doses of allergen were used, all patients would develop a late reaction (Solley *et al.* 1976). The cumulative effect of natural exposure to allergen and late reactions may be important in the pathogenesis of allergic rhinitis. While the immediate reaction is characterized by sneezing, rhinorrhoea and to a lesser extent nasal congestion, the dominant symptom in the late reaction is nasal congestion, suggesting different mechanisms may be involved. This is supported by the pattern of mediator release which occurs.

Levels of many mediators, including histamine, TAME, LTB_4 and kinins, increase during the late-phase reaction (about 3–10 hours after the initial challenge), having declined after the early reaction. However, the level of PGD_2 does not rise (Naclerio *et al.* 1983a). Since mast cells release both histamine and PGD_2, whereas basophils release histamine but not PGD_2, it seems likely that basophils are responsible for the histamine released in the late reaction.

RECHALLENGE PHASE

The nasal mucosa is hypersensitive to rechallenge with allergen 12–24 hours after the initial challenge. There is also increased sensitivity to non-specific stimuli, such as histamine. A rapid rise in mediators, with the same pattern as in the immediate reaction, occurs but the response (both symptoms and mediator release) is augmented in many patients.

Relationship between allergen-induced specific and non-specific reactions

The relationship between allergen-induced specific and non-specific reactions has been studied in patients with seasonal allergic rhinitis, who underwent nasal challenge with histamine and then three successive doses of allergen on the first day (Andersson *et al.* 1989). The next day they were rechallenged with histamine and the lowest dose of allergen. An increase in nasal symptoms and TAME activity in nasal secretions occurred on day 2 compared with day 1 for both the specific (allergen) and non-specific (histamine) challenges. A close correlation was found between the allergen-induced increase in both specific and non-specific reactivity. An influx of eosinophils and basophils to the nasal mucosal surface occurred at the time of increased nasal reactivity. Treatment with topical corticosteroids blocked the increase in both specific and non-specific nasal reactivity.

Effect of steroids on mediator release

The effect of systemic steroids on the nasal response to allergen is different from that of topical steroids. Pretreatment with systemic steroids markedly reduces symptoms and mediator release in the late and rechallenge phases, but has little or no effect on the immediate reaction. Oral prednisolone (60 mg daily for 2 days) before a pollen challenge will not affect the immediate sneezing but significantly reduces the symptom in the late phase (Pipkorn *et al.* 1987a). Similarly, many mediators (histamine, kinin, TAME) are reduced in the late phase, but there is no reduction in the early-phase mediators, except for kinin.

Topical steroids in the nose (200 mg flunisolide daily for 7 days) pre-challenge reduce symptoms and mediator release in the immediate as well as the late and rechallenge phases (Pipkorn *et al.* 1987b). Pretreatment with topical steroids blocks the influx of basophils into the nose in the late phase. A reduction in the numbers of eosinophils, neutrophils and mononuclear cells in the late phase was also seen.

The concentration of steroid activity in the nose is higher after topical application than after an oral dose. It is not known whether larger oral doses for longer periods would also block the immediate reaction. It is possible that topical nasal steroids exert their effects by reducing the numbers of mast cells in the nasal mucosa (Lavker and Schechter 1985).

Mediator release during natural allergen exposure

Studies to monitor the inflammatory response in the nasal mucosa by measuring mediator release have been extended to patients undergoing natural exposure to allergen. This model should better reflect the disease state than the artificial nasal allergen challenge, in which much larger doses of allergen are administered — at least 10 000 ragweed pollen grains are needed to induce an immediate reaction in the nose, whereas during the ragweed pollen season a subject will inhale about 150 grains per hour (Marsh 1975). In patients with birch pollen allergy, in whom daily nasal lavage was performed during the pollen season, increased levels of TAME were found in the lavage fluid (Andersson *et al.* 1988). The high TAME levels correlated with nasal symptoms and with pollen counts.

Effects of mediators

In order to determine the clinical significance of different mediators in allergic rhinitis, these have been used to challenge the nose, while symptoms have been monitored. Histamine is the only mediator which produces all the major symptoms of rhinitis: sneezing, nasal blockage and secretions. Histamine applied locally to the nose will induce all three symptoms to about the same extent as allergen. Leukotriene D_4 increases nasal secretions and blockage, but does not induce sneezing. Platelet-activating factor and substance P do not produce the typical allergic symptoms. No single mediator, when applied to the nose, has been able to induce a late-phase response.

Histamine causes increased vascular permeability, capillary dilation, increased secretions and smooth-muscle contraction. Prostaglandin D_2 also increases vascular permeability and contracts smooth muscle. Leukotrienes C_4, D_4 and E_4 (the slow-reacting substance of anaphylaxis) are potent constrictors of smooth muscle, and induce pronounced and prolonged nasal obstruction. Leukotriene B_4 attracts leucocytes and has potent inflammatory effects. Kinins cause vasodilation, contribute to oedema and stimulate nerves.

Eosinophils

Local eosinophilia is a major feature of allergic rhinitis. During the pollen season, an increase in eosinophils on the surface of the nasal mucosa occurs in hay fever patients, with a direct time relationship to pollen exposure. Likewise, after allergen is applied to the nasal mucosa, an influx of eosinophils begins after about an hour, with a peak after several hours. Degranulation is seen, most marked in the nasal epithelium. Allergen challenge of the nose induces increase in the levels of the eosinophil-derived proteins, eosinophil-derived neurotoxin (EDN), eosinophil cationic protein (ECP) and major basic protein (MBP) (Bascom *et al.* 1989; Bisgaard *et al.* 1990). The time course of release of these proteins is compatible with the development of a late-phase reaction.

There is evidence to suggest that the eosinophil granule contents contribute to tissue injury in allergic rhinitis. Eosinophil peroxidase (EPO)-rich and MBP-rich fractions, obtained from soluble extracts from eosinophils, have been shown to impair ciliary movement of nasal cells *in vitro* (Liu and Okuda 1988). Another study, using purified eosinophil granule products, has shown that both an EPO–hydrogen peroxide–halide system and MBP are toxic to cultured human nasal epithelium *in vitro*, causing cell lysis (Ayars *et al.* 1988).

Much more is known about the relationship of the eosinophil to asthma, where there is a body of evidence to suggest that these cells are important for the development of the late reaction (De Monchy *et al.* 1985). It is probable that this also applies in allergic rhinitis, but further study is required.

It has been assumed that the ability of normal and allergic subjects to recruit eosinophils to the site of IgE-mediated reactions is similar, e.g. the Prausnitz–Küstner reaction is usually performed in normal subjects. While it is true that challenge with high concentrations of anti-IgE will produce immediate weal-and-flare reactions as well as late cutaneous reactions, which are morphologically similar, in both normal and allergic subjects (Umemoto *et al.* 1976), there is now evidence to suggest that the underlying cellular response is quite different in these two groups. After intracutaneous injection of PAF, a striking accumulation of degranulated eosinophils occurs in allergic subjects, while these cells are almost absent in normal subjects (Henocq and Vargaftig 1986). Similarly, in another study, where immediate and late cutaneous reactions were induced by anti-IgE challenge, significant eosinophil accumulation occurred in atopic subjects but not in normal subjects (Henocq and Rihoux 1990). It therefore appears that atopic eosinophils behave differently from normal cells *in vivo* during anti-IgE challenge, and in response to agonists such as PAF. The reasons for this difference are not clear, but the increased number of mast cells or increased activity of mast cells in atopics is a possibility. The mast cells of allergic subjects may be able to produce more eosinophil chemotactic factors, such as interleukin 5 (IL-5), than those of normal individuals.

Neutrophils

The role of neutrophils in nasal allergy is not clear. While eosinophils are frequently seen in nasal smears, less attention has been paid to neutrophils and their presence has often been attributed to coincident local infection. There are, however, reports of neutrophils in nasal smears of patients with allergic rhinitis who do not have infection. There is evidence to suggest that neutrophil chemotactic activity (NCA) may be involved in the pathogenesis of allergic rhinitis. Elevated levels of serum NCA have been reported in patients with house dust mite rhinitis, during natural exposure to allergen (McHugh and Ewan 1989). The NCA levels fell to normal with clinically effective allergen immunotherapy. It has also been shown that resected nasal turbinates, from similar patients, when challenged *in vitro* with house dust mite, release both high-molecular-weight NCA and histamine (Nagakura *et al.* 1989). These mediators were released together, with the same time course, in an allergen dose-dependent fashion, suggesting they were released by the same cell. Pretreatment with nasal sodium cromoglycate blocked the release of NCA and histamine.

T cells

Antigen-specific T cell proliferation in atopic subjects has been reported by several groups, although others have found no difference between atopics and normal subjects. The discrepancy is possibly due to different culture conditions (personal observation). However, more recent studies clearly demonstrate an antigen-specific T cell response in allergic subjects. Rawle *et al.* (1984) showed that the majority of house dust mite-allergic patients demonstrated T cell proliferation to the major allergen, *Der p* I, whereas this did not occur in non-allergic subjects. The responding cells were shown to be T cells, mainly T helper cells, and there was a progressive increase in the percentage of Leu 3a +ve cells in culture by the time of the maximum proliferate response. The production of IL-2 in the cultures was maximal 2 days before the peak proliferation. Although no significant difference in the T cell responses was found in different *Dermatophagoides pteronyssinus* allergic disorders (e.g. rhinitis or asthma or eczema), the weakest responses were in the rhinitis group. In this study a correlation between the titre of *Der p* I IgE and the degree of T cell proliferation was found. McHugh *et al.* (1992a) have also reported increased T proliferative responses to *D. pteronyssinus* in house dust mite allergic patients, and increased IL-2 production.

In ragweed allergy, T cell proliferation to antigen E has been reported (Phillips *et al.* 1987). However, because the response at 7 days was very weak, long-term culture and a second *in vitro* boost with antigen E were required to demonstrate a marked (20–50-fold over background) proliferative response, which occurred only in subjects with ragweed allergy. Again, the responding cells were shown to be mainly helper T cells. Clones derived from ragweed donors were antigen-specific.

Studies in patients with laboratory animal allergy, allergic to mouse urine, have also shown T cell proliferation to the major allergen, MA-1 (Gurka *et al.* 1987, 1988). Allergen-specific (MA-1) major histocompatibility complex (MHC)-restricted T cell clones were generated from these patients. Most clones were phenotyped as CD3 +ve, CD4 +ve. On stimulation with MA-1 together with irradiated antigen-presenting cells, they released IL-2, with peak levels 24 hours before maximum T cell proliferation. The clones, responsive to MA-1, were found to cross-react with a related rat protein RA2UG. Using these clones, it was shown that, in this model, a single dominant epitope was required for T cell activation.

Immunotherapy may also have an effect on T cells. House dust mite-allergic patients have been shown to produce more IL-2 than normal in response to mite antigen (Hsieh 1985). After immunotherapy with a house dust mite extract, the IL-2 production fell to normal. Immunotherapy has also been shown to increase antigen-specific suppressor T cells. Such cells have been demonstrated after ragweed and rye-grass immunotherapy (Rocklin *et al.* 1980; Nagaya 1985). In the ragweed system, these suppressor cells were shown to have histamine receptors. It has been postulated that the lack of these cells in untreated allergic patients may reflect a deficiency of suppressor cell activity, necessary to inhibit IgE production.

There have been many studies of T cell subsets in peripheral blood in atopic diseases, with conflicting results. Although most recent studies show consistent abnormalities in atopic dermatitis, with an increase in the CD4 +ve/CD8 +ve ratio in peripheral blood and an increase in CD4 +ve cells in biopsies of active skin lesions, and there is evidence of activation and recruitment of T cells into the lung in acute severe asthma, there are few data on allergic rhinitis.

Cytokines

T cells may have important effects in allergic disease through the production of a number of lymphokines. Cytokines have regulatory effects on both IgE and IgG responses to allergens, and may activate cells involved in the type I reaction. Interleukin 4 has been shown to stimulate both IgE and IgG production, *in vivo* and *in vitro* (Coffman and Carty 1986; Finkelman *et al.* 1986). Studies with recombinant IL-4 in mice have shown that the effect of IL-4 is complex and the dose- and time-course response differs for different isotypes. Recombinant IL-4 can induce IgE synthesis in normal human peripheral blood mononuclear cells (PBMC), and this effect is inhibited by interferon gamma (IFN-γ). Recombinant IFN-γ inhibits the expression of IL-4 receptors on human lymphocytes. Many other cytokines have effects likely to be important in type I reactions. These include IL-2, which up-regulates IFN-γ production, IL-3, which activates mast cells, and IL-5, which stimulates eosinophil production and activation. These cytokines have multiple, and sometimes synergistic or antagonistic, effects, so that their interactions *in vivo* are complex.

It was established in the mouse that T cell clones are divided into T_H1 cell clones which secrete exclusively IL-2 and IFN-γ, and T_H2 clones which produce IL-4, IL-5 and IL-6, amongst others (Mossman *et al.* 1986). It can be seen that a predominantly T_H2 type response, with IL-4, IL-5 and IL-6 production will lead to IgE production and activation and/or increased production of eosinophils and mast cells. In contrast a T_H1 response would inhibit IgE production.

It has not been straightforward to establish whether T_H1 and T_H2 subsets also occur in man, but this has recently become generally accepted (Weirenga *et al.* 1990; Kapsenberg *et al.* 1991; Romagnani 1991). *Dermatophagoides pteronyssinus*-specific T cell clones from allergic patients have been shown to have a preferential ability to produce IL-4 rather than IFN-γ, compared with clones from non-atopic donors, which produce IFN-γ but little or no IL-4 (Weirenga *et al.* 1990; Yssel *et al.* 1990). In keeping with these observations, work with PBMC from allergic patients has shown normal IFN-γ production by cells stimulated with mitogen but grossly impaired IFN-γ production from cells stimulated with specific antigen (*D. pteronyssinus*) (Ewan *et al.* 1990). These findings suggest that an imbalance between the production of IL-4 and IFN-γ may be involved in the generation of the high IgE levels seen in allergic disease, i.e. that atopic subjects have a predominantly T_H2-type response. Abnormalities of IL-6 and IL-2 production have also been described in allergic patients (McHugh *et al.* 1992b) and other cytokines are likely to be important.

There is evidence that within the same atopic individual the pattern of cytokine response varies according to the type of antigen presenting to the immune system. Work with T cell clones shows that stimulation with antigen leads to a predominantly T_H1-type response (delayed hypersensitivity response), whereas stimulation with allergen leads to a T_H2-type response (Weirenga *et al.* 1990; Del Prete *et al.* 1991). Further, it has been shown that addition of cytokines to peripheral blood mononuclear cells early in culture before clonal selection, could alter the cytokine secretion of the resulting T cell clones. Thus preincubation of atopic cells with IFN-γ before clonal selection, suppressed the development of T_H2-type clones and lead to the secretion of T_H1 type cytokines (Maggi *et al.* 1992).

Clearly, cytokines play an important and complex role in the pathogenesis of allergic disease. Our understanding of this area has increased rapidly in recent years but much more information is needed.

Priming

It was found that, if allergic subjects were challenged daily with allergen, lower doses were required on successive days to produce the same reaction in the nose (Connell 1968). Initially, the amount of pollen required to induce hay fever symptoms on nasal challenge greatly exceeded the amounts inhaled on natural exposure in the pollen season. However, after several days of challenge, the amount of pollen required to induce a reaction decreased, approaching levels similar to those encountered during seasonal exposure. This phenomenon was defined by Connell as priming. Connell went on to show that priming was specific for the side of the nose challenged, disappeared when exposure was stopped, occurred during seasonal exposure and was not specific for the antigen inhaled (Connell 1969). The latter point is clearly demonstrated clinically: during the hay fever season some patients also react to a second allergen, such as cats, to which they exhibit no clinical response out of the pollen season.

The mechanism of nasal priming has been investigated in ragweed hay fever patients given successive nasal challenges with ragweed pollen (Wachs *et al.* 1989). Whereas 10 000 grains of pollen were required to induce sneezing initially, after priming a reduced dose (1000 grains or in some patients as little as 100 grains) induced an increased response. Mediator release into nasal lavage fluid was shown to increase on priming. A significant increase in histamine release occurred first, but later increases in TAME, kinins and PGD_2 occurred. A considerable increase in the number of white blood cells in the lavage fluid was found before the challenge on the priming days, neutrophils, eosinophils and alcian-blue +ve cells all being increased. The pattern of mediator release suggested that the alcian-blue-staining cells were basophils, which infiltrated the nose early, followed later by a subpopulation of mast cells.

Migration of basophils and mast cells

A rise in the number of mast cells in the nasal mucosa has been reported during the grass pollen season (Viegas *et al.* 1987). Other studies suggest there may be little change in the total number of nasal mast cells but that mast cells are redistributed into the nasal epithelium as part of the mucosal response in hay fever (Enerback *et al.* 1986), migrating from the connective tissue to the more superficial layers, from which they can be recovered by surface 'imprints'. Alternatively, mast cells and/or basophil precursors may have trafficked from the blood to the nasal mucosa. This is suggested by several studies. For example, in allergic patients during the ragweed pollen season, the peripheral blood basophil count rises, the number of circulating metachromatic cell precursors falls and the number of formalin-sensitive (i.e. mucosal mast cell-like) nasal mast cells rises (Otsuka *et al.* 1986).

The migration of mast cells appears to be related to the start of the pollen season, and in one study mast cells began to appear in imprints of the nasal mucosa after 4–5 days of pollen exposure (Pipkorn *et al.* 1988a). However, another study by the same group failed to show a rise in the number of nasal mast cells in mucosal imprints and redistribution into the epithelium (Pipkorn *et al.* 1988b). These observations need to be clarified, with particular attention to the staining techniques used to identify cells. The latter study did show a correlation between histamine content and symptoms and a fall in mast cell numbers without a reduction in histamine content, suggesting the appearance of a non-mast cell pool of cells in the nasal mucosa.

Nasal anatomy and physiology

Because of the prominence of the turbinates, the airspace in each nasal cavity is reduced to a small slit, only 2–4 mm wide. This facilitates a number of functions of the nose, which include heating, humidification and filtration of inhaled air. There is high mucosal blood flow, which is under neurological control, but which can also change quickly in response to humoral factors. Large amounts of blood can be shunted through the arteriovenous anastomoses of the turbinates, bypassing the capillary bed, so that the degree to which inspired air is warmed can be rapidly adjusted. Air at room temperature, inhaled through the nose, is warmed to 30°C by the time it reaches the pharynx, and is almost saturated with water. When air at 0°C is inhaled, it is warmed to about 25°C when it reaches the pharynx. The nose also retains about 99% of inhaled water-soluble gases. This means that gases such as sulphur dioxide and ozone, which are powerful irritants, only reach the lower airways in extremely small quantities.

The nose is an important filter: the bending of the airstream, as it passes through the nose, allows particles to impinge on the nasal mucosa, and turbulence promotes particle deposition. The nose filters large volumes of air each day, and most of the large particles (>10 μm) are impacted and do not pass through. These particles include pollen grains 15–30 μm in diameter, which also impact on the conjunctiva. Smaller particles (<2 μm), such as moulds, pass through the nose and reach the lungs. When nasal obstruction develops, and there is a switch to mouth breathing, this filtering effect is impaired. This may be harmful, not only because more particles reach the lungs, but also because bronchial heat and water loss may occur.

Particles deposited on the nasal mucosa are cleared by mucociliary transport within 10–30 minutes and taken back towards the pharynx, where they are swallowed. Soluble protein, however, is eluted from some particles very rapidly and can either be passed through the basement membrane to be presented to lymphocytes to stimulate antibody formation or, in sensitized subjects, induce an allergic reaction.

There is no smooth muscle in the nose, and vascular congestion is thought to be the major cause of nasal obstruction. Nasal hyper-reactivity, however, can occur, but this is a less well-defined phenomenon than in the lung. Histamine or metacholine challenges in the nose can be used to differentiate groups of allergic rhinitis patients from healthy subjects, but there is considerable overlap and they are not useful clinically. The relationship between the nasal late reaction and allergen-induced nasal hyper-reactivity is not clear.

Bronchial reactivity in allergic rhinitis

Most patients with seasonal allergic rhinitis do not have clinical asthma. However, these patients have an increased bronchial reactivity during the pollen season as shown by an increased bronchoconstrictor response to metacholine challenge (Gerblich *et al.* 1986; Madonini *et al.* 1987). The patients with hay fever who do have an associated asthma usually develop their asthma symptoms later in the season than their rhinitis; one explanation is that they may be responding to repeated exposure to allergen. The implications of these observations are not clear, but it is well known that in asthmatics an increase in non-specific bronchial activity occurs after challenge with allergen. Whether similar changes in non-specific reactivity in the nose occur regularly or are important is less clear, but an increase in non-specific (histamine) responsiveness has been demonstrated after nasal allergen challenge (Andersson *et al.* 1989).

Clinical features

The history is of great importance in the diagnosis of allergic rhinitis, and often gives clues to the likely causative allergen(s). Tests for specific IgE antibodies cannot be interpreted without a detailed history.

Patients with allergic rhinitis have three main symptoms: sneezing, nasal discharge and nasal congestion. Sneezing and watery discharge predominate in seasonal rhinitis, whereas congestion is more likely to be the major problem in a perennial rhinitis, such as house dust mite allergy. Nasal congestion can vary in severity from mild nasal stuffiness to complete nasal obstruction with mouth breathing, and is one of the most difficult symptoms to treat. Some patients also have conjunctivitis (which less commonly occurs alone) and complain of discomfort, itching and grittiness of the eyes, sometimes with redness and watering. Less often, and in more severe cases, conjunctival oedema, ulcerative blepharitis, inflammation of the tarsal plate or periorbital oedema may occur. Patients may also complain of itching of the palate, pharynx or external auditory meaths. Some patients have other allergic problems, particularly asthma or eczema, but occasionally urticaria or angio-oedema.

Allergic rhinitis usually begins in children or young adults, and an onset in later life is more suggestive of a non-allergic cause.

The timing of symptoms and factors provoking symptoms help to elucidate the cause. In perennial rhinitis, symptoms occur throughout the year; however, symptoms need not be constant and spontaneous fluctuations in severity may occur. There may also be seasonal exacerbations, showing a pattern over several years, due to an additional seasonal allergy. The commonest causes of perennial allergic rhinitis are house dust mite (*Dermatophagoides* species) and animal dander (usually cats and dogs). These can often be distinguished on the basis of the history (e.g. timing — house dust mite allergy is typically worst on waking and may improve during the day; effects of exposure to large quantities of allergen — hoovering, bedmaking or close contact with a pet, etc.) but can be more difficult to diagnose clinically when both allergies occur together.

Seasonal allergies vary from country to country

and a knowledge of the season of different allergens is essential for diagnosis. In the United Kingdom, grass pollen is the commonest cause of seasonal rhinitis and the grass pollen season extends from early to mid-June to late July, but varies with the location and climate. Tree pollens occur in the spring (with a peak in March and April, although some occur in early May). Flower and shrub pollens appear later in the summer, usually after the grass pollen season.

There is a broad correlation between hay fever symptoms and pollen counts, but symptoms do not usually begin until the pollen count rises above the initial very low levels. Thus the duration of symptoms is usually less than the length of the pollen season and patients with less severe forms of hay fever may only have symptoms for 2–4 weeks of a 6-week pollen season. It has been shown that, by the time the pollen count reaches 50 grains per cubic metre, all patients who are going to develop symptoms will have done so (R.R. Davies, pers. comm.). Asthma symptoms appear later in the pollen season.

Examination reveals nasal mucosal hypertrophy with swelling over the turbinates, encroaching on the narrow airways. Secretions are usually watery and more profuse in a seasonal rhinitis, and more viscous or mucoid in perennial allergies. The conjunctiva may be inflamed or there may be signs of more severe ocular problems.

Perennial allergic rhinitis has to be differentiated from non-allergic (vasomotor) rhinitis and from repeated episodes of nasal infection. Measurement of specific IgE antibodies will be helpful, but some clues can be obtained from the history. In vasomotor rhinitis, symptoms are normally perennial but intermittent, and completely asymptomatic periods occur. The main symptoms are nasal obstruction and post-nasal drip. There should be no history of exacerbations after exposure to dust or animals, but commonly patients complain of increased nasal congestion in poorly ventilated, smoky or stuffy atmospheres, and on change of temperature or environment. In nasal infection the secretions should be more purulent and episodes are more likely to be discreet. There may be associated chronic sinusitis.

Chronic rhinitis can be distressing and interfere with concentration or efficiency at work or at school. The morbidity and economic consequences are considerable. A survey in 1975 in the USA found that, as a result of allergic rhinitis in 1 year alone, sufferers were restricted in their activities for 28 million days, were bedridden for 6 million days and lost 2 million school days (Young 1980). The cost of medical services for allergic rhinitis for 1 year in the USA was 500 million dollars.

Investigations

From the history alone, it is often possible to tell whether rhinitis is allergic or non-allergic, and, if allergic, to pin-point putative allergens. The diagnosis can then be confirmed by measuring specific IgE antibodies, which can be detected either by skin prick tests or in the serum, most commonly by radio-allergosorbent tests (RAST). Skin prick tests are simple, quick and relatively cheap and have the advantage of providing the result while the patient is still in the clinic. An aqueous solution of allergen extract is pricked into the skin with a stylet, and the appearance of a weal and flare within 10–15 minutes indicates that allergen has bound to the relevant specific IgE antibody on cutaneous mast cells and triggered histamine release. A number of allergens can be tested simultaneously, and it is important to include positive (histamine) and negative (saline) controls. A dry skin prick testing system is also available, using lancets with tips coated with allergen. The quality of extracts for skin testing is improving, and a number of standardized extracts are now available.

Specific IgE in the serum has traditionally been measured by RAST, where the allergen is coupled to paper discs, and a radio-immunoassay is performed (Wide *et al.* 1967). The results of RAST correlate well with the results of skin tests, but the skin test is more often positive than the RAST and of those with a positive skin test and negative RAST up to one-third have been reported to have positive provocation tests (Berg and Johansson 1974). The RAST is expensive and time-consuming and requires good laboratory facilities, but can be helpful if skin tests are not available or require corroboration. It is also useful in patients who have extensive skin disease or are taking drugs which might impair the skin response.

Other systems are available to measure specific IgE in the serum. The ImmunoCAP utilizes a capsulated hydrophilic carrier polymer as solid phase, which is able to bind more allergen than conventional systems. This assay is quicker than the RAST, since the reaction between test IgE and bound allergen takes place within 20 minutes. Good correlation has been demonstrated between the ImmunoCAP test and RAST, but the ImmunoCAP showed greater sensitivity, identifying more positive tests than RAST and approximating more closely with the skin prick test (Ewan and Coote 1990).

These tests for specific IgE indicate atopy and should not automatically be equated with disease, since only a proportion of atopic subjects develop clinical allergy. The tests need to be interpreted in conjunction with the history, and are never, by themselves, an indication for treatment. The severity of symptoms in allergic rhinitis does not necessarily relate to the titre of specific IgE (Nickelson *et al.* 1986).

Measurement of the total serum IgE is not helpful in the diagnosis of allergic rhinitis, since specific IgE antibodies can be present without a rise in total IgE. A normal level would therefore not exclude hay fever. In vasomotor rhinitis, an extremely low total IgE (<10 IU/ml) would usually be found, but there would be no need to measure this if skin tests to a range of common allergens were negative.

Tests for specific IgE are not essential in hay fever if the diagnosis is clear from the history, unless immunotherapy is to be given. They are much more helpful in patients with perennial rhinitis, where it can be difficult from the history alone to distinguish allergic from non-allergic causes, to be sure if there is a seasonal exacerbation or to confirm coexisting allergies. They are helpful in patients who are uncertain of the timing of their symptoms or the circumstances in which exacerbations or remissions occur. Precise identification of allergens is worth while, since it may lead to improvements in therapy. In the case of seasonal allergens, patients can be warned when to expect the onset of symptoms, and thus introduce treatment early when it is easier to gain effective control. It may also be possible to reduce exposure to allergens.

Treatment

Allergic rhinitis

Topical corticosteroids or sodium cromoglycate and oral antihistamines — the established treatments for allergic rhinitis — have all been compared extensively with placebo and shown to be effective.

STEROIDS

Steroids have a variety of actions. Part of their effect results from the activation of cytoplasmic steroid receptors, leading to transcription of messenger ribonucleic acid (RNA) to produce a family of polypeptides, including lipocortin (or calpactin). Within 2 hours of a single dose of 100 mg hydrocortisone intravenously in man, huge increases in lipocortin 1 in peripheral monocytes and on the surface of mononuclear cells occur (Goulding *et al.* 1990). Lipocortin inhibits the conversion of phospholipids to prostaglandins, leukotrienes and PAF (Flower 1988). Steroids also have potent anti-inflammatory effects, inhibiting local recruitment and activation of granulocytes and lymphocytes and suppressing mediator release from inflammatory cells. They cause vasoconstriction and reduced permeability of mucosal capillaries, so reducing airway microvascular leakage and secretions. Both oral and inhaled steroids block the late-phase reaction on allergen challenge and the increased bronchial hyper-responsiveness which follows allergen challenge. The immediate reaction can also be blocked by inhaled steroids, providing pretreatment is given for a week or more. This is thought to be due to effects on mast cell recruitment and differentiation.

Topical steroids are highly effective in the treatment of allergic rhinitis. In normal dosage, systemic absorption is extremely small and of no clinical importance. No significant side-effects have been reported after years of treatment. A variety of nasal sprays are available: beclomethasone diproprionate, budesonide, flunisolide and betamethasone sodium phosphate. Beclomethasone is the most widely studied. There is probably little to choose between the various preparations; for example, beclomethasone and flunisolide have been found to have comparable effects in a number of clinical trials (Sipila *et al.* 1983).

Topical steroids are effective in the vast majority of patients, providing: (i) the nose is patent, allowing effective application so that the drug reaches most of the nasal mucosa; and (ii) that the treatment is used regularly. The propellant in aerosols can cause sneezing in some patients, but this can be overcome by the use of aqueous preparations.

Systemic steroids should be avoided and the annual use of a depot steroid injection for hay fever should be discouraged. Very disabling symptoms occasionally justify the use of oral steroids for short periods — for example, in students taking important examinations.

SODIUM CROMOGLYCATE

Sodium cromoglycate has been in clinical use since 1968 and, although it was identified at an early stage to be a mast cell stabilizer, its mechanism of action in immediate hypersensitivity reactions remains unclear. Although it is a weak mast cell stabilizer *in vitro*, drugs which are more potent have been found to have negligible therapeutic effects. It has inhibitory effects on eosinophils, macrophages and platelets, and may thus inhibit the inflammatory response. It also has neural effects, blocking afferent discharges along non-myelinated nerves. In challenge studies, it can block both the early and the late reaction (Hutson *et al*. 1988).

Topical sodium cromoglycate is available in a variety of formulations for the nose (Rynacrom), and aqueous preparations cause less irritation than the powder. In studies comparing nasal steroids and cromoglycate, steroids are generally found to be superior (Frankland and Walker 1975; Brown *et al*. 1981), although some show equal efficacy. This impression is borne out in clinical practice, where more patients have a poor response to cromoglycate than to steroids. A study which showed beclomethasone aqueous suspension and flunisolide to be more effective than cromoglycate in the treatment of ragweed rhinitis also demonstrated that all of these nasal treatments considerably reduced the symptoms of seasonal asthma (Welsh *et al*. 1987).

ANTIHISTAMINES

Antihistamines block only the histamine-mediated component of the type I reaction; however, this is important in rhinitis, particularly in seasonal rhinitis. The usefulness of these drugs has been increased by the introduction of the non-sedative antihistamines, which cross the blood–brain barrier to only a limited extent. Since the introduction of terfenadine (Triludan) and astemizole (Hismanal), a number of other non-sedative antihistamines have been marketed, including acrivastine (Semprex), cetirizine (Zirtek) and loratadine (Clarityn). These all cause less sedation and psychomotor impairment. However, the older, sedative antihistamines, such as chlorpheniramine maleate (Piriton), do not cause sedation in all patients, are more effective in some and are much cheaper.

Astemizole has the disadvantage of a slower onset of action over 7 days, and a long half-life, so that its effects may persist for up to 4 weeks after withdrawal of the drug. The effects of terfenadine and the other non-sedative antihistamines are of rapid onset and shorter duration, and this is more appropriate to the intermittent or short-term use, which is often required in the management of seasonal rhinitis. All of the non-sedative antihistamines have been shown to be effective, particularly in the control of rhinorrhoea and sneezing. They are less effective for nasal congestion.

A question of practical importance is whether there is any clear difference in efficacy of nasal steroids and non-sedative antihistamines. Many allergists feel that nasal steroids are superior. However, the choice of drug has to be tailored to the individual patient, since this will be influenced by other factors, such as the presence of nasal obstruction and the extent of the disease; for example, an antihistamine will be helpful if there is itching of the eye, palate or external auditory meatus in addition to the rhinitis. In a comparative study of astemizole tablets and beclomethasone nasal spray, both treatments were equally effective for rhinitis but astemizole was superior in the control of eye symptoms (Wood 1986). However, intranasal steroids are often effective in relieving mild allergic conjunctivitis, and this has been confirmed in a formal study (Welsh *et al*. 1987).

NASAL DECONGESTANTS

Nasal obstruction is the most difficult symptom to treat and, if marked, interferes with the efficacy of topical steroids, since they can only be delivered to a reduced area of mucosa. In such patients, it can help to prescribe a topical nasal decongestant (such as ephedrine nasal drops) in addition to a topical nasal steroid for up to 3 days only. The nasal steroid is then continued alone. Prolonged or regular use of decongestants should be avoided since they lead to rebound congestion.

Allergic conjunctivitis

Sodium cromoglycate eyedrops or oral antihistamines are effective treatments for allergic conjunctivitis. Cromoglycate eyedrops can cause initial stinging and, ideally, they should be introduced early, before the eyes become very inflamed. More severe forms of allergic conjunctivitis may require steroid eyedrops, but only a short course should be given and, once the conjunctivitis is controlled, cromoglycate eyedrops should be used for maintenance therapy. Patients with more complex eye problems or those who require longer-term steroids must be seen by an ophthalmologist. The prolonged use of steroid eyedrops may cause glaucoma, so the intraocular pressure must be measured.

Drug selection

The most appropriate drug will depend on the severity, site(s) and nature of the symptoms. In the majority of patients where rhinitis is the only or major problem, nasal steroids are highly effective. They also have the advantage, over antihistamines, of being preventative, of blocking the late reaction and of reducing inflammation. It is important to first check that the nose is patent, so that adequate application can be achieved. Patients must be taught the correct technique for use of nasal steroids and understand the need for regular (prophylactic) therapy. Cromoglycate is a useful alternative in a minority of patients, including those who develop epistaxes or nasal soreness when using steroids.

Antihistamines are particularly effective either when there are symptoms at multiple sites (e.g. rhinitis, conjunctivitis and itching of the palate or external auditory meatus) or when intermittent or short-term therapy is required.

Reducing exposure to allergen

Although it is not possible to avoid exposure to airborne allergens, such as pollens, understanding of some of the factors determining pollen counts can lead to ways of reducing allergen exposure. Within a city pollen counts are highest in parks and open areas, and much lower in built-up areas. However, there are variations within built-up areas due to turbulence, and counts are usually higher at the top of a building than at street level. Simple measures such as avoiding parks and areas of freshly cut grass, and closing car windows when driving through the countryside may reduce the degree of pollen exposure.

The pollen count varies with the time of day, and the mean daily counts mask peaks and troughs which occur during the day. It is best to open windows in the morning when pollen counts are lowest, and close them by midday as the pollen count rises during the afternoon and evening. There is very little pollen in the air at night. There are further variations as a result of the weather.

A variety of measures can be taken to reduce exposure to house dust mite. Hoovering, including the mattress, damp dusting, frequent washing of bedding, and the use of synthetic fillings in quilts and pillows are amongst measures often recommended. There is evidence to suggest that such measures lead neither to a reduction in dust exposure in the bedroom nor to a reduction in symptoms (Burr *et al.* 1980; Korsgaard 1982). More extreme manoeuvres — for example, where house dust mite-allergic asthmatics slept in the almost dust-free environment of hospital side-rooms for several weeks — have been shown to lead to clinical benefit (Platts-Mills *et al.* 1982). Similarly, more aggressive measures in the home, involving removing carpets from bedrooms, covering mattresses with plastic and frequent hot washing of bedding, have been shown to result in clinical improvement (Sarsfield *et al.* 1974; Walshaw and Evans 1986). It seems that less stringent measures used in the home may not reduce levels of *Der p* I below a critical threshold for a reduction in symptoms (Platts-Mills *et al.* 1986). The practicality of these measures needs to be considered in relation to the severity of the allergy and the family situation. While they are appropriate for patients with moderate to severe asthma, they may not be for a patient with rhinitis.

Chemicals, which can be applied to mattresses and carpets, to eradicate mites are available, but their effects are disappointing. Natamycin, an antifungal antibiotic which kills the fungus on which the house dust mite depends, does not seem particularly effective (Colloff *et al.* 1989; Reiser *et al.*

1990). Acarosan, a derivative of benzylbenzoate, kills the mites and, because it contains acrylate polymers, is said to 'clump' the mites together so that they can be more effectively removed from mattresses by hoovering. Initial clinical studies have not been properly controlled and results are anecdotal (Bischoff *et al*. 1986; Morrow Brown and Merrett 1990). A recent controlled study suggesting Acarosan was of benefit (Kniest *et al*. 1991) has some methodological problems and involved small numbers of patients (Godfrey 1991). Further studies are therefore needed before this treatment could be recommended.

Liquid nitrogen is effective in killing mites, but a practicable system of delivery needs to be devised.

Allergen immunotherapy

Allergen immunotherapy or hyposensitization consists of a series of injections of allergen extract given over months or years, with the aim of reducing the patient's sensitivity to that allergen. This type of treatment has been widely used since its introduction in 1911 by Noon, and yet it remains controversial. Practice varies in different countries and the role of immunotherapy has been reviewed by the European Academy of Allergology and Clinical Immunology (EAACI 1988).

Immunotherapy is most effective in the treatment of bee and wasp venom allergy, where an 'improvement' rate of 90% or more can be achieved against an improvement of about 40% in the placebo-treated group (Hunt *et al*. 1978). However, results must be interpreted in the light of a considerable spontaneous improvement rate in untreated patients (P.W. Ewan 1984, and in preparation). Immunotherapy is also effective in grass, ragweed and birch pollen allergies (Frankland and Augustin 1954; Patterson *et al*. 1978; EAACI 1988). Although efficacy has been demonstrated for other allergens, such as house dust mite (Ewan *et al*. 1988a) and cat dander (Hedlin *et al*. 1986), more controlled studies are needed before immunotherapy could be recommended for these allergies. There are no or few controlled studies of the many mixed allergen extracts which are in widespread use. These should be avoided.

Although immunotherapy can be effective, there are problems with many of the studies carried out: the allergen extracts have often been crude and unstandardized, no allowance has been made for variation in patient sensitivity within groups and most studies are short-term. Another major problem has been the risk of serious anaphylactic reactions and death. Although fatalities are rare, the report of a number of deaths in the UK led the Committee for Safety in Medicines to issue guidelines on immunotherapy which effectively preclude its use in general practice and, by recommending a 2-hour observation period after each injection, make it difficult to carry out in hospital (CSM Update 1986). Deaths have almost always occurred when inexperienced doctors have administered immunotherapy, and it is recognized by allergists that only trained staff should give this form of treatment. The very serious reactions usually occur within minutes of injection, and when generalized reactions occur later they are usually mild (Ewan *et al*. 1988a, b; Ewan and Stewart 1992). However, prospective studies of reactions suggest that less serious generalized reactions are commoner than is usually perceived (Ewan *et al*. 1988b; Ewan and Stewart 1992).

The mechanism of immunotherapy is not clear. For many years this has been thought to be due to the production of IgG ('blocking') antibody, which prevents binding of allergen to IgE on mast cells. This seems to be a factor in bee and wasp venom allergy (Golden *et al*. 1982) and in bee venom immunotherapy, where the administration of hyperimmune serum together with allergen can reduce the incidence of adverse reactions (Müller *et al*. 1986; Bousquet *et al*. 1987). However, the titre of IgG antibody does not always correlate well with clinical improvement (Ewan *et al*. 1992), particularly in allergy to inhaled allergens. Two more recent studies of house dust mite immunotherapy do show a rise in specific IgG levels in patients treated with clinically effective extracts (Nakagawa *et al*. 1987; McHugh *et al*. 1990). In one of these, in which both standardized allergen extracts and sensitive IgG assays were used, IgG levels rose only in the group who improved and who had been treated with a potent extract (McHugh *et al*. 1990). This, however, does not of necessity imply that IgG levels are responsible for the clinical effect. Studies of IgG subclasses suggest IgG-4 levels rise with immunotherapy, but again it is difficult to know whether this relates to efficacy or whether this is a consequence of repeated immunization with a potent antigen (Aalberse *et al.* 1983; Nakagawa *et al.* 1987; McHugh *et al.* 1990). The ratio of specific IgG to IgE may be relevant.

The lack of a clear relationship between IgG antibody and clinical improvement suggests that other factors may be important. Immunotherapy has been shown to reduce the late asthmatic reaction (Warner *et al.* 1978; van Bever *et al.* 1988) and abolish the generation of eosinophil and neutrophil chemotactic activity (Rak *et al.* 1987; McHugh and Ewan 1989), effects compatible with blocking of mast cell activation or possibly with alteration of T cell responsiveness. Immunotherapy leads to a reduced lymphocyte proliferative response to allergen (Rawle *et al.* 1984; personal observation), and the fall in specific IgE levels seen late in immunotherapy may reflect the induction of antigen-specific suppressor T cells (Rocklin *et al.* 1980).

Despite these problems, it is clear that this form of treatment can be effective. The availability of safe and effective drug treatments, such as topical corticosteroids, makes them the preferred first-line therapy. Immunotherapy may, however, be indicated in a small number of carefully selected patients. In deciding whether to use immunotherapy, one must balance the variable degree of efficacy against the risk of allergic reaction. There is a greater risk of serious reaction in patients with a history of asthma. Immunotherapy should only be given by doctors experienced in its use, and this will not only reduce the incidence of reactions but also result in prompt recognition and treatment of reactions, and so improve safety.

There are not many studies comparing immunotherapy with drug therapy, but one study showed an alum-adsorbed grass pollen preparation (of only moderate potency) to have the same effect as topical sodium cromoglycate (Andersen *et al.* 1987). A study looking at the effect of grass pollen immunotherapy in patients with hay fever who had been poorly controlled by conventional drug therapy in previous years showed immunotherapy to be significantly more effective than placebo (Varney *et al.* 1991). There is, however, little information on the care patients received in earlier years, and it is possible that some were simply given a prescription without adequate instruction or follow-up. More studies comparing immunotherapy directly with drug therapy are needed.

The future of immunotherapy is uncertain at present, but, with the development of new types of vaccine which are both safe and effective, this type of therapy may be an important option in the management of allergic disease in the future.

References

Aalberse, R.C., van der Gaag, R. and Leeuwen, J.V. (1983). Serologic aspects of IgG antibodies. I. Prolonged immunization results in an IgG_4-restricted response. *J. Immunol.* **130**, 722–6.

Aberg, N. (1989). Birth season variation in asthma and allergic rhinitis. *Clin. Exp. Allergy* **19**, 643–8.

Andersen, N.H., Jeppesen, F., Schioler, T. *et al.* (1987). Treatment of hay fever with sodium cromoglycate, hyposensitisation or a combination. *Allergy* **42**, 343–51.

Andersson, M., Svensson, C., Andersson, P. and Pipkorn, U. (1988). Objective monitoring of the allergic inflammatory response of the nasal mucosa in patients with hay fever during natural allergen exposure. *Ann. Rev. Respir. Dis.* **139**, 911–14.

Andersson, M., Andersson, P. and Pipkorn, U. (1989). Allergen-induced specific and non-specific nasal reactions: reciprocal relationship and inhibition by topical glucocorticoids. *Acta Otolaryngol. (Stockholm)* **107**, 270–7.

Andrae, S., Axelson, O., Bjorksten, F., Fredricksson, M. and Kjellman, N.-I.M. (1988). Symptoms of bronchial hyperreactivity and asthma in relation to environmental factors. *Arch. Dis. Child.* **63**, 473–8.

Asherson, G.L. and Webster, A.D.B. (1980). Wiskott–Aldrich syndrome. In *Diagnosis and Treatment of Immunodeficiency Diseases*, p. 240, Blackwell Scientific Publications, Oxford.

Ayars, G.H., Altman, L.C., McManus, M.M. *et al.* (1988). Injurious effect of the eosinophil peroxide–hydrogen peroxide–halide system and major basic protein on human nasal epithelium *in vitro*. *Am. Rev. Respir. Dis.* **140**, 125–31.

Ball, L.M. and Harper, J.I. (1987). Atopic eczema and HIV positive haemophiliacs. *Lancet* **ii**, 627 (letter).

Bascom, R., Pipkorn, U., Proud, D. *et al.* (1989). Major basic protein and eosinophil-derived neurotoxin concentrations in nasal-lavage fluid after antigen challenge: effect of systemic corticosteroids and relationship to eosinophil influx. *J. Allergy Clin. Immunol.* **84**, 338–46.

Berg, T.L.O. and Johansson, S.G.O. (1974). Allergy diagnosis with the radioallergosorbent test. *J. Allergy Clin. Immunol.* **54**, 209–21.

Bischoff, E., Krause-Michael, B. and Nolte, G. (1986). Zur Bekampfung der Haussaubmilben in Haushalten von Patienten mit Milbenasthma. *Allergologie* **9**, 448–57.

Bisgaard, H., Grønborg, H., Mygind, N., Dahl, R., Lindqvist, N. and Venge, P. (1990). Allergen-induced increase of eosinophilic cationic protein in nasal lavage fluid: effect of the glucocorticoid budesonide. *J. Allergy Clin. Immunol.* **85**, 891–5.

Björksten, F. and Suoniemi, I. (1976). Dependence of immediate hypersensitivity on the month of birth. *Clin. Allergy* **6**, 165–71.

Björksten, F., Suoniemi, I. and Koski, V. (1980). Neonatal birch pollen contact and subsequent allergy to birch pollen. *Clin.*

Allergy **10**, 585–91.

Blair, H. (1974). The incidence of asthma, hay fever and infantile eczema in an East London Group Practice of 9,145 patients. *Clin. Allergy* **4**, 389.

Bousquet, J., Fontez, A., Aznar, R., Robinet-Levey, M. and Michel, F.B. (1987). Combinations of passive and active immunization in honey bee venom immunotherapy. *J. Allergy Clin. Immunol.* **79**, 947–54.

Brown, H.M., Engler, G. and English, J.R. (1981). A comparative trial of flunisolide and sodium cromoglycate nasal sprays in the treatment of seasonal allergic rhinitis. *Clin. Allergy* **11**, 169.

Burr, M.L., Dean, V.B., Merrett, T.G., Neale, E., St Leger, A.S. and Verrier-Jones, E.R. (1980). Effects of anti-mite measures on children with mite-sensitive asthma: a controlled trial. *Thorax* **35**, 506–12.

Coffman, R.L. and Carty, J. (1986). A T cell activity that enhances polyclonal IgE production and its inhibition by interferon-gamma. *J. Immunol.* **136**, 949–56.

Cogswell, J.J., Mitchell, E.B. and Alexander, J. (1987). Parental smoking, breast feeding and respiratory infection in development of allergic disease. *Arch. Dis. Child.* **62**, 338–44.

Colloff, M.J., Lever, R.S. and McSharry, C. (1989). A controlled trial of house dust mite eradication using natamycin in homes of patients with atopic dermatitis: effect on clinical status and mite populations. *Br. J. Dermatol.* **121**, 199–208.

Connell, J.T. (1968). Quantitative intranasal pollen challenge. II. Effect of daily pollen challenge, environmental pollen exposure, and placebo challenge on the nasal membrane. *J. Allergy* **41**, 123–39.

Connell, J.T. (1969). Quantitative intranasal pollen challenge. III. The proming effect in allergic rhinitis. *J. Allergy* **43**, 33–44.

CSM Update (1986). Desensitising vaccines. *Br. Med. J.* **293**, 948.

De Monchy, J.G.R., Kauffman, H.F., Venge, P. *et al.* (1985). Bronchoalveolar eosinophils during allergen-induced late asthmatic reactions. *Am. Rev. Respir. Dis.* **131**, 373–6.

Del Prete, G.F., De Carli, M., Mastromauro, C. *et al.* (1991). Purified protein derivative of *Mycobacterium tuberculosis* and excretory-secretory antigen(s) of *Toxocara canis* expand *in vitro* human T cells with stable and opposite (type 1 helper or type 2 helper) profile of cytokine production. *J. Clin. Invest.* **88**, 346–50.

Dvoracek, J.E., Yunginger, J.W., Kern, E.B., Hyatt, R.E. and Gleich, G.J. (1984). Induction of nasal late-phase reactions by insufflation of ragweed-pollen extract. *J. Allergy Clin. Immunol.* **73**, 363–8.

EAACI Immunotherapy Sub-committee (1988). Immunotherapy position paper (ed. H.-J. Malling). *Allergy* **43** (suppl. 6), 1–33.

Enerback, L., Pipkorn, U. and Granerus, G. (1986). Intraepithelial migration of nasal mucosal mast cells in hay fever. *Int. Arch. Allergy Appl. Immunol.* **80**, 44–54.

Ewan, P.W. (1984). Clinical features, natural history and immunological studies in insect sting allergy. *Q. J. Med.* **52**, 542–43.

Ewan, P.W. and Coote, D. (1990). Evaluation of a capsulated hydrophilic carrier polymer (the ImmunoCAP) for measurement of specific IgE antibodies. *Allergy* **45**, 22–9.

Ewan, P.W. and Stewart, A.G. (1992). A prospective study of systemic reactions to venom immunotherapy. *Clin. Exp. Allergy* (in press).

Ewan, P.W., Deighton, J., Wilson, A.B. and Lachmann, P.J. (1992). Venom specific IgG antibodies in bee and wasp allergy: lack of correlation with protection from stings. Submitted.

Ewan, P.W., Alexander, M.M., Snape, C., Ind, C., Agrell, B. and Dreborg, S. (1988a). Effective hyposensitisation in allergic rhinitis using a potent partially purified extract of house dust mite. *Clin. Allergy* **18**, 501–8.

Ewan, P.W., Lavelle, B.M., Snape, C., Alexander, M.M., Agrell, B. and Dreborg, S. (1988b). An analysis of reactions to three house dust mite desensitisation regimens. *Allergy* **43** (suppl. 7), 43.

Ewan, P.W., McHugh, S.M. and Romero, C. (1990). Defective interferon-gamma production in house dust mite allergy. *Clin. Exp. Allergy* **20** (suppl. 1), 50.

Finkelman, F.D., Katona, I.M., Urban, J.F., Jr, Snapper, C.M., Ohara, J. and Paul, W.E. (1986). Suppression of *in vivo* polyclonal IgE responses by monoclonal antibody to the lymphokine B-cell stimulatory factor I. *Proc. Nat. Acad. Sci. (USA)* **83**, 9675–80.

Fleming, D.M. and Crombie, D.L. (1987). Prevalence of asthma and hay fever in England and Wales. *Br. Med. J.* **294**, 279–83.

Flower, R.J. (1988). Lipocortin and the mechanism of action of the glucocorticoids. *Br. J. Pharmacol.* **94**, 987–1015.

Frankland, A.W. and Augustin, R. (1954). Prophylaxis of summer hay fever and asthma. *Lancet* **i**, 1054–57.

Frankland, A.W. and Walker, S.R. (1975). A comparison of intranasal betamethasone valerate and sodium cromoglycate in seasonal allergic rhinitis. *Clin. Allergy* **5**, 295.

Freeland, J., Pipkorn, U., Proud, D. *et al.* (1989). Leukotriene B4 and a mediator of early and late reactions to antigen in humans: the effect of specific glucocorticoid treatment *in vivo*. *J. Allergy* **83**, 634–42.

Frick, O.L., German, D.F. and Mills, J. (1979). Development of allergy in children. I. Association with virus infection. *J. Allergy Clin. Immunol.* **63**, 228–41.

Gerblich, A.A., Schwartz, H.J. and Chester, E.H. (1986). Seasonal variation of airway function in allergic rhinitis. *J. Allergy Clin. Immunol.* **77**, 676–81.

Godfrey, K. (1991). House dust mite avoidance — the way forward. *Clin. Exp. Allergy* **21**, 1–2.

Golden, D.B., Myers, D.A., Kagey-Sobotka, A., Valentine, M.D. and Lichtenstein, L.M. (1982). Clinical relevance of the venom-specific immunoglobulin G antibody level during immunotherapy. *J. Allergy Clin. Immunol.* **69**, 489–93.

Goulding, N.J., Godolphin, J.L., Sharland, P.R. *et al.* (1990). Anti-inflammatory lipocortin 1 production by peripheral blood leucocytes in response to hydrocortisone. *Lancet* **335**, 1416–18.

Gurka, G., Ohman, J. and Rosenwasser, L.J. (1987). Human T cell clones specific for a mouse urinary protein allergen. *J. Allergy Clin. Immunol.* **79**, 179 (abstract).

Gurka, G., Kalluri, A., McDonald, B., Ohman, J. Jr, Feigelson, P. and Rosenwasser, L.J. (1988). Allergen specific T cell clones can be utilized to map allergenic epitopes for T cell activation. *J. Allergy Clin. Immunol.* **81**, 195 (abstract).

Hedlin, G., Graff-Lonnevig, V., Heilborn, H. *et al.* (1986). Immunotherapy with cat- and dog-dander extracts: *in vivo* and *in vitro* immunologic effects observed in a 1-year double-blind placebo study. *J. Allergy Clin. Immunol.* **77**, 488–96.

Henocq, E. and Rihoux, J.-P. (1990). Does reversed-type anaphylaxis in healthy subjects mimic a real allergic reaction? *Clin. Exp. Allergy* **20**, 269–72.

Henocq, E. and Vargaftig, B.B. (1986). Accumulation of eosinophils in response to intracutaneous PAF-acether and allergens in man. *Lancet* **i**, 1378–9.

Hsieh, K.H. (1985). Altered interleukin-2 (IL-2) production and responsiveness after hyposensitization to house dust. *J. Allergy Clin. Immunol.* **76**, 188–94.

Hunt, K.J., Valentine, M.D., Sobotka, A.K., Benton, A.W., Amodio, F.J. and Lichtenstein, L.M. (1978). A controlled trial of immunotherapy in insect hypersensitivity. *N. Engl. J. Med.* **299**, 157.

Hutson, P.A., Holgate, S.T. and Church, M.K. (1988). The effect of cromolyn sodium and albuterol on early and late phase broncho constriction and airway leukocyte infiltration after allergen challenge on non-anaesthetized guinea pigs. *Am. Rev. Respir. Dis.* **138**, 1157–63.

Johnsen, N.J. and Mygind, N. (1978). Incidence of latent and clinical respiratory allergy in medical students. *Ugeskrift Laeger* **140**, 597.

Kapsenberg, M.L., Weirenga, E.A., Bos, J.D. and Jansen, H.M. (1991). Functional subsets of allergen-reactive human CD4+ T cells. *Immunol. Today* **12**, 392–5.

Kjellman, N.-I.M. (1976). Predictive value of high IgE in children. *Acta Paediatr. Scand.* **65**, 463.

Kjellman, N.-I.M. (1988). Epidemiology and prevention of allergy. *Allergy* **43** (suppl. 8), 39–40.

Kniest, F.M., Young, E., Van Praag, M.C.G. *et al.* (1991). Clinical evaluation of a double-blind dust-mite avoidance trial with mite-allergic rhinitic patients. *Clin. Exp. Allergy* **21**, 39–48.

Korsgaard, J. (1982). Preventative measures in house dust allergy. *Am. Rev. Respir. Dis.* **125**, 80–84.

Lavker, R.M. and Schechter, N.M. (1985). Cutaneous mast cell depletion results from topical steroid usage. *J. Immunol.* **135**, 2868–73.

Liu, C.M. and Okuda, M. (1988). Injurious effect of eosinophil extract on the human nasal mucosa. *Rhinology* **26**, 121–32.

McHugh, S.M. and Ewan, P.W. (1989). Reduction of increased serum neutrophil chemotactic activity following effective hyposensitisation in house dust mite allergy. *Clin. Exp. Allergy* **19**, 327–31.

McHugh, S.M., Lachmann, P.J. and Ewan, P.W. (1992a). Peripheral blood mononuclear cells from house dust mite allergic patients produce IL-2 in response to specific allergen challenge. *Clin. Exp. Allergy* (in press).

McHugh, S.M., Wilson, A.B., Deighton, J., Lachmann, P.J. and Ewan, P.W. (1992b). IL-2, IL-6 and IFN-γ profiles from peripheral blood mononuclear cells of house dust mite allergic patients: a major role for IL-6 in allergic disease. Submitted.

McHugh, S.M., Lavelle, B., Kemeny, D.M., Patel, S. and Ewan, P.W. (1990). A placebo-controlled trial of immunotherapy with two extracts of *Dermatophagoides pteronyssinus* in allergic rhinitis, comparing clinical outcome with changes in antigen-specific IgE, IgG and IgG subclasses. *J. Allergy Clin. Immunol.* **86**, 521–31.

Madonini, E., Briatico-Vangosa, G., Pappacoda, A., Maccagni, G., Cardani, A. and Saporiti, F. (1987). Seasonal increase of bronchial reactivity in allergic rhinitis. *J. Allergy Clin. Immunol.* **79**, 358–63.

Maggi, E., Parronchi, P., Manetti, R. *et al.* (1992). Reciprocal regulatory effects of IFN-γ and IL-4 on the *in vitro* development of human T_H1 and T_H2 clones. *J. Immunol.* **148**, 2142–7.

Marsh, D.E. (1975). Allergens and the genetics of allergy. In *The Antigens*, ed. M. Sela, vol. III, pp. 271–359, Academic Press, New York.

Meltzer, E.O., Zeiger, R.S., Schatz, M. and Jalowayski, A. (1983). Chronic rhinitis in infants and children: etiologic, diagnostic, and therapeutic considerations. *Pediatr. Clin. North Am.* **30**, 847–71.

Miadonna, A., Tedeschi, A., Leggieri, E., Lorini, M., Folco, G. and Saia, A. (1987). Behaviour and clinical relevance of histamine and leukotrienes C_4 and B_4 in grass pollen-induced rhinitis. *Am. Rev. Respir. Dis.* **136**, 357–62.

Morrow Brown, H. and Merrett, T.G. (1990). The indirect effects of acarosan on mite allergic patients — a clinical study. *Clin. Exp. Allergy* **20** (suppl. 1), 118 (abstract).

Mosmann, T.R., Cherwinski, H., Bond, M.M., Giedin, M.A. and Coffman, R.L. (1986). Two types of murine helper T cell clone: 1. Definition according to the profiles of lymphokine activities and secreted proteins. *J. Immunol.* **136**, 2348–57.

Müller, U.R., Morris, T., Bishof, M. *et al.* (1986). Combined active and passive immunotherapy in honey bee immunotherapy. *J. Allergy Clin. Immunol.* **78**, 115.

Naclerio, R.M., Meier, H.L., Adkinson, N.F., Jr *et al.* (1983a). *In vivo* demonstration of inflammatory mediator release following nasal challenge with antigen. *Eur. J. Respir. Dis.* **64** (suppl. 128), 26.

Naclerio, R.M., Meier, H.L., Kagey-Sobotka, A. *et al.* (1983b). Mediator release after nasal airway challenge with allergen. *Am. Rev. Respir. Dis.* **128**, 597–602.

Nagakura, T., Iikura, Y., Onda, T. *et al.* (1989). Release of high-molecular-weight neutrophil chemotactic activity from resected human nasal turbinate after antigen challenge. *J. Allergy Clin. Immunol.* **83**, 656–62.

Nagaya, H. (1985). Induction of antigen-specific suppressor cells in patients with hay fever receiving immunotherapy. *J. Allergy Clin. Immunol.* **75**, 388–96.

Nakagawa, T., Kozeki, H., Katagiri, J. *et al.* (1987). Changes of house dust mite-specific IgE, IgG and IgG subclass antibodies during immunotherapy in patients with perennial rhinitis. *Int. Arch. Allergy Appl. Immunol.* **82**, 95–9.

Nickelson, J.A., Georgitis, J.W. and Reisman, R.E. (1986). Lack of correlation between titers of serum allergen-specific IgE and symptoms in untreated patients with seasonal allergic rhinitis. *J. Allergy Clin. Immunol.* **77**, 43–8.

Noon, L. (1911). Prophylactic innoculation against hay fever. *Lancet* **i**, 1572–3.

Otsuka, H., Dolovich, J., Befus, A.D., Telizyn, S., Bienenstock, J. and Denburg, J.A. (1986). Basophilic cell progenitors, nasal metachromatic cells and peripheral blood basophils in ragweed allergic patients. *J. Allergy Clin. Immunol.* **78**, 365–71.

Parkin, J.M., Eales, L.J., Galazka, A.R. and Pinching, A.J. (1987). Atopic manifestations in the acquired immunodeficiency syndrome: response to recombinant interferon gamma. *Br Med. J.* **294**, 1185–6.

Patterson, R., Lieberman, P., Irons, S.S. *et al.* (1978). Immunotherapy. In *Allergy: Principles and Practice*, ed. E. Middleton, C.E. Reed and E.F. Ellis, pp. 877–898, C.V. Mosby, Missouri.

Phillips, L., Chambers, C., Underdown, B.J. and Zimmerman, B. (1987). Lymphocyte proliferation to antigen E: demonstration of the restriction of antigen E-specific T cells to ragweed-allergic donors. *J. Allergy Clin. Immunol.* **79**, 933–1001.

Pipkorn, U., Proud, D., Kagey-Sobotlea, A., Wormen, P.S. Lichtenstein, L.M. and Neclerio, R.M. (1987a). Effect of short-term systemic glucocorticoid treatment on human nasal mediator release after antigen challenge. *J. Clin. Invest.* **80**, 957–61.

Pipkorn, U., Proud, D. and Lichtenstein, L.M. *et al.* (1987b). Topical nasal steroid pretreatment inhibits mediator release *in vivo*. *N. Engl. J. Med.* **316**, 1506–10.

Pipkorn, U., Karlsson, G. and Enerbäck, L. (1988a). The cellular response of the human allergic mucosa to natural allergen exposure. *J. Allergy Clin. Immunol.* **82**, 1046–54.

Pipkorn, U., Karlsson, G. and Enerbäck, L. (1988b). Secretory activity of nasal mucosal mast cells and histamine release in hay fever. *Int. Arch. Allergy Appl. Immunol.* **87**, 349–60.

Platts-Mills, T.A.E., Tovey, E.R., Mitchell, E.B., Moszoro, M.H., Nock, P. and Wilkins, S.R. (1982). Reduction of bronchial hyperreactivity during prolonged allergen avoidance. *Lancet*, **ii**, 675–8.

Platts-Mills, T.A.E., Hayden, M.L., Chapman, M.D. and Wilkins, S.R. (1986). Seasonal variation in dust mite and grass pollen allergens in dust from the houses of patients with asthma. *J. Allergy Clin. Immunol.* **79**, 781–91.

Rak, S., Hakansson, L. and Venge, P. (1987). Eosinophil chemotactic activity in allergic patients during the birch pollen season: the effect of immunotherapy. *Int. Arch. Allergy Appl. Immunol.* **82**, 349–50.

Rantakallio, P. (1978). Relationship of maternal smoking to morbidity and mortality of the child up to age five. *Acta Paediatr. Scand.* **67**, 621–31.

Rawle, F.C., Mitchell, E.B. and Platts-Mills, T.A.E. (1984). T cell responses to the major allergen from the house dust mite *Dermatophagoides pteronyssinus*, antigen P1: comparison of patients with asthma, atopic dermatitis, and perennial rhinitis. *J. Immunol.* **133**, 195–201.

Reiser, J., Ingram, D., Mitchell, E.B. and Warner, J.O. (1990). House dust mite allergen levels and an anti-mite mattress spray (Natamycin) in the treatment of childhood asthma. *Clin. Exp. Allergy* **20**, 561–7.

Rocklin, R.E., Sheffer, A.L., Greineder, D.R. and Melmon, K.L. (1980). Generation of antigen-specific suppressor cells during allergy desensitization. *N. Engl. J. Med.* **302**, 1213–19.

Romagnani, S. (1991). Human T_H1 and T_H2 subsets: doubt no more. *Immunol. Today* **12**, 256–7.

Sarsfield, J.K., Gowland, G., Toy, R. and Normal, A.L. (1974). Mite-sensitive asthma of childhood: trial of avoidance measures. *Arch. Dis. Child.* **49**, 711–16.

Shaw, R.J., Fitzharris, P., Cromwell, O., Wardlaw, A.J. and Kay, A.B. (1985). Allergen-induced release of sulphidopeptide leukotrienes (SRS-A) and LTB_4 in allergic rhinitis. *Allergy* **40**, 1–6.

Sibbald, B. and Rink, E. (1991). Labelling of hay fever and rhinitis. *Thorax* **5**, 378–81.

Sipila, P., Sorni, M., Ojala, K. (1983). Comparative trial of flunisolide and beclomethasone dipropionate nasal sprays in patients with seasonal allergic rhinitis. *Allergy*, **38**, 303.

Solley, G.O., Gleich, G.J., Jordon, R.E. and Schroeter, A.L. (1976). The late phase of the immediate wheal and flare skin reaction: its dependence upon IgE antibodies. *J. Clin. Invest.* **58**, 408–20.

Umemoto, L., Poothullil, J., Dolovich, J. and Hargreave, F.E. (1976). Factors which influence late cutaneous allergic responses. *J. Allergy Clin. Immunol.* **58**, 60–8.

van Bever, H.P., Bosmans, J., De Clerck, L.S. and Stevens, W.J. (1988). Modification of the late asthmatic reaction by hyposensitisation in asthmatic children allergic to house dust mite (*Dermatophagoides pteronyssinus*) or grass pollen. *Allergy* **43**, 378–85.

Varney, V.A., Gaga, M., Frew, A.J., Aber, V.R., Kay, A.B. and Durham, S.R. (1991). Usefulness of immunotherapy in patients with severe summer hay fever uncontrolled by anti-allergic drugs. *Br. Med. J.* **302**, 265–9.

Viegas, M., Gomez, E., Brooks, J. and Davies, R.J. (1987). Changes in nasal mast cell numbers in and out of the pollen season. *Int. Arch. Allergy Appl. Immunol.* **82**, 275–6.

Wachs, M., Proud, D., Lichtenstein, L.M., Kagey-Sobotka, A., Norman, P.S. and Naclerio, R.M. (1989). Observations on the pathogenesis of nasal priming. *J. Allergy Clin. Immunol.* **84**, 492–501.

Walshaw, M.J. and Evans, C.C. (1986). Allergen avoidance in house dust mite-sensitive adult asthma. *Quart. J. Med.* **58**, 199–215.

Warner, J.O., Price, J.F., Soothill, J.F. and Hay, E.N. (1978). Controlled trial of hyposensitisation to *Dermatophagoides pteronyssinus* in children with asthma. *Lancet* **ii**, 912–5.

Weirenga, E.A., Snoek, M., de Groot, C. *et al.* (1990). Evidence for compartmentalization of functional subsets of CD4+ T lymphocytes in atopic patients. *J. Immunol.* **144**, 4651–6.

Welliver, R.C., Wong, D.T., Sun, M., Middleton, E., Jr, Vaughan, R.S. and Ogra, P.L. (1981). The development of respiratory syncytial virus-specific IgE and the release of histamine in nasopharyngeal secretions after infection. *N. Engl. J. Med.* **305**, 841–6.

Welsh, P.W., Stricker, W.E., Chu, C.-P., Naessens, J.M., Reese, M.E. and Reed, C.E. (1987). Efficacy of beclomethasone nasal solution, flunisolide and cromolyn in relieving symptoms of ragweed allergy. *Mayo Clin. Proc.* **62**, 125–34.

WHO report (1986). The prevention of allergic diseases: epidemiological and socio-economic aspects of allergic diseases. *Clin. Allergy* **16** (suppl.), 11–7.

Wide, L., Bennich, H. and Johansson, S.G.O. (1967). Diagnosis of allergy by an *in vitro* test for allergen antibodies. *Lancet* **ii**, 1105–7.

Wood, S.F. (1986). Oral antihistamine or nasal steroid in hay fever: a double-blind double-dummy comparative study of once daily oral astemizole vs twice daily nasal beclomethasone dipropionate. *Clin. Allergy* **16**, 195–201.

Young, P. (1980). *Asthma and Allergies: an Optimistic Future.* US Department of Health and Human Services, US Public Health Service, National Institutes of Health, DIHN, 80–388.

Yssel, H., Gasean, H., Schneider, P.V. *et al.* (1990). *Der p* I specific T cell clones selectively produce extremely high levels of IL-4 which is associated with enhanced IgE synthesis. *Clin. Exp. Allergy* **20** (suppl. 1), 6.

56: Food Allergy and Intolerance

M.H. Lessof

Introduction

Food allergy is now recognized as an immunologically determined form of specific food intolerance. Allergic and other immunological responses are not, however, the only mechanisms involved in protecting the integrity of the gastrointestinal mucosal barrier, and adverse reactions to food may depend on a wide range of other factors. Both immunological and non-immunological mechanisms can also provoke adverse effects in other parts of the body.

In terms of the sheer bulk of its lymphoid tissue, the gastrointestinal tract is the body's largest immunological organ. The gut may have to handle about 100 tons of food during a lifetime (Johansson *et al.* 1984) and its lymphoid tissue therefore has an outstanding role in host defence. The specialized epithelium on the surface of its lymphoid aggregates can sample both the particulate and the soluble antigens which are present in the lumen. Microfold (M) cells present antigen to the underlying macrophages and trigger both T cell and B cell activity, resulting in the release of a number of products, including secretory immunoglobulin A (IgA) (Targan 1987). Antigen-activated Peyer's patch T and B cells proliferate, migrate through the lymphatics to the bloodstream, and after terminal differentiation finally seed themselves back into the mucosal lymphoid tissues.

Apart from secretory IgA, IgE responses also play a prominent part in the gastrointestinal tract, notably in parasitic infections and in gastrointestinal allergy. About 2% of intestinal B cells produce IgE and the intestinal IgE response is known to be stimulated by T cell factors. Atopic individuals may inherit a suppressor cell defect which prevents them from down-regulating IgE-mediated responses (Geha 1985).

There is a sharp rise in both circulating eosinophils and serum IgE levels in human infection with *Trichinella spiralis* and other parasites. When anti-IgE is administered to *Trichinella*-infected rats, both the eosinophil response and the control of the parasitic infection have been shown to be impaired (Capron *et al.* 1986). There is, however, a distinction between the responses to micro-organisms or parasites, on the one hand, and food antigens, on the other. There is clear evidence that orally administered antigens can induce tolerance by inducing suppressor T cells, especially within the Peyer's patch (Titus and Chiller 1981), but questions remain about the conditions which determine this type of response. Although little is known about most of the factors involved, a failure of antigen exclusion (see Table 56.1) can affect the response and has been studied in some detail.

The mucous coat in the microvillous border is an important physical barrier to bacterial attachment and acts as a sieve, excluding large molecules or trapping particles non-specifically. Several mucus constituents interfere with the ability of bacteria to bind to mucosal cells, notably by offering harmless attachment sites, not only for bacteria and other pathogens but also for lectins and toxins. In IgE-mediated disease, the release of mast cell histamine leads to a further release of mucus from goblet cells. In addition, leucotrienes and mast cell mediators stimulate gut motility and so diminish the period of exposure during which antigen penetration might otherwise occur, especially in conditions in which mucous membrane permeability has been increased by malnutrition, infection or gastrointestinal disease.

In spite of this defensive system, food antigens have been shown to penetrate the mucosal barrier of normal, healthy subjects. The classical experiments of Brunner and Walzer (1928) showed that the serum of fish-allergic individuals could be used to transfer skin sensitivity to healthy volunteers and that 62 out of 65 individuals who were sensitized in this way developed a weal and flare response at the sensitized site within an hour of eating raw fish. This suggests that some antigens gain access to the circulation by crossing the gut mucous membrane and evading the mechanisms whereby antigens provoke immune complex formation and are removed by Kupffer cell phagocytosis in the liver.

Adverse reactions to foods

Adverse reactions to foods include IgE-mediated and other immunological reactions as well as a wide range of toxicological, pharmacological and other disorders. Adverse effects which involve gastrointestinal motility lead to symptoms which are not sufficiently specific to provide a clear indication of the mechanisms involved. Even features such as asthma and urticaria, which suggest an IgE-mediated sensitivity, do not always imply an immunological cause. Asthma can be provoked by the direct toxic effect of inhaled sulphur dioxide, arising from foods which have been preserved by metabisulphite. Pharmacological effects can also occur, as in the vasodilator action of nitrite additives. Several other adverse effects of food additives have been reported, without evidence of an immunological cause, and even in conditions like gluten enteropathy (see Chapter 105) the presence of immunological abnormalities can be accompanied by a non-immunological type of food intolerance — in this case intolerance to disaccharides caused by microvillous damage and the enzyme deficiencies which result from this. Test methods which rely exclusively on demonstrating an IgE response or some other immunological abnormality may therefore be inadequate for diagnostic purposes.

Table 56.1. Intestinal tract: causes of failure of antigen exclusion

Immaturity
Hypogammaglobinaemias (notably IgA deficiency)
Protein malnutrition
Allergic reactions
Inflammatory bowel disease and gluten enteropathy
Effects of toxins and drugs

Pathogenesis of food allergies

The gastrointestinal tract is normally able to discriminate between food antigens, which induce tolerance, and toxic or infective agents, which provoke a whole range of immunological reactions and inflammatory responses. This discriminating ability depends on the genetic make-up and nutritional status of the individual and on the intact state of the mucosal barrier. It can be influenced by the effects of lectins, infection or toxins and by the nature of the antigen. It can probably also be influenced by the route of entry of the allergen, since allergy to ingested eggs can accompany the occupational development of respiratory allergy to avian proteins (Hoffman and Guenther 1988). In neonates factors such as immaturity, a family history of atopy, and infective gastroenteritis all predispose to a relatively high prevalence of cow's milk protein intolerance, which has been identified in between 0.3% and 12% of various groups of children (Bahna and Heiner 1978). It has been reported that hypersensitivity reactions are more likely to occur in infants who have a transient IgA deficiency (Taylor *et al.* 1973), an observation which accords with other suggestive evidence that allergic reactions are more common in immunodeficient individuals. It has also been noted very frequently that the symptoms of cow's milk intolerance can appear for the first time after a bout of infective gastroenteritis (Hager *et al.* 1987). This has led to increasing caution in the reintroduction of cow's milk feeding after bouts of gastroenteritis in infants.

The nature of the antigen itself can be crucial, as has been shown by studies of infants with immediate reactions to untreated or pasteurized cow's milk who, on skin testing and challenge tests, elicit no reaction to cow's milk protein hydrolysate (Host and Samuelsson 1988). Protein hydrolysates may not offer a complete answer, however. When hospital-treated infants with gastroenteritis were deliberately given a protein hydrolysate formula for 6 weeks after their admission to hospital, secondary cow's milk protein hypersensitivity still occurred in two cases out of 24 infants so treated (Hager *et al.* 1987).

The protective effect of breast milk can be important in infants. Immunoglobulin A, which is less readily digested than other immunoglobulins, is present in very high concentrations in milk, and breast milk also contains lymphocytes and nonspecific immune factors such as macrophages, lysozyme, lactoferrin and complement components. Breast milk therefore has advantages over bottled feeds, not only in sterility but also as an anti-infective agent.

About a third of children with cow's milk protein hypersensitivity have reactions which develop within about 45 minutes (Firer *et al.* 1987). All but four of the 15 children with immediate reactions studied by Firer had high IgE antibody levels to cow's milk but — apart from children with eczema — there was no evidence that late reactions were IgE-mediated. The lack of evidence of an IgE reaction in many cases has led to a search for other mechanisms.

In children (but not in adults) there is good evidence that cow's milk can cause small intestinal mucosal damage, and this has been demonstrated by serial small intestinal biopsies before and after dietary exclusion and food challenge (Walker-Smith 1986). Egg, soya, rice, chicken and fish can all cause a similar hypersensitive enteropathy, which is patchy and accompanied by an increase in intraepithelial lymphocytes and by damage to the microvilli but is generally much less severe than in gluten enteropathy.

The nature of the atopic mucosal changes in the small bowel following exposure to cow's milk is still unclear (Iyngkaran *et al.* 1979) and it is possible that, in a few such cases, mucosal damage may precede the development of cow's milk protein intolerance. The mucosal changes described are usually non-specific, and apart from the more grossly atrophic changes there is generally an increase in crypt depth and some blunting of the villi. It still remains to be established whether they relate directly to reactions involving reaginic, cytotoxic, immune complex or T-cell-mediated hypersensitivity.

Food intolerance is also an important cause of infantile colitis. In one study of eight infants with continuing bloody diarrhoea associated with inflammatory infiltration in the lamina propria and mild ulceration, the replacement of milk feeds with soya milk resulted in a prompt recovery (Jenkins *et al.* 1984).

Many of the more general observations that have been made concerning intolerant reactions to foods have been extrapolated from the childhood example of cow's milk protein intolerance to the adult population. This also applies to those gastrointestinal symptoms which, in the adult, are often grouped together as the irritable bowel syndrome. When adults with alactasia are unable to break down lactose, it reaches the colon as an unabsorbed food residue and is there fermented by gas-producing bacteria, forming propionic acid and other irritant substances. Lactose intolerance is less common in infants and, when Donovan and Torres-Pinedo (1987) investigated children with persistent diarrhoea following gastroenteritis, they found evidence that the persistence of this diarrhoea was due to the use of a soya protein formula containing sucrose and dextromaltose. These adverse reactions could be prevented when these sugars were replaced by lactose, suggesting that other disaccharides may cause more problems than lactose itself. There is other evidence that, except in cow's milk-sensitive subjects, soya-based compounds have no advantages — and may have disadvantages — in infant feeding (Miskelly *et al.* 1988), but this appears to be the first evidence that the non-lactose sugars used in these preparations can increase the incidence of complications.

Food antigens

Most allergic reactions to food appear to involve a limited number of food substances — cow's milk, egg, nuts, fish and shellfish, soya and wheat. The allergens involved appear to share a number of characteristics (Metcalfe 1984). They are generally heat- and acid-stable glycoproteins with a molecular weight in the range of 18 000 to 36 000 daltons. Their clinical importance varies with the food habits of each particular society. Peanut hypersensitivity is relatively common in Britain and the United States but not in Sweden. Rice hypersensitivity is not uncommon in Japan but rare in Western countries. The foods which are most commonly involved have been summarized in Table 56.2. While lists of this kind can be helpful by drawing attention to foods which are capable of causing very severe reactions that might not otherwise be suspected (for example, celery, mustard, sesame seeds), it should be recognized that exclusion diets (discussed below) may need to eliminate not only the main ingredients which have been identified, but also a number of immunologically related substances or substances which contain a widely used additive.

Cross-reactions between related food substances are not uncommon. Soy bean and peanut are both legumes, and peanut-sensitive individuals frequently report an associated intolerance to other legumes or to other nuts. Attempts have been made to identify major component proteins which may be chiefly responsible for food-allergic responses and, since soy bean is used in many commercial foods, detailed studies have been carried out on the antigenic components of soy bean (Burks *et al.* 1988). Although soy bean trypsin inhibitor has been incriminated in one patient's severe allergic reactions to soya (Moroz and Yang 1980), it is clear that there is considerable cross-reactivity between different globulins present and that no single antigenic component can account for allergenic responses in all individuals. Examination of the antigens in milk and in egg (Clinton *et al.* 1986) has led to similar evidence for the presence of several antigenic components in a single food.

Table 56.2. Foods provoking intolerant reactions

Common
Milk, egg, fish and shellfish, nuts and peanuts
Wheat (and other cereals, flour, yeast)
Soya. Pork, bacon, tenderized meats. Food additives (colours and preservatives). Chocolate, coffee, tea
Citrus fruits

Other
Apple and other fruits (banana, berries, chestnut, mango, peach, strawberries)
Aniseed and other seeds (carraway, dill, millet, sesame, poppy, sunflower)
Herbs and spices (bay leaf, cinnamon, clove, garlic, ginger, mint, mustard, nutmeg, sage, thyme)

When food reactions are based on an immunological response, the component involved is usually a protein. Reactions induced by food additives often involve low-molecular-weight substances, however. Sodium nitrite can have vasodilator effects and high concentrations of monosodium glutamate may possibly act as an oesophageal irritant (Smith *et al.* 1982).

Clinical features

There has been a wide discrepancy between the public perception of allergy to food and food additives and the medical profession's view of the problem. A population survey carried out by Young *et al.* (1987) indicated that, of 30 000 people covered by a postal survey, 2890 (9.6%) perceived themselves to have allergy or sensitivity to specific foods, while 1372 (4.6%) thought they were sensitive to food additives. In order to investigate food additive sensitivity, attempts were made at a special clinic to assess those individuals with a suggestive history and, where appropriate, to use challenge tests with five mixtures of food additives. When assessed both clinically and by measuring blood and urine levels of histamine and prostanoids, the diagnosis of intolerance to food additives could be confirmed in only three cases. Subsequently, two additional individuals were shown to have metabisulphite-induced asthma, which was not tested in the original survey (E. Young, personal communication). While accepting that challenge tests may sometimes give falsely negative results, the discrepancy between public perception and confirmed disease was very substantial.

Leaving aside false perceptions about the nature

of a specific food-intolerant reaction, a firm diagnosis is made more difficult by the wide range of symptoms which may be provoked. A diagnosis of food allergy is easily made if a man's lips swell, his mouth and throat tingle, and he develops blebs of mucosal swelling on the inside of the cheeks within minutes of eating a meal. As Amlot (1985) has shown, this 'oral allergy syndrome' correlates closely with the presence of IgE antibodies to the food concerned, and so do other clinical features such as urticaria, asthma, anaphylaxis (less specifically), nausea and vomiting (see Table 56.3). Those with immediate allergic problems of this kind usually make their own diagnosis and often solve their problems without medical help. Those with symptoms of late onset, however, seldom have evidence of an IgE reaction, as judged by skin prick test or radio-allergosorbent test. It is in these cases particularly that it may be difficult to establish whether there is an association of symptoms with a particular food. These are the cases in which an elimination diet is most useful, followed by the reintroduction of foods and a formal challenge test in those cases in which a recurrence of symptoms appears to be food-related.

Of those whose symptoms are reproducible, not all have problems caused by the food itself. Similar symptoms can be caused by repeated episodes of food poisoning or by the toxins which are naturally present in foods — glycoalkaloids present in certain potatoes, cyanogenic glycosides in Lima beans and millet sprouts, or toxins present in badly stored mackerel or other scombroid fish. The pharmacological effects of caffeine include irritability, tachycardia and sleep disturbance. Caffeine stimulates gastric secretion and can provoke oesophageal reflux, nausea, vomiting and diarrhoea (Turnberg 1978). As a diuretic, caffeine can also affect the consistency of the faeces and provoke colic and bloating. The clinician who wishes to concentrate on a study of the immunological aspects of food intolerance may therefore find that the differential diagnosis of reproducible food reactions cannot easily be confined to the immunological response.

Table 56.3. Clinical features of food-induced reactions

Gastrointestinal
Lip swelling, mucosal blebs, tingling of mouth and throat
Vomiting, diarrhoea, pain, bloating
Constipation
Steatorrhoea
Haemorrhagic colitis (infants)

Remote effects
Anaphylaxis, asthma
Rhinorrhoea, urticaria, angio-oedema
Headache, migraine, joint pains

Gastrointestinal symptoms also arise as a result of lactase deficiency, which affects up to 80% or more of many Asian and African communities, 5–20% or North American Caucasians and 3% of Danes (Gray 1980). The fermentation of unabsorbed lactose in the lower bowel produces lactic and propionic acid. Because of their irritant and osmotic effects, there follows the intestinal hurry, bloating and malabsorption which are sometimes seen in the irritable bowel syndrome. Similar symptoms have been linked in other cases with intolerance to cereal grains, coffee, tea, eggs and citrus fruits. Many of these patients have increased numbers of bacteria in their stool, suggesting that, in this case too, bacterial fermentation may play a part (Alun Jones 1985).

Some of the gastrointestinal symptoms which arise may be secondary to the loss of brush border enzymes, which occurs when the gastrointestinal mucosa is denuded by infectious diarrhoea, giardiasis or cow's milk protein reactions (Iyngkaran *et al*. 1979). In severe cases of mucosal damage, in conditions ranging from cholera and kwashiorkor to gluten enteropathy and tropical sprue, it appears that not only lactase but also sucrase and maltase may be deficient (Gray 1980).

Remote manifestations of food intolerance

Migraineurs who suffer headache after eating cheese or chocolate have evidence of an allergic reaction in some cases, while others may be responding to various platelet-activating factors which are present in a number of foods. Remote manifestations such as asthma can also occur either because of an immunological reaction or through the irritant effect of inhaled sulphur dioxide on hyper-reactive bronchi (Allen and Delohery 1985). The ability to achieve similar end-organ effects by both immunological and non-immunological mechanisms is also seen in the skin as exemplified by urticaria, which can be provoked not only by allergic mechanisms, but also by the enzyme-inhibitory effects of aspirin, or by temperature changes, local trauma and other physical mechanisms. Few of these mechanisms have been studied in any detail; they are poorly understood.

Asthma can also be provoked by more than one mechanism, and it is not always clear whether it is initiated by the inhalational or the alimentary route. The smell of fish can induce an immmediate asthmatic attack in fish-allergic individuals and there are other examples of this kind. Nevertheless, when asthma is provoked by foods containing sodium metabisulphite as a preservative, there is evidence that the sulphur dioxide which is released at a concentration of 1–3 ppm is sufficient to provoke bronchospasm in susceptible asthmatics because of its irritant effect (Allen and Delohery 1985). Some preserved foods, for example sulphited lettuce (Taylor *et al.* 1988), seem to be much more likely to provoke asthma than others. Most wines contain at least 100 mg/l of sulphur dioxide, but, of two individuals studied by Gershwin *et al.* (1985) who had reproducible asthma after drinking 4 oz. of white wine, one reacted to alcohol solution without sulphur dioxide (suitably disguised) while the other reacted only when metabisulphite was added. There are also many cases in which the provocation of an attack of asthma by the inhalational route seems unlikely because of the time interval, and in such cases preservatives are less likely to be involved. Several patients with milk intolerance have been described who have developed asthmatic reactions up to an hour or more after drinking cow's milk but who have negative IgE tests for cow's milk allergy and low total IgE levels (Lessof *et al.* 1980; Papageorgiou *et al.* 1983).

In addition to the reactions listed, there are a few conditions affecting other organs of the body which are sometimes — but not usually — provoked by food intolerance. An example is the nephrotic syndrome, in which there may occasionally be evidence of an IgE-mediated reaction to food, sometimes with a remission following the exclusion of such foods as cow's milk and a relapse following their reintroduction (Lagrue *et al.* 1987; Laurent *et al.* 1987; Williams 1987).

In some cases, the observations which have been made remain unexplained, for example the observation of Genova *et al.* (1987) that in 10 out of 12 cases in which the nephrotic syndrome appeared to be associated with food intolerance there was a massive submucosal lymphocytic infiltration on small bowel biopsy, sometimes associated with a reduced villus crypt ratio and submucosal fibrinogen deposits.

Arthralgia and, in exceptional cases, transient joint swellings can also be provoked by food (Denman 1987) but it is rare to find clear evidence that foods such as cow's milk can exacerbate more severe inflammatory joint diseases such as rheumatoid arthritis (Parke and Hughes 1981).

The similarity between immunological and non-immunological food reactions lies chiefly in their ability to produce the same end-organ effects through the release of inflammatory mediators. There is persuasive evidence that less potent inflammatory mediators are synthesized on a diet supplemented by fish oil as compared with a diet rich in animal fats (Lee *et al.* 1985) and this has encouraged a further examination of the influence of diet on joint disease. Nevertheless, the use of low-fat elimination diets have given disappointing results in rheumatoid arthritis (Denman *et al.* 1983).

Food intolerance in infancy and childhood

Reactions to cow's milk now provide the most studied examples of food intolerance. Whether they present with gastrointestinal symptoms, eczema, anaphylactic shock or even cot death, these conditions present considerable diagnostic problems. Although cow's milk protein hypersensitivity is recognized with increasing frequency, the affected infants and children are not a homogeneous group. Out of the 15 affected children reported by Firer *et al.* (1987) to have reactions of rapid onset which were thought to be IgE-mediated, 12 had an accompanying urticaria and another had asthma. The majority of children, however, developed their symptoms much later and had no clinical or laboratory evidence to suggest an IgE-mediated reaction.

Reactions in the skin can be difficult to analyse precisely. Those which develop within 1–2 hours tend to be urticarial and to be associated with an IgE response. Eczematous reactions are much more complex. Meara (1965) studied 29 children who had both eczema and a positive skin test to egg. Eleven improved on an egg-free diet but the reintroduction of egg caused urticaria in eight subjects and eczema in only two.

The mechanism by which skin reactions progress to eczema requires further study but, in patients with atopic eczema and high IgE levels, patch tests with antigens to which the patient is sensitive appear to provoke a local infiltration with basophils (Mitchell *et al.* 1982) and eosinophils (Bruynzeel-Koomen *et al.* 1988). In the epidermis, where activated eosinophils are present within 24 hours, electron-microscopic pictures show that there is close contact between some eosinophils and dendritic cells, suggesting a cell–cell interaction.

In childhood eczema occurring in the first year of life, the exacerbating effect of food may be especially important. The onset is sometimes related to the introduction of cow's milk, wheat or eggs, and the initial symptom may be pruritis or urticaria, followed by erythematous skin changes and then by typical eczema. In one study of a selected group of eczematous patients, an erythematous rash developed in about half of the subjects after double-blind food challenges, and elimination of the relevant foods led to an improvement in their eczema (Sampson 1983).

Additional reactions which may occur include angio-oedema, wheezing or even acute anaphylaxis. Reactions to egg and cow's milk can occur in entirely breast-fed infants, who have presumably become sensitized by egg and cow's milk antigens in breast milk, but this is not common (Matsumura *et al.* 1976; Björksten and Saarinen 1978). Controlled studies have shown the advantages of breast-feeding in infants of atopic families and it has been claimed that a controlled diet for the mother during lactation also has a highly protective effect (Businco *et al.* 1983). The problem of hypersensitivity to milk and eggs is not necessarily a lasting one, since allergy which develops in infancy does not always persist. Of six children with a previous allergy to eggs studied by Hattevig and colleagues (1987), only two retained their sensitivity by the age of 7 years.

When older asthmatic children were studied in a community survey, they seldom reported that food provoked coughing or wheezing. However, nearly three-quarters of children attending a hospital asthma clinic noted that wheezing could be precipitated by at least one food (Wilson 1985), especially milk, egg, nuts and iced or fizzy drinks. The symptoms tended to occur at night. It has been suggested that the mechanism may be an indirect one in some cases and that, in childhood asthma, food can often provoke an increase in bronchial reactivity rather than directly provoking an asthmatic episode (Wilson and Silverman 1985).

One other controversial claim has been made, that certain foods, artificial colours and preservatives may exacerbate or provoke behaviour disorders in children, who become over-active, destructive, impulsive and excitable (Egger *et al.* 1985). Price (1987) has reviewed the evidence which suggests that there is often a family history of similar behaviour problems and either evidence of developmental delay or of 'minimal brain dysfunction'. Tartrazine and other food colours have attracted much attention, but most double-blind studies either have given negative results (Mattes and Gittelman 1981) or have suggested that in only a few younger children is there an improvement on a restricted diet (Harley *et al.* 1978a, b). David (1987) studied 24 children who had been placed on an additive-free diet because their parents suspected a disturbed behavioural response to a food additive (usually tartrazine). After being given drinks containing first 50 mg and then 250 mg of tartrazine, followed by benzoate in some cases, none were found to react adversely and most resumed a normal diet without incident. Six children showed a disturbed pattern of behaviour that was unrelated to the challenge procedure. Nevertheless, three sets of parents refused the evidence of the tests and continued to impose dietary restrictions. At least some of these anomalous claims have been explained by the finding that there are parents who become obsessed by the belief that their healthy child suffers from food allergy when the problems are largely psychological and social. In some cases of 'Munchausen's disease by proxy' fanciful symptoms may be either imagined or fabricated (Warner and Hathaway 1984).

Clinical management

Diagnosis

For the purpose of clinical diagnosis, it is necessary to establish that a problem is food-related before considering whether it arises through immunological or other mechanisms. A double- or single-blind placebo-controlled oral food challenge remains the only definitive procedure for the diagnosis of food intolerance (Sampson *et al.* 1987).

Food allergy is diagnosed when, in addition, there is evidence that this food intolerance is based on an immunological reaction (see Table 56.4). Immunoglobulin E antibodies can nevertheless occur in the absence of clinical symptoms or persist after clinical sensitivity has been lost. Furthermore, individuals with clear evidence of an IgE-mediated sensitivity can have a negative response on one occasion but a life-threatening anaphylactic response on another, for example when exercise is taken after the ingestion of food.

In a study of children with atopic dermatitis, Sampson (1988b) showed that skin prick tests with commercially available preparations of egg, peanut, milk, wheat and chicken were almost totally reliable in excluding IgE-mediated food reactions when the test was negative but, because of the relatively frequent occurrence of positive reactions in individuals who had no symptoms, could merely be regarded as suggestive when a positive result was obtained. In screening patients with a suggestive history of food allergic reactions, it is nevertheless useful to carry out a battery of skin tests using these materials together with extracts of fish, shellfish, soya, mixed nuts and common inhaled allergens (e.g. grass pollen, dust mite, birch pollen and cat). In Sampson's study radioallergosorbent tests, whether taken alone or in combination with skin prick tests, could not provide a better prediction of clinical hypersensitivity than the skin test alone. In patients with an immediate reaction to foods, some support for the diagnosis may therefore be obtained from a positive skin prick test. Radioallergosorbent tests appear to have little to offer except in cases where there is extensive skin disease or skin tests have been invalidated by the previous administration of antihistamines.

Since subclinical reactions can escape detection under challenge test conditions, tests have also been proposed which measure inflammatory mediator release on exposure to foods *in vitro* or *in vivo* or which measures change in bronchial reactivity after food is given. These have the further advantage that they do not depend solely on the presence of an IgE-mediated response. Such test methods have been developed over a number of years. May and Remigio (1982) at first suggested that the basophils of children with food sensitivity release histamine spontaneously to an extent which is not observed in other atopic subjects. Others have made similar observations, and peripheral blood mononuclear cells from food-allergic individuals have been reported to produce a factor which activates basophils from other food-allergic individuals (Sampson 1988a). Nevertheless, leucocyte histamine release studies, either with or without exposure to the appropriate food, have not yet led to the development of a useful diagnostic test. In research studies, Reiman (1985) has provided an alternative approach by showing that the direct application of a specific food to the gastric mucosa of food-sensitive subjects provokes histamine release from the gastric mucosal mast cells. Similar changes have been observed in individuals who are sensitive to tartrazine (Schaubschlager *et al.* 1987), and the *in vitro* application of tartrazine to gastric biopsy samples from these patients has also caused mast cell degranulation. In an attempt to develop less invasive methods, Murdoch *et al.* (1987b) have shown that food additive-induced urticaria — or even ery-

Table 56.4. Criteria for distinguishing food intolerance and food aversion

	Challenge tests		Immunological abnormality
	Open	Double-blind	
Food allergy	+	+	+
Other food intolerance — toxins, pharmacological effects, enzyme deficiencies, fermentation of unabsorbed residues	+	+	0
Food aversion or avoidance	±	0	0

Based on Joint Report (1984).

thema or itching in the absence of urticaria — can be accompanied by a rise in plasma and urine histamine and prostanoid levels. Tests of this type have the advantage that they do not depend on the presence of an IgE-mediated mechanism, for which there is little evidence in the case of food additive-induced reactions. They can, however, cause difficulties in interpretation as shown by the nine out of 10 volunteers who had no symptoms but had a rise in plasma histamine after being given 150 mg tartrazine (Murdoch *et al.* 1987a). Since the fluctuations in histamine output in healthy subjects have yet to be defined, this cannot be taken as clear evidence of a potentially toxic effect or of an adverse reaction. More work is indicated in this area.

Other attempts to develop diagnostic tests have been less fruitful. Immunoglobulin G antibodies to food and IgG subclass antibodies are present in healthy subjects and, despite claims to the contrary, their measurement cannot discriminate between food-sensitive individuals and others. The relatively high IgG antibody level to gluten in patients with egg allergy and the relatively low levels in patients with coeliac disease on a gluten-free diet (as compared with untreated coeliac disease) provide supporting evidence for the view that such antibodies may represent a secondary response to proteins which cross a damaged mucous membrane (Kemeny *et al.* 1986).

Of the remaining diagnostic tests which have been investigated, the presence of circulating immune complexes containing food antigen has been demonstrated in normal individuals as well as in those with food allergy (Paganelli and Levinsky 1980). The discriminating value of circulating immune complexes containing IgE and antigen does not appear to be any greater (Carini *et al.* 1987). T cell activation markers, tests with autologous mixed lymphocytes, and leucocyte migration inhibition tests also fail to discriminate between allergic and other subjects (Dirienzo *et al.* 1987; Vanto *et al.* 1987).

Challenge tests

Food reactions which occur within an hour and are associated with a positive skin prick test or other evidence of an IgE-mediated reaction are relatively easy to diagnose and to confirm. From the patient's point of view, it is also important to test for reactions which might reflect the presence of a more delayed immune response or a non-immunological defect. If the patient is symptom-free but has a history which suggests the involvement of one or two major foods — and especially if a positive skin test is obtained — an open challenge test may be sufficient to establish the diagnosis, and, since the elimination of one or two foods is relatively simple to arrange, the finding of a positive challenge test can justify an appropriate dietary restriction for a period of 2 to 3 months, after which there should be a clinical reassessment of the response to treatment. Where there appear to be positive challenge test responses to several foods — especially if they are unrelated — the results are, however, suspect. In that case, if dietary restrictions are to be considered, it is important that double-blind, placebo-controlled food challenges should first be carried out (see Table 56.5). For the purpose of blind challenge tests the food and the control substance should be made up in a similarly flavoured form and should also be made to look the same (for example, by adding tomato). Oral challenge is to be preferred to a nasogastric tube, which is unpleasant and may bypass some of the receptor areas which can trigger a response. Such challenge tests are in fact seldom necessary and mainly serve the purpose of providing reassurance to the patient.

If the patient is not symptom-free at the time of study, it is necessary to establish the relationship of food to the patient's symptoms by eliminating the suspect substances and showing that the patient's symptoms remit. Lack of response to an elimination diet within 2–3 weeks usually means that food allergy can be excluded. In a few patients it may be justifiable to introduce further empirical dietary changes (Table 56.6) or an even more restricted diet — for example, lamb, pears and mineral water.

Since life-threatening anaphylactic reactions can occur during food challenge (David 1987), patients who have a past history of severe reactions should either avoid challenge tests entirely or else be given extremely small doses of the suspect food while under close observation. Adrenaline and resuscitation facilities should be available.

Where the symptoms are subjective only, the differential diagnosis includes that of the hyperventilation syndrome — perhaps one of the most underdiagnosed conditions in medicine. Patients

Table 56.5. Outline of challenge test procedure

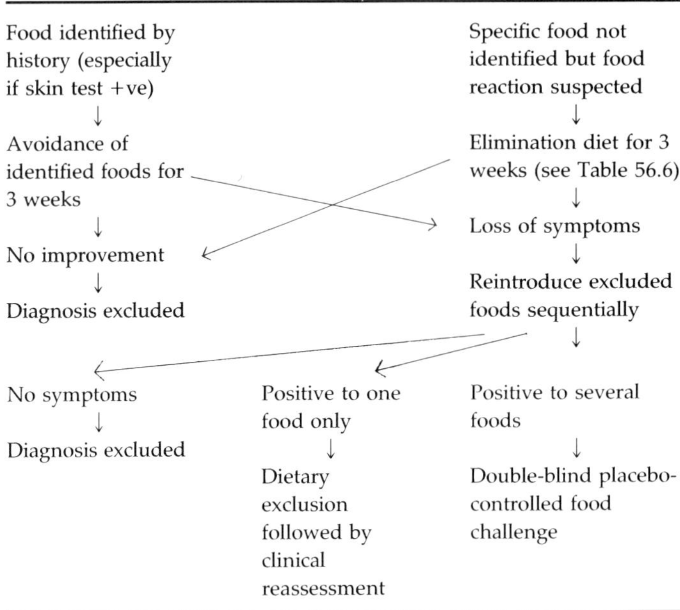

Table 56.6. Simple exclusion diet (modified from a diet used at Northwick Park Hospital)

1 Permitted (weeks 1–2)	**2** Alternative to **1** (weeks 3–4)	Major exclusions
Lamb or mutton	Beef or chicken	Other meat and poultry. Fish
Gluten-free bread rice (and Rice Krispies)	Rye crispbread maize (and cornflakes)	Other bread, cakes, biscuits, pasta, cereals
Vegetarian margarine (e.g. Tomor or Golden Rose)	No change	Milk, butter and dairy products, eggs
Fresh fruit and vegetables	Exclude citrus fruits, apples beans, peas, soya	Strawberries, nuts, preserves and commercially frozen food
Tea, coffee, sugar, juice	Water or spring water	Wines and fruit. Spirits
Barley sugar	Corn syrup	Confectionery
Olive oil	Corn oil, sunflower seed oil or cotton seed oil	Other cooking oils

who attend with the self-diagnosis of food allergy not infrequently complain of paraesthesiae, muscle weakness or faintness, palpitations or chest pain. Forced hyperventilation, for a period of up to 2–3 minutes, often reproduces similar sensations, which the patient will recognize and accept as evidence that these symptoms are provoked by hyperventilation, which it is within the patient's power to prevent. If, in these circumstances, the patient does not accept simple explanation and reassurance, blind challenge tests may carry conviction by demonstrating that it is the apprehension associated with a particular food which provokes symptoms, whereas the food itself can be taken without problems. The diagnosis of the hyperventilation syndrome does not, however, exclude the possibility of associated organic disease.

Treatment

When a diagnosis of food allergy or intolerance has been firmly made, the only proved method of treatment is the avoidance of those foods which provoke symptoms. There may, however, be a difference between those with immediate, IgE-mediated sensitivity and those with food intolerance of other types. In the latter case, an obsessional avoidance of all traces of the offending food may not be necessary. Patients may themselves observe that large quantities of a food taken on two or three successive days will provoke symptoms whereas small quantities at less frequent intervals can be tolerated without any problem. Patients may also be able to tolerate heat-denatured proteins — for example, cow's milk or egg incorporated in a cake — while reacting to raw foods containing cow's milk or partly cooked egg. When there is intolerance to a number of immunologically related substances or to a widely used additive, additional care may be necessary. Those who are sensitive to silver birch tree pollen can have cross-reacting sensitivities to a number of soft fruits, nuts and root vegetables (Halmepuro and Björksten 1985). Those who have ragweed allergy sometimes have an associated hypersensitivity to melon and banana (Andersson *et al.* 1970). In addition, sensitivity to tenderized meats may depend not on the meat protein but on an IgE-mediated reaction to papain or other enzymes used as tenderizers (Mansfield *et al.* 1985).

When the reaction is immunological, the material causing problems is usually a protein, so those who are sensitive to soya protein may nevertheless be able to eat commercial soya oils added to margarine (Bush *et al.* 1985). Nut oils can also be tolerated by those who are sensitive to nuts (Taylor *et al.* 1981).

With the more restricted diets, and especially when cow's milk is removed from a child's diet, there is a need for a dietetic analysis to ensure that the diet is nutritionally adequate in protein, calcium and vitamins. Children with cow's milk protein intolerance may nevertheless tolerate protein hydrolysates or milk products from a goat or a sheep. Otherwise vegetable proteins, notably soya, can be substituted with appropriate calcium and vitamin supplementation.

Since food sensitivity frequently diminishes with time, some reassurance may be justified. Of 67 children followed by Sampson (1988a), one-third had lost their sensitivity when rechallenged 1–2 years later. In an earlier study Sampson (1985) showed that, out of 28 children with atopic dermatitis and egg hypersensitivity who were rechallenged after maintaining an egg-free diet for a year, eight were able to tolerate eggs and to eat them freely, despite the fact that repeat skin testing before the second challenge showed no obvious loss of sensitivity. It appeared that the loss of clinical hypersensitivity was more frequent with soya but less common with peanut, wheat, egg and milk.

The response of patients with atopic dermatitis to dietary measures is much more difficult to establish than for most other types of food reaction, perhaps because of the complications introduced by associated factors such as contact sensitization to other antigens and the secondary effects of scratching. The avoidance of non-specific irritants, including soap, the prevention of dehydration by the use of emulsifying creams, the use of antihistamines and, when necessary, the brief use of topical steroid may all be necessary.

There is at present no scientific evidence to support the claims made for immunotherapy with food antigens in the treatment of food hypersensitivity. Nevertheless, the fact that a remission of symptoms can occur spontaneously suggests that this method of treatment warrants re-examination.

Eosinophilic gastroenteritis

Eosinophilic gastroenteritis involves diffuse eosinophilic infiltration in the gastrointestinal tract, most commonly in the stomach or pyloric region. It is usually associated with peripheral blood eosinophilia, in the absence of any evidence of intestinal parasites, vasculitis, neoplasm or any other recognized local cause. Most cases have shown some mucosal eosinophilic infiltration but there is a more pronounced eosinophilic involvement of the deeper layers of the gut wall, sometimes with mucosal oedema and ascites. Thickening of the gut wall can be sufficient to produce proximal small bowel obstruction and vomiting. About half of the patients have associated atopic diseases, such as asthma or allergic rhinitis (Caldwell *et al.* 1978), and a number of patients have been reported who have an associated food intolerance with a very clear response to intestinal challenge (Caldwell *et al.* 1975; Nelson *et al.* 1979).

The eosinophilic infiltration that is characteristic of the disease is sometimes almost entirely confined to the deeper layers of the gut and may spare the mucosa or cause only patchy mucosal changes. A negative intestinal biopsy — or even multiple biopsies — cannot always, therefore, exclude the condition, which, in cases associated with intestinal obstruction, may be detectable only at laparotomy. Exceptionally, there may be an associated lymphadenopathy, hepatomegaly and protein-losing gastroenteropathy or steatorrhoea (Kettelhut and Metcalfe 1988).

The mechanism which provokes eosinophilic accumulation in the gut is still unknown but is presumed to result from the release of eosinophilic chemotactic factors. Food antigens and specific IgE-mediated hypersensitivity reactions do not always seems to be involved. However, the identification of an associated food allergy, if present, can clearly be of importance, since in children under the age of 1 the identification of cow's milk intolerance and its withdrawal can lead to a remission (Katz *et al.* 1984) and dietary control has been of value in several cases. Even so, corticosteroids may be needed in addition to dietary restriction (Caldwell *et al.* 1975).

Apart from the treatment of individual patients, the fact that an occasional food-induced reaction can lead to death (Salmon and Paulley 1967) provides a reminder that, in exceptional cases, food allergies can be sufficiently severe to be life-threatening and to require initial treatment by elemental diet.

References

Allen, D. and Delohery, J. (1985). Metabisulfite induced asthma. *J Allergy Clin. Immunol.* **75**, 145.

Alun Jones, V.A. (1985). Irritable bowel syndrome. In *Food and the Gut* ed. J.O. Hunter and V.A. Alun Jones, pp. 208–20, Baillière, Tindall, London.

Amlot, P.L., Urbanek, R., Youlten, L.J.F., Kemeny, D.M., Lessof, M.H. (1985). Type 1 allergy to egg and milk proteins: comparison of skin prick tests with nasal, buccal and gastric provocation test. *Int. Arch. Allergy Appl. Immunol.* **77**, 171–3.

Andersson, L.B., Dreyfuss, E.M., Logan, J., Johnstone, D.E., Glaser, J. (1970). Melon and banana sensitivity coincident with ragweed pollinosis. *J Allergy* **45**, 310–19.

Bahna, S.L. and Heiner, D.C. (1978). Cows' milk allergy. Adv. *Pediatr* **25**, 1–37.

Björksten, F. and Saarinen, U.M. (1978). IgE antibodies to cow's milk in infants fed breast milk and milk formulae. *Lancet* **ii**, 624–5.

Brunner, M. and Walzer, M. (1928). Absorption of undigested proteins in human beings: the absorption of unaltered fish protein in adults. *Arch. Intern. Med.* **42**, 173–9.

Bruynzeel-Koomen, C.A.F.M., van Wicken, D.F., Spry, C.J.F. *et al.* (1988). *Br. J. Dermatol.* **118**, 229–38.

Burks, A.W. Brooks, J.R. and Sampson, H.A. (1988). Allergenicity of major component proteins of soybean determined by enzyme linked immunosorbent assay (ELISA) and immunoblotting in children with atopic dermatitis and positive soy challenges. *J. Allergy Clin. Immunol.* **81**, 1135–42.

Bush, R.K., Taylor, J.L., Nordlee, J.A., Busse, W.W. (1985). Soybean oil is not allergenic to soybean-sensitive individuals. *J. Allergy Clin. Immunol.* **76**, 242–5.

Businco, L., Marchetti, F., Pelligrini, G., Cantani, A. and Perlini, R. (1983). Prevention of atopic disease in 'at risk' newborns by prolonged breast feeding. *Ann. Allergy* **51**, 296–9.

Caldwell, J.H., Tennenbaum, J.I. and Bronstein, H.A. (1975). Serum IgE in eosinophilic gastroenteritis. *N. Engl. J. Med.* **292**, 1388–90.

Caldwell, J.H., Mekhjian, H.J., Hurtubige, P.E. *et al.* (1978). Eosinophilic gastroenteritis with obstruction — immunological studies of seven patients. *Gastroenterology* **74**, 825–9.

Capron, A., Dessanto, J.P., Capron, M., Joseph, M., Amerisen, J.C. and Tonnel, A.B. (1986). From parasites to allergy: a second receptor for IgE. *Immunol. Today* **7**, 15–18.

Carini, C., Brostoff, J. and Wraith, D.G. (1987). IgE complexes in food allergy. *Ann. Allergy* **59**, 110–17.

Clinton, P.M., Kemeny, D.M., Amlot, P.L., Urbanek, R. and Lessof, M.H. (1986). Histamine release from peripheral blood leucocytes in egg-allergic patients. *Clin. Allergy* **16**, 345–54.

David, T.J. (1987). Reactions to dietary tartrazine. *Arch. Dis. Child.* **62**, 119–22.

Denman, A.M. (1987). Allergy and joint complaints. In *Allergy: an International Textbook*, ed. M.H. Lessof, T.H. Lee and D.M. Kemeny, pp. 567–75, John Wiley & Sons, Chichester.

Denman, A.M., Mitchell, B. and Ansell, B.M. (1983). Joint complaints and food allergic disorders. *Ann. Allergy* **51**, 260–3.

Dirienzo, W., Ciprandi, G., Caria, M., Scordamaglia, A., Bagnasco, M. and Canonica, G.W. (1987). T cell activation surface markers and autologous mixed lymphocyte reaction do not differ in true and pseudo food allergy. *Int. Arch. Allergy Appl. Immunol.* **83**, 193–7.

Donovan, G.K. and Torres-Pinedo, R. (1987). Chronic diarrhea and soy formulas. *Am. J. Dis. Child.* **141**, 1069–71.

Egger, J., Carter, C.M., Graham, P.J., Gumley, D. and Soothill, J.F. (1985). Controlled total of oligoantigenic treatment in the hyperkinetic syndrome. *Lancet* **i**, 540–2.

Firer, M.A., Hoskings, C.S. and Hill, D.J. (1987). Humoral immune response to cow's milk in children with cow's milk allergy. *Int. Arch. Allergy Appl. Immunol.* **84**, 173–7.

Geha, R.S. (1985). Human IgE. *J. Allergy Clin. Immunol.* **74**, 109–20.

Genova, R., Sanfilippo, M., Rossi, M.E. and Vierucci, A. (1987). Food allergy in steroid-resistant nephrotic syndrome. *Lancet* **i**, 1315–16.

Gershwin, M.E., Ough, C. and Bock, A. (1985). Grand rounds: adverse reactions to wine. *J. Allergy Clin. Immunol.* **75**, 411–20.

Gray, G.M. (1980). Absorption and malabsorption of dietary carbohydrate. In *Nutrition and Gastroenterology*, ed. M. Winicle, pp. 43–53, John Wiley & Sons, New York.

Hager, C., Faber, J., Kaczuni, A., Goldstein, R., Levy, E. and Freier, S. (1987). Prevalence of postenteritis cow's milk protein intolerance. *Israel J. Med. Sci.* **23**, 1129–31.

Halmepuro, L. and Björksten, F. (1985). Immunological partial identity between pollen and food allergens. *Allergy* **3**, 70–1.

Harley, J.P., Ray, R.S., Tomas, L. *et al.* (1978a). Hyperkinesis and food additives: testing the Feingold hypothesis. *Pediatrics* **61**, 818–28.

Harley, J.P., Matthews, C.G. and Eichman, C. (1978b). Synthetic food colors and hyperactivity in children: a double-blind challenge experiment. *Pediatrics* **62**, 975–83.

Hattevig, G., Kjellman, B. and Björksten, B. (1987). Clinical symptoms and IgE responses to common food proteins and inhalants in the first 7 years of life. *Clin. Allergy* **17**, 571–8.

Hoffman, D.R. and Guenther, D.M. (1988). Occupational allergy to avian proteins presenting as allergy to ingestion of egg yolk. *J. Allergy Clin. Immunol.* **81**, 484–8.

Host, A. and Samuelsson, E.G. (1988). Allergic reactions to raw, pasteurized and homogenized/pasteurized cow's milk: a comparison. *Allergy* **43**, 113–18.

Iyngkaran, N., Davis, K., Robinson, M.H., Bosy, C.G., Sumithran, E. and Yadav, M. (1979). Cow's milk protein sensitive enteropathy: an important contributory cause of secondary sugar intolerance in young infants with acute infective enteritis. *Arch. Dis. Child.* **54**, 39–43.

Iyngkaran, N., Robinson, M.J., Prathap, K., Sunnithran, E. and Yadav, M. (1978). Cow's milk protein sensitive enteropathy — combined clinical and histological criteria for diagnosis. *Arch. Dis. Child.* **53**, 20–6.

Jenkins, H.R., Pincott, J.R., Soothill, J.F., Milla, P.J. and Harries, J.T. (1984). *Arch. Dis. Child.* **59**, 326–9.

Johansson, S.G.O., Dannaeus, A. and Lilja, G. (1984). The relevance of anti-food antibodies for the diagnosis of food allergy. *Ann. Allergy* **53**, 665–70.

Joint Report (1984). Food intolerance and food aversion. *J. Roy. Coll. Physicians* **18**, 83–123.

Katz, A.J., Twarog, F.J., Zeiger, R.S., Falchuk, Z.M. (1984). Milk-sensitive and eosinophilic gastroenteropathy — similar clinical features with contrasting mechanisms and clinical course. *J. Allergy Clin. Immunol.* **74**, 72–8.

Kemeny, D.M., Urbanek, R., Amlot, P.L. *et al.* (1986). Sub-class of IgG in allergic disease. 1. IgG subclass antibodies in immediate and non-immediate food allergy. *Clin. Allergy* **16**, 571–82.

Kettelhut, B.V. and Metcalfe, D.D. (1988). Adverse reactions to food. In *Allergy, Principles and Practice*, ed. F. Middleton, Jr, C.E. Reed, E.F. Ellis, N.F. Adkinson and J.W. Younger, vol. II, pp. 1481–502, C.V. Mosby, St Louis.

Lagrue, G., Laurent, J., Rostoker, G. and Lang, P. (1987). Food allergy in idiopathic nephrotic syndrome. *Lancet* **ii**, 277.

Laurent, J., L'Héritier, M., Gilson-Henry, P. and Lagrue, G. (1987). Rôle de l'hypersensibilité alimentaire masquée dans la néphrose lipoidique. *Rév. Fr. Allergol* **27**, 79–80.

Lee, T.H., Hoover, R.L.R.L., Williams, J.D. *et al.* (1985). Dietary enrichment with eicosapentaenoic and docosahexaenoic acids in human subjects impairs *in vitro* neutrophils and monocyte function and leukotriene generation. *N. Engl. J. Med.* **312**, 1217–24.

Lessof, M.H. and Challacombe, S. (1987). Gastrointestinal allergy. In *Allergy: an International Textbook*, eds. M.H. Lessof, T.H. Lee and D.M. Kemeny, pp. 455–80, John Wiley & Sons, Chichester.

Lessof, M.H., Wraith, D.G., Merrett, T.G. *et al.* (1980). Food allergy and intolerance in 100 patients — local and systemic effects. *Quart. J. Med.* **195**, 259–71.

Mansfield, L.E., Ting, S., Haverley, R.W. and Yoo, T.J. (1985). The incidence and clinical implications of hypersensitivity to papain in an allergic population, confirmed by blinded oral challenge. *Ann. Allergy* **55**, 541–3.

Moroz, L.A. and Yang, W.H. (1980). Kunitz soybean trypsin-inhibitor: a specific allergen in food anaphylaxis. *N. Engl. J. Med.* **302**, 1126–8.

Matsumura, T., Kuroume, T., Oguri, M., Iwasaki, I., Kanbe, Y. and Yamada, T. (1976). Egg sensitivity and eczematous manifestations in breast-fed newborns with particular reference to intrauterine sensitization. *Ann. Allergy* **35**, 221–9.

Mattes, J.A. and Gittelman, R. (1981). Effects of artificial food colourings in children with hyperactive symptoms. *Arch. Gen. Psychiatry* **38**, 714–18.

May, C.D. and Remigio, L. (1982). Observations on high spontaneous release of histamine from leucocytes *in vitro*. *Clin. Allergy* **12**, 229–41.

Meara, R.H. (1965). Skin reactions in atopic eczema. *J. Dermatol.* **67**, 60–4.

Metcalfe, D.D. (1984). Food hypersensitivity. *J. Allergy Clin. Immunol.* **73**, 749–62.

Miskelly, F.G., Burr, M.L., Vaughan-Williams, E., Fehily, A.M., Butland, B.K. and Merrett, T.G. (1988). Infant feeding and allergy. *Arch. Dis. Child.* **63**, 388–93.

Mitchell, E.B., Crow, J., Chapman, M.D., Jouhal, S.S., Pope, F.M. and Platts-Mills, T.A.E. (1982). Basophils in allergen-induced patch test sites in atopic dermatitis. *Lancet* **i**, 127–30.

Murdoch, R.D., Pollock, I. and Naeem, S. (1987a). Tartrazine induced histamine release *in vivo* in normal subjects. *J. Roy. Coll. Physicians* **21**, 257–61.

Murdoch, R.D., Pollock, I., Young, E. and Lessof, M.H. (1987b). Food additive-induced urticaria: studies of mediator release during provocation tests. *J. Roy. Coll. Physicians* **21**, 262–6.

Nelson, T.L., Klein, G.L. and Galant, S.P. (1979). Severe eosinophilic gastroenteritis successfully treated with an elemental diet. *J. Allergy Clin. Immunol.* **63**, 198A.

Paganelli, R. and Levinsky, R. (1980). Solid-phase radioimmunassay for detection of circulating food protein antigens in human serum. *J. Immunol. Methods* **37**, 333–41.

Papageorgiou, N., Lee, T.H., Nagakura, T., Cromwell, O., Wraith, D.G. and Kay, B.A. (1983). Neutrophil chemotactic activity in milk induced asthma. *J. Allergy Clin. Immunol.* **72**, 75–83.

Parke, H.L. and Hughes, G.R.V. (1981). Rheumatoid arthritis and food: a case study. *Br. Med. J.* **282**, 2027–8.

Price, J.F. (1987). Paediatric allergy. In *Allergy: an International Textbook*, ed. M.H. Lessof, T.H. Lee and D.M. Kemeny, pp. 423–53, John Wiley & Sons, Chichester.

Reiman, H.-J., Ring, J., Ultsch, B. and Wendt, P. (1985). Intragastral provocation under endoscopic control (IPEC) in food allergy: mast cell and histamine changes in gastric mucosa. *Clin. Allergy* **15**, 195–202.

Salmon, P.L. and Paulley, J.W. (1967). Eosinophilic granuloma of the gastrointestinal tract. *Gut* **8**, 8–14.

Sampson, H.A. (1983). Role of immediate food sensitivity in the pathogenesis of atopic dermatitis. *J. Allergy Clin. Immunol.* **71**, 473–80.

Sampson, H.A. (1985). Persistence of food hypersensitivity in children with atopic dermatitis. *J. Allergy Clin. Immunol.* **75**, 179A.

Sampson, H.A. (1988a). IgE mediated food intolerance. *J. Allergy Clin. Immunol.* **81**, 495–504.

Sampson, H.A. (1988b). The role of food allergy and mediator release in atopic dermatitis. *J. Allergy Clin. Immunol.* **81**, 635–45.

Sampson, H.A., Buckley, R.H. and Metcalfe, D.D. (1987). Food allergy. *JAMA* **258**, 2886–9.

Schaubschläger, W.W., Zabel, P. and Schlaak, M. (1987). Tartrazine-induced histamine release from gastric mucosa. *Lancet* **ii**, 800–1.

Smith, S.J., Markandu, N.D., Rotellar, C. *et al.* (1982). A new or old Chinese restaurant syndrome. *Br. Med. J.* **285**, 205.

Targan, S.R. (1987). Immunologic mechanisms in intestinal diseases. *Ann. Intern. Med.* **106**, 859–62.

Taylor, B., Norman, A.P., Orgel, H.A. *et al.* (1973). Transient IgA deficiency and pathogenesis of infantile atropy. *Lancet* **ii**, 111–13.

Taylor, S., Busse, W.W., Sachs, M.I., Parker, J.L., Yunginger, J.W. (1981). Peanut oil is not allergenic to peanut-sensitive individuals. *J. Allergy Clin. Immunol.* **68**, 372–5.

Taylor, S.L., Bush, R.K., Selner, J.C., Nordlee, J.A., Wiener, M.B. and Holden, K. (1988). Sensitivity to sulfited foods among sulfite-sensitive subjects with asthma. *J. Allergy Clin. Immunol.* **81**, 1159–67.

Titus, R.G. and Chiller, J.M. (1981). Orally induced tolerance: definition at the cellular level. *Int. Arch. Allergy Appl. Immunol.* **65**, 323–38.

Turnberg, L.E. (1978). Coffee and the gastrointestinal tract. *Gastroenterology* **75**, 529–30.

Vanto, T., Smogorzewska, M., Viander, M., Kalimo, K. and Koivikko, A. (1987). Leukocyte migration inhibition test in children with cow milk allergy. *Allergy* **42**, 612–18.

Walker-Smith, J.A. (1986). Milk intolerance in children. *Clin. Allergy* **16**, 183–90.

Warner, J.O. and Hathaway, M.J. (1984). Allergic form of Meadow's syndrome (Munchausen by proxy). *Arch. Dis. Child.* **59**, 151–6.

Williams, D.G. (1987). Allergy and the kidney. In: *Allergy: an International Textbook*, ed. M.H. Lessof, T.H. Lee and D.M. Kemeny, pp. 553–63, John Wiley and Sons, Chichester.

Wilson, N.M. (1985). Food related asthma — a difference between two ethnic groups. *Arch. Dis. Child.* **60**, 861–5.

Wilson, N.M. and Silverman, M. (1985). The diagnosis of food sensitivity in childhood asthma. *J. Roy. Soc. Med.* **78**, (suppl. 5), 11.

Young, E., Patel, S., Stoneham, M., Rona, R. and Wilkinson, J.D. (1987). The prevalence of reaction to food additives in a survey population. *J. Roy. Coll. Physicians* **21**, 241–7.

57: Paediatric Allergy

J.O. Warner and J.A. Warner

Introduction

Allergic diseases affect between 15 and 20% of the child population and cause a third of all school absences due to chronic disease (Schiffer and Hunt 1963). They are occasionally life-threatening and have a considerable impact on health, development, education, examination performance and academic attainment. Furthermore, there is some evidence that the prevalence of allergic disease is increasing in the population (Burr *et al.* 1989a; Fleming and Crombie 1987). Thus, much attention is inevitably focused on possible explanations for this (Table 57.1).

Paediatricians have the opportunity to witness the development of the hypersensitivity response and to identify underlying defects that allow allergy and allergic disease to evolve. They can also observe the rapid changes that occur in the pattern of allergic diseases with increasing age. Thus, food intolerance with either gastrointestinal or dermatological manifestations predominates in infancy, whereas inhalant allergies associated with diseases in the respiratory tract predominate in later childhood and adolescence.

Inheritance

When the term atopy was first introduced by Coca and Cooke (1923) to describe asthma and hay fever, it was already apparent that the problem ran in families. Indeed, Maimonides in the eleventh century recognized the familial nature of asthma (Muntner 1963). Cooke and Van der Veer (1916) proposed a dominant mode of inheritance for atopy in identifying that offspring of families where both parents were atopic had a 75% chance of developing atopy. The risk was 50% if only one parent was atopic and only 14% if neither was atopic. Subsequent studies have suggested that the percentage is slightly smaller and therefore the inheritance might be dominant with incomplete

Table 57.1. Possible predisposing factors in allergy

Genetic	Immunological	Environmental
Ir genes	IgA deficiency	Diet in infancy
IgE regulator genes (R′r)	Opsonization defect	Aeroallergen load
HLA link with diseases	C2 deficiency	Month of birth
? Autosomal dominant	Reduced T suppressor cells	Pets
	Cystic fibrosis	Cigarette smoke
		Infection
		Air pollution

penetrance (Schwartz 1952). However, with the identification of the causal relationship between the presence of immunoglobulin E (IgE) antibodies and type 1 hypersensitivity, it has been possible to make a more accurate assessment of inheritance, and again this lends support to the idea that simple autosomal dominant inheritance is involved (Cookson and Hopkin 1988).

Whilst a simple Mendelian inheritance pattern may explain the presence of atopy, it does not explain the variations in the expression of atopic disease. Concordance for asthma is greater in monozygotic than dizygotic twins but even for monozygotic pairs is less than 20% (Edfors-Lubs 1974). Thus, whilst genetic factors influence the development of atopy, other factors may be more important in relation to the manifestation of allergy. This may be an independently inherited characteristic, such as bronchial hyper-reactivity in asthma (Sibbald and Turner-Warwick 1979), or an influence of the environment.

Interleukin 4 (IL-4) is an inducer of IgE production with IL-5 and 6, whilst interferon γ (IFN-γ) down-regulates this response. IL-5 with IL-3 and granulocyte-macrophage colony stimulating factor (GM-CSF) promotes terminal differentiation of eosinophils and enhances survival and effector function of these cells. T cell clones from atopic individuals selectively produce IL-4 and 5 when stimulated (T_H2) while non-atopic T cell clones produce IL-2 and IFN-γ (T_H1) (Weirenga *et al.* 1990). We have shown that stimulated cord blood T cells from infants who subsequently developed eczema and asthma produced less IFN-γ than those of infants who had so far not developed atopic disease (Warner *et al.* 1992). Thus variations in the cytokine repertoire of T cells may be fundamental to the development of atopic disease.

Host defects

A number of primary immunological defects are associated with an increased prevalence of atopy. Indeed, atopy could be the commonest manifestation of immunodeficiency. Eczema is, for instance, a feature of Wiskott–Aldrich syndrome and has been described in patients with X-linked agammaglobulinaemia. In 1970, Kauffman and Hobbs noted an increase in IgA deficiency amongst atopic individuals. More recent associations with the development of atopy have included the presence of the yeast opsonization defect, which is one of the more common abnormalities, affecting 5% of the population but 27% of a group of children with eczema and adults with hay fever (Turner *et al.* 1978). Deficiency of the second component of complement has been observed in 18% of adults with hay fever. However, C2 deficiency and opsonization defects in hay fever are mutually exclusive (Turner *et al.* 1978). Immunoglobulin G-2 subclass deficiency has been linked with severe childhood asthma (Loftus *et al.* 1988).

Inevitably attention has focused on the influence of the T cell in the regulation of IgE production. Some workers have proposed that there is a genetically determined defect in T lymphocytes of atopic subjects which leads to an imbalance of helper and suppressor cells (Strannegard and Strannegard 1978). There is some support for this hypothesis in that infants with a family history of atopy who have a relative deficiency of suppressor T cells subsequently have a higher incidence of eczema and allergic rhinitis than similar infants without the T cell defect (Juto and Strannegard 1979; Chandra and Baker 1983).

Children with cystic fibrosis have a higher prevalence of atopy involving inhalant allergens, although the range of sensitivities is greater to

Aspergillus fumigatus and other moulds than to the more common inhalant allergens such as house dust mite (Warner *et al.* 1976a). Furthermore, there is some suggestion that atopy might be more common in the parents of cystic fibrosis children, who are obligate heterozygotes (Warner *et al.* 1976b). As no primary defect of immune response has been identified in cystic fibrosis, this might suggest that other defects also predispose to sensitization. Cystic fibrosis patients are susceptible to severe lower respiratory tract infection and this may be due to a defect of antigen exclusion at mucosal surfaces, which would also promote the development of allergy.

It is possible that maturational defects of immune response may also be important. One study demonstrated lower levels of serum IgA at 3 months of age in infants of allergic parents who subsequently developed eczema and positive skin tests, compared with children who did not become atopic (Taylor *et al.* 1973). Furthermore, defective yeast opsonization has been identified in cord blood and associated with a higher incidence of both infection and atopy than controls with normal yeast opsonization in the cord blood, even when carefully matched for date of birth, sex, parental atopy, smoking and infant feeding practices. Many of the infants, who had the defects at birth, had normal activity by 1 year of age (Richardson *et al.* 1983). Both these studies suggest that the presence of an immune defect at a critical stage in infancy may be sufficient to lead to atopy and might explain why most atopic individuals subsequently have no identifiable underlying immunological defect.

Genetics

Asthma is very much more frequent in males than females during childhood, although the sex ratio changes dramatically during adolescence (McNicol and Williams 1973a). Furthermore, males have a higher geometric mean IgE level than females throughout life (Burr *et al.* 1989). The IgE levels increase through childhood to reach a maximum just after puberty and thereafter decline (Merrett *et al.* 1980; Berciano *et al.* 1987). Suppressor T cell activity may determine this variation through life.

Twin studies show that IgE levels are very similar in monozygotic, but not dizygotic, pairs (Bazaral *et al.* 1974). This has led to the postulate that the IgE phenotype is controlled by a single regulator locus R'r (Marsh *et al.* 1981). The dominant R allele occurs in people producing only low levels of IgE and the homozygote recessive rr would correspond to a high IgE phenotype. The computed gene frequency for the r allele must be 0.5 to account for the frequency of atopy in the community (Gerrard *et al.* 1978). Whilst some authors have also suggested a recessive allele determining high IgE levels, others have suggested a dominant allele or polygenic inheritance (Cookson and Hopkin 1988). Indeed these authors have suggested that the dominant gene for atopy is on the long arm of chromosome 11 (Cookson *et al.* 1989). There are numerous ways in which the gene product might exert its effect. It could influence T cell regulation, differentiation of B cells into IgE-producing plasma cells or the number of different IgE-forming cell clones that can respond to stimulation (Willcox and Marsh 1978).

Animal studies have demonstrated specific immune responses which were determined by immune response genes (Ir genes) linked to the major histocompatibility complex. The first evidence that Ir genes exist in man came from a study in seven families in which all of the atopic members who had positive skin tests to antigen E of ragweed also had the same human leucocyte antigen (HLA) haplotypes (Levine *et al.* 1972). The most interesting observation has been in atopics with low total IgE levels who have the tightest association between IgE antibody production and a particular HLA type. Thus allergy to Ra3 (now known as Amb A III — a component of ragweed) is associated with HLA-A2 in 93% of subjects but with only a 55% overall association for those with high IgE levels. This may be because persons with low IgE levels have HLA associations with only a few Ir genes, whilst high IgE-producing atopics have so many Ir genes that no particular HLA association will be obvious (Marsh *et al.* 1981). Most of the striking associations have been with reactions to low-molecular-weight allergens, where there are presumably a limited number of allergenic determinants. Ra5 (Amb A V), an allergen of ragweed, consists of a single peptide chain of 45 amino acids. Studies have revealed that DR2 DW2 is an excellent marker for the immune response to this allergen. Immunotherapy with Ra5 allergen produces higher IgG responses in ragweed-sensitive individuals who possess DW2 than in those who do not (Marsh *et al.* 1982). This suggests that similar epitopes on these antigens are recognized by the same immune-associated (HLA-D) molecule during antigen presentation. It is possible that characterization of HLA-A and HLA-D genes might predict which allergens are most likely to sensitize individuals, which, in turn, could lead to the institution of effective avoidance regimens or immunotherapy (Marsh *et al.* 1987).

Several studies have looked at HLA antigen linkage with particular atopic manifestations. Human leucocyte antigen haplotype A1B8 has been noted in higher than expected frequency in children with severe asthma and in babies with immediate skin sensitivity or eczema in the first year of life (Thorsby *et al.* 1971; Soothill *et al.* 1976). Antigens A3, A9 but not A1, B8 occurred more frequently in adults with atopic dermatitis (Krain and Terasaki 1973). Turner *et al.* (1977) identified HLA A1 B8 to be increased in eczematous patients with either asthma or hay fever and HLA A3, B7 more frequently in patients with hay fever and asthma. However, there are other studies that failed to identify HLA haplotype associations (Bruce *et al.* 1976). It is nevertheless of interest to note that HLA A1 B8 is associated with other diseases, such as chronic active hepatitis and coeliac disease, and thus this may be a marker of non-specific hypersensitivity.

Cord blood immunoglobulin E

The level of the total IgE in the cord blood has been shown to predict the development of atopy in several studies (Kjellman 1976; Michel *et al.* 1980; Businco *et al.* 1983; Chandra *et al.* 1985; Burr *et al.* 1989). In a 7-year follow-up study, obvious atopic disease developed in 19.9% of children, of whom 58% had a raised cord blood of IgE and 14% a low cord blood IgE (Kjellman and Croner 1984). As a result of such studies, it has been recommended that a combination of a family history and cord blood IgE level could generate a family allergy score which would give a probability for the development of atopy. Individuals with a high score could then be studied in various preventive regimens. However more recent and longer follow-up studies have failed to support the predictive value of cord blood IgE (Ruiz *et al.* 1991).

Environment

Whilst primary defects of immune response may be inherent and have a major influence upon allergic status, there is much less influence on the manifestation of the allergy. Recent epidemiological studies suggest a very considerable increase in the prevalence of allergic disease in populations where there has been no change in genetic stock (Fleming and Crombie 1987). Indeed the prevalence of asthma, eczema and hay fever has doubled in 12-year-olds between 1973 and 1988, in the same S. Wales community (Burr *et al.* 1989). Asthma with house dust mite allergy has appeared for the first time in small village communities at high altitude in New Guinea (Dowse *et al.* 1985) and asthma appears much more common in second-generation West Indian immigrants than in their parents who were born overseas (Smith *et al.* 1971). This suggests that environmental influences play an important role in the manifestations of the allergy. Much attention has focused on allergen load, particularly during susceptible periods in early infancy when a maturational defect of immune response may be present.

Dietary allergens and the development of atopy

Thirty-five years ago an American study suggested that there was a low incidence of atopic disease amongst infants fed on breast or soya milk, rather than cow's milk (Glaser and Johnstone 1953). More recent studies have suggested a reduced incidence of allergic disease in breast-fed (Matthew *et al.* 1977; Saarinen *et al.* 1979, Businco *et al.* 1983; Chandra *et al.* 1985) compared with bottle-fed infants, although other studies have failed to show this (Hide and Guyer 1981; Krammer and Moroz 1981). It is also possible that the early introduction of diverse solids to the infant may decrease the incidence of eczema (Fergusson *et al.* 1981) but not asthma (Fergusson *et al.* 1983). The suggestion that soya milk is less allergenic than cow's milk has not been confirmed. Furthermore, there is now evidence that the allergenicity of cow's milk may be reduced by heat treatment or hydrolysis as used in the preparation of new infant formulae based on cow's milk (McLaughlin *et al.* 1981). The variations in antigenicity of different cow's milk formulae might account for the discrepant observations of the protective effect of these formulae, compared with breast milk. Older studies using relatively unaltered cow's milk formulae have produced a higher incidence of atopy than breast-feeding, whilst more recent studies with newer infant formulae appear to have much lower incidences (Taylor *et al.* 1984). Furthermore, food intolerance and allergy can occur even in fully breast-fed infants from antigen ingestion by the mother which penetrates into breast milk (Shannon 1921; Warner 1980), and it is well known that the human placenta is permeable to food antigens which could lead to sensitization of the fetus *in utero* (Matsumura *et al.* 1975; Chandra *et al.* 1986; Zeiger *et al.* 1986). Indeed, food-specific IgE antibodies have occasionally been found in cord blood samples and fetal cells have been shown to be capable of producing IgE from mid-pregnancy onwards (Michel *et al.* 1980). We have shown that high levels of T lymphocyte proliferation to milk allergen (β lactoglobulin) and low IFN-γ production in the cord blood is strongly associated with the subsequent development of milk-induced eczema. This observation was supported by the finding of high levels of memory (CD45RO+) cells in the cord blood, and suggests *in utero* priming (Warner *et al.* 1992).

These latter observations have led to the suggestion that maternal diet during pregnancy and lactation may influence the development of atopy (Chandra *et al.* 1986). There is, however, an alternative opinion, arising from animal studies, which suggests that food hyposensitization, in other words increased food exposure during pregnancy and lactation (via the mother), may be a way of preventing atopic disease in the infant (Kleinman *et al.* 1983; Jarrett and Hall 1984). These postulates have been investigated in control studies. A randomized prospective trial of maternal abstention from cow's milk and egg for the third trimester of pregnancy showed that, whilst maternal IgG antibodies to cow's milk diminished during the dietary period, there was no difference in cord blood IgE levels and subsequent atopic disease between abstention and non-abstention groups (Falth-Magnusson and Kjellman 1987). It remains to be seen whether longer follow-up will show any effect. This is possible, as a prospective study of allergy in high-risk children only began to reveal relationships between high cord blood IgE and wheeze after the 4th year of life (Burr *et al.* 1989b). Alternatively, diet only in the third trimester may not have been adequate as T cell activation may occur earlier in pregnancy (Hayward 1983). However, for the present there is no evidence to support the recommendation of dietary abstention during pregnancy to reduce atopy.

The alternative suggestion from animal studies that exposure to antigen under protection of maternal antibodies may be part of the normal development of tolerance has been investigated in another randomized prospective study of mother/baby pairs, comparing a high maternal intake of cow's milk and egg during pregnancy with a low intake. So far, the only results available are of cord blood IgG and E antibodies to cow's milk and egg, which show no difference in the two groups (Lilja *et al.* 1988). Again, it remains to be seen whether subsequent manifestation of atopy is affected.

One open prospective, but uncontrolled, study investigated the combined effect of dieting during the last trimester of pregnancy and lactation. The regimen was an 'idealized strategy' in which mothers avoided cow's milk, egg and peanuts from the 28th week of gestation onwards and also restricted the intake of wheat, soy and citrus fruits. There was a delay in introduction of highly allergenic foods to the babies and environmental control, including the avoidance of smoke and pets and reduction of house mite levels. Despite this enormous undertaking, the cumulative incidence of allergic disease to 3 years of age appeared no different from that which would have been predicted from population studies (Zeiger *et al.* 1986). However, there may have been some problems with compliance with the regimen, which might account for failure. One prospective controlled study has demonstrated a lower incidence of atopic eczema up to 6 months of age when their breast-feeding mothers avoided egg, cow's milk and fish. Unfortunately, the protective effect of maternal diet did not last beyond 6 months, either for atopic dermatitis or other atopic manifestations or for the number of positive skin tests to egg, cow's milk or fish (Hattevig *et al.* 1989). However, the overall conclusion at present must be that dietary manipulations during pregnancy are of no value but that there may be some benefit in recommending restriction of highly allergenic foods from the mother during lactation and in delaying the introduction of those allergenic foods once the infant is weaned.

Aeroallergen exposure and the development of atopy

Most studies to date have focused on diets and the evolution of eczema. This has occurred because it is easier to monitor diet and to document the presence or absence of eczema. Furthermore, this condition is likely to evolve within the first few years of life. The prospective controlled study which showed the greatest protective effect of breast-feeding which extended well beyond the period of dietary control in fact also employed other environmental manipulations, which included reducing exposure to common aeroallergens such as house dust mite and animal danders (Matthew *et al.* 1977).

Studies from Papua New Guinea would suggest that increasing exposure to house dust mite is a particularly important factor in the increased prevalence of asthma (Dowse *et al.* 1985). The results of this study suggest that, although bronchial hyper-reactivity may be independently, genetically inherited, it is not revealed until the lung has received an allergen-induced inflammatory insult (Britton *et al.* 1986). The same is almost certainly true in Europe, and studies of individuals raised at high altitude, where house dust mite exposure is extremely low, have revealed a lower prevalence of asthma than in similar ethnic groups living at sea-level (Vervloet *et al.* 1982).

Indirect information that aeroallergenic exposure may be important in infancy comes from month-of-birth studies, particularly in relation to birch pollen allergy. Bjorksten *et al.* (1980) correlated the highest skin reactivity to birch pollen in infants born just before the peak of the birch pollen season. This exposure influenced the development of pollen allergy for 20 years. These authors estimated that allergy to birch pollen could be reduced by 28% if individuals were not born in the month of February to April. These findings were confirmed in a second study, but the seasonal influence was limited to babies with elevated cord blood IgE (Croner and Kjellman 1986). Furthermore, there are significant differences in month-of-birth distribution in patients with mould sensitivity from studies done in Strasburg (Quoix *et al.* 1988). House mite-sensitive asthmatics, compared with asthmatics not sensitive to this allergen, have significantly different months of birth, which correlates with the height of the house mite dust season in London, England (Warner and Price 1978). Studies in Rome, Italy, have similarly revealed different months of birth for both house mite-sensitive and pollen-sensitive individuals (Búsinco *et al.* 1988). Similar associations have been observed for exposure to cat (Suoniemi *et al.* 1981) and dog (Vanto *et al.* 1983) dander in infancy and subsequent cat or dog allergy. However, not all studies of month of birth and atopic diseases have revealed such striking associations (Reed 1958; Kemp 1979; David and Beards 1985).

The differences in month of birth in relation to house mite sensitivity is difficult to explain on the basis of studies done by the Platts-Mills group (Tovey *et al.* 1981). They found that in an undisturbed room airborne mite allergen cannot be detected when using sampling rates of 17 litres per minute for up to 8 hours. Most of the house mite allergen found in the air during vigorous domestic disturbance was in particles of greater than 10 μm. Thus, it would be unlikely that such particles would penetrate the airways, particularly of small infants with a tidal minute volume of only 2–3 litres per minute. Furthermore, a study attempting to estimate the likely exposure of infants to house dust mite allergen using an infant respiratory pump only detected very minute quantities during bed-making when the apparatus was held extremely close to the blankets. In other situations no allergen was detected (Carswell *et al.* 1982). This being the case, the month of birth associations must be spurious.

We have recently investigated the potential aeroallergen exposure in homes of asthmatic children in the month after their month of birth, provided they have not moved homes. Air sampling was performed using a low-volume sampler equivalent to the minute tidal volume of the new-born baby. We have been able to detect significant quantities of aeroallergen by low-volume sampling in rooms during normal domestic activity (Price *et al.* 1990). Furthermore, correlates with a degree of sensitivity to the allergen strongly suggest that early allergenic exposure is important (Warner *et al.* 1991) (Table 57.2). It remains to be seen in prospective studies whether primary aeroallergen avoidance will alter the incidence or natural history of manifestations of respiratory allergy. However, the weight of evidence supports the idea that exposure to allergen

Table 57.2. Comparison of aeroallergens detected in 68 homes with patient skin test reactions. The association between aeroallergens' presence or absence in the room air of asthmatic children's homes and a positive or negative skin test response to those allergens in the same children

Aeroallergen in homes	Relationship with SPT
Der p 1	$P < 0.001$
Fel d 1	$P < 0.001$
Tree pollen	$P < 0.01$
Grass pollen	$P < 0.77$
3 Common fungi	$P < 0.45$

Source: Warner *et al.* 1991.

in early infancy has a considerable influence on the pattern of sensitivities which develop in susceptible individuals.

Other environmental influences

Currently there is considerable interest in the influence of passive smoking of infants and young children in relation to the subsequent development of allergy and asthma. Many studies have identified that children of smoking parents and, in particular, smoking mothers have a higher frequency of respiratory illnesses (Holt and Turner 1984). More recent studies have shown a highly significant increase in wheezing, coughing and respiratory infections in children with smoking mothers and that this effect is directly proportional to the number of cigarettes smoked by the mother (Kershaw 1987). This effect may also be apparent with antenatal smoking, where the influence cannot be on the airways directly but may affect both immunological maturation and perhaps lung growth (Taylor and Wadsworth 1987). Studies have shown that children of parents who smoke have an increased prevalence of eczema (Rantakallio 1978) and higher IgE levels than those of parents who do not smoke (Kjellman 1981). Furthermore, antenatal maternal smoking increases the cord blood IgE of the resulting offspring (Magnusson 1986).

Cigarette smoking obviously increases the risk of certain respiratory illnesses and, in particular, infection with the respiratory syncytial virus in infancy. Following this illness, recurrent coughing and wheezing over the next 4–5 years is a frequent occurrence (Pullan and Hey 1982). However, there is some dispute as to whether this is associated with an increased family history of atopy or a greater likelihood of full-blown atopic asthma. Some studies show no greater incidence of atopy, although there is a continued increase in bronchial hyper-reactivity even 10 years after recovery from the original illness (Pullan and Hey 1982). However, in other studies a higher family history of atopy has been apparent in infants who have developed bronchiolitis following respiratory syncytial infection, and therefore these individuals subsequently have a higher than expected incidence of asthma (Zweiman *et al.* 1966). Similar observations have been made in relation to whooping cough due to infection with *Bordetella pertussis* (Johnston *et al.* 1986). These and other infections are common trigger factors for bronchial obstruction and can induce IgE production.

Other forms of environmental air pollution have long been identified as triggers of attacks in asthmatic individuals. However, animal studies suggest that such factors may also compound the development of asthma and other atopic diseases in the first place (Gershwin *et al.* 1981). Such factors as sulphur dioxide, chemical pollution from new building materials, low temperature and high relative humidity may be important. Mould colonization in damp homes is associated with an increase in symptoms in the upper and lower respiratory tract and in an increased frequency of allergy (Waegemaekers *et al.* 1989). However, to what extent the dampness and allergy are causally related because of mould, house mite, bacteria or other factors is not clear. Large prospective studies will be required to identify the relative importance of each factor. A hypothetical link between the many factors associated with the development of allergy and allergic disease is shown in Fig. 57.1.

Asthma

Epidemiology

Asthma is the commonest chronic disease of childhood. It is eminently treatable in virtually all cases and yet remains commonly underdiagnosed and undertreated. Studies in schoolchildren have shown that less than half of those who have had recurrent wheezing in the previous year have been diagnosed as having asthma. The diagnosis of

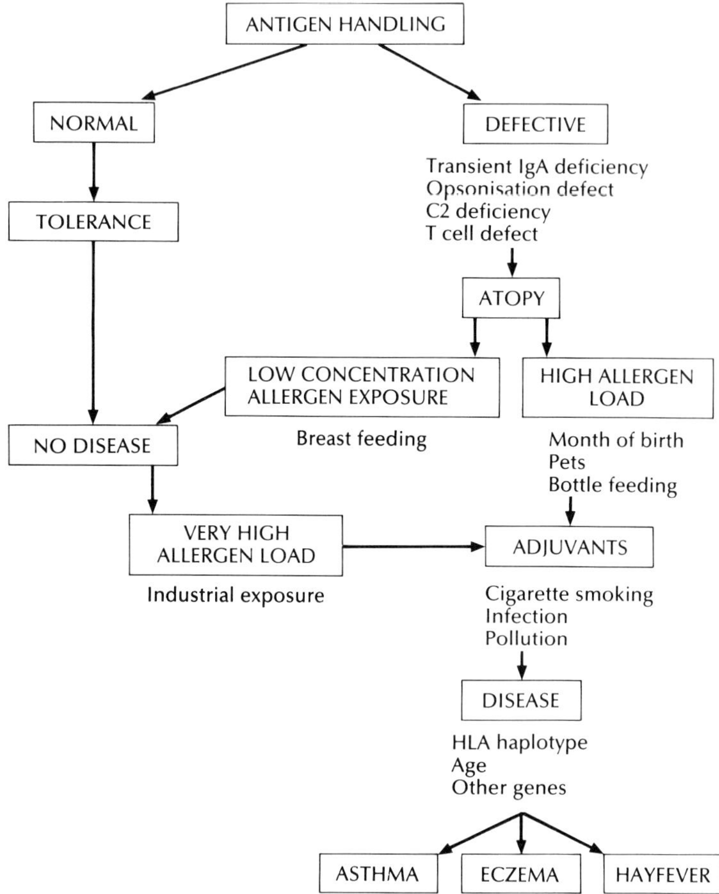

Fig. 57.1. Hypothetical links between the various predisposing factors associated with the development of allergy and allergic disease.

asthma has usually been associated with the use of appropriate anti-asthma treatment whilst conversely a lack of diagnosis in a recurrently wheezy child has been associated with an absence of use of bronchodilators and other appropriate anti-asthma therapies (Speight *et al.* 1983). The consequence has inevitably been considerable school absences, which can be reduced by the use of appropriate treatment (Colver 1984). The overall prevalence of asthma from studies done in Great Britain has ranged between 10 and 15% in mid-childhood (Hill *et al.* 1989). However, figures as high as 25% have been quoted from some studies, whereas, in rural Africa and amongst Canadian Eskimos, there is an extremely low prevalence (Gregg 1983).

Deaths from asthma in childhood are rare but 40–45 children die each year in England and Wales from this disease and there has been no diminution in the death-rate in the last 20 years. Indeed, there was an increase in mortality in the 10- to 14-year-old age-group during the mid-1960s, which paralleled the increase in adult asthma deaths. The cause of this epidemic has been discussed at length and, even today, remains unresolved, although there are strong suggestions of a relationship between inappropriate use of bronchodilators rather than anti-inflammatory prophylactic compounds such as steroids. The same has been suggested for the more recent epidemic of asthma deaths in New Zealand with regular use of inhaled β-agonists more than three times daily being implicated as a factor contributing to increased morbidity and mortality. (Sears *et al.* 1990). At the same time, there has been an enormous increase in hospital admissions for asthma in all age-groups. This is more likely to be explained by a shift in the balance in care, with increasing reliance on hospital rather than primary medical care. Nevertheless, despite this, there has not been an improvement in outcome (Storr *et al.* 1988).

Natural history

It is repeatedly stated that childhood asthma is a self-limiting disorder which tends to improve spontaneously during adolescence. However, this is a misleading and inaccurate generalization (Kelly *et al.* 1987). The Melbourne prospective study of asthma provides the most complete data on its natural history. Mild episodic wheezing of mid-childhood is predominantly self-limiting, with up to 12% of the Melbourne child population falling into this group. The 5% of all children who have more frequent earlier-onset asthma were more likely to have persistent symptoms through adolescence, and the chronic severe perennial asthmatic very rarely remitted (McNicol and Williams 1973a). Prognosis was less favourable with an early age of onset, frequent severe or prolonged attacks in the first year after onset and the presence of infantile eczema (Blair 1977). The sex ratio progressed from a male to female ratio of 1:1 for mild episodic asthma to 4:1 for chronic severe perennial asthma (McNicol and Williams 1973a). As the ratio for severe asthma is closer to 1:1 in adults, there must be more males who improve or remit and more females who have persistent problems or develop asthma for the first time in adolescence (Kelly *et al.* 1987). This has not yet been clearly documented. Smoking in adolescence decreases the probability of an improvement in asthmatic symptoms amongst patients who have wheezed since early childhood (Martin *et al.* 1982).

Whilst treatment has greatly reduced the morbidity from asthma, no studies have yet identified whether any therapy alters the natural history of the condition. Indeed, the only long-term follow-up study suggested that undertreatment in early adolescence did not influence the severity of asthma at the age of 21 (Martin *et al.* 1982). The relationship between chronic obstructive lung disease in the adult and childhood asthma has yet to be established. Epidemiological studies addressing this problem have, unfortunately, not separated other causes of lower respiratory tract illness from asthma.

Bronchial hyper-responsiveness

The *sinae qua non* of asthma is bronchial hyper-responsiveness. The very definition incorporates this concept in stating that rapid variations in airflow limitation are the characteristic feature of the disease. Only smooth muscle spasm can produce such rapid changes but this cannot explain the chronicity of the condition nor the intense inflammatory response in the airways which is characteristic of severe asthma and a typical finding at post mortem. Nevertheless, bronchial hyper-reactivity is present in most childhood asthmatics and tends to subside during adolescence when asthma is remitting (Balfour-Lynn *et al.* 1981). Bronchial hyper-reactivity, however, occurs in non-asthmatic conditions such as cystic fibrosis and following viral respiratory tract infections. Furthermore, there are considerable inconsistencies in the way non-specific bronchial responses are modified by drugs compared with the response to such drugs clinically (Warner and Boner 1988).

Allergy

Allergy occurs commonly in childhood asthma with 93% of asthmatic children beyond the age of 5 having positive prick skin tests (Russell and Jones 1976). Raised serum IgE and detectable IgE antibodies to allergens is commonly associated with asthma (Foucard 1973). Asthma is more severe in individuals who have had atopic eczema (McNichol and Williams 1973b).

These facts point to a more fundamental role of allergy in the pathogenesis of asthma. However, below the age of 5, allergy is relatively less easily demonstrated and viral respiratory infection is a far more common precipitant of wheezing (Weiss *et al.* 1985). In addition, wheezing can be exacerbated by factors such as exercise, cold air and irritants, such as cigarette smoke and sulphur dioxide (Silverman and Wilson 1985). Gastro-oesophageal reflux may occasionally increase bronchial hyper-reactivity (Wilson *et al.* 1985) and emotional stress is also important (Cohen and Lask 1983). However, only allergy and infection have a significant and prolonged influence on bronchial hyper-responsiveness.

Direct bronchial challenge with allergen has been used in the study of bronchial asthma for many years. It produces the final arbiter for a precise allergy diagnosis (Warner 1977). The initial response to allergen is similar to that of other non-specific provoking agents, such as histamine and methacholine. However, the response is slightly

Table 57.3. Comparison of characteristics of natural and laboratory allergen-induced asthma

	Laboratory allergen challenge		Natural allergen-induced asthma
	Immediate reaction	Dual — immediate and late reaction	
Allergen	Soluble		Particulate
Exposure	Short duration		Prolonged or repeated
Other precipitants	Partially controlled		Many
Response	Short duration self-timing	Prolonged	May be prolonged
Bronchodilator response	Excellent	Poor	Variable
Steroid response	No effect	Excellent	Excellent
Severity of reaction	No correlation with clinical features	Occurs in patients with severe asthma	—

slower to develop and is of somewhat longer duration, being up to 1 hour. There are several difficulties in relating this response to naturally induced asthma. The allergen bronchial challenge in the laboratory utilizes a soluble extract administered over a short period of time. This distributes the allergen diffusely in large airways in a high total dose compared with natural exposure. However, in natural exposure particulate material is inhaled and, at the point where these particles sediment on mucosal surfaces, the concentration of antigen release is extremely high (Platts-Mills *et al.* 1984). This would produce an intense immunological response in a small area, which may be amplified by neurogenic and immunological mechanisms (Chung 1986). Furthermore, natural exposure occurs continuously, or repeatedly, over long periods. Thus, it is not surprising that the laboratory-induced reaction is of short duration, self-limiting and totally abolished by bronchodilators, whereas natural asthma can be severe prolonged and sometimes unresponsive to bronchodilators (Table 57.3).

Allergen challenge is not only followed by an immediate response; between 50 and 75% of asthmatics also have a late reaction (Warner 1976; Price *et al.* 1982; Bierman 1984). This develops 3–4 hours after challenge and lasts for at least 12 and sometimes 48 hours. The late reaction is usually more severe than the immediate reaction and its lung function characteristics are those of severe asthma. The presence of an immediate and late reaction to allergen is associated with more severe clinical disease (Warner 1976). Furthermore, the late reaction is less responsive to bronchodilators but completely abolished by pretreatment with steroids. Sodium cromoglycate has a variable effect on both responses, sometimes preventing both and on other occasions having no effect on either (Booij-Noord and De Vries 1971). Thus, the response to drugs is rather more similar to that of severe asthma and suggests that the late reaction is associated with airway inflammation, as well as bronchospasm.

In adults the allergen-induced dual bronchial response is associated with an enhancement of bronchial hyper-reactivity (Cockcroft *et al.* 1977). Our own studies on children with seasonal asthma due to grass pollen sensitivity demonstrated enhancement of histamine responses only in those with dual reaction to pollen inhalation, and not in those who had an isolated immediate reaction to pollen (Warner and Boner 1988). However, there is some controversy as to whether bronchial hyper-reactivity can be enhanced after an isolated allergen-induced immediate bronchial response (Thorpe *et al.* 1987). The bronchial hyper-reactivity can persist for a long time after recovery from the allergen-induced reaction and is associated with repeated dips in lung function for 2–4 weeks after a single allergen challenge (Cartier *et al.* 1982). This is comparable to the clinical situation in pollen-sensitive asthmatics, who develop increased bronchial hyper-reactivity during the course of the pollen season (Boulet *et al.* 1983).

The mechanism of the late bronchial reaction is unknown. In the skin it occurs more frequently the higher the dose of antigen and the larger the immediate skin reaction. The frequency of dual bronchial or nasal reactions has not been associated with the magnitude of the immediate reaction and has often occurred with a very low dose of antigen (Price *et al.* 1983). In some studies a high IgE level to antigen has been associated with late responses, which suggests that the dual reaction is related to a greater degree of allergy (Boulet *et al.* 1984). The presence of IgG-4 antibodies has not been associated with the presence or absence of a dual response, and it is unlikely that the late reaction is due to type 3 hypersensitivity as it is not associated with fever or complement consumption (Price *et al.* 1983).

Allergens

House dust mite sensitivity is the commonest allergy in asthmatics in most parts of the world (Warner 1978). Unfortunately, attempts to reduce exposure to this agent have predominantly been a failure in UK (Burr *et al.* 1980) but not in other countries (Murray and Ferguson 1983). The warm humid conditions which exist in the bedclothes are ideal for mite replication. Most simple hygiene measures are ineffective whilst the use of sprays which kill the mite do not eliminate enough of the allergen to be effective clinically and even new bedding will be recolonized by mites within 1–2 months (Reiser *et al.* 1990). However, there are some promising developments in this area (Green *et al.* 1989). The admission of house dust mite-sensitive asthmatics to hospital, where there are few, if any, house dust mites, has been shown to produce a decrease in bronchial hyper-reactivity over 3 months in adults (Platts-Mills *et al.* 1982). We have also shown this in asthmatic children resident at high altitude for 9 months, where the humidity is low and house mite exposure is zero. In these conditions there is a progressive decrease in asthma symptoms and in bronchial hyper-reactivity (Warner and Boner 1988).

Banishing the much-loved family pet is difficult but should be recommended if it is shown to be a cause of problems, but it will take at least 3 months for the dander to be totally eliminated from the dust (Warner *et al.* 1991). Avoidance of seasonal aeroallergens is impossible without an air compressor, filter and helmet, but exposure can be reduced by keeping windows shut in the home and by installation of air-conditioners.

It is rare for children to have a clear history of asthma precipitated by food or drink, although the relative importance of ingestants has not been well studied. If such a history does exist, avoidance is indicated. Assessment of the importance of food and food additives can be very complicated because the ingestants may not produce a direct asthmatic response but may increase bronchial hyper-reactivity, as has been demonstrated with oral tartrazine challenge in children (Hariparsad *et al.* 1984). The difficulty in diagnosis, the problems in maintaining a nutritious and attractive diet if food avoidance is recommended and the efficacy of pharmacotherapy irrespective of allergic status render consideration of food intolerance superfluous in the majority of cases.

Diagnostic tests

There is considerable confusion as to the relative value of allergy investigations in the clinical situation. As most children will respond to simple pharmacotherapy, irrespective of allergic status, allergy investigation might be considered unnecessary. However, it is important to search for causes and sometimes simple avoidance regimens can reduce reliance on pharmacotherapy.

Skin prick tests remain the principal aid to allergy diagnosis, but great care is required in performing the test, with appropriate positive and negative controls and the use of well-characterized allergen extracts (Dreborg 1987). It is unnecessary to use a large number of allergens, and for the diagnosis of atopy alone this can be restricted to three (house dust mite, cat fur and grass pollen) (Russell and Jones 1976). In general, the larger the weal reaction, together with the presence of a late skin reaction, the more likely the sensitivity is to be of relevance. However, correlation with bronchial allergen challenge can sometimes be poor (Warner 1977).

Immunoglobulin E antibody measurement correlates well with bronchial provocation tests but reliability depends on the quality of the allergen extracts employed. In routine clinical practice, bronchial provocation test is only marginally more accurate than a well-taken clinical history with skin prick test and IgE antibody measurements to those factors considered to be important (Aas 1970). Further studies will only be necessary in those individuals where drastic allergen avoidance measures are likely to be recommended or where immunotherapy is being considered.

Immunotherapy

The only specific therapy available is immunotherapy, sometimes known as hyposensitization. This treatment has been used extensively since it was first demonstrated in 1911 that injection of boiled grass pollen extracts produced a reduction in conjunctival sensitivity and in symptoms of hay fever (Freeman 1911; Noon 1911). At that time, no other treatments were available for allergic patients and thus this approach was appropriate. Now that we have highly effective and safe pharmacotherapies, the role of immunotherapy has been questioned. Particularly in asthma, it has resulted in death from both anaphylaxis and provocation of severe asthma (Warner and Kerr 1987). Sixteen of the 26 deaths from hyposensitization reported by the Committee on Safety of Medicines were in asthmatic patients, although this should be balanced against the 25 000 patients with asthma who have died because 'medicine' has failed them over the same period.

There is good evidence of efficacy of house dust mite immunotherapy in childhood asthma (Warner *et al.* 1978), although not in adult asthma (Warner 1984). One trial of house dust mite hyposensitization in a group of children with moderately severe asthma demonstrated by bronchial challenge showed considerable clinical benefit. There was a highly significant and large reduction in requirement for standard anti-asthma therapies in the actively treated group (Warner *et al.* 1978). There was, however, no change in immediate skin or bronchial response to house dust mite and also no change in IgE or IgG antibodies to house mite (Price *et al.* 1984; Turner *et al.* 1984). However, a significant number of actively treated patients lost their late bronchial response after the treatment and this did not occur in the placebo-treated group. The greatest clinical improvements occurred in those patients who lost their late bronchial reaction (Price *et al.* 1984). These observations have been substantiated by one or two other studies published recently (Van Bever and Stevens 1990; Fling *et al.* 1989). This establishes the importance of allergy in relation to asthma and indicates that the late, rather than the immediate, reaction is the principal factor in this relationship. Unfortunately, children with the most severe asthma do not benefit from this therapy and, furthermore, symptoms recur as soon as the treatment is stopped, which suggests that this treatment is little different from any other prophylactic remedy (Warner 1986).

Anti-asthma therapy

The treatment of asthma involves a multidisciplinary approach, including an appreciation of the importance of psychosocial factors, counselling and education. Avoidance of obvious precipitants may be possible but in the end the employment of pharmacotherapy will be necessary. Drugs should be prescribed in a rational sequence (Fig. 57.2). Beta-2 agonists will be used for mild episodic wheezing, sodium cromoglycate for mild to moderate asthma and inhaled steroids for moderate to severe asthma. Xanthines, ipratropium bromide

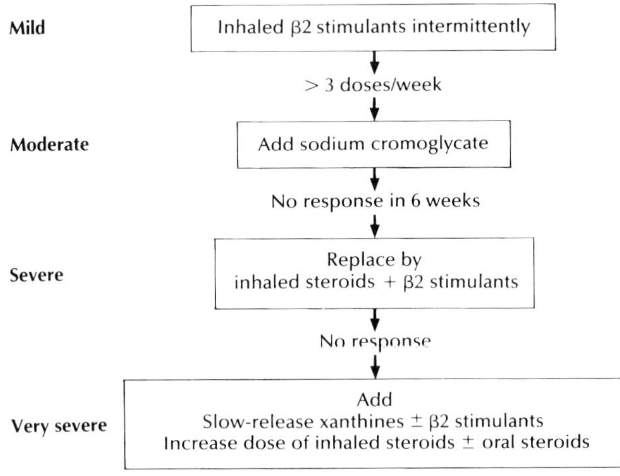

Fig. 57.2. Algorithm for asthma therapy.

and oral steroids have their place in more persistent and severe cases (Warner *et al.* 1989). In general, the inhaled route is preferred for the administration of therapies, although there are practical difficulties to be overcome in the very young child (Reiser and Warner 1986). Thus, under 18 months, only nebulized inhalation therapy will be possible. Between 18 months and 5 years of age, the use of valved reservoir spacer inhalers is to be recommended. Beyond 5, either dry powder or metered-dose inhalers can be employed, although with the latter there are commonly errors of usage which compromise control of the disease.

It should be possible to return all but a tiny minority of children to a normal life style, which includes active participation in sports.

Allergic rhinitis

Allergic rhinitis is also a very common disorder, occurring in approximately 10% of children and in up to 20% of adolescents and young adults (Smith 1984). It occurs in 75% of children with asthma and, like asthma, is frequently underdiagnosed (Viner and Jackman 1976). Its importance as a cause of morbidity is grossly underestimated. It has a profound effect on school performance and, in this respect, underachievement at examinations, which are often inappropriately held during the height of the pollen season, is common. Seasonal allergic rhinitis is estimated to occur in 5–9% of children but is quite rare under the age of 5 (Emanuel 1988). Isolated perennial rhinitis occurs in 3% of children, but in association with perennial asthma it is very common.

Like asthma, individuals with allergic rhinitis have non-specific irritability of the affected organ. Thus symptoms of nasal congestion, sneezing, itching and rhinorrhoea can be triggered by non-specific irritants such as cigarette smoke and strong paint fumes or odours, as well as exposure to allergens (Krayenbuhl *et al.* 1988). Noisy breathing and irritating sniffing, coughing and throat-clearing often lead to social isolation at school and discord at home. Itching of the pharynx and palate, hearing loss and anosmia may also occur. Particularly in seasonal allergic rhinitis, an associated conjunctivitis is common. At least 20% of children also have middle ear abnormalities with hearing deficit, leading to learning difficulties and speech delay (Bernstein *et al.* 1981).

The distribution of allergen sensitivities is very similar in allergic rhinitis to that for asthma, and the tests employed to identify them are equally similar. Intranasal challenge can be performed even in small children. Anterior rhinomanometry to detect changes in resistance can be used in children down to the age of 4. Posterior rhinomanometry and nasal peak inspiratory flow require more patient co-operation and are usually reproducible beyond the ages of 6 or 7. On the whole, nasal challenge is only a research tool. Utilizing this technique, it is possible to demonstrate late allergic responses. In a study of nasal provocation in atopic children, symptomatic rhinitis was strongly associated with late, rather than immediate, nasal reactions, which is equivalent to observations made with bronchial challenge (Price *et al.* 1982).

Therapy for allergic rhinitis follows similar lines to that for asthma. Allergen avoidance should be recommended if possible. It is also important to avoid non-specific irritants, such as paint fumes, dust, cigarette smoke and exhaust fumes. Hot and spicy foods may exacerbate already pre-existing rhinitis. However, food intolerance as a cause of this condition is relatively rare. There is little to no evidence that milk, or indeed any other food, is a particularly common cause of rhinitis.

Immunotherapy has a rather more established place in the treatment of this condition than in asthma. Pollen immunotherapy for one or more years has been associated with significant clinical improvements and reduction in requirements for other therapy (Freeman 1911; Frankland and Augustin 1954; Sadan *et al.* 1969; Lichtenstein *et al.* 1971). Furthermore, in the absence of asthma, it is likely to be a safer therapy. So far, only subcutaneous immunotherapy injections have an established place in treatment of seasonal allergic rhinitis and conjunctivitis. Oral and sublingual immunotherapy is of very dubious efficacy (Cooper *et al.* 1984). House dust mite immunotherapy has also been shown to be of greater benefit than placebo (Warner *et al.* 1978), but perennial house mite-induced allergic rhinitis is usually very easily controlled with simple pharmacotherapy.

Pharmacotherapy has included nasal decongestant, antihistamines, cromoglycate and topical steroids. In general, decongestants are not recommended in this condition. Antihistamines form the mainstay of treatment, with a new generation of non-sedative specific H1 receptor antagonists being preferred. They are more effective when used prophylactically rather than awaiting the development of symptoms, and long-term use may even have a small anti-asthma effect. Sodium cromoglycate has been shown to be more effective than placebo, provided a dose frequency of up to six times a day is maintained. However, inhaled corticosteroids have been found to be superior in the relief of symptoms, although rather more for nasal obstruction than for sneezing and rhinorrhoea. They are effective when administered only twice daily and have a good record of safety. Antihistamines and ocular sodium cromoglycate are the most appropriate therapy for allergic conjunctivitis. At present, the combination of an H1-specific antagonist, nasal steroids and ocular cromoglycate has been shown to be the best combination for the treatment of allergic rhinoconjunctivitis (Simons 1988). It is unfortunate that patients with allergic rhinitis tend to be submitted to ear, nose and throat (ENT) surgery more frequently than the rest of the population, because there is no evidence that this approach to treatment has any value (Sanderson and Warner 1987).

Atopic dermatitis (eczema)

Children with eczema are usually atopic. Most have positive immediate skin tests and high levels of total serum IgE. Twenty per cent to 50% go on to develop asthma and up to 50% have allergic rhinitis (Stifler 1965). In Britain the incidence appears to be increasing. In a 1970 cohort of children 12.3% were reported by their parents to have eczema, which is more than double the prevalence that had been noted 12 years previously (Taylor *et al.* 1984).

The pathogenesis of the condition and, indeed, its management are much less well sorted out than for respiratory allergic disease. Whilst atopy is common in the condition, the role of IgE in the aetiology is uncertain. Allergens can be demonstrated to produce weal-and-flare reactions in atopic individuals but they do not usually produce the skin lesions of eczema. However, it is possible to replicate lesions by patch testing with house dust mite in house dust mite-sensitive individuals (Mitchell *et al.* 1982). To date, most of the studies plotting the evolution of atopic diseases have associated dietary variations with the development of eczema and have monitored indices of type 1 hypersensitivity, all of which points to IgE-mediated mechanisms being important (Matthew *et al.* 1977; Krammer and Moroz 1981; Fergusson *et al.* 1983; Chandra *et al.* 1986; Hattevig *et al.* 1989). Furthermore, resolution of the disease, either spontaneously or after long-term treatment with steroids, is associated with a fall in IgE.

It is now well accepted that reactions to foods are important in childhood eczema, both in initiating the disease and in causing exacerbations (Atherton 1982). It has been suggested that this occurs because of enhanced absorption of antigen across the gut mucosa. Mediators are released from sensitized gut mast cells on exposure to food allergens which increase gut permeability, leading to greater antigen absorption, systemic sensitization and allergic manifestations (Paganelli *et al.* 1981). However, positive skin tests and IgE antibody measurements do not accurately predict which foods are likely to be involved in exacerbating eczema (Sampson and Albergo 1984); thus, the pathophysiological relationship between food intolerance and eczema has not been elucidated.

Eighty per cent of patients with eczema present by 1 year of age and more than 90% by the age of 5. Seventy-five per cent of those with milder disease will clear over the first few years of life, whilst those with more severe problems are more likely to have a chronic course. The pattern changes with age. In infancy it is characterized by dry red scaly plaques, usually appearing after 3 months and before 12 months of age, and confined to cheeks, abdomen and extensive surfaces of limbs. Beyond 2 years of age, it is characterized by papules and plaque, with excoriations often restricted to flexural areas. In late childhood and adolescence, the most common location for the rash is on the hands and feet, with often pustular-like lesions. It is also present on upper eyelids and skin flexures (Atherton 1982).

Defective cell-mediated immunity has been identified in individuals with eczema (McGeady and Buckley 1975; Byrom and Timlin 1979). This is very apparent, because eczematous children are particularly susceptible to varicelliform infections. Thus, vaccinia virus can produce devastatingly severe general disease and death. Herpes simplex virus can produce generalized lesions with eczema herpeticum, and eczematous children are particularly prone to molluscum contagiosum. Patients with eczema have a higher than normal incidence of cutaneous anergy to common antigens such as *Candida* (Krafchik 1983). The condition has been associated with decreased lymphocyte proliferation to mitogens, reduced chemotaxis of monocytes (McGeady and Buckley 1975) and polymorphonuclear cells, decreased number of circulating suppressor cells and the presence of IgG anti-IgE autoantibodies (Ito *et al.* 1983).

Some children with eczema improve on diet. This has been established on double-blind crossover studies, particularly in relation to cow's milk and egg antigen avoidance (Atherton *et al.* 1978). In this, as in other studies, there was no correlation between positive skin prick tests to egg and milk and the response to the diet (Broadbent and Sampson 1988). However, this may relate to the quality of food extracts used in skin testing and in IgE antibody assays. The use of fresh-food skin prick tests gives more accurate information for some foods, particularly vegetables and fruits (Ortolani *et al.* 1989). Elemental diets have sometimes been employed in patients with very severe disease, with some benefit (Hill and Lynch 1982). Whilst the use of diets for childhood eczema has been amply justified, the long-term results are often disappointing. Diet can be nutritionally incomplete and impose an immense financial burden on children and parents. Even in highly motivated families with severe eczema associated with food intolerance, up to 20% of children under the age of 3 and 50% over the age of 3 will be unable to maintain the diet, despite worsening of the disease (Hathaway and Warner 1983). At present, it is suggested that only simple diets, such as dairy product and hen's egg avoidance, should be recommended for a therapeutic trial.

Other allergens, including contactants and inhalants, might also be involved, and thus avoidance of house dust mite and animal danders may also be important. As with all other allergic conditions, local irritation by non-specific factors also exacerbates the condition. This will particularly relate to clothing, the washing-powders used to clean the clothes, soaps, perfumes, shampoos and other cosmetics. The presence of lanolin (wool fat) and other skin sensitizers may be particularly important. Many of the topical preparations used to treat the condition contain skin-sensitizing chemicals. Often a trial-and-error approach to the topical preparations is required to establish which are acceptable.

Antihistamine preparations, particularly those which have sedative effects, can reduce pruritus and sleep disturbance. Only topical corticosteroids have a dramatic effect on the condition, but they are potentially dangerous, particularly in young children. They can cause skin atrophy, striae and adrenal suppression. Thus low-potency preparations should be preferred, avoiding the fluorinated corticosteroids. Any skin sepsis should be treated both with topical and systemic antibiotics and may subsequently be prevented by the employment of antiseptics, both on the skin and in the bath water.

Angio-oedema and urticaria

Urticaria and angio-oedema are most frequently seen after acute illnesses such as β-haemolytic streptococcal tonsillitis (Voss *et al.* 1982) or *Campylobacter* enteritis (Lopez-Brea 1984). The symptoms can usually be controlled with antihistamines and will resolve spontaneously within 4–6 weeks. This condition is extremely common in the population, although its prevalence has not been estimated. In some patients it is more persistent or recurrent, and causes include physical factors such as heat, cold and exercise or allergens such as animal danders, drugs and sometimes foods (Twarog 1983). In childhood, chronic persistent urticaria is relatively less common than in adults. Severe angio-oedema, particularly if familial, has very occasionally been associated with C1 esterase inhibitor deficiency. However, in up to 40–50% of patients, a cause cannot be identified from clinical history or standard investigation. In such patients, we have found that up to 75% will improve on diets free of artificial food additives, including azo dyes and benzoate preservatives. However, on subsequent double-blind challenge with these compounds, only about 50% actually react to the compounds. Thus, the frequency of food additive intolerance in more chronic persistent urticaria of childhood is in the region of 35% (Supramaniam and Warner 1986). This matches very closely with the experience of Juhlin (1981), who attributed a third of recurrent urticarias in adults to food additive reactions. The exact mechanism of this reaction is unclear. It is associated with an unexpectedly low frequency of conventional atopic problems. There is no evidence to confirm the presence of specific antibodies, and, if mediator release occurs, then it may well be due to a non-immunological phenomenon (Murdoch *et al.* 1987). Follow-up of food additive intolerance in children has indicated that the problem is transient in the majority (Pollock and Warner 1987).

In contrast, atopic urticaria and angio-oedema associated with reactions to foods (such as dairy products, nuts or fish) are rather more likely to be persistent. For egg allergy, at least 50% persist through to adult life (Ford and Taylor 1982), and for peanut allergy virtually 100% (Bock and Atkins 1989). Antibiotic allergy is relatively rare, though commonly misreported (Graff-Lonnevig *et al.* 1988), but when associated with urticaria or angio-oedema is more likely to be genuine (*Lancet* editorial 1989). The basic treatment is avoidance. However, it is sometimes possible to protect against the reactions to foods by pretreatment with oral sodium cromoglycate (Church and Warner 1985).

Other forms of food intolerance

Food intolerance has acquired a dubious reputation and has become a highly topical subject with regular features in the lay media. This has tended to polarize medical opinion to either complete dismissal or extravagant claims of relationship to a vast number of ill-defined conditions. Unfortunately, most genuine reactions to food cannot yet be identified to have an immunological basis and thus must be termed food intolerance rather than food allergy. It must be distinguished from various forms of food aversion and psychological intolerance, where reactions will not be reproducible when the food is given in a disguised form (Royal College of Physicians/British Nutrition Foundation Committee 1984).

Estimates of prevalence vary widely, depending on the methods of ascertainment. Up to 20% of the community perceive themselves as reacting to foods, whereas the number who can be demonstrated to react on subsequent double-blind challenge is infinitely smaller. Cow's milk protein intolerance, the most common intolerance in childhood, has a prevalence of between 0.2 and 7.5% (Warner 1985). The prevalence of food intolerance appears to diminish progressively and rapidly with age over the first few years of life, and there is no evidence that children treated by dietary manipulations improve any more rapidly or completely than those receiving no such treatment. Eczema, urticaria and angio-oedema would appear to be the commonest manifestations of food intolerance, but failure to thrive, diarrhoea, vomiting, gastrointestinal blood loss, asthma and allergic rhinitis can also be associated. The associations with migraine, epilepsy, infantile colic and hyperactivity, or hyperkinesis, remain highly controversial. Furthermore, it has become apparent that the condition of Munchausen by proxy (a condition where children are presented by their mothers with a variety of fabricated disorders, resulting in extensive and unnecessary investigation and treatment) sometimes presents with apparent food intolerance. These cases are particularly difficult to manage (Warner and Hathaway 1984).

Gastrointestinal reactions present in two forms. Some foods, such as milk, eggs, nuts and fish, can produce an immediate rapid-onset reaction with vomiting and abdominal pain and, within an hour or two, diarrhoea. Such patients may also have other obvious atopic manifestations. The reactions are usually IgE-mediated, with strongly positive skin tests and IgE antibodies. The slower-onset reactions, which are probably more common, may take hours or days to evolve. In such situations, abdominal distension and pain, diarrhoea, gastrointestinal blood loss and failure to thrive may occur. Sometimes there is evidence of an enteropathy, with small-bowel biopsies revealing patchy villous atrophy. This condition is best studied for cow's milk enteropathy but can also occur in association with egg, soy, gluten, rice, chicken and fish intolerance (Hutchins and Walker-Smith 1982). Food intolerance may also lead to infantile colitis with chronic bloody diarrhoea. Whilst there is superficial ulceration of the mucosa, unlike ulcerative colitis there is no abnormality of crypt architecture. Inflammatory cells within the lamina propria mainly consist of plasma cells and eosinophils (Jenkins *et al.* 1984). In all these conditions, food avoidance results in dramatic improvements in the condition.

Migraine and epilepsy

The association of migraine and epilepsy with food intolerance still requires confirmation. There has been one double-blind placebo controlled trial in children with severe migraine who were intolerant to food. Children successfully treated with diets no longer developed migraine to a variety of recognized non-specific stimuli, and other symptoms such as abdominal pain and eczema were also improved (Egger *et al.* 1983). There was a reduction in epileptic fits in a few of the patients. It remains to be seen whether these observations can be replicated in other studies, and, indeed, whether the reaction is immunologically based. Evidence from adults suggests that there can be several provoking factors for migraine which are not necessarily the same in all people who have this condition and pharmacological mechanisms may be involved (Moneret-Vautrin 1983).

Hyperactivity (Hyperkinesis)

The term 'hyperactivity' is used very loosely. In the United Kingdom it is considered to be rare and often associated with defects of neurological function. However, in the United States, it is commonly diagnosed in relatively normal children who have behaviour disorders and learning problems. It is all too easy to collude with parents who cannot accept a psychosocial explanation for their child's disruptive behaviour, by suggesting that the child is suffering from food intolerance. The use of the Feingold diet, which is essentially free from additives and natural salicylates, has been extensively encouraged by lay organizations representing hyperactive children (Feingold 1975). The Nutrition Foundation in the United States concluded (1980) that therapeutic claims were based only on anecdotal reports and double-blind studies have given equivocal results which tend to refute the claim that food additives are responsible for hyperactivity. One controlled trial in London has shown that diets may improve behaviour in some children with severe hyperactivity (Egger *et al.* 1985). Our own recent studies have suggested that unnaturally high doses of food additives can produce a small adverse effect on childhood behaviour, but this phenomenon is not reproducibly detected by the parents during double-blind challenge procedures. Thus, the parents' perception of food as an obvious cause of aberrent behaviour in their children was usually incorrect (Pollock and Warner, 1990). Our studies would suggest that the phenomenon is pharmacologically, rather than immunologically, based. It has been demonstrated that high doses of food additives can produce histamine release, both *in vivo* and *in vitro* (Murdoch *et al.* 1987). Chronic urticarial individuals are intolerant to histamine, possibly because of deficiency of diamine oxidase (Murdoch and Pollock 1989). Similar abnormalities could occur in patients with other manifestations of food additive and food intolerance.

DIAGNOSIS AND TREATMENT

In the absence of reliable objective diagnostic tests, dietary manipulations are the only method of establishing a diagnosis and treatment of food intolerance or allergy. A series of diets may be employed. Initially, a simple exclusion diet may be employed, and subsequently it may be necessary to resort to drastic exclusions, using so-called oligo-antigenic diets. Each diet is employed for a fixed period in order to establish whether an improvement in the condition can be achieved. If not, alternative therapeutic approaches should be employed. If there is a significant improvement, the eliminated foods are sequentially reintroduced one per week in appropriate quantities, at least as large as in the normal diet. This enables parents to produce a short list of foods which appear to have produced reaction (Warner 1985). Thereafter, rechallenging is done on a double-blind basis in order to establish unequivocally that the foods are associated with symptoms (Fig. 57.3). Ideally, the double-blind challenge should be performed on three occasions in order to establish beyond doubt the association (Goldman *et al.* 1985). However, in clinical situations, this is often not possible. Furthermore, great care is required during challenge, as occasional children may have a severe generalized reaction on rechallenge after a period of abstinence (David 1984). Subsequently, a stable exclusion diet can be established. The whole procedure requires careful supervision by a dietitian to ensure the nutritional soundness of the regime. Thereafter, the diet is maintained for a minimum of 12 months. It may then be possible to reintroduce offending foods. It must be clear that, if diets fail, then food intolerance is not a cause of the problem or, if the rigours of the diet are more intrusive than the disease, alternative treatment must be sought.

Apart from symptomatic treatment, the only other valid pharmacological approach to food in-

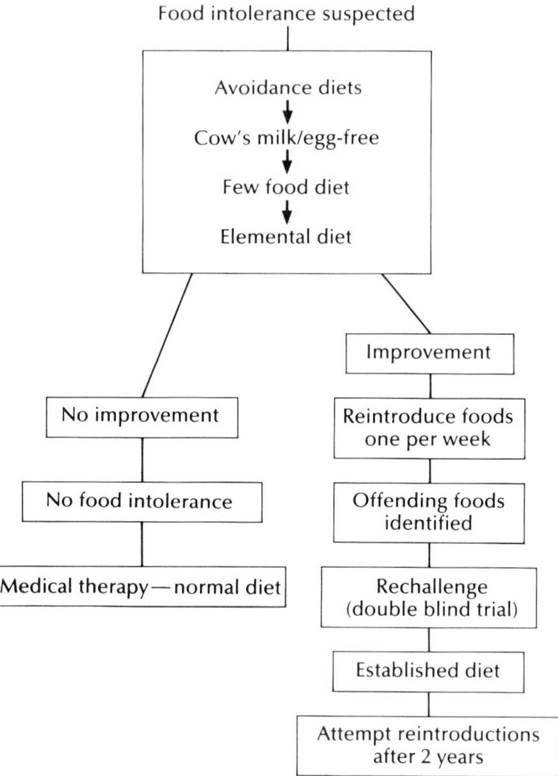

Fig. 57.3. Flow diagram of management of suspected food intolerance.

tolerance has been the use of large doses of sodium cromoglycate taken orally before food. This is occasionally effective, although usually only for IgE-mediated reactions. There is no convincing evidence that immunotherapy, either by injection or orally, has any role in the management of food allergy (Warner 1985).

References

Aas, K. (1970). Bronchial provocation tests in asthma. *Arch. Dis. Child* **45**, 221–8.

Atherton, D.J. (1982). Atopic eczema. In *Food Allergy*, ed. J. Brostoff and S.J. Challacombe. *Clin. Immunol Allergy* **2**, 77–100.

Atherton, D.J., Sewell, M., Soothill, J.F., Wells, R.S. and Chilvers, C.E.D. (1978). A double-blind controlled crossover trial of an antigen avoidance diet in atopic eczema. *Lancet* **i**, 401–3.

Balfour-Lynn, L., Tooley, M. and Godfrey, S. (1981). Relationship of exercise-induced asthma to clinical asthma in childhood. *Arch. Dis. Child.* **56**, 450–4.

Bazaral, M., Orgel, H.A. and Hamburger, R.N. (1974). Genetics of IgE and allergy: serum IgE levels in twins. *J. Allergy Clin. Immunol.* **54**, 288–304.

Berciano, F.A., Crespo, M., Bao, C.G. and Alvarez, F.V. (1987). Serum levels of total IgE in non-allergic children. *Allergy* **42**, 276–83.

Bernstein, J.M., Ellis, E. and Li, P. (1981). The role of IgE mediated hypersensitivity in other media with effusion. *Otolaryngol. Head Neck Surg.* **89**, 874–8.

Bierman, C.W. (1984). A comparison of late reactions to antigen and exercise. *J. Allergy Clin. Immunol.* **73**, 654–9.

Bjorksten, F., Suoniemi, I. and Koski, V. (1980). Neonatal birch-pollen contact and subsequent allergy to birch pollen. *Clin. Allergy* **10**, 581–91.

Blair, H. (1977). Natural history of childhood asthma: 20 year follow-up. *Arch. Dis. Child.* **52**, 613–19.

Bock, S.A. and Atkins, F.M. (1989). The natural history of peanut allergy. *J. Allergy Clin. Immunol.* **83**, 900–4.

Booij-Noord, H. and De Vries, K. (1971). Immediate and late bronchial obstructive reaction to inhalation of house-dust and protective effects of disodium cromoglycate and prednisolone. *J. Allergy Clin. Immunol.* **48**, 344–54.

Boulet, L.P., Cartier, A., Thomson, N.C., Roberts, R.S., Dolovich, J. and Hargreave, F.E. (1983). Asthma and increases in non-allergic bronchial responsiveness from seasonal pollen exposure. *J. Allergy Clin. Immunol.* **71**, 399–406.

Boulet, L.R., Roberts, R.S., Dolovich, J. and Hargreave, F.E. (1984). Prediction of late asthmatic responses to inhaled allergen. *Clin. Allergy* **14**, 379–85.

Britton, W.J., Woolcock, A.J., Peat, J.K., Lloyd, D.M. and Leader, S.R. (1986). Prevalence of bronchial responsiveness in children: the relationship between asthma and skin reactivity to allergens in two communities. *Int. J. Epidemiol.* **15**, 202–9.

Broadbent, J.B. and Sampson, H.A. (1988). Food hypersensitivity and atopic dermatitis. *Pediatr. Clin. North Am.* **35**, 1115–30.

Bruce, C.A., Bias, W.B., Norman, P.S., Lichtenstein, L.M. and Marsh, D.G. (1976). Studies of HLA antigen frequencies, IgE levels, and specific allergic sensitivities in patients having ragweed hayfever, with or without asthma. *Clin. Exp. Immunol.* **25**, 67.

Burr, M.L., Dean, B.V., Merrett, T.G., Neale, E., St Leger, A.S. and Verrier-Jones, E.R. (1980). Effects of antimite measures on children with mite-sensitive asthma: a controlled trial. *Thorax* **35**, 506–12.

Burr, M.L., Butland, B.H., King, S., Vaughan-Williams, E. (1989a). Changes in asthma prevalence: two studies 15 years apart. *Arch. Dis. Child* **64**, 1452–6.

Burr, M.L., Merrett, T.G., Merrett, J., Butland, B.K. and Miskelly, F.G. (1989b). A prospective study of allergy in high-risk children. *Adv. Biosci.* **74**, 239–55.

Businco, L., Marchetti, F., Pellegrini, G. and Perlini, R. (1983). Predictive value of cord blood IgE levels in 'at risk' newborn babies and influence of type of feeding. *Clin. Allergy* **13**, 503–8.

Businco, L., Cantani, A., Farinella, F. and Businco, E. (1988). Month of birth and grass pollen or mite sensitisation in children with respiratory allergy: a significant relationship. *Clin. Allergy* **18**, 269–74.

Byrom, N.A. and Timlin, D.M. (1979). Immune status in atopic eczema: a survey. *Br. J. Dermatol.* **100**, 491–8.

Carswell, F., Clarke, J., Robinson, D.W. and Platts-Mills, T.A.E. (1982). Bristol house dust mites. *Mod. Prob. Paediatr.* **21**, 86–93.

Cartier, A., Thomson, N.C., Frith, P.A., Roberts, R. and

Hargreaves, F.E. (1982). Allergen-induced increase in bronchial responsiveness to histamine: relationship to the late asthmatic response and change in airway calibre. *J. Allergy Clin. Immunol.* **70**, 170–7.

Chandra, R.K. and Baker, M. (1983). Numerical and functional deficiency of suppressor T cells precedes development of atopic eczema. *Lancet* **i**, 1393–4.

Chandra, R.K., Puri, S. and Cheema, P.S. (1985). Predictive value of cord blood IgE in the development of atopic disease and role of breast-feeding in its prevention. *Clin. Allergy* **15**, 517–22.

Chandra, R.K., Puri, S., Suraiya, C. and Cheema, P.S. (1986). Influence of maternal food antigen avoidance during pregnancy and lactation on incidence of atopic eczema in infants. *Clin. Allergy* **16**, 563–9.

Chung, K.F. (1986). Role of inflammation in the hyper-reactivity of the airways in asthma. *Thorax* **41**, 657–62.

Church, M.K. and Warner, J.O. (1985). Sodium cromoglycate and related drugs. *Clin. Allergy* **15**, 311–20.

Coca, A.F. and Cooke, R.A. (1923). On the classification of the phenomena of hypersensitiveness. *J. Immunol.* **8**, 163.

Cockcroft, D.W., Ruffin, R.E., Dolovich, J. and Hargreave, F.E. (1977). Allergen-induced increase in non-allergic bronchial activity. *Clin. Allergy* **7**, 503–13.

Cohen, S.I. and Lask, B. (1983). Psychological factors. In *Asthma*, 2nd edn, ed. T.J.H. Clarke and S. Godfrey, pp. 184–201, Chapman Hall, London.

Colver, A.F. (1984). Community campaign against asthma. *Arch. Dis. Child.* **59**, 449–52.

Committee on Safety of Medicines (1986) CSM Update. Desensitizing vaccines. *Brit. Med. J.* **293**, 148.

Cooke, R.A. and Van der Veer, A. (1916). Human sensitisation. *J. Immunol.* **1**, 201–239.

Cookson, W.O.C.M. and Hopkin, J.M. (1988). Dominant inheritance of atopic immunoglobin-E responsiveness. *Lancet* **i**, 86–8.

Cookson, W.O.C.M., Faux, J.A., Sharp, P.A., Hopkin, J.M. (1989). Linkage between immunoglobulin E responses underlying asthma and rhinitis and chromosome 11q. *Lancet* **i**, 1292–4.

Cooper, P.J., Darbyshire, J., Nunn, A.J. and Warner, J.O. (1984). A controlled trial of oral hyposensitisation in pollen asthma and rhinitis in children. *Clin. Allergy* **14**, 541–50.

Croner, S. and Kjellman, N.-I.M. (1986). Predictors of atopic disease: cord blood IgE and month of birth. *Allergy* **41**, 68–70.

David, T.J. (1984). Anaphylactic shock during elimination diets for severe atopic dermatitis. *Arch. Dis. Child.* **59**, 983–6.

David, T.J. and Beards, S.C. (1985). Asthma and the month of birth. *Clin. Allergy* **15**, 391–5.

Dowse, G., Turner, K.J., Stewart, G.A., Alpers, M.P. and Woolcock, A.J. (1985). The association between *Dermatophagoides* mites and the increasing prevalence of asthma in village communities within the Papua New Guinea highlands. *J. Allergy Clin. Immunol.* **75**, 75–83.

Dreborg, S. (1987). The skin prick test: methodological studies and clinical application. *Linkoping Univ. Med. Dissertations*, no. 239.

Edfors-Lubs, M. (1974). Allergy in 7000 twin pairs. *Acta Allergol.* **26**, 249–85.

Egger, J., Carter, C.M. and Graham, P.J. (1985). Controlled trial of oligoantigenic: treatment in the hyperkinetic syndrome. *Lancet* 540–5.

Egger, J., Carter, C.M., Wilson, J., Turner, M.W. and Soothill, J.F. (1983). Is migraine food allergy? *Lancet* **ii**, 865–9.

Emanuel, M.B. (1988). Hayfever, a post industrial revolution epidemic: a history of its growth during the 19th century. *Clin. Allergy* **18**, 295–304.

Falth-Magnusson, K. and Kjellman, N.-I.M. (1987). Development of atopic disease in babies whose mothers were on exclusion diet during pregnancy — a randomised study. *J. Allergy Clin. Immunol.* **80**, 868–75.

Falth-Magnusson, K., Oman, H. and Kjellman, N.-I.M. (1987). Maternal abstention from cow's milk and egg in allergy risk pregnancies: effect on antibody production in the mother and the newborn. *Allergy* **42**, 64–73.

Feingold, B. (1975). Hyperkinesis and learning disabilities linked to artificial food flavours and colours. *Am. J. Nursing* **75**, 797–803.

Ferguson, D.M., Horwood, L.J., Bentrais, A.L., Shannon, F.T. and Taylor, B. (1981). Eczema and infant diet. *Clin. Allergy* **11**, 325–31.

Ferguson, D.M., Horwood, L.J. and Shannon, F.T. (1983). Asthma and infant diet. *Arch. Dis. Child.* **58**, 48–51.

Fleming, D.M. and Crombie, D.L. (1987). Prevalence of asthma and hayfever in England and Wales. *Br. Med.J.* **294**, 279–83.

Fling, J.A., Ruff, M.E., Parker, W.A., Whisman, B.A., Martin, M.E., Moss, R.B. and Reid, M.J. (1989). Suppression of the late cutaneous response by immunotherapy. *J. Allergy Clin. Immunol.* **83**, 101–9.

Ford, R.P.K. and Taylor, B. (1982). Natural history of egg hypersensitivity. *Arch. Dis. Child.* **57**, 644–52.

Foucard, T. (1973). A follow-up study of children with asthmatoid bronchitis. 1. Skin test reactions and IgE antibodies to common allergens. *Acta Paediatr. Scand.* **62**, 633–44.

Frankland, A.W. and Augustin, R. (1954). Prophylaxis of summer hayfever and asthma. *Lancet* **i**, 1055–7.

Freeman, J. (1911). Further observations on the treatment of hayfever by hypodermic inoculations of pollen vaccine. *Lancet* **ii**, 814–7.

Gerrard, J.W., Rao, D.C. and Morton, N.E. (1978). A genetic study of immunoglobulin E. *Am. J. Hum. Genet.* **30**, 46–58.

Gershwin, L.J., Osebold, J.W. and Zee, Y.C. (1981). Immunoglobulin E containing cells in mouse lung following allergen inhalation and ozone exposure. *Int. Arch. Allergy Appl. Immunol.* **65**, 266–77.

Glaser, J. and Johnstone, D.E. (1953). Prophylaxis of allergic disease in newborns. *JAMA* **153**, 620–2.

Goldman, A.S., Anderson, D.W. and Sellars, W.A. (1985). Milk allergy. 1. Oral challenge with milk and isolated milk proteins in allergic children. *Pediatrics* **19**, 154–62.

Graff-Lonnevig, V., Hedlin, G. and Lindfors, A. (1988). Penicillin allergy — a rare paediatric condition. *Arch. Dis. Child.* **63**, 1342–6.

Green, W.F., Nicholas, N.R., Salome, C.M. and Woolcock, A.J. (1989). Reduction of house dust mite and mite allergens: effects of spraying carpets and blankets with Allersearch DMS, an acaride combined with an allergen reducing agent. *Clin. Exp. Allergy* **19**, 203–7.

Gregg, I. (1983). Epidemiological aspects: In *Asthma*, 2nd edn, ed. T.J.H. Clarke and S. Godfrey, pp. 242–84. Chapman and Hall Medical, London.

Hariparsad, D., Wilson, N., Dixon, C. and Silverman, M. (1984). Oral tartrazine challenge in childhood asthma: effect of bronchial reactivity. *Clin. Allergy* **14**, 81–5.

Hathaway, M.J. and Warner, J.O. (1983). Compliance problems in the dietary management of eczema. *Arch. Dis. Child.* **58**, 463–4.

Hattevig, G., Kjellman, B., Sigurs, N., Bjorksten, B. and Kjellman, N.-I.M. (1989). Effect of maternal avoidance of eggs, cow's milk and fish during lactation upon allergic manifestations in infants. *Clin. Exp. Allergy* **19**, 27–32.

Hayward, A.R. Development of immunity mechanism. (1983). In *Paediatric Immunology* ed. J.F. Soothill, A.R. Hayward and C.B.S. Wood, Blackwell Scientific Publications, Oxford, pp. 48–55.

Hide, D.W. and Guyer, B.M. (1981). Clinical manifestations of allergy related to breast and cow's milk feeding. *Arch. Dis. Child.* **56**, 172–5.

Hill, D.C. and Lynch, B.C. (1982). Elemental diet in the management of severe eczema in childhood. *Clin. Allergy* **12**, 313–15.

Hill, R.A., Standen, P.J. and Tattersfield, A.E. (1989). Asthma, wheezing and school absence in primary schools. *Arch. Dis. Child.* **64**, 246–51.

Holt, P.G. and Turner, K.J. (1984). Respiratory symptoms in the children of smokers: an overview. *Eur. J. Respir. Dis.* **65** (suppl. 133), 109–20.

Hutchins, P. and Walker-Smith, J.A. (1982). The gastrointestinal system. *Clin. Immunol. Allergy* **2**, 43–76.

Ito, S., Shinomiya, K. and Mikawa, H. (1983). Suppressive effect of IgE soluble immune complex on neutrophil chemotaxis. *Clin. Exp. Immunol.* **51**, 407–12.

Jarrett, E.E. and Hall, E. (1984). The devèlopment of IgE-suppressive immunocompetence in young animals: influence of exposure to antigen in the presence or absence of maternal immunity. *Immunology* **53**, 365–73.

Jenkins, H.R., Pincott, J.R., Soothill, J.F., Milla, P.J. and Haries, J.F. (1984). Food allergy: the major cause of infantile colitis. *Arch. Dis. Child.* **59**, 326–9.

Johnston, I.D.A., Bland, J.M., Ingram, D., Anderson, H.R., Warner, J.O. and Lambert H.P. (1986). Effect of whooping cough in infancy on subsequent lung function and bronchial reactivity. *Am. Rev. Respir. Dis.* **134**, 270–5.

Juhlin, L. (1981). Recurrent urticaria: clinical investigation of 330 patients. *Br. J. Dermatol.* **104**, 369–81.

Juto, P. and Strannegard, O. (1979). T-lymphocytes and blood eosinophils in early infancy in relation to heredity for allergy and type of feeding. *J. Allergy Clin. Immunol.* **64**, 38–42.

Kauffman, H.S. and Hobbs, J.R. (1970). Immunoglobulin deficiencies in an atopic population. *Lancet* **ii**, 1061.

Kelly, W.J.W., Hudson, I., Phelan, P.D., Pain, M.F. and Olinsky, O. (1987). Childhood asthma in adult life: a further study at 28 years of age. *Br. Med. J.* **294**, 1059–62.

Kemp, A.S. (1979). Relationship between the time of birth and the development of immediate hypersensitivity to grass pollen antigens. *Med. J. Aust.* **1**, 263–4.

Kershaw, C.R. (1987). Passive smoking, potential atopy and asthma in the first five years. *J. Roy. Soc. Med.* **80**, 683–8.

Kjellman, N.-I.M. (1976). Predictive value of high IgE levels in children. *Acta Paediatr. Scand.* **65**, 465–71.

Kjellman, N.-I.M. (1981). Effect of parental smoking on IgE levels in children. *Lancet* **i**, 993–4.

Kjellman, N.-I.M. and Croner, S. (1984). Cord blood IgE determination for allergy prediction — a follow-up to seven years of age in 1651 children. *Ann. Allergy* **53**, 167–71.

Kleinman, R.E., Harmatz, P.R., Jacobsson, L.A., Udall, J.N., Bloch, K.J. and Walker, W.A. (1983). Passive transplacental immunization: influence of the detection of enteric antigen in the systemic circulation. *Pediatr. Res.* **17**, 449–51.

Krafchik, B.R. (1983). Atopic dermatitis. *Pediatr. Clin. North Am.* **30**, 669–85.

Krain, L.S. and Terasaki, P. (1973). HLA types in atopic dermatitis. *Lancet* **i**, 1059–64.

Krammer, M.S. and Moroz, B. (1981). Do breast-feeding and delayed introduction of solid foods protect against subsequent atopic eczema? *J. Pediatr.* **98**, 546–50.

Krayenbuhl, M.C., Hudspith, B.N., Scadding, G.K. and Brostoff, J. (1988). Nasal response to allergen and byperosmolar challenge. *Clin. Allergy* **18**, 157–64.

Lancet editorial (1989). Penicillin allergy in childhood. *Lancet* **i**, 420.

Levine, B.B., Stember, R.H. and Fotins, M. (1972). Ragweed hayfever: genetic control and linkage to HLA haplotypes. *Science* **178**, 1201–3.

Lichtenstein, C.M., Norman, P.J. and Winkenwerder, W.L. (1971). A single year of immunotherapy for ragweed hayfever. *Ann. Intern. Med.* **75**, 663–71.

Lilja, G., Dannaeus, A., Falth-Magnusson, K. *et al.* (1988). Immune response of the atopic woman and foetus: effects of high and low dose food allergen intake during late pregnancy. *Clin. Allergy* **18**, 131–42.

Loftus, B.G., Price, J.F., Lobo-Yeo, A. and Vergani, D. (1988). IgG subclass deficiency in asthma. *Arch. Dis. Child.* **63**, 1434–7.

Lopez-Brea, M. (1984). Urticaria associated with *Campylobacter* enteritis *Lancet* **i**, 1354.

McGeady, S.J. and Buckley, R.H. (1975). Depression of cell mediated immunity in atopic eczema. *J. Allergy Clin. Immunol.* **56**, 393–406.

McLaughlin, P., Anderson, K.J., Widdowson, E.M. and Coombs, R.A. (1981). Effect of heart on the anaphylactic-sensitising capacity of cow's milk, goat's milk and various infant formulae fed to guinea pigs. *Arch. Dis. Child.* **56**, 165–71.

McNicol, K.N. and Williams, H.E. (1973a). Spectrum of asthma in children. 1. Clinical and physiological components. *Br. Med. J.* **4**, 7–11.

McNicol, K.N. and Williams, H.E. (1973b). Spectrum of asthma in children. 2. Allergic components. *Br. Med. J.* **4**, 12–16.

Magnusson, C.G.M. (1986). Maternal smoking influences cord serum IgE and IgD levels and increases the risk for subsequent infant allergy. *J. Allergy Clin. Immunol.* **78**, 898–904.

Marsh, D.G., Meyers, D.A. and Bias, W.B. (1981). The epidemiology and genetics of atopic allergy. *N. Engl. J. Med.* **305**, 1551–9.

Marsh, D.G., Meyers, D.A., Friedhoff, L.R. *et al.* (1982). HLA-DW2: a genetic marker for human immune response to short ragweed pollen allergen Ra5. 2. Response after ragweed immunotherapy. *J. Exp. Med.* **155**, 1452.

Marsh, D.G., Zwollo, P. and Ansari, A.A. (1987). Toward a total human immune response fingerprint: the allergy model. *Adv. Biosci.* **74**, 65–82.

Martin, A.J., Landau, L.I. and Phelan, P.D. (1982). Predicting the course of asthma in children. *Aust. Paediatr. J.* **18**, 84–7.

Matsumura, T., Kuroume, T., Oguri, M. *et al.* (1975). Egg sensitivity and eczematous manifestations in breast-fed newborns with particular reference to intra-uterine sensitisation. *Ann. Allergy* **35**, 221.

Matthew, D.J., Taylor, B., Norman, A.P., Turner, M.W. and Soothill, J.F. (1977). Prevention of eczema. *Lancet* **i**, 321–4.

Merrett, T.G., Burr, M.L., Saint Leger, A.S. and Merrett, J. (1980) Circulating IgE levels in the over-seventies. *Clin. Allergy* **10**, 433–9.

Michel, F.B., Bousquet, J., Greillier, P., Robinet-Leucy, M. and Coulomb, Y. (1980). Comparison of cord blood immunoglobulin E concentrations and maternal allergy for the prediction of atopic diseases in infancy. *J. Allergy Clin. Immunol.* **65**, 422–30.

Mitchell, E.B., Crow, J., Chapman, M.D., Jouhal, S.S., Pope, F.M., Platts-Mills, T.A.E. (1982). Basophils in allergen-induced patch test sites in atopic dermatitis. *Lancet* **i**, 127–30.

Moneret-Vantrin, D.A. (1983). False food allergies: non-specific reactions to foodstuffs. In *Clinical Reactions to Food*, ed M.H. Lessof, pp. 135–53, John Wiley & Sons, Chichester.

Muntner, M. (1963). *Treatise of Asthma — Maimonides, M.* Lippincott, Philadelphia.

Murdoch, R.D. and Pollock, I. (1989). Plasma histamine and clinical tolerance to infused histamine in normal atopic and urticarial subjects. *Clin. Exp. Allergy* **1**, 103 (abstract 52/2).

Murdoch, R.D., Pollock, I., Young, E. and Lessof, M.H. (1987). Food additive induced urticaria: studies of mediator release during provocation tests. *J. Roy. Coll. Physicians* **4**, 262–6.

Murray, A.B. and Ferguson, A.C. (1983). Dust-free bedrooms in the treatment of asthmatic children with house dust mite allergy: a controlled trial. *Pediatrics* **71**, 418.

National Advisory Committee on Hyperkinesis and Food Additives (1980). Final Report to the Nutrition Foundation, New York. The Nutrition Foundation.

Noon, L. (1911). Prophylactic inoculation for hayfever. *Lancet* **i**, 1572–3.

Ortolani, C., Ispano, M., Pastorello, E.A., Ansaloni, R. and Magri, G.C. (1989). Comparison of results of skin prick tests (with fresh foods and commercial food extracts) and RAST in 100 patients with oral allergy syndrome. *J. Allergy Clin. Immunol.* **83**, 683–90.

Paganelli, R., Levinsky, R.J. and Atherton, D.J. (1981). Detection of specific antigen within circulating immune complexes: validation of the assay and the application to food antigen–antibody complexes found in health and food allergic subjects. *Clin. Exp. Immunol.* **46**, 44–53.

Platts-Mills, T.A.E., Tovey, E.R., Mitchell, E.B., Moszoro, H., Nock, P. and Wilkins, S.R. (1982). Reduction of bronchial hyper-reactivity during prolonged allergen avoidance. *Lancet* **ii**, 675–8.

Platts-Mills, T.A.E., Mitchell, E.B., Tovey, E.R., Chapman, M.D. and Wilkins, S.R. (1984). Airborne allergen exposure, allergen avoidance and bronchial hyper-reactivity. In *Asthma: Physiology, Immunotherapy and Treatment*, ed. A.B. Kay and K.F. Austen, pp. 297–311, Academic Press, London.

Pollock, I. and Warner, J.O. (1987). A follow-up study of childhood food additive intolerance. *J. Roy. Coll. Physicians* **21**, 248–50.

Pollock, I. and Warner, J.O. (1990). The effect of artificial food colours on behaviour. *Arch. Dis. Child.* **65**, 74–7.

Price, J.A., Pollock, I., Little, S.A., Longbottom, J.L. and Warner, J.O. (1990). Measurement of airborne mite antigen in homes of asthmatic children. *Lancet* **336**, 895–7.

Price, J.F., Hey, E.N. and Soothill, J.F. (1982). Antigen provocation to the skin, nose and lung in children with asthma: immediate and final hypersensitivity reactions. *Clin. Exp. Immunol.* **47**, 587–94.

Price, J.F., Turner, M.W., Warner, J.O. and Soothill, J.F. (1983). Immunological studies in asthmatic children undergoing antigen provocation in the skin, lump and nose. *Clin. Allergy* **13**, 419–26.

Price, J.F., Warner, J.O., Hey, E.N., Turner, M.W. and Soothill, J.F. (1984). A controlled trial of hyposensitisation with adsorbed tyrosine *Dermatophagoides pteronyssinus* antigen in childhood asthma: *in vivo* aspects. *Clin. Allergy* **14**, 209–19.

Pullan, C.R. and Hey, E.N. (1982). Wheezing, asthma and pulmonary dysfunction ten years after infection with respiratory syncitial virus in infancy. *Br. Med. J.* **284**, 1665–9.

Quoix, E., Bessot, J.C., Kopperschmitt-Kubler, M.C., Fraisse, P. and Panli, G. (1988). Positive skin tests to aeroallergen and month of birth. *Allergy* **43**, 127–31.

Rantakallio, P. (1978). Relationship of maternal smoking to morbidity and mortality of the child up to the age of five. *Acta Paediatr. Scand* **67**, 621–31.

Reed, C.E. (1958). The failure of antepartum or neonatal exposure to grass pollen to influence later development of grass sensitivity. *J. Allergy* **29**, 300–1.

Reiser, J. and Warner, J.O. (1986). Inhalation treatment for asthma. *Arch. Dis. Child.* **61**, 88–94.

Reiser, J., Ingram, D., Mitchell, E.B. and Warner, J.O. (1990). House dust mite allergen levels and an anti-mite mattress spray (Natamycin) in the treatment of childhood asthma. *Clin. Exp. Allergy* **20**, 561–7.

Richardson, V.F., Larcher, V.F. and Price, J.F. (1983). A common congenital immunodeficiency predisposing to infection and atopy in infancy. *Arch. Dis. Child.* **58**, 799–802.

Royal College of Physicians/British Nutrition Foundation Committee (1984). Food intolerance and aversion. *J. Roy. Coll. Physicians* **18**, 83–123.

Russell, G. and Jones, S.P. (1976). Selection of skin tests in childhood asthma. *Br. J. Dis. Chest* **70**, 104–6.

Ruiz, R.G.G., Richards, D., Kemeny, D.M. and Price, J.F. (1991). Neonatal IgE: a poor screen for atopic disease. *Clin. Exp. Allergy* **21**, 467–72.

Saarinen, U.M., Kajosaari, M., Bachman, A. and Siimes, M.A. (1979). Prolonged breast feeding as prophylaxis for atopic disease. *Lancet* **ii**, 163–6.

Sadan, N., Rhyne, M.B., Mellits, E.D., Goldstein, E.O., Levy, D.A. and Lichtenstein, L.M. (1969). Immunotherapy of pollinosis in children: an investigation of the immunological basis of clinical improvement. *N. Engl. J. Med.* **280**, 623–7.

Sampson, H.A. and Albergo, R. (1984). Comparison of results of skin tests, RAST and double-blind placebo controlled food challenges in children with atopic dermatitis. *J. Allergy Clin. Immunol.* **74**, 26–33.

Sanderson, J. and Warner, J.O. (1987). Previous ear, nose and throat surgery in children presenting with allergic perennial rhinitis. *Clin. Allergy* **17**, 113–17.

Schiffer, C.G. and Hunt, E.P. (1963). *Illness among Children*. Children's Bureau Publication No. 405, US Dept of Health Education and Welfare, Washington DC.

Schwartz, M. (1952). Heredity in bronchial asthma. *Acta Allergol.* **5** (suppl. 2), 1–288.

Sears, M.R., Taylor, D.R., Print, C.G. *et al.* (1990). Regular inhaled beta-agonist treatment in bronchial asthma. *Lancet* **336**, 1391–6.

Shannon, W.R. (1921). Demonstration of food proteins in human breast milk by anaphylactic experiments on guinea pigs. *Am. J. Dis. Child.* **22**, 223.

Sibbald, B. and Turner-Warwick, M. (1979). Factors influencing the prevalence of asthma in first degree relatives of extrinsic and intrinsic asthmatics. *Thorax* **34**, 332–7.

Silverman, M. and Wilson, N. (1985). Bronchial responsiveness in children: a clinical view. In *Neonatal and Pediatric Respiratory Medicine*, ed. A.D. Milner and R.J. Martin, pp. 161–89. Butterworths, London.

Simons, F.E.R. (1988). Allergic rhinitis: recent advances. *Pediatr. Clin. North Am.* **35**, 1053–74.

Smith, J.M. (1984). The epidemiology of allergic rhinitis. In *Rhinitis: New England Regional Allergy Proceedings*, ed. G.A. Settipane, pp. 86–91. Oceanside Publications, New York.

Smith, J.M., Harding, L.K. and Cumming, G. (1971). The changing prevalence of asthma in school children. *Clin. Allergy* **1**, 57–61.

Soothill, J.F., Stokes, C.R., Turner, M.W., Norman, A.P. and Taylor, B. (1976). Predisposing factors and the development of reaginic allergy in infancy. *Clin. Allergy* **6**, 305–8.

Speight, A.N.P., Lee, D.A. and Hey, E.N. (1983). Underdiagnosis and undertreatment of asthma in childhood. *Br. Med. J.* **286**, 1253–6.

Stifler, W.C. (1965). A twenty-one year follow-up of infantile eczema. *J. Pediatr.* **66**, 166–7.

Storr, J., Barrell, E. and Lenney, W. (1988). Rising asthma admissions and self-referral. *Arch. Dis. Child.* **63**, 774–9.

Strannegard, O. and Strannegard, I.L. (1978). T-lymphocyte numbers and function in human IgE-mediated allergy. *Immunol. Rev.* **41**, 149.

Suoniemi, I., Bjorksten, F. and Haahtela, T. (1981). Dependence of immediate hypersensitivity in the adolescent period on factors encountered in infancy. *Allergy* **36**, 263–8.

Supramaniam, G. and Warner, J.O. (1986). Artificial food additive intolerance in patients with angio-oedema and urticaria. *Lancet* **i**, 907–9.

Taylor, B. and Wadsworth, J. (1987). Maternal smoking during pregnancy and lower respiratory tract illness in early life. *Arch. Dis. Child.* **62**, 76–9.

Taylor, B., Norman, A.P., Orgel, H.A., Stokes, C.R., Turner-Warwick, M. and Soothill, J.F. (1973). Transient IgA deficiency and pathogenesis of infantile atopy. *Lancet* **ii**, 111–13.

Taylor, B., Wadsworth, J., Wadsworth, M. and Peckham, C. (1984). Changes in the reported prevalence of childhood eczema since the 1939–45 war. *Lancet* **ii**, 1255–7.

Thorpe, J.E., Steinberg, D., Bernstein, I.L. and Murlas, C.G. (1987). Bronchial reactivity increases soon after the immediate response in dual responding asthmatic subjects. *Chest* **91**, 21–5.

Thorsby, E., Engeset, A. and Lie, S.O. (1971). HLA antigens and susceptibility to diseases: a study of patients with acute lympholastic leukaemia, Hodgkins disease and childhood asthma. *Tissue Antigens* **1**, 147–159.

Tovey, E.R., Chapman, M.D. and Platts-Mills, T.A.E. (1981). The distribution of dust mite allergen in the houses of patients with asthma. *Am. Rev. Respir. Dis.* **124**, 630–5.

Turner, M.W., Brostoff, J., Wells, R.S., Stokes, C.R. and Soothill, J.F. (1977). HLA in eczema and hayfever. *Clin. Exp. Immunol.* **27**, 43–47.

Turner, M.W., Mowbray, J.F., Harvey, B.A.M., Brostoff, J., Wells, R.S. and Soothill, J.F. (1978). Defective yeast opsonisation and C2 deficiency in atopic patients. *Clin. Exp. Immunol.* **34**, 253–9.

Turner, M.W., Yalcin, I., Soothill, J.F. *et al.* (1984). *In vitro* investigations in asthmatic children undergoing hyposensitisation with tyrosine-adsorbed *Dermatophagoides pteronyssinus* antigen. *Clin. Allergy* **14**, 221–31.

Twarog, F.J. (1983). Urticaria in childhood: pathogenesis and management. *Pediatr. Clin. North Am.* **30**, 887–98.

Van Bever, H.P. and Stevens, W.J. (1990). Evolution of the late asthmatic reaction during immunotherapy and after stopping immunotherapy. *J. Allergy Clin. Immunol.* **86**, 141–6.

Vanto, T., Viander, M. and Koivikko, A. (1983). Humoral and cell-mediated immune response to dog dander and hair in asthmatic children. *Allergy* **38**, 103–12.

Vervloet, D., Pernaud, A., Razzouk, H. *et al.* (1982). Altitude and house dust mite. *J. Allergy Clin. Immunol.* **69**, 290–6.

Viner, A.S. and Jackman, N. (1976). Retrospective survey of 1271 patients diagnosed as perennial rhinitis. *Clin. Allergy* **6**, 251–9.

Voss, M.J., O'Connell, E.S. and Hall, J.F. (1982). Association of acute urticaria in children with respiratory tract infections. *J. Allergy Clin. Immunol.* **69**, 134 (abstract 166).

Waegemaekers, M., Van Wageningen, N., Brunekreef, B. and Boleij, J.S.M. (1989). Respiratory symptoms in damp homes. *Allergy* **44**, 192–8.

Warner, J.A., Little, J.A., Pollock, I., Longbottom, J.L. and Warner, J.O. (1991). The influence of exposure to house dust mite, cat, pollen and fungal allergens in the home on primary sensitization in asthma. *Pediatr. Allergy Immunol.* **1**, 79–86.

Warner, J.A., Miles, E.A., Quint, D.J. and Warner, J.O. (1992). Gamma interferon production by allergen triggered cord blood cells in the prediction of allergy. *J. Allergy Clin. Immunol.* **89** (in press).

Warner, J.O. (1976). The significance of late reactions following bronchial challenge with house dust mite. *Arch. Dis. Child* **51**, 905–11.

Warner, J.O. (1977). Bronchial provocation tests. *Arch. Dis. Child.* **52**, 750–1.

Warner, J.O. (1978). Mites and asthma in children (review article). *Br. J. Dis. Chest* **72**, 79–87.

Warner, J.O. (1980). Food allergy in fully breast-fed infants. *Clin. Allergy* **10**, 133–6.

Warner, J.O. (1984) Immunotherapy. In *Allergy: Immunological and Clinical Aspects*, ed. M.H. Lessof, pp. 447–64, John Wiley and Sons Ltd, Chichester.

Warner, J.O. (1985). Intolerance and food allergy. *Maternal Child Health* **10**, 40–6.

Warner, J.O. (1986). Immunotherapy: yesterday's treatment. In *Proceedings of the XIIth ICACI*, ed. C.E. Reed, pp. 323–6, C.V.

Mosby Co., St Louis.

Warner, J.O., Boner, A.L. (1988). Allergy and childhood asthma. *Clin. Immunol. Allergy* **2**, 217–29.

Warner, J.O. and Hathaway, M.J. (1984). Allergic form of Meadow's syndrome (Munchausen by proxy). *Arch. Dis. Child.* **59**, 151–6.

Warner, J.O. and Kerr, J.W. (1987). Hyposensitization. *Br. Med. J.* **294**, 1179–80.

Warner, J.O. and Price, J.F. (1978). House mite sensitivity in childhood asthma. *Arch. Dis. Child.* **53**, 710–13.

Warner, J.O., Norman, A.P. and Soothill, J.F. (1976a). Cystic fibrosis heterozygosity in the pathogenesis of allergy. *Lancet* **i**, 990–1.

Warner, J.O., Taylor, B.W., Norman, A.P. and Soothill, J.F. (1976b). Association of cystic fibrosis with allergy. *Arch. Dis. Child.* **51**, 507–11.

Warner, J.O., Price, J.F., Soothill, J.F. and Hey, E.N. (1978). Controlled trial of hyposensitisation to *Dermatophagoides pteronyssinus* in children with asthma. *Lancet* **ii**, 912–15.

Warner, J.O., Gotz, M., Landau, I. *et al.* (1989). Management of asthma: a consensus statement. *Arch. Dis. Child.* **64**, 1065–79.

Weiss, S.T., Tager, I.B., Munoz, A. and Speizer, F.E. (1985). The relationship of respiratory infections in early childhood to the occurrence of increased levels of bronchial responsiveness and atopy. *Am. Rev. Respir. Dis.* **131**, 573–8.

Weirenga, E.A., Snoek, M., De Groot, C. *et al.* (1990). Evidence for compartmentalization of functional subsets of CD4+ T lymphocytes in atypic patients. *J. Immunol.* **144**, 4651–6.

Willcox, H.N.A. and Marsh, D.G. (1978). Genetic regulation of antibody heterogeneity: its possible significance in human allergy. *Immunogenetics* **6**, 209–215.

Wilson, N.M., Charette, L., Thomson, A.H. and Silverman, M. (1985). Gastro-oesophageal reflux and childhood asthma: the acid test. *Thorax* **40**, 592–7.

Zeiger, R.S., Heller, S., Mellon, M., O'Connor, R. and Hamburger, R.N. (1986). Effectiveness of dietary manipulation in the prevention of food allergy in infants. *J. Allergy Clin. Immunol.* **78**, 224–38.

Zweiman, B., Schoenwetter, W.F. and Hildreth, E.A. (1966). The relationship between bronchiolitis and allergic asthma: a prospective study with allergy evaluation. *J. Allergy* **37**, 48–53.

58: Cell Interactions in Allergic Inflammation

A.J. Frew and A.B. Kay

Introduction

This chapter is concerned with the pathophysiology of allergic tissue reactions in atopic individuals and, in particular, with the cellular interactions which are thought to take place at such sites. In recent years considerable progress has been made towards understanding the biology of allergic inflammation: a picture is now emerging of a complex and ordered sequence of events, initiated by the recognition of allergen by immunoglobulin E (IgE), and possibly also by T cells, leading to the selective recruitment of inflammatory effector cells. These processes seem to be regulated at several points by the co-ordinated release of intercellular mediators.

Of all the cells involved in the atopic allergic response, and indeed in any immune reaction, it is only the T and B lymphocytes which are inherently antigen-specific. The actions of mast cells, neutrophils, eosinophils and mononuclear phagocytes are only specific in so far as their activities are focused by interactions between surface receptors and specific immunoglobulin or complement molecules bound to target surfaces. In addition, their activation and efficiency appear to be regulated, at least in part, by soluble products released from T lymphocytes and other cells.

It is now generally accepted that atopic hypersensitivity reactions are IgE-dependent. This is certainly and obviously true for the immediate hypersensitivity reaction and is probably, but not entirely, proved in the case of the allergen-induced late-phase reaction (LPR). In patients with allergic diseases such as extrinsic asthma and rhinitis, affected tissues are characterized histologically by oedema and infiltration by a mixture of leucocytes. Additional features, such as mucus hypersecretion, epithelial desquamation, smooth-muscle contraction and exudative fluid loss, may be present at mucosal surfaces.

Cellular consequences of antigen–immunoglobulin E interaction

Cross-linking of IgE molecules bound to the surface of mast cells leads rapidly to an elevation in intracellular calcium concentrations and thence to degranulation. A wide range of preformed and newly generated substances (mediators) are released, which are believed to act: on endothelial cells to induce leakage of plasma, oedema and adherence of leucocytes; on epithelial glands to discharge mucus; on smooth-muscle cells to cause bronchoconstriction; and on secondary inflammatory cells to promote local accumulation of leucocytes. *In vitro*, histamine is released in large amounts from sensitized mast cells following challenge with specific allergen, as are various arachidonic acid metabolites, principally prostaglandin D_2 (PGD_2), thromboxane A_2 (TXA_2) and leukotriene B-4 (LTB_4). Leukotriene C-4 and platelet activating factor (PAF) are also elaborated *in vitro* during IgE-dependent reactions, but their precise cellular origins remain to be established. The detailed mechanism of IgE-dependent activation of mast cells and the nature of mast cell-associated mediators are discussed elsewhere (see Chapter 52).

Mast cell actions on other cell types

Histamine has a complex array of actions mediated by specific H_1, H_2 and H_3 receptors. In atopic allergy the pro-inflammatory H_1 effects predominate and include, in general, contraction of non-vascular smooth muscle and relaxation of vascular smooth muscle. Histamine also acts on vascular endothelium, inducing leakage of plasma proteins and fluid, leading in turn to the formation of oedema. Other spasmogenic, vasoactive and chemotactic mediators released by mast cells and by other IgE-bearing ($Fc_\varepsilon R$ +ve) cells (see below) include LTC_4/D_4, LTB_4, TXA_2, PGD_2, $PGF_{2\alpha}$ and PAF. Several of these mediators (i.e. histamine, PAF and LTC_4) induce mucus secretion, both directly and indirectly through autonomic reflexes.

In addition to inducing extravasation of plasma fluid, endothelial cell alterations lead to local increases in the adhesion of leucocytes to endothelial cells. Margination of neutrophils and eosinophils can be seen histologically within 5 minutes following allergen or anti-IgE challenge. Subsequently, the granulocytes start to emigrate through the vascular endothelium (diapedesis), a process which is generally considered to occur under the influence of chemotactic gradients. Chemotactic factors released during immediate, IgE-dependent hypersensitivity reactions include LTB_4 and PAF, which are active on both neutrophils and eosinophils (Wardlaw *et al.* 1986). A number of weaker peptide and lipid chemotactic factors have also been described, with variable degrees of target cell specificity (reviewed by Wardlaw and Kay 1988).

While there is no doubt that mast cell-derived chemotactic factors are released following exposure to relevant allergens, it is less clear whether these cells are the only cells responsible for the cellular infiltration seen in the LPR. Within individuals, the magnitude of the weal and the cutaneous LPR are partially related to the serum concentration of allergen-specific IgE and to the amount of allergen administered. However, between individuals there is only a modest correlation between the magnitudes of the early reaction and the LPR (Umemoto *et al.* 1976; Frew and Kay 1988a), indicating that additional factors must regulate the development of the LPR.

Basophils

Another cell with high-affinity $Fc_\varepsilon R$ is the basophil. While basophils are probably not involved in the acute IgE-dependent response in the skin, increased numbers of basophils have been observed in the nasal mucosa and in nasal secretions, both following pollen exposure and during the pollen season. Basophil infiltration has also been observed in an experimental model of allergic inflammation in the guinea-pig, termed cutaneous basophil hypersensitivity (Richerson *et al.* 1970). In this model, animals are sensitized with hapten–carrier conjugates in incomplete Freund's adjuvant and, on challenge, a delayed skin response is seen which is infiltrated by lymphocytes, eosinophils and basophils. This phenomenon is T-cell-dependent and has some histological similarities to dermatitic lesions induced experimentally by patch testing with extracts of aeroallergens (Mitchell *et al.* 1982).

Basophils may thus participate directly (via $Fc_\varepsilon R$) in allergic reactions at sites repeatedly exposed to allergen. The clearest evidence implicating basophils in allergic tissue inflammation comes from studies of the profile of mediators released in the nose after allergen challenge. Histamine is released in a biphasic manner during such reactions, with an early peak which parallels the acute symptoms of allergic rhinitis. This early peak is accompanied by elevated concentrations of PGD_2 and is thus attributable to mast cells. In contrast, the secondary peak in histamine release, 4–8 hours after challenge, is not accompanied by PGD_2 release; it seems likely therefore that the secondary-phase histamine release comes from basophils and not from mast cells (Naclerio *et al.* 1985). The mechanism inducing late-phase degranulation of basophils is uncertain. If specific IgE–antigen interaction is involved, this would imply that antigen must persist at the site of challenge. Immunoglobulin E-independent mechanisms may be important here: there is considerable circumstantial evidence which suggests that histamine-releasing factors (HRF) are released from T lymphocytes and may trigger the late-phase release of histamine.

Histamine-releasing factors are a heterogeneous group of factors which can induce histamine release from basophils and/or mast cells by non-cytotoxic mechanisms. They have been described in biological fluids (Warner *et al.* 1986) and in supernatants from cultured mononuclear cells (Kaplan *et al.* 1985) and platelets (Orchard *et al.* 1986). A number of well-characterized cytokines, including granulocyte–macrophage colony-stimulating factor (GM-CSF), have HRF activity but most HRF have yet to be characterized. Some HRF are of small molecular size (<5000 Da), while others are associated with molecular weights of 17–30 kD. The mechanisms by which HRF induce histamine release vary within certain limits, but all HRF are temperature- and calcium-dependent. Some HRF seem to induce release directly (i.e. presumably via a specific receptor for the HRF) while others appear to function only in the presence of cytophilic IgE. Indeed, not all IgE-containing sera are equally active in these assays, implying the existence of functional variants of IgE (MacDonald *et al.* 1987).

From the theoretical point of view, HRF may influence the threshold of stimuli which activate the immediate atopic allergic reaction and may also play a role in cellular activation and inflammation in the allergic LPR. The observations that allergic subjects are more likely to respond to HRF after seasonal exposure to allergen (MacDonald and Lichtenstein 1990) and that injection immunotherapy attenuates the production of HRF *in vitro* (Kuna *et al.* 1988) both indicate the possible clinical relevance of HRF in allergic disease.

Until recently it was assumed that all IgE-dependent reactions were initiated by mast cells or basophils and that other inflammatory cells were attracted into allergic reaction sites and then activated by mediators released from the $Fc_\varepsilon R$-bearing cells. It has now become apparent that a lower-affinity receptor for IgE ($Fc_\varepsilon RII$) is present on the platelet, macrophage, eosinophil, B cell and activated T cell (Melewicz and Spiegelberg 1980; Capron *et al.* 1981; Joseph *et al.* 1986; Prinz *et al.* 1988). The fact that $Fc_\varepsilon RII$ can be divided into two types, with identical extracellular regions and different N-terminal cytoplasmic portions, implies alternative messenger ribonucleic acid (mRNA) splicing from a single gene (Yokota *et al.* 1988). These $Fc_\varepsilon RII$ seem to be functionally relevant in that passively sensitized alveolar macrophages have been shown to release leucotrienes when stimulated by anti-IgE (Fuller *et al.* 1986) and eosinophils can exhibit cytotoxicity and LTC_4 release through IgE-dependent mechanisms (Moqbel *et al.* 1988). It would thus seem possible that $Fc_\varepsilon RII$-bearing cells may participate directly in IgE-dependent reactions without a requirement for mast cells or basophils.

Eosinophils

Considerable attention has been paid to the role of the eosinophil in allergic inflammation. It has long been recognized that blood and tissue eosinophilia is a feature of subjects with atopic allergic disease. Over the years a number of theories have been put forward regarding the role of eosinophils. These have included ideas that eosinophils inactivate mast cell mediators or that they play a part in repair processes (Ramesh *et al.* 1985). The recognition that the cationic proteins of the eosinophil granule could damage respiratory epithelium *in vitro* (Frigas and Gleich 1986) and that toxic concentrations of the eosinophil major basic protein were present in the sputum of patients with chronic asthma (Frigas *et al.* 1981) has favoured a deleterious role for the eosinophil. Other documented pro-inflammatory properties of the eosinophil include the elaboration of substantial amounts of LTC_4 (Shaw *et al.* 1985) and PAF (Jörg *et al.* 1982).

In biopsies from experimentally induced allergic

skin reactions in man, activated eosinophils can clearly be demonstrated (Frew and Kay 1988b). Increased numbers of eosinophils were also found in bronchoalveolar lavage (BAL) performed 6 hours after allergen inhalation. The magnitude of this BAL eosinophilia correlated with the degree of bronchoconstriction observed during the late asthmatic response (LAR). Furthermore, elevated concentrations of eosinophil cationic protein were detected in BAL supernatant, indicating that eosinophil degranulation had occurred during the LAR (De Monchy *et al.* 1985). Further support for a pathogenic role of the eosinophil comes from the demonstration that non-specific bronchial hyper-responsiveness correlates with blood eosinophil counts (Durham and Kay 1984) and with BAL concentrations of the eosinophil major basic protein (Wardlaw *et al.* 1988a).

There is now strong evidence that the bone marrow production of eosinophils is regulated by T lymphocyte products, whether eosinophilia is induced by allergen exposure, parasitic infestation or malignant disease or exists in isolation, as in the idiopathic hypereosinophilic syndrome. *In vitro*, the lymphokines interleukin 3 (IL-3) and GM-CSF act on myeloid precursors to promote the development of both eosinophil and neutrophil promyelocytes, while IL-5 stimulates the terminal differentiation of committed eosinophil precursors. *In vivo*, additional T-lymphocyte-derived eosinophil colony-stimulating factors have been identified in the serum of patients with the hypereosinophilic syndrome (Kern *et al.* 1987; Raghavachar *et al.* 1987).

Although the majority of eosinophils develop in the bone marrow, it has been suggested that eosinophils and basophils may differentiate and proliferate locally at sites of allergic inflammation. Certainly, eosinophil and basophil precursors have been demonstrated in allergic nasal polyps; it has been shown that colony-stimulating factors can be elaborated *in vitro* by cultured nasal epithelial cells and it appears that this process is T-lymphocyte-dependent (Ohnishi *et al.* 1988).

Neutrophils

The role of the neutrophil in allergic inflammation remains controversial. Neutrophil infiltration is a feature of many different forms of inflammation (Henson and Johnston 1987). Neutrophils and eosinophils share many effector functions and surface receptors; both cells are capable of releasing proteolytic enzymes and partial reduction products of oxygen, as well as the lipid mediators LTB_4 and PAF.

Animal experiments have implicated the neutrophil in the development of bronchial hyper-responsiveness, one of the cardinal features of asthma (Lee *et al.* 1977; O'Byrne *et al.* 1984; Chung *et al.* 1985). The requirement for granulocytes in these experiments has been established by depletion studies using nitrogen mustard, and by depletion followed by selective replacement of neutrophils (Murphy *et al.* 1986). On the other hand, it would appear that certain animal models of bronchial hyper-responsiveness are less dependent on neutrophils. For example, in a guinea-pig model of antigen-induced bronchoconstriction, both neutrophils and eosinophils infiltrated the airways after allergen inhalation challenge, but pretreatment with nedocromil prevented bronchoconstriction but did not affect the influx of neutrophils (Church *et al.* 1988).

In man, BAL studies indicate that neutrophils are part of the resident population of the large airways in asthmatic and non-asthmatic subjects (Wardlaw *et al.* 1988a). Biopsies of asthmatic airways show infiltration by neutrophils (Laitinen *et al.* 1985), and neutrophil influx is observed in the skin following allergen challenge (Solley *et al.* 1976; Frew and Kay 1988b). In exercise- and allergen-induced asthmatic reactions in man, increased numbers of 'activated' neutrophils were detected in the peripheral blood (as shown by enhanced complement rosette formation) (Papageorgiou *et al.* 1983; Carroll *et al.* 1984).

Whether neutrophils actually participate in the development of allergic inflammation remains unanswered, but the circumstantial evidence is certainly strong enough to warrant the further investigation of factors which may alter neutrophil function.

Allergic inflammation: the need for a model

While useful information can be obtained from biopsis of affected sites in patients with chronic allergic asthma and rhinitis, most of our knowledge of the pathophysiology of allergic tissue responses comes from experimental models, in which allergen is administered to the skin, nose or lungs of sensitized individuals. The histopathology of allergic inflammation in man has largely been studied in the skin. In addition, a few key studies have used bronchial biopsy and lavage to supply corroborative evidence to support the extrapolation of skin study findings to the airways; however, allergen inhalation has mainly been used to obtain physiological and pharmacological data in allergic asthma and rhinitis.

The introduction of allergen extracts into the skin of atopic subjects provokes an immediate reaction with itching, oedema (weal) and erythema (flare). Histologically, this is accompanied by mast cell degranulation, retraction of endothelial cell processes and interstitial oedema (Ting *et al.* 1980). Subsequently, some but not all subjects will experience an LPR, characterized macroscopically by oedema and erythema; in addition, itching may occasionally be present. Biopsies from LPR show cellular infiltration: initially neutrophils and eosinophils but by 24 hours mononuclear cells predominate.

Analogous immediate reactions and LPR occur in the lungs (as airways obstruction), nose (as blockage and itching) and conjunctiva (as oedema and itching) after exposure to relevant allergens. Pharmacologically and physiologically, these LPR resemble more closely the clinical disorders of allergic asthma, rhinitis and conjunctivitis than do immediate responses to allergen. Thus antihistamine drugs, which are partially effective in preventing the immediate response to allergen exposure, are of limited use in treating clinical asthma. On the other hand, glucocorticosteroids are extremely effective in the treatment of asthma and ablate the LPR, without affecting the immediate allergic response when given as a single dose before allergen challenge.

The precise mode of action of corticosteroids in these situations remains unknown. Corticosteroids have a number of properties which might account, at least in part, for their anti-inflammatory effects and which might be relevant to their efficacy in atopic allergy and asthma. The more important of these can be summarized as follows: (i) inhibition of lymphocyte proliferation and lymphokine release; (ii) inhibition of macrophage activation and mediator release; (iii) inhibition of eosinophil colony formation (Butterfield *et al.* 1986) and eosinophil chemotaxis; (iv) inhibition of human basophil (but not mast cell) mediator release (Lichtenstein and MacGlashan 1986); (v) decrease in the number of mast cells (Otsuka *et al.* 1991) and eosinophils (Lichtenstein and MacGlashan 1986) in the nasal mucosa after prolonged treatment; and (vi) decreased bronchial hyper-reactivity after prolonged treatment with inhaled corticosteroids (Kerrebijn *et al.* 1987).

Moreover, patients who experience LPR tend to have worse symptoms than those who only experience early reactions (Warner 1976). For these reasons, many investigators have used the LPR as a convenient model in which to analyse the component parts of allergic inflammation.

At present, the pathogenesis of the LPR remains unresolved. The expression of the LPR is associated with the release of a variety of chemical mediators, e.g. leucotrienes, prostaglandins and kinins (Zweiman 1988), which may come from several cell types, including mast cells, resident inflammatory cells and cells attracted as a result of the immediate IgE-dependent response. Many chemical mediators and mast cell products (PAF, LTC_4, kallikrein, etc.) can induce macroscopic LPR in the skin of man or experimental animals (Dor *et al.* 1983; Archer *et al.* 1985) but the LPR does not appear to be attributable to the actions of a single mediator.

Since the early 1970s, it has been generally accepted that LPR are induced through IgE-dependent mechanisms. The evidence for this comes from experiments showing that passive cutaneous sensitization with IgE-containing sera confers the ability to mount LPR to subsequent challenge with relevant allergens of anti-IgE antisera (Dolovich *et al.* 1973; Solley *et al.* 1976). This activity can be removed by depleting the serum of IgE by affinity chromatography. Furthermore, LPR to common airborne allergens (e.g. pollens, danders, moulds and dust mites) are almost invariably preceded by a weal-and-flare reaction, indicating that these patients have allergen-specific IgE.

In a recent immunohistological study of the human late-phase skin reaction (LPSR), monoclonal antibodies and immunocytochemistry were used to assess the cellular component of these reactions and to obtain evidence of eosinophil and T lymphocyte activation (Frew and Kay 1988b). Numerous neutrophils were present in biopsies obtained 6 hours after allergen challenge (as shown by staining for the neutrophil-specific enzyme elastase). By 24 hours, the number of neutrophils had fallen by 64% while at 48 hours few neutrophils remained. It is noteworthy that there was no association between the magnitude of the LPSR and the numbers of neutrophils detected in the tissue sections.

Numerous eosinophils were present at allergen-challenged sites. The kinetics of eosinophil accumulation differed from those of the neutrophils in that eosinophils persisted in the tissues for up to 48 hours. The majority of these eosinophils were activated, as demonstrated by staining with the monoclonal antibody EG2 (Tai *et al.* 1984), which recognizes an epitope on the secreted form of the eosinophil cationic protein. Activated eosinophils persisted at allergen-challenged sites for at least 48 hours. There was no association between the number of eosinophils and the size of the LPR at 6 hours, but at 24 hours a modest association began to emerge between the number of eosinophils and the size of the preceding LPR (measured at 6 hours), which was statistically significant at 48 hours. The implication of these findings is that common and/or proportional mechanisms are involved in the expression of the macroscopic LPR and in the persistence of activated eosinophils in allergen-challenged tissue.

Increased numbers of T lymphocytes were seen in and around small blood-vessels at the site of LPSR and this T lymphocyte infiltrate persisted for at least 48 hours. The majority of the infiltrating T lymphocytes were CD4 +ve (helper/inducer subset) and the infiltration appeared to be specific in that CD4 +ve/CD8 +ve ratio of cells in the skin was substantially increased compared with peripheral blood. A small number of cells expressed the IL-2 receptor, providing evidence of T cell activation. Supporting this observation, there was increased expression of human leucocyte antigen (HLA)-DR by endothelial cells and of CD4 antigen by epidermal Langerhans cells, both phenomena providing indirect evidence of interferon gamma (IFN-γ) secretion from activated T cells (Miossec and Ziff 1986; Walsh *et al.* 1987). There was no clear association between the numbers of infiltrating T cells and the size of the LPSR, but there was a striking association of CD4+ve T cell numbers with the number of activated eosinophils at 24 hours and to a lesser extent 48 hours (Frew and Kay 1988b).

Late asthmatic reactions

In numerical terms, asthma is the single most important disorder associated with reaginic hypersensitivity. Allergic reactions are clearly important in episodes of acute extrinsic asthma, such as occur when sensitive individuals are exposed acutely to animals or to grass pollen. It has also been proposed, but is less widely accepted, that recurrent exposure to allergens may be important in the development and maintenance of airways inflammation in chronic asthma (Cockcroft 1983). Various aspects of this hypothesis have been studied in the experimentally induced asthmatic reactions provoked by inhalation of relevant allergens. Late asthmatic reactions are conventionally defined as a 20% fall in FEV_1 (or 50% fall in specific airways conductance) 3–12 hours after a standardized allergen inhalation challenge which evoked an early asthmatic response equivalent to a 20% fall in FEV_1. Using this operational 'definition', LAR occur in about 50% of atopic asthmatic subjects (Booij-Noord *et al.* 1971).

Several groups have used BAL to study cellular infiltration in the human LAR. As previously discussed, De Monchy *et al.* (1985) showed that eosinophils are present in BAL 6 hours after allergen challenge. In another study of the LAR, Diaz *et al.* (1989) found no difference in total BAL cell counts in subjects with dual asthmatic responses (DAR) compared to single early responders (SER) after allergen inhalation. However, BAL eosinophils, lymphocytes and neutrophils were increased in the DAR group. The majority of subjects in both the SER and DAR groups had elevated BAL concentrations of eosinophil basic proteins, confirming that eosinophil activation is a feature of the LAR.

Alterations in bronchoalveolar T lymphocyte subsets following allergen challenge were found, which supports the concept that T cells are involved in the expression of the allergen-induced asthmatic LPR in man. For instance, relative increases in CD8 +ve cells were found in BAL in SER, as compared with DAR (Gonzalez *et al.* 1987). In another study, segmental bronchial allergen challenge was performed via the fibre optic bronchoscope and a selective increase in CD4 +ve cells in lavage fluid was observed 48 hours after challenge in subjects who had previously been shown to experience DAR (Metzger *et al.* 1987). These findings are consistent with the decrease in

CD4+ve cells in the peripheral blood which has been reported following allergen inhalation (Gerblich *et al*. 1984). Taken together, these observations suggest that a process of selective recruitment and retention of CD4+ve T lymphocytes is occurring in the lungs during the LAR.

We have studied allergen-induced accumulation of T cells in the bronchi, using a guinea-pig model of the LAR (Frew *et al*. 1990). Following allergen inhalation, an elevation of T lymphocyte numbers in the bronchial mucosa and adventitia was detected. The kinetics of this T cell accumulation paralleled the changes in airways resistance. The numbers of T cells and eosinophils were significantly correlated preceding the peak of the late phase of bronchoconstriction. Subset analysis showed that the majority of the infiltrating T cells were CD3+ve, CD8−ve (i.e. putative T helper cells). In contrast to the striking changes observed in the tissues, analysis of BAL and blood T cell subsets did not show any significant changes in this model.

It is clearly of considerable importance to determine the mechanisms through which inflammatory cells are attracted and the extent to which cellular interactions modulate their activity after arrival at the inflammatory site.

Leucocyte accumulation/adherence reactions

Granulocyte adhesion to endothelial cells seems largely to depend on interactions between leucocyte surface proteins and their specific ligands on leucocytes and endothelial cells. For the neutrophil and eosinophil, the most important adhesion molecule seems to be the CR3 complement receptor molecule (also known as Mac-1). CR3 is one of a family of leucocyte adhesion receptors (lymphocyte function-associated antigen (LFA)-1, Mac-1 and p150,95). Each has a heterodimer structure, consisting of a unique alpha chain and a common beta chain (CD18). The alpha chains of Mac-1, LFA-1 and p150,95 are recognized by CD11b, CD11a and CD11c monoclonal antibodies respectively.

Although originally described as a receptor for inactivated C3b, it is now clear that CR3 has a more general role in intercellular adhesion. Expression of CR3 can be up-regulated by PAF and other chemotactic mediators but this could not on its own account for the localization of granulocytes at inflammatory sites. It seems more likely that the initial events in granulocyte adhesion are effected by up-regulation of endothelial adhesion molecules, whose expression appears largely to be regulated by local secretion of cytokines.

Lymphocyte adherence to endothelial cells seems to be largely mediated via the LFA-1 molecule (CD11a/CD18). Lymphocyte function-associated antigen 1 binds specifically to a molecule known as ICAM-1 (intercellular adhesion molecule 1), whose expression on endothelial cells is inducible by the cytokines IFN-γ and tumour necrosis factor (TNF). There is a wide variation in the kinetics of induction of endothelial adhesion molecules by different cytokines. It is clear, for example, that IFN-γ-induced ICAM-1 expression peaks after 24 hours, while peak induction by TNF is achieved within 6 hours (Lapierre *et al*. 1988). Additional mechanisms must presumably operate to regulate the accumulation of T lymphocytes in the first few hours after allergen exposure.

The initial adhesion of eosinophils at inflammatory sites is probably due to local effects of mast cell mediators on endothelial cells, which cause exudation of plasma proteins and render the endothelial surface adhesive. As regards directional migration, *in vitro* experiments show that neutrophils and eosinophils respond differently to chemotactic mediators. The most potent eosinophil chemotactic factor thus far described is the lipid mediator PAF. Leukotriene B_4 is a potent neutrophil chemotactic factor but has a relatively weak action on eosinophils, while histamine and the eosinophil chemotactic factor of anaphylaxis (ECF-A) tetrapeptides (Val−Gly−Ser−Glu and Ala−Gly−Ser−Glu) have trivial activity compared with PAF (Wardlaw *et al*. 1988b).

Skin chamber studies have revealed the release of LTB_4 and PAF at allergen-induced LPSR sites. The precise source of these mediators is unclear, since human mast cells, unlike those of the rat, do not generate significant quantities of PAF. Other cells are also capable of elaborating chemotactic factors: neutrophils make PAF and LTB_4, eosinophils make PAF and LTC_4, monocytes and macrophages can elaborate LTB_4 and PAF, while lymphocytes produce a number of chemotactic cytokines (Maestrelli *et al*. 1988). These chemotactic products may well be important in the maintenance and development of allergic tissue infiltrates and, in chronically inflamed tissue, may participate directly in the events which follow allergen exposure.

Once arrived at the site of inflammation, eosinophils become activated, as can be shown in allergen-induced LPSR by the expression of epitopes associated with activation on eosinophils (Frew and Kay 1988b). A host of stimuli have been shown to activate eosinophils *in vitro* but to date it is less clear which of these actually operate *in vivo*. *In vitro*, the lipid mediators LTB_4 and PAF, the complement fragments C5a and C3a, the bacterial analogue fMet–Leu–Phe, opsonized zymosan and calcium ionophore all give impressive enhancement of eosinophil function (Gleich and Adolphson 1986). Each of these stimuli is an effective activator of neutrophil function and thus none can account for the apparently selective accumulation and activation of eosinophils which is seen in allergic inflammation. One of the few mediators which selectively activate eosinophil function is the T cell product IL-5, which can enhance antibody-dependent cytotoxic capacity, superoxide generation, degranulation (Lopez *et al*. 1988) and adherence (Walsh *et al*. 1990). Interleukin-5 has also been reported to be weakly chemotactic for eosinophils, although this effect was weak and has not yet been confirmed (Kurihara *et al*. 1988; Yamaguchi *et al*. 1988).

In the absence of a clearly selective attractant for eosinophils, attention has turned to factors regulating the persistence of eosinophils at inflammatory sites. *In vitro*, eosinophils survive in culture for only a few days, but their survival can be prolonged by the addition of IL-3, IL-5 or GM-CSF, especially if fibroblasts or endothelial cells are also present (Owen *et al*. 1987; Rothenburg *et al*. 1988). Such a mechanism might account for the persistence of activated eosinophils at LPSR sites, and for the association of eosinophil persistence with the intensity of T lymphocyte accumulation.

T lymphocytes and allergic inflammation

Until quite recently, it was generally considered that the main role of T lymphocytes in IgE-dependent hypersensitivity was the induction and regulation of IgE production by B lymphocytes. The intensive application of monoclonal antibodies and recombinant deoxyribonucleic acid (DNA) technology has led to a reappraisal of the breadth of T lymphocyte function (Fig. 58.1). It is clear that T cells are capable of operating as pro-inflammatory cells in their own right, as well as orchestrating B cell proliferation and differentiation. In addition, T lymphocytes have a clearly defined role in recruiting and activating other effector cells (Miyajima *et al*. 1988). Co-ordination

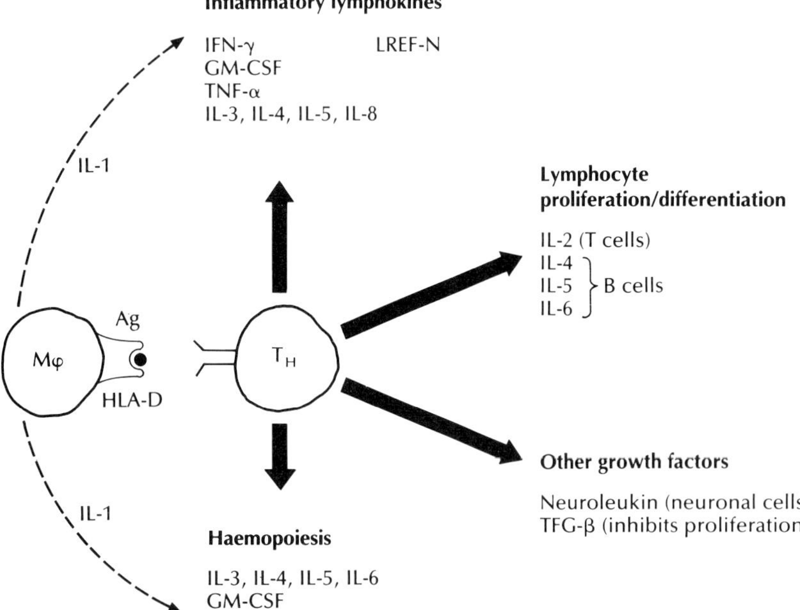

Fig. 58.1. The range of cytokines which may be released by T lymphocytes following specific antigen challenge and their possible contributions to allergic inflammation.

of these various effector functions is achieved by the secretion of lymphokines by T cells in response to stimulation with specific antigen.

The cytokines IL-4 and IFN-γ have important roles in the regulation of IgE production (Teale and Abraham 1987), while IL-5 is also implicated in the mouse but thus far apparently not in man (Sanderson *et al.* 1988). These cytokines are also active on macrophages, eosinophils and endothelial cells, and allergen-specific T lymphocytes attracted following allergen challenge will presumably release these various cytokines at the site of allergic inflammation. Thus there are a number of important and fundamental questions about the functional properties of T cells which recognize allergens.

It is of particular importance to determine the amount and proportions of cytokines secreted by T cells which recognize allergenic determinants. In the mouse it has been possible to divide CD4 +ve T lymphocytes into two distinct subsets on the basis of their profile of lymphokine production. Both subsets secrete IL-3 and GM-CSF; one subset of T lymphocytes (Th1 cells) produces IL-2 and IFN-γ and mediates delayed-type hypersensitivity reactions, while the other subset (Th2 cells) secretes IL-4 and IL-5, but not IL-2 or IFN-γ, and supports immunoglobulin production (Mosmann *et al.* 1986).

In man, it seems that atopic individuals have an increased proportion of circulating T lymphocytes which elaborate IL-4 following activation (Maggi *et al.* 1988). This is consistent with their tendency to produce increased amounts of IgE, but it remains uncertain whether this increase in the numbers of IL-4-producing cells is confined to allergen-specific cells or whether IL-4-producing cells can recognize non-allergenic epitopes.

The functional repertoire of a limited number of allergen-specific human T lymphocyte clones has been studied in detail, and it has been shown that individual T cell clones can provide support for IgE production which is at least partially mediated via IL-4 (O'Hehir *et al.* 1988). These same cells also elaborate substantial quantities of pro-inflammatory lymphokines, including lymphokines which attract and activate neutrophils (Maestrelli *et al.* 1988; Tsai *et al.* 1988).

The relative absence of monocyte infiltration in the human LPSR is also consistent with the hypothesis that a different subset of T lymphocytes is attracted in this model, as compared with other forms of cell-mediated hypersensitivity.

Novel lymphokines

The majority of the lymphokines that have thus far been characterized were first described in terms of their activity in T or B cell growth and differentiation assays. The two exceptions are TNF and IFN-γ, whose effects were initially thought to be specific for macrophages. As time has progressed, it has become clear that each lymphokine can have several different effects and that, broadly speaking, several lymphokines are active in any given assay system. Given the provenance of the currently available lymphokines, it is not really surprising that none of them are particularly active in the chemotaxis and activation of granulocytes. By focusing on the ability of T cell products to modulate granulocyte function, two novel lymphokines have recently been characterized. One of these is a 12−15 kD protein which is chemotactic for neutrophils (Maestrelli *et al.* 1988) and the other is a 35 kD protein which activates neutrophils and enhances neutrophil production of the lipid mediator LTB_4 (Tsai *et al.* 1988). Both these factors are released by lymphocytes specifically stimulated with antigen or non-specifically with the lectin phythaemagglutinin or anti-CD3 monoclonal antibodies and are distinct from the lymphokines IL-1, IL-2, IL-3, IL-5, GM-CSF and TNF.

Although both these lymphokines have greater effects on neutrophils than on eosinophils, they illustrate the importance of using appropriate assay systems to study lymphokine effects on inflammatory cells. It seems likely that other cytokines will be described in the future whose primary effects are on granulocytes.

The revised model (Figs 58.2 and 58.3)

Putting together the established facts and the new information generated in this work, it is possible to see T lymphocytes playing a central regulatory role in allergic responses.

Allergens entering a sensitized epithelium bind to mast cells, triggering the release of preformed and newly generated mediators. The expression of the early reaction to allergen can be attributed to the vasoactive and spasmogenic actions of these soluble mediators. Other $Fc_{\varepsilon}R$-bearing cells may

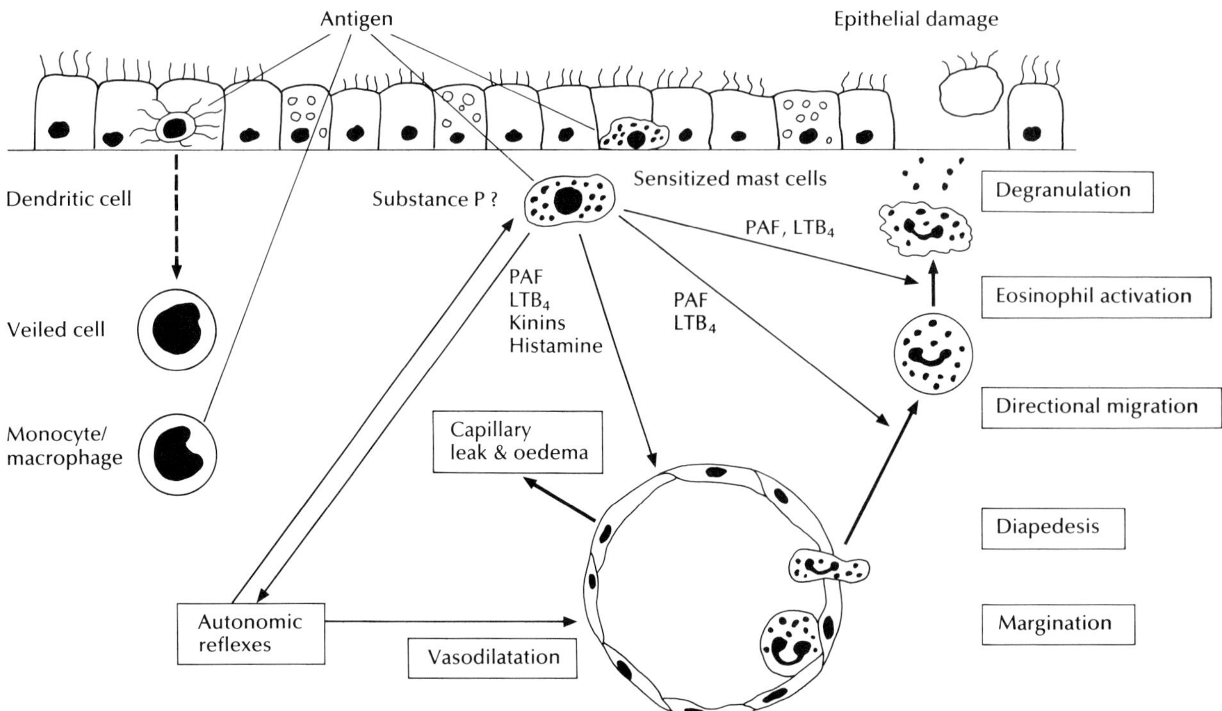

Fig. 58.2. Immunological events in the early phases of IgE-dependent allergic reactions. Mechanisms of oedema formation, granulocyte recruitment and activation, and antigen handling by mononuclear phagocytes.

also contribute to this phase if already present in the epithelium.

Simultaneously, allergen is collected by dendritic and phagocytic cells for presentation to resident and migratory T lymphocytes. This may lead ultimately to the boosting of specific antibody production. In addition, T cells will act directly as pro-inflammatory cells, by secreting lymphokines capable of recruiting and activating other leucocytes. It is postulated that the time-scale of this latter process would make it unlikely that T-cell-derived soluble factors contribute directly to the expression of the early response.

In addition to producing endothelial leakage, mast cell mediators augment granulocyte adhesion to endothelial cells, by local effects on the endothelial cells and systemic effects on circulating granulocytes. Diapedesis and migration are regulated by local chemotactic gradients, PAF and LTB_4 probably being the most active. Once at the inflammatory site, granulocyte function is upregulated by a combination of lipid mediators and acute-phase proteins.

During the preceding phases, T lymphocytes will be recruited in response to locally altered endothelial cells, either through non-specific adhesion to 'sticky' cells or possibly by IL-1 secretion. Antigen-presenting cells will meet T cells reactive against the allergen and induce activation, proliferation and lymphokine secretion. Interferon-γ secretion will enhance endothelial cell Class II major histocompatibility complex (MHC) expression and antigen-presenting activity. The increase in IL-1 secretion (from mononuclear phagocytes and epidermal cells) will cause endothelial cells to release IL-6, which will in turn facilitate the proliferation of locally activated T cells (Wong and Clark 1988).

Selective survival of eosinophils and local differentiation of granulocyte precursors may then be regulated by IL-3, IL-5 and GM-CSF, while mature eosinophils will be activated by IL-5. Basophil precursors are also present at allergic reaction sites and these will be driven to differentiate by IL-3. Interleukin 6 from endothelial cells may contribute to the local production of granulocytes by stimulating haemopoietic precursors to enter the cell cycle.

Depending on the balance of pro-inflammatory and counter-inflammatory forces, chronic allergic

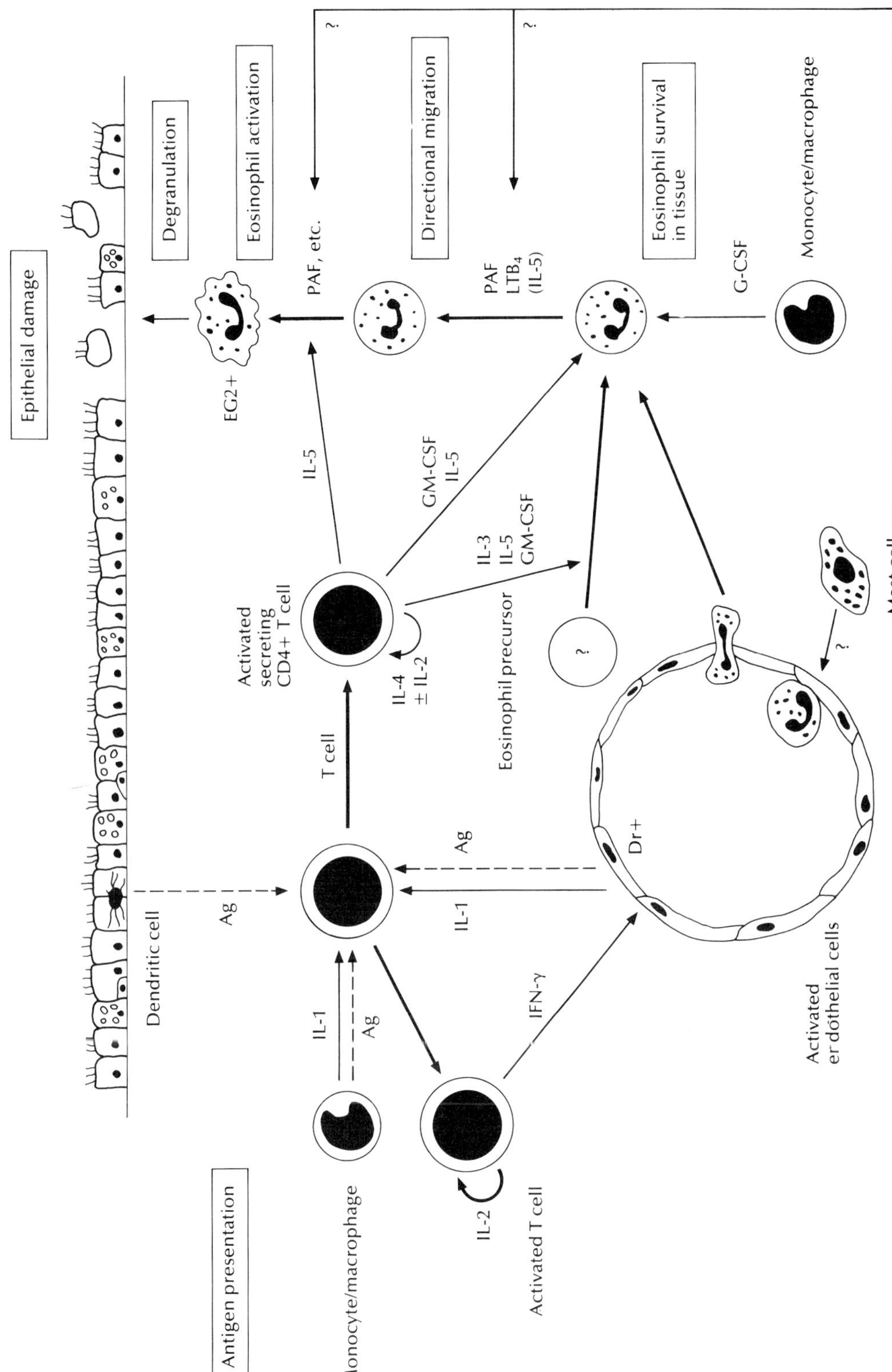

Fig. 58.3. Possible interactions between T lymphocytes and eosinophils in the chronic phase of atopic allergic inflammation.

inflammation may then be self-sustaining or gradually disappear.

Summary

Allergic inflammation presents a unique pattern of cellular infiltration and activation: the complexity of some of its constituent parts is gradually being unravelled by applying techniques of cellular and molecular biology. This review has stressed the T cell dependence of the different processes which contribute to atopic allergic inflammation. Further proof and determination of the details of this process will be obtained through experiments with cloned T lymphocytes, and by the assessment of T lymphocyte function using *in situ* hybridization techniques. It is to be hoped that investigations in this area will lead in time to a better understanding of the genetic basis of atopy; thence to a clearer definition of the pathogenic mechanisms of asthma and rhinitis; and ultimately to novel approaches to the therapy of these common and important disorders.

References

Archer, C.B., Page, C.P., Paul, W., Morley, J. and Macdonald, D.M. (1985). Inflammatory cell accumulation in response to intracutaneous Paf-acether: a mediator of acute and persistent inflammation. *Br. J. Dermatol.* **113** (suppl. 28), 133–5.

Booij-Noord, H., Orie, N.G.M. and DeVries, K. (1971). Immediate and late bronchial obstructive reactions to inhalation of house dust and protective effects of disodium cromoglycate and prednisolone. *J. Allergy Clin. Immunol.* **48**, 344–54.

Butterfield, J.H., Ackerman, S.J., Weller, D., Eisenberg, A.B. and Gleich, G.J. (1986). Effects of glucocorticoids on eosinophil colony growth. *J. Allergy Clin. Immunol.* **78**, 450–7.

Capron, M., Capron, A., Dessaint, J.P. *et al.* (1981). Fc receptors for IgE on human and rat eosinophils. *J. Immunol.* **126**, 2087–92.

Carroll, M.P., Durham, S.R., Walsh, G.M. and Kay, A.B. (1984). Activation of neutrophils and monocytes after allergen and histamine induced bronchoconstriction. *J. Allergy Clin. Immunol.* **75**, 290–6.

Chung, K.F., Becker, A.B., Lazarus, S.C., Frick, O.L., Nadel, J.A. and Gold, W.M. (1985). Antigen-induced airway hyperresponsiveness and pulmonary inflammation in allergic dogs. *J. Appl. Physiol.* **58**, 1347–53.

Church, M.K., Hutson, P. and Holgate, S.T. (1988). Comparison of nedocromil sodium and albuterol against late-phase bronchoconstriction and cellular inflammation in guinea pigs. *Am. Rev. Respir. Dis.* **137**, A136.

Cockcroft, D.W. (1983). Mechanism of perennial allergic asthma. *Lancet* **ii**, 253–6.

De Monchy, J.G.R., Kauffman, H.F., Venge, P. *et al.* (1985). Bronchoalveolar eosinophilia during allergen-induced late asthmatic reactions. *Am. Rev. Respir. Dis.* **131**, 373–6.

Diaz, P., Gonzalez, M.C., Galleguillos, F.R., Ancic, P., Cromwell, O., Shepherd, D. *et al.* (1989). Leucocytes and mediators in bronchoalveolar lavage during allergen-induced late asthmatic reactions. *Am. Rev. Respir. Dis.* **139**, 1383–9.

Dolovich, J., Hargreave, F.E., Chalmers, R., Shier, K.J., Gauldie, J. and Bienenstock, J. (1973). Late cutaneous allergic responses in isolated IgE-dependent reactions. *J. Allergy Clin. Immunol.* **52**, 38–46.

Dor, P.J., Vervloet, D., Sapene, M., Andrac, L., Bonerandi, J.J. and Charpin, J. (1983). Induction of late cutaneous reaction by kallikrein injection: comparison with allergic-like late response to compound 48/80. *J. Allergy Clin. Immunol.* **71**, 363–70.

Durham, S.R. and Kay, A.B. (1985). Eosinophils, bronchial hyperreactivity and late-phase asthmatic reactions. *Clin. Allergy* **15**, 411–8.

Frew, A.J. and Kay, A.B. (1988a). The pattern of human allergic cutaneous late-phase responses. *J. Allergy Clin. Immunol.* **81**, 1117–21.

Frew, A.J. and Kay, A.B. (1988b). The relationship between infiltrating CD4+ lymphocytes, activated eosinophils and the magnitude of the allergen-induced late phase cutaneous reaction in man. *J. Immunol.* **141**, 4158–64.

Frew, A.J., Moqbel, R., Azzawi, M., Hartnell, A., Barkans, J., Jeffery, P.K. *et al.* (1990). T-lymphocytes and eosinophils in allergen-induced late asthmatic reactions in the guinea pig. *Am. Rev. Respir. Dis.* **141**, 407–13.

Frigas, E. and Gleich, G.J. (1986). The eosinophil and the pathophysiology of asthma. *J. Allergy Clin. Immunol.* **77**, 527–37.

Frigas, E., Loegering, D.A., Solley, G.O., Farrow, G.M. and Gleich, G.J. (1981). Elevated levels of the eosinophil granule major basic protein in the sputum of patients with bronchial asthma. *Mayo Clin. Proc.* **56**, 345–53.

Fuller, R.W., Morris, P.K., Richmond, R. *et al.* (1986). Immunoglobulin E-dependent stimulation of human alveolar macrophages: significance in type I hypersensitivity. *Clin. Exp. Immunol.* **65**, 416–26.

Gerblich, A.A., Campbell, A. and Schuyler, M. (1984). Changes in T lymphocyte subpopulations after antigenic bronchial provocation in asthmatics. *N. Engl. J. Med.* **310**, 1349–52.

Gleich, G.J. and Adolphson, C.R. (1986). The eosinophil leukocyte: structure and function. *Adv. Immunol.* **39**, 177–253.

Gonzalez, M.C., Diaz, P., Galleguilos, F.R., Ancic, P., Cromwell, O. and Kay, A.B. (1987). Allergen-induced recruitment of bronchoalveolar helper (OKT4) and suppressor (OKT8) T-cells in asthma. *Am. Rev. Respir. Dis.* **136**, 600–4.

Henson, P.M. and Johnston, R.B. (1987). Tissue injury in inflammation: oxidants, proteinases and cationic proteins. *J. Clin. Invest.* **79**, 669–74.

Jörg, A., Henderson, W.R., Murphy, R.C. and Klebanoff, S.J. (1982). Leukotriene generation by eosinophils. *J. Exp. Med.* **155**, 390–402.

Joseph, M., Capron, A., Ameisen, J.C. *et al.* (1986). The receptor for IgE on blood platelets. *Eur. J. Immunol.* **16**, 306–12.

Kaplan, A.P., Haak-Frendscho, M., Fauci, A., Dinarello, C. and Halbert, E. (1985). A histamine releasing factor from activated human mononuclear cells. *J. Immunol.* **135**, 2027–32.

Kern, P., Horstmann, R.D. and Dietrich, M. (1987). Eosinophil production in human bone marrow cultures induced by 80–85 kDa serum components of patients with eosinophilia. *Br. J. Haematol.* **66**, 165–72.

Kerrebijn, K.F., van Essen-Zandvliet, E.E.M. and Neijens, H.J. (1987). Effect of long term treatment with inhaled corticosteroids and beta-agonists on the bronchial responsiveness in children in asthma. *J. Allergy Clin. Immunol.* **79**, 653–9.

Kuna, P., Alam, R., Kuszminska, B. and Rozniecki, J. (1988). Effect of immunotherapy on the production of histamine releasing factors by mononuclear cells from asthmatic patients. *J. Allergy Clin. Immunol.* **81**, 291 (abstract).

Kurihara, K., Wardlaw, A.J., Maestrelli, P., Tsai, J.-J. and Kay, A.B. (1988). IL-1, IL-2, TNF, IFN-gamma, GM-CSF and PHA-stimulated leukocyte supernatants have negligible eosinophil chemotactic activity compared with platelet activating factor. *FASEB J.* **2**, A1449.

Laitinen, L.A., Heino, M., Laitinen, A., Kava, T. and Haahtela, T. (1985). Damage of the airway epithelium and bronchial reactivity in patients with asthma. *Am. Rev. Respir. Dis.* **131**, 599–606.

Lapierre, L.A., Fiers, W. and Pober, J.S. (1988). Three distinct classes of regulatory cytokines control endothelial major histocompatibility complex antigen expression. *J. Exp. Med.* **167**, 794–804.

Lee, L.Y., Bleecker, E.R. and Nadel, J.A. (1977). Effect of ozone on bronchomotor response to inhaled histamine aerosol in dogs. *J. Appl. Physiol.* **43**, 626–31.

Lichtenstein, L.M. and MacGlashan, D.W. (1986). The concept of basophil releasibility. *J. Allergy Clin. Immunol.* **77**, 291–4.

Lopez, A.F., Sanderson, C.J., Gamble, J.R., Campbell, H.D., Young, I.G. and Vadas, M.A. (1988). Recombinant human interleukin-5 is a selective activator of human eosinophil function. *J. Exp. Med.* **167**, 219–24.

MacDonald, S.M. and Lichtenstein, L.M. (1990). Histamine releasing factors: heterogeneity of IgE. *Springer Semin. Immunopathol.* **12**, 415–28.

MacDonald, S.M., Lichtenstein, L.M., Proud, D., Plaut, M., Naclerio, R.M. and Kagey-Sobotka, A. (1987). Studies of IgE-dependent histamine releasing factors: heterogeneity of IgE. *J. Immunol.* **137**, 506–12.

Maestrelli, P., Tsai, J.-J., Cromwell, O. and Kay, A.B. (1988). The identification and partial characterisation of a human mononuclear cell-derived neutrophil chemotactic factor apparently distinct from IL-1, IL-2, GM-CSF, TNF and IFN-gamma. *Immunology* **64**, 219–25.

Maggi, E., Del Prete, G., Macchia, D. *et al.* (1988). Profiles of lymphokine activities and helper function for IgE in human T cell clones. *Eur. J. Immunol.* **18**, 1045–50.

Melewicz, F.M. and Spiegelberg, H.L. (1980). Fc receptors for IgE on a subpopulation of human peripheral blood monocytes. *J. Immunol.* **125**, 1026–31.

Metzger, W.J., Zavala, D., Richerson, H.B. *et al.* (1987). Local allergen challenge and bronchoalveolar lavage of allergic asthmatic lungs: description of the model and local airway inflammation. *Am. Rev. Respir. Dis.* **135**, 433–40.

Miossec, P. and Ziff, M. (1986). Immune interferon enhances the production of interleukin 1 by human endothelial cells stimulated with lipopolysaccharide. *J. Immunol.* **137**, 2848–52.

Mitchell, E.B., Crow, J., Chapman, M.D., Jonhal, S.S., Pope, F.M. and Platts-Mills, T.A.E. (1982). Basophils in allergen induced patch test sites in atopic dermatitis. *Lancet* **i**, 127–30.

Miyajima, A., Miyatake, S., Schreurs, J. *et al.* (1988). Coordinate regulation of immune and inflammatory responses by T cell derived lymphokines. *FASEB J.* **2**, 2462–73.

Moqbel, R., Macdonald, A.J. and Kay, A.B. (1988). IgE-dependent release of leukotriene C4 from human low density eosinophils. *J. Allergy Clin. Immunol.* **81**, 208 (abstract).

Mosmann, T.R., Cherwinski, H., Bond, M.W., Giedlin, M.A. and Coffman, R.L. (1986). Two types of murine helper T cell clone. 1. Definition according to profiles of lymphokine activities and secreted proteins. *J. Immunol.* **136**, 2348–57.

Murphy, K.R., Wilson, M.C., Irvin, C.G. *et al.* (1986). The requirement for polymorphonuclear leukocytes in the late asthmatic response and heightened airways reactivity in an animal model. *Am. Rev. Respir. Dis.* **134**, 62–8.

Naclerio, R.M., Proud, D., Togias, A.G. *et al.* (1985). Inflammatory mediators in late antigen-induced rhinitis. *N. Engl. J. Med.* **313**, 65–70.

O'Byrne, P.M., Walters, E.H., Gold, B.D. *et al.* (1984). Neutrophil depletion inhibits airway hyperresponsiveness induced by ozone exposure. *Am. Rev. Respir. Dis.* **130**, 214–19.

O'Hehir, R.E., Bal, V., Quint, D. *et al.* (1988). IgE induction by human cloned T lymphocytes specific for house dust mite is IL-4 dependent. *FASEB J.* **2**, A1442.

Ohnishi, M., Ruhno, J., Bienenstock, J., Milner, R., Dolovich, J. and Denburg, J.A. (1988). Human nasal polyp epithelial basophil/mast cell and eosinophil colony stimulating activity: the effect is T-cell dependent. *Am. Rev. Respir. Dis.* **138**, 560–4.

Orchard, M.A., Kagey-Sobotka, A., Proud, D. and Lichtenstein, L.M. (1986). Basophil histamine release induced by a substance from stimulated human platelets. *J. Immunol.* **136**, 2240–4.

Otsuka, H., Mezawa, A., Ohnishi, M., Okubo, K., Seki, H. and Okuda, M. (1991). Changes in nasal metachromatic cells during allergen immunotherapy. *Clin. Exp. Allergy* **21**, 115–19.

Owen, W.F., Rothenburg, M.E., Silberstein, D.S. *et al.* (1987). Regulation of human eosinophil viability, density and function by granulocyte–macrophage colony stimulating factor in the presence of 3T3 fibroblasts. *J. Exp. Med.* **166**, 129–41.

Papageorgiou, N., Carroll, M., Durham, S.R. *et al.* (1983). Complement receptor enhancement as evidence of neutrophil activation after exercise-induced asthma. *Lancet* **ii**, 1220–3.

Prinz, J.C., Baur, X., Ring, J., Endres, N. and Rieber, E.P. (1988). Allergen induced Fc receptors for IgE on human T lymphocytes. *J. Allergy Clin. Immunol.* **81**, 304 (abstract).

Raghavachar, A., Fleischer, S., Frickhofen, N., Heimpel, H. and Fleischer, B. (1987). T lymphocyte control of human eosinophilic granulopoiesis: clonal analysis of an idiopathic hypereosinophilic syndrome. *J. Immunol.* **139**, 3753–8.

Ramesh, K.S., Pincus, S.H. and Rocklin, R.E. (1985). Human lymphocyte–eosinophil interactions. 1. Modulation of phytohaemagglutinin-induced lymphocyte proliferation by eosinophils. *Cell. Immunol.* **92**, 366–75.

Richerson, H.B., Dvorak, H.F. and Leskowitz, S. (1970). Cutaneous basophil hypersensitivity. 1. A new look at the Jones–Mote reaction, general characteristics. *J. Exp. Med.* **132**, 546–57.

Rothenburg, M.E., Owen, W.F., Silberstein, D.S. *et al.* (1988). Human eosinophils have prolonged survival, enhanced functional properties and become hypodense when exposed to human interleukin-3. *J. Clin. Invest.* **81**, 1986–92.

Sanderson, C.J., Campbell, H.D. and Young, I.G. (1988). Molecular and cellular biology of eosinophil differentiation factor (interleukin-5) and its effect on human and mouse B cells. *Immunol. Rev.* **102**, 29–50.

Shaw, R.J., Walsh, G.M., Cromwell, O., Moqbel, R., Spry, C.J.F. and Kay, A.B. (1985). Activated human eosinophils generate SRS-A leukotrienes following physiological (IgG-dependent) stimulation. *Nature* **316**, 150–2.

Solley, G., Gleich, G.J., Jordon, R. and Schroeter, A.L. (1976). The late phase of the immediate weal and flare skin reaction: its dependence upon IgE antibodies. *J. Clin. Invest.* **58**, 408–20.

Tai, P.-C., Spry, C.J.F., Peterson, C., Venge, P. and Olsson, I. (1984). Monoclonal antibodies distinguish between storage and secreted forms of eosinophil cationic protein. *Nature* **309**, 182–4.

Teale, J.M. and Abraham, K.M. (1987). The regulation of antibody class expression. *Immunol. Today* **8**, 122–6.

Ting, S., Dunsky, E.H., Lavker, R.M. and Zweiman, B. (1980). Patterns of mast cell alterations and *in vivo* mediator release in human allergic skin reactions. *J. Allergy Clin. Immunol.* **66**, 417–23.

Tsai, J.J., Maestrelli, P., Cromwell, O., Moqbel, R., Fitzharris, P. and Kay, A.B. (1988). A T-lymphocyte-derived factor that enhances IgE-dependent release of leukotriene B4 from human neutrophils. *Immunology* **65**, 449–56.

Umemoto, L., Poothullil, J., Dolovich, J. and Hargreave, F.E. (1976). Factors which influence late cutaneous allergic responses. *J. Allergy Clin. Immunol.* **58**, 60–8.

Walsh, G.M., Hartnell, A., Wardlaw, A.J., Kurihara, K., Sanderson, C.J. and Kay, A.B. (1990). IL-5 enhances the *in vitro* adhesion of human eosinophils but not neutrophils in a leucocyte integrin (CD11/18)-dependent manner. *Immunology* **71**, 258–65.

Walsh, L.J., Parry, A., Scholes, A. and Seymour, G.J. (1987). Modulation of CD4 antigen on human gingival langerhans cells by gamma interferon. *Clin. Exp. Immunol.* **70**, 379–82.

Wardlaw, A.J. and Kay, A.B. (1988). Neutrophil and eosinophil chemotaxis and cutaneous inflammatory reactions. In *Pharmacology of the Skin*, ed. M.W. Greaves and S. Shuster, vol. I, ch. 24, pp. 395–408, Springer Verlag, Berlin.

Wardlaw, A.J., Moqbel, R., Cromwell. O. and Kay, A.B. (1986). Platelet activating factor: a potent chemotactic and chemokinetic factor for human eosinophils. *J. Clin. Invest.* **78**, 1701–6.

Wardlaw, A.J., Dunnette, S., Gleich, G.J., Collins, J.V. and Kay, A.B. (1988a). Eosinophils and mast cells in bronchoalveolar lavage in subjects with mild asthma: relationship to bronchial hyperreactivity. *Am. Rev. Respir. Dis.* **137**, 62–9.

Wardlaw, A.J., Kurihara, K., Maestrelli, P., Tsai, J.J. and Kay, A.B. (1988b). Relative eosinophil and neutrophil chemotactic activities. *J. Allergy Clin. Immunol.* **81**, 207.

Warner, J.A., Pienkowski, M.M., Plaut, M., Norman, P.S. and Lichtenstein, L.M. (1986). Identification of histamine releasing factor(s) in the late phase of cutaneous IgE-mediated reactions. *J. Immunol.* **136**, 2583–7.

Warner, J.O. (1976). Significance of late reactions after bronchial challenge with house dust mite. *Arch. Dis. Child.* **51**, 905–11.

Wong, G.G. and Clark, S.C. (1988). Multiple actions of interleukin-6 within a cytokine network. *Immunol. Today* **9**, 137–9.

Yamaguchi, Y.. Havashi, Y., Sugama, Y. *et al.* (1988). Highly purified murine interleukin-5 stimulates eosinophil function and prolongs *in vitro* survival: IL-5 as a chemotactic factor. *J. Exp. Med.* **167**, 1737–42.

Yokota, A., Kikutani, H., Tanaka, T. *et al.* (1988). Two species of human Fc epsilon receptor II (FceRII/CD23): tissue-specific and IL-4-specific regulation of gene expression. *Cell* **55**, 611–18.

Zweiman, B. (1988). Mediators of allergic inflammation in the skin. *Clin. Allergy* **18**, 419–33.

Section 7
Connective Tissue Disease

59: Sjögren's Syndrome

P.J.W. Venables

Introduction

Sjögren's syndrome (SS) is a systemic autoimmune rheumatic disease characterized by inflammation and destruction of exocrine glands (Sjögren 1933). The salivary and lachrymal glands are principally involved, giving rise to dry eyes and mouth, although other exocrine glands, including those of the pancreas, sweat glands and mucus-secreting glands of the bowel, bronchial tree and vagina, may be affected. It was originally described as the triad of dry eyes, dry mouth and rheumatoid arthritis (RA) (Sjögren 1933) although it is now classified as (i) primary SS, where the disease exists on its own, and (ii) secondary SS, where it is associated with another autoimmune rheumatic disease such as RA or systemic lupus erythematosus (SLE).

Sjögren's syndrome may affect up to 3% of the population (Jacobson *et al.* 1989). The exact prevalence is not known as there are thought to be many sufferers whose symptoms are so mild that they do not seek medical advice. It is nine times commoner in women than men and its onset is at any age from 15 to 65. The patients complain of a gritty sensation in the eyes, soreness, photosensitivity or intolerance of contact lenses. The dry mouth is often manifest as inability to swallow dry food without fluid, or the need to wake up in the night to take sips of water.

Keratoconjunctivitis sicca can be detected by Schirmer's test, tear breakup time and Rose Bengal staining (Manthorpe *et al.* 1981) and xerostomia by observing a diminished salivary pool, by a reduced parotid salivary flow rate and by reduced uptake and clearance on isotope scans (Daniels *et al.* 1975; Manthorpe *et al.* 1981). The majority of patients have a raised erythrocyte sedimentation rate (ESR), often associated with a mild normocytic anaemia, hypergammaglobulinaemia and rheumatoid factors (RFs). Antibodies to Ro (SS-A) are found in about 85% of patients and La (SS-B) in 60%.

For the diagnosis of SS in epidemiological studies, the recent criteria of Fox *et al.* (1986a) are probably the most practical but may miss early disease. Four were proposed: (i) dry eyes (by Schirmer's and by Rose Bengal or fluorescein staining); (ii) dry mouth (symptoms and decreased salivary flow rate); (iii) lymphocytic infiltrates on lip biopsy; (iv) demonstration of serum autoantibodies antinuclear antibodies, Ro or La antibodies). Four criteria represent 'definite' and three 'possible' SS.

Systemic features of Sjögren's syndrome

Arthritis, Raynaud's phenomenon and a purpuric vasculitis on the lower legs are the commonest extraglandular features of primary SS. A high incidence of pulmonary function abnormalities has been described, although these are rarely clinically significant. A wide range of neurological diseases, including central nervous system disorders resembling multiple sclerosis, have been noted in some centres (Alexander *et al.* 1986) although these appear to be rare in unselected populations. Interstitial nephritis, leading to renal tubular acidosis or nephrogenic diabetes insipidus, occurs in about 30% of patients. These lesions are usually subclinical but may lead to hypokalaemia, causing muscular weakness or, occasionally, nephrocalcinosis (reviewed in Venables, in press). Lymphomas, almost always of B cell lineage, are a characteristic but unusual feature of SS. They occur in about 5% of patients in referral units and are particularly found in patients with high levels of immunoglobulins, autoantibodies and cryoglobulins. As the lymphoma develops, the immunoglobulin levels often fall and the autoantibodies become negative. The development of lymphomas may reflect the long-standing stimulation of B cells as an underlying pathogenic feature of SS (Tzioufas *et al.* 1987).

In secondary SS the features are those of the associated disease, the commonest being RA and SLE. In RA the patients with SS tend to have more severe disease, with frequent extra-articular manifestations, and the vasculitis is more manifest as digital infarcts and subcutaneous ulcers (Maini 1987). In SLE, those with SS have a lower frequency of renal disease and a relatively good prognosis. Primary biliary cirrhosis and scleroderma, although rare in themselves, are frequently complicated by SS. Other autoimmune diseases which have been described in association with SS include polymyositis, mixed connective tissue disease, chronic active hepatitis and Hashimoto's thyroiditis (Morrow and Isenberg 1987).

Immunogenetics

Primary SS is strongly associated with human leucocyte antigen (HLA) B8, DR3, DRW 52, DQ2 2 and C4A null gene (reviewed in Harley *et al.* 1986; Papasteriades *et al.* 1988). All of the antigens in this haplotype are in strong linkage disequilibrium so that it is too difficult to establish which of the genes contains the locus conferring the risk. The fact that DR5 rather than DR3 is the commonest susceptibility gene for Greek patients with SS (Papasteriades 1988) suggests that DR3 itself is not the risk factor. While DRW 52, linked to DR3 and DR5, could carry the risk, the very high frequency of DRW 52 in the general population (over 50%) suggests that its contribution as a predisposing factor would be low. Alternatively, it is possible that a short amino acid sequence common to DR3 and DR5, analogous to the EQKRAA sequence present on both DR1 and DR4 which prediposes to RA (Chapter 60), may be the major factor, although no such sequence has been identified in SS.

The immune response genes may be more strongly linked to autoantibody specificity than to diagnostic entities. Over 90% of West European Caucasian patients with anti-La and anti-Ro antibodies are HLA-DR3 +ve, and the frequency is also increased (to 60%) in anti-Ro/La +ve black patients (Arnett *et al.* 1989). Interestingly, the variant of DR3 (defined by restriction fragment polymorphism) in this subgroup of Blacks is predominantly of the type found in Caucasians (Arnett *et al.* 1989). One study using ELISA has suggested that high levels of anti-Ro in the absence of anti-La are primarily associated with both DQ1 and DQ2 antigens, with DQ1 and DQ2 heterozygosity conferring the highest relative risk (Harley *et al.* 1986). It is important to recognize that DQw 1.2 and 2 are linked to DR2 and DR3 respectively and, at present, the evidence that the important loci are in or near the DQ locus, rather than DR, is weak. Also, the anti-La −ve anti-Ro +ve patients tend towards the SLE part of the spectrum or have SLE. This means the contribution of more than one immune response gene may reflect the different clinical manifestations of SLE rather than heterozygosity being directly linked with anti-Ro antibody production.

It is not known how DR3 or its linked genes could contribute to the pathogenesis of SS. It is possible that the association between the haplotype and anti-La antibodies is due to DR3 conferring a direct predisposition to the production of anti-La. Some evidence in support of this concept was the demonstration that stimulated lymphocytes from DR3 +ve healthy subjects secreted more anti-La antibody than those from DR3 −ve subjects whereas antibodies to other autoantigens were not increased (Venables *et al.* 1988a). A second possibility is that the C4 null gene, by leading to a relative deficiency of complement, is associated with impaired clearance of immune complexes, which in turn leads to immune complex-mediated tissue damage. Additional clearance defects due to impaired Fc receptor function found both in patients with SS and in DR3 +ve healthy subjects (reviewed in Venables *et al.* 1988a) would explain the high frequency of cryoglobulins and immune complexes (Morrow and Isenberg 1987) and their association with vasculitis in SS. However, it is difficult to envisage how circulating immune complexes could account for pathological changes within the exocrine glands themselves.

Class II major histocompatibility complex (MHC) expression within salivary epithelium is a more direct mechanism whereby HLA antigens could be involved in exocrine glandular destruction (Lindahl *et al.* 1985). This phenomenon, first described in autoimmune thyroid disease (Botazzo *et al.* 1983), could be responsible for antigen presentation by epithelial cells within the gland. There is good evidence that epithelial Class II MHC expression is mediated principally by interferon-γ, and this in turn could be due to virus infection. The Class II MHC antigens could also be presenting either viral antigens or autoantigens and these could be directing a cytotoxic attack against the salivary epithelium itself.

Autoantibodies in Sjögren's syndrome: antibodies to Ro and La

Over 25 years ago, Bloch *et al.* (1965) described precipitating antibodies termed SjT and SjD, now thought to be La and Ro (Tan 1982), that were found in primary sicca syndrome but not in SS/RA. Antibodies to the Ro and La antigens, described a few years later (Clark *et al.* 1969; Reichlin and Mattioli 1974), were thought to be more a feature of SLE than of SS. Alspaugh *et al.* (1976) then independently described anti-SS-A and anti-SS-B, both of which occurred in primary SS and not in SS/RA. They also described a third antibody, anti-SS-C, which occurred in SS/RA but not in other forms of SS. Much of the confusion of different antigens became resolved when Alspaugh and Maddison demonstrated conclusively that Ro and SS-A were the same, as were La and SS-B (Tan 1982). It is now agreed that anti-La antibodies are found in 40–60% and anti-Ro in 50–85% of patients with primary SS, with the frequency rising to over 95% by enzyme-linked immunosorbent assay (ELISA) with purified antigens (Harley *et al.* 1986). However, the significance of such a high frequency of these antibodies becomes reduced when it is realized that with these highly sensitive assays autoantibodies are detected in normal sera.

The apparent discrepancy between the previously reported diagnostic associations of the antibodies (Ro and La with SLE, as opposed to SS-A and SS-B with SS) was subsequently reconciled by the recognition that the antibodies were associated with SS/SLE overlap syndromes (Fig. 59.1) (Pease *et al.* 1989), that anti-Ro +ve SLE patients had evidence of SS on salivary gland biopsy and that the extraglandular features of primary SS resemble SLE (Moutsopoulos *et al.* 1980). This has led to the proposal of three types of SS: primary disease, SS/SLE and SS/RA (Table 59.1) (Maini 1987; Venables 1988). Sjögren's syndrome/RA, being DR4 +ve and anti-Ro/La −ve, now appears quite distinct, whereas primary SS and SLE share both clinical and immunogenetic features and form

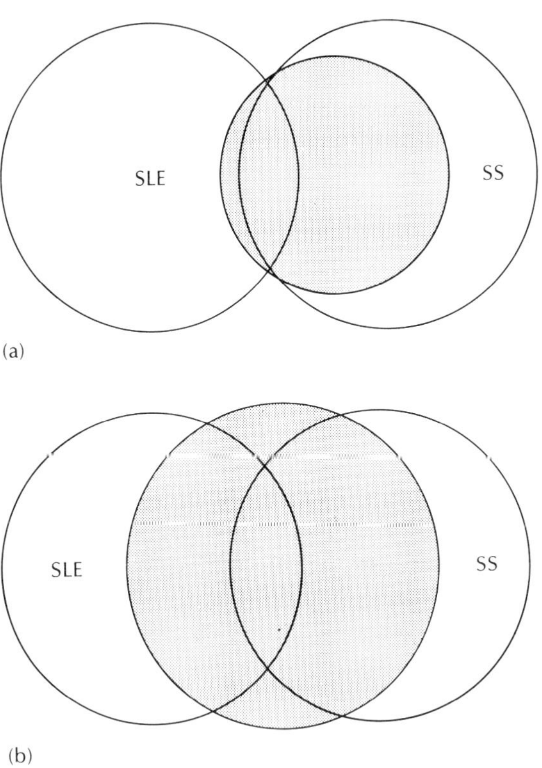

Fig. 59.1. Venn-type diagram showing overlap between systemic lupus erythematosus (SLE) and Sjögren's syndrome and their relationship to antibodies (a) La and (b) Ro shown as shaded areas.

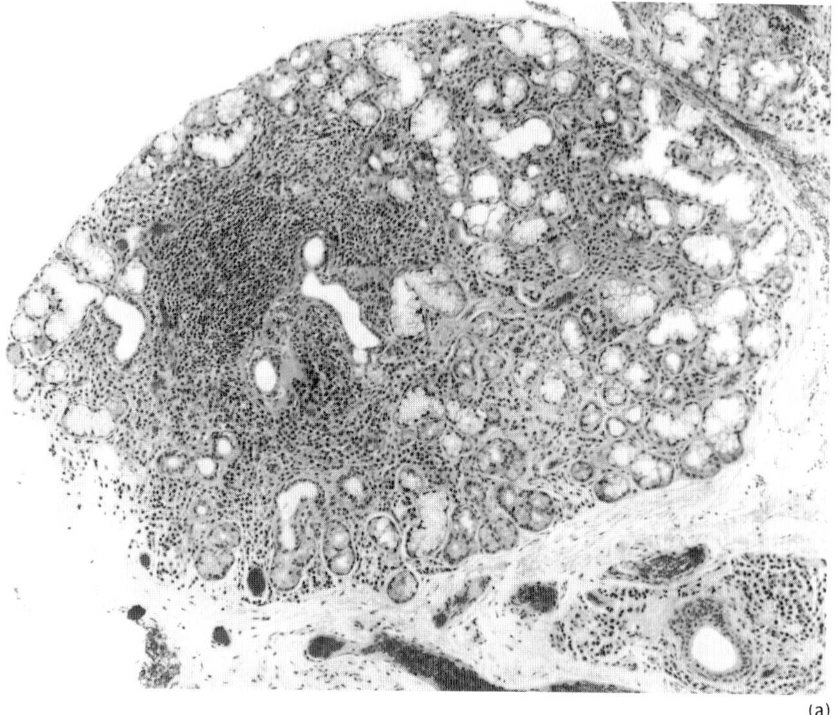
(a)

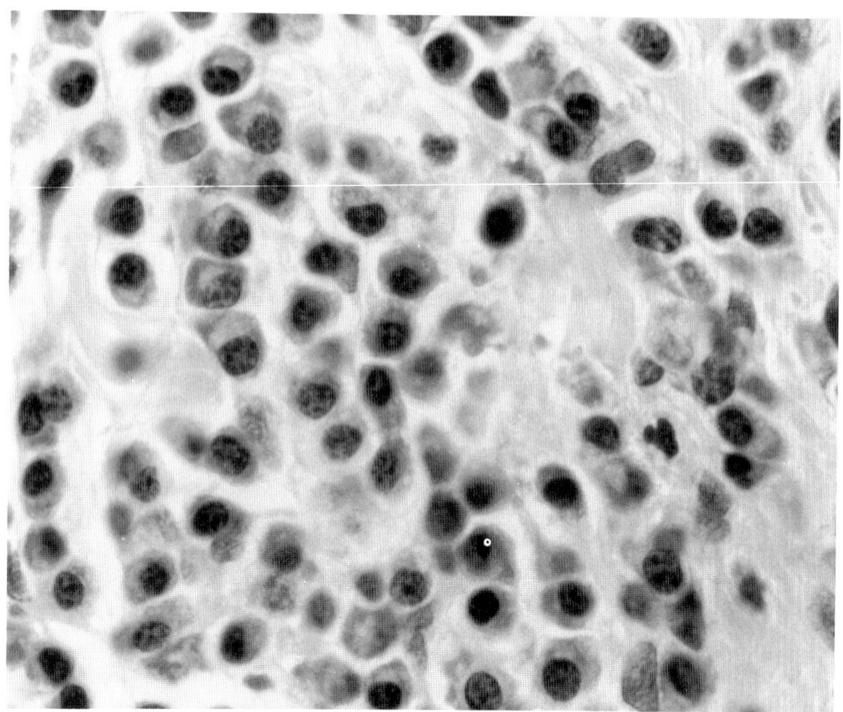
(b)

Fig. 59.2. Haematoxylin- and eosin-stained photomicrograph of a salivary gland biopsy.

a spectrum of overlapping diseases, with anti-La and anti-Ro being found at the point of overlap. Anti-Ro, being less specific for SS than is anti-La, spreads rather further into the SLE part of the spectrum.

Now there are known to be at least four isoforms of Ro: 60 and 52 kD in nucleated cells and 60 and 54 kD in erythrocytes (Rader *et al*. 1989) (see also Chapter 61). The search is therefore on for diagnostically specific subsets of anti-Ro antibodies.

Table 59.1. Clinical, serological and immunogenetic features of primary Sjögren's syndrome, SS/SLE overlap and secondary SS with RA

	Primary SS	SS/SLE	SS/RA
Arthritis	Non-erosive	Non-erosive	Erosive
Raynaud's	++	+++	±
Purpura	++	++	±
Digital infarcts	−	±	++
Subcutaneous ulcers	−	±	++
Leucopenia	++	+++	−
Rheumatoid factors	++	+	++
Anti-Ro	++	++	±
Anti-La	++	++	−
DR3[a]	63%	60%	30%
DR4[a]	24%	20%	68%

a Data from author's unit.

So far none have emerged, apart from one report of a close association between anti-52 kD Ro and congenital heart block (Buyon *et al.* 1989). A detailed account of the structure and molecular biology of Ro and La is given in Chapter 61.

Anti-SS-C has not stood the test of time as a diagnostically useful antibody in SS. When the antibody was found to be equally common in rheumatoid arthritis without SS, its name was changed to RAP (rheumatoid arhritis precipitin) and subsequently to anti-RANA (rheumatoid arthritis nuclear antigen) (Alspaugh *et al.* 1979). The main reactive epitope on RANA is now known to be part of the Epstein–Barr virus (EBV) nuclear antigen (Venables *et al.* 1988b) and it is this relationship to the virus which is of much more interest than the diagnostic use of the antibody. Anti-salivary gland antibodies, detected as a reaction with salivary gland epithelium on indirect immunofluorescence (Feltcamp and Rossum 1968b), occur in 60% of SS/RA patients and were originally thought to be useful in defining this subset of the disease. However, the occurrence of the antibody in about 20% of uncomplicated RA patients as well as 20% of patients with primary SS (Youinou and Pennec 1987) has resulted in the assay being discontinued in most laboratories. Antinuclear, anti-perinuclear, anti-cytoskeletal and anti-Golgi apparatus antibodies have also been described in SS (reviewed in Fox *et al.* 1984; Youinou and Pennec 1987). Although not diagnostic, they are indicative of an autoimmune process, which may help to distinguish SS from other causes of kerato-conjunctivitis sicca. Indeed, antinuclear antibodies (other than La) are now included among the diagnostic criteria for SS (Fox *et al.* 1986a), and in one recent study (Pease *et al.* 1989) were found in over 60% of SS patients negative for anti-Ro and anti-La.

Rheumatoid factors, as measured by routine assays, occur in at least 80% of SS. Detected by ELISA, immunoglobulin A (IgA) RFs are characteristic (Elkon *et al.* 1983; Fox *et al.* 1984), possibly reflecting the mucosal involvement in the disease. The germline gene-derived 17–109 idiotype is found on a high proportion of these RFs, with the concentration increasing as the patients develop B cell lymphomas, suggesting oligoclonal proliferation evolving into monoclonal proliferation followed by malignant transformation (reviewed in Tzioufas *et al.* 1987). Rheumatoid factors do not distinguish SS/RA from other forms of SS, and their detection in primary SS is a common reason for misdiagnosing such patients as RA.

Immunohistopathology

The cardinal pathological features of SS are inflammation and destruction of salivary gland tissue (Greenspan *et al.* 1974; Fox *et al.* 1984; Leroy *et al.* 1989). The inflammatory infiltrates consist of focal aggregates of lymphocytes, mainly localized around ducts (Fig. 59.2). Occasionally lymphocytes can be seen within duct epithelium itself (Leroy *et al.* 1989). Scattered interstitial plasma cells are commonly found, although these are not disease-specific and are also found in glands from healthy individuals. The destructive changes are predominantly duct dilatation, acinal atrophy and interstitial fibrosis. These findings have also been described in biopsies from people without SS, particularly in the elderly, and are not regarded as diagnostically specific (Leroy *et al.* 1989).

Within the gland, the majority of the lymphocytes are of the CD4 (Fox *et al.* 1984; Morrow and Isenberg 1987; Youinou and Pennec 1987) phenotype with a relative paucity of CD8 (suppressor/cytotoxic) cells. The recent descriptions of Class II MHC-restricted, CD4+ve cytotoxic T cells (De Berardinis *et al.* 1989) raise the possibility that many of the lymphocytes are directly involved in the destruction of the salivary epithelium. If the CD4 cells are similar to those in RA synovium (see

Chapter 60) and bear the 4B4 helper/inducer phenotype, it is likely that T cell help, rather than cytotoxicity, predominates and that the inflamed salivary gland is a site of antigen presentation and induction of autoantibodies. About 10% of the lymphocytes are B cells. There are also plentiful plasma cells whose cytoplasm contains IgA. Horsfall *et al.* (1988, 1989) have demonstrated anti-La idiotypes within these plasma cells as well as specific concentration of IgA anti-La and IgA RFs in saliva, supporting the concept of local production of autoantibodies within the gland. Natural killer cells and macrophages are rare (Elkon *et al.* 1983; Fox *et al.* 1984; Morrow and Isenberg 1987).

It is generally agreed that the infiltrating cells, both T and B (Youinou and Pennec 1987), are activated. Virtually all of the T cells are Class II MHC +ve and produce high levels of interleukin (IL)-2 *in vitro* (Fox *et al.* 1985). Interferon-γ has been detected immunohistochemically in SS biopsies (Morrow and Isenberg 1987) and is thought to be the primary stimulus for the induction of Class II MHC expression on the epithelial cells. This phenomenon has also been demonstrated *in vitro*, using an epithelial cell line from an SS lymphoma which expressed class II MHC when treated with interferon-γ (Fox *et al.* 1986b). A recent study showed that, in sialadinitis complicating graft-versus-host disease, lymphocytic infiltrates antedated Class II MHC expression, suggesting that lymphocytes trafficking to the gland was an early event and that interferon-γ production and Class II MHC expression occurred subsequently (Lindhal *et al.* 1989).

Within the blood the most striking abnormality is the presence of an increased number of B cells bearing the CD5 antigen (Plater-Zyberk *et al.* 1985). The CD5 marker, present in much greater density on T cells, is also found on B cells from patients with chronic lymphocytic leukaemia and in fetal blood, implying primitive ontogeny and suggesting an intriguing link with B cell malignancy. These cells secrete immunoglobulins with autoantibody specificities, particularly those with the characteristics of natural antibodies. The antibodies tend to be of IgM class, polyreactive and often with RF activity, and they bear the unmutated phenotypes of germline genes. The regulation of CD5 B cells is unknown, but the coordinate expansion of T cells bearing γδ (as opposed to the more abundant αβ) receptors (Brennan *et al.* 1989) suggests that they interact with CD5 +ve B cells. Alternatively genetic factors or simply the presence of inflammation may promote the expansion of both cell types.

It is possible that the CD5 +ve B cell may play a role, not only in the autoimmunity of SS, but also in the lymphomas that occasionally complicate it. Analysis of immunoglobulin gene rearrangements and cellulose acetate electrophoresis of serum immunoglobulins (Moutsopoulos *et al.* 1983) show a high frequency of oligoclonal and monoclonal B cell activation, even in patients with no evidence of lymphoma. Whether the CD5 B cell is responsible for this phenomenon remains unknown. Its participation in events in the salivary gland is also unknown because of technical problems posed by the relative paucity of B cells and by the high density of CD5 on the T cells in such tissue.

Abnormalities in circulating lymphocyte numbers in SS are similar to those in SLE (Chapter 61) and may reflect the frequent overlap between the two diseases. Lymphopenia is found in about 50% of patients, with a marked reduction in CD8 cells and a relative increase in B cells (Fox *et al.* 1982). An increased proportion of all cell types bear activation markers such as Class II MHC or the transferrin receptor (Fox *et al.* 1984). Unlike SLE, functional studies do not show evidence of impaired suppression (Moutsopoulos and Fauci 1980). There is, however, a decreased response of cells to mitogens (Miyasaka *et al.* 1980), decreased autologous mixed lymphocytes reaction and, in contrast to events within the gland, impaired IL-2 production (Fox *et al.* 1985). It is difficult to envisage how these events within the circulation could contribute to autoimmunity in SS although Youinou and Pennec (1987) suggested that the CD8 deficiency and defective IL-2 response could lead to impairment of cytotoxic T cell function with a resultant increase in virus-infected cells. These cells could then drive an autoimmune response by any of the mechanisms discussed below.

Viruses and Sjögren's syndrome

It has long been thought that autoimmune disease could result from a virus acting as a trigger on the background of immune response genes (HLA tissue type) within the appropriate hormonal environment (oestrogens). Sjögren's syndrome is a particularly strong candidate for a viral aetiology for the following reasons:

1 The main site of pathology, the salivary gland, is a site of latency for a number of viruses.

2 The interferon-γ and epithelial Class II MHC expression within ducts and acini could be caused by viruses.

3 La antigen is involved in the processing of viral ribonucleic acids (RNAs).

The viruses which are the most likely agents are those which are sialotropic, accounting for sialadinitis, and lymphotropic, leading to immunological disregulation and autoimmunity. Such viruses include three from the herpesvirus group, EBV, cytomegalovirus (CMV) and human herpesvirus 6 (HHV-6). The retroviruses are also under investigation, although their localization to salivary gland has not been well documented.

In general, serological studies of the herpesvirus group have been inconclusive. Whereas elevated titres of antibodies to all three viruses have been claimed in some studies (Shillitoe *et al.* 1982; Biberfeld *et al.* 1988; Yamaoka *et al.* 1988), others have found that antibody prevalence and titre were normal in SS for CMV (Venables *et al.* 1985), EBV (Venables *et al.* 1985, 1989) and HHV-6 (Baboonian *et al.* 1990). The disagreement between studies may be due to lack of age- and sex-matched controls and allowing for possible interference by RFs. In spite of the negative serological findings, there is other evidence for involvement of the herpesvirus group in SS, EBV being the best studied to date.

Using deoxyribonucleic acid (DNA) hybridization techniques, EBV has been detected in parotid gland and in labial biopsies (Fox *et al.* 1986c; Venables *et al.* 1989b). Salivary epithelium can contain up to 50 copies of EBV DNA per cell in healthy people without inducing an immune response, suggesting that the gland is an important site of persistence (Venables *et al.* 1989b). The extent of EBV infection load in salivary gland in SS is still controversial, with one report finding it increased (Fox *et al.* 1986c) and one decreased (Venables *et al.* 1989b). Other studies have implicated EBV indirectly. These include case reports of patients with infectious mononucleosis developing SS (Whittingham *et al.* 1985) and, more recently, a study which showed that B cells from SS patients transformed into continuous cell lines more easily than controls (Yamaoka *et al.* 1988). Although the evidence remains indirect and contradictory, EBV is still considered a major candidate for involvement in the pathogenesis of SS.

There is no direct evidence for the involvement of retroviruses in SS, although the abnormalities in lymphocyte subset numbers, the link between SS and lymphoma and the description of parotitis and keratoconjunctivitis sicca in patients with acquired immune deficiency syndrome (AIDS), (Itescu *et al.* 1989) suggest that they merit investigation. More recent evidence is provided by a preliminary study which found antibodies to p24 gag protein in 30% of patients with SS (Talal 1989) and by a study which showed that transgenic mice with the human T cell lymphotrophic virus (HTLV)-1 tax gene develop an exocrinopathy resembling SS (Green *et al.* 1989). Retrovirus infection could also cause SS by interacting with a herpesvirus. There is evidence that HHV-6, EBV and CMV can activate human immunodeficiency virus (HIV) *in vitro* (Luso *et al.* 1989) and *in vivo* in lymphomas, hairy leucoplakia and AIDS (Luso *et al.* 1989; Webster *et al.* 1989).

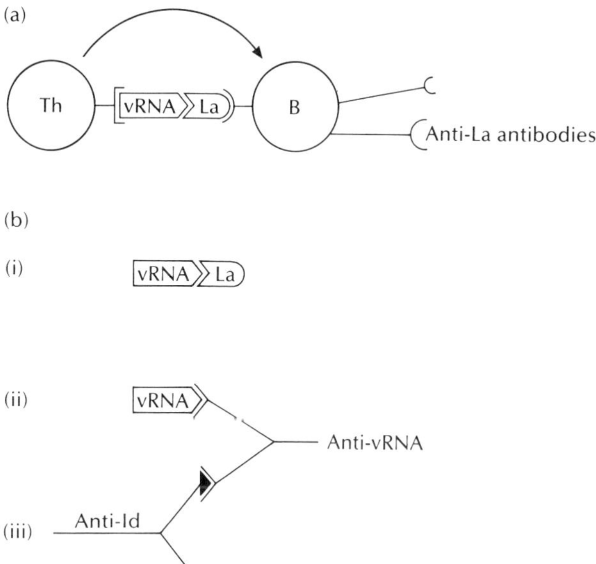

Fig. 59.3. Possible mechanisms whereby the interaction of viral RNA and La could lead to the generation of anti-La autoantibodies. (a) Self + X hypothesis. T cells binding to determinants on viral RNA provide help to B cells recognizing La. (b) Idiotype network hypothesis (Plotz 1983). Antibodies to the La binding site on viral RNA induce anti-idiotypes. Internal image anti-idiotypes react with the RNA binding site of La.

The involvement of La in the processing of viral RNAs including the RNAs of EBV, herpes simplex and adenovirus (Tan 1982) could represent a clue to the involvement of viruses in the aetiology or pathogenesis of SS. It is possible that the interaction between host (La) and virus (viral RNA) is a mechanism for tolerance bypass (Fig. 59.3(a)). This was suggested (Mathews and Bernstein 1983) for the ribonucleoprotein Jo-1, which is known to be involved in the aminoacylation of enteroviruses with histidine (see also Chapter 63). A problem with this hypothesis in relation to the La antigen is that viral RNAs have not been shown to be immunogenic. A second mechanism, suggested

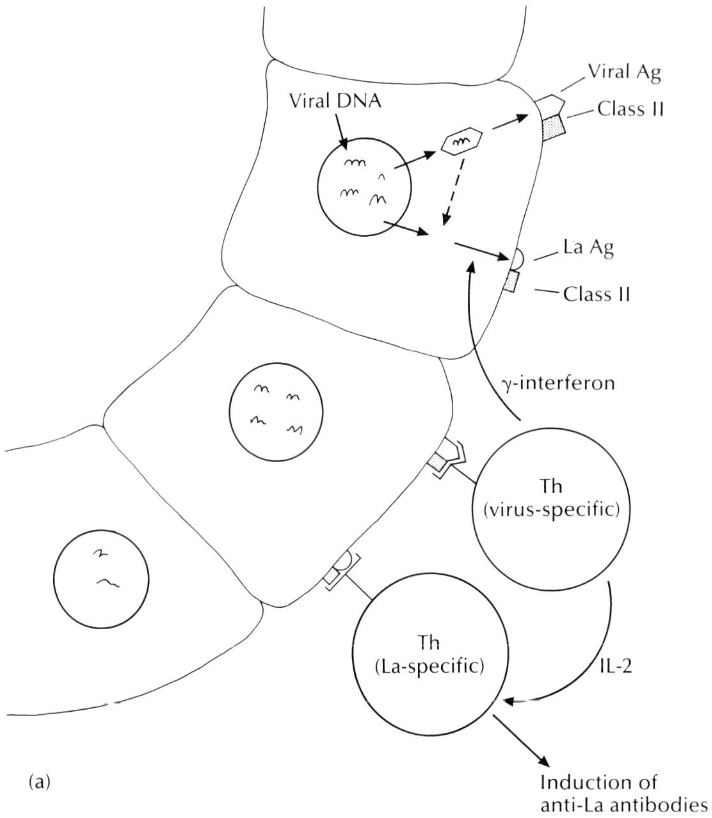

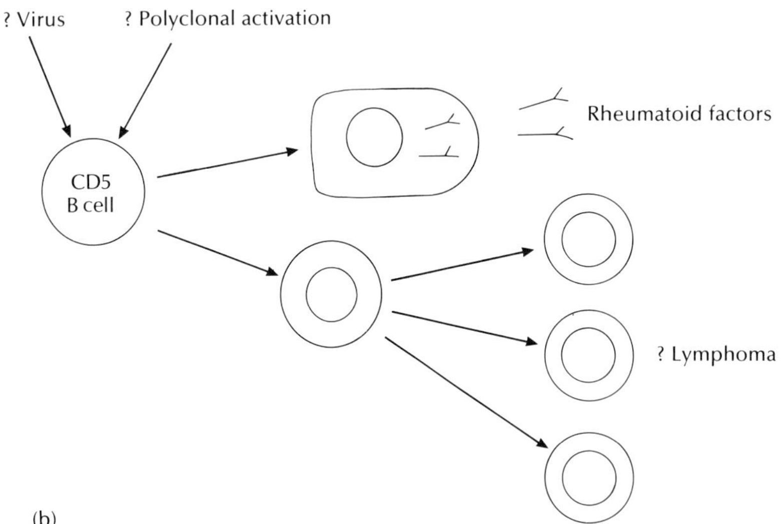

Fig. 59.4. Possible mechanisms whereby virus infection of salivary gland and lymphocytes could lead to the pathological features of Sjögren's syndrome. (a) In salivary gland. Virus infection of epithelial cells leads to surface expression of La, partly as a result of the virus itself and partly due to an effect of interferon-γ (Baboonian *et al.* 1989). Co-expression of Class II MHC antigens leads to induction of anti-La antibodies within the gland. The presence of viral antigens would further increase the inflammatory response and possibly direct an immune attack on the epithelium. (b) In B cells. Virus infection leads to stimulation of B cells (perhaps those bearing the CD5 phenotype), resulting in polyclonal activation with the production of rheumatoid factors. Some clones eventually undergo malignant transformation and become lymphomatous.

by Plotz (1983), is also based on the La/virus interaction, although he suggested that antibodies to viral RNA could result in an anti-idiotype response which would include antibodies reactive with La (Fig. 59.3(b)). This hypothesis also suffers from the absence of an immune response to viral RNAs. In addition, it would predict that the predominant immune response to La would be directed against the RNA binding site, whereas epitope mapping has shown that antibodies react with epitopes stretched along the whole length of the polypeptide (St Clair *et al.* 1989). A third mechanism is suggested by the finding that virus infection of epithelial cells causes La to migrate from the nucleus to the cytoplasm and the surface of epithelial cells *in vitro* (Baboonian *et al.* 1989). A similar phenomenon occurring in salivary epithelium or infiltrating inflammatory cells could be the basis of an antigen-driven mechanism for the generation of anti-La antibodies or it could represent a target for damage by antibody or cytotoxic T cells. It is likely that the Ro antigen is also expressed on the surface of virally infected cells, but the lack of usable monoclonal anti-Ro antibodies has made it difficult to study. However, the demonstration of Ro on the surface of keratinocytes irradiated with ultraviolet light (LeFeber *et al.* 1984) shows that, like La, Ro antigen is capable of translocation to the cell membrane.

All these findings suggest that the disease starts with a persistent virus infection of salivary epithelium which, mediated by interferon-γ, induces Class II MHC together with the expression of viral and host antigens such as Ro and La. The cellular response, predominantly of the CD4 phenotype and unchecked by the deficient suppressor cells, leads to an immune attack on salivary epithelium and the production of anti-Ro and anti-La antibodies (Fig. 59.4(a)). A second mechanism, polyclonal activation, either as a direct result of virus infection or secondary to lymphokine production, could then lead to the expansion of CD5+ve B cells and the secretion of RFs and other autoantibodies (Fig. 59.4(b)). Both mechanisms would then result in the formation of immune complexes, which in turn lead to the extraglandular features of the disease.

References

Alexander, E.L., Malinow, K., Lijewski, J.E., Jerdan, M.S., Provost, T.T. and Alexander, G.E. (1986). Primary Sjögren's syndrome with central nervous system dysfunction mimicking multiple sclerosis. *Ann. Intern. Med.* **104**, 323–30.

Alspaugh, M.A., Talal, N. and Tan, E.M. (1976). Differentiation and characterization of autoantibodies and their antigens in Sjögren's syndrome. *Arthritis Rheum.* **19**, 216–22.

Alspaugh, M.A., Jensen, F.C., Rabin, H. and Tan, E.M. (1979). Lymphocytes transformed by EB virus: induction of nuclear antigen reactive with antibody in rheumatoid arthritis. *J. Exp. Med.* **147**, 1018–27.

Arnett, F.C., Bias, W.B. and Reveilli, J.D. (1989). Genetic studies in Sjögren's syndrome and systemic lupus erythematosus. *J. Autoimmunity* **2**, 403–13.

Baboonian, C., Venables, P.J.W., Booth, J., Williams, D.W., Roffe, L. and Maini, R.N. (1989). Virus infection induces redistribution and membrane localisation of the nuclear antigen La (SS-B): a possible mechanism for autoimmunity. *Clin. Exp. Immunol.* **78**, 454–9.

Baboonian, C., Venables, P.J.W., Kangro, H.O. and Maini, R.N. (1990). Antibodies to human herpes virus-6 in Sjögren's syndrome. *Arthritis Rheum.* **33**, 1749–50.

Biberfeld, P., Petren, A.L., Eklund, A. *et al.* (1988). Human herpes virus-6 (HHV-6) in sarcoidosis and lymphoproliferative disorders. *J. Virol. Methods* **21**, 49–59.

Bloch, K.H., Buchanan, W.W., Wohl, M.J. and Bunim, J.J. (1965). Sjögren's syndrome: a clinical, pathological and serological study of sixty-two cases. *Medicine (Baltimore)* **44**, 187–231.

Botazzo, G.F., Pujol-Borrel, R., Hanafusa, T. and Feldmann, M. (1983). Role of aberrant HLA expression in the induction of endocrine autoimmunity. *Lancet* **ii**, 1115–18.

Brennan, F., Plater-Zyberk, C., Maini, R.N. and Feldmann, M. (1989). Coordinate expansion of fetal type lymphocytes (TCR $\gamma\delta$+ and CD5+B) in rheumatoid arthritis and primary Sjögren's syndrome. *Clin. Exp. Immunol.* **77**, 175–8.

Buyon, J.P., Ben-Chetrit, E., Karp, S. *et al.* (1989). Acquired congenital heart block: pattern of maternal antibody response to biochemically defined antigens of the SS-A/Ro–SS-B/La system in neonatal lupus. *J. Clin. Invest.* **84**, 627–34.

Clark, G., Reichlin, M. and Tomasi, J.R. (1969). Characterisation of a soluble cytoplasmic antigen reactive with sera from patients with systemic lupus erythematosus. *J. Immunol.* **102**, 117–22.

Daniels, T.E., Silverman, S., Michalski, J.P., Greenspan, J.S., Sylvester, R.A. and Talal, N. (1975). The oral component of Sjögren's syndrome. *Oral Surg.* **39**, 875–85.

De Berardinis, P., Londei, M., James, R.F.L., Lake, S.P., Wise, P.H. and Feldmann, M. (1989). Do CD4-positive cytotoxic T cells damage islet β cells in type 1 diabetes? *Lancet* **ii**, 823–4.

Elkon, K.B., Ghavari, A.E., Patel, B.M., Hughes, G.R.V. and Frankel, A. (1983). IgA and IgM rheumatoid factors in serum, saliva and other secretions: relationship to immunoglobulin ratios in systemic sicca syndrome and rheumatoid arthritis. *Clin. Exp. Immunol.* **52**, 75–81.

Feltcamp, T.E.W. and Rossum, A.L. (1968). Antibodies to salivary duct cells and other autoantibodies in patients with Sjögren's syndrome and other idiopathic autoimmune diseases. *Clin. Exp. Immunol.* **3**, 1–16.

Fox, R.I., Carstens, S.A., Robinson, S.A., Howel, F. and Vaughan, J.H. (1982). Use of monoclonal antibodies to analyse peripheral blood and salivary gland subsets in Sjögren's syndrome. *Arthritis Rheum.* **25**, 419–26.

Fox, R.I., Howel, F.V., Bone, R.C. and Michelson, P. (1984). Primary Sjögren's syndrome: clinical and immunopathologic features. *Semin. Arthritis Rheum.* **14**, 77–105.

Fox, R.I., Theofilopoulos, A.N. and Altman, A. (1985). Production of interleukin 2 by salivary gland lymphocytes in Sjögren's syndrome: detection of reactive cells by using antibody directed to synthetic peptides of interleukin 2. *J. Immunol.* **135**, 3109–15.

Fox, R.I., Robinson, C., Kozin, F. and Howell, F.V. (1986a). Sjögren's syndrome: proposed criteria for classification. *Arthritis Rheum.* **29**, 577–86.

Fox, R.I., Bumol, T., Fantozzi, R., Bone, R. and Schreiber, R. (1986b). Expression of histocompatibility antigen HLA-DR by salivary gland epithelial cells in Sjögren's syndrome. *Arthritis Rheum.* **29**, 1105–11.

Fox, R.I., Pearson, G. and Vaughan, J.H. (1986c). Detection of Epstein–Barr virus associated antigens and DNA in salivary gland biopsies from patients with Sjögren's syndrome. *J. Immunol.* **137**, 3162–8.

Green, J.E., Hinrichs, S.H., Vogel, J. and Jay, G. (1989). Exocrinopathy resembling Sjögren's syndrome in transgenic mice. *Nature* **341**, 72–4.

Greenspan, J.S., Daniels, T.E., Talal, N. and Sylvester, R.A. (1974). The histopathology of Sjögren's syndrome in labial gland biopsies. *Oral Surg.* **27**, 217–29.

Harley, J.B., Reichlin, M., Arnett, F.C., Alexander, E.L., Bias, W.B. and Provost, T.T. (1986). Gene interaction at HLA-DQ enhances antoantibody production in primary Sjögren's syndrome. *Science* **232**, 1145–7.

Horsfall, A.C., Venables, P.J.W., Allard, S.A. and Maini, R.N. (1988). Coexistent anti-La antibodies and rheumatoid factors bear distinct idiotypic markers. *Scand. J. Rheumatol.* **75**, (suppl.) 84–8.

Horsfall, A.C., Rose, L.M. and Maini, R.N. (1989). Autoantibody synthesis in salivary glands of Sjögren's syndrome patients. *J. Autoimmunity* **2**, 559–68.

Itescu, S., Brancato, L., Dalton, J., Perdue, R. and Winchester, R. (1989). Phenotypic analysis of lymphocyte subsets in the diffuse infiltrative lymphocytosis syndrome associated with HIV infection. *Arthritis Rheum.* **32**, S86.

Jacobsson, L.T.H., Axel, T.E., Hansen, B.U. *et al.* (1989). Dry eyes or mouth — an epidemiological study in Swedish adults, with special reference to primary Sjögren's syndrome. *J. Autoimmunity* **2**, 521–7.

LeFeber, W.P., Norris, D.A., Ryan, S.R. *et al.* (1984). Ultraviolet light induces binding of antibodies to selected nuclear antigens on cultured human keratinocytes. *J. Clin. Invest.* **74**, 1545–51.

Leroy, J.P., Pennec, Y.L., Jouquan, J., Lelong, A. and Youinou, P. (1989). Relations of the histopathology of sublingual and labial salivary glands to the clinical presentation in primary Sjögren's syndrome. *Clin. Exp. Rheumatol.* **7**, 171–4.

Lindahl, G., Hedfors, E., Klareskog, L. and Forsum, U. (1985). Epithelial HLA-DR expression and T lymphocyte subsets in salivary glands in Sjögren's syndrome. *Clin. Exp. Immunol.* **61**, 475–82.

Lindhal, G., Lonnquist, B. and Hedfors, E. (1989). Lymphocytic infiltrations of lip salivary glands in bone marrow recipients: a model for the development of the histopathology changes in Sjögren's syndrome? *J. Autoimmunity* **2**, 579–83.

Luso, P., Ensoli, B., Markham, P.D. *et al.* (1989). Productive dual infection of human CD4+ T lymphocytes by HIV-1 and HHv6. *Nature* **337**, 370–3.

Maini, R.N. (1987). The relationship of Sjögren's syndrome to rheumatoid arthritis. In *Sjögren's Syndrome: Clinical and Immunological Aspects*, ed. N. Talal, H.M. Moutsopoulos and S.S. Kassan, pp. 15–24, Springer-Verlag, Berlin.

Manthorpe, R., Frost-Larsen, K., Isager, H. and Prause, J.U. (1981). Sjögren's syndrome: a review with emphasis on immunological features. *Allergy* **36**, 139–53.

Mathews, M.B. and Bernstein, R.M. (1983). Myositis antibody inhibits histidyl-T-RNA synthetase: a model for autoimmunity. *Nature* **304**, 177–9.

Miyasaka, N., Sauvezie, B., Pierce, D.A., Daniels, T.E. and Talal, N. (1980). Decreased mixed lymphocyte reaction in Sjögren's syndrome. *J. Clin. Invest.* **66**, 928–33.

Morrow, J. and Isenberg, D. (1987). Sjögren's syndrome. In *Autoimmune Rheumatic Diseases*, ed. J. Morrow and D. Isenberg, Blackwell Scientific Publications, Oxford.

Moutsopoulos, H.M. and Fauci, A.S. (1980). Immunoregulation in Sjögren's syndrome: influence of serum factors on T cell populations. *J. Clin. Invest.* **65**, 519–28.

Moutsopoulos, H.M., Klippel, J.H., Pavilidis, N., Steinberg, A.D., Chu, F.C. and Tarpley, T.M. (1980). Correlative histologic and serologic abnormalities of sicca syndrome in systemic lupus erythematosis. *Arthritis Rheum.* **23**, 36–40.

Moutsopoulos, H.M., Steinberg, A.D., Fauci, A.S., Lane, H.C. and Papadopoulos, N.M. (1983). High incidence of monoclonal lambda light chains in the sera of patients with Sjögren's syndrome. *J. Immunol.* **130**, 2663–5.

Papasteriades, C., Skopouli, F.N., Drosos, A.A., Andronopoulos, A.P. and Moutsopoulos, H.M. (1988). HLA alloantigen associations in Greek patients with Sjögren's syndrome. *J. Autoimmunity* **1**, 85–90.

Pease, C.T., Shattles, W., Charles, P.J., Venables, P.J.W. and Maini, R.N. (1989). Clinical, serological and HLA phenotype subsets in Sjögren's syndrome. *Clin. Exp. Rheumatol.* **7**, 185–90.

Plater-Zyberk, C., Maini, R.N., Lam, K., Kennedy, T.D. and Janossy, G. (1985). A rheumatoid arthritis B cell subset expresses a phenotype similar to that in chronic lymphatic leukemia. *Arthritis Rheum.* **28**, 971–6.

Plotz, P.H. (1983). Autoantibodies are anti-idiotypes to antiviral antibodies. *Lancet* **ii**, 824–6.

Rader, M.D., Codding, C. and Reichlin, M. (1989). Differences in the fine specifity of anti-Ro (SS-A) in relation to the presence of other precipitating autoantibodies. *Arthritis Rheum.* **32**, 1563–71.

Reichlin, M. and Mattioli, M. (1974). Antigens and antibodies characteristic of systemic lupus erythematosus. *Bull. Rheum. Dis.* **24**, 756–60.

St Clair, E.W., Talal, N., Moutsopoulos, H.M. *et al.* (1989). Epitope specificity of anti-La antibodies from patients with Sjögren's syndrome. *J. Autoimmunity* **2**, (suppl.) 335–44.

Shillitoe, E.J., Daniels, T.E., Whitcher, J.P., Strand, C.V., Talal, N. and Greenspan, J.S. (1982). Antibody of cytomegalovirus in patients with Sjögren's syndrome as detected by enzyme-linked immunosorbent assay. *Arthritis Rheum.* **25**, 260–5.

Sjögren, H. (1933). Zur Kenntnis der Keratoconiunctivitis sicca (Keratitis filiformis bei Hypunfuntion der Tränendrusen). *Acta Ophthalmol* **11**, 1–15.

Talal, N. (1989). Introduction. *J. Autoimmunity*, 309–10.

Tan, E.M. (1982). Autoantibodies to nuclear antigens (ANA): their immunobiology and medicine. *Adv. Immunol.* **33**, 167–240.

Tzioufas, A.G., Moutsopoulos, H.M. and Talal, N. (1987). Lymphoid malignancy and monoclonal proteins. In *Sjögren's Syndrome: Clinical and Immunological Aspects*, ed. N. Talal, H.M. Moutsopoulos and S.S. Kassan, pp. 15–24, Springer-Verlag, Berlin.

Venables, P.J.W. (1988). Sjögren's syndrome: differential diagnosis, immunopathology and genetics. *Rep. Rheum. Dis.* series 2, no. 10.

Venables, P.J.W. (in press). Sjögren's syndrome and overlap syndromes. In *Oxford Textbook of Nephrology*, ed. S. Cameron.

Venables, P.J.W., Ross, M.G.R., Charles, P.J., Melsom, R.D., Griffiths, P.D. and Maini, R.N. (1985). A seroepidemiological study of cytomegalovirus and Epstein–Barr virus in rheumatoid arthritis and sicca syndrome. *Ann. Rheum. Dis.* **44**, 742–6.

Venables, P.J.W., Rigby, S. and Mumford, P.A. (1988a). Autoimmunity to La (SS-B) *in vitro* is related to HLA DR3 in healthy subjects. *Ann. Rheum. Dis.* **47**, 22–7.

Venables, P.J.W., Pawlowski, T., Mumford, P.A., Brown, C., Crawford, D.H. and Maini, R.N. (1988b). Reaction of antibodies to rheumatoid arthritis nuclear antigen with a synthetic peptide corresponding to part of Epstein–Barr nuclear antigen 1. *Ann. Rheum. Dis.* **47**, 270–9.

Venables, P.J.W., Baboonian, C. and Maini, R.N. (1989a). Normal serological response to Epstein–Barr virus in Sjögren's syndrome. *Arthritis Rheum.* **32**, 811.

Venables, P.J.W., Teo, C.G., Baboonian, C., Hughes, R.A., Griffin, B.E. and Maini, R.N. (1989). Persistence of EBV in salivary gland biopsies from patients with Sjögren's syndrome and healthy controls. *Clin. Exp. Immunol.* **75**, 359–64.

Webster, A., Lee, C.A., Cook, D.G. *et al.* (1989). Cytomegalovirus infection and progression towards AIDS in haemophiliacs with human immunodeficiency virus infection. *Lancet* **ii**, 63–6.

Whittingham, S., McNeilage, J. and McKay, I.R. (1985). Primary Sjögren's syndrome after infectious mononucleosis. *Ann. Intern. Med.* **102**, 490–7.

Yamaoka, K., Miyasaka, N. and Yamamoto, K. (1988). Possible involvement of Epstein–Barr virus in polyclonal activation in Sjögren's syndrome. *Arthritis Rheum.* **31**, 1014–21.

Youinou, P. and Pennec, Y. (1987). Immunological features of primary Sjögren's syndrome. *Clin. Exp. Rheumatol.* **5**, 173–84.

60: Rheumatoid Arthritis

G.J. Silverman and D.A. Carson

Introduction

The pathogenesis of rheumatoid arthritis (RA) has remained an enigma, despite decades of intensive investigation. It is a common disorder, and in the United States most surveys estimate that between 1 and 2% of the population are affected, with a similar prevalence throughout the world (Mitchell 1985). While RA initially affects the joints, it may progress to vasculitis and involve many organs of the body, with potential to cause life-threatening complications. The clinical course is therefore highly variable. Most rheumatologists agree that there are distinct subsets of RA patients. Different clinical presentations and demographic profiles are associated with features prognostic for extent and severity of disease (Halla *et al.* 1987).

Most studies of RA have used the clinical criteria of the American Rheumatism Association (ARA) (Ropes 1959; Arnett *et al.* 1988). However, the polyarticular process occurring in patients with 'definite' or 'classic' RA (by ARA criteria) may be different from that in patients with less extensive or more recent-onset disease. Studies of the most severely affected patients have yielded insight into the pathophysiology of longstanding RA; however, the earliest events in the disease remain largely unknown. At present, it appears likely that the initiation and perpetuation of synovitis occur by separate mechanisms.

Immunogenetics and susceptibility to rheumatoid arthritis

The first-degree relatives of patients with RA

are at an increased risk of developing disease (Lawrence 1970). Familial concordance is strongest when disease onset is at an early age (Wasmuth *et al.* 1972). Studies of twins provide the best evidence of a genetic contribution to RA susceptibility. In a review of published clinical series, Lawrence (1970) found a concordance of disease expression in 23% of monozygotic twins and in 5% of dizygotic twins, with the strongest association in patients seropositive for rheumatoid factor (RF). In a more recent Finnish study, a comparable pattern of concordance was also reported (Aho *et al.* 1986).

Multiple genetic factors have been analysed for disease association. The first evidence of a specific genetic linkage was reported by Astorga and Williams (1969), who reported that the peripheral blood lymphocytes from unrelated patients with RA were frequently mutually non-stimulatory in mixed lymphocyte cultures. Stastny (1976) subsequently revealed the basis of this finding when he reported that Caucasians with seropositive RA have an increased frequency of expression of the cell surface human leucocyte antigen (HLA), DR4. Studies of multi-index families have since corroborated a strong association of this HLA haplotype with RA (Grennan *et al.* 1983; del Jungo *et al.* 1984; Walker *et al.* 1987). As determined by serotyping of B cell alloantigens, DR4 is expressed by 70% of seropositive RA patients in northern European populations, compared with 30% of controls (Stastny 1978). It has been suggested that an individual that is heterozygous for DR4 has greater than an eightfold relative risk for developing RA, while DR4 homozygotes have a 36-fold risk factor (Legrand *et al.* 1984; Nepom *et al.* 1984).

As HLA expression has been shown to vary in different populations, studies have been performed to establish whether all ethnic groups have the same RA susceptibility determinants. While the DR4 haplotype is generally less common in American blacks and Mexicans, this haplotype still carries an increased relative risk for seropositive RA in these groups (Karr *et al.* 1980; Stastny 1980; Ueno *et al.* 1981; Alarif *et al.* 1983). Japanese patients also display a strong association of DR4 with disease susceptibility (Nakai *et al.* 1981; Ueno *et al.* 1981; Ohta *et al.* 1982). However, while the DR4/Dw4 and Dw14 alleles are common in Caucasians with RA, the Dw15 allele of DR4 is most common amongst Japanese (Stastny 1978). In contrast, analyses of Asian Indians with RA and of Israeli Jews revealed an increased occurrence of HLA-DR1 (Stastny 1980; Woodrow *et al.* 1981; Schiff *et al.* 1982). Therefore, there is obvious HLA allelic variation between RA groups of different ethnic backgrounds.

It should be mentioned that almost every report of a DR4 linkage with RA patients has come from a tertiary care centre, while a community-based study by De Jongh *et al.* (1986) failed to find any unique DR association. Hospital-based studies may be biased towards more severely affected patients, and these patients may be representative of the RA subset that is predominantly associated with the DR4 haplotype. In support of this notion, DR4 has been reported to be more prevalent in definite and classic RA than in possible and probable RA (by ARA criteria) (Brackeretz and Wernet 1980). Further, patients expressing DR4 generally have a worse prognosis (Jaraquemada *et al.* 1979), and they may develop disease at an earlier age (Legrand *et al.* 1984). Extra-articular manifestations such as vasculitis and Felty's syndrome also seem to occur more often in these patients (Dinant *et al.* 1980; Scott *et al.* 1981; Klouda *et al.* 1986). In fact, many patients with the most severe disease are DR4 homozygotes (Brackeretz and Wernet 1980; Klouda *et al.* 1986). Similar trends have also been reported in juvenile-onset rheumatoid arthritis. The Nepom group (1984) have identified a near-identical DR4 occurrence in a paediatric subpopulation with severe seropositive polyarthritis.

The pathological mechanism by which DR4 expression predisposes to RA is unclear. DR4 was reported in one study to be a genetic marker for individuals with increased cellular reactivity to type II collagen (Solinger and Stobo 1981; Solinger *et al.* 1981). Although the results have never been confirmed, *in vitro* studies have shown RA patients to have increased T cell reactivity to collagen, and anti-collagen antibodies in serum and synovial fluid (Klareskog *et al.* 1982b). Several studies have examined whether inheritance of the DR4 haplotype is linked to increased RF production. From their own work and a review of the literature, Gran and Husby concluded that the severe erosive disease associated with HLA-DR4 occurs in both seronegative and seropositive patients (Gran *et al.* 1984). Similarly, several studies of *in vitro* B cell stimulation found that RF production was independent of HLA status (Alarcon *et al.* 1982a;

Rodriguez *et al.* 1983). In contrast, Olsen *et al.* (1987) reported that, if suppressor T cells are removed, even normal DR4 +ve individuals have an increased *in vitro* capacity for mitogen-induced immunoglobulin M (IgM) RF production. However, this finding is apparently unrelated to spontaneous *in vivo* RF production, as women with circulating RF without disease do not have increased occurrence of the DR4 haplotype (Engleman *et al.* 1978).

The association between seronegative RA and HLA-DR4 is controversial (Gran and Husby 1987; Masi 1988). While one Austrian study found an equivalent DR4 frequency in seropositive and seronegative patients (Scherak *et al.* 1980), most studies have found that seronegative patients have the same DR4 occurrence as normal controls (Panayi and Wooley 1977; Gibofsky *et al.* 1978; Stastny 1980; Alarcon *et al.* 1982b). Others have reported that seronegative patients have an increased occurrence of DR1 (Swiss Federal Commission 1981; Bardin *et al.* 1985). Separate genetic factors have also been suggested to predispose to seronegative disease (Rossen *et al.* 1980). Definite conclusions are difficult, as uniform criteria for seropositivity and seronegativity have not been utilized (Gran and Husby 1987). Available data suggest that RF seropositive and seronegative patients represent two separate types of chronic symmetric polyarthritis that may be influenced by different genetic factors and possibly different mechanisms of aetiopathogenesis (Alarcon *et al.* 1982b).

Molecular biology of the major histocompatibility complex gene locus

An understanding of the molecular biology of HLA expression has provided a basis for speculation on the pathogenesis of RA (Nepom *et al.* 1987). The HLA-DR glycoproteins associated with RA susceptibility were originally shown to influence 'immune activation', and therefore these proteins are also referred to as Ia antigens. In humans, the cell surface proteins are encoded by the Class II genes of the major histocompatibility complex (MHC) locus. This locus has at least 14 different genes on the sixth chromosome, most of which are found in three major subregions, designated DP, DQ and DR. The DR region has one functional α gene and two functional β (β1 and β3) genes. The protein products of an α and β gene can non-covalently associate to form heterodimers that are expressed on the surface of the cell. In general, the β genes are the most polymorphic, and they are primarily responsible for the allelic diversity in different populations.

Electrophoretic analysis of DR4 molecules has characterized six distinct allelic variants (Nepom *et al.* 1983). By use of oligonucleotide probes of restriction enzyme-digested deoxyribonucleic acid (DNA) fragments, DR4 polymorphism (together with disease susceptibility) has been linked to the β1 chain (Nepom *et al.* 1983, 1987; McDaniel *et al.* 1987). Only the Dw4, Dw14 and Dw15 alleles are associated with RA, while Dw10 and Dw13 are not (Panayi *et al.* 1978; Stastny 1978; Nepom *et al.* 1984, 1987). Following the isolation and cloning of the various β1 alleles by Cairns *et al.* (1985) and Gregersen *et al.* (1986), sequence analysis demonstrated that disease predisposition is tied to variation in amino acid positions 69–74 in the third hypervariable region (Gregersen *et al.* 1987) (Fig. 60.1). Allelic diversity is postulated to have occurred due to a series of mutational and gene conversion events (Fig. 60.2).

Certain DR1 and DR4 alleles have been shown to share antigenic determinants. A possible structural basis for such a shared epitope was suggested when it was demonstrated that the DR1 β1 chain allele has a sequence in the third hypervariable region identical to that of the DR4/DRw4 and DR4/DRw14 alleles (Bell *et al.* 1985; Gregersen *et al.* 1987) (see Table 60.1). This homology is of particular relevance, since the third hypervariable region of the β chain is a site involved in the recognition of Class II MHC molecules by T cell receptors (Braunstein and Germain 1987; Ronchese *et al.* 1987).

Human leucocyte antigen testing showed that over 93% of seropositive RA patients at tertiary referral centres express either the DR1 or the DR4 β-chain alleles (McDermott and McDevitt 1989). This suggests why there is allelic diversity of HLA-DR expression in different seropositive RA groups. It is apparent that each RA-associated DR haplotype occurs in an RA disease population in proportion to its frequency in that ethnic group, i.e. DR4/Dw4 and Dw14 alleles are common in Caucasians (Zoschke and Segall 1986), the DR1 allele in Israelis and Ashkenazı Jews (Schiff *et al.* 1982) and DR4/Dw15 in Japanese (Maeda *et al.*

Table 60.1. Light chain amino acid sequence comparison of Humkv325 and kv325-encoded human autoantibodies, including Vk gene-encoded and Jk-encoded regions

Humkv325		CRI				CDR1		
		PSL2	PSL3	1 E I V L T Q S P G T	L S L S P G E R A T	24 30A L S C R A S Q S V S	34 S S Y L A W Y Q Q K	P C Q A P R L L I Y
RFs								
1–4	CUR, FLO, GAR, GLO							
5	GOT	++	++	----------	----------	---------R	----------	----------
6	PAY	++	++	----------	----------	----------	---------R	----------
7	BOR	++	+	----------	----------	----------	----------	----------
8	SIE	++	++	----------	----------	----------	N---------	----------
9	NEU	++	+	----------	----------	----------	-R--------	----------
10	WOL	++	−	----------	----------	----------	-G--G-----	----------
11	KAS	+	++	D---------	----------	--------L-	-T--------	----------
12	GOL	++	++	----------	----------	------ALLS-	RG--------	---------M-
Cold agglutinins								
1	AJ	++	−	---------D-	----------	----------	end of the published sequence	
2	DRE	nd		----------	----------	----------	------end	
3	GJ	nd		----------	---------V-	------end		
4	MA	nd		----------	----------	----------	end	
5	NIC	nd		----------	----------	----------	end	
6	PER	nd		-----Z----	------Z---	------Zend		
7	STE	nd		----------	----------A	--end		
8	TAK	nd		-----Z----	------Z-V-	----------	?----end	
Anti-low density lipoprotein antibody								
1	SON	++	++	----------	----------	----------	----------	----------
Anti-intermediate filament antibody								
1	PIE	++	++	----------	----------	----------	----------	----------
Germline Vk genes								
1	Humkv305			--------A-	----------	---G------	----------	--L-------
2	Humkv328			---M----A-	--V-------	----------	- N. -------	----------
3	Humkv3g			--------A-	----------	----------	. ---------	----------
4	Humkv3g''			--------A-	----------	-------G--	. ---------	----------
5	Humkv3h			---M----P-	--------V-	----------	----T-----	----------

			CDR2				CDR3		
			50 56			89	95	96	Jk
Humkv325			GASSRATGIP	DRFSGSGSGT	DFTLTISRLE	PEDFAVYYCQ	QYGSSP		
RFs						R1, Y2,	Y2,	L1	
1–4	CUR, FLO, GAR, GLO								
		Difference							
5	GOT	1	----------	----------	----------	----------	------	R	2
6	PAY	1	----------	----------	----------	----------	------	L	1
7	BOR	2	----------	----------	----------	----V-----	---N--	Q	1
8	SIE	2	----------	----------	----------	-D--------	------	Q	1
9	NEU	4	----------	---T------	-----V----	----------	---A--	C	2
10	WOL	4	----------	----------	----------	----------	----LG	R	1
11	KAS	5	--------V-	----------	----------	----------	------	F	4
12	GOL	7	----------	----------	----------	----------	------	R	1
Anti-low density lipoprotein antibody									
1	SON	1	----------	N---------	----------	----------	------	PY	4
Anti-intermediate filament antibody									
1	PIE	0	----------	----------	----------	----------	------	W	2
Germline Vk genes									
1	Humkv305		D---------	----------	----------	----------	------		
2	Humkv328		---T------	A---------	E------S-Q	S---------	--MNW-		
3	Humkv3g		D--N------	A---------	-------S--	----------	-RSNW-		
4	Humkv3g''		D--N------	A------P--	-------S--	----------	-RSNWH		
5	Humkv3h		---T---S--	A---------	-------S-Q	----------	-DHNL-		

Amino acid differences from Humkv325 are given for the first 95 residues. The PSL2 and PSL3 cross-reactive idiotype (CRI) represents reactivities of antipeptide antisera to portions of the second and third hypervariable regions of a Humkv325-encoded light chain, respectively. Residues identical to Humkv325 are indicated by dashes and gaps by dots. One-letter amino acid code Z represents either glutamine or glutamic acid residue. Taken from Edman and Cooper (1968), Gergely *et al.* (1970), Andrews and Capra (1981), Pons-Estel *et al.* (1984), Goni *et al.* (1985), Radoux *et al.* (1986) and Chen *et al.* (1987a).

Class II Allele	Beta 1 Chain Amino Acid Sequence			
	65	70 74	80	
HLA DR1	K D L L E	Q R R A A	V D T Y C R	RA associated haplotypes
HLA Dw4	K D L L E	Q K R A A	V D T Y C R	
HLA Dw14	K D L L E	Q R R A A	V D T Y C R	
HLA Dw15	K D L L E	Q R R A A	V D T Y C R	
HLA Dw13	K D L L E	Q R R A E	V D T Y C R	no RA association
HLA Dw10	K D I L E	D E R A A	V D T Y C R	

Fig. 60.1. The rheumatoid arthritis (RA) susceptibility determinant QKRAA/QRRAA is present on the third hypervariable region of the DR β1 chain in the HLA-Dw4 and HLA-Dw14, HLA-Dw15 and HLA-DR1 haplotypes, but not in the HLA-Dw13 and HLA-Dw10 haplotypes. The lysine (K) to arginine (R) substitution represents a conservative change. Taken from Roudier *et al.* (1989).

1981; Ohta *et al.* 1982; Gregersen *et al.* 1987).

Alternative hypotheses of RA predisposition have also been explored. Winchester and co-workers have suggested that RA predisposition in Caucasian and Mexican populations is most accurately defined by the 109d6 monoclonal antibody (Lee *et al.* 1984). Recent studies have correlated this antibody reactivity with the β1 and β2 alleles in the DRw10 and DRw53 allospecificities, respectively. By transfection experiments this epitope has been linked to a portion of the third hypervariable region (Merryman *et al.* 1988).

In another study, RA was found to be linked to the co-expression of a certain DQ allele in association with DR4 in a 'superhaplotype' in four of five multi-index families (Wallin *et al.* 1988). Rheumatoid arthritis patients with Felty's syndrome have also been found to have an increased prevalence of both DR4 and a complement-null allele (Thomson *et al.* 1988). It has also been suggested that genetic predisposition to RA is conferred by a separate gene in linkage disequilibrium with DR4. In this regard, juvenile-onset RA patients commonly express the DQw3 haplotype in association with both DR4/Dw4 and DR4/Dw14 specificities. However, DQw3 also occurs with the DR4 alleles unassociated with arthritis (Duqesnoy *et al.* 1984; Nepom *et al.* 1987). Based on serological reactivity and restriction length polymorphism analysis, the DQw3.1 allele has been suggested as preferentially associated with RA and Felty's syndrome (Singal *et al.* 1987; So *et al.* 1988). In summary, recent advances have provided a better understanding of the genetic basis of seropositive RA. Genetic predisposition is determined by the presence of a specific sequence in the expressed HLA-DR β1 genes. It is possible, however, that other genes may also contribute to disease susceptibility.

Hypotheses concerning the molecular basis of rheumatoid arthritis susceptibility

Recent progress in understanding the interaction between Class II MHC antigens and T cell receptors has generated several new hypotheses on the

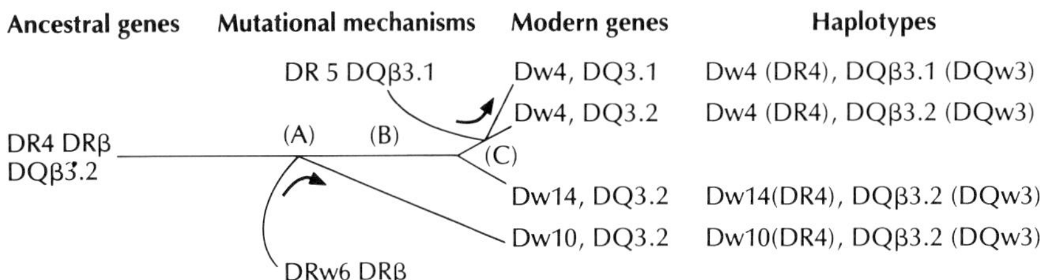

Fig. 60.2. A model for the development of DR4 +ve genes associated with RA. A postulated ancestral DR4 +ve haplotype undergoes a number of mutational events which lead to alterations of DR β gene or DQ β genes, resulting in the formation of distinct DR4 +ve haplotypes. (A) A postulated gene conversion event from a donor DRw6 sequence results in DR β changes which yield a Dw10 +ve gene, lacking the 'RA susceptibility' genetic information. (B) Less substantial mutational changes lead to a two-amino acid alteration in DR β, resulting in a Dw14 +ve gene, which retains its contribution to RA susceptibility. (C) Recombination with a DQ3.1 +ve haplotype (e.g. DR5 +ve) leads to the exchange of the DQ3.2 gene for DQ3.1, creating a new DR4 +ve haplotype but not altering the DR genes. This haplotype also retains its contribution to RA susceptibility. Taken from Nepom *et al.* (1987).

mechanisms of RA aetiopathogenesis. Class II proteins of the MHC locus have two known functions: they are important structures for interaction with T cell receptors, and they act as receptors for presentation of processed protein antigens to T cells (Babbitt *et al.* 1985; Guillet *et al.* 1987). The identification of the nucleotide and amino acid sequences in Class II MHC molecules associated with RA susceptibility suggests at least three potential disease initiation mechanisms:

1 Inheritance of a particular DR haplotype may influence thymic selection of T cell clones during development, such that clones with the potential for autoreactivity may arise at higher frequency (defect in clonal deletion).

2 The expression of specific DR molecules may allow the presentation of a foreign antigen that results in a cross-reactivity of certain T cells to a self antigen, causing an autoimmune inflammatory process.

3 Class II MHC molecules may themselves resemble an exogenous epitope. Exposure of an individual with this haplotype to the exogenous epitope may trigger T cells that cross-react with any cell bearing this Class II MHC molecule.

Human leucocyte antigen D allospecific T cell clones reactive with cells from patients with RA have been characterized by Goronzy, Fathman and their co-workers (Goronzy *et al.* 1986; Weyand and Goronzy 1987). By cross-blocking experiments they determined that cross-reactive determinants were shared by different DR β1 chains. These experiments support the hypothesis that certain DR1 and DR4 alleles are functionally similar in their interaction with T cells, and that these DR molecules may interact with the same T cell subsets.

Rheumatoid arthritis and the Epstein–Barr virus

As not all individuals with the relevant DR4/DR1 HLA haplotypes develop seropositive RA, a second genetic (Go *et al.* 1987) and/or environmental factor must also contribute to the development of overt disease. In a search for potential environmental factors, Roudier *et al.* (1989) reviewed computer data bases for proteins with sequences related to the disease-associated DR β1 molecule. Significantly, the HLA DR/Dw4 third hypervariable region sequence perfectly matches a six amino acid sequence, EQKRAA, in the Epstein–Barr virus (EBV) glycoprotein gp110 that is part of the viral capsid or envelope (Pellet *et al.* 1985; Gong *et al.* 1987) (Fig. 60.3). Computer analysis of this sequence predicts a secondary structure of an α helix — a motif common in peptides bound by Class II MHC molecules. Furthermore, high titres of antibodies to the gp110 protein are present in the circulation of most individuals with evidence of EBV exposure (Luka *et al.* 1984). Importantly, following clinical EBV infection T cells arise that are reactive with synthetic peptides with this sequence, while individuals without serological evidence of EBV exposure do not recognize these epitopes (Roudier *et al.* 1989). These data are consistent with the hypothesis that, in genetically predisposed individuals, EBV infection may occasionally initiate a T cell-mediated autoimmune reaction.

The EBV has many properties that make it a particularly attractive candidate for a role in triggering RA (Venables 1988). It is lymphotropic, as most B cells express the complement receptor, CR2, used as a receptor by this virus. The virus may persist indefinitely in a subset of infected B cells. It stimulates antigen-independent production of immunoglobulins, commonly referred to as polyclonal activation. As part of this process, many of the stimulated B cells produce antibodies directed against self antigens (including rheumatoid factors). As most adults have been infected with EBV, seropositive RA patients without evidence of EBV exposure are very rare. Significantly, RA patients have higher titres of antibodies to certain EBV-encoded proteins than do normal controls (Alspaugh *et al.* 1981; Rhodes *et al.* 1985). There is also extensive evidence that RA patients have an elevated frequency of EBV-infected cells, possibly due to a defect in control by T lymphocytes of virally infected B cells (Depper *et al.* 1981;

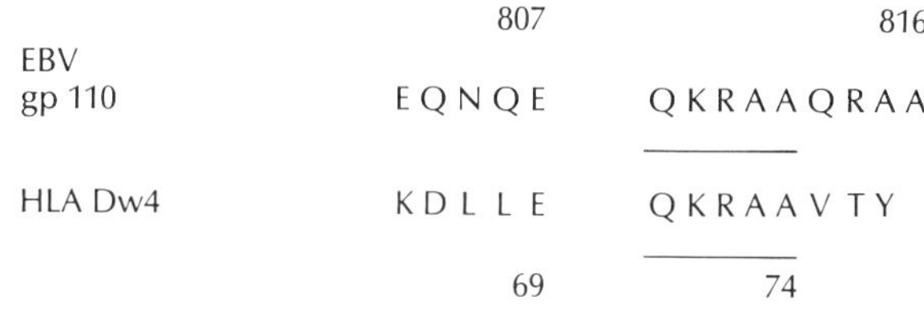

Fig. 60.3. The β1 chain of the HLA-DR4/Dw4 allele shares a five-amino acid sequence with an EBV capsular glycoprotein, gp110.

Hasler *et al.* 1983a, b; Tosato *et al.* 1984; Konttinen *et al.* 1986; Lotz *et al.* 1986a).

The observations of Roudier *et al.* (1989) are consistent with the pathogenic model described above, in which the disease-associated DR antigen itself is the target for cross-reactive T cells. According to this hypothesis, exposure to EBV may cause T cell sensitization to the gp110 protein. A cross-reactive state with the β1 chain would then occur in many individuals that express certain DR4/DR1 alleles. Thereafter, cells bearing these DR molecules would be the targets of an autoimmune response. Lymphocytes that identify the QKRAA self moiety would then elaborate cytokines and activate and enlist other lymphocyte and monocyte subsets into the inflammatory response. This process may then be the basis for a chronic process which histologically resembles an autologous mixed lymphocyte reaction.

In an alternative hypothesis, during ontogeny T cell clones that identify the DR4/DR1 sequence on self molecules may be deleted in the thymus. Subsequently, this epitope would not be recognized even in the context of the gp110 EBV envelope glycoprotein. Without the normal T cell control, infected cells would then proliferate. The gp110 protein and/or other viral products would be produced intermittently, resulting in antibody production and immune complex deposition in the joints and extravascular sites. However, to date neither infectious virus nor viral DNA has been detected in synovial tissues of patients with RA. Therefore, although both processes are plausible, there is currently inadequate evidence to support either theory.

Heat-shock protein and adjuvant arthritis

Adjuvant arthritis (AA) is an animal model of chronic synovitis induced by intradermal injection with an emulsion of killed *Mycobacterium tuberculosis* (Mtb) in mineral oil. In certain strains of rats, immunization causes a rheumatoid-like process with development of pannus, cellular infiltrates and erosions (Pearson and Wood 1959). The disease can be transmitted by T cell lines or clones that recognize a mycobacterial antigen, and that cross-react with a self antigen in joint cartilage (van Eden *et al.* 1985). The epitope recognized by the synovial fluid-derived T cells is on a ubiquitous 65 kD Mtb heat-shock protein that is produced during growth at high temperatures, or following cell injury (Res *et al.* 1988). Significantly, lymphocytes from patients with chronic arthritis have an increased proliferative response to an identical recombinant protein. Also, in each individual with arthritis, lymphocytes from synovial fluid are more reactive than those from peripheral blood. This reactivity has been demonstrated in patients with seropositive and seronegative RA, as well as in other forms of chronic arthritis.

The DR4 haplotype has been reported to confer immune responsiveness to certain Mtb antigens in RA patients and normal controls, but the response to this 65 kD heat-shock protein is not Class II MHC-restricted (Lamb *et al.* 1988; Palacios-Boix *et al.* 1988). The structure of heat-shock proteins has been highly conserved throughout evolution, and there is considerable homology between these proteins from prokaryotes and eukaryotes (Thole *et al.* 1988). Therefore, even if an autoreactive state can be triggered by this mechanism, Mtb may not necessarily be the initiating agent, and this pathogenesis may not be unique to RA.

Rheumatoid factor

Pathophysiology

Rheumatoid factors are antibodies that bind to the Fc portion of IgG. They are present in high concentration in the circulation of over 85% of patients with RA. Although initially thought to be unique to RA, they arise during a variety of infectious and inflammatory disorders, and are also prevalent in the aged (Carson *et al.* 1981).

Experimental studies have demonstrated that RF may be produced by at least two distinct mechanisms. *In vivo* RF may be generated from antigen-independent B lymphocyte stimulation (i.e. polyclonal activation). Alternatively, RFs may arise after antigen-driven, T cell-dependent immunization.

Coulie and van Snick (1985) delineated the cellular requirements in mice for RF synthesis during the secondary immune response to antigen–antibody complexes. Adoptive transfer studies showed that RF production required T cells reactive with the immunizing antigen. Immunoglobulin G aggregates, or irrelevant antigen–antibody complexes, did not induce RF production. The RF precursor B cells could originate from naïve or immunodeficient mice. In either case, the B cells produced RF mainly specific for the IgG subclass in the antigen–antibody complex (Coulie and Van Snick 1985). Taken together, these data imply that RF synthesis is apparently regulated by T cells specific for the antigens in the immune complexes (Fig. 60.4) (Nemazee 1985).

In humans, RF precursors are common in the circulation of normal individuals (Slaughter *et al.* 1978; Koopman and Schrohenloher 1980), and these cells increase in frequency several-fold after a booster immunization with tetanus toxoid (Welch *et al.* 1983). In fact, RF is the principal if not the sole autoantibody produced during anamnestic immune responses. If inhibitory influences are removed, *in vitro* production of RFs can be demonstrated from peripheral or bone marrow lymphocytes from most, if not all, people (Fong *et al.* 1985a). Rheumatoid factor B cell precursors are also present in umbilical cord blood, suggesting that RFs are part of the physiological B cell repertoire. For reasons that are still unknown, there is little affinity maturation or class switching of RFs during normal immune responses.

Preliminary data suggest that RF precursor cells are common in the marginal and mantle zones of spleen, sites active in antigen processing (Brown *et al.* 1973; MacLennan *et al.* 1982). Cells from these areas are believed to be important for the clearance and processing of circulating antigen–antibody complexes. Thus, RF precursor cells may play a critical role in normal physiology. Rheumatoid factor on the surface of B cells can bind immune complexes, leading to subsequent antigen processing and presentation to immune reactive T cells (Van Snick *et al.* 1978). Although originally considered as purely pathogenic, from these studies RFs are now appreciated to be 'natural' autoantibodies.

Rheumatoid factors in rheumatoid arthritis

In RA the presence of high concentrations of circulating RFs, especially early after the onset of articular symptoms, is a predictor of severe disease and poor outcome (Ohta *et al.* 1982). Patients with high titres of RFs more frequently develop joint erosions and extra-articular disease (Masi *et al.* 1976; Feigenbaum and Masi 1978; Alarcon *et al.* 1982b; Gran *et al.* 1984; Tuomi *et al.* 1988).

Synovial immune complexes (ICs) have been detected early in the rheumatoid process. These complexes have been extensively analysed, but the identity of the initiating antigen is unknown. Various antibodies, including those reactive with microbial antigen and cartilage collagen, have been detected in these ICs (Mottonen *et al.* 1988), but none has been proved to initiate synovitis. As synovial RFs have been detected only after the appearance of ICs, the production of these autoantibodies may represent a secondary event. However, since RFs may be 'hidden' within the ICs, this interpretation could be flawed (Aho *et al.* 1987). Generally, RFs are only detected in the peripheral circulation much later (Masi *et al.* 1976; Jones *et al.* 1982). During established disease the synovium is quite active in RF production, and 10% or more of synovial plasma cells produce RFs (Smiley *et al.* 1968; Munthe and Natvig 1972). Taken together, the data suggest that during the development of rheumatoid synovitis there is a preferential clonal expansion of RF B cell precursors in the synovium.

Synovial fluid assays and analyses of *in vitro* stimulated lymphocytes have suggested that

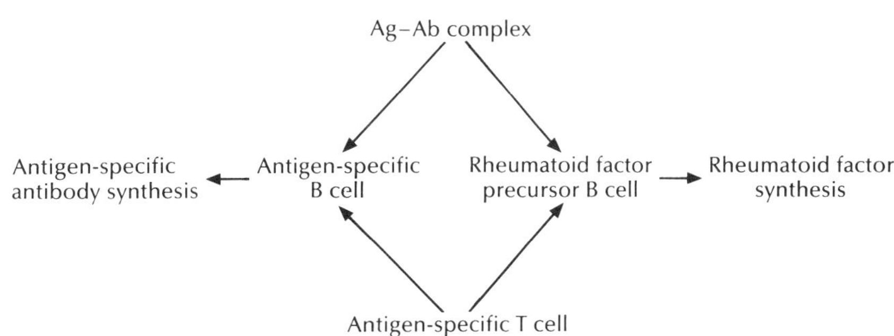

Fig. 60.4. Model for the induction of rheumatoid factor synthesis by antigen (Ag)–antibody (Ab) complexes. The Ag–Ab complexes bind to rheumatoid factor precursor B cells. Then, antigen in conjunction with surface membrane Class II MHC (Ia) antigens is presented to antigen-specific T cells. T cells sensitized to the antigen then trigger specific antibody and rheumatoid factor synthesis.

locally produced immunoglobulin and ICs are often enriched in the IgG-3 subclass (Munthe and Natvig 1972; Hoffman *et al*. 1982; Mellbye *et al*. 1984). In RA the synovial RFs bind IgG-3, but RFs in the peripheral circulation do not (Robbins and Wistar 1985). Speculatively, this finding is consistent with local antigenic stimulation of RF synthesis, and local deposition of IgG-3–RF ICs. The preferential reactivity of synovial RFs with the IgG-3 subclass is also of particular interest, since IgG-3 may be preferentially expressed in the immune response to certain viral infections (Sundquist *et al*. 1984).

The RFs in RA are characteristically polyclonal, and probably have higher affinity for IgG than monoclonal RF paraproteins. The polyclonal RFs are heterogeneous, and may bind to several distinct determinants in the Fc region (Natvig *et al*. 1972). A proportion of RFs from RA patients also bind IgG from different mammalian species (Butler and Vaughan 1965). This cross-reactive binding is, in fact, the basis of the classic Rose–Waaler test for RA, i.e. the agglutination by human serum of sheep red cells or latex beads sensitized with rabbit IgG.

Immunoglobulin M–RFs and IgG–RFs are a major component of circulating and synovial fluid ICs in RA patients. The autoantibodies also represent a significant proportion (10–20%) of synovial immunoglobulin production (Natvig and Munthe 1975). Immunoglobulin G–RFs have the unique ability to form intra- and extracellular IgG–IgG complexes (Pope *et al*. 1975). They have also been detected in low concentrations in the synovial fluid ICs of 'seronegative' juvenile rheumatoid arthritis (Bluestone *et al*. 1969; Arnett *et al*. 1988).

Both IgM– and IgG–RFs contribute to complement activation and inflammation within the joint (Winchester 1975; Brown *et al*. 1982). By immunofluorescent staining, cytoplasmic granules of phagocytic synoviocytes and neutrophils have been shown to contain RFs, immunoglobulins and various complement components (Hollander *et al*. 1965; Vaughan *et al*. 1968). The activated complement products, C3a and C5a, are potent anaphylatoxins that cause vasodilation and increased capillary permeability. C5a attracts neutrophils, eosinophils and monocytes, and stimulates the release of their lysosomal enzymes. These activated leucocytes have been observed invading the pannus–cartilage interface where proteolytic destruction of the matrix occurs. Monocyte production of interleukin 1 (IL-1) and tumour necrosis factor (TNF) may be augmented by C5a. Among its other effects, this cytokine promotes protease release and prostaglandin E_2 (PGE_2) synthesis. Although protease inhibitors are present in the synovial fluid (Hadler *et al*. 1981), it is likely that cartilage degradation by lysosomal enzymes nevertheless occurs at the sites of local release.

Rheumatoid factors are uncommon in diseases associated with transient arthritis. During many infections, including Lyme arthritis and early hepatitis B infection, there is synovial deposition of antigens and/or ICs, but the associated inflammation is only transient. However, in RA there is continued local antibody synthesis and IC deposition accompanied by mononuclear infiltration. Therefore, circumstantial evidence suggests that the interaction of RFs with synovial ICs contributes to the chronic synovitis of RA. After the initial trigger, class switch of RF precursors to high-affinity IgG RF autoantibodies appears to be an integral part of the process that perpetuates the synovial inflammation of RA.

Immunogenetics of rheumatoid factor

As discussed, although RFs are important in the pathophysiology of RA, they are also detectable in other diverse infectious and lymphoproliferative conditions (Silverman *et al*. 1987b; Fong *et al*. 1988). Monoclonal RFs from patients with essential mixed cryoglobulinaemia have been used to investigate the structural basis of RF activity. Kunkel first demonstrated that carefully adsorbed sera from rabbits immunized with certain monoclonal RFs selectively identified RFs from unrelated patients (Kunkel *et al*. 1973). The basis of this shared antigen reactivity, commonly referred to as a cross-reactive idiotype (CRI), was demonstrated when the heavy (H) and light (L) chain sequences from these RFs were compared. Members of the largest subset of these RFs, identified as the Wa CRI, were shown to use identical, or near-identical, L chains (Pons-Estel *et al*. 1984; Goni *et al*. 1985; reviewed in Chen *et al*. 1988). In our laboratory the variable (V) gene segment that encodes these L chains has been isolated and sequenced, and designated Humkv325. A comparison of the Wa L chains encoded by the Humkv325 gene demon-

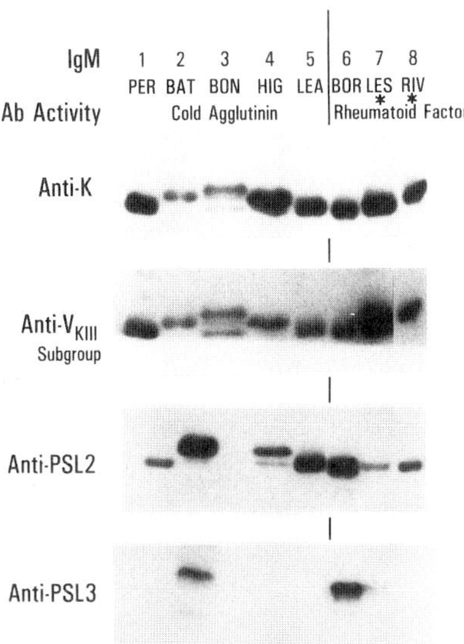

Fig. 60.5. Characterization of light chains from human monoclonal autoantibodies by Western immunoblotting. Proteins were alkylated and reduced, and light and heavy chains separated by polyacrylamide gel electrophoresis. After transfer to nitrocellulose and blocking of non-specific binding sites, replicate blots were treated with a series of antipeptide antisera. Anti-κ recognizes the sequence VFIFPPSDEQLKSGTASVVC in the first domain of the kappa constant region. Anti-κIII recognizes the sequence TLSLSPGERATLSC, in the first framework region of VκIII gene family-derived proteins (Silverman *et al*. 1986). The products of the Humkv325 genes are recognized by anti-PSL2 (YGASSRATGIPDR) and anti-PSL3 (CQQYGSSPETFG) that were taken from portions of the second and third hypervariable regions, respectively (Fong *et al*. 1985b). These five cold agglutinins all bind epitopes of the developmentally regulated carbohydrate I system. Most of the cold agglutinins are shown to derive from the Humkv325 gene. Taken from Silverman *et al*. (1988b).

strated that these L chains are expressed without somatic mutation in some RFs (Table 60.1).

Antibodies with specificities other than RF have been shown to also use L chains derived from the Humkv325 gene (Pons-Estel *et al*. 1984; Silverman *et al*. 1988b). In order to evaluate the structural diversity within H chains of these Humkv325-derived antibodies, antipeptide antibodies were generated that could distinguish variable regions from the three major H chain subgroups (Silverman *et al*. 1988a). In a panel of 30 RFs with Humkv325-derived L chains, 77% (22/30) used H chains of the V_HI gene family (Silverman *et al*. 1988b). Almost every one of these H chains was also identified by a monoclonal anti-idiotype, designated G6 (Silverman *et al*. 1988a). By sequence comparison, it is highly likely that these RF H chains are encoded by the germline V_H gene, termed 51P1 or 783, that is preferentially used during early ontogeny (Newkirk *et al*. 1987; Schroeder *et al*. 1987).

Autoantibodies to red cell epitopes (cold agglutinins) are as common as RFs amongst IgM paraproteins (Duggan and Schattner 1986). The majority of cold agglutinins reactive with the I carbohydrate epitope on red cells use L chains from the KIII family (Gergely *et al*. 1970; Capra *et al*. 1972; Feizi *et al*. 1976) (Fig. 60.5 and Table 60.1). In a panel of ten KIII cold agglutinins, sequence analysis and/or idiotypic markers showed that six were encoded by the kv325 gene (Silverman *et al*. 1988b). Serological evaluation with the H chain subgroup reagents suggested that all ten used V_H IV-derived heavy chains that probably derived from the V_H4.21 germline gene (Silverman *et al*. 1988b; Silberstein *et al*. 1991; unpublished observations) (Fig. 60.6). In contrast, three autoantibodies against low-density lipoprotein and one against cytomegalovirus that all had kv325-derived L chains, used V_HIII H chains (Newkirk *et al*. 1988; unpublished observations). The collected results suggest that the Humkv325 gene can be used in different antibodies, and that binding specificity in these antibodies is largely defined by the H chain partner. These studies of human H and L chains were the first to demonstrate a relationship between H chain V region and autoantibody specificity. The correlation of function with V_H usage has recently been found to be common amongst antibodies (Kabat and Wu 1991).

Amongst monoclonal RFs a second major subset has recently been defined. These RFs react with a monoclonal murine anti-idiotype, designated 6B6.6, which identifies structurally related KIIIa L chains (Crowley *et al*. 1988). Sequence comparisons have suggested that these L chains are highly homologous, and may all derive from the germline Humkv328 gene, or a nearly identical gene (Chen *et al*. 1987b). In contrast to the V_HI association of the KIIIB–Humkv325 RFs, this second set of autoantibodies display their own unique H–L chain pairing pattern. No KIIIa RF has been shown to use H chains bearing the G6 or V_H4 markers. Of nine KIIIa RFs characterized, seven use V_H4 subgroup H chains, and two use V_HIII-derived H chains. Further, six or seven V_HII subgroup

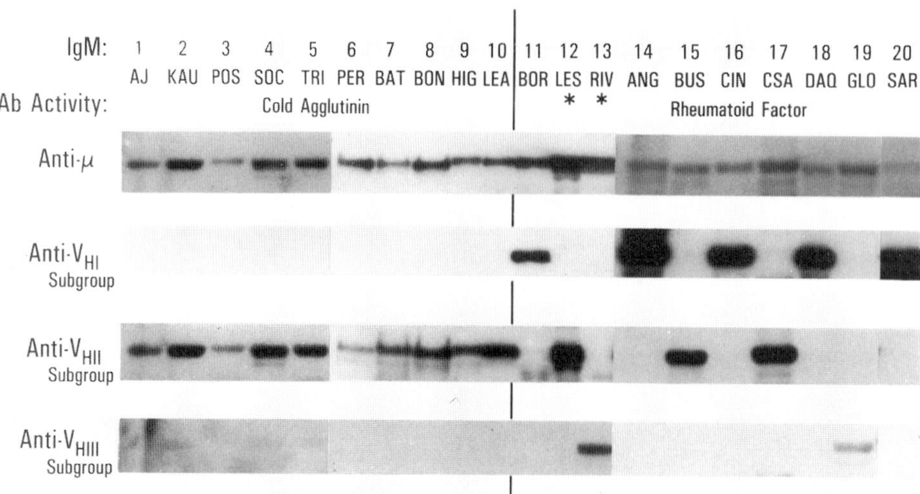

Fig. 60.6. Western blot analysis of the heavy chains of human monoclonal autoantibodies. Technique as described in Fig. 60.5. Here, the heavy chains of ten anti-I cold agglutinins, eight rheumatoid factors that use Humkv325-derived light chains and two other rheumatoid factors (Les and Riv) are displayed. The anti-μ reagent recognizes the sequence SASAPTLFPLVSC in the μ constant region. The anti-V_HI and anti-V_HIII subgroup antisera recognize heavy chain variable region first-framework sequences AEVKKPGASVKVSC and GGLVQPGGSLRLSC, respectively. The anti-V_HII subgroup sequence, PGLVKPSETLSLTC, was deduced from the first framework of the V_HIV gene, 71-2. Here, all of the anti-cold agglutinins are shown to use V_HII subgroup proteins, which derive from one V_HIV genes, V_H4.21 (Silberstein *et al.* 1991). The majority (5/8) of Humkv325-encoded rheumatoid factors use V_HI heavy chains. Taken from Silverman *et al.* (1988b).

RF H chains are identified by the LC1 antibody (Silverman *et al.* 1990). Immunoglobulins bearing the LC1 idiotype have been reported to be increased in the sera of RA patients (Ono *et al.* 1987). To date neither 6B6.6 nor LC1 reactivity has been detected in cold agglutinins, or in any non-RF antibody of known specificity. Therefore, the LC1 antibody identifies RFs that use a sub-subgroup of H chains, and these proteins probably all derive from a subset of the minor V_HIV family (or perhaps a single V_HIV gene) that is distinct from those used by anti-I cold agglutinins (unpublished observation). Certain V_HIV genes have extensive homology with members of the 36–60 murine gene family, which are preferentially expressed in the neonatal mouse repertoire (Riley *et al.* 1986).

The proteins bearing these RF-linked CRIs are prevalent within human monoclonal IgMs, probably due to the fact that these proteins arise with little or no somatic mutation during lymphoproliferative processes (Kipps *et al.* 1988). Many normal donors have low concentrations of immunoglobulins bearing these markers in their circulation, and their B cells can also be stimulated to produce idiotype +ve proteins (Bonagura *et al.* 1982; Silverman *et al.* 1987a). However, most of the immunoglobulins bearing these defined CRI markers lack autoantibody activity. This result is not surprising considering that RF activity requires specific H–L chain pairing.

Rheumatoid arthritis and cross-reactive idiotypes

As noted earlier, in RA the RFs are polyclonal and structurally diverse. Some plasma cells in rheumatoid synovium do elaborate RFs that express the same CRIs associated with monoclonal RFs (Bonagura *et al.* 1982). However, the RFs in the circulation of each RA patient have many 'private' idiotypes that are not found in the sera of other individuals (Nelson *et al.* 1987). In our laboratory we have found that RFs from the peripheral circulation of RA patients have multiple subpopulations expressing a variety of H- and L-chain CRIs (Fong *et al.* 1986). Collectively, these observations suggest that the RFs produced in RA are derived from many H- and L-chain V genes. This evidence is consistent with a model of RF induction in RA that is driven by antigenic selection that results in somatic diversification (Table 60.2). Prolonged immune stimulation may cause mutations that erase idiotypic markers of germline V gene origins,

Table 60.2. Comparison of two proposed types of (auto) antibodies

	Germline-encoded (part of the preimmune repertoire)	Somatically generated
Occurrence in IgM paraproteins and hybridomas	Common	Rare
Expression of cross-reactive idiotypes	Present	Absent
Occurrence in normal individuals	Common	Rare
Isotype	IgM	All isotypes
Affinity	Low	High
Specificity	Often polyspecific	Monospecific
Frequency of B cell precursors	High	Low
Clonality	Often mono- or oligoclonal	Polyclonal
Activity	May have physiological function	Antigen-specific
Examples of autoantibodies	Rheumatoid factors Cold agglutinins Anti-ssDNA Anti-myelin-associated glycoprotein	Anti-Sm Anti-RNP Anti-La Anti-Ro Anti-RNP Anti-Jo-1 Organ-specific antibodies

and/or B cells may be recruited that did not initially have RF activity.

Rheumatoid factors and CD5 B cells

B cells bearing the CD5 (Leu-1) marker have been described as a self-replenishing lymphocytic lineage (reviewed in Calvert *et al*. 1988). They represent about 20% of the circulating and splenic B cells, and contribute much of the IgM in the peripheral circulation (Casali *et al*. 1987; Hardy *et al*. 1987). These cells are present in rheumatoid synovial fluid, but they are not enriched compared with the peripheral circulation (Sowden *et al*. 1987). In a recent study, the percentage of total peripheral B cells that express the CD5 marker was concordant in identical twins and remained constant with time. This was true, whether or not the twins were concordant or discordant for RA (Kipps and Vaughan 1987). However, since expression of CD5 can be increased by treatment of B cells with phorbol esters (Miller and Gralow 1984), this marker may not accurately represent a specific B cell lineage. Even so, incubation with other polyclonal activators does not stimulate CD5 expression.

Epstein–Barr-virus-transformed cell lines from human CD5 B cells have been created that produce polyreactive, low-affinity antibodies. Many of these antibodies react with self determinants, including ssDNA, insulin, thyroglobulin and the Fc portion of IgG (Casali *et al*. 1987). More recently a subpopulation of these cells has been shown to produce monoreactive high-affinity RFs (Burastero *et al*. 1988). We have found that some RFs from CD5-derived cell lines have markers of the Humkv325 gene (unpublished observation). Although the physiological role of these cells is undefined, there is evidence that the CD5 B cell population may be expanded in certain RA patients (Plater-Zyberk *et al*. 1985; Hardy *et al*. 1987; Taniguchi *et al*. 1987; Burastero *et al*. 1988).

Structure of the synovium

Synovial histology

The normal diarthrodial joint is lined with a layer of synoviocytes that is one to three cells thick. No basement membrane separates these cells from the subsynovium. Structural and functional studies have distinguished three major cell types of synovial lining cells (Barland *et al.* 1962). The type A synoviocytes have macrophage function, and are replenished from monocytes in the blood (Barland *et al.* 1962; Dreher 1982). Characteristically, they have heterochromatic nuclei, multiple lysosomes, undeveloped rough endoplasmic reticulum and protruding filopodia. A larger proportion of synoviocytes have been termed type B, and they resemble fibroblasts with pale nuclei, well-developed Golgi apparatus and prominent rough endoplasmic reticulum. The remaining, type C, synoviocytes have intermediate properties (Fassbender 1975).

The subsynovium is a loose stroma of collagen fibres and proteoglycans interspersed with rare fibroblasts, fat cells and other unclassified cells. This tissue is penetrated by an abundant complex of blood vessels and lymphatics. This vasculature has unique post-capillary venules with specialized endothelium, called high endothelial venules (HEV). There is preferential binding of lymphocytes at these sites, which is enhanced by IL-1, TNF and interferon gamma. The high endothelial venules are thought to facilitate the entrance of blood lymphocytes into the synovium (Cavender *et al.* 1987).

The joint capsule and synovium are well innervated with mechanoreceptors and unmyelinated nerves. It has been postulated that the distribution of afferent nerve fibres of varying type may influence the pattern of joint involvement in RA (Thompson and Bywaters 1962). For example, in hemiplegic patients, the paralysed joints have less severe synovitis. Many afferent sensory nerves contain pro-inflammatory neuropeptides, such as substance P (SP). Substance P stimulates synoviocytes to proliferate and produce collagenase and PGE_2 (Lotz *et al.* 1987). In monocytes, SP enhances release of IL-1, TNF and IL-6. This neuromediator is believed to be active in the inflammation of osteoarthritis, RA and other chronic arthritides.

The synovium in early rheumatoid arthritis

Even early in the course of RA, evidence of injury to the subsynovial vasculature is prominent (Schumacher and Kitridou 1972; Schumacher 1975; Konttinen *et al.* 1986). During the first few weeks of disease there is congestion, erythrocyte extravasation and lumenal obliteration. Fibrin deposition occurs throughout the synovium. Endothelial cells are swollen and exhibit phagocytic activity. Electron microscopy has revealed gaps between the endothelial cells. Neutrophils appear in the superficial synovium, often as perivascular infiltrates. Lymphocytes are rare, and plasma cells and germinal follicles are uncommon or absent. Synovial lining cell proliferation is prominent, even before the appearance of mononuclear cells. However, these changes are not specific for RA as identical lesions can also be observed in other chronic arthritides or even in self-limited synovitis. In addition, early in disease synovial histology is a poor predictor of short-term prognosis, and inflammation does not necessarily increase with disease duration.

The chronic synovitis of rheumatoid arthritis

There are many detailed evaluations of synovial histopathology in chronic, well-established RA. Grossly, the synovium of RA is pale and oedematous with slender villous projections protruding into the joint cavity. In the established pannus, synovial hyperplasia is massive, with 100- to 1000-fold weight increases (Smiley *et al.* 1985). The synovial lining cells are swollen and up to 100 layers thick. These lining cells have enhanced phagocytic capacity (Lewis and Ziff 1966). Underneath, there is proliferation of subsynovial fibroblasts. The hyperplastic synovial tissue, which is responsible for the joint destruction in RA, has an extensive vascular network. Vascular abnormalities are common, and consist of venous distension, areas of capillary obstruction, thrombosis and haemorrhage. Koch *et al.* (1986) demonstrated that a subpopulation of macrophages is responsible for the neovascularization, probably by elaboration of necessary factors. Likely candidates include IL-1, IL-6, TNF and other monokines that have the ability to promote the growth of blood-vessels (Malone *et al.* 1984b). Tumour necrosis factor alpha

(TNF-α) has been well studied; it is readily detectable in RA synovial fluid (Hopkins 1989), and *in vivo* it stimulates neovascularization and leucocyte infiltration (Frater-Schroder *et al.* 1987).

Monocytes/macrophages serve a critical role in the inflamed synovium, and are responsible for much of the destruction of cartilage and bone (Zvaifler 1973; Krane *et al.* 1982). Also, macrophage-like cells bearing Class II MHC molecules are interdigitated within the lymphocyte-predominant regions of the synovium, often with long cytoplasmic processes (Duke *et al.* 1982; Klareskog *et al.* 1982a). These cells are important stimulators of mixed lymphocyte reactions. Other necessary cells have been termed dendritic cells, due to the morphology that these cells acquire after *in vitro* culture. The origins of these cells are unclear, as they are devoid of the cell surface markers and cytoplasmic lysosomal granules associated with the monocyte/macrophage lineage. However, due to their great prevalence in the synovial membrane and fluid, and the high density of surface MHC molecules, it has been suggested that they are important antigen-presenting cells (Winchester and Burmester 1981; reviewed in Waalen 1988).

Lymphocytic infiltrates in the synovium

At biopsy, most rheumatoid synovia have a prominent mononuclear infiltrate. Experimental models have suggested that the development of proliferative synovitis requires invasion by inflammatory cells from the peripheral circulation and bone marrow (Dreher 1982; Edwards and Willoughby 1982). Although non-specific for RA, early in their course many patients will have lymphocytic perivascular infiltrates. Later, dramatic mononuclear infiltrates may represent half of the mass of the synovium (Smiley *et al.* 1985). These cells are predominantly T cells and macrophages (Van Boxel and Paget 1975; Bankhurst *et al.* 1976).

By use of immunoelectron microscopy Ziff and co-workers have described a histological pattern which is apparently common in RA (Ishikawa and Ziff 1976; Kurosaka and Ziff 1983). The great majority of infiltrating lymphocytes bear T cell markers, while others express surface IgG and other B cell antigens (Bankhurst *et al.* 1976; Konttinen *et al.* 1981). Most of the lymphocytic infiltrate is perivascular, and here the ratio of T cell subsets is comparable to the patients' peripheral blood, i.e. there is an equal or greater number of CD4 (helper/inducer) than CD8 (suppressor/cytotoxic)-bearing T cells (Froland and Abrahamsen 1979; Janossy *et al.* 1981; Duke *et al.* 1982; Forre *et al.* 1982; Klareskog *et al.* 1982b). In these regions the CD4-bearing cells are often clustered and small; true lymphoblasts are uncommon. Cells with dendritic morphology and prominent expression of Class II MHC antigens are common in close apposition with lymphocytes, and have the appearance of accessory cells involved in antigen presentation (Galili *et al.* 1979; Palacios 1982). Many synovial T cells bear activation markers; most of these have the CD4 phenotype (Poulter *et al.* 1985). Peripheral to the lymphocyte-predominant regions, CD8 +ve lymphocytes are more prevalent than CD4 +ve cells. The CD8 lymphocytes are larger, often with a blast appearance (Forre *et al.* 1982). Adjacent to these transitional areas are regions rich in plasma cells.

A separate and common pattern of synovial involvement in RA entails the appearance of germinal follicles within the lymphocytic infiltrates (Young *et al.* 1984). Here, clusters of B cells are capped by scattered T cells bearing the CD4 marker. While this architecture has been likened to the organization of lymph nodes during an inflammatory response (Klareskog *et al.* 1981), some investigators have suggested that the nodular collections of small lymphocytes in the synovial membrane may represent a more quiescent and less destructive variety of synovitis (Muirden and Mills 1971). Other studies have described biopsies with mononuclear infiltrate that are primarily subsynovial and more scattered, with CD4 cells predominating (Meijer *et al.* 1982). Still other rheumatoid synovia have been described with CD4 and CD8 T cells scattered throughout the synovium in roughly equal numbers (Lindblad *et al.* 1983; Malone *et al.* 1984a).

The severity of articular disease does not correlate with the organization or severity of synovial infiltration. In many biopsies from severely affected individuals there are rare lymphocytes and plasma cells, and only a thin synovial lining layer and extensive fibrosis (Vaughan 1978). Therefore, clinicopathological correlation of synovial histological patterns is difficult and controversial.

The degree of sampling variation within a joint may make accurate interpretation difficult (Rooney *et al.* 1988). However, a histological pattern with sparse infiltrates has consistently been described in immunosuppressed patients treated with remittive agents (Young *et al.* 1984; Gaston *et al.* 1988). More recently Rooney *et al.* have presented evidence that response to therapy was correlated with decreases in T and B cell infiltration in serial biopsies (Rooney *et al.* 1989).

While it is possible that the various histological patterns represent individual variation determined by an unknown genetic or environmental factor, it is more likely that they reflect a common progression within the joint. In the early phases of disease, lymphocytes infiltrate and proliferate selectively to form the characteristic histological patterns (Ishikawa and Ziff 1976). However, in the chronic phase, a lymphocyte-mediated immune response may be less important. Cartilage and bone have only limited regenerative abilities, and various processes, including release of neuropeptides from damaged nerves and the presence of local tissue breakdown products, may facilitate the inflammation that occurs even in patients treated with immunosuppressive agents. Synovial biopsies with either dense or sparse lymphocytic infiltrates both frequently have nests of synoviocytes and polymorphonuclear leucocytes at the pannus–cartilage junction, the site of cartilage destruction. These clusters of cells may be observed to penetrate damaged cartilage (Kobayashi and Ziff 1975; Mohr *et al.* 1981; Muirden 1982), and here synovial collagenase can be detected (Woolley *et al.* 1977).

Cellular content of rheumatoid synovial fluid

In general, the cellular content within the synovial fluid does not correlate with the degree of inflammation within a synovial biopsy. While lymphocytes predominate in the synovial membrane, within rheumatoid synovial fluid 65–90% of the cells are polymorphonuclear neutrophils. Only in very early RA is there a predominance of lymphocytes in the synovial fluid. Further, while the CD4 marker identifies the majority of T cells in the synovium and peripheral blood of RA patients, in synovial fluid there is a relative enrichment for the CD8 (suppressor/cytotoxic) phenotype (Duclos *et al.* 1982; Fox *et al.* 1982; Poulter *et al.* 1985; Feldman *et al.* 1988). Several hypotheses have been presented to explain the different CD4/CD8 ratios present in synovial tissue and fluid. The discrepancy could reflect the selective homing of activated CD8 cells to the synovial fluid (Fox *et al.* 1982), the chronicity of the effusion, and/or the longer lifespan of CD8 T cells compared with CD4 cells (Kurosaka and Ziff 1983; Bergroth *et al.* 1985). *In vitro* culture has corroborated that most proliferating lymphocytes in synovial fluid bear the CD8 phenotype (Bergroth *et al.* 1985). In addition, growth factors present in synovial fluids may foster the predominance of CD8 cells. Significantly, synovial fluid enrichment of CD8 T cells occurs in other chronic inflammatory effusions, and thus is not specific for RA.

Cytokine profiles and immune response in rheumatoid arthritis

Activation markers and interleukins

The study of cytokines and cell surface molecules has allowed the dissection of immunoregulation into distinct steps. Experimental models have indicated that T cell activation results in an increase in the surface density of Class II MHC (Ia) molecules, the IL-2 receptors (Tac) and transferrin receptor (CD9). There is subsequent appearance of the very late activation markers (VLA-1 and VLA-2). Activated T cells also release cytokines such as IL-2, IL-3 and interferon gamma (Burmester *et al.* 1984). In normal subjects only 3% of T cells in the peripheral circulation bear Class II MHC (Ia) antigens, while in RA 15–20% of peripheral lymphocytes and 20–40% of synovial lymphocytes bear these activation markers (Yu *et al.* 1980; Fox *et al.* 1982). Most Ia-bearing T cells are of the CD8 phenotype (Burmester *et al.* 1981). The mechanism of cell surface Ia induction is unclear, as synovial fluid T cells release only small amounts of IL-2 *in vitro*, and little IL-2 is detected in fresh synovial fluid specimens (Malone *et al.* 1984a; Bergroth *et al.* 1985; Combe *et al.* 1985; Lotz *et al.* 1986b).

Synovial monocytes in RA also have an increased density of Class II MHC antigens (Firestein and Zvaifler 1987b). However, while interferon gamma is the most potent macrophage activator and inducer of Class II MHC antigens, little of this cytokine is detectable in fresh joint fluid or in synovial cell cultures (Firestein and Zvaifler 1987a). During early rheumatoid disease and during flares, both synovial and circulating T cells (mostly CD4) have elevated levels of transferrin receptor (Salmon *et al.* 1985). In contrast, few synovial T cells bear IL-2 receptors or VLA. Similarly, explanted synovial lymphocytes undergo only limited mitogen-induced proliferation. At least *in vitro*, these defects can be reversed by the addition of growth factors (Helmer *et al.* 1986). One interpretation of these results is that during the rheumatoid inflammatory process many T cells become blocked in a particular stage of activation.

Increased local production of IL-1 has been documented in the joints of patients with RA and other inflammatory arthritides (Fontana *et al.* 1982; Ise *et al.* 1982; Wood *et al.* 1983; Nouri *et al.* 1984; Miossec *et al.* 1986; Miyasaka *et al.* 1988). The exact cellular source of the increased synovial IL-1 is unknown, as macrophages, endothelial and other cell types are all capable of IL-1 production. Interleukin 1 has diverse biological and immunoregulatory activities that are consistent with a role for this cytokine in rheumatoid arthritis. *In vitro* IL-1 causes fibroblasts to proliferate and to produce collagen (Schmidt *et al.* 1982), and also stimulates vascular endothelial cells to secrete colony-stimulating factor (Bagby *et al.* 1986). Interleukin 1 is also a potent chemoattractant for neutrophils and lymphocytes, and it enhances their adhesion to vascular endothelium (Waddel and Ullman 1983; Bevilacqua *et al.* 1985; Miossec *et al.* 1986). *In vivo* IL-1 accelerates the synovial lymphocytic infiltration and fibroblast proliferation in collagen-induced arthritis (Hom *et al.* 1988). Bone resorption by osteoclasts is also stimulated *in vitro* by IL-1 (Pope *et al.* 1984; Gowen and Mundy 1986). Interleukin 1 may cause T lymphocytes to release IL-2 (Durum *et al.* 1985), and other cells to release IL-6 (see below) (Guerne *et al.* 1989). Further, IL-1 can induce IL-2 receptor expression on T cells. It seems likely that IL-1 contributes to joint destruction, as it can stimulate synoviocytes and macrophages to produce PGE_2 and collagenase (Krane *et al.* 1982; Dayer *et al.* 1986).

It appears that the full inflammatory potential of IL-1 is modulated in the rheumatoid pannus. At least *in vitro* the effects of IL-1 are dampened by a specific interleukin inhibitor of IL-1 that may be locally secreted by macrophages (Lotz *et al.* 1986b). Some of this inhibition may be attributed to transforming growth factor-beta (TGF-β), as this pleiotropic growth factor has been shown to block IL-1-dependent proliferation of T and B cells (Shalaby and Ammann 1988; Wahl *et al.* 1988). Furthermore, in culture TGF-β also blocks the release of neutral proteases by IL-1-treated chondrocytes (Chandrasekhar and Harvey 1989). The contribution of IL-1 to rheumatoid synovitis has been clinically documented in patients treated with total lymphoid irradiation. Responders have been found to have dramatic decreases in synovial production of IL-1 and in CD4 +ve T cells in the blood, even though IgM RF titres did not change appreciably (Gaston *et al.* 1988; Solovera *et al.* 1988).

It is conceivable that inhibitors of IL-1 may also be responsible for the relative lack of IL-2 in the synovial membrane and joint fluid (Husby and Williams 1985). Since T cell activation is a coordinated process, IL-1 inhibitors may block IL-2 production. There is also evidence of a specific inhibitor of IL-2 in rheumatoid synovium (Miossec *et al.* 1987) that may contribute to the apparent maturational arrest of synovial T cells.

Clinical correlative studies have confirmed that T lymphocytes in the synovium and peripheral blood usually have impaired responsiveness to mitogens and antigens during active or severe rheumatoid disease (Reynolds and Abdou 1973; Abrahamsen *et al.* 1978; Combe *et al.* 1985). Decreased accessory activity of rheumatoid monocytes during T cell activation induced by mitogenic antibodies against the CD3 receptor or T cells has also been reported (Lotz *et al.* 1986b). Taken together, the various studies suggest that the intensity of the synovitis of RA is tempered by a balance between many cell types and the interactions of multiple cytokines.

Interleukin 6 and rheumatoid arthritis

As discussed, humoral immunity appears to play an important part in the synovial inflammation of seropositive (and perhaps seronegative) RA. Studies of the regulation of B cell maturation have suggested that at least three specific activities or factors are required at different stages (reviewed in Kishimoto and Hirano 1988). The terminal differentiation to B cells capable of secretion of large quantities of immunoglobulins requires interferon gamma and/or BSF-2 (B cell stimulating factor 2), also known as IL-6. Interleukin 6 is produced by lymphocytes and fibroblasts (Yasukawa *et al*. 1987), and recently Guerne, Lotz and co-workers (1989) showed that synoviocytes and chondrocytes are also capable of significant IL-6 synthesis. Very high levels of IL-6 are detected in synovial fluids (>500 ng/ml), exceeding the concentration of any other known cytokine or growth factor. The IL-6 produced by synoviocytes in RA may be responsible for the local production of immunoglobulins and RFs that contribute to immune complex formation, and for the accumulation of plasma cells that is characteristic of the rheumatoid synovium.

At present the inducers of synovial IL-6 production are unknown. Although IL-1 is a potent inducer of IL-6 *in vitro*, the levels of this cytokine in synovial fluid are insufficient to account for the abundant IL-6. It is possible, however, that the membrane-bound form of IL-1 plays a role as an IL-6 inducer in the direct cell-to-cell interactions that occur in the inflamed synovium. Tumour necrosis factor, other growth factors (such as PDGF or FGF), immune complexes or complement products are also possible inducers of IL-6.

Interleukin 6 does not contribute to the local inflammatory milieu by inducing collagenase and PGE_2 production. However, it probably contributes to constitutional symptoms in severe disease, such as fever, fatigue, weight loss and anaemia. Interleukin 6 is a potent hepatocyte stimulatory factor, and induces the production of acute-phase reactants (Gauldie *et al*. 1987). The high IL-6 levels in synovial fluid may also have an impact on T cell function and phenotype. Interleukin 6 is a co-stimulant for human T cell proliferation, and part of this effect is independent of the IL-2/IL-2 receptor pathway. Recent findings suggest that IL-6 may preferentially promote proliferation of the CD8 +ve subset of T cells rather than the CD4 +ve helper cells (M. Lotz, pers. comm.). This finding is consistent with the effects of IL-6 on CD8 +ve T cell-mediated cytotoxicity and suppression, and may explain the decreased CD4/CD8 ratios in synovial fluid. However, increased IL-6 is not unique to rheumatoid synovitis, as comparable synovial levels are also seen in other inflammatory arthropathies unassociated with autoimmune phenomena (Guerne *et al*. 1989). Although IL-6 is likely to be a major driving force in RF production, these observations illustrate that other factors, perhaps specific to RA, activate B cells to become sensitive to the IL-6 inductive pathway.

Autologous mixed lymphocyte reaction

The prominence of activated macrophage-like cells in close apposition to CD4-bearing T cells (helper/inducer cells) in the synovium has suggested to many researchers similarities with the *in vitro* autologous mixed lymphocyte reaction (AMLR). This response occurs in the presence of a high ratio of autologous non-T stimulator cells rich in surface Ia to T cells (Chiorazzi *et al*. 1976; Kurosaka and Ziff 1983). To display the immune defect in RA, cells must be handled without exposure to xenoantigens, such as fetal bovine serum or sheep red cells. In this case, there is a poor AMLR if synovial T cells are used as responders and synovial non-T cells as stimulators. In contrast, when non-T cells from the synovium and T cells from the peripheral circulation are cultured together, T cell proliferation may exceed normal values by several-fold (reviewed in Firestein *et al*. 1987). This effect appears to be due to the enrichment of synovial fluid with dendritic stimulator cells, compared with the peripheral circulation.

Although an AMLR reaction typically induces copious production of interferon gamma and IL-2, the rheumatoid synovial cells release scant amounts of these cytokines following culture with non-T cells (Hasler *et al*. 1983a; Manthorpe and Prause 1986; Firestein and Zvaifler 1987a, b). Hence, IL-4, IL-6 and the recently described growth factor for CD4 +ve T cells (Van Snick *et al*. 1989) may be the true T cell growth factors in the rheumatoid joint. The synovial proliferative response in rheumatoid patients may also be controlled by macrophage colony-stimulating factor (CSF-1) and/or granulocyte–macrophage-stimulating factor (GM-CSF), which are both prominent in rheumatoid synovium (Firestein *et al*. 1988; Xu *et al*. 1989).

The *in vitro* AMLR has been reported to induce the generation of autoreactive cytotoxic T cells (Goto and Zvaifler 1983). Cells with similar function and phenotype can also be induced by treatment of peripheral blood mononuclear cells with IL-2. In the synovial fluid of RA patients similar mononuclear cells have been detected that can lyse a broad variety of target cells (Goto and Zvaifler 1985). These cells are phenotypically distinct from conventional natural killer cells, as they are devoid of Fc receptor. In the mouse, natural killer cells have been shown to lyse activated dendritic cells (Shah *et al*. 1985). Although the function of the autologous cytotoxic cells within the inflamed joint is unclear, they may conceivably regulate T cell proliferation by interaction with synovial dendritic cells.

Summary

Genetic factors predispose a large segment of the population to RA and they are now being characterized. Certain HLA-DR4 and DR1 β alleles contribute to disease susceptibility, and this association appears to be linked to a short amino acid primary sequence in the third hypervariable region of the DR β1 chain. What initiates RA is unknown, but this structural correlation may be critical as Class II MHC proteins are involved in both self-recognition and antigen presentation.

Extensive studies have shown that RFs contribute to intra-articular pathology, and that seropositive patients clearly have a tendency toward more severe disease. Although detectable in some normal subjects, RFs are produced in excess in most patients with RA, probably due to a regulatory defect. These autoantibodies may contribute to the development of chronic synovitis, via their ability to form immune complexes. However, during normal physiology RFs are beneficial, and they function in the clearance of immune complexes and in antigen processing. Genes that encode RF autoantibodies appear to be inherited by all humans, and they represent part of the preimmune repertoire.

The synovitis of long-standing RA probably represents a smouldering inflammatory response, which may be sustained by processes entirely different from those that triggered the disease. How different cell types and cytokines interact in the joint to produce synovitis is still not entirely clear, although the field is progressing rapidly. Since many inflammatory joint diseases are similar in the chronic state, a common final pathway of connective tissue destruction may occur in several different forms of chronic arthritis.

Acknowledgements

We appreciate the invaluable suggestions of Drs Martin Lotz, Jean Roudier and Pierre-Andre Guerne. We thank BCR Word Processing for clerical assistance. G.J. Silverman is a recipient of the National Institutes of Health (NIH) Physician-Scientist Award. This work was supported in part by grants AI00866, AR25443 and AI24466 from the NIH. This is publication number 5792-BCR from the Research Institute of Scripps Clinic.

References

Abrahamsen, T.G., Froland, S.S. and Natvig, J.B. (1978). *In vitro* mitogen stimulation of synovial fluid lymphocytes from rheumatoid arthritis and juvenile rheumatoid arthritis patients: dissociation between the response to antigens and polyclonal mitogens. *Scand. J. Immunol.* **7**, 81–90.

Aho, K., Koskenvuo, M., Tuominen, J. and Kaprio, J. (1986). Occurrence of rheumatoid arthritis in a nationwide series of twins. *J. Rheumatol.* **13**, 899–902.

Aho, K., Palosuo, T., Raunio, V. and Tuomi, T. (1987). The timing of rheumatoid factor seroconversions. *Arthritis Rheum.* **30**, 719–20.

Alarcon, G.S., Koopman, W.J. and Schroenloher, R.E. (1982a). Differential patterns of *in vitro* IgM rheumatoid factor synthesis in seronegative and seropositive rheumatoid arthritis. *Arthritis Rheum.* **25**, 150–5.

Alarcon, G.S., Koopman, W.J., Acton, R.T. and Barger, B.O. (1982b). Seronegative rheumatoid arthritis. *Arthritis Rheum.* **25**, 502–7.

Alarif, L.I., Ruppert, G.B., Wilson, R., Jr and Barth, W.F. (1983). HLA-DR antigens in blacks with rheumatoid arthritis and systemic lupus erythematosus. *J. Rheumatol.* **10**, 297–300.

Alspaugh, M.A., Henle, G., Lennette, E.T. and Henle, W. (1981). Elevated levels of antibodies to Epstein–Barr virus antigens in sera and synovial fluids of patients with rheumatoid arthritis. *J. Clin. Invest.* **67**, 1134–40.

Andrews, D.W. and Capra, J.D. (1981). Amino acid sequence of the variable regions of heavy chains from two idiotypically cross-reactive human IgM anti-gammaglobulins of the Wa group. *Biochemistry* **20**, 5816–22.

Arnett, F.C., Edworthy, S.M., Bloch, D.A. *et al.* (1988). The American Rheumatism Association 1987 revised criteria for the classification of rheumatoid arthritis. *Arthritis Rheum.* **31**, 315–24.

Astorga, G.P. and Williams, R.C., Jr (1969). Altered reactivity in mixed lymphocyte culture of lymphocytes from patients with rheumatoid arthritis. *Arthritis Rheum.* **12**, 547–54.

Babbitt, B.P., Allen, P.M., Matsueda, G., Haber, E. and Unanue, E.R. (1985). Binding of immunogenic peptides to Ia histocompatibility molecules. *Nature* **317**, 359–61.

Bagby, G.C., Jr, Dinarello, C.A., Wallace, P., Wagner, C., Hefeneider, S. and McCall, E. (1986). Interleukin 1 stimulates granulocyte macrophage colony-stimulating activity release by vascular endothelial cells. *J. Clin. Invest.* **78**, 1316–23.

Bankhurst, A.D., Husby, G. and Williams, R.C., Jr (1976). Predominance of T cells in the lymphocytic infiltrates of synovial tissue in rheumatoid arthritis. *Arthritis Rheum.* **19** (3), 555–62.

Bardin, T., Legrand, L., Naveau, B. *et al.* (1985). HLA antigens and seronegative rheumatoid arthritis. *Ann. Rheum. Dis.* **44**, 50–3.

Barland, P., Novikoff, A.B. and Hamerman, D. (1962). Electron microscopy of the human synovial membrane. *J. Cell Biol.* **14**, 207–14.

Bell, J.I., Estess, P., St John, T. *et al.* (1985). DNA sequence and characterization of human class II major histocompatibility complex B chains from the DR1 haplotype. *Proc. Nat. Acad. Sci. (USA)* **82**, 3495–509.

Bergroth, V., Konttinen, Y.T., Nykanen, P., von Essen, R. and Koota, K. (1985). Proliferating cells in the synovial fluid in rheumatic disease. *Scand. J. Immunol.* **22**, 383–8.

Bevilacqua, M.P., Pober, J.S., Wheeler, M.E., Cotran, R.S. and Gimbrone, M.A., Jr (1985). Interleukin 1 acts on cultured human vascular endothelium to increase the adhesion of polymorphonuclear leukocytes, monocytes, and related leukocyte cell lines. *J. Clin. Invest.* **76**, 2003–11.

Bluestone, R., Goldberg, L.S. and Cracchiolo, A., III (1969). Hidden rheumatoid factor in seronegative nodular rheumatoid arthritis. *Lancet* **ii**, 878–9.

Bonagura, V.R., Kunkel, H.G. and Pernis, B. (1982). Cellular localization of rheumatoid factor idiotypes. *J. Clin. Invest.* **69**, 1356–65.

Brackeretz, D. and Wernet, P. (1980). Genetic analysis of rheumatoid arthritis: population and family studies. *Arthritis Rheum.* **23**, 656.

Braunstein, N. and Germain, R.N. (1987). Allele specific control of Ia molecule surface expression and conformation: implications for a general model of Ia structure function relationships. *Proc. Nat. Acad. Sci. (USA)* **84**, 2921–5.

Brown, J.C., Harris, G., Papamichail, M., Sljivic, V.S. and Holborow, E.J. (1973). The localization of aggregated human gammaglobulin in the spleens of normal mice. *Immunology* **24**, 955–68.

Brown, P.B., Nardella, F.A. and Mannik, M. (1982). Human complement activation by self-associated IgG rheumatoid factors. *Arthritis Rheum.* **25**, 1101–7.

Burastero, S.E., Casali, P., Wilder, R.L. and Notkins, A.L. (1988). Monoreactive high affinity and polyreactive low affinity rheumatoid factors are produced by CD5+ B cells from patients with rheumatoid arthritis. *J. Exp. Med.* **168**, 1979–92.

Burmester, G.R., Yu, D.T.Y., Irani, A.-M., Kunkel, H.G. and Winchester, R.J. (1981). Ia+ T cells in synovial fluid and tissues of patients with rheumatoid arthritis. *Arthritis Rheum.* **24**, 1370–6.

Burmester, G.R., John, B., Gramatzki, M., Zacher, J. and Kalden, J.R. (1984). Activated T cells *in vivo* and *in vitro*: divergence in expression of Tac and Ia antigens in the nonblastoid small T cells of inflammation and normal T cells activated *in vitro*. *J. Immunol.* **133**, 1230–4.

Butler, V.P., Jr and Vaughan, J.H. (1965). The reaction of rheumatoid factor with animal gammaglobulins: quantitative considerations. *Immunology* **8**, 144–59.

Cairns, J.S., Curtsinger, J.M., Dahl, C.A., Freeman, S., Alter, B.J. and Bach, F.H. (1985). Sequence polymorphism of HLA DRB1 alleles relating to T-cell-recognized determinants. *Nature* **317**, 166–8.

Calvert, J.E., Duggan-Keen, M.F., Smith, S.W.G., Givan, A.L. and Bird, P. (1988). The CD5+ B Cell: a B cell lineage with a central role in autoimmune disease? *Autoimmunity* **1**, 223–40.

Capra, J.D., Kehoe, J.M., Williams, R.C., Jr, Feizi, T. and Kunkel, H.G. (1972). Light chain sequences of human IgM cold agglutinins. *Proc. Nat. Acad. Sci. (USA)* **69**, 40–3.

Carson, D.A., Pasquali, J.-L., Tsoukas, C.D. *et al.* (1981). Physiology and pathology of rheumatoid factors. *Springer Semin. Immunopathol.* **4**, 161–79.

Casali, P., Burastero, S.E., Nakamura, M., Inghirami, G. and Notkins, A.L. (1987). Human lymphocytes making rheumatoid factor and antibody to ssDNA belong to Leu-1+ B-cell subset. *Science* **236**, 77–81.

Cavender, D., Haskard, D., Lu, C. *et al.* (1987). Pathways to chronic inflammation in rheumatoid arthritis. *Fed. Proc.* **46**, 116–18.

Chandrasekhar, S. and Harvey, A.K. (1988). Transforming growth factor is a potent inhibitor of IL-1 induced protease activity and cartilage proteoglycan degradation. *Biochem. Biophys. Res. Commun.* **157**, 1352–9.

Chen, P.P., Albrandt, K., Kipps, T.J., Radoux, V., Liu, F.-T. and Carson, D.A. (1987a). Isolation and characterization of human VkIII germline genes: implications for the molecular basis of human VkIII light chain diversity. *J. Immunol.* **139**, 1727–33.

Chen, P.P., Robbins, D.L., Jirik, F.R., Kipps, T.J. and Carson, D.A. (1987b). Isolation and characterization of a light chain variable region gene for human rheumatoid factors. *J. Exp. Med.* **166**, 1900–5.

Chen, P.P., Fong, S., Goni, F. *et al.* (1988). Cross-reacting idiotypes on cryoprecipitating rheumatoid factor. *Springer Semin. Immunopathol.* **10**, 35–55.

Chiorazzi, N., Fu, S.M. and Kunkel, H.G. (1976). Induction of polyclonal antibody synthesis by human allogeneic and autologous helper factors. *J. Exp. Med.* **149**, 1543–8.

Combe, B., Pope, R.M., Fischbach, M., Darnell, B., Baron, S. and Talal, N. (1985). Interleukin-2 in rheumatoid arthritis: production of and response to interleukin-2 in rheumatoid synovial fluid, synovial tissue and peripheral blood. *Clin. Exp. Immunol.* **59**, 520–8.

Coulie, P.G. and Van Snick, J. (1985). Rheumatoid factor (RF) production during anamnestic immune responses in the mouse. III. Activation of RF precursor cells is induced by their interaction with immune complexes and carrier-specific helper T cells. *J. Exp. Med.* **161**, 88–97.

Crowley, J.J., Goldfien, R.D., Schrohenloher, R.E. *et al.* (1988). Incidence of three cross-reactive idiotypes on human rheumatoid factor paraproteins. *J. Immunol.* **140**, 3411–18.

Dayer, J.-M., de Rochemonteix, B., Burrus, B., Demczuk, S. and Dinarello, C.A. (1986). Human recombinant interleukin 1 stimulates collagenase and prostaglandin E-2 production by human synovial cells. *J. Clin. Invest.* **77**, 645–8.

De Jongh, B.M., Westedt, M.-L., De Vries, R.R.P., Valkenburg, H.A. and Cats, A. (1986). Genetic heterogeneity of rheumatoid arthritis. *Dis. Markers* **4**, 29–33.

del Jungo, D.J., Luthra, H.S., Annegers, J.F., Worthington, J.W. and Kurland, L.T. (1984). The familial aggregation of rheumatoid arthritis and its relationship to the HLA-DR4 association. *Am. J. Epidemiol.* **119**, 813–29.

Depper, J.M., Bluestein, H. and Zvaifler, N. (1981). Impaired regulation of Epstein–Barr virus induced lymphocyte proliferation in rheumatoid arthritis is due to a T cell defect. *J. Immunol.* **127**, 1899–902.

Dinant, H.J., Hissink, M.W., van den Berg-Loonen, E.M., Nijenhuis, L.E. and Engelfried, C.P. (1980). HLA-DRw4 in Felty's syndrome. *Arthritis Rheum.* **23**, 1336–6.

Dreher, R. (1982). Origin of synovial type A cells during inflammation: an experimental approach. *Immunobiology* **161**, 232–45.

Duclos, M., Zeidler, H., Liman, W., Pichler, W.J., Rieber, P. and

Peter, H.H. (1982). Characterization of blood and synovial fluid lymphocytes from patients with rheumatoid arthritis and other joint diseases by monoclonal antibodies (OKT series) and acid alpha-naphthyl esterase staining. *Rheumatol. Int.* **2**, 75–82.

Duggan, D.B. and Schattner, A. (1986). Unusual manifestations of monoclonal gammopathies. *Am. J. Med.* **81**, 864–70.

Duke, O., Panayi, G.S., Janossy, G. and Poulter, L.W. (1982). An immunohistological analysis of lymphocyte subpopulations and their microenvironment in the synovial membranes of patients with rheumatoid arthritis using monoclonal antibodies. *Clin. Exp. Immunol.* **49**, 22–30.

Duqesnoy, R.J., Marrari, M., Hackbarth, S. and Zeevi, A. (1984). Serological and cellular definition of a new HLA-DR associated determinant, MC1, and its association with rheumatoid arthritis. *Hum. Immunol.* **10**, 165–76.

Durum, S.K., Schmidt, J.A. and Oppenheim, J.J. (1985). Interleukin 1: an immunological perspective. *Ann. Rev. Immunol.* **3**, 263–87.

Edman, P. and Cooper, A.G. (1968). Amino acid sequence at the N-terminal end of a cold agglutinin kappa chain. *FEBS Lett.* **2**, 33–5.

Edwards, J.C.W. and Willoughby, D.A. (1982). Demonstration of bone marrow-derived cells in synovial lining by means of giant intracellular granules as genetic markers. *Ann. Rheum. Dis.* **41**, 177–82.

Engleman, E.G., Sponzilli, E.E., Batey, M.E., Ramcharan, S. and McDevitt, H.O. (1978). Mixed lymphocyte reaction in healthy women with rheumatoid factor. *Arthritis Rheum.* **21**, 690–3.

Fassbender, H.G. (1975). In *Pathology of Rheumatic Diseases*, ed. G. Loewi p. 1, Springer-Verlag, Berlin, FRG.

Feigenbaum, S.L. and Masi, A.T. (1978). Prognosis in rheumatoid arthritis. *Am. J. Med.* **66**, 377–84.

Feizi, T., Lecomte, J., Childs, R. and Solomon, A. (1976). Kappa chain (V kappa III) subgroup-related activity in an idiotypic anti-cold agglutinin serum. *Scand. J. Immunol.* **5**, 629–36.

Feldmann, M., Londei, M., Leech, Z., Brennan, F., Savill, C. and Maini, R.N. (1988). Analysis of T cell clones in rheumatoid arthritis. *Springer Semin. Immunopathol.* **10**, 157–67.

Firestein, G.S. and Zvaifler, N.J. (1987a). Peripheral blood and synovial fluid monocyte activation in inflammatory arthritis. I. A cytofluorographic study of monocyte differentiation antigens and class II antigens and their regulation by gamma-interferon. *Arthritis Rheum.* **30**, 857–63.

Firestein, G.S. and Zvaifler, N.J. (1987b). Peripheral blood and synovial fluid monocyte activation in inflammatory arthritis. II. Low levels of synovial fluid and synovial tissue interferon suggest that gamma-interferon is not the primary macrophage activating factor. *Arthritis Rheum.* **30**, 864–71.

Firestein, G.S., Tsai, V. and Zvaifler, N.J. (1987). Cellular immunity in the joints of patients with rheumatoid arthritis and other forms of chronic arthritis. *Rheum. Clin. North Am.* **13**, 191–213.

Firestein, G.S., Xu, W.-D., Townsend, K. *et al.* (1988). Cytokines in chronic inflammatory arthritis. I. Failure to detect T cell lymphocytes (interleukin 2 and interleukin 3) and presence of macrophage colony-stimulating factor (CSF-1) and a novel mast cell growth factor in rheumatoid synovitis. *J. Exp. Med.* **168**, 1573–86.

Fong, S., Gilbertson, T.A., Hueniken, R.J., Singhal, S.K., Vaughan, J.H. and Carson, D.A. (1985a). IgM rheumatoid factor autoantibody and immunoglobulin producing precursor cells in the bone marrow of humans. *Cell. Immunol.* **95**, 157–72.

Fong, S., Chen, P.P., Gilbertson, T.A., Fox, R.I., Vaughan, J.H. and Carson, D.A. (1985b). Structural similarities in the kappa light chains of human rheumatoid factor paraproteins and serum immunoglobulins bearing a cross-reactive idiotype. *J. Immunol.* **135**, 1955–60.

Fong, S., Chen, P.P., Gilbertson, T.A., Weber, J.R., Fox, R.I. and Carson, D.A. (1986). Expression of three cross reactive idiotypes on rheumatoid factor autoantibodies from patients with autoimmune diseases and seropositive adults. *J. Immunol.* **137**, 122–8.

Fong, S., Chen, P.P., Fox, R.I. *et al.* (1988). The diversity and idiotypic pattern of human rheumatoid factors in disease. *Concepts Immunopathol.* **5**, 168–91.

Fontana, A., Hengartner, H., Weber, E., Fehr, K., Grob, P.J. and Cohen, G. (1982). Interleukin 1 activity in the synovial fluid of patients with rheumatoid arthritis. *Rheumatol. Int.* **2**, 49–53.

Forre, O., Thoen, J., Lea, T. *et al.* (1982). *In situ* characterization of mononuclear cells in rheumatoid tissues, using monoclonal antibodies: no reduction of T8-positive cells or augmentation in T4-positive cells. *Scand. J. Immunol.* **16**, 315–19.

Fox, R.I., Fong, S., Sabharwal, N., Carstens, S.A., Kung, P.C. and Vaughan, J.H. (1982). Synovial fluid lymphocytes differ from peripheral blood lymphocytes in patients with rheumatoid arthritis. *J. Immunol.* **128**, 351–4.

Frater-Schroder, M., Risau, W., Hallman, R., Gautschi, P. and Bohlen, P. (1987). Tumor necrosis factor type a, a potent inhibitor of endothelial cell growth in vitro, is angiogenic *in vivo*. *Proc. Nat. Acad. Sci. (USA)* **84**, 5277–81.

Froland, S.S. and Abrahamsen, T.G. (1979). Lymphocyte populations in blood, synovial fluid, and synovial tissue in rheumatoid arthritis. In *Immunopathogenesis of Rheumatoid Arthritis*, ed. G.S. Panayi and P.M. Johnson, p. 25, Reedbooks, Chertsey, Surrey, England.

Galili, U., Rosenthal, L., Galili, N. and Klein, E. (1979). Activated T cells in the synovial fluid of arthritic patients: characterization and comparison with *in vitro* activated human and murine T cells in cooperation with monocytes in cytotoxicity. *J. Immunol.* **122**, 878–83.

Gaston, J.S.H., Strober, S., Solovera, J.J. *et al.* (1988). Dissection of the mechanisms of immune injury in rheumatoid arthritis, using total lymphoid irradiation. *Arthritis Rheum.* **31** (1), 21–30.

Gauldie, J., Richards, C., Harnish, D., Lansdorp, P. and Baumann, H. (1987). Interferon beta-2/B cell stimulatory factor type 2 shares identity with monocyte-derived hepatocyte-stimulating factor and regulates the major acute phase protein response in liver cells. *Proc. Nat. Acad. Sci. (USA)* **84**, 7251–5.

Gergely, J., Wang, A.C. and Fudenberg, H.H. (1970). Chemical analyses of variable regions of heavy and light chains of cold agglutinins. *Vox Sang.* **24**, 432–40.

Gibofsky, A., Winchester, R.J., Patarroyo, M., Fotino, M. and Kunkel, H.G. (1978). Disease associations of the Ia-like human alloantigens: contrasting patterns in rheumatoid arthritis and systemic lupus erythematosus. *J. Exp. Med.* **148**, 1728–32.

Go, R.C.P., Alarcon, G.S., Acton, R.T., Koopman, W.J., Vittor, V.J. and Barger, B.O. (1987). Analyses of HLA linkage in white families with multiple cases of seropositive rheumatoid arthritis. *Arthritis Rheum.* **30**, 1115–23.

Gong, M., Ooka, T., Matsuo, T. and Kieff, E. (1987). Epstein–Barr virus glycoprotein homologous to herpes simplex virus gB. *J. Virol.* **61**, 499–508.

Goni, F., Chen, P.P., Pons-Estel, B., Carson, D.A. and Frangione, B. (1985). Sequence similarities and cross-idiotypic specificity of L chains among human monoclonal IgM-K with anti-gammaglobulin activity. *J. Immunol.* **135**, 4073–9.

Goronzy, J., Weyand, C.M. and Fathman, C.G. (1986). Shared T cell recognition sites on human histocompatibility leukocyte antigen class II molecules of patients with seropositive rheumatoid arthritis. *J. Clin. Invest.* **77**, 1042–9.

Goto, M. and Zvaifler, N.J. (1983). Characterization of the killer cell generated in the autologous mixed leukocyte reaction. *J. Exp. Med.* **157**, 1309–23.

Goto, M. and Zvaifler, N.J. (1985). Characterization of the natural killer-like lymphocytes in rheumatoid synovial fluid. *J. Immunol.* **134**, 1483–6.

Gowen, M. and Mundy, G.R. (1986). Actions of recombinant interleukin 1, interleukin 2, and interferon-gamma on bone resorption *in vitro*. *J. Immunol.* **136**, 2478–82.

Gran, J.T. and Husby, G. (1987). Seronegative rheumatoid arthritis and HLA-DR4: proposal for criteria. *J. Rheumatol.* **14**, 1079–82.

Gran, J.T., Husby, G. and Thorsby, E. (1984). HLA antigens in palindromic rheumatism, nonerosive rheumatoid arthritis and classical rheumatoid arthritis. *J. Rheumatol.* **11**, 136–40.

Gregersen, P.K., Shen, M., Song, Q.-L. *et al.* (1986). Molecular diversity of HLA-DR4 haplotypes. *Proc. Nat. Acad. Sci. (USA)* **83**, 2642–6.

Gregersen, P.K., Silver, J. and Winchester, R.J. (1987). The shared epitope gypothesis — an approach to understanding the molecular genetics of susceptibility to rheumatoid arthritis. *Arthritis Rheum.* **30**, 1205–13.

Grennan, D.M., Dyer, P.A., Clague, R., Dodds, W., Smeaton, I. and Harris, R. (1983). Family studies in RA — the importance of HLA-DR4 and of genes for autoimmune thyroid disease. *J. Rheumatol.* **10**, 584–9.

Guerne, P.-A., Zuraw, B.L., Vaughan, J.H., Carson, D.A. and Lotz, M. (1989). Synovium as a source of interleukin-6 *in vitro*: contribution to local and systemic manifestations of arthritis. *J. Clin. Invest.* **83**, 585–92.

Guillet, J.-G., Lai, M.-Z., Briner, T.J. *et al.* (1987). Immunological self, nonself discrimination. *Science* **235**, 865–70.

Hadler, N.M., Johnson, A.M., Spitznagel, J.K. and Quinet, R.J. (1981). Protease inhibitors in inflammatory synovial effusions. *Ann. Rheum. Dis.* **40**, 55–9.

Halla, J.T., Hardin, J.G. and Fallahi, S. (1987). The nature of the onset of rheumatoid arthritis: a reassessment. *Rheumatol. Int.* **7**, 169–71.

Hardy, R.R., Hayakawa, K., Shimizu, M., Yamasaki, K. and Kishimoto, T. (1987). Rheumatoid factor secretion from human Leu-1+ B cells. *Science* **236**, 81–3.

Hasler, F., Bluestein, H.G., Zvaifler, N.J. and Epstein, L.B. (1983a). Analysis of the defects responsible for the impaired regulation of Epstein–Barr virus-induced B cell proliferation by rheumatoid arthritis lymphocytes. I. Diminished gamma interferon production in response to autologous stimulation. *J. Exp. Med.* **157**, 173–88.

Hasler, F., Bluestein, H.G., Zvaifler, N.J. and Epstein, L.B. (1983b). Analysis of the defects responsible for the impaired regulation of EBV-induced B cell proliferation by rheumatoid arthritis lymphocytes. II. Role of monocytes and the increased sensitivity of rheumatoid arthritis lymphocytes to prostaglandin E. *J. Immunol.* **131**, 768–72.

Helmer, M.E., Glass, D., Coblyn, J.S. and Jacobson, J.G. (1986). Very late activation antigens on rheumatoid synovial fluid T lymphocytes: association with stages of T cell activation. *J. Clin. Invest.* **78**, 696–706.

Hoffman, W.L., Goldberg, M.S. and Smiley, J.D. (1982). Immunoglobulin G-3 subclass production by rheumatoid synovial tissue cultures. *J. Clin. Invest.* **69**, 136–44.

Hollander, J.L., McCarty, D.J., Jr, Astorga, G. and Castro-Murillo, E. (1965). Studies on the pathogenesis of rheumatoid joint inflammation. I. The 'R.A. cell' and a working hypothesis. *Ann. Intern. Med.* **62**, 271–80.

Hom, J.T., Bendele, A.M. and Carlson, D.G. (1988). *In vivo* administration with IL-1 accelerates the development of collagen-induced arthritis in mice. *J. Immunol.* **141** (3), 834–41.

Hopkins, S.J. and Meager, A. (1988). Cytokines in synovial fluid: II The presence of tumor necrosis factor and interferon. *Clin. Exp. Immunol.* **73**, 88–92.

Husby, G. and Williams, R.C., Jr (1985). Immunohistochemical studies of interleukin-2 and gamma-interferon in rheumatoid arthritis. *Arthritis Rheum.* **28**, 174–81.

Ise, K., Nakamura, S., Ohkawara, S. and Yoshinaga, M. (1982). DNA synthesis-potentiating activity on mouse thymocytes of synovial fluid of rheumatoid arthritis patients. *Acta Pathol. Jap.* **32**, 491–503.

Ishikawa, H. and Ziff, M. (1976). Electron microscopic observations of immunoreactive cells in the rheumatoid synovial membrane. *Arthritis Rheum.* **19** (1), 1–14.

Janossy, G., Panayi, G., Duke, O., Bofill, M., Poulter, L.W. and Goldstein, G. (1981). Rheumatoid arthritis: a disease of T-lymphocyte/macrophage immunoregulation. *Lancet* **ii**, 839–41.

Jaraquemada, D., Pachoula-Papasteriadis, C., Festenstein, H. *et al.* (1979). HLA-D and DR determinants in rheumatoid arthritis. *Transplant. Proc.* **11**, 1306.

Jones, V.E., Jacoby, R.K., Cowley, P.J. and Warren, C. (1982). Immune complexes in early arthritis. II. Immune complex constituents are synthesized in the synovium before rheumatoid factors. *Clin. Exp. Immunol.* **49**, 31–40.

Kabat, E.A. and Wu, T.T. (1991). Identical V region amino acid sequences and segments of sequences in antibodies of different specificities. *J. Immunol.* **147**, 1709–19.

Karr, R.W., Rodney, G.E., Lee, T. and Schwartz, B.D. (1980). Association of HLA-DRw4 with rheumatoid arthritis in black and white patients. *Arthritis Rheum.* **23**, 1241–5.

Kipps, T.J. and Vaughan, J.H. (1987). Genetic influence on the levels of circulating CD5 B lymphocytes. *J. Immunol.* **139**, 1060–4.

Kipps, T.J., Tomhave, E., Chen, P.P. and Carson, D.A. (1988). Autoantibody-associated kappa light chain variable region gene expressed in chronic lymphocytic leukemia with little or no somatic mutation: implications for etiology and immunotherapy. *J. Exp. Med.* **167**, 840–52.

Kishimoto, T. and Hirano, T. (1988). Molecular regulation of B lymphocyte response. *Ann. Rev. Immunol.* **6**, 485–512.

Klareskog, L., Forsum, U., Tjernlund, M., Kabelitz, D. and Wigren, A. (1981). Appearance of anti-HLA-DR-reactive cells in normal and rheumatoid synovial tissue. *Scand. J. Immunol.* **14**, 183–92.

Klareskog, L., Forsum, U., Kabelitz, D. *et al.* (1982a). Immune functions of human synovial cells: phenotypic and T cell regulatory properties of macrophage-like cells that express HLA-DR. *Arthritis Rheum.* **25**, 488–501.

Klareskog, L., Forsum, U., Scheynius, A., Kabelitz, D. and Wigzell, H. (1982b). Evidence in support of a self-perpetuating HLA-DR-dependent delayed-type cell reaction in rheumatoid arthritis. *Proc. Nat. Acad. Sci. (USA)* **79**, 3632–6.

Klouda, P.T., Corbin, S.A., Bidwell, J.L., Bradley, B.A., Ahern, M.J. and Maddison, P.J. (1986). Felty syndrome and HLA-DR antigens. *Tissue Antigens* **27**, 112–13.

Kobayashi, I. and Ziff, M. (1975). Electron microscopic studies of the cartilage–pannus junction in rheumatoid arthritis. *Arthritis Rheum.* **18** (5), 475–83.

Koch, A.E., Polverini, P.J. and Leibovich, S.J. (1986). Stimulation of neovascularization by human rheumatoid synovial tissue macrophages. *Arthritis Rheum.* **29**, 471–9.

Konttinen, Y.T., Reitamo, S., Hayry, P., Kankaanapaa, U. and Wegelius, O. (1981). Characterization of the immunocompetent cells of rheumatoid synovium from tissue sections and eluates. *Arthritis Rheum.* **24**, 71–9.

Konttinen, Y.T., Bluestein, H.G. and Zvaifler, N.J. (1986). Regulation of the growth of Epstein–Barr virus-infected B cells: temporal profile of the *in vitro* development of three distinct cytotoxic cells. *Cell. Immunol.* **103**, 84–95.

Koopman, W.J. and Schrohenloher, R.E. (1980). *In vitro* synthesis of IgM rheumatoid factor by lymphocytes from healthy adults. *J. Immunol.* **125**, 934–9.

Krane, S., Golding, S.R. and Dayer, J.M. (1982). Interactions among lymphocytes, monocytes and other synovial cells in the rheumatoid synovium. *Lymphokines* **7**, 75–89.

Kunkel, H.G., Agnello, V., Joslin, F.G., Winchester, R.J. and Capra, J.D. (1973). Cross-idiotypic specificity among monoclonal IgM proteins with anti-gammaglobulin activity. *J. Exp. Med.* **137**, 331–42.

Kurosaka, M. and Ziff, M. (1983). Immunoelectron microscopic study of the distribution of T cell subsets in rheumatoid synovium. *J. Exp. Med.* **158**, 1191–210.

Lamb, J.R., Rees, A.D.M., Bal, V. *et al.* (1988). Prediction and identification of an HLA-DR-restricted T cell determinant in the 19 kDa protein of *Mycobacterium tuberculosis*. *Eur. J. Immunol.* **18**, 973–6.

Lawrence, J.S. (1970). Rheumatoid arthritis — nature or nurture? *Ann. Rheum. Dis.* **29**, 357–78.

Lee, S.H., Gregersen, P.K., Shen, H., Nunez-Roldan, A., Silver, J. and Winchester, R.J. (1984). Strong association of rheumatoid arthritis with the presence of a polymorphic Ia epitope defined by a monoclonal antibody: comparison with the allodeterminant DR4. *Rheumatol. Int.* **4** (suppl.), 17–23.

Legrand, L., Lathrop, G.M., Marcelli-Barge, A. *et al.* (1984). HLA-DR genotype risks in seropositive rheumatoid arthritis. *Am. J. Hum. Genet.* **36**, 690–9.

Lewis, D.C. and Ziff, M. (1966). Intra-articular administration of gold salts. *Arthritis Rheum.* **9**, 682–92.

Lindblad, S., Klareskog, L., Hedfors, E., Forsum, U. and Sundstrom, C. (1983). Phenotypic characterization of synovial tissue cells *in situ* in different types of synovitis. *Arthritis Rheum.* **26**, 1321–32.

Lotz, M., Tsoukas, C.D., Fong, S., Dinarello, C.A., Carson, D.A. and Vaughan, J.H. (1986a). Release of lymphokines after infection with Epstein–Barr virus *in vitro*. II. A monocyte-dependent inhibitor of interleukin-1 downregulates the production of interleukin-2 and interferon-gamma in rheumatoid arthritis. *J. Immunol.* **136**, 3643–8.

Lotz, M., Tsoukas, C.D., Robinson, C.A., Dinarello, C.A., Carson, D.A. and Vaughan, J.H. (1986b). Basis for defective responses of rheumatoid arthritis synovial fluid lymphocytes to anti-CD3 (T3) antibodies. *J. Clin. Invest.* **78**, 713–21.

Lotz, M., Carson, D.A. and Vaughan, J.H. (1987). Substance P activation of rheumatoid synoviocytes: neural pathway in the pathogenesis of arthritis. *Science* **235**, 893–5.

Luka, J., Chase, R.C. and Pearson, G.R. (1984). A sensitive enzyme-linked immunosorbent assay (ELISA) against the major EBV-associated antigens. I. Correlations between ELISA and immunofluorescence titers using purified antigens *J. Immunol. Methods* **67**, 145–56.

McDaniel, D.O., Barger, B.O., Reveille, J.D., Alarcon, G.S., Koopman, W.J. and Acton, R.T. (1987). Analysis of restriction fragment length polymorphisms in rheumatic diseases. *Rheum. Dis. North Am.* **13**, 353–67.

McDermott, M. & McDevitt, H.O. (1988). The immunogenetics of rheumatic diseases. *Bull. Rheum. Dis.* **38**, 1–10.

MacLennan, I.C.M., Gray, D., Kumaratne, D.S. and Bazin, H. (1982). The lymphocytes of splenic marginal zones: a distinct B cell lineage. *Immunol. Today* **3**, 305–7.

Maeda, H., Juji, T., Mitsui, H., Sonozaki, H. and Okitsu, K. (1981) HLA DR4 and rheumatoid arthritis in Japanese people. *Ann. Rheum. Dis.* **40**, 299–302.

Malone, D.G., Wahl, S.M., Tsokos, M., Cattell, H., Decker, J.L. and Wilder, R.L. (1984a). Immune function in severe, active rheumatoid arthritis: a relationship between peripheral blood mononuclear cell proliferation to soluble antigens and synovial tissue immunohistologic characteristics. *J. Clin. Invest.* **74**, 1173–85.

Malone, D.G., Wahl, S.M. and Wilder, R.L. (1984b). Spontaneous production of fibroblast activating factor(s) (FAF) by synovial inflammatory cells. *Arthritis Rheum.* **27**, S35.

Manthorpe, R. and Prause, J. (1986). Proceedings of the First International Seminar on Sjogren's Syndrome. *Scand. J. Rheumatol.* **61**, 17–31.

March, L.M. (1987). Dendritic cells in the pathogenesis of rheumatoid arthritis. *Rheumatol. Int.* **7**, 93–100.

Masi, A.T. (1988). Rheumatoid factor negative (seronegative) rheumatoid arthritis: evolving clinical classification and immunogenetic associations. *J. Rheumatol.* **15**, 4–6.

Masi, A.T., Maldonado-Cocco, J.A., Kaplan, S.B., Feigenbaum, S.L. and Chandler, R.W. (1976). Prospective study of the early course of rheumatoid arthritis in young adults: comparison of patients with and without rheumatoid factor positivity at entry and identification of variables correlating with outcome. *Semin. Arthritis Rheum.* **5**, 299–326.

Meijer, C.J.L.M., Lafeber, G.J.M., Cnossen, J., Damsteeg, M.G.M. and Cats, A. (1982). T lymphocyte subpopulations in rheumatoid arthritis. *J. Rheumatol.* **9**, 18–24.

Mellbye, O.J., Vartal, F. and Dobloug, J.H. (1984). Subclasses of IgG produced in the rheumatoid synovium. *Rheumatol. Int.* **4** (suppl.), 49–52.

Merryman, P., Gregersen, P.K., Lee, S. *et al.* (1988). Nucleotide sequence of a DRw10 beta chain cDNA clone. *J. Immunol.* **140**, 2447–52.

Miller, R.A. and Gralow, J. (1984). The induction of Leu-1 antigen expression in human malignant and normal B cells by phorbol myristic acetate. *J. Immunol.* **133**, 3408–14.

Miossec, P., Dinarello, C.A. and Ziff, M. (1986a). Interleukin-1 lymphocyte chemotactic activity in rheumatoid arthritis synovial fluid. *Arthritis Rheum.* **29**, 461–70.

Miossec, P., Kashiwado, T. and Ziff, M. (1987). Inhibitor of interleukin-2 in rheumatoid synovial fluid. *Arthritis Rheum.* **30**, 121–9.

Mitchell, D. (1985). Epidemiology. In *Rheumatoid Arthritis*, ed. P.D. Utsinger, N.J. Zvaifler and G.E. Ehrlich, p. 133, J.B. Lippincott Co., Philadelphia, Pennsylvania.

Miyasaka, N., Sato, K., Goto, M. *et al.* (1988a). Augmented interleukin-1 production and HLA-DR expression in the synovium of rheumatoid arthritis patients. *Arthritis Rheum.* **31** (4), 480–6.

Mohr, W., Westerhellweg, H. and Wessinghage, D. (1981). Polymorphonuclear granulocytes in rheumatic tissue destruction. III. An electron microscopic tissue study of PMNs at the pannus–cartilage junction in rheumatoid arthritis. *Ann. Rheum. Dis.* **40**, 396–9.

Mottonen, T., Hannonen, P., Oka, M. *et al.* (1988). Antibodies against native type II collagen do not precede the clinical onset of rheumatoid arthritis. *Arthritis Rheum.* **31**, 776–9.

Muirden, K.D. (1982). Electron microscopy studies of the synovial cartilage junction in rheumatoid arthritis. *Eur. J. Rheumatol. Inflamm.* **5**, 30–8.

Muirden, K.D. and Mills, K.W. (1971). Do lymphocytes protect the rheumatoid joint? *Br. Med. J.* **23**, 219–21.

Munthe, E. and Natvig, J.B. (1972). Immunoglobulin classes, subclasses and complexes of IgG rheumatoid factor in rheumatoid plasma cells. *Clin. Exp. Immunol.* **12**, 55–77.

Nakai, Y., Wakisaka, M., Aizawa, M., Itakura, K., Nakai, H. and Ohashi, A. (1981). HLA and rheumatoid arthritis in the Japanese. *Arthritis Rheum.* **24**, 722.

Natvig, J.B. and Munthe, E. (1975). Self-associating IgG rheumatoid factor represents a major response of plasma cells in rheumatoid inflammatory tissue. *Ann. NY Acad. Sci.* **256**, 88–95.

Natvig, J.B., Gaarder, P.I. and Turner, M.N. (1972). IgG antigens of the C-gamma-2 and C-gamma-3 homology regions interacting with rheumatoid factors. *Clin. Exp. Immunol.* **12**, 177–83.

Nelson, J.L., Nardella, F.A., Oppliger, I.R. and Mannik, M. (1987). Rheumatoid factors from patients with rheumatoid arthritis possess private repertoires of idiotypes. *J. Immunol.* **138**, 1391–6.

Nemazee, D.A. (1985). Immune complexes can trigger specific, T cell-dependent, autoanti-IgG antibody production in mice. *J. Exp. Med.* **161**, 242–56.

Nepom, B.S., Nepom, G.T., Mickelson, E., Antonelli, P. and Hansen, J.A. (1983). Electrophoretic analysis of human HLA-DR antigens from HLA-DR4 homozygous cell lines: correlation between beta-chain diversity and HLA-D. *Proc. Nat. Acad. Sci. (USA)* **80**, 6962–6.

Nepom, B.S., Nepom, G.T., Mickelson, E., Schaller, J.G., Antonelli, P. and Hansen, J.A. (1984). Specific HLA-DR4-associated histocompatibility molecules characterize patients with seropositive juvenile rheumatoid arthritis. *J. Clin. Invest.* **74**, 287–91.

Nepom, G.T., Hansen, J.A. and Nepom, B.S. (1987). The molecular basis for HLA Class II associations with rheumatoid arthritis. *J. Clin. Immunol.* **7**, 1–7.

Newkirk, M.M., Mageed, R.A., Jefferis, R., Chen, P.P. and Capra, J.D. (1987). Complete amino acid sequences of variable regions of two human IgM rheumatoid factors, BOR and KAS of the Wa idiotypic family, reveal restricted use of heavy and light chain variable and joining region gene segments. *J. Exp. Med.* **166**, 550–64.

Newkirk, M.M., Gram, H., Heinrich, G.F., Ostberg, L., Capra, J.D. and Wasserman, R.L. (1988). Complete protein sequences of the variable regions of the cloned heavy and light chains of a human anti-cytomegalovirus antibody reveal a striking similarity to human monoclonal rheumatoid factors of the Wa idiotype family. *J. Clin. Invest.* **81**, 1511–18.

Nouri, A.M.E., Panayi, G.S. and Goodman, S.M. (1984). Cytokines and the chronic inflammation of rheumatic disease. I. The presence of interleukin-1 in synovial fluids. *Clin. Exp. Immunol.* **55**, 295–302.

Ohta, N., Nishimura, Y.K., Tanimoto, M.K. *et al.* (1982). Association between HLA and Japanese patients with rheumatoid arthritis. *Hum. Immunol.* **5**, 123–32.

Olsen, N.J., Stastny, P. and Jasin, H.E. (1987). High levels of *in vitro* IgM rheumatoid factor synthesis correlate with HLA-DR4 in normal individuals. *Arthritis Rheum.* **30**, 841–8.

Ono, M., Winearls, C.G., Amos, N. *et al.* (1987). Monoclonal antibodies to restricted and cross-reactive idiotopes on monoclonal rheumatoid factors and their recognition of idiotope-positive cells. *Eur. J. Immunol.* **17**, 343–9.

Palacios, R. (1982). Mechanism of T cell activation: role and functional relationship of HLA antigens and interleukins. *Immunol. Rev.* **63**, 73–111.

Palacios-Boix, A.A., Estrada-G., I., Colston, M.H. and Panayi, G.S. (1988). HLA-DR4 restricted lymphocyte proliferation to a *Mycobacterium tuberculosis* extract in rheumatoid arthritis and healthy subjects. *J. Immunol.* **140**, 1844–50.

Panayi, G.S. and Wooley, P.H. (1977). B lymphocyte alloantigens in the study of the genetic basis of rheumatoid arthritis. *Ann. Rheum. Dis.* **36**, 365–8.

Panayi, G.S., Wooley, P. and Batchelor, J.R. (1978). Genetic basis of rheumatoid disease: HLA antigens, disease manifestations and toxic reactions to drugs. *Br. Med. J.* **2**, 1326–8.

Pearson, C.M. and Wood, F.D. (1959). Studies of polyarthritis and other lesions induced in rats by injection of mycobacterial adjuvant. I. General clinical and pathologic characteristics and some modifying factors. *Arthritis Rheum.* **2**, 440–59.

Pellet, P., Biggin, M., Barrel, B. and Roizman, B. (1985). Epstein–Barr virus genome may encode a protein showing significant amino acid and predicted secondary structure homology with glycoprotein B of herpes simplex virus. *J. Virol.* **56**,

807–13.

Plater-Zyberk, C., Maini, R., Lam, K., Kennedy, T.D. and Janossy, G. (1985). A rheumatoid arthritis B cell subset expresses a phenotype similar to that in chronic lymphocytic leukemia. *Arthritis Rheum.* **28**, 971–6.

Pons-Estel, B., Goni, F., Solomon, A. and Frangione, B. (1984). Sequence similarities among kIIIb chains of monoclonal human IgMk autoantibodies. *J. Exp. Med.* **160**, 893–904.

Pope, R.M., Teller, D.C. and Mannik, M. (1975). The molecular basis of self-association of IgG rheumatoid factors. *J. Immunol.* **115**, 365–73.

Pope, R.M., McChesney, L., Talal, N. and Fischbach, M. (1984). Characterization of the defective autologous mixed lymphocyte response in rheumatoid arthritis. *Arthritis Rheum.* **27**, 1234–44.

Poulter, L.W., Duke, O., Panayi, G.S., Hobbs, S., Raftery, M.J. and Janossy, G. (1985). Activated T lymphocytes of the synovial membrane in rheumatoid arthritis and other arthropathies. *Scand. J. Immunol.* **22**, 683–90.

Radoux, V., Chen, P.P., Sorge, J.A. and Carson, D.A. (1986). A conserved human germline Vk gene directly encodes rheumatoid factor light chains. *J. Exp. Med.* **164**, 2119–24.

Res, P.C.M., Breedveld, F.C., van Embden, J.D.A., Schaar, C.G., van Eden, I.R. and De Vries, R.R.P. (1988). Synovial fluid T cell reactivity against 65 kD heat shock protein of mycobacteria in early chronic arthritis. *Lancet* **ii**, 478–82.

Reynolds, M.D. and Abdou, N.I. (1973). Comparative study of the *in vitro* proliferative responses of blood and synovial fluid leukocytes of rheumatoid arthritis patients. *J. Clin. Invest.* **52**, 1627–31.

Rhodes, G., Carson, D.A., Valbracht, J., Houghten, R. and Vaughan, J.H. (1985). Human immune responses to synthetic peptides from the Epstein–Barr nuclear antigen. *J. Immunol.* **134**, 211–16.

Riley, S.C., Connors, S.J., Klinman, N.R. and Ogata, R.T. (1986). Preferential expression of variable region heavy chain gene segments by predominant 2,4-dinitrophenyl-specific Balb/c neonatal antibody clonotypes. *Proc. Nat. Acad. Sci. (USA)* **83**, 2589–93.

Robbins, D.L. and Wistar, R., Jr (1985). Comparative specificities of serum and synovial cell 19s IgM rheumatoid factors in rheumatoid arthritis. *J. Rheumatol.* **12**, 437–43.

Rodriguez, M.A., Bankhurst, A.D., Williams, R.C., Jr, Troup, G.M. and Stastny, P. (1983). Studies on the relationship between HLA-DR4 and *in vitro* IgM rheumatoid factor production. *Clin. Immunol. Immunopathol.* **27**, 96–109.

Ronchese, F., Schwartz, R.H. and Germain, R.M. (1987). Functionally distinct subsites on a class II major histocompatibility complex molecule. *Nature* **329**, 254–6.

Rooney, M., Condell, D., Quinlan, W. *et al.* (1988). Analysis of the histologic variation of synovitis in rheumatoid arthritis. *Arthritis Rheum.* **31**, 956–63.

Rooney, M., Whelan, A., Feighery, C. and Bresnihan, B. (1989). Changes in lymphocyte infiltration of the synovial membrane and the clinical course of rheumatoid arthritis. *Arthritis Rheum.* **32**, 361–9.

Ropes, M.W. (1959). Diagnostic criteria for rheumatoid arthritis — 1958 revision. *Ann. Rheum. Dis.* **18**, 49–53.

Rossen, R.D., Brewer, E.J., Sharp, R.M., Ott, J. and Templeton, J.W. (1980). Linkage of HLA to disease susceptibility locus in four families where proband presented with juvenile rheumatoid arthritis. *J. Clin. Invest.* **65**, 629–42.

Roudier, J., Petersen, J., Rhodes, G.H., Luka, J. and Carson, D.A. (1989). Susceptibility to rheumatoid arthritis maps to a T cell epitope shared by the HLA-DW4 β1 chain and the Epstein–Barr virus glycoprotein gp110. *Proc. Nat. Acad. Sci.* **86**, 5104–8.

Salmon, M., Bacon, P.A., Symmons, D.P.M. and Blann, A.D. (1985). Transferrin receptor bearing cells in the peripheral blood of patients with rheumatoid arthritis. *Clin. Exp. Immunol.* **62**, 346–52.

Scherak, O., Smolen, J.S. and Mayr, W. (1980). Rheumatoid arthritis and B lymphocyte alloantigen HLA-DRw4. *J. Rheumatol.* **7**, 9–12.

Schiff, B., Mizrachi, Y., Orgad, S., Yaron, M. and Gazit, E. (1982). Association of HLA-Aw31 and HLA-DR1 with adult rheumatoid arthritis. *Ann. Rheum. Dis.* **41**, 403–4.

Schmidt, J.A., Mizel, S.B., Cohen, D. and Green, I. (1982). Interleukin 1, a potential regulator of fibroblast proliferation. *J. Immunol.* **128**, 2177–82.

Schroeder, H.W., Jr, Hillson, J.L. and Perlmutter, R.M. (1987). Early restriction of the human antibody repertoire. *Science* **238**, 791–3.

Schumacher, H.R., Jr (1975). Synovial membrane and fluid morphologic alterations in early rheumatoid arthritis: microvascular injury and virus-like particles. *Ann. NY Acad. Sci.* **256**, 39–64.

Schumacher, H.R., Jr and Kitridou, R.C. (1972). Synovitis of recent onset: a clinicopathologic study during the first month of disease. *Arthritis Rheum.* **15**, 465–83.

Scott, D.G.I., Bacon, P.A. and Tribe, C.R. (1981). Systemic rheumatoid vasculitis: a clinical and laboratory study of 50 cases. *Medicine* **60**, 282–97.

Shah, P.D., Gilbertson, S.M. and Rowley, D.A. (1985). Dendritic cells that have interacted with antigen are targets for natural killer cells. *J. Exp. Med.* **162**, 625–36.

Shalaby, M.R. and Ammann, A.J. (1988). Suppression of immune cell function *in vitro* by recombinant human transforming growth factor-beta. *Cell. Immunol.* **112**, 343–50.

Silberstein, L.E., Jefferies, L.C., Goldman, J. *et al.* (1991). Variable region gene analysis of pathologic human autoantibodies to the related i and I red blood cell antigens. *Blood* (in press).

Silverman, G.J., Carson, D.A., Solomon, A. and Fong, S. (1986). Human kappa light chain subgroup analysis with synthetic peptide-induced antisera. *J. Immunol. Methods* **95**, 249–57.

Silverman, G.J., Carson, D.A., Patrick, K., Vaughan, J.H. and Fong, S. (1987a). Expression of a germline human kappa chain associated cross reactive idiotype after *in vitro* and *in vivo* infection with Epstein–Barr virus. *Clin. Immunol. Immunopathol.* **43**, 403–41.

Silverman, G.J., Fong, S., Chen, P.P. and Carson, D.A. (1987b). Clinical update: cross reactive idiotypes and the genetic origin of rheumatoid factors. *J. Clin. Lab. Anal.* **1**, 129–35.

Silverman, G.J., Goldfien, R.D., Chen, P. *et al.* (1988a). Idiotypic and subgroup analysis of human monoclonal rheumatoid factors: implications for structural and genetic basis of autoantibodies in humans. *J. Clin. Invest.* **82**, 469–75.

Silverman, G.J., Goni, F., Chen, P.P., Fernandez, J., Frangione, B. and Carson, D.A. (1988b). Distinct patterns of heavy chain variable region subgroup use by human monoclonal autoantibodies of different specificity. *J. Exp. Med.* **168**, 2361–6.

Silverman, G.J., Schrohenloher, R.E., Aeavitti, M.A., Koopman, W.J. and Carson, D.A. (1990). Structural characterization of the second major cross-reactive idiotype group of human rheumatoid factors. Association with the VH4 gene family. *Arthritis Rheum.* **33**, 1347–60.

Singal, D.P., Reid, B., Kassam, Y.B., D'Souza, M., Bensen, W.G. and Adachi, J.D. (1987). HLA-DQ beta-chain polymorphism in HLA-DR4 haplotypes associated with rheumatoid arthritis. *Lancet* **i**, 1118–19.

Slaughter, L., Carson, D.A., Jensen, F.C., Holbrook, T.L. and Vaughan, J.H. (1978). *In vitro* effects of Epstein–Barr virus on peripheral blood mononuclear cells from patients with rheumatoid arthritis and normal subjects. *J. Exp. Med.* **148**, 1429–34.

Smiley, J.D., Sachs, C. and Ziff, M. (1968). *In vitro* synthesis of immunoglobulin by rheumatoid synovial membrane. *J. Clin. Invest.* **47**, 624–32.

Smiley, J., Hoffman, W., Moore, S. and Paradies, L. (1985). The humoral immune response of the rheumatoid synovium. *Semin. Arthritis Rheum.* **14**, 151–62.

So, A.K.L., Warner, C.A., Sansom, D. and Walport, M.J. (1988). DQ-beta polymorphism and genetic susceptibility to Felty's syndrome. *Arthritis Rheum.* **31** (8), 990–4.

Solinger, A.M. and Stobo, J.D. (1981). Regulation of immune reactivity to collagen in human beings. *Arthritis Rheum.* **24** (8), 1057–63.

Solinger, A.M., Bhatnagar, R. and Stobo, J.D. (1981). Cellular, molecular, and genetic characteristics of T cell reactivity to collagen in man. *Proc. Nat. Acad. Sci. (USA)* **78** (6), 3877.

Solovera, J.J., Farinas, M.C. and Strober, S. (1988). Changes in B lymphocyte function in rheumatoid arthritis and lupus nephritis after total lymphoid irradiation. *Arthritis Rheum.* **31**, 1481–1.

Sowden, J.A., Roberts-Thomson, P.J. and Zola, H. (1987). Evaluation of CD5-positive B cells in blood and synovial fluid of patients with rheumatic diseases. *Rheumatol. Int.* **7**, 255–9.

Stastny, P. (1976). Mixed lymphocyte cultures in rheumatoid arthritis. *J. Clin. Invest.* **57**, 1148–57.

Stastny, P. (1978). Association of the B-cell alloantigen DRw4 with rheumatoid arthritis. *N. Engl. J. Med.* **298**, 869–71.

Stastny, P. (1980). Joint report on rheumatoid arthritis. In *Histocompatibility Testing 1980*, ed. P.I. Terasaki, p. 681, UCLA Tissue Typing Laboratory, Los Angeles, California.

Sundquist, V.A., Linde, G.A. and Wahren, B. (1984). Virus-specific immunoglobulin G subclasses in herpes simplex and varicells zoster virus infections. *J. Clin. Microbiol.* **20**, 94–8.

Swiss Federal Commission for the Rheumatoid Diseases (1981). HLA-DR antigens in rheumatoid arthritis. *Rheumatol. Int.* **1**, 111–13.

Taniguchi, O., Miyajimma, H., Hirano, T. *et al.* (1987). The Leu-1 B cell subpopulation in patients with rheumatoid arthritis. *J. Clin. Immunol.* **7**, 441–8.

Thole, J.E.R., Hindersson, P., de Bruyn, J. *et al.* (1988). Antigenic relatedness of a strongly immunogenic 65 kDa mycobacterial protein antigen with a similar sized ubiquitous bacterial common antigen. *Microbiol. Pathogenesis* **4**, 71–83.

Thompson, M. and Bywaters, E.G.L. (1962). Unilateral rheumatoid arthritis following hemiplegia. *Ann. Rheum. Dis.* **21**, 370–7.

Thomson, W., Sanders, P.A., Davis, M., Davidson, J., Dyer, P.A. and Grennan, D.M. (1988). Complement C4B-null alleles in Felty's syndrome. *Arthritis Rheum.* **31**, 984–9.

Tosato, G., Steinberg, A.D., Yarchoan, R. *et al.* (1984). Abnormally elevated frequency of Epstein–Barr virus-infected B cells in the blood of patients with rheumatoid arthritis. *J. Clin. Invest.* **73**, 1789–95.

Tuomi, T., Aho, K., Palosuo, T. *et al.* (1988). Significance of rheumatoid factors in an eight-year longitudinal study on arthritis. *Rheumatol. Int.* **8**, 21–6.

Ueno, Y., Iwaki, Y., Terasaki, P.I. *et al.* (1981). HLA-DR4 in Negro and Mexican rheumatoid arthritis patients. *J. Rheumatol.* **8**, 804–7.

Van Boxel, J.A. and Paget, S.A. (1975). Predominantly T-cell infiltrate in rheumatoid synovial membranes. *N. Engl. J. Med.* **293**, 517–20

van Eden, W., Holoshitz, J., Nevo, Z., Frenkel, A., Klajman, A. and Cohen, I.R. (1985). Arthritis induced by a T-lymphocyte clone that responds to *Mycobacterium tuberculosis* and to cartilage proteoglycans. *Proc. Nat. Acad. Sci. (USA)* **82**, 5117–20.

Van Snick, J.L., Van Roost, E., Markowetz, B., Cambiaso, C.L. and Masson, P.L. (1978). Enhancement by IgM rheumatoid factor of *in vitro* ingestion of macrophages and *in vivo* clearance of aggregated IgG or antigen–antibody complexes. *Eur. J. Immunol.* **8**, 279–85.

Van Snick, J.L., Goethals, A., Renauld, J.-C. *et al.* (1989). Cloning and characterization of a cDNA for a new mouse T cell growth factor (P40). *J. Exp. Med.* **169**, 363–8.

Vaughan, J.H. (1978). Autoimmune and histocompatibility (HLA)-associated diseases: general considerations. In *Immunological Diseases*, 3rd edn, ed. M. Samter, pp. 1029–37, Little, Brown & Company, Boston, Massachusetts.

Vaughan, J.H., Barnett, E.V., Sobel, M.V. and Jacox, R.F. (1968). Intracytoplasmic inclusions of immunoglobulins in rheumatoid arthritis and other diseases. *Arthritis Rheum.* **11**, 125–33.

Venables, P. (1988). Epstein–Barr virus infection and autoimmunity in rheumatoid arthritis. *Ann. Rheum. Dis.* **47**, 265.

Waalen, K., Farre, O. and Natvig, J.B. (1988). Dendritic cells in rheumatoid inflammation. *Springer Semin. Immunopathol.* **10**, 141–56.

Waddell, D. and Ullman, B. (1983). Characterization of a cultured human T-cell line with genetically altered ribonucleotide reductase activity. *J. Biol. Chem.* **258**, 4226.

Wahl, S.M., Hunt, D.A., Wong, H.L. *et al.* (1988). Transforming growth factor-beta is a potent immunosuppressive agent that inhibits IL-1 dependent lymphocyte proliferation. *J. Immunol.* **140**, 3026–32.

Walker, D.J., Burn, J., Griffiths, I.D., Roberts, D.F. and Stephenson, A.M. (1987). Linkage studies of HLA and rheumatoid arthritis in multicase families. *Arthritis Rheum.* **30**, 31–5.

Wallin, J., Carlsson, B., Strom, H. and Moller, E. (1988). A DR4-associated DR-DQ haplotype is significantly associated with rheumatoid arthritis. *Arthritis Rheum.* **31**, 72–9.

Wasmuth, A.G., Veale, A.M.O., Palmer, D.G. and Highton, T.C. (1972). Prevalence of rheumatoid arthritis in families. *Ann. Rheum. Dis.* **31**, 85–91.

Welch, M.J., Fong, S., Vaughan, J.H. and Carson, D.A. (1983). Increased frequency of rheumatoid factor precursor B lymphocytes after immunization of normal adults with tetanus toxoid. *Clin. Exp. Immunol.* **51**, 299–305.

Weyand, C. and Goronzy, J. (1987). Shared conformational T cell epitopes on DR-molecules of the HLA-DR1 and DR4 haplotypes associated with rheumatoid arthritis. *Arthritis Rheum.* **30**, S25.

Winchester, R.J. (1975). Characterization of IgG complexes in patients with rheumatoid arthritis. *Ann. NY Acad. Sci.* **256**, 73–81.

Winchester, R.J. and Burmester, G.R. (1981). Demonstration of Ia antigens on certain dendritic cells and on a novel elongate cell found in human synovial tissue. *Scand. J. Immunol.* **14**, 439–44.

Wood, D.D., Ihrie, E.J., Dinarello, C.A. and Cohen, P.L. (1983). Isolation of an interleukin-1-like factor from human joint effusions. *Arthritis Rheum.* **26**, 975–83.

Woodrow, T.C., Nichol, F.E. and Zaphiropoulos, G. (1981). DR antigens and rheumatoid arthritis: a study of two populations. *Br. Med. J.* **283**, 1287–8.

Woolley, D.E., Crossley, M.J. and Evanson, J.M. (1977). *Arthritis Rheum.* **20**, 1231–9.

Xu, W.-D., Firestein, G.S., Taetle, R., Kaushansky, K. and Zvaifler, N.J. (1989). Cytokines in chronic inflammatory arthritis. II. Granulocyte macrophage colony-stimulating factor (GM-CSF) in rheumatoid synovial effusions. *J. Clin. Invest.* **83**, 876–82.

Yasukawa, K., Hirano, T., Watanabe, Y. *et al.* (1987). Structure and expression of human B cell stimulatory factor-2 (BSF-2/IL-6) gene. *EMBO J.* **6**, 2939–45.

Young, C.L., Adamson, T.C., III, Vaughan, J.H. and Fox, R.I. (1984). Immunohistologic characterization of synovial membrane lymphocytes in rheumatoid arthritis. *Arthritis Rheum.* **27**, 32–9.

Yu, D.T.Y., Winchester, R.J., Fu, S.M., Gibofsky, A., Ko, H.S. and Kunkel, H.G. (1980). Ia+ cell. *J. Exp. Med.* **151**, 91.

Zoschke, D. and Segall, M. (1986). Dw subtypes of DR4 in rheumatoid arthritis: evidence for a preferential association with Dw4. *Hum. Immunol.* **15**, 118–24.

Zvaifler, N.J. (1973). The immunopathology of joint inflammation in rheumatoid arthritis. *Adv. Immunol.* **16**, 265–36.

61: Systemic Lupus Erythematosus

M.J. Walport

Introduction

The clinical manifestations of systemic lupus erythematosus (SLE) are highly variable but the unifying serological feature is the presence of autoantibodies, expressing binding reactivity to cellular antigens, including nucleic acids, molecules involved in the transcription and translation of nucleic acids, and constituents of cell membranes. Because of the great polymorphism of disease, definition of SLE in humans has depended on the application of disease classification criteria (Tan *et al*. 1982). The aetiology is unknown, although certain disease-susceptibility genes have been identified. It is likely that the causes of SLE are heterogeneous and that disease expression represents the consequences of a final common immunopathological pathway, initiated by a variety of environmental insults, combined with genes conferring susceptibility to disease. A large number of papers have described the clinical features of SLE, which fall outside the scope of this review, but a few references containing original descriptions of large series of patients are given here (Harvey *et al*. 1954; Dubois and Tuffanelli 1964; Estes and Christian 1971; Lee *et al*. 1977; Hochberg *et al*. 1985).

It is generally accepted that the clinical manifestations of SLE result from activation of inflammatory pathways as a consequence of autoimmunity. Many workers believe that immune complexes formed by autoantibodies binding to autoantigens are the main stimulus to inflammation. This view still merits critical examination and the evidence that immune complexes containing autoantibodies cause inflammation will be considered in detail below. It is noteworthy that transfusion of autoantibodies from patients with SLE into other humans does not cause disease. It is very uncommon for infants born to mothers with SLE to suffer from any clinical signs of SLE themselves, with the exceptions of congenital heart block, rashes and thrombocytopenia, which are considered below. Beck and Rowell (1963) measured the half-life of antinuclear antibodies in serum, taken serially from the infant of a mother with SLE, to be 17 days, which is similar to the half-life of normal immunoglobulin G (IgG). Infusion of plasma from patients with SLE into subjects suffering from advanced malignancies did not cause overt clinical manifestations of SLE, although the LE test became positive for 2–3 weeks after the infusions (Bencze *et al*. 1958; Marmont 1965). These data show that the presence of autoantibodies in plasma is not sufficient to cause disease.

Antigens bound by autoantibodies

The majority of autoantibodies from patients with SLE bind to nucleic acids and the proteins concerned with the intracellular transcriptional and translational machinery. Many of these autoantibodies bind to very minor intracellular components and have been extremely useful reagents for the elucidation of basic aspects of cell biology. Three complexes of nucleic acids and proteins within cells appear to provide the major antigenic stimuli for the production of autoantibodies — nucleosomes, small nuclear ribonucleoproteins (snRNP) particles and small cytoplasmic ribonucleoproteins (scRNP) (Hardin 1986). Patients usually have antibodies to one or two of these three complexes and the antibodies usually react with more than one component of each complex. This latter observation implies that the relevant immunogen may be the entire complex of nucleic acid and proteins. The antigens recognized by antinuclear antibodies have been the subject of two recent comprehensive reviews by Tan (1989a, b).

Nucleosome: nucleic acids and histones

The first, well-characterized, autoantibodies from patients with SLE were those that bound deoxyribonucleic acid (dsDNA) and histones, although these are not present in all patients. Antibodies to histones are probably responsible for the LE cell phenomenon (reviewed in Rubin and Waga 1987). Histones form the scaffolding for the supercoiling of DNA and the basic packing unit of DNA is the nucleosome, comprising 146 base pairs of dsDNA wound around an octameric core of histones (two molecules each of H2A, H2B, H3 and H4). Nucleosomes are linked by stretches of approximately 60 base pairs of DNA and tightly packed together, in part by histone protein H1, which is located outside the core. Autoantibodies are commonly found to both dsDNA and histones — an observation that has led to the hypothesis that the immunogen may be nucleosomes (Hardin and Thomas 1983).

Anti-dsDNA antibodies have been the subject of several recent reviews (Schwartz and Stollar 1985; Emlen *et al*. 1986; Zouali *et al*. 1988). nDNA exists in two major forms, bDNA with a right-handed helical structure and zDNA, rich in guanine and cytosine, with a left-handed helical structure. Autoantibodies which bind selectively to bDNA or zDNA have been found in sera from patients with SLE (Lafer *et al*. 1983). Antibodies which bind to ssDNA, synthetic polynucleotides, ribonucleic acid (ssRNA), dsRNA and polyadenosine diphosphate (ADP-ribose) are also commonly found in sera from patients (reviewed in Schwartz and Stollar 1985).

The anti-histone autoantibody response has been analysed in great detail — the C terminus of H1 and the trypsin-sensitive N terminus of H2B are the dominant antigenic determinants in SLE (Thomas *et al*. 1984; Rubin and Waga 1987). However autoantibodies may also be found to the trypsin-sensitive N and C termini of H2A and H3 and the N terminus of H4 (Thomas *et al*. 1984), and to the complex of H2A/H2B (reviewed in Rubin and Waga 1987). Autoantibodies have recently been described which bind to ubiquinated-H2A (Plaué *et al*. 1989). Immunization of rabbits with purified histones elicits a rather different antibody response, which is directed mainly against trypsin-insensitive portions of histones. A possible explanation for the difference between the autoantibody response and the antibody response to purified histones is that autoantibodies are directed against epitopes of histones which are displayed by nucleosomes (Hardin and Thomas 1983).

Small nuclear ribonucleoproteins

The snRNP complexes are a series of small RNA species, named U1 to U6 (U standing for uridine-rich) (Fig. 61.1). Each RNA is complexed to a number of proteins, which are the major targets for the anti-Sm and anti-RNP autoantibody responses (Lerner and Steitz 1979). The U RNP complexes direct the removal of introns from pre-messenger RNA (mRNA) transcripts to form mature mRNA (Lerner *et al*. 1980; Padgett *et al*. 1983). The anti-RNP response is mediated by antibody responses to the 70 kD A and C proteins, which precipitate U1 RNP alone. In contrast, anti-Sm antibodies bind the B, B′ and D proteins and precipitate U1, U2, U4/6 and U5 RNP particles. It is usual in SLE for anti-Sm to be found concurrently with anti-RNP antibodies. However, anti-RNP antibodies may be found unaccompanied by anti-Sm antibodies, often in very high titres, and are associated with a syndrome which has been called mixed connective tissue disease (MCTD) (see below).

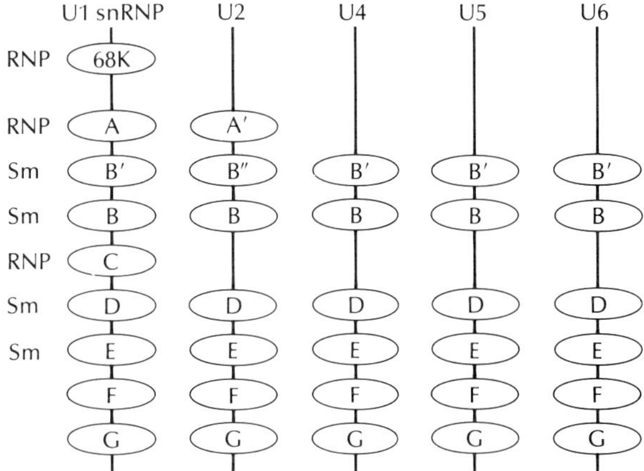

Fig. 61.1. Polypeptide binding of anti-RNP and anti-Sm.

Ro and La

Two common autoantibodies recognize the Ro and La RNP particles, which were originally identified as scRNP species, but which are also present in the nucleus. Anti-Ro and anti-La are identical with the independently described anti-SS-A (Sjögren's syndrome A) and anti-SS-B. La is a 48 kD protein that binds to a series of RNA species that are the products of RNA polymerase III. These include transfer RNA (tRNA), 5S ribosomal RNA, human cytoplasmic (hY) RNA, and U6 RNA. La protein appears to be involved in the termination of transcription (Gottlieb and Steitz 1989). A number of viral RNA species, including some from adenovirus (Lerner *et al*. 1981a) and Epstein–Barr virus (Lerner *et al*. 1981b), associate with La protein. These observations have stimulated speculation that anti-La antibody production may be stimulated by complexes of host proteins with viral DNA (Lerner *et al.* 1981b).

Anti-Ro antibodies bind to two closely related proteins of 60 and 52 kD (Venables *et al.* 1983; Ben-Chetrit *et al.* 1988) (each of which has two different isoforms expressed in erythrocytes and lymphocytes (Rader *et al.* 1989)), which bind to a series of five hY RNAs (Hendrick *et al.* 1981). The precise isoform recognized by anti-Ro antibodies varies between different patients and can be assayed by Western blotting (Rader *et al.* 1989). Antibodies reacting solely with the human Ro protein associated with the hY5 RNA have recently been described (Boire and Craft 1989). The Ro and La proteins are frequently associated in a multimolecular complex through their common binding to hY RNAs (Wolin and Steitz 1984), and this association may explain the common coexistence of anti-Ro and anti-La antibodies (Mattioli and Reichlin 1974) — further evidence that multimolecular complexes of nucleic acids and proteins may be immunogenic.

Phospholipids

Antibodies to phospholipids (reviewed in Harris *et al.* 1988; Mackworth-Young *et al.* 1989) may be identified in patients with SLE by three assays, which measure populations of antibodies with partially overlapping specificities. These are: (i) the Venereal Diseases Reference Laboratory (VDRL) reagent, developed for detection of infection by *Treponema pallidum*, which is a flocculation assay using carbon particles coated with cholesterol, lecithin (phosphatidylcholine) and cardiolipin; (ii) the lupus anticoagulant assay, a prolongation of the kaolin partial thromboplastin time (KPTT), which is not corrected by addition of normal plasma; and (iii) immunoassays using cardiolipin or another negatively charged phospholipids as antigens. The common structural denominator of the phospholipids recognized by antibodies from patients with SLE is a negatively charged phosphate group, present in cardiolipin, phosphatidic acid, phosphatidylserine and phosphatidylinositol (Harris *et al.* 1985b). Many patients with syphilis (Mouritsen *et al.* 1989) and leprosy (Furukawa *et al.* 1986) also have anti-cardiolipin antibodies, which are not associated with presence of a lupus anticoagulant (Johansson and Lassus 1974). Anti-phospholipid antibodies, when found in patients with SLE and related diseases, are associated with a range of pathology, including thrombosis and recurrent abortion (see below). However, it is not known what the binding properties of anti-phospholipid antibodies are that render them pathogenic in patients with SLE.

It was initially proposed that antibodies to dsDNA and to cardiolipin may be one and the same, an idea that came from observations of cross-reactive binding to these two antigens by monoclonal antibodies derived from mice with lupus (Lafer *et al.* 1981). However, the majority of data suggest that the high-affinity IgG anti-dsDNA and anti-cardiolipin antibodies derived from the sera of patients with SLE show very little antigenic cross-reactivity (Harris *et al.* 1985a; Eilat *et al.* 1986).

Membrane antigens

Many autoantibodies reactive with cell surfaces have been found in patients with SLE and are thought to be the main cause of leucopenia, thrombocytopenia and haemolytic anaemia, which are common features of SLE. There are only limited data on the antigens bound by these autoantibodies because many are IgM antibodies of low affinity and have been difficult to use in immunoprecipitation and immunoblotting studies. Three types of autoantibodies reacting with cell surfaces have been characterized: (i) cross-reacting antinuclear antibodies (ANA); (ii) antibodies thought to be primarily directed against cell surface antigens; and (iii) antibodies bound to cell surfaces indirectly as immune complexes attached to receptors.

CROSS-REACTING ANTINUCLEAR ANTIBODIES

The hypothesis that ANA might be pathogenic by binding to cell surface structures was supported by initial experiments which showed that antibodies derived from serum reacted with intact nucleosomes and also with cell surfaces of lymphocytes and neutrophils. It was discovered that the relevant antibody specificity was directed against histones (Rekvig and Hannestad 1980). The screening for such cross-reactivities has become easier since the advent of monoclonal antibodies. Certain monoclonal human autoantibodies, which bound DNA, were found to react as cold and warm lymphocytotoxins also (Shoenfeld *et al*. 1985). A series of studies have been reported by Jacob and his collaborators (Jacob *et al*. 1985, 1987) of monoclonal antibodies and serum-derived antibodies, from humans and mice with lupus, which bound to dsDNA and proteins on membranes of lymphocytes, erythrocytes, platelets, glomerular cells and neuronal cells. They have named the protein, which is assayed as 5 polypeptides of 14 to 34 kD, lupus-associated membrane protein (LAMP).

ANTIBODIES REACTING PRIMARILY WITH CELL SURFACE ANTIGENS

Antigens on cell surfaces which have been characterized as targets for autoantibodies in SLE include β-2-microglobulin (Revillard *et al*. 1979; Yamada *et al*. 1985); Class II major histocompatibility complex (MHC) (Okudaira *et al*. 1982); 55 kD, 70 kD and 105–110 kD antigens on T cells (Minota and Winfield 1987); different CD45 isoforms (Mimura *et al*. 1990); interleukin (IL)-2 receptor (Sano *et al*. 1986); complement receptor type 1 (CR1) (Wilson, J.G. *et al*. 1985); and DNA receptors (Bennett *et al*. 1987). Glycolipid and phospholipid antigens on cell surfaces have been much harder to characterize and their role as autoantigens in patients with SLE has not been rigorously explored.

Many cell types have been identified as possible binding sites for autoantibodies, including almost all the cellular elements of peripheral blood (reviewed by Budman and Steinberg 1977), marrow precursors (Fitchen *et al*. 1979), endothelial cells (Cines *et al*. 1984), epidermal cells (Lee *et al*. 1989) and neurones (reviewed in Zvaifler and Bluestein 1982; How *et al*. 1985). Many anti-cell surface antibodies may cross-react with a number of different cell types, for example some anti-lymphocyte antibodies also bound to neuronal cells (Bluestein and Zvaifler 1976; Bresnihan *et al*. 1979).

RECEPTOR-MEDIATED BINDING OF AUTOANTIBODIES TO CELLS

Fc and complement receptors on many cell types are implicated in the clearance of immune complexes. Erythrocytes and platelets bind, but do not internalize, immune complexes, and complexes attached to these cells may mediate clearance of cells as well as immune complexes in the fixed mononuclear phagocytic system. There is little evidence that this is an important cause of red cell turnover in patients with SLE, but it is possible that some of the thrombocytopenia is due to this cause. A possible role for DNA receptors, present on most leucocytes, in localizing DNA–anti-DNA immune complexes to cell surfaces has been explored by Bennett and his co-workers (1985, 1986).

Cytoskeletal proteins

The cytoskeleton comprises: (i) three types of filaments: microfilaments, containing actin; microtubules, containing tubulin; and intermediate filaments, comprising vimentin, prekeratin, desmin, glial filaments and neurofilaments; and (ii) anchoring structures, such as centrioles and centromeres. Autoantibodies to many of the proteins of the cytoskeleton have been described and show little disease specificity (reviewed in Senecal *et al*. 1985). Approximately 50% of patients with SLE have been found to have autoantibodies that react with intermediate filaments (Senecal *et al*. 1985), in particular vimentin (Alcover *et al*. 1984), and a smaller number have antibodies to microfilaments (Senecal *et al*. 1985). Antibodies to two of three proteins comprising the tissue-specific intermediate filaments, neurofilaments, have been correlated with the presence of central nervous system (CNS) disease (Robbins *et al*. 1988) (see below). Many monoclonal human autoantibodies show cross-reactive binding to DNA and cytoskeletal proteins, but about 40% of monoclonal antibodies with anti-cytoskeletal activity do not bind DNA (Senecal and Rauch 1988).

Heat-shock proteins

A great deal of attention has been paid recently to autoimmune responses to heat-shock proteins (HSP), a heterogeneous group of highly conserved intracellular proteins (Lindquist 1986), expressed in all cells and increased at sites of inflammation (Polla 1988). Cell-mediated responses to HSP with similar structures in prokaryotes and eukaryotes have been found in patients with rheumatoid arthritis and reactive arthritis (see chapter 60).

Autoantibody responses to three HSP have been described in patients with SLE: to ubiquitin (Muller *et al.* 1988); to the constitutively expressed 73 kD protein of the HSP70 family of molecules (Minota *et al.* 1988a); and to HSP90 (Minota *et al.* 1988b).

Other antigens

PROLIFERATING CELL NUCLEAR ANTIGEN

Autoantibodies are found in 3% of patients with SLE to an antigen named proliferating cell nuclear antigen (PCNA) because of its variation in expression during the cell cycle (Miyachi *et al.* 1978). This antigen was found to be identical with the protein cyclin (Mathews *et al.* 1984), independently named for a similar reason. The antigen has recently been characterized as DNA polymerase-δ auxiliary protein (Bravo *et al.* 1987; Prelich *et al.* 1987), whose function is necessary for DNA synthesis and progression through the cell cycle.

KU

The Ku autoantigen comprises two proteins of 70 kD and 80 kD which bind to the ends of dsDNA (Mimori and Hardin 1986). Autoantibodies to this antigen have been found amongst a subset of patients with a scleroderma–polymyositis overlap syndrome (Mimori *et al.* 1981) and in between 10% (Francoeur *et al.* 1986) and 40% (Reeves 1985) of patients with SLE. The physiological activity of these proteins has not been elucidated, although it has been suggested that they may play a role in the repair of DNA. Anti-Ku antibodies inhibit the binding of the protein complex to DNA (Mimori and Hardin 1986). The 70 kD protein has recently been cloned (Reeves and Sthoeger 1989) and has similarities with other DNA-binding proteins.

RIBOSOMAL PHOSPHOPROTEINS

About 12% of patients with SLE have antibodies reactive with a shred epitope on the C terminus of three phosphoproteins (P proteins), P0, P1 and P2, of the 60S large ribosomal subunit (Bonfa and Elkon 1986; Elkon *et al.* 1986). Presence of these antibodies was correlated with the presence of anti-Sm antibodies, but this was not explained by a shared epitope (Elkon *et al.* 1989).

POLY(ADENOSINE DIPHOSPHATE-RIBOSE) POLYMERASE

The enzyme, poly(ADP-ribose) polymerase, catalyses poly(ADP-ribosyl)ation of many proteins, including some important in DNA repair (reviewed in Ueda and Hayaishi 1985). Autoantibodies to this enzyme (Yamanaka *et al.* 1988) and to poly(ADP-ribose) (Kanai *et al.* 1977) are present in some patients with SLE.

Antigens in drug-induced lupus

The characteristic autoantibody response in lupus induced by hydralazine or procainamide is to histones (reviewed in Rubin and Waga 1987). Procainamide-induced disease is associated with anti-H1 and anti-H2A/H2B antibodies, which are predominantly IgM (Gohill *et al.* 1985), and hydralazine-induced lupus with anti-H3 and anti-H4 antibodies (Portanova *et al.* 1987). In contrast to idiopathic SLE, where the histone epitopes are trypsin-sensitive, in both procainamide- and hydralazine-induced disease the epitopes on the histones are resistant to trypsin (Portanova *et al.* 1987). It was argued above that the antibody response in SLE is dictated by the conformation of histones in the nucleosome. The observation that different epitopes are bound in drug-induced compared with idiopathic disease implies that histones may be presented to the immune system in different configurations.

Epitopes on autoantigens

Analysis of the epitopes within self proteins that function as autoantigens might help to explain the mechanisms of autoimmunity. The autoantibody response of rabbits immunized with rabbit cytochrome c in Freund's adjuvant was directed to three major epitopes, located in regions of the molecule which showed considerable sequence variability when compared with other mammalian cytochrome c molecules (Jemmerson and Margoliash 1979). This observation led to formulation of a hypothesis of evolving tolerance of the immune system to self — i.e. no immunity should arise against ancient structural portions of molecules; but, in contrast, newly evolved structures could act as autoimmunity epitopes (Jemmerson and Margoliash 1979).

An interesting feature of autoantibodies found in patients with SLE and related diseases is the almost total violation of this hypothesis; in fact, the most conserved structures within autoantigens often appear to be the most antigenic. A few examples that demonstrate this are: (i) anti-histone autoantibodies bound chicken histones (Thomas *et al.* 1984); (ii) anti-ribosomal P protein antibodies bound to the P proteins of a brine shrimp, *Artemia salina* (Elkon *et al.* 1988); and (iii) anti-Sm and anti-RNP antibodies immunoprecipitated snRNPs from frogs and arthropods (Lerner and Steitz 1979). There are exceptions: certain antibodies to Ro react with the Ro protein of the hY5 RNA complex, but not with Ro proteins from other species (Boire and Craft 1989). It may not be a general rule that antibody responses following immunization are directed against non-conserved epitopes: Elkon and colleagues (1988) found that immunization of mice with chicken ribosomes gave rise to an antibody response to ribosomal P proteins that mimicked the autoimmune response, with recognition of conserved sequences.

A further observation that illustrates the general rule that autoantibodies bind determinants that are conserved throughout phylogeny is that autoantibodies frequently inhibit a major functional activity of their antigens, usually a property of a structural element that is conserved. Examples that illustrate this are: (i) the binding of Ku proteins to DNA by anti-Ku (Mimori and Hardin 1986); (ii) aminoacylation by anti-aminoacyl tRNA synthetase enzymes (Bunn *et al.* 1986); and (iii) pre-mRNA splicing by anti-Sm and anti-RNP antibodies (Padgett *et al.* 1983). Functional activity is usually located within conserved domains of proteins. Such inhibition is a useful attribute of the autoantibody to the cell biologist, probably irrelevant to the pathogenesis of disease (as antibodies cannot penetrate viable cells), and an unexplained enigma to those interested in the origin of the autoantibody response.

The nature of autoantibodies in systemic lupus erythematosus

There are a number of important questions about the nature of the autoantibodies from patients with SLE: (i) What are the germline genes that encode them and do these show inherited polymorphisms? (ii) How much somatic mutation is contained in rearranged autoantibody genes? (iii) Are autoantibodies produced by a distinct lineage of B lymphocytes? (iv) What are the idiotypic relationships between autoantibodies?

The development of monoclonal antibodies and simplification of techniques for sequencing of immunoglobulin genes has allowed these questions to be addressed and some preliminary answers are available. However, the progress of such studies in humans has been limited by two major impediments: (i) suitable fusion partners for the production of human monoclonal antibodies have been elusive; and (ii) it is not certain that the human monoclonal antibodies that have been produced are representative of the B cell repertoire as a whole.

Monoclonal autoantibodies

The most striking feature of many of the monoclonal autoantibodies that have been derived from mice and humans with lupus is their polyreactivity. For example, monoclonal anti-DNA antibodies derived from mice cross-reacted with a range of synthetic polynucleotides and with phospholipids (Lafer *et al.* 1981). Large numbers of similar monoclonal antibodies derived from humans have been characterized and have been designated 'natural' autoantibodies by some authors. These show wide cross-reactivity to autoantigens, including DNA and many cytoskeletal proteins, and have a high precursor rate in the spleens of neonatal animals (Dighiero *et al.* 1985) and in peripheral blood lymphocytes of normal humans (Seigneurin *et al.* 1988). Many of these antibodies also bind to surface structures on bacteria; for example, a Waldenstrom's IgM-λ reacted with capsular polysaccharides of group B meningococci and *Escherichia coli* and also bound to a variety of polynucleotides (Kabat *et al.* 1986); several murine monoclonal anti-dsDNA antibodies cross-reacted with *Streptococcus faecalis* (Carroll *et al.* 1985).

Many patients with SLE have anti-dsDNA, anticardiolipin and anticytoskeletal antibodies. A hypothesis was therefore formulated that polyreactive monoclonal antibodies were representative of the autoantibodies found *in vivo* in patients with SLE and that the spectrum of autoantigens in the disease might be explained by their possession of cross-reacting epitopes.

Unfortunately there are major flaws in this

attractive hypothesis. These have been revealed by detailed studies of the binding characteristics of polyclonal autoantibodies derived from sera from patients with SLE. These antibodies bind to their antigens with high affinity and do not show the same cross-reactivities as monoclonal autoantibodies; for example, anti-dsDNA and anti-cardiolipin antibodies from patients are not usually cross-reactive (Harris *et al.* 1985a,b; Eilat *et al.* 1986). Additional evidence that polyreactive autoantibodies are not directly pathogenic came from the observation that, despite the finding of polyreactive anti-DNA antibodies in sera from patients with SLE, antibodies eluted from renal biopsies bound monospecifically to DNA (Matsiota *et al.* 1987). However, these observations do not exclude the possibility that cross-reactive autoantibodies may represent the precursors of mature, high-affinity, non-cross-reactive autoantibodies, and evidence in favour of this hypothesis is presented below.

The interpretation of many of the studies demonstrating wide antigenic cross-reactivity of monoclonal antibodies is subject to an important additional caveat. Enzyme-linked immunosorbent assays performed using concentrations of 3–10 μg/ml of hybridoma-derived monoclonal antibody may measure binding affinities as low as 2×10^4 M^{-1}, which are likely to be of no physiological consequence. Klinman and colleagues (1988) demonstrated that antigen-specific anti-phosphorylcholine antibodies (which bind to phosphorylcholine with an affinity of 10^7 M^{-1}) showed the same type of low-affinity cross-reactions to a panel of autoantigens as a group of monoclonal autoantibodies. However, a small number of IgG monoclonal autoantibodies have been characterized which bind to their cognate antigens with high affinity and do not cross-react with other autoantigens (Nakamura *et al.* 1988). These may be representative of the autoantibodies associated with disease pathogenesis.

Cellular origins of autoantibodies

Much attention has focused on B cells bearing the CD5 surface antigen as a source of autoantibodies (reviewed in Hayakawa and Hardy 1988). CD5 +ve B lymphocytes are prominent early in development and represent up to 75% of B lymphocytes in umbilical cord blood (Hardy *et al.* 1987), compared with ~20% in peripheral blood from adults (Casali *et al.* 1987; Hardy *et al.* 1987). Lymphocytes of this phenotype appear to be the commonest source of monoclonal autoantibodies which show cross-reactive binding. These include rheumatoid factors (Casali *et al.* 1987; Hardy *et al.* 1987), anti-ssDNA (Casali *et al.* 1987) and anti-phosphatidylcholine antibodies (Mercolino *et al.* 1988). Chronic lymphatic leukaemia is a tumour of CD5 +ve B lymphocytes (reviewed in Hayakawa and Hardy 1988), and 50% or more of these were found to produce antibodies reactive with IgG, ss- or ds-DNA (Sthoeger *et al.* 1989). It is not known for certain whether CD5 +ve B lymphocytes are a separate lineage of B lymphocytes or whether they are a stage in the maturation of mature B cells. Some evidence from studies of mice favours the former explanation whilst some evidence from studies in humans supports the latter hypothesis (Caligaris-Cappio *et al.* 1989). Immunoglobulin M anti-tetanus toxoid production was limited to CD5 +ve B cells, whereas IgG anti-tetanus toxoid was produced by CD5 −ve B lymphocytes (Casali and Notkins 1989).

Idiotypic and genetic analysis of autoantibodies

Estimates may be made of the relationships between antibodies by measurements of idiotypic cross-reactivity. A number of anti-idiotypic antibodies to autoantibodies have been characterized which show interesting patterns of cross-reactivity. One such is an antibody to an idiotype named 16/6, raised originally to an anti-ssDNA monoclonal antibody derived from a patient with SLE (Shoenfeld *et al.* 1983). Anti-16/6 antibodies bind to anti-dsDNA antibodies in humans (Madaio *et al.* 1986), but also bind to antibodies with other antigenic specificities, including antibodies which bind to RNP, Sm and Ro (Kaburaki and Stollar 1987) and to bacteria, such as *Klebsiella* (Naparstek *et al.* 1985). A possible role for 16/6-bearing antibodies in the pathogenesis of SLE was implied by detection of 16/6 +ve material in biopsies from inflamed kidneys (Isenberg and Collins 1985). Two 16/6 +ve DNA-binding monoclonal antibodies were sequenced and found to be encoded by identical heavy-chain variable (V_H) genes (Dersimonian *et al.* 1987); this gene was almost identical to the published sequence of a germline V_H gene, VH26 (Matthyssens and Rabbitts 1980). Other cross-reactive idiotypes have been described on anti-DNA antibodies (Solomon *et al.* 1983), including one that is present on human and murine anti-DNA antibodies (Eilat *et al.* 1985).

Similar idiotypic relationships have been described for anti-Sm antibodies; the Y2 idiotype, present on a murine anti-Sm antibody, was expressed on murine and human anti-Sm antibodies, and on antibodies which did not bind to Sm from SLE patients (Takei *et al.* 1987). A closely related idiotype, 4B4, was defined on a human, Y2 +ve, monoclonal anti-Sm antibody (Takei *et al.* 1988), and the V_H sequence of this antibody (Sanz *et al.* 1989) was identical to a previously published germline V_H sequence (Schroeder *et al.* 1987).

Polyreactive autoantibodies may be the precursors of antibodies to foreign antigens

The finding that germline V genes encode antibodies with broadly cross-reactive binding, which includes binding to bacteria, is not surprising on teleological grounds. It might be expected that the inherited antibody repertoire is directed against common, environmental, pathogenic bacteria. It has been shown that such polyreactive antibodies may be the precursors of high-affinity antibodies selected by injection of foreign antigens such as the hapten, *p*-azophenyl arsonate (Naparstek *et al.* 1986). It has similarly been shown, by analysis of anti-dsDNA monoclonal autoantibodies from mice, that autoantibodies appear to undergo affinity maturation by the process of somatic mutation (Shlomchik *et al.* 1987). Antibodies to phosphoryl choline are encoded by germline immunoglobulin genes in mice; it was observed that a murine anti-DNA antibody differed by a single amino acid from an anti-phosphorylcholine antibody (Eilat *et al.* 1984). Mutation at a single point in a myeloma protein converted it from a phosphorylcholine-binding to a DNA- and cardiolipin-binding antibody (Diamond and Scharff 1984).

The autoantibody response is driven by antigen

The majority of the evidence from humans with SLE shows that autoantibody production is stimulated by antigen, and there are experimental findings which show that unselective activation of B lymphocytes does not occur (Gharavi *et al.* 1988). The data showing that autoantibody production is stimulated by antigen are as follows: (i) individual autoantibodies form a disproportionately large fraction of total immunoglobulins present in patients' sera — up to 30 g/litre of anti-Ro (Harley *et al.* 1986), 8 g/litre of anti-RNP (Maddison and Reichlin 1977) and 15 g/litre of anti-Sm (Eisenberg *et al.* 1985); (ii) autoantibodies are polyclonal and their immunoglobulin class and subclass distribution is similar to that following immunization; (iii) diverse epitopes are recognized on target autoantigens, again as seen following immunization with exogenous antigen; and (iv) some autoantigens are immunogenic in experimental systems.

The autoantibody response to individual autoantigens is polyclonal

A characteristic of antibody production stimulated by antigen is that the response is polyclonal, which appears to be the case for the majority of autoantibodies in SLE. Autoantibodies to Sm, RNP, Ro and La have been shown to be polyclonal, using the technique to isoelectric focusing (Eisenberg *et al.* 1985). A possible exception appears to be anti-dsDNA antibodies, which were predominantly monoclonal or biclonal in 15 of 20 patients (Stott *et al.* 1986). Similarly, in mice the anti-dsDNA response was found to be predominantly oligoclonal, with clonal expansion associated with ageing, the latter a characteristic expected of an antigen-driven response.

Diverse epitopes are recognized by autoantibodies

The observation that multiple, non-cross-reactive, epitopes are recognized on autoantigens is in favour of an antigen-driven antibody response. Two distinct epitopes in La (Chan *et al.* 1986) and PCNA (Ogata *et al.* 1987) for the binding of lupus autoantibodies were demonstrated, using peptides which were derived from these proteins by digestion with V8 protease. Elkon and colleagues (1988) mapped in great detail, using synthetic peptides, epitopes on ribosomal P2 protein bound by lupus autoantibodies and found considerable variation in the fine specificity of binding between different sera. A rapidly increasing number of autoantigens have recently become available which have been prepared by recombinant technology, and these have been used for epitope mapping of autoantibodies. The recognition of multiple epitopes appears to be a general rule and has been shown, using the following recombinant proteins: PCNA, Ku, La, U1 RNP (68/70 kD), Sm B′/B, histidyl-tRNA synthetase and CENP-B (reviewed in Huff *et al.* 1990).

Autoantigens are immunogenic

The hypothesis that the autoimmune response in SLE is driven by antigen leads to the prediction that the autoantigens should themselves be immunogenic. This has proved extremely difficult to demonstrate in the case of nDNA. It has not been possible to directly immunize normal mice or lupus-prone mice with nDNA and to obtain anti-nDNA antibodies resembling those found in disease (Steinberg *et al.* 1971; Stollar 1981; Madaio *et al.* 1984). Synthetic polynucleotides and denatured DNA, in contrast to nDNA, stimulate strong immune responses against their cognate antigens, but, even when these are administered to lupus-prone mice, do not stimulate an anti-nDNA response (Madaio *et al.* 1984). The majority of workers who have attempted to immunize animals with DNA have used purified nDNA, and it may be that this is the wrong form of antigen. There is a moderately strong association between the presence of anti-nDNA antibodies and anti-histone autoantibodies (Hardin and Thomas 1983), which has stimulated speculation that it is the entire nucleosome that may be immunogenic (reviewed in Hardin 1986; Fournie 1988).

Autoantibodies to RNP antigens have been easier to generate. Monoclonal and polyclonal autoantibodies to Ro and La (Bachmann *et al.* 1986) and to Sm and RNP (Reuter and Luhrmann 1986) have been obtained by immunization of normal mice with purified antigens. Similarly it was shown that immunization of young MRL mice with Sm antigen induced an anti-Sm response resembling the spontaneous anti-Sm antibodies that these mice develop later in life (Shores *et al.* 1986).

Immunity to foreign antigens in systemic lupus erythematosus

Humoral immunity

The antibody response to foreign antigens is normal or slightly reduced in patients with SLE. A slightly reduced primary response to *Brucella* was found, together with lower levels of naturally occurring antibodies to *E. coli*, compared with control subjects (Baum and Ziff 1969). Pre- and post-immunization titres to influenza vaccine were slightly reduced in one study (Williams *et al.* 1978), but normal in another (Brodman *et al.* 1978), and there were very similar findings of slightly reduced response to immunization with tetanus toxoid (Sarkany 1961; Abe and Homma 1971). Disease activity did not increase after immunization with influenza vaccine (Williams *et al.* 1978).

Cell-mediated immunity

There is a consensus that cutaneous, cell-mediated, responses to delayed-type hypersensitivity (DTH) antigens are reduced in patients with active SLE. Cutaneous anergy to purified protein derivative (PPD) alone (Block *et al.* 1968), PPD and *Trichophyton* (Hahn *et al.* 1973) and to a whole panel of DTH antigens (Horwitz 1972) were described. Delayed-type hypersensitivity responses improved after treatment of disease (Rosenthal and Franklin 1975) and the degree of impairment of reactivity correlated with disease activity (Horwitz and Cousar 1975).

Pathophysiology of disease

Do autoantibodies cause disease?

Although autoantibodies are the most striking immunological feature of SLE, their role in causing disease is not established beyond all doubt. Transfer of disease across the placenta is the strongest evidence that IgG antibodies cause disease in humans, e.g. neonatal myasthenia gravis. However, neonatal lupus (see below) is uncommon (prevalence of less than 5%) and has restricted features — a rash resembling that of subacute cutaneous lupus erythematosus (SCLE), congenital heart block, leucopenia and occasional thrombocytopenia or haemolytic anaemia. The autoantibodies most strongly associated with the first two of these abnormalities are anti-Ro and anti-La, usually in association with anti-La, and, very occasionally, solely anti-U1 RNP antibodies have been found (Provost *et al.* 1987). No disease has been attributed to the transfer of anti-DNA antibodies across the placenta, and nephritis is not a feature of neonatal lupus.

Transfusion of plasma from patients with SLE into patients with terminal malignancies was not followed (fortunately) by any adverse effects, although LE cells were detectable in recipient blood for up to 3 weeks (Bencze *et al.* 1958; Marmont 1965). Despite evidence of certain ANA cross-reacting with cell surface components *in vitro* (see above), this may not occur to any significant effect *in vivo*. Antinuclear antibodies were observed to clear from the circulation of an infant born to a mother with SLE with the half-life of normal IgG (Beck and Rowell 1963), showing no evidence of accelerated clearance of antibody. These data imply that, in normal subjects, antigen is not available to the majority of autoantibodies in the extracellular fluid. The normal growth of cells *in vitro* in medium supplemented with sera from patients with SLE (Lachmann 1961) suggests that autoantibodies cannot penetrate into the cytoplasm of living cells. Two exceptions to this have been reported. Alarcon-Segovia and colleagues (1978) found that anti-RNP antibodies from patients with MCTD could enter Fc_γ receptor-bearing T cells and inhibit their activity. These observations were not confirmed by another group (Okudaira *et al.* 1982b), who did, however, find that immunoglobulins could penetrate viable lymphocytes via a route independent of Fc receptors. This material was correlated with the presence of lymphocytotoxic antibodies.

Anti-deoxyribonucleic acid antibodies

The probable role of anti-DNA antibodies in causing disease has recently been reviewed (Fournie 1988). Deoxyribonucleic acid and anti-DNA antibodies were found in renal tissue (Koffler *et al.* 1967; Krishnan and Kaplan 1967) and in skin (Tan and Kunkel 1966; Landry and Sams 1973). Anti-DNA antibodies could be eluted from renal tissue (Krishnan and Kaplan 1967) and were concentrated compared with their levels in serum (Koffler *et al.* 1967). Most workers found correlations between the levels in sera of antibodies to dsDNA and disease activity, in both cross-sectional and longitudinal studies, although almost everyone identified some patients with very high levels of anti-dsDNA and apparently inactive disease and vice versa (Schur and Sandson 1968; Pincus *et al.* 1969; Bardana *et al.* 1975; Cameron *et al.* 1976).

It remains unclear how anti-dsDNA antibodies localize to tissues and several possibilities have been considered: (i) that complexes comprising anti-dsDNA/dsDNA are deposited from plasma; (ii) that dsDNA is deposited in tissues and immune complexes form *in situ* (Izui *et al.* 1976); and (iii) that anti-dsDNA antibodies bind to other cross-reacting antigens in tissues, such as LAMP, (Jacob *et al.* 1985, 1987), or proteoglycan heparan sulphate, which is a normal constituent of glomerular basement membrane (Faaber *et al.* 1984).

The occurrence in plasma of patients with SLE of immune complexes containing DNA and anti-dsDNA is controversial. Both DNA and anti-dsDNA antibodies were identified in sera and plasma by Tan and colleagues (1966). DNA and anti-dsDNA were both identified as constituents of cryoglobulins (Davis, J.S. *et al.* 1978; Adu *et al.* 1981). Treatment of plasma with deoxyribonuclease (DNase) caused an increase in the levels of measurable anti-dsDNA antibodies (Harbeck *et al.* 1973). However, this observation cannot be reconciled easily with the more recent observation that anti-dsDNA antibodies may protect short stretches of complexed DNA from digestion with DNase (Burdick and Emlen 1985). Others have failed to find DNA/anti-dsDNA immune complexes in sera from patients (Izui *et al.* 1977). Difficulty in the demonstration of such immune complexes in the circulation either may reflect their very rapid transit time, which has been demonstrated experimentally in mice (Emlen and Mannik 1982), or alternatively may indicate that such immune complexes form *in situ*.

The pathogenicity of anti-dsDNA antibodies (reviewed by Hahn 1982) has been correlated with IgG class and the ability to fix complement (Rothfield and Stollar 1967; Tojo and Friou 1968; Sontheimer and Gilliam 1978). The avidity and charge of anti-dsDNA antibodies may also be important. Antibodies of high avidity were eluted from renal tissue of patients with active nephritis, although serum antibodies from the same subjects were of low avidity, suggesting selective renal binding (Winfield *et al.* 1977). Another study failed to find significant correlation between the avidity of circulating anti-dsDNA antibodies and the presence of renal disease (Tron and Bach 1977).

There have been several studies of whether increased pathogenicity of anti-dsDNA antibodies may be related to alkaline pI. Glomerular basement membrane bears fixed, negatively charged (anionic) sites, particularly sulphated glycosaminoglycans containing heparan sulphate, and these may hinder the passage through basement membrane of cationic molecules. Immune complexes containing cationic immunoglobulins or antigens were found to selectively deposit in subepithelial and subendothelial sites in glomeruli of mice (Gallo *et al.* 1981). Serum anti-dsDNA antibodies had a broad spread of pI with a tendency towards high pI amongst mice of different strains with SLE, but anti-dsDNA antibodies eluted from renal tissue were concentrated in the high pI range (Ebling and Hahn 1980). However, Yoshida and colleagues (1985) found no correlation between the pI range of serum anti-dsDNA antibodies in mice and the presence of renal disease. Although there was a predominance of alkaline bands amongst anti-dsDNA antibodies derived from human serum (Fischbach *et al.* 1981), there was no link between high pI and the presence of nephritis.

Anti-phospholipid antibodies

These antibodies are associated with an unusual spectrum of pathology — recurrent venous and arterial thromboses, spontaneous abortions (often in the second trimester), thrombocytopenia and haemolytic anaemia (reviewed in Harris *et al.* 1988). Their causal role in these events is far from proved and a number of hypotheses are being pursued. The interference of these antibodies with tests of coagulation *in vitro* implied the possibility of a similar interaction *in vivo*. Anti-phospholipid antibodies inhibit coagulation *in vitro* by interfering with the binding of vitamin K-dependent coagulation proteins to the phospholipid component of the prothrombin activator complex. This inhibition can be overcome by the use of platelets as a source of phospholipid and anti-phospholipid antibodies are correlated *in vivo* with thrombosis, rather than anticoagulation. It has been proposed that anti-phospholipid antibodies may promote thrombosis by: (i) binding and activating platelets; (ii) binding to endothelium and inhibiting prostacyclin release (Carreras and Vermylen 1982); and (iii) inhibiting the interactions of thrombomodulin and protein C, thereby inhibiting fibrinolysis (Freyssinet and Cazenave 1987). However there has been no convincing demonstration of the binding of anti-phospholipid antibodies to any intact cell membrane, and conflicting results have been obtained pertaining to the other possible modes of action of these antibodies *in vivo* (Hasselaar *et al.* 1988; Coade *et al.* 1989).

Lymphocytotoxins and disordered immunoregulation

LYMPHOCYTOTOXINS

It was discovered during the screening of sera for alloreactive antibodies to human leucocyte antigen (HLA) products that cold-reactive lymphocytotoxic autoantibodies were common in sera from patients with SLE (Mittal *et al.* 1970; Terasaki *et al.* 1970). In addition to complement-mediated cell lysis, these antibodies were shown to cause antigenic modulation at 37°C (Winfield *et al.* 1986). The presence of cold-reactive lymphocytotoxins was correlated with lymphopenia, predominantly of T cells (Messner *et al.* 1973), disease activity and reduced C3 levels (Butler *et al.* 1972).

Warm-reactive IgG autoantibodies to lymphocytes have also been characterized (Wernet and Kunkel 1973; Sagawa and Abdou 1979). These were able to mediate antibody-dependent cell-mediated cytotoxicity (ADCC) against T lymphocytes (Kumagai *et al.* 1981). Certain IgG lymphocytotoxic antibodies reacted with activation antigens expressed only on lymphocytes treated with mitogens (Litvin *et al.* 1983).

Observations were made in parallel with the characterization of normal subsets of T and B lymphocytes that anti-lymphocyte autoantibodies showed restricted specificities. Depression of CD4 and CD8 subsets of lymphocytes has been identified. Antibodies were characterized that reacted with 'suppressor' T lymphocytes identified by function (Sagawa and Abdou 1979; Sakane *et al.* 1979), the presence of Fc_{γ} receptors (Fauci *et al.* 1978) and CD8 (Morimoto *et al.* 1980). Similarly, reduction has been observed in peripheral blood of CD4 +ve (Winfield *et al.* 1987) and of CD4 +ve, CD45R +ve 'suppressor−inducer' T cells (Morimoto *et al.* 1987; Tanaka *et al.* 1989). There was a correlation between the ratio *in vivo* of CD4 +ve to CD8 +ve T cells and the reactivity *in vitro* of cold-reactive lymphocytotoxic antibodies reactive with these lymphocyte subsets (Morimoto *et al.* 1984). It has recently been found that certain IgM cold lymphocytotoxins have specificity for different isoforms of CD45 (Mimura *et al.* 1990).

Data have been presented showing a correlation between the pattern of lymphopenia and the clinical expression of SLE. Reduced CD4 : CD8 ratio was correlated with severe renal disease and thrombocytopenia, increased CD4 : CD8 ratio with multisystem disease and lymphadenopathy, and a normal ratio with the most severe pattern of disease (Smolen *et al.* 1982).

IMMUNOREGULATORY ABNORMALITIES

Lymphocytotoxic antibodies are associated with lymphopenia *in vivo*, which in turn can be correlated with abnormalities of immunological function *in vitro*. These abnormalities include: (i) decreased suppressor function (Abdou *et al.* 1976; Bresnihan and Jasin 1977; Sakane *et al.* 1978a); (ii) increased spontaneous production of IgG by B cells (Jasin and Ziff 1975; Abdou *et al.* 1976; Budman *et al.* 1977), and a decreased response to pokeweed mitogen (Fauci *et al.* 1978; Ginsburg *et al.* 1979); (iii) decreased autologous mixed lymphocyte responses (Sakane *et al.* 1978b); (iv) decreased helper cell activity (Delfraissy *et al.* 1980); (v) reduced T cell cytotoxicity in assays of cytotoxic T lymphocytes (CTL) (Charpentier *et al.* 1979) and ADCC (Schneider *et al.* 1975; Scheinberg and Cathcart 1976); and (vi) increased numbers of spontaneously activated circulating T cells (Yu *et al.* 1980). However, it remains quite uncertain whether these abnormalities have any causal role in the pathogenesis of SLE. It is possible that deficiency of T cell 'suppressor' activity, induced by autoantibodies, could allow polyclonal activation of B lymphocytes. It is equally plausible that the changes in lymphocytes are secondary to autoantibodies produced as part of the disease process and are irrelevant to the pathogenesis of SLE. The truth may lie somewhere in between.

Other autoantibodies

The role of other autoantibodies in the mediation of inflammation in patients with SLE is very uncertain. In order to cause damage, the relevant antigen must be exposed on cell surfaces or released from dying tissue and participate in the extracellular formation of immune complexes. The association of anti-Ro and anti-La antibodies with neonatal lupus is persuasive evidence that they, or an unidentified associated autoantibody, directly mediate pathology. There is evidence for the expression on cell surfaces of Ro (LeFeber *et al.* 1984), reviewed below. Anti-Ro antibodies were enriched compared with serum in eluates from kidneys of two patients who died of SLE with nephritis (Maddison and Reichlin 1979). There is no unequivocal evidence for the participation in inflammation of other autoantibodies, such as anti-RNP and anti-Sm.

Immune complexes

Systemic lupus erythematosus is often considered to be the prototype of a disease mediated by immune complexes. Many tests to identify soluble immune complexes in serum and plasma have been devised and sera from patients with lupus almost invariably provide a test bed for such assays. The results of immune complex assays up to 1979 were reviewed comprehensively by Theofilopoulos and Dixon (1979). Probable circulating immune complexes were first detected in sera from patients with SLE as cryoglobulins, containing IgG, IgM and complement proteins (Christian *et al.* 1963; Hanauer and Christian 1967a). The identification of the specificity of antibodies and antigens within such cryoglobulins has been difficult, and the presence (Davis, J.S. *et al.* 1978; Adu *et al.* 1981) or absence of DNA (Stastny and Ziff 1969; Izui *et al.* 1977) remains controversial.

The ability of C1q and rheumatoid factors to bind aggregated IgG has been used by many workers to study immune complexes. Using a fluid-phase C1q-binding assay, there were correlations between immune complex levels and serum complement levels and between disease activity and levels of anti-DNA antibodies (Nydegger *et al.* 1974; Zubler *et al.* 1976). Similar correlations were reported for the solid-phase C1q-binding assay (Hay *et al.* 1976; Abrass *et al.* 1980; Tung *et al.* 1981). However, there was a poor correlation between fluid-phase and solid-phase C1q-binding assays (Abrass *et al.* 1980). Agnello and colleagues (1971) found that C1q precipitins in sera from lupus patients were of high (18S) and low (7S) molecular weight. The existence of C1q-binding material with a sedimentation coefficient of monomeric IgG was confirmed by later workers (Robinson *et al.* 1979; Tung *et al.* 1981). This raised the suspicion that such material might represent autoantibodies to C1q, which has recently been confirmed (Antes *et al.* 1988; Uwatoko and Mannik 1988). It appears that the majority of the IgG binding to C1q in the solid phase may be explained by autoantibodies to the collagenous portion of C1q (Wener *et al.* 1989).

Other assays for immune complexes have suffered from artefacts. The Raji cell assay (Theofilopoulos *et al.* 1976), dependent on binding of immune complexes to Fc receptors and CR2, may yield false positives due to antibodies to Raji cells (Anderson and Stillman 1980). Possibly the most reliable assays for immune complexes are those that detect combinations of neo-antigens of complement proteins and immunoglobulins, such as the conglutinin assay (Casali *et al.* 1977; Eisenberg *et al.* 1977) and more recent assays using monoclonal antibodies to neo-antigens expressed in C3b, iC3b and C3dg (Aguado *et al.* 1985). These assays all produce positive results in sera from SLE patients, which in general correlate with disease activity. The overall conclusion that can be drawn from a very large number of studies is that small amounts of circulating immune complexes, of largely unknown composition, may be found in patients with SLE.

The role of complement

There is general agreement that complement activity in sera from patients with SLE is reduced, related to disease activity (Townes *et al.* 1963; Schur and Sandson 1968; Lloyd and Schur 1981) and improves with treatment (Vaughan *et al.* 1951). Complement deposition has also been identified in inflamed tissues (Lachmann *et al.* 1962; Tan and Kunkel 1966). Levels of the classical pathway proteins, C1q, C2 and C4, are often markedly reduced (Morse *et al.* 1962; Hanauer and Christian 1967b; Schur and Sandson 1968). C3 levels are less frequently abnormal, and reduction of C3 is often an indication of severe disease (Lloyd and Schur 1981; Weinstein *et al.* 1983). Sera from patients with low C3 levels usually show evidence of activation of the alternative pathway, reflected by reduced factor B levels (Hunsicker *et al.* 1972; Perrin *et al.* 1973). However, studies of cohorts of patients with SLE show weak correlations only (albeit highly significant) between disease activity and reductions in the levels of individual complement proteins (Cameron *et al.* 1976; Valentijn *et al.* 1985). A partial explanation for this observation came from studies of the turnover *in vivo* of radiolabelled complement proteins in patients with SLE (Alper and Rosen 1967; Hunsicker *et al.* 1972; Sliwinski and Zvaifler 1972). Protein concentrations are a function of synthetic and catabolic rates. Increased turnover rates of complement proteins were usually observed, commensurate with increased catabolism associated with disease activity. However, there was great variability in synthetic rates, which in different patients were reduced, normal or increased. This variation in synthetic rates of complement proteins may mask hypercatabolism; for example, a normal C3 antigenic level will be measured in a patient with hypercatabolism and hypersynthesis of C3.

In order to overcome this problem, assays were devised to measure products of complement activation, levels of which might reflect directly the increased catabolism of complement following disease activity. Measurements of levels of C3d and Ba (Perrin *et al.* 1975), iC3b (Negoro *et al.* 1989), C1inh−C1s, C1r complexes (Sturfelt and Sjöholm 1984), C3bP complexes (Mayes *et al.* 1984), C3a (Hopkins *et al.* 1988) and neo-antigens of the membrane attack complex (Falk *et al.* 1985; Gawryl *et al.* 1988) correlate with disease activity. Increased expression of the complement receptor, CR3, on neutrophils has also been reported to correlate with disease activity (Buyon *et al.* 1988). However, even using these approaches to measure complement activation, no single assay of complement activity provides anything beyond an approximate correlation with disease activity.

Another explanation for the poor correlation between measures of complement activation and disease activity is the presence in some patients of an autoantibody that directly stimulates activation of the classical pathway of complement. This classical pathway 'nephritic factor' is an autoantibody that stabilizes the C4b2b C3 convertase enzyme, and allows unregulated classical pathway activation (Daha *et al.* 1983).

Many problems beset the measurement of complement in tissues. There are poor correlations between the presence of immunoglobulin and complement proteins and histological evidence of inflammatory damage (Pohle and Tuffanelli 1968; Gilliam *et al.* 1974; Biesecker *et al.* 1981). A positive lupus band test, i.e. deposits of antibody and complement at the dermoepidermal junction, is commonly found in skin from patients with SLE, which shows no clinical or histological evidence of inflammation. Measurement of neo-antigens of the membrane attack complex may provide a better index of the deposition of complement proteins correlated with inflammation (Biesecker *et al.* 1981, 1982).

Acute-phase response

The rise in acute-phase proteins that accompanies most forms of inflammation is atypical in patients with SLE. Active disease is frequently accompanied by fever and elevated erythrocyte sedimentation rate (ESR), but by only modest elevations in the concentrations of C-reactive protein (CRP) (Honig *et al.* 1977; Pepys *et al.* 1978) and serum amyloid A (SAA) protein (De Beer *et al.* 1982). As a corollary amyloidosis is an extremely rare complication of SLE (Huston *et al.* 1981; Ridley *et al.* 1984). The capacity of patients to produce CRP and SAA appears normal, in that plasma concentration of both of these proteins increases in response to infection and tissue necrosis (Honig *et al.* 1977; Becker *et al.* 1980; De Beer *et al.* 1982). This unusual pattern of acute-phase response was observed amongst caucasoid and Chinese patients (Hind *et al.* 1985) with SLE. Mice of the (NZB × NZW)F_1 strain show a similar abnormality and express very low levels of serum amyloid P (an acute-phase protein in mice, but not humans) in the presence of active disease (Rordorf *et al.* 1982). There have been few studies of other acute-phase proteins in patients with SLE; one group reported correlations between α_1-antichymotrypsin, α_1-antitrypsin and orosomucoid levels with disease activity (Sturfelt and Sjöholm 1984). Outstanding questions about the acute-phase response in patients with SLE include: (i) does the abnormality encompass all hepatic acute-phase proteins? and (ii) does the abnormality result from the nature of the inflammation in SLE, or is it inherited, and possibly a disease-susceptibility gene?

Specific organ involvement

The pattern of organ involvement varies greatly between different patients with SLE. The basis for this heterogeneity in not understood. The pathogenesis of lesions in skin, kidneys and the CNS is discussed.

Skin disease

There is a discordance in many organs between the presence of immune deposits and the occurrence of inflammation. Antibody and complement proteins are frequently seen by direct immunofluorescence at the dermoepidermal junction in the absence of rash (positive lupus band test). In skin and kidneys the presence of the membrane attack complex of complement is correlated with the presence of inflammation (Biesecker *et al.* 1981, 1982). Ultraviolet irradiation plays a clear role in initiating rash in some patients, and this suggests that a combination of two or more injurious stimuli may be needed to cause rash in SLE. The possibility that anti-Ro binds directly to epidermal cells and mediates rash is suggested by experiments in which affinity-purified antibodies localized to human epidermal cells in skin grafts on immunodeficient mice (Lee *et al.* 1989). Photosensitivity is almost universal in patients with SCLE, and observations of enhanced binding of anti-Ro antibodies to irradiated keratinocytes may be relevant to this (LeFeber *et al.* 1984).

Neurological disease

Central nervous system disease in SLE is extremely heterogeneous (Hughes 1987) and its pathogenesis is ill understood. Cerebral vasculitis with inflammation is uncommon, found in only 10–15% of patients studied by necropsy (Johnson and Richardson 1968; Ellis and Verity 1979). Much commoner, in 40–50% of subjects, was disease of the small cerebral vessels with endothelial proliferation, hyaline changes and scant lymphocytic infiltration. Immune complex disease, mediated by complement and neutrophils, is therefore unlikely to explain many cases of CNS disease, whose pathogenesis remains largely mysterious. The choroid plexus, with a similar structure to glomeruli, is a common site of deposition of antibodies and complement (Atkins *et al.* 1972), but there is no evidence that this is directly relevant to CNS disease. Studies of cerebrospinal fluid (CSF) protein levels have shown only minor impairment of the blood–brain barrier in most patients (Zvaifler and Bluestein 1982; Winfield *et al.* 1983); however, there is evidence of intrathecal immunoglobulin synthesis, with oligoclonal IgG synthesis (Winfield *et al.* 1983). A variety of autoantibodies have a raised prevalence in patients with CNS disease, including: (i) cross-reacting lymphocytotoxic antibodies (Bluestein and Zvaifler 1976; Bresnihan *et al.* 1979); (ii) antineuronal autoantibodies (reviewed in Zvaifler and Bluestein 1982; How *et al.* 1985) — some evidence has been presented for the local synthesis of these in the CNS (Bluestein *et al.* 1981); (iii) anti-cardiolipin antibodies — associated with cerebral vascular disease and possibly chorea; (iv) antiribosomal P antibodies — associated with lupus psychosis (Bonfa *et al.* 1987); and (v) anti-neurofilament antibodies (Robbins *et al.* 1988). There are many doubts about the significance of these observations. How do these antibodies gain access to the CNS and cause adverse effects? Despite the lack of inflammatory vasculitis, there is some evidence of complement activation within the CNS. The cerebrospinal fluid of 11 patients with CNS disease showed very reduced levels of C4 compared with control patients with SLE (Petz *et al.* 1971), and elevated levels of the C5b−9 complex were measured in CSF of three patients with cerebral lupus (Sanders *et al.* 1986).

Renal disease

Particular attention has been paid to elucidation of the pathogenesis of renal disease in patients with SLE because the presence of severe nephritis is a serious adverse prognostic feature. Glomerulonephritis in SLE is common, and a morphological classification has been prepared by a committee of the World Health Organization (Table 61.1). The differences between grades I to IV of nephritis may represent quantitative differences in inflammation; however, several qualitatively different patterns of inflammation have been identified in renal tissue which probably have differing aetiologies. Amongst these are membranous nephritis, intraglomerular thrombosis and tubulointerstitial disease.

Table 61.1. World Health Organization classification of systemic lupus erythematosus nephritis

I	Normal
IIA	Mesangial deposits
IIB	Mesangial hypercellularity
III	Focal-segmental glomerulonephritis
IV	Diffuse glomerulonephritis
V	Membranous glomerulonephritis

A causal role for autoantibodies and complement in renal inflammation seems very likely, and many groups have found correlations between the severity of nephritis and systemic complement activation and levels of anti-dsDNA antibodies (Koffler *et al.* 1967; Steinman *et al.* 1977; Hill *et al.* 1978) — although all of these correlations are weak and have little predictive values for the development of nephritis in individual patients. The pathogenic features of anti-dsDNA antibodies (complement fixation, high avidity, cationic charge) which may be associated with the presence of nephritis have been reviewed above. Further evidence that only certain subsets of anti-dsDNA antibodies may be involved in nephritis comes from measurement of levels of an idiotype, IdGN2, in renal tissue and sera from patients with SLE. This idiotype, defined by an anti-idiotypic antibody raised against anti-dsDNA antibodies eluted from the glomeruli of mice with lupus, was found to be enriched in the immunoglobulins eluted from renal biopsies from certain patients with SLE nephritis (Kalunian *et al.* 1989).

The location of immune deposits in glomeruli seems to be important in determining the nature of the associated inflammatory change. Membranous nephritis, associated with heavy proteinuria, is defined by subepithelial deposits of immunoglobulin and complement and little cellular infiltration. An animal model of membranous nephritis (Heymann nephritis) has been extensively characterized, mediated by antibodies to a glycoprotein on the surface of tubular epithelial cells. Immune complexes form, which move from the surface of epithelial cells to the subepithelial space. The development of proteinuria in this model requires subepithelial deposition of the membrane attack complex of complement, which stimulates local prostaglandin synthesis. A similar hypothesis is being pursued to account for membranous nephritis in humans, but the relevant antigen has not yet been defined. An alternative hypothesis is that autoantigens or certain autoantibodies may be 'non-specifically' trapped beneath glomerular basement membrane by virtue of particular properties of size or charge.

Many mechanisms of injury appear to contribute to glomerular injury. Intraglomerular thrombosis is commonly found in patients with focal and diffuse proliferative glomerulonephritis and is associated with deposition of complement and immune complexes, and with thrombocytopenia (Kant *et al*. 1981). Glomerular thrombosis may also be found in patients with the lupus anticoagulant and in this circumstance is associated with much less glomerular inflammation (Kant *et al*. 1981). The majority of studies of inflammation in SLE have concentrated on humoral and neutrophil-mediated mechanisms. However, the development of mesangial hypercellularity and cellular crescents emphasizes a role for mononuclear cells (Cole *et al*. 1985).

Tubulointerstitial disease is a common finding in SLE and severe disease at this site appears to be an important determinant of subsequent renal failure (Magil *et al*. 1984; Parichatikanond *et al*. 1986; Esdaile *et al*. 1989). Immune deposits are commonly present and the presence of the membrane attack complex of complement has been correlated with the presence of tissue inflammation. Lymphocytes, natural killer (NK) cells and mononuclear phagocytes are also present and may also mediate inflammation (Caligaris-Cappio *et al*. 1985; Alexopoulos *et al*. 1990), which may be independent of immunoglobulin and complement deposition.

Subsets of disease

There have been many attempts to subclassify various disease subsets of SLE. It is not known whether the variation in clinical expression of SLE is due to variation in host responsiveness to a single aetiological stimulus, or whether different patterns of disease are responses to different aetiological agents. Evidence for the former hypothesis comes from studies of families in whom one member may suffer from discoid lupus, whilst another has SLE which is fully expressed. Subclassification of disease has led to the realization that certain autoantibodies appear to be associated with particular pattern of illness, e.g. anti-Ro with cutaneous disease, anti-phospholipid antibodies with thrombosis. Subclassification has also allowed the designation of variants of SLE with a favourable prognosis.

Subacute cutaneous lupus erythematosus

Subacute cutaneous lupus erythematosus is

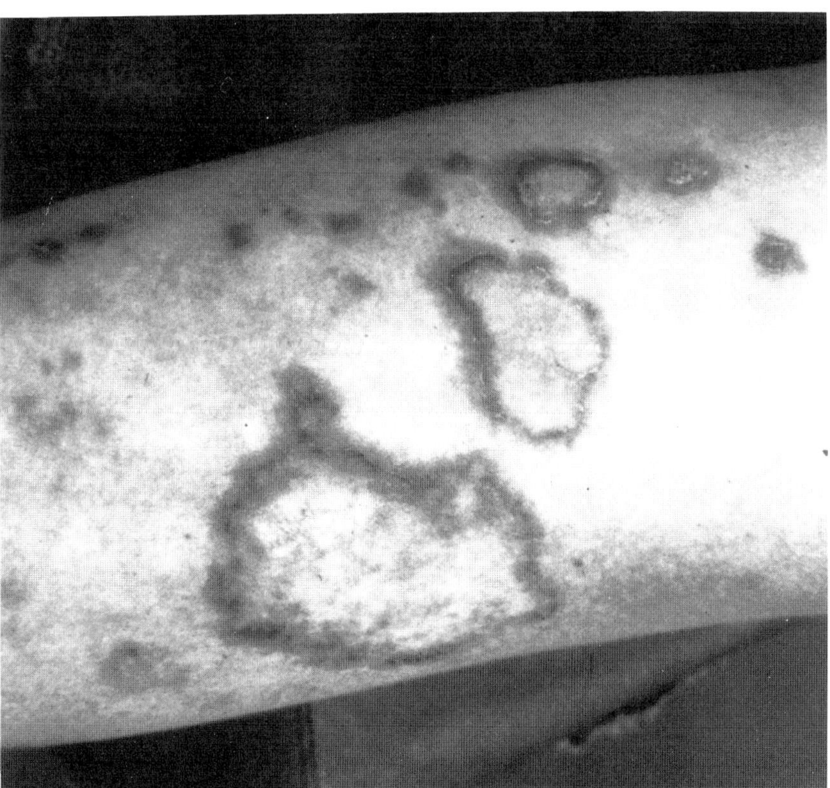

Fig. 61.2. Rash of subacute cutaneous lupus erythematosus.

characterized by annular (Fig. 61.2) or psoriaform, photosensitive eruptions associated with mild systemic features (Sontheimer *et al.* 1979, 1982). Characteristic serological abnormalities include antibodies to Ro and La, rheumatoid factor, and hyperglobulinaemia. There is a strong association of this subtype of disease with HLA-B8, DR3 (reviewed in Sontheimer 1989). However, the homogeneity of the serological associations with this type of rash has been questioned (Callen and Klein 1988). The serological profile of SCLE is similar to that of primary Sjögren's syndrome and there is overlap between these conditions.

Antinuclear antibody-negative lupus

Approximately 5% of patients with a syndrome closely resembling SLE had negative ANA results using sections of rodent liver and kidney as substrates for their detection (Fessel 1978). Subsequent investigations showed that the majority of patients with 'ANA −ve' SLE had anti-Ro and anti-La antibodies (Maddison *et al.* 1981). Amongst such subjects a negative ANA result is usually a consequence of the use of an insensitive substrate for the detection of ANA; almost all these patients have a positive ANA using the HEp-2 (human epithelial) cell line as substrate. The clinical features of 'ANA −ve' lupus are identical to those of SCLE.

Primary Sjögren's syndrome

Primary Sjögren's syndrome is considered in chapter 59. The characteristic autoantibodies of primary Sjögren's syndrome are anti-Ro, anti-La and rheumatoid factors. The clinical features of SLE and primary Sjögren's syndrome overlap considerably (Provost *et al.* 1988) and the MHC haplotype, HLA-A1, B8, DR3, C4AQ0, C4B1, BfS, C2-1, has a raised prevalence amongst patients with both diseases. 'Secondary' Sjögren's syndrome has been reported to have a prevalence of approximately 20% amongst patients with SLE (Watson *et al.* 1984); this is also associated with anti-Ro and anti-La antibodies and the immunogenic background of SLE. It is unknown whether SLE and primary Sjögren's syndrome are part of the spectrum of a single disease or have different aetiologies but share disease susceptibility genes.

Neonatal lupus

One of the surprising features of SLE, apparently mediated by IgG autoantibodies, is the rarity of neonatal disease (Watson *et al.* 1984; Lockshin *et al.* 1988). The cutaneous manifestations of neonatal lupus closely resemble those of SCLE and both show extremely strong associations with autoantibodies to Ro and La (Watson *et al.* 1984). There are equally strong associations between antibodies to Ro and La and congenital cardiac disease (Scott *et al.* 1983), although the prevalence of congenital cardiac disease in children born of mothers with anti-Ro antibodies in less than 5% (Watson *et al.* 1984; Lockshin *et al.* 1988). The role of these antibodies in the causation of fetal myocarditis progressing to congenital heart block and, occasionally, generalized cardiac fibrosis has not been established, although immunoglobulin deposits have been described in cardiac tissue (Litsey *et al.* 1985). Analysis of the polypeptides bound by sera from mothers of 20 patients with congenital heart block showed that no single autoantibody specificity could be singled out to account for congenital disease (Buyon *et al.* 1989). The strongest association was with antibodies to the 48 kD La and 52 kD Ro polypeptides (see above), and large quantities of these proteins were found in fetal hearts. However, two infants with neonatal lupus and anti-U1 RNP antibodies, but not anti-Ro and anti-La antibodies, have been described (Provost *et al.* 1987).

Anti-phospholipid syndrome

The clinical features of the anti-phospholipid syndrome variant of SLE are venous and arterial thrombosis, recurrent spontaneous abortion, thrombocytopenia, livedo reticularis and cardiac valvular lesions. The nature of anti-phospholipid antibodies and hypotheses to explain the associated immunopathology have been explored above. A causal role for anti-phospholipid antibodies in the aetiology of these lesions has not been established, but there is strong epidemiological evidence for a true association. The prevalence of anti-phospholipid antibodies amongst patients who fulfil the American Rheumatism Association (ARA) classification criteria for SLE has been estimated to up to 50% (Sturfelt *et al.* 1987). A subgroup of patients have been identified who have the clinical features associated with presence of anti-phospholipid antibodies, but who do not have other features of SLE and who do not fulfil the ARA classification criteria. These patients have been designated by some authors as suffering from the 'primary anti-phospholipid syndrome'. There is little merit in pursuit of the argument as to whether the primary anti-phospholipid syndrome is part of the spectrum of SLE or represents a discrete disease.

Discoid lupus

There is considerable evidence of overlap between discoid and systemic lupus erythematosus (reviewed in Rowell 1986). Up to 15% of patients with SLE have cutaneous discoid lesions (Estes and Christian 1971), which are indistinguishable by histopathological techniques from the lesions in patients with isolated discoid lupus (Clark *et al.* 1973). Families have been described containing members with chronic discoid lupus and SLE (Rothfield *et al.* 1983). Amongst two large series of SLE patients, 6% (Rothfield *et al.* 1963) and 12% (Scott and Rees 1959) had discoid lupus for a variable number of years before the onset of systemic disease. There is evidence of systemic disturbance of immune function in patients with chronic discoid lupus as judged by the presence of several autoantibodies and findings of increased activation of peripheral blood B lymphocytes (Wangel *et al.* 1984; Kind *et al.* 1986) and hyperglobulinaemia (Beck and Rowell 1966). Antinuclear antibodies are commonly found, with estimates of prevalence varying from 6% to 50% (Weir *et al.* 1961; Rothfield *et al.* 1983; Shrank and Doniach 1963; Beck and Rowell 1966; Wangel *et al.* 1984). The finding of LE cells is uncommon and estimates have varied from 0% (Weir *et al.* 1961) to 5% (Rothfield *et al.* 1963), presumably reflecting an absence of anti-histone antibodies in these patients (Rubin and Waga 1987). Anti-phospholipid antibodies, assayed as a false-positive Wassermann reaction, have been measured in 5% of patients with chronic discoid lupus (Beck and Rowell 1966; Rothfield *et al.* 1983). Other abnormalities indicating systemic autoimmunity include mild leucopenia (Rothfield *et al.* 1963; Beck and Rowell 1966), thrombocytopenia (Beck and Rowell 1966) and rheumatoid factors (Beck and Rowell 1966). Despite the clear evidence of overlap of many of the features of chronic discoid and systemic lupus, there are important clinical differences. The sex ratio of discoid lupus (2 females : 1 male) is much less biased towards females than the systemic form, and less than 5% of patients with discoid lupus progress to systemic disease (Cannon and Curtis 1958; Rothfield *et al.* 1963; Shrank and Doniach 1963; Beck and Rowell 1966).

Lupus panniculitis/lupus erythematosus profundus

Lupus panniculitis/lupus erythematosus profundus is similar to discoid lupus in its relationship to SLE (Peters and Su 1989). About 2% of patients with SLE have the lesions of lupus panniculitis and only a small percentage of patients who present with lupus panniculitis develop systemic illness. Characteristic pathology in fat includes hyaline necrosis and lymphoid germinal centres. Similar serological abnormalities occur in patients with lupus profundus to those seen in patients with discoid lupus, e.g. a positive lupus band test in otherwise normal skin (Tuffanelli 1971).

Mixed connective tissue disease

Antibodies to RNP have been associated with an overlap between SLE, myositis and scleroderma — 'MCTD' (Sharp *et al.* 1972). Nosological aspects of this condition have been extensively debated and arguments as to whether it is a separate disease entity are sterile until more is known of the aetiology of SLE. In low titre, anti-RNP antibodies are found in up to 30% of all SLE patients. In high titre, and in the absence of antibodies to dsDNA, they are associated with MCTD, whose most consistent clinical feature is severe Raynaud's phenomenon. An erosive polyarthritis with prominent swelling of fingers is another common clinical feature of MCTD, distinguishing patients from those with classical SLE (Bennett and O'Connell 1978; Halla and Hardin 1978; Rasmussen *et al.* 1987). Patients with MCTD seem to have a slightly different spectrum of reactivity to the proteins of U1 RNP from that of patients with SLE. Antibodies to the 68 kD protein are much commoner in MCTD than in SLE (Pettersson *et al.* 1986; Habets *et al.* 1989). Antibodies to RNP certainly do not define a unique subset of disease and the clinical features of the original series of patients described with MCTD evolved into those found in a variety of diseases, including SLE, scleroderma and rheumatoid arthritis (Nimelstein *et al.* 1980).

Drug-induced lupus

The lupus-like illness associated with the ingestion of certain drugs (reviewed in Lee and Chase 1975), especially procainamide and hydralazine, provides evidence for heterogeneity in the aetiology of SLE in humans. The autoantibody response associated with drug-induced disease is different from idiopathic SLE. Anti-dsDNA antibodies are rare in drug-induced disease, in contrast to anti-histone antibodies, which are common. There is some evidence for heterogeneity of autoantibody response according to drug type, hydralazine and procainamide being associated with antibodies to histones H2A–H2B, whereas chlorpromazine, and to a lesser extent procainamide (Davis *et al.* 1978), are associated with the development of lupus anticoagulant activity (though probably not the clinical manifestations of the 'anti-phospholipid syndrome'). The genetic predisposition to hydralazine-induced lupus appears to differ from that of 'idiopathic' SLE. A raised prevalence of HLA-DR4 was found in two groups of patients with hydralazine-induced lupus (Batchelor *et al.* 1980; Mitchell *et al.* 1987) although these findings were not confirmed amongst a group of Australian patients (Brand *et al.* 1984). The metabolic pathway of both hydralazine and procainamide includes acetylation, and there is strong evidence that the moiety which induces disease is the native drug and not its acetylated metabolite (Sonnhag *et al.* 1979; Kluger *et al.* 1981). There is an inherited polymorphism of the drug-metabolizing acetyltransferase enzyme and lupus is much more prevalent amongst slow acetylators than fast. Similarly, acetylprocainamide has been administered safely to patients who had previously suffered from procainamide-induced lupus. Both procainamide and hydralazine induce ANA production very commonly, but overt disease only develops in a small percentage of patients treated with these agents. The mechanism of induction of disease by drugs is unknown and a number of hypotheses have been explored, which include: (i) direct interaction of drug with DNA, resulting in modified antigenicity (Dubroff and Reid 1980; Thomas and Messner 1986); (ii) inhibition of DNA methylation altering T cell reactivity (Cornacchia *et al.* 1988); (iii) nucleophilic inactivation of complement C4, causing acquiring C4 deficiency (Sim *et al.* 1984).

Disease-susceptibility genes

Approximately 5% of patients with SLE have a relative with the same disease (Estes and Christian 1971). Although this observation does not discriminate between genetic and environmental factors predisposing to disease, the results of studies of twins provided strong evidence for the presence of genes conferring susceptibility to SLE. Monozygotic twins had 57% concordance for SLE, compared with a much lower rate in dizygotic twins, similar to that of other first-degree relatives (Block *et al.* 1975, 1976; Arnett and Shulman 1976). The observation that the concordance rate for SLE amongst monozygotic twins was 57%, rather than 100%, also implicated environmental factors as determinants of expression of disease.

There is evidence in humans for heterogeneity of disease-susceptibility genes for the development of SLE. The majority of SLE patients are females of reproductive age, suggesting the involvement of sex hormones. However, families have been described amongst whom SLE showed a male inheritance pattern (Lahita *et al.* 1983a), similar to that of a murine lupus-prone strain, the BXSB mouse.

The strongest disease-susceptibility genes of all to be identified in humans are those encoding deficiencies of proteins of the classical pathway of complement, especially C1q, C2 and C4. Although patients with such complete, inherited deficiencies of complement proteins only account for a tiny minority of patients with SLE, their description has stimulated detailed studies of complement proteins encoded within the MHC. These studies have led to the identification of null alleles (associated with no expressed protein) of one of the two isotypic variants of C4, C4A, as a putative disease-susceptibility gene present in the majority of patients with SLE. Possible physiological explanations for the association of complement deficiency with SLE are considered below.

The role of environmental factors was established by observations of a raised prevalence of serological abnormalities amongst spouses of SLE patients (DeHoratius and Messner 1975; DeHoratius *et al.* 1975; Lowenstein and Rothfield 1977) and amongst laboratory workers exposed to the sera of patients with SLE (Carr *et al.* 1975; DeHoratius *et al.* 1979). The timing of the onset of disease within a given family also suggested a role for environmental factors; identical twins developed disease within a mean of 2 years of each other; siblings, with a mean age of difference of 9 years, developed disease within a mean of 3 years (Arnett and Shulman 1986). Systemic lupus erythematosus-like disease associated with drugs, such as hydralazine and procainamide, represents a further example of disease that is induced by exposure of a genetically susceptible subject to an exogenous factor.

Racial variation in disease expression

Both the prevalence and severity of expression of SLE differ between races. Systemic lupus erythematosus has a higher prevalence and greater severity in black (prevalence: Siegel and Lee 1973; Fessel 1974; severity: Hochberg *et al.* 1985; Harris *et al.* 1989), oriental and Asian (prevalence: Serdula and Rhoads 1979; severity: Kaslow and Masi 1978; Kaslow 1982) compared with caucasoid patients. Many factors may contribute to differential mortality of patients in widely varying environments and it is not certain that race *per se* has a direct influence. A large number of studies have compared the difference in the prevalence of autoantibodies between different races. The most striking difference observed consistently appears to be the prevalence of anti-Sm antibodies, which is around 25% in black (Arnett *et al.* 1988), Chinese (Boey *et al.* 1988) and Japanese (Yokohari and Tsunematsu 1985) patients compared with approximately 10% in caucasoid subjects (Bernstein *et al.* 1984; Arnett *et al.* 1988).

Major histocompatibility complex associations

It is still not certain what the relevant MHC gene/genes are which confer increased susceptibility to the development of SLE, despite the very large number of studies performed (reviewed in Walport *et al.* 1982). The two groups of genes encoded within the MHC that have attracted the greatest interest are the Class II genes and the Class III complement genes, particularly those encoding C4A, C4B (the two isotypes of C4) and C2. Initial studies of Class II MHC antigens showed a raised prevalence of HLA-DR2 and of HLA-DR3 amongst caucasoid SLE patients, although the relative risk of disease associated with possession of these antigens was only two- to threefold (reviewed in Walport *et al.* 1982). Subsequent studies confirmed a significant association between B8 and DR3 and SLE (Reveille *et al.* 1983; Bell *et al.* 1984). Family studies demonstrated that the haplotype HLA-A1, B8, DR3 was increased in prevalence in SLE (Fielder *et al.* 1983). This haplotype is also associated with a number of other autoimmune diseases, e.g. Graves' disease, autoallergic Addison's disease, juvenile diabetes mellitus, chronic active hepatitis and coeliac disease.

The second candidates within the MHC as disease-susceptibility genes for the development of SLE are the Class III complement genes: the arguments in favour of these being relevant disease-susceptibility genes are considered below, and follow from the observed strong association of complete hereditary complement deficiencies with SLE.

A large number of additional genes have recently been discovered within the MHC, including the genes for tumour necrosis factor (TNF)-α and β (Spies *et al.* 1986) and for a collagen disease, an HSP gene and in excess of 30 other genes encoding unidentified products. No polymorphisms of these genes or proteins have yet been fully characterized in humans, but inherited variation in TNF expression would represent another candidate for a disease-susceptibility gene for SLE, especially in view of the abnormal acute-phase response in patients with SLE. The findings of reduced TNF-α production in (NZB × NZW)F_1 mice (Jacob and McDevitt 1988) are particularly intriguing in this respect. It has recently become apparent that HSP represent common targets for autoimmunity, and it is conceivable that inherited variation of these may be important.

The finding of strong correlations between the presence of HLA-B8 and HLA-DR3 and autoantibodies to Ro and La (Bell and Maddison 1980; Manthorpe *et al.* 1982; Wilson *et al.* 1984) led some workers to suggest that there are 'immune response genes' in the MHC controlling production of these particular autoantibodies (Bell and Maddison 1980). However, a strong piece of evidence against this idea comes from studies of patients with inherited complement deficiencies (Meyer *et al.* 1985), which showed that the most common autoantibody in patients with SLE and hereditary complement deficiency was anti-Ro. No particular MHC haplotype was associated with disease amongst these individuals, except in the case of C2 deficiency, which is predominantly inherited within the haplotype, HLA-A10, B18, DR2. The study of Harley and co-workers (1986a) suggested an alternative role for the haplotype encoding HLA-B8, DR3 in influencing antibody responses to Ro and La. They found that levels of these autoantibodies were much higher amongst HLA-DR3 +ve patients, but that their presence was not exclusively restricted to HLA-DR3 +ve subjects. HLA-DR4, associated with disease susceptibility to rheumatoid arthritis, has an increased prevalence in patients with anti-U1 RNP antibodies (Genth *et al.* 1987). These antibodies are associated with MCTD, in which an erosive arthropathy is a prominent clinical feature (see above).

Complement deficiency

The strongest disease-susceptibility genes for the development of SLE are inherited homozygous deficiencies of the classical pathway of complement proteins C1q, C2 or C4 (Schifferli *et al.* 1986a), although patients with such deficiencies account for only a tiny minority of cases of SLE. The arguments that suggest that the deficient complement protein is itself the predisposing factor to immune complex disease have recently been reviewed (Lachmann and Walport 1987). These can be summarized as follows: (i) SLE is found in association with inherited complement deficiencies encoded in different parts of the genome; (ii) inherited complement deficiencies are hardly ever encountered amongst normal populations, excluding ascertainment artefact as the explanation for the association of deficiency with SLE; and (iii) acquired complement deficiency states, such as those which are associated with inherited C1 inhibitor deficiency and C3 nephritic factor, are also associated with a raised prevalence of autoimmunity. These observations suggest that there is a causal pathophysiological link between the complement deficiency and the development of SLE.

Null alleles of complement genes encoded in the major histocompatibility complex

Because of the strong association of inherited homozygous complement deficiencies with SLE-like disease, the hypothesis was tested of an association between SLE and partial inherited deficiencies of complement proteins. Heterozygous C2 deficiency was found at increased prevalence in patients with SLE and juvenile chronic arthritis (Glass *et al.* 1976). There is an extensive polymorphism of both the C4A and the C4B genes, which includes null genes (with no expressed protein, denoted by the symbol Q0, quantity 0). These null genes are moderately common amongst caucasoid subjects with an overall prevalence of approximately 55% (30% with one or more AQ0 genes and 25% BQ0). A markedly raised prevalence of C4AQ0 genes (Christiansen *et al.* 1983; Fielder *et al.* 1983; Reveille *et al.* 1985; Howard *et al.* 1986; Kemp *et al.* 1987) was found amongst caucasoid patients with SLE (reviewed in Ng and Walport 1988). However, the majority of these C4AQ0 alleles were encoded on haplotypes bearing HLA-DR3 and the commonest haplotype was: HLA-A1, B8, DR3, C4AQ0, C4B1, BfS, C2-1 (Fielder *et al.* 1983; Reveille *et al.* 1985; Kemp *et al.* 1987). It was therefore impossible to disentangle the relative contributions of HLA-DR3 and of C4AQ0 to disease susceptibility, or indeed to exclude the possibility that a further disease-susceptibility gene was encoded within this haplotype.

Two approaches have been taken to identify the relevant disease-susceptibility gene or genes within the MHC. One has been to study the prevalence of C4 null alleles amongst caucasoid patients with SLE who do not carry HLA-DR3. One such study showed an increased prevalence amongst these subjects of both C4AQ0 and C4BQ0 alleles (Batchelor *et al.* 1987). The second approach has been to study the prevalence of C4 null alleles in patients of other racial groups. Black (Howard *et al.* 1986), Chinese (Dunckley *et al.* 1987; Hawkins *et al.* 1987) and Japanese patients with SLE (Dunckley *et al.* 1987) have all been found to have an increased prevalence of C4AQ0 alleles unaccompanied by an increase in HLA-DR3. However, not all groups have confirmed the raised prevalence of C4AQ0 alleles in patients with SLE (C. Alper, pers. comm.).

It is not obvious how deficiency of only one of

four expressed C4 genes is sufficient to increase disease susceptibility to SLE. C4 is an acute-phase protein and levels of C4 vary quite widely between different individuals. Several groups have found that it is impossible to ascertain whether a C4 null allele is present simply by measuring the C4 concentration in the subject's serum. The effects of null alleles on C4 concentration can only be clearly seen at a population level (Welch *et al.* 1985), with the mean C4 level being correlated with the number of expressed C4 genes.

There is a difference between the functional activities of the two C4 isotypes. The internal thiolester bond of C4A is more susceptible to nucleophilic attack by amine groups with the formation of covalent amide bonds, whereas C4B is more susceptible to attack by hydroxyl groups with production of ester bonds (Isenman and Young 1984; Law *et al.* 1984). Free amine groups are frequent in proteins, whereas hydroxyl groups predominate in carbohydrates. C4B is haemolytically more active than C4A, presumably reflecting an abundance of cell surface carbohydrate residues. C4A is more active in binding to protein-containing immune complexes (Schifferli *et al.* 1986b). Since partial deficiency of C4A is more strongly associated with SLE than deficiency of C4B, the difference in binding specificities may provide a clue to the mechanism of this putative disease-susceptibility gene.

Complement receptor type 1

Erythrocytes from patients with SLE showed defective immune adherence, suggesting dysfunction or deficiency of CR1 (Miyakawa *et al.* 1981). This finding was confirmed using antibodies to the receptor (Iida *et al.* 1982; Wilson *et al.* 1982; Walport *et al.* 1985a), and a reduction in CR1 numbers on red cells was demonstrated. An inherited numerical polymorphism of CR1 on erythrocytes was shown by family studies of immune adherence (Klopstock *et al.* 1965) and later by direct enumeration of CR1 (Wilson *et al.* 1982). A restriction-fragment length polymorphism (RFLP) of the CR1 gene was identified, which correlated with the CR1 numerical polymorphism (Wilson *et al.* 1986). There has been some controversy about the relative contributions of inherited and environmental factors in the reduction of CR1 on erythrocytes of SLE patients (reviewed in Walport and Lachmann 1988). Most of the evidence suggests that the reduction of CR1 is acquired as a consequence of disease: (i) family studies showed that patients had low phenotypic expression of CR1 in the presence of genotypically high family members (Walport *et al.* 1985a); (ii) the frequencies of the two alleles segregating with high and low expression of CR1 were not significantly different between SLE patients and normal subjects in English (Moldenhauer *et al.* 1987) and French populations (Cohen *et al.* 1989) (although there was a slight excess of heterozygotes in a Boston population (Wilson *et al.* 1987); (iii) CR1 numbers correlated with serological parameters of disease activity (Iida *et al.* 1982; Ross *et al.* 1985; Hammond *et al.* 1989); (iv) transfused erythrocytes lost CR1 expression in the circulation of patients with SLE who had low CR1 numbers; and (v) low CR1 numbers have been described on erythrocytes of patients with a variety of diseases, including autoimmune haemolytic anaemias, paroxysmal nocturnal haemoglobinuria, acquired immune dificiency syndrome (AIDS) and lepromatous leprosy (reviewed in Walport and Lachmann 1988).

Immunoglobulin and T cell receptor genes

Obvious candidate genes for encoding disease susceptibility are those for immunoglobulins and T cell receptors. The investigation of inherited variation of V genes encoding these molecules is at an extremely early stage, and the results are likely to be extremely complex due to the large number of tandemly duplicated genes. Disease susceptibility could also be due to somatic selection of particular T cell repertoires within the thymus.

There is considerable polymorphic variation of the constant (C) region genes for these molecules, but the results of studies of associations of their allotypic variants with expression of SLE have been inconsistent. Four studies of Gm allotypes have been reported, two in caucasoid populations (Whittingham *et al.* 1983; Schur *et al.* 1985), one in an American black population (Fedrick *et al.* 1983) and one in a Japanese population (Nakao *et al.* 1980). All found associations between SLE and particular Gm haplotypes, particularly when expressed in heterozygous combinations. However, no two studies gave the same results, although the differences may be explained by the different ethnic origins of the populations studied. The lack of very significant associations of polymorphisms of C region genes with disease is not surprising — antibodies and T cell receptors are encoded within very large stretches of DNA (up to 4000 kilobases for the immunoglobulin heavy chain), and there is no evidence of crossover suppression within this DNA. Therefore it is unlikely that study of the C region genes would give useful information about unlinked V genes encoding disease susceptibility.

Two studies have been reported examining the prevalence of RFLPs of T cell receptor genes amongst patients with SLE. No associations were found between the gene frequency of T cell receptor α-, β- (Fronek *et al.* 1986) and γ-chain DNA polymorphic variants and SLE (Dunckley *et al.* 1988).

Acetylator and hydroxylator phenotypes

There is no evidence for any alteration in the prevalence of slow acetylators amongst patients with idiopathic SLE (reviewed in Baer *et al.* 1986a), in contrast to the situation in hydralazine- and procainamide-induced disease.

Hormones

The predominance of SLE in females of reproductive age, coupled with observations that the outcome of murine lupus in the NZB/W F_1 strain could be manipulated using sex hormones (Roubinian *et al.* 1977), stimulated studies of sex hormone metabolism in humans with SLE. There are several case reports of the association of SLE with Klinefelter's syndrome; however, it is not clear whether this link is physiological or due to biased ascertainment. Alterations in sex hormone metabolism in patients of both sexes with SLE have been identified. The family of oestrogen molecules are metabolized by a family of cytochrome P-450 monoxygenase enzymes in the liver. Oestrone is primarily metabolized by 2-hydroxylation, leading to the inactive product 2-hydroxy-oestrone. A quantitatively smaller pathway of 16α-hydroxylation leads to the production of 16α-hydroxy-oestrone, a precursor for the production of oestriol, which retains oestrogenic activity. Patients of both sexes with SLE were found to have increased 16α-hydroxylation and decreased 2-hydroxylation, the combination of which might augment peripheral oestrogen activity (Lahita *et al.* 1979, 1981). Testosterone levels were reduced in females, though not in males, with SLE and this may be explained in part by observations of accelerated testosterone oxidation in females with SLE (Jungers *et al.* 1982; Lahita *et al.* 1983b). It is not clear whether the abnormalities of oestrogen are primary or secondary to active disease. The abnormality of testosterone metabolism has been correlated with disease activity and is probably a secondary effect (Jungers *et al.* 1982). Related to these results are observations of the activity of certain polymorphic drug-metabolizing enzymes that have been studied in patients with SLE. There is a single report of an increased prevalence of poor 4-hydroxylation of debrisoquine, catalysed by a P-450 cytochrome enzyme, in caucasoid patients (Baer *et al.* 1986b) compared with normal controls, but again it is not known whether this defect was attributable to disease activity or to the known inherited polymorphism of activity of this enzyme amongst normal subjects.

Animal models

There is a voluminous literature describing SLE-like illnesses in dogs and mice and several comprehensive reviews are available (Theofilopoulos and Dixon 1981, 1985; Steinberg *et al.* 1984). Perhaps the most important messages from these studies are: (i) that lupus in animals is characterized by the production of autoantibodies to the same range of antigens found in human disease; and (ii) that animal models of lupus are extremely heterogeneous in their aetiology and disease can be stimulated by a variety of disparate insults to the immune system. An abbreviated summary of some of these models of disease follows — only selected references are supplied as more comprehensive bibliographies are published in the reviews cited above.

Dogs

A breeding colony of alsations and poodles with disease closely resembling human SLE was established by Lewis and Schwartz (1971). It was observed that cell-free filtrates from the spleens of these animals induced the production of LE cells, ANA and sometimes anti-dsDNA antibodies in recipient dogs and mice, although disease was not transmitted (Lewis *et al.* 1973).

Mice

1 Disease may be transmitted by transplantation of bone marrow from lupus-prone strains of mice to their normal, irradiated, counterparts. This shows that expression of the disease-susceptibility gene/genes within cells arising from haemopoietic stem cells is sufficient to induce disease.

2 There is marked genetic heterogeneity amongst the several strains of mice that develop lupus. Four types of genes controlling disease in mice have been recognized:

(a) Disease-susceptibility genes, which may be dominant or recessive. Two genes causing lymphoproliferation, *lpr* (lymphoproliferation) and *gld* (generalized lymphoproliferative disease), are examples of such genes whose expression is sufficient to cause disease — introduction of these genes into normal strains of mice leads to the development of SLE.

(b) Disease-accelerating genes. These hasten the onset of disease in genetically susceptible mice and include: (i) those determining sex-hormone production in NZB/W mice; (ii) a Y chromosome gene in the BXSB mouse; and (iii) the *lpr* gene in MRL mice.

(c) Genes controlling individual manifestations of disease. Studies of recombinant inbred strains of mice have shown that individual features of autoimmunity, e.g. anti-erythrocyte antibodies, anti-ssDNA antibodies, raised levels of IgM, thymocytotoxic antibodies, behave as though they are under the control of individual genes, some of which are linked to each other. These are separate from the genes encoding overall disease susceptibility.

(d) Protective genes which inhibit the development of disease, e.g. *xid* (X-linked immunodeficiency) (see below).

3 There are environmental as well as genetic accelerating factors that hasten or delay the onset of disease in lupus-prone animals. Viral (e.g. Gross virus or lymphocytic choriomeningitis virus) and bacterial infection accelerate the onset of disease. Of particular interest is a virus, lactate dehydrogenase (LDH) virus, that inhibits disease development (Oldstone and Dixon 1972); it has been discovered that this virus uses Class II MHC molecules as its receptor (Inada and Mims 1985; Mims 1986) and thereby may enter and inhibit the activities of antigen-presenting cells.

4 There is no evidence that distinct allotypic variants of antibodies, T cell receptors or autoantigens are involved in disease susceptibility. However, there is some evidence for selective usage of certain immunoglobulin V gene families in the formation of autoantibodies (Bona 1988), although there is evidence that these gene families are present in normal as well as lupus-prone mice (Trepicchio *et al.* 1987). Similarly there is evidence that a particular lineage of B lymphocytes, bearing the Ly-1 antigen (CD5 in humans), may preferentially express autoantibodies (reviewed in Hayakawa and Hardy 1988). These B lymphocytes are usually expressed early in ontogenesis and are only present in small numbers in mature animals. In New Zealand mice they are present in mature animals as a high proportion of circulating lymphocytes. The gene, *xid*, which is associated with an immunodeficiency syndrome in normal mouse strains and with suppression of disease in lupus-prone strains, is found associated with normal numbers of Ly-1 +ve B cells when expressed in NZB mice. However, Ly-1 +ve B cells are expressed in normal numbers in MRL/l mice, which develop an accelerated form of SLE. This observation casts doubt on a universally important role for Ly-1 +ve B cells in murine lupus.

5 The single abnormality of immune cellular function common to all strains of lupus-prone mice is excessive activation of B lymphocytes. It is not yet clear whether this is due to their excessive sensitivity to normally derived signals from lymphokines or whether they are stimulated excessively by abnormal production of lymphokines from other activated cells of the lymphon. In the case of the MRL strain of mice, the *lpr*, disease-accelerating, gene is associated with proliferation of T lymphocytes of helper phenotype and it is tempting to believe that these accelerate disease by the excessive secretion of B cell helper factors. Normal strains of mice into which the *lpr* and *gld* genes had been introduced developed autoimmunity, with evidence of polyclonal activation (Izui *et al.* 1984; Ishigatsubo *et al.* 1988).

6 There appear to be major differences between the genetics of murine and human SLE. The role of MHC-linked disease-susceptibility genes amongst inbred mice is less well established than amongst outbred humans. The various lupus-prone strains of mice do not share a particular MHC haplotype. A gene in, or linked to, the H-2^z

haplotype of NZW mice, appears to be the dominant disease-susceptibility gene in promoting high levels of anti-DNA antibodies and early nephritis in (NZB × NZW)F_1 hybrids (Kotzin and Palmer 1987). There is little evidence that inherited complement deficiency plays an important role in disease susceptibility to murine lupus, in contrast to the situation in humans.

It was recently reported that NZW and (NZB × NZW)F_1 mice show impaired production of TNF-α (encoded within the MHC), and regular injections of TNF-α ameliorated nephritis and prolonged the life of these mice (Jacob and McDevitt 1988). An RFLP of the TNF-α gene was characterized which was present in many lupus-prone mice, but also found in some normal strains.

7 A number of models of disease produced by deliberate manipulation of the immune system of normal mice have been described:

(a) Immunization of mice with a human monoclonal autoantibody bearing the 16/6 cross-reactive idiotype. Normal C3H.SW mice were injected with a human monoclonal anti-dsDNA antibody of the 16/6 idiotype in adjuvant and made autoantibodies to polynucleotides, histones, Ro, La, Sam, RNP and cardiolipin, accompanied by development of systemic inflammatory disease (Mendlovic *et al.* 1988). Similar disease could be induced using a murine monoclonal anti-idiotypic antibody to the 16/6 idiotype (Mendlovic *et al.* 1989). Further experiments showed that a 16/6 +ve monoclonal antibody to Sm, which did not bind to DNA, also induced disease, whereas a 16/6 −ve monoclonal anti-DNA antibody did not cause any abnormality in recipient mice (Blank *et al.* 1990).

(b) Graft-versus-host disease. Two models of SLE in mice have been induced by graft-versus-host responses. Injection of DBA/2 spleen and lymph node cells into (DBA/2 × C57BL/10)F_1 recipients was followed by a production of the typical spectrum of autoantibodies of SLE, accompanied by development of nephritis (Gleichmann *et al.* 1982). A number of studies of this animal model of disease demonstrated that these autoantibodies were not produced as a result of random polyclonal B cell activation (Van Rappard-Van Der Veen *et al.* 1984a, b). Similarly, BALB/c mice developed hyperglobulinaemia and autoantibodies following neonatal injection with C57BL/6 × BALB/c)F_1 spleen cells (Goldman *et al.* 1983). Autoantibodies in this model were produced exclusively by F_1 donor B cells (Luzuy *et al.* 1986), which were activated by host T cells (Merino *et al.* 1989).

8 There is some variation between strains in the clinical manifestations of disease. NZB mice have marked haemolytic anaemia but not the severe sytemic disease of (NZB × NZW)F_1 mice. (NZW × BXSB)F_1 develop severe systemic vasculitis and coronary arteritis (Hang *et al.* 1981). MRL/*lpr* mice develop vasculitis and also develop an arthropathy, accompanied by the presence of rheumatoid factors. Sjögren's syndrome is a feature of disease in (NZB × NZW)F_1 mice and PN mice, and the immunohistology of T cells infiltrating the salivary glands of these animals is very similar to that seen in humans (Hoffman *et al.* 1984; Jonsson *et al.* 1987).

Aetiological hypotheses

The message of all of these studies in animals is that SLE is a syndrome with similar final pathways of disease expression, but may have diverse causes. The processes which initiate disease may well be different from those that perpetuate it. Five groups of hypotheses proposing explanations for the aetiology of SLE in humans will be considered: (i) failure of the mononuclear phagocytic system to clear immune complexes, leading to stimulation of autoimmunity by autoantigens; (ii) aberrant polyclonal activation of B lymphocytes, resulting in autoantibody production; (iii) abnormality of 'idiotypic networks'; (iv) the breaking of tolerance to autoantigens by antigenic mimicry by microbial antigens or by the interaction of viral antigens with host intracellular molecules; and (v) viruses as a cause of disease.

Is systemic lupus erythematosus due to failure of the physiological clearance mechanisms of immune complexes?

The idea that dysfunction of the mononuclear phagocytic system may result in failure of clearance of immune complexes and their deposition in many organs first dates to experimental studies demonstrating 'reticuloendothelial saturation'. The hypothesis has been extended by observations that the strongest disease-susceptibility genes characterized for the development of SLE are null genes for complement proteins C1q, C2 and C4 (see above). Failure of the physiological disposal mechanisms of immune complexes may follow from abnormalities in any of the steps involved in this process, which are depicted diagrammatically in Fig. 61.3. Each of these is considered below.

COMPLEMENT AND COMPLEMENT RECEPTOR TYPE 1

A possible pathophysiological mechanism for the association of complement deficiency with SLE is shown in Fig. 61.3. The interaction of immune complexes with complement results in modification of the lattice structure to prevent their precipitation from solution and to solubilize immune complexes deposited in tissues (Schifferli *et al*. 1986a). C3b, iC3b and C4b bound to complexes are ligands for complement receptors leading to: (i) opsonization for phagocytosis; (ii) binding to CR1 on erythrocytes; and (iii) binding of immune complexes to antigen-presenting and to B cells. It follows that defective binding of C4 and C3 to immune complexes may impair each of these activities, and abnormal lattice structure, reduced phagocytosis of immune complexes and impaired binding to erythrocyte CR1 may impair clearance of immune complexes and their removal from tissues (Lachmann and Walport 1987).

In support of this hypothesis, abnormal clearance was observed of IgA-containing immune complexes, which fixed complement poorly (Waxman *et al*. 1986), and also of immune complexes injected into the circulation of decomplemented baboons (Waxman *et al*. 1984). Similarly, there was abnormal clearance of tetanus toxoid/anti-tetanus toxoid immune complexes in patients with hypocomplementaemia (Schifferli *et al*. 1988).

Only a very small minority of SLE patients have total, inherited deficiency of a complement protein, and it is harder to explain a physiological link between heterozygous deficiency of C4A, apparently the commonest disease-susceptibility gene to SLE, and impaired immune complex handling *in vivo*. It has been shown that as little as 1% of C4A is sufficient to allow normal inhibition of immune precipitation of immune complexes *in vitro* (Schifferli *et al*. 1986b) and normal adherence of immune complexes to erythrocytes (Schifferli *et al*. 1987). However, complement functions as an extravascular as well as an intravascular triggered enzyme cascade, and it is possible therefore that C4A levels are lower in this compartment in heterozygote subjects, which may allow the triggering of SLE. Once the process of immune complex formation is started, activation of the classical and alternative pathways of complement leads to increased turnover and reduced levels of complement proteins. This may be a factor which perpetuates disease, by further impairing the mechanisms of disposal of immune complexes.

Immune complexes and heat-aggregated IgG bound to CR1 on erythrocytes when injected into baboons (Cornacoff *et al*. 1983), chimpanzees (Lobatto *et al*. 1987) and humans (Lobatto *et al*. 1987; Schifferli *et al*. 1988), showing that this molecule may play a part in the disposal of certain immune complexes from the circulation. Reduced CR1 numbers and reduced binding of immune complexes to erythrocytes were factors correlating

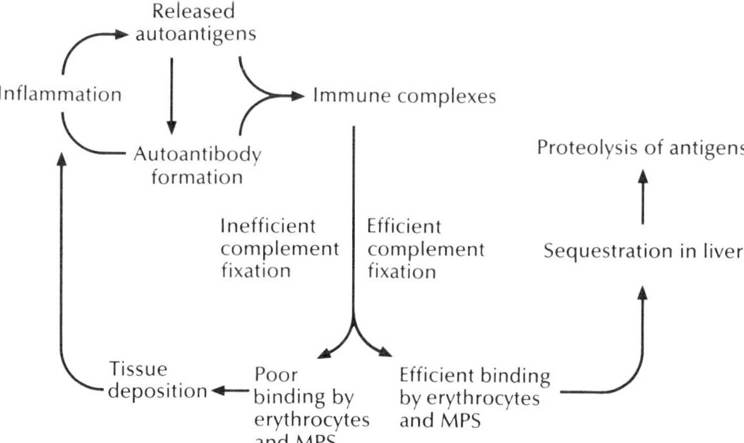

Fig. 61.3. Hypothesis linking abnormal complement function with development of SLE.

with abnormal clearance of tetanus toxoid/anti-tetanus toxoid immune complexes in humans (Schifferli *et al*. 1989). It is possible that the acquired reduction of CR1 on erythrocytes in patients with SLE may contribute to disease persistence in a similar manner to reduced C4 levels (Walport and Lachmann 1988).

ABNORMAL MONONUCLEAR PHAGOCYTIC SYSTEM FUNCTION

The concept of saturation of the mononuclear phagocytic system (previously known as the reticuloendothelial system) followed experiments of Biozzi on the fate of large doses of colloidal carbon particles injected into the circulation of rabbits (Biozzi *et al*. 1953). Possible relevance of these observations to immune complex disease came from the finding that immune complexes injected into rabbits showed saturable uptake into the liver, followed by spillover into other organs, including kidneys (Haakenstad and Mannik 1974). It remains debatable whether this is a factor in human disease, due to the obvious difficulty of repeating this type of experiment in humans. The first probes of function of Fc and complement receptor function of the mononuclear cell phagocytic system *in vivo* in humans were designed to study the pathophysiology of haemolytic anaemias (Frank *et al*. 1983). Radiolabelled erythrocytes coated with IgG antibodies, which did not fix complement, were found to clear from the circulation in the spleen, with clearance times related to the density of the IgG coating. In contrast, cells coated with IgM which fixed complement were retained transiently in the liver, and released back into the circulation with normal or increased lifespans.

These cells have been extensively used as probes of the mononuclear phagocytic system in humans and the conclusions of these studies may be summarized as follows: IgG-coated erythrocytes were cleared more slowly from the circulation of patients with SLE and there were correlations between the amount of delay with disease activity and, in some studies, with levels of circulating immune complexes (Frank *et al*. 1983).

There are important differences between particulate immune complexes and soluble immune complexes which cloud the extrapolation of results from one to the other. More than 90% of soluble immune complexes were cleared in the hepatic circulation of primates (Cornacoff *et al*. 1983), compared with the almost exclusively splenic clearance of IgG-coated red cells. An important factor in the clearance of the latter appears to be splenic blood flow (Walport *et al*. 1985b), and this alone may explain some of the disease-associated abnormalities in clearance of coated cells.

Is systemic lupus erythematosus due to polyclonal activation of lymphocytes?

One hypothesis for the development of SLE is that polyclonal activation of B lymphocytes leads to unregulated proliferation of all antibody-producing cells (reviewed in Fauci 1980; Klinman and Steinberg 1987), including those producing autoantibodies. This could follow from extrinsic activation of lymphocytes, e.g. stimulated by viral infection, or from breakdown of intrinsic control mechanisms, e.g. loss of function of 'suppressor' T lymphocytes (Abdou *et al*. 1976). Experimental evidence that SLE may be due to polyclonal activation of B lymphocytes comes from studies performed in mice by Steinberg and his collaborators, in which they found that the immune response to autoantigens (such as DNA, actin and T cells) and external antigens (such as ovalbumin and keyhole limpet haemocyanin (TNP−KLH)) was qualitatively the same in autoimmune strains of mice and normal mice, but quantitatively different (Klinman and Steinberg 1987). A similar increase in the prevalence of plaque forming cells to TNP and other extrinsic antigens has been found in humans with SLE (Budman *et al*. 1977; Morimoto *et al*. 1977). However, other studies of human lupus (reviewed above) have provided strong evidence that the autoantibody response is selective and driven by antigen and that there is no polyclonal activation of all B cells. These latter data do not exclude the possibility that the early phase of SLE is initiated by polyclonal B cell activation, with a secondary antigen-specific phase in which disease is expressed.

Disturbances of idiotypic networks

The finding of cross-reactive idiotypes on autoantibodies, some of which are represented on several of the characteristic lupus autoantibodies has led to the hypothesis that a disturbance of the network of idiotypes and anti-idiotypes may stimulate autoantibody production (Cooke *et al.* 1983; Schwartz and Stollar 1985; Zouali *et al.* 1988). The evidence for the existence *in vivo* of networks of autoantibodies and anti-idiotypes is very limited, although a number of groups have found anti-idiotypic antibodies to anti-DNA antibodies in sera from patients, particularly from those with inactive disease (Abdou *et al.* 1981; Nasu *et al.* 1982; Muryoi *et al.* 1988; Sasaki *et al.* 1988).

The hypothesis that antibody production may be regulated by anti-idiotypes has therapeutic implications. It has been tested by Hahn and Ebling (1984), who attempted to suppress expression of a cross-reactive idiotype borne by murine anti-dsDNA antibodies, using a monoclonal anti-idiotypic antibody. Although the idiotype could be suppressed, with transient therapeutic benefit, this was soon overcome by the development of large quantities of anti-dsDNA antibodies bearing other idiotypes. This result is strongly in favour of the hypothesis of an antigen-driven immune response. An augmentation of idiotype production was found when MRL mice were administered polyclonal anti-idiotypic antibodies (Teitelbaum *et al.* 1984). Much of the evidence that may be used to argue against the hypothesis that polyclonal activation is the cause of autoantibody production can be used to counter the hypothesis that a disturbance of idiotypic networks is responsible for the stimulation of autoantibodies. In particular, the spectrum of SLE autoantigens and the recognition on these by autoantibodies of multiple epitopes would be difficult to reconcile with a disturbed idiotypic network.

Cross-reaction of autoantibodies with other structures

A further hypothesis for the generation of autoantibodies is that the initial stimulus to antibody production is a foreign antigen containing epitopes that show sequence or conformational similarities to auto-antigens. Cross-reacting antibodies are produced and the immune response may then be perpetuated by the antoantigen without the need for persistence of foreign antigen. Cross-reactivities of polyreactive autoantibodies with bacterial antigens *in vitro* were reviewed above. Immunization of MRL/*lpr* mice with a polymer of glutamic acid–tyrosine (GT) led to the production of antibodies which cross-reacted with GT, DNA and Sm with approximately equal binding constants (Bailey *et al.* 1989).

Viruses as a cause of systemic lupus erythematosus

Viruses could, in theory, cause SLE by: (i) infecting lymphoid cells and perturbing their function; (ii) interacting with host machinery for the replication of nucleic acids and creating neo-antigens which could break immunological tolerance (Mathews and Bernstein 1983); (iii) stimulating the production of anti-idiotypic antibodies which could interact with receptors for viruses on cells (Plotz 1983); (iv) direct cross-reactions between viral and host antigens (Query and Keene 1987); or (v) infection of non-lymphoid cells causing prolonged release of autoantigens. There is a virtually total lack of evidence in support of any of these hypotheses.

The occurrence of antibodies to C-type retroviruses in NZB mice raised the possibility that such viruses may play an aetiological role in murine lupus (Mellors *et al.* 1969). Antibodies to the viral *env* gene product, GP70, are produced in large amounts in these animals and immune complexes comprising GP70–anti-GP70 have been shown to participate in the lesions of glomerulonephritis. However, expression of retroviral antigens is not essential for the development of murine lupus. The expression of xenotropic virus is genetically controlled. Analysis of F_1, F_2 and backcross progeny of NZB mice crossed with SWR (a strain homozygous for recessive alleles of viral expression) showed that expression of retroviral antigens could be dissociated from that of autoimmune disease (Datta and Schwartz 1978).

There is very little evidence for the participation of retroviruses in human SLE (reviewed by Pincus 1982). Both *gag*-like proteins and antibodies reactive with $p30^{gag}$ have been identified in renal biopsy material from SLE patients (Mellors and Mellors 1976, 1978; Reynolds and Panem 1981). Antibodies binding in immunoblotting reactions to products of murine leukaemia virus *gag* gene have been identified in patients with antibodies to Sm, RNP and La (Rucheton *et al.* 1985). However, both the stimulus for their production and their binding specificity need to be considered with caution. Antibodies with apparent specificity for the *env* product GP70 may actually react with cellular carbohydrates, and not epitopes encoded by viruses (Barbacid *et al.* 1980; Snyder and Fleissner 1980).

The cloning and sequencing of autoantigens has allowed the searching of data bases for sequences of similarity. Query and Keene (1987) identified a sequence of similarity between the 70 kD protein associated with U1 RNP and murine leukaemia virus group specific antigen, $p30^{gag}$. Antibodies raised against the $p30^{gag}$ protein bound to the native 70 kD protein. Although this is an attractive experimental result, the search for sequence similarity is a procedure fraught with the potential for artefactual results. As the number of published protein sequences increases, so the probability of randomly occurring similarities increases; an analysis of the Dayhoff Protein Sequence Database which illustrates this point has been published (Wilson I.A. *et al.* 1985).

Conclusions

Evidence gathered from studies of humans and mice with SLE supports the hypothesis that SLE is a syndrome in which disease is caused by a final common pathway of inflammation initiated by many different stimuli. Both the genetic susceptibility to disease and provocative environmental stimuli appear to be heterogeneous. The presence of high titres of autoantibodies accompanied by evidence of complement activation is the most striking abnormality to be identified in patients with SLE. However, it is clear that the presence of autoantibodies is not sufficient for the development of inflammation, although it is probable that they are necessary. A role for cell-mediated mechanisms for disease has been suggested by some studies and more work is needed to define these.

References

Abdou, N.I., Sagawa, A., Pascual, E., Hebert, J. and Sadeghee, S. (1976). Suppressor T cell abnormality in idiopathic systemic lupus erythematosus. *Clin. Immunol. Immunopathol.* **6**, 192.

Abdou, N.I., Wall, H., Lindsley, H.B., Halsey, J.F. and Suzuki, T. (1981). Network theory in autoimmunity: *in vitro* suppression of serum anti-DNA antibody binding to DNA by anti-idiotypic antibody in systemic lupus. *J. Clin. Invest.* **67**, 1297.

Abe, T. and Homma, M. (1971). Immunologic reactivity in patients with systemic lupus erythematosus: humoral antibody and cellular immune responses. *Acta Rheumatol. Scand.* **17**, 35.

Abrass, C.K., Nies, K.M., Louie, J.S., Border, W.A. and Glassock, R.J. (1980). Correlation and predictive accuracy of circulating immune complexes with disease activity in patients with systemic lupus erythematosus. *Arthritis Rheum.* **23**, 273.

Adu, D., Dobson, J. and Williams, D.G. (1981). DNA–anti-DNA circulating complexes in the nephritis of systemic lupus erythematosus. *Clin. Exp. Immunol.* **43**, 605.

Agnello, V., Koffler, D., Eisenberg, J.W., Winchester, R.J. and Kunkel, H.G. (1971). C1q precipitins in the sera of patients with systemic lupus erythematosus and other hypocomplementemic states: characterisation of high and low molecular weight types. *J. Exp. Med.* **134**, 228S.

Aguado, M.T., Lambris, J.D., Tsokos, G.C. *et al.* (1985). Monoclonal antibodies against complement 3 neoantigens for detection of immune complexes and complement activation: relationship between immune complex levels, state of C3, and numbers of receptors for C3b. *J. Clin. Invest.* **76**, 1418.

Alarcon-Segovia, D., Ruiz-Arguelles, A. and Fishbein, E. (1978). Antibody to nuclear ribonucleoprotein penetrates live human mononuclear cells through Fc receptors. *Nature* **271**, 67.

Alcover, A., Molano, J., Renart, J., Gil-Aguado, A., Nieto, A. and Avila, J. (1984). Antibodies to vimentin intermediate filaments in sera from patients with systemic lupus erythematosus. *Arthritis Rheum.* **27**, 922.

Alexopoulos, E., Seron, D., Hartley, R.B. and Cameron, J.S. (1990). Lupus nephritis: correlation of interstitial cells with glomerular function. *Kidney Int.* **37**, 100.

Alper, C.A. and Rosen, F.S. (1967). Studies of the *in vivo* behavior of human C′3 in normal subjects and patients. *J. Clin. Invest.* **46**, 2021.

Anderson, C.L. and Stillman, W.S. (1980). Raji assay for immune complexes: evidence for detection of Raji-directed immunoglobulin G antibody in sera from patients with systemic lupus erythematosus. *J. Clin. Invest.* **66**, 353.

Antes, U., Heinz, H.P. and Loos, M. (1988). Evidence for the presence of autoantibodies to the collagen-like portion of C1q in systemic lupus erythematosus. *Arthritis Rheum.* **31**, 457.

Arnett, F.C. and Shulman, L.E. (1976). Studies in familial systemic lupus erythematosus. *Medicine (Baltimore)* **55**, 313.

Arnett, F.C., Hamilton, R.G., Roebber, M.G., Harley, J.B. and Reichlin, M. (1988). Increased frequencies of Sm and nRNP autoantibodies in American blacks compared to whites with systemic lupus erythematosus. *J. Rheumatol.* **15**, 1773.

Atkins, C.J., Kondon, J.J., Quismorio, F.P. and Friou, G.J. (1972). The choroid plexus in systemic lupus erythematosus. *Ann. Intern. Med.* **76**, 65.

Bachmann, M., Mayet, W.J., Schroder, H.C. *et al.* (1986). Association of La and Ro antigens with intracellular structures in HEp-2 carcinoma cells. *Proc. Nat. Acad. Sci. (USA)* **83**, 7770.

Baer, A.N., Woosley, R.L. and Pincus, T. (1986a). Further evidence for the lack of association between acetylator phenotype and systemic lupus erythematosus. *Arthritis Rheum.* **29**, 508.

Baer, A.N., McAllister, C.B., Wilkinson, G.R., Woosley, R.L. and Pincus, T. (1986b). Altered distribution of debrisoquine oxidation phenotypes in patients with systemic lupus erythematosus. *Arthritis Rheum.* **29**, 843.

Bailey, N.C., Fidanza, V., Mayer, R., Mazza, G., Fougereau, M. and Bona, C. (1989). Activation of clones producing self-reactive antibodies by foreign antigen and antiidiotypic antibodies carrying the internal image of the antigen. *J. Clin. Invest.* **84**, 744.

Barbacid, M., Bolognesi, D. and Aaronson, S.A. (1980). Humans have antibodies capable of recognizing oncoviral glycoproteins: demonstration that these antibodies are formed in response to cellular modification of glycoproteins rather than as consequence of exposure to virus. *Proc. Nat. Acad. Sci. (USA)* **77**, 1617.

Bardana, E.J., Jr, Harbeck, R.J., Hoffman, A.A., Pirofsky, B. and Carr, R.I. (1975). The prognostic and therapeutic implications of DNA : anti-DNA immune complexes in systemic lupus erythematosus (SLE). *Am. J. Med.* **59**, 515.

Batchelor, J.R., Welsh, K.I., Tinoco, R.M. *et al.* (1980). Hydralazine-induced systemic lupus erythematosus: influence of HLA-DR and sex on susceptibility. *Lancet* **i**, 1107.

Batchelor, J.R., Fielder, A.H., Walport, M.J. *et al.* (1987). Family study of the major histocompatibility complex in HLA DR3 negative patients with systemic lupus erythematosus. *Clin. Exp. Immunol.* **70**, 364.

Baum, J. and Ziff, M. (1969). Decreased 19S antibody response to bacterial antigens in systemic lupus erythematosus. *J. Clin. Invest.* **48**, 758.

Beck, J.S. and Rowell, N.R. (1963). Transplacental passage of antinuclear antibody. *Lancet* **i**, 134.

Beck, J.S. and Rowell, N.R. (1966). Discoid lupus erythematosus: a study of the clinical features and biochemical and serological abnormalities in 120 patients with observation. *Quart. J. Med.* **35**, 119.

Becker, G.J., Waldburger, M., Hughes, G.R. and Pepys, M.B. (1980). Value of serum C-reactive protein measurement in the investigation of fever in systemic lupus erythematosus. *Ann. Rheum. Dis.* **39**, 50.

Bell, D.A. and Maddison, P.J. (1980). Serologic subsets in systemic lupus erythematosus: an examination of autoantibodies in relationship to clinical features of disease and HLA. *Arthritis Rheum.* **23**, 1268.

Bell, D.A., Rigby, R., Stiller, C.R., Clark, W.F., Harth, M. and Ebers, G. (1984). HLA antigens in systemic lupus erythematosus: relationship to disease severity, age at onset, and sex. *J. Rheumatol.* **11**, 475.

Ben-Chetrit, E., Chan, E.K., Sullivan, K.F. and Tan, E.M. (1988). A 52-kD protein is a novel component of the SS-A/Ro antigenic particle. *J. Exp. Med.* **167**, 1560.

Bencze, G., Cserhati, S., Kovacs, J. and Tiboldi, T. (1958). Production of L.E. cells *in vivo* by transfusion of systemic lupus erythematosus plasma. *Ann. Rheum. Dis.* **17**, 426.

Bennett, R.M. and O'Connell, D.J. (1978). The arthritis of mixed connective tissue disease. *Ann. Rheum. Dis.* **37**, 397.

Bennett, R.M., Gabor, G.T. and Merritt, M.M. (1985). DNA binding to human leukocytes: evidence for a receptor-mediated association, internalization, and degradation of DNA. *J. Clin. Invest.* **76**, 2182.

Bennett, R.M., Davis, J. and Merritt, M. (1986). Anti-DNA antibodies react with DNA expressed on the surface of monocytes and B lymphocytes. *J. Rheumatol.* **13**, 679.

Bennett, R.M., Kotzin, B.L. and Merritt, M.J. (1987). DNA receptor dysfunction in systemic lupus erythematosus and kindred disorders: induction by anti-DNA antibodies, antihistone antibodies, and antireceptor antibodies. *J. Exp. Med.* **166**, 850.

Bernstein, R.M., Bunn, C.C., Hughes, G.R., Francoeur, A.M. and Mathews, M.B. (1984). Cellular protein and RNA antigens in autoimmune disease. *Mol. Biol. Med.* **2**, 105.

Biesecker, G., Katz, S. and Koffler, D. (1981). Renal localization of the membrane attack complex in systemic lupus erythematosus. *J. Exp. Med.* **154**, 1779.

Biesecker, G., Lavin, L., Ziskind, M. and Koffler, D. (1982). Cutaneous localization of the membrane attack complex in discoid and systemic lupus erythematosus. *N. Engl. J. Med.* **306**, 264.

Biozzi, B., Benacerraf, B. and Halpern, B.N. (1953). Quantitative study of granulopectic activity of reticulo-endothelial system; study of granulopectic activity of R.E.S. in relation to dose of carbon injected: relationship between weight of organs and their activity. *Br. J. Exp. Pathol.* **34**, 441.

Blank, M., Krup, M., Mendlovic, S. *et al.* (1990). The importance of the pathogenic 16/6 idiotype in the induction of SLE in naive mice. *Scand. J. Immunol.* **31**, 45.

Block, S.R., Gibbs, C.B., Stevens, M.B. and Shulman, L.E. (1968). Delayed hypersensitivity in systemic lupus erythematosus. *Ann. Rheum. Dis.* **27**, 311.

Block, S.R., Winfield, J.B., Lockshin, M.D., D'Angelo, W.A. and Christian, C.L. (1975). Studies of twins with systemic lupus erythematosus: a review of the literature and presentation of 12 additional sets. *Am. J. Med.* **59**, 533.

Block, S.R., Lockshin, M.D., Winfield, J.B. *et al.* (1976). Immunologic observations on 9 sets of twins either concordant or discordant for SLE. *Arthritis Rheum.* **19**, 545.

Bluestein, H.G. and Zvaifler, N.J. (1976). Brain-reactive lymphocytotoxic antibodies in the serum of patients with systemic lupus erythematosus. *J. Clin. Invest.* **57**, 509.

Bluestein, H.G., Williams, G.W. and Steinberg, A.D. (1981). Cerebrospinal fluid antibodies to neuronal cells: association with neuropsychiatric manifestations of systemic lupus erythematosus. *Am. J. Med.* **70**, 240.

Boey, M.L., Peebles, C.L., Tsay, G., Feng, P.H. and Tan, E.M. (1988). Clinical and autoantibody correlations in Orientals with systemic lupus erythematosus. *Ann. Rheum. Dis.* **47**, 918.

Boire, G. and Craft, J. (1989). Biochemical and immunological heterogeneity of the Ro ribonucleoprotein particles: analysis with sera specific for the Roh Y5 particle. *J. Clin. Invest.* **84**, 270.

Bona, C.A. (1988). V genes encoding autoantibodies: molecular and phenotypic characteristics. *Ann. Rev. Immunol.* **6**, 327.

Bonfa, E. and Elkon, K.B. (1986). Clinical and serologic associations of the antiribosomal P protein antibody. *Arthritis Rheum.* **29**, 981.

Bonfa, E., Golombek, S.J., Kaufman, L.D. *et al.* (1987). Association between lupus psychosis and antiribosomal P protein antibodies. *N. Engl. J. Med.* **317**, 265.

Brand, C., Davidson, A., Littlejohn, G. and Ryan, P. (1984). Hydralazine-induced lupus: no association with HLA-DR4, *Lancet* **i**, 462 (letter).

Bravo, R., Frank, R., Blundell, P.A. and MacDonald-Bravo, H. (1987). Cyclin/PCNA is the auxiliary protein of DNA polymerase-δ. *Nature* **326**, 515.

Bresnihan, B. and Jasin, H.E. (1977). Suppressor function of peripheral blood mononuclear cells in normal individuals and in patients with systemic lupus erythematosus. *J. Clin.*

Invest. **59**, 106.

Bresnihan, B., Oliver, M., Williams, B. and Hughes, G.R. (1979). An antineuronal antibody cross-reacting with erythrocytes and lymphocytes in systemic lupus erythematosus. *Arthritis Rheum.* **22**, 313.

Brodman, R., Gilfillan, R., Glass, D. and Schur, P.H. (1978). Influenzal vaccine response in systemic lupus erythematosus. *Ann. Intern. Med.* **88**, 735.

Budman, D.R., Steinberg, A.D. *et al.* (1977). Hematologic aspects of systemic lupus erythematosus: current concepts. *Ann. Intern. Med.* **86**, 220.

Budman, D.R., Merchant, E.B., Steinberg, A.D. *et al.* (1977). Increased spontaneous activity of antibody-forming cells in the peripheral blood of patients with active SLE *Arthritis Rheum.* **20**, 829.

Bunn, C.C., Bernstein, R.M. and Mathews, M.B. (1986). Autoantibodies against alanyl-tRNA synthetase and tRNAAla coexist and are associated with myositis. *J. Exp. Med.* **163**, 1281.

Burdick, G. and Emlen, W. (1985). Effect of antibody excess on the size, stoichiometry, and DNAse resistance of DNA anti-DNA immune complexes. *J. Immunol.* **135**. 2593.

Butler, W.T., Sharp, J.T. and Rossen, R.D. (1972). Relationship of the clinical course of systemic lupus erythematosus to the presence of circulating lymphocytotoxic antibodies. *Arthritis Rheum.* **15**, 231.

Buyon, J.P., Shadick, N., Berkman, R. *et al.* (1988). Surface expression of Gp 165/95, the complement receptor CR3, as a marker of disease activity in systemic lupus erythematosus. *Clin. Immunol. Immunopathol.* **46**, 141.

Buyon, J.P., Ben-Chetrit, E., Karp, S. *et al.* (1989). Acquired congenital heart block: pattern of maternal antibody response to biochemically defined antigens of the SSA/Ro−SSB/La system in neonatal lupus. *J. Clin. Invest.* **84**, 627.

Caligaris-Cappio, F., Bergui, L., Tesio, L., Ziano, R. and Camussi, G. (1985). HLA-DR+ T cells of the Leu 3 (helper) type infiltrate the kidneys of patients with systemic lupus erythematosus. *Clin. Exp. Immunol.* **59**, 185.

Caligaris-Cappio, F., Riva, M., Tesio, L., Schena, M., Gaidano, G. and Bergui, L. (1989). Human normal CD5+ B lymphocytes can be induced to differentiate to CD5− B lymphocytes with germinal center cell features. *Blood* **73**, 1259.

Callen, J.P. and Klein, J. (1988). Subacute cutaneous lupus erythematosus: clinical, serologic, immunogenetic, and therapeutic consideration in seventy-two patients. *Arthritis Rheum.* **31**, 1007.

Cameron, J.S., Lessof, M.H., Ogg, C.S., Williams, B.D. and Williams, D.G. (1976). Disease activity in the nephritis of systemic lupus erythematosus in relation to serum complement concentrations: DNA-binding capacity and precipitating anti-DNA antibody. *Clin. Exp. Immunol.* **25**, 418.

Cannon, E.F. and Curtis, A.C. (1958). A survey of lupus erythematosus in the University of Michigan Hospital since 1948. *Arch Dermatol.* **78**, 196.

Carr, R.I., Hoffmann, A.A. and Harbeck, R.J. (1975). Comparison of DNA binding in normal population, general hospital laboratory personnel, and personnel from laboratories studying SLE. *J. Rheumatol.* **2**, 178.

Carreras, L.O. and Vermylen, J.G. (1982). 'Lupus' anticoagulant and thrombosis — possible role of inhibition of prostacyclin formation. *Thromb. Haemostasis* **48**, 38.

Carroll, P., Stafford, D., Schwartz, R.S. and Stollar, B.D. (1985). Murine monoclonal anti-DNA autoantibodies bind to endogenous bacteria. *J. Immunol.* **135**, 1086.

Casali, P. and Notkins, A.L. (1989). Probing the human B-cell repertoire with EBV polyreactive antibodies and CD5+ B lymphocytes. *Ann. Rev. Immunol.* **7**, 513.

Casali, P., Bossus, A., Carpenter, N.A. and Lambert, P.H. (1977). Solid phase immunoassay or radioimmunoassay for the detection of immune complexes based on their recognition by conglutinin: conglutinin binding test: a comparative study with 125-I labelled C1q binding and Raji cell RIA tests. *Clin. Exp. Immunol.* **29**, 342.

Casali, P., Burastero, S.E., Nakamura, M., Inghirami, G. and Notkins, A.L. (1987). Human lymphocytes making rheumatoid factor and antibody to ssDNA belong to Leu-1+ B-cell subset. *Science* **236**, 77.

Chan, E.K., Francoeur, A.M. and Tan, E.M. (1986). Epitopes, structural domains, and asymmetry of amino acid residues in SS-B/La nuclear protein. *J. Immunol.* **136**, 3744.

Charpentier, B., Carnaud, C. and Bach, J.-F. (1979). Selective depression of the xenogeneic cell-mediated lympholysis in systemic lupus erythematosus. *J. Clin. Invest.* **64**, 351.

Christian, C.L., Hatfield, W.B. and Chase, P.H. (1963). Systemic lupus erythematosus: cryoprecipitation of sera. *J. Clin. Invest.* **42**, 823.

Christiansen, F.T., Dawkins, R.L., Uko, G., McCluskey, J., Kay, P.H. and Zilko, P.J. (1983). Complement allotyping in SLE: association with C4A null. *Aust. NZ J. Med.* **13**, 483.

Cines, D.B., Lyss, A.P., Reeber, M.B. and Dehoratius, R.J. (1984). Presence of complement-fixing anti-endothelial cell antibodies in systemic lupus erythematosus. *J. Clin. Invest.* **73**, 611.

Clark, W.H., Reed, R.J. and Mihm, M.C. (1973). Lupus erythematosus: histopathology of cutaneous lesions. *Hum. Pathol.* **4**, 157.

Coade, S.B., Van Haaren, E., Loizou, S., Walport, M.J., Denman, A.M. and Pearson, J.D. (1989). Endothelial prostacyclin release in systemic lupus erythematosus. *Thromb. Haemostasis* **61**, 97.

Cohen, J.H., Caudwell, V., Levi Strauss, M., Bourgeois, P. and Kazatchkine, M.D. (1989). Genetic analysis of CR1 expression on erythrocytes of patients with systemic lupus erythematosus. *Arthritis Rheum.* **32**, 393.

Cole, E.H., Schulman, J., Urowitz, M., Keystone, E., Williams, C. and Levy, G.A. (1985). Monocyte procoagulant activity in glomerulonephritis associated with systemic lupus erythematosus. *J. Clin. Invest.* **75**, 861.

Cooke, A., Lydyard, P.M. and Roitt, I.M. (1983). Mechanisms of autoimmunity: a role for cross-reactive idiotypes. *Immunol. Today* **4**, 170.

Cornacchia, E., Golbus, J., Maybaum, J., Strahler, J., Hanash, S. and Richardson, B. (1988). Hydralazine and procainamide inhibit T cell DNA methylation and induce autoreactivity. *J. Immunol.* **140**, 2197.

Cornacoff, J.B., Hebert, L.A., Smead, W.L., Vanaman, M.E., Birmingham, D.J. and Waxman, F.J. (1983). Primate erythrocyte-immune complex-clearing mechanism. *J. Clin. Invest.* **71**, 236.

Daha, M.R., Hazevoet, H.M. and Van Es, L.A. (1983). Regulation of immune complex-mediated complement activation by autoantibodies (F-42) isolated from sera of patients with systemic lupus erythematosus. *Clin. Exp. Immunol.* **53**, 541.

Datta, S.K. and Schwartz, R.S. (1978). Xenotropic virus and autoimmunity in NZB mice. *Arthritis Rheum.* **21**, S113.

Davis, J.S., IV, Godfrey, S.M. and Winfield, J.B. (1978). Direct evidence for circulating DNA/anti-DNA complexes in systemic lupus erythematosus. *Arthritis Rheum.* **21**, 17.

Davis, S., Furie, B.C., Griffin, J.H., Furie, B. and Willey, R. (1978). Circulating inhibitors of blood coagulation associated with procainamide-induced lupus erythematosus. *Am. J. Hematol.* **4**, 401.

De Beer, F.C., Mallya, R.K., Fagan, E.A., Lanham, J.G., Hughes, G.R. and Pepys, M.B. (1982). Serum amyloid-A protein concentration in inflammatory diseases and its relationship to the incidence of reactive systemic amyloidosis. *Lancet* **ii**, 231.

DeHoratius, R.J. and Messner, R.P. (1975). Lymphocytotoxic antibodies in family members of patients with systemic lupus erythematosus. *J. Clin. Invest.* **55**, 1254.

DeHoratius, R.J., Pillarisetty, R., Messner, R.P. and Talal, N. (1975). Anti-nucleic acid antibodies in systemic lupus erythematosus patients and their families: incidence and correlation with lymphocytotoxic antibodies. *J. Clin. Invest.* **56**, 1149.

DeHoratius, R.J., Rubin, R.L., Messner, R.P. and Carr, R.I. (1979). Lymphocytotoxic antibodies in laboratory personnel exposed to SLE sera. *Lancet* **ii**, 1141 (letter).

Delfraissy, J.F., Segond, P., Galanaud, P., Wallon, C., Massias, P. and Dormont, J. (1980). Depressed primary *in vitro* antibody response in untreated systemic lupus erythematosus: T helper cell defect and lack of defective suppressor cell function. *J. Clin. Invest.* **66**, 141.

Dersimonian, H., Schwartz, R.S., Barrett, K.J. and Stollar, B.D. (1987). Relationship of human variable region heavy chain germ-line genes to genes encoding anti-DNA autoantibodies. *J. Immunol.* **139**, 2496.

Diamond, B. and Scharff, M.D. (1984). Somatic mutation of the T15 heavy chain gives rise to an antibody with autoantibody specificity. *Proc. Nat. Acad. Sci. (USA)* **81**, 5841.

Dighiero, G., Lymberi, P., Holmberg, D., Lundquist, I., Coutinho, A. and Avrameas, S. (1985). High frequency of natural autoantibodies in normal newborn mice. *J. Immunol.* **134**, 765.

Dubois, E.L. and Tuffanelli, D.L. (1964). Clinical manifestations of systemic lupus erythematosus: computer analysis of 520 cases. *JAMA* **190**, 104.

Dubroff, L.M. and Reid, R.J., Jr (1980). Hydralazine–pyrimidine interactions may explain hydralazine-induced lupus erythematosus. *Science* **208**, 404.

Dunckley, H., Gatenby, P.A., Hawkins, B., Naito, S. and Serjeantson, S.W. (1987). Deficiency of C4A is a genetic determinant of systemic lupus erythematosus in three ethnic groups. *J. Immunogenet.* **14**, 209.

Dunckley, H., Gatenby, P.A. and Serjeantson, S.W. (1988). T-cell receptor and HLA class II RFLPs in systemic lupus erythematosus. *Immunogenetics* **27**, 393.

Ebling, F. and Hahn, B.H. (1980). Restricted subpopulations of DNA antibodies in kidneys of mice with systemic lupus: comparison of antibodies in serum and renal eluates. *Arthritis Rheum.* **23**, 392.

Eilat, D., Hochberg, M., Pumphrey, J. and Rudikoff, S. (1984). Monoclonal antibodies to DNA and RNA from NZB/NZW F1 mice antigenic specificities and NH2 terminal amino acid sequences. *J. Immunol.* **133**, 489.

Eilat, D., Fischel, R. and Zlotnick, A. (1985). A central anti-DNA idiotype in human and murine systemic lupus erythematosus. *Eur. J. Immunol.* **15**, 368.

Eilat, D., Zlotnick, A.Y. and Fischel, R. (1986). Evaluation of the cross-reaction between anti-DNA and anti-cardiolipin antibodies in SLE and experimental animals. *Clin. Exp. Immunol.* **65**, 269.

Eisenberg, R.A., Theofilopoulos, A.N. and Dixon, F.J. (1977). Use of bovine conglutinin for the assay of immune complexes. *J. Immunol.* **118**, 1428.

Eisenberg, R.A., Dyer, K., Graven, S.Y., Fuller, C.R. and Yount, W.J. (1985). Subclass restriction and polyclonality of the systemic lupus erythematosus marker antibody anti-Sm. *J. Clin. Invest.* **75**, 1270.

Elkon, K.B., Skelly, S., Parnassa, A. *et al.* (1986). Identification and chemical synthesis of a ribosomal protein antigenic determinant in systemic lupus erythematosus. *Proc. Nat. Acad. Sci. (USA)* **83**, 7419.

Klkon, K.B., Bonfa, E., Llovet, R., Danho, W., Weissbach, H. and Brot, N. (1988). Properties of the ribosomal P2 protein autoantigen are similar to those of foreign protein antigens. *Proc. Nat. Acad. Sci. (USA)* **85**, 5186.

Elkon, K.B., Bonfa, E., Llovet, R. and Eisenberg, R.A. (1989). Association between anti-Sm and anti-ribosomal P protein autoantibodies in human systemic lupus erythematosus and MRL/lpr mice. *J. Immunol.* **143**, 1549.

Ellis, S.G. and Verity, M.A. (1979). Central nervous system involvement in systemic lupus erythematosus: a review of neuropathologic findings in 57 cases, 1955–1977. *Semin. Arthritis Rheum.* **8**, 212.

Emlen, W. and Mannik, M. (1982). Clearance of circulating DNA-anti-DNA immune complexes in mice. *J. Exp. Med.* **155**, 1210.

Emlen, W., Pisetsky, D.S. and Taylor, R.P. (1986). Antibodies to DNA: a perspective. *Arthritis Rheum.* **29**, 1417.

Esdaile, J.M., Levinton, C., Federgreen, W., Hayslett, J.P. and Kashgarian, M. (1989). The clinical and renal biopsy predictors of long-term outcome in lupus nephritis: a study of 87 patients and review of the literature. *Quart. J. Med.* **72**, 779.

Estes, D. and Christian, C.L. (1971). The natural history of systemic lupus erythematosus by prospective analysis. *Medicine (Baltimore)* **50**, 85.

Faaber, P., Capel, P.J., Rijke, G.P., Vierwinden, G., Van de Putte, L.B. and Koene, R.A. (1984). Cross-reactivity of anti-DNA antibodies with proteoglycans. *Clin. Exp. Immunol.* **55**, 502.

Falk, R.J., Dalmasso, A.P., Kim, Y., Lam, S. and Michael, A. (1985). Radioimmunoassay of the attack complex of complement in serum from patients with systemic lupus erythematosus. *N. Engl. J. Med.* **312**, 1594.

Fauci, A.S. (1980). Immunoregulation in autoimmunity. *J. Allergy Clin. Immunol.* **66**, 5.

Fauci, A.S., Steinberg, A.D., Haynes, B.F. and Whalen, G. (1978). Immunoregulatory aberrations in systemic lupus erythematosus. *J. Immunol.* **121**, 1473.

Fedrick, J.A., Pandey, J.P., Chen, Z., Fudenberg, H.H. and Ainsworth, S.K. (1983). Gm allotypes in blacks with systemic lupus erythematosus. *Hum. Immunol.* **8**, 177.

Fessel, W.J. (1974). Systemic lupus erythematosus in the community: incidence, prevalence, outcome, and first symptoms, the high prevalence in black women. *Arch. Intern. Med.* **134**, 1027.

Fessel, W.J. (1978). ANA-negative systemic lupus erythematosus. *Am. J. Med.* **64**, 80.

Fielder, A.H., Walport, M.J., Batchelor, J.R. *et al.* (1983). Family study of the major histocompatibility complex in patients with systemic lupus erythematosus: importance of null alleles of C4A and C4. *Br. Med. J.* **286**, 425.

Fischbach, M., Rabbie, J. and Talal, N. (1981). Comparison of different antinucleic acid antibody spectrotypes in spontaneous, induced, and murine lupus. *J. Clin. Invest.* **68**, 1036.

Fitchen, J.J., Cline, M.J., Saxon, A. and Golde, D.W. (1979). Serum inhibitors of hematopoiesis in a patient with aplastic anemia and systemic lupus erythematosus: recovery after exchange plasmapheresis. *Am. J. Med.* **66**, 537.

Fournie, G.J. (1988). Circulating DNA and lupus nephritis. *Kidney Int.* **33**, 487.

Francoeur, A.M., Peebles, C.L., Gompper, P.T. and Tan, E.M. (1986). Identification of Ki (Ku, p70/p80) autoantigens and analysis of anti-Ki autoantibody reactivity. *J. Immunol.* **136**, 1648.

Frank, M.M., Lawley, T.J., Hamburger, M.I. and Brown, E.J. (1983). Immunoglobulin G Fc receptor-mediated clearance in autoimmune diseases. *Ann. Intern. Med.* **98**, 206.

Freyssinet, J.M. and Cazenave, J.P. (1987). Lupus-like anticoagulants, modulation of the protein C pathway and thrombosis. *Thromb. Haemostasis* **58**, 679.

Fronek, Z., Lentz, D., Berliner, N. *et al.* (1986). Systemic lupus erythematosus is not genetically linked to the beta chain of the T cell receptor. *Arthritis Rheum.* **29**, 1023.

Furukawa, F., Kashihara, M., Imamura, S., Ohshio, G. and Hamashima, Y. (1986). Evaluation of anti-cardiolipin antibody and its cross-reactivity in sera of patients with lepromatous leprosy. *Arch. Dermatol. Res.* **278**, 317.

Gallo, G.R., Caulin-Glaser, T. and Lamm, M.E. (1981). Charge of circulating immune complexes as a factor in glomerular basement membrane localization in mice. *J. Clin. Invest.* **67**, 1305.

Gawryl, M.S., Chudwin, D.S., Langlois, P.F. and Lint, T.F. (1988). The terminal complement complex, C5b-9, a marker of disease activity in patients with systemic lupus erythematosus. *Arthritis Rheum.* **31**, 188.

Genth, E., Zarnowski, H., Mieran, R., Wohltmann, D. and Hartl, P.W. (1987). HLA-DR4 and Gm(1,3;5,21) are associated with U1-nRNP antibody positive connective tissue disease. *Ann. Rheum. Dis.* **46**, 189.

Gharavi, A.E., Chu, J.L. and Elkon, K.B. (1988). Autoantibodies to intracellular proteins in human systemic lupus erythematosus are not due to random polyclonal B cell activation. *Arthritis Rheum.* **31**, 1337.

Gilliam, J.N., Cheatum, D.E., Hurd, E.R., Stastny, P. and Ziff, M. (1974). Immunoglobulin in clinically uninvolved skin in systemic lupus erythematosus: association with renal disease. *J. Clin. Invest.* **53**, 1434.

Ginsburg, W.W., Finkelman, F.D. and Lipsky, P.E. (1979). Circulating and pokeweed mitogen-induced immunoglobulin-secreting cells in systemic lupus erythematosus. *Clin. Exp. Immunol.* **35**, 76.

Glass, D., Raum, D., Gibson, D., Stillman, J.S. and Schur, P.H. (1976). Inherited deficiency of the second component of complement: rheumatic disease associations. *J. Clin. Invest.* **58**, 853.

Gleichmann, E., Van Elven, E.H. and Van der Veen, J.P.W. (1982). A systemic lupus erythematosus (SLE)-like disease in mice induced by abnormal T-B cooperation: preferential formation of autoantibodies characteristic of SLE. *Eur. J. Immunol.* **12**, 152.

Gohill, J., Cary, P.D., Couppez, M. and Fritzler, M.J. (1985). Antibodies from patients with drug-induced and idiopathic lupus erythematosus react with epitopes restricted to the amino and carboxyl termini of histone. *J. Immunol.* **135**, 3116.

Goldman, M., Feng, H.M., Engers, H., Hochman, A., Louis, J. and Lambert, P.H. (1983). Autoimmunity and immune complex disease after neonatal induction of transplantation tolerance in mice. *J. Immunol.* **131**, 251.

Gottlieb, E. and Steitz, J.A. (1989). Function of the mammalian La protein: evidence for its action in transcription termination by RNA polymerase III. *EMBO J.* **8**, 851.

Haakenstad, A.O. and Mannik, M. (1974). Saturation of the reticuloendothelial system with soluble immune complexes. *J. Immunol.* **112**, 1939.

Habets, W.J., Hoet, M.H., Sillekens, P.T., De Rooij, D.J., Van de Putte L.B. and Van Venrooij, W.J. (1989). Detection of autoantibodies in a quantitative immunoassay using recombinant ribonucleoprotein antigens. *Clin. Exp. Immunol.* **76**, 172.

Hahn, B.H. (1982). Characteristics of pathogenic subpopulations of antibodies to DNA. *Arthritis Rheum.* **25**, 747.

Hahn, B.H. and Ebling, F.M. (1984). Suppression of murine lupus nephritis by administration of an anti-idiotypic antibody to anti-DNA. *J. Immunol.* **132**, 187.

Hahn, B.H., Bagby, M.K. and Osterland, C.K. (1973). Abnormalities of delayed hypersensitivity in systemic lupus erythematosus. *Am. J. Med.* **55**, 25.

Halla, J.T. and Hardin, J.G. (1978). Clinical features of the arthritis of mixed connective tissue disease. *Arthritis Rheum.* **21**, 497.

Hammond, A., Rudge, A.C., Loizou, S., Bowcock, S.J. and Walport, M.J. (1989). Reduced numbers of complement receptor type 1 on erythrocytes are associated with increased levels of anticardiolipin antibodies: findings in patients with systemic lupus erythematosus and the antiphospholipid syndrome. *Arthritis Rheum.* **32**, 259.

Hanauer, L.B. and Christian, C.L. (1967a). Studies of cryoproteins in systemic lupus erythematosus. *J. Clin. Invest.* **46**, 400.

Hanauer, L.B. and Christian, C.L. (1967b). Clinical studies of hemolytic complement and the 11S component. *Am. J. Med.* **42**, 882.

Hang, L.M., Izui, S. and Dixon, F.J. (1981). (NZW × BXSB)F1 hybrid: a model of acute lupus and coronary vascular disease with myocardial infarction. *J. Exp. Med.* **154**, 216.

Harbeck, R.J., Bardana, E.J., Kekker, P.F. and Carr, R.I. (1973). DNA: anti-DNA complexes: their detection in systemic lupus erythematosus sera. *J. Clin. Invest.* **52**, 789.

Hardin, J.A. (1986). The lupus autoantigens and the pathogenesis of systemic lupus erythematosus. *Arthritis Rheum.* **29**, 457.

Hardin, J.A. and Thomas, J.O. (1983). Antibodies to histones in systemic lupus erythematosus: localization of prominant autoantigens in H1 and H2B. *Proc. Nat. Acad. Sci. (USA)* **80**,

7410.

Hardy, R.R., Hayakawa, K., Shimizu, M., Yamasaki, K. and Kishimoto, T. (1987). Rheumatoid factor secretion from human Leu-1+ B cells. *Science* **236**, 81.

Harley, J.B., Alexander, E.L., Bias, W.B. *et al.* (1986a). Anti-Ro (SS-A) and anti-La (SS-B) in patients with Sjögren's syndrome. *Arthritis Rheum.* **29**, 196.

Harley, J.B., Reichlin, M., Arnett, F.C., Alexander, E.L., Bias, W.B. and Provost, T.T. (1986b). Gene interaction at HLA-DQ enhances autoantibody production in primary Sjögren's syndrome. *Science* **232**, 1145.

Harris, E.N., Gharavi, A.E., Loizou, S. *et al.* (1985a). Cross-reactivity of antiphospholipid antibodies. *J. Clin. Lab. Immunol.* **16**, 1.

Harris, E.N., Gharavi, A.E., Tincani, A. *et al.* (1985b). Affinity purified anti-cardiolipin and anti-DNA antibodies. *J. Clin. Lab. Immunol.* **17**, 155.

Harris, E.N., Asherson, R.A. and Hughes, G.R. (1988). Antiphospholipid antibodies — autoantibodies with a difference. *Ann. Rev. Med.* **39**, 261.

Harris, E.N., Williams, E., Shah, D.J. and De Ceulaer, K. (1989). Mortality of Jamaican patients with systemic lupus erythematosus. *Br. J. Rheumatol.* **28**, 113.

Harvey, A.M., Shulman, L.E., Tumulty, P.A., Conley, C.L. and Schoenrich, E.H. (1954). Systemic lupus erythematosus: review of the literature and clinical analysis of 138 cases. *Medicine (Baltimore)* **33**, 291.

Hasselaar, P., Derksen, R.H., Blokzijl, L. and De Groot, P.G. (1988). Thrombosis associated with antiphospholipid antibodies cannot be explained by effects on endothelial and platelet prostanoid synthesis. *Thromb. Haemostasis* **59**, 80.

Hawkins, B.R., Wong, K.L., Wong, R.W., Chan, K.H., Dunckley, H. and Serjeantson, S.W. (1987). Strong association between the major histocompatibility complex and systemic lupus erythematosus in southern Chinese. *J. Rheumatol.* **14**, 1128.

Hay, F.C., Nineham, L.J. and Roitt, I.M. (1976). Routine assay for the detection of immune complexes of known immunoglobulin class using solid phase C1q. *Clin. Exp. Immunol.* **24**, 396.

Hayakawa, K. and Hardy, R.R. (1988). Normal, autoimmune, and malignant CD5+ B cells: the Ly-1 B lineage, *Ann. Rev. Immunol.* **6**, 197.

Hendrick, J.P., Wolin, S.L., Rinke, J., Lerner, M.R. and Steitz, J.A. (1981). Ro small cytoplasmic ribonucleoproteins are a subclass of La ribonucleoproteins: further characterization of the Ro and La small ribonucleoproteins from uninfected mammalian cells. *Mol. Cell Biol.* **1**, 1138.

Hill, G.S., Hinglais, N., Tron, F. and Bach, J.F. (1978). Systemic lupus erythematosus: morphologic correlations with immunologic and clinical data at the time of biopsy. *Am. J. Med.* **64**, 61.

Hind, C.R., Ng, S.C., Feng, P.H. and Pepys, M.B. (1985). Serum C-reactive protein measurement in the detection of intercurrent infection in Oriental patients with systemic lupus erythematosus. *Ann. Rheum. Dis.* **44**, 260.

Hochberg, M.C., Boyd, R.E., Ahearn, J.M. *et al.* (1985). Systemic lupus erythematosus: a review of clinico-laboratory features and immunogenetic markers in 150 patients with emphasis on demographic subsets. *Medicine (Baltimore)* **64**, 285.

Hoffman, R.W., Alspaugh, M.A., Waggie, K.S., Durham, J.B. and Walker, S.E. (1984). Sjögren's syndrome in MRL/l and MRL/n mice. *Arthritis Rheum.* **27**, 157.

Honig, S., Gorevic, P. and Weissmann, G. (1977). C-reactive protein in systemic lupus erythematosus. *Arthritis Rheum.* **20**, 1065.

Hopkins, P., Belmont, H.M., Buyon, J., Philips, M., Weissmann, G. and Abramson, S.B. (1988). Increased levels of plasma anaphylatoxins in systemic lupus erythematosus predict flares of the disease and may elicit vascular injury in luus cerebritis. *Arthritis Rheum.* **31**, 632.

Horwitz, D.A. (1972). Impaired delayed hypersensitivity in systemic lupus erythematosus. *Arthritis Rheum.* **15**, 353.

Horwitz, D.A. and Cousar, J.B. (1975). A relationship between impaired cellular immunity, humoral suppression of lymphocytes function and severity of systemic lupus erythematosus. *Am. J. Med.* **58**, 829.

How, A., Dent, P.B., Liao, S.K. and Denburg, J.A. (1985). Antineuronal antibodies in neuropsychiatric systemic lupus erythematosus. *Arthritis Rheum.* **28**, 789.

Howard, P.F., Hochberg, M.C., Bias, W.B., Arnett, F.C., Jr and McLean, R.H. (1986). Relationship between C4 null genes, HLA-D region antigens, and genetic susceptibility to systemic lupus erythematosus in Caucasian and black Americans. *Am. J. Med.* **81**, 187.

Huff, J.P., Roos, G., Peebles, C.L., Houghten, R., Sullivan, K.F. and Tan, E.M. (1990). Insights into native epitopes of proliferating cell nuclear antigen using recombinant DNA protein products. *J. Exp. Med.* **172**, 419.

Hughes, G.R.V. (1987). *Connective Tissue Diseases*, 3rd edn. Blackwell Scientific Publications, Oxford.

Hunsicker, L.G., Ruddy, S., Carpenter, C.B. *et al.* (1972). Metabolism of third complement component (C3) in nephritis: involvement of the classic and alternate (properdin) pathways for complement activation. *N. Engl. J. Med.* **287**, 835.

Huston, D.P., McAdam, K.P.W.J., Balow, J.E., Bass, R. and Delellis, R.A. (1981). Amyloidosis in systemic lupus erythematosus. *Am. J. Med.* **70**, 320.

Iida, K., Mornaghi, R. and Nussenzweig, V. (1982). Complement receptor (CR1) deficiency in erythrocytes from patients with systemic lupus erythematosus. *J. Exp. Med.* **155**, 1427.

Inada, T. and Mims, C.A. (1985). Pattern of infection and selective loss of Ia positive cells in suckling and adult mice inoculated with lactic dehydrogenase virus. *Arch. Virol.* **86**, 151.

Isenberg, D.A. and Collins, C. (1985). Detection of cross-reactive anti-DNA antibody idiotypes on renal tissue-bound immunoglobulins from lupus patients. *J. Clin. Invest.* **76**, 287.

Isenman, D.E. and Young, J.R. (1984). The molecular basis for the difference in immune hemolysis activity of the Chido and Rodgers isotypes of human complement component C4. *J. Immunol.* **132**, 3019.

Ishigatsubo, Y., Steinberg, A.D. and Klinman, D.M. (1988). Autoantibody production is associated with polyclonal B cell activation in autoimmune mice which express the lpr or gld genes. *Eur. J. Immunol.* **18**, 1089.

Izui, S., Lambert, P.H. and Miescher, P.A. (1976). *In vitro* demonstration of a particular affinity of glomerular basement membrane and collagen for DNA: a possible basis for a local formation of DNA-anti-DNA complexes in systemic lupus erythematosus. *J. Exp. Med.* **144**, 428.

Izui, S., Lambert, P.H. and Miescher, P.A. (1977). Failure to detect circulating DNA–anti DNA complexes by four radioimmunological methods in patients with systemic lupus erythematosus. *Clin. Exp. Immunol.* **30**, 384.

Izui, S., Kelley, V.E., Masuda, K., Yoshida, H., Roths, J.B. and Murphy, E.D. (1984). Induction of various autoantibodies by mutant gene *lpr* in several strains of mice. *J. Immunol.* **133**, 227.

Jacob, C.O. and McDevitt, H.O. (1988). Tumour necrosis factor-alpha in murine autoimmune 'lupus' nephritis. *Nature*, **331**, 356.

Jacob, L., Lety, M.-A., Louvard, D. and Bach, J.-F. (1985). Binding of a monoclonal anti-DNA autoantibody to identical protein(s) present at the surface of several human cell types involved in lupus pathogenesis. *J. Clin. Invest.* **75**, 315.

Jacob, L., Lety, M.-A., Choquette, D. *et al.* (1987). Presence of antibodies against a cell-surface protein, cross-reactive with DNA, in systemic lupus erythematosus: a marker of the disease. *Proc. Nat. Acad. Sci. (USA)* **84**, 2956.

Jasin, H.E. and Ziff, M. (1975). Immunoglobulin synthesis by peripheral blood cells in systemic lupus erythematosus. *Arthritis Rheum.* **18**, 219.

Jemmerson, R. and Margoliash, E. (1979). Specificity of the antibody response of rabbits to a self-antigen. *Nature*, **282**, 468.

Johansson, E.A. and Lassus, A. (1974). The occurrences of circulating anticoagulants in patients with syphilitic and biologically false positive antilipoidal antibodies. *Ann. Clin. Res.* **6**, 105.

Johnson, R.T. and Richardson, E.P. (1968). The neurological manifestations of systemic lupus erythematosus: a clinical-pathologic study of 24 cases and review of the literature. *Medicine (Baltimore)* **47**, 337.

Jonsson, R., Tarkowski, A., Backman, K. and Klareskog, L. (1987). Immunohistochemical characterization of sialadenitis in NZB × NZW F1 mice. *Clin. Immunol. Immunopathol.* **42**, 93.

Jungers, P., Nahoul, K., Pelissier, C., Dougados, M., Tron, F. and Bach, J.-F. (1982). Low plasma androgens in women with active or quiescent systemic lupus erythematosus. *Arthritis Rheum.* **25**, 454.

Kabat, E.A., Nickerson, K.G., Liao, J. *et al.* (1986). A human monoclonal macroglobulin with specificity for alpha(2–8)-linked poly-*N*-acetyl neuraminic acid, the capsular polysaccharide of group B meningococci and *Escherichia coli* K1, which crossreacts with polynucleotides and with denatured DNA. *J. Exp. Med.* **164**, 642.

Kaburaki, J. and Stollar, B.D. (1987). Identification of human anti-DNA, anti-RNP, anti-Sm, and anti-SS-A serum antibodies bearing the cross-reactive 166 idiotype. *J. Immunol.* **139**, 385.

Kalunian, K.C., Panosian-Sahakian, N., Ebling, F.M. *et al.* (1989). Idiotypic characteristics of immunoglobulins associated with systemic lupus erythematosus: studies of antibodies deposited in glomeruli of humans. *Arthritis Rheum.* **32**, 513.

Kanai, Y., Kawaminami, Y., Miwa, M., Matsushima, T. and Sugimura, T. (1977). Naturally-occurring antibodies to poly(ADP-ribose) in patients with systemic lupus erythematosus. *Nature* **265**, 175.

Kant, K.S., Pollak, V.E., Weiss, M.A., Glueck, H.I., Miller, A.N. and Hess, E.V. (1981). Glomerular thrombosis in systemic lupus erythematosus: prevalence and significance. *Medicine (Baltimore)* **60**, 71.

Kaslow, R.A. (1982). High rate of death caused by systemic lupus erythematosus among U.S. residents of Asian descent. *Arthritis Rheum.* **25**, 414.

Kaslow, R.A. and Masi, A.T. (1978). Age, sex, and race effects on mortality from systemic lupus erythematosus in the United States. *Arthritis Rheum.* **21**, 473.

Kemp, M.E., Atkinson, J.P., Skanes, V.M., Levine, R.P. and Chaplin, D.D. (1987). Deletion of C4A genes in patients with systemic lupus erythematosus. *Arthritis Rheum.* **30**, 1015.

Kind, P., Lipsky, P.E. and Sontheimer, R.D. (1986). Circulating T- and B-cell abnormalities in cutaneous lupus erythematosus. *J. Invest. Dermatol.* **86**, 235.

Klinman, D.M. and Steinberg, A.D. (1987). Systemic autoimmune disease arises from polyclonal B cell activation. *J. Exp. Med.* **165**, 1755.

Klinman, D.M., Banks, S., Hartman, A. and Steinberg, A.D. (1988). Natural murine autoantibodies and conventional antibodies exhibit similar degrees of antigenic cross-reactivity. *J. Clin. Invest.* **82**, 652.

Klopstock, A., Schartz, J., Bleiberg, Y., Adam, A., Szeinberg, A. and Schlomo, J. (1965). Hereditary nature of the behaviour of erythrocytes in immune adherence — haemagglutination phenomenon. *Vox Sang.* **10**, 177.

Kluger, J., Drayer, D.E., Reidenberg, M.M. and Lahita, R. (1981). Acetylprocainamide therapy in patients with previous procainamide-induced lupus syndrome. *Ann. Intern. Med.* **95**, 18.

Koffler, D., Schur, P.H. and Kunkel, H.G. (1967). Immunological studies concerning the nephritis of systemic lupus erythematosus. *J. Exp. Med.* **126**, 607.

Kotzin, B.L. and Palmer, E. (1987). The contribution of NZW genes to lupus-like disease in (NZB × NZW)F1 mice. *J. Exp. Med.* **165**, 1237.

Krishnan, C. and Kaplan, M.H. (1967). Immunopathologic studies of systemic lupus erythematosus. II. Anti-nuclear reaction of gamma-globulin eluted from homogenates and isolated glomeruli of kidneys from patients with lupus nephritis. *J. Clin. Invest.* **46**, 569.

Kumagai, S., Steinberg, A.D. and Green, I. (1981). Antibodies to T cells in patients with systemic lupus erythematosus can induce antibody-dependent cell-mediated cytotoxicity against human T cells. *J. Clin. Invest.* **67**, 605.

Lachmann, P.J. (1961). An attempt to characterize the lupus erythematosus cell antigen. *Immunology* **4**, 153.

Lachmann, P.J. and Walport, M.J. (1987). Deficiency of the effector mechanisms of the immune response and autoimmunity. In *Autoimmunity and Autoimmune Disease: Ciba Foundation Symposium #129*, ed. J. Whelan, p. 149, Wiley Ltd., Chichester.

Lachmann, P.J., Muller-Eberhard, H.J., Kunkel, H.G. and Paronetto, F. (1962). The localization of *in vivo* bound complement in tissue sections. *J. Exp. Med.* **115**, 63.

Lafer, E.M., Rauch, J., Andrzejewski, C., Jr *et al.* (1981). Polyspecific monoclonal lupus autoantibodies reactive with both polynucleotides and phospholipids. *J. Exp. Med.* **153**, 897.

Lafer, E.M., Valle, R.P., Moller, A. *et al.* (1983). Z-DNA-specific antibodies in human systemic lupus erythematosus. *J. Clin.*

Invest. **71**, 314.

Lahita, R.G., Bradlow, H.L., Kunkel, H.G. and Fishman, J. (1979). Alterations of estrogen metabolism in systemic lupus erythematosus. *Arthritis Rheum.* **22**, 1195.

Lahita, R.G., Bradlow, H.L., Kunkel, H.G. and Fishman, J. (1981). Increased 16 alpha-hydroxylation of estradiol in systemic lupus erythematosus. *J. Clin. Endocrinol. Metab.* **53**, 174.

Lahita, R.G., Chiorazzi, N., Gibofsky, A., Winchester, R.J. and Kunkel, H.G. (1983a). Familial systemic lupus erythematosus in males. *Arthritis Rheum.* **26**, 39.

Lahita, R.G., Kunkel, H.G. and Bradlow, H.L. (1983b). Increased oxidation of testosterone in systemic lupus erythematosus. *Arthritis Rheum.* **26**, 1517.

Landry, M. and Sams, W.M. (1973). Systemic lupus erythematosus: studies of the antibodies bound to skin. *J. Clin. Invest.* **52**, 1871.

Law, S.K., Dodds, A.W. and Porter, R.R. (1984). A comparison of the properties of two classes, C4A and C4B, of the human complement component C4. *EMBO J.* **3**, 1819.

Lee, L.A., Gaither, K.K., Coulter, S.N., Norris, D.A. and Harley, J.B. (1989). Pattern of cutaneous immunoglobulin G deposition in subacute cutaneous lupus erythematosus is reproduced by infusing purified anti-Ro (SSA). *J. Clin. Invest.* **83**, 1556.

Lee, P., Urowitz, M.B., Bookman, A.A. *et al.* (1977). Systemic lupus erythematosus: a review of 110 cases with reference to nephritis, the nervous system, infections, aseptic necrosis and prognosis. *Quart. J. Med.* **46**, 1.

Lee, S.L. and Chase, P.H. (1975). Drug-induced systemic lupus erythematosus: a critical review, *Semin. Arthritis Rheum.* **5**, 83.

LeFeber, W.P., Norris, D.A., Ryan, S.R. *et al.* (1984). Ultraviolet light induces binding of antibodies to selected nuclear antigens on cultured human keratinocytes. *J. Clin. Invest.* **74**, 1545.

Lerner, M.R. and Steitz, J.A. (1979). Antibodies to small nuclear RNAs complexed with proteins are produced by patients with systemic lupus erythematosus. *Proc. Nat. Acad. Sci. (USA)* **76**, 5495.

Lerner, M.R., Boyle, J.A., Mount, S.M., Wolin, S.L. and Steitz, J.A. (1980). Are snRNPs involved in splicing? *Nature* **283**, 220.

Lerner, M.R., Boyle, J.A., Hardin, J.A. and Steitz, J.A. (1981a). Two novel classes of small ribonucleoproteins detected by antibodies associated with lupus erythematosus. *Science* **211**, 400.

Lerner, M.R., Andrews, N.C., Miller, G. and Steitz, J.A. (1981b). Two small RNAs encoded by Epstein–Barr virus and complexed with protein are precipitated by antibodies from patients with systemic lupus erythematosus. *Proc. Nat. Acad. Sci. (USA)* **78**. 805.

Lewis, R.M. and Schwartz, R.S. (1971). Canine systemic lupus erythematosus: genetic analysis of an established breeding colony. *J. Exp. Med.* **134**, 417.

Lewis, R.M., Andre-Schwartz, J., Harris, G.S., Hirsch, M.S., Black, P.H. and Schwartz, R.S. (1973). Canine systemic lupus erythematosus: transmission of serologic abnormalities by cell-free filtrates. *J. Clin. Invest.* **52**, 1893.

Lindquist, S. (1986). The heat-shock response. *Ann. Rev. Biochem.* **55**, 1151.

Litsey, S.E., Noonan, J.A., O'Connor, W.N., Cottrill, C.M. and Mitchell, B. (1985). Maternal connective tissue disease and congenital heart block: demonstration of immunoglobulin in cardiac tissue. *N. Engl. J. Med.* **312**, 98.

Litvin, D.A., Cohen, P.L. and Winfield, J.B. (1983). Characterization of warm-reactive IgG anti-lymphocyte antibodies in systemic lupus erythematosus: relative specificity for mitogen-activated T cells and their soluble products. *J. Immunol.* **130**, 181.

Lloyd, W. and Schur, P.H. (1981). Immune complexes, complement, and anti-DNA in exacerbations of systemic lupus erythematosus (SLE). *Medicine (Baltimore)* **60**, 208.

Lobatto, S., Daha, M.R., Voetman, A.A. *et al.* (1987). Clearance of soluble aggregates of immunoblobulin G in healthy volunteers and chimpanzees. *Clin. Exp. Immunol.* **68**, 133.

Lockshin, M.D., Bonfa, E., Elkon, K. and Druzin, M.L. (1988). Neonatal lupus risk to newborns of mothers with systemic lupus erythematosus. *Arthritis Rheum.* **31**, 697.

Lowenstein, M.B. and Rothfield, N.F. (1977). Family study of systemic lupus erythematosus: analysis of the clinical history, skin immunofluorescence, and serologic parameters. *Arthritis Rheum.* **20**, 1293.

Luzuy, S., Merino, J., Engers, H., Izui, S. and Lambert, P.H. (1986). Autoimmunity after induction of neonatal tolerance to alloantigens: role of B cell chimerism and F1 donor B cell activation. *J. Immunol.* **136**, 4420.

Mackworth-Young, C.G., Loizou, S. and Walport, M.J. (1989). Antiphospholipid antibodies and disease. *Quart. J. Med.* **72**, 767.

Madaio, M.P., Hodder, S., Schwartz, R.S. and Stollar, B.D. (1984). Responsiveness of autoimmune and normal mice to nucleic acid antigens. *J. Immunol.* **132**, 872.

Madaio, M.P., Schattner, A., Shattner, M. and Schwartz, R.S. (1986). Lupus serum and normal human serum contain anti-DNA antibodies with the same idiotypic marker. *J. Immunol.* **137**, 2535.

Maddison, P.J. and Reichlin, M. (1977). Quantitation of precipitating antibodies to certain soluble nuclear antigens in SLE. *Arthritis Rheum.* **20**, 819.

Maddison, P.J. and Reichlin, M. (1979). Deposition of antibodies to a soluble cytoplasmic antigen in the kidneys of patients with systemic lupus erythematosus. *Arthritis Rheum.* **22**, 858.

Maddison, P.J., Provost, T.T. and Reichlin, M. (1981). Serological findings in patients with 'ANA-negative' systemic lupus erythematosus. *Medicine (Baltimore)* **60**, 87.

Magil, A.B., Ballon, H.S., Chan, V., Lirenman, D.S., Rae, A. and Sutton, R.A. (1984). Diffuse proliferative lupus glomerulonephritis: determination of prognostic significance of clinical, laboratory and pathologic factors. *Medicine (Baltimore)* **63**, 210.

Manthorpe, R., Teppo, A.M., Bendixen, G. and Wegelius, O. (1982). Antibodies to SS-B in chronic inflammatory connective tissue diseases: relationship with HLA-Dw2 and HLA-Dw3 antigens in primary Sjögren's syndrome. *Arthritis Rheum.* **25**, 662.

Marmont, A. (1965). The transfusion of active LE plasma into nonlupus recipients, with a note on the LE-like cell. *Ann. NY Acad. Sci.* **124**, 838.

Mathews, M.B. and Bernstein, R.M. (1983). Myositis autoantibody inhibits histidyl-tRNA synthetase: amodel for autoimmunity. *Nature* **304**, 177.

Mathews, M.B., Bernstein, R.M., Franza, B.R., Jr and Garrels, J.I. (1984). Identity of the proliferating cell nuclear antigen and cyclin. *Nature* **309**, 374.

Matsiota, P., Druet, P., Dosquet, P., Guilbert, B. and Avrameas, S. (1987). Natural autoantibodies in systemic lupus erythematosus. *Clin. Exp. Immunol.* **69**, 79.

Matthyssens, G. and Rabbitts, T.H. (1980). Structure and multiplicity of genes for the human immunoglobulin heavy chain variable region. *Proc. Nat. Acad. Sci. (USA)* **77**, 6561.

Mattioli, M. and Reichlin, M. (1974). Heterogeneity of protein antigens reactive with sera of patients with systemic lupus erythematosus. *Arthritis Rheum.* **17**, 421.

Mayes, J.T., Schreiber, R.D. and Cooper, N.R. (1984). Development and application of an enzyme-linked immunosorbent assay for the quantitation of alternative complement pathway activation in human serum. *J. Clin. Invest.* **73**, 160.

Mellors, R.C. and Mellors, J.W. (1976). Antigen related to mammalian type-C viral p30 proteins is located in renal glomeruli in human systemic lupus erythematosus. *Proc. Nat. Acad. Sci. (USA)* **73**, 233.

Mellors, R.C. and Mellors, J.W. (1978). Type C virus-specific antibody in human systemic lupus erythematosus demonstrated by enzymoimmunoassay. *Proc. Nat. Acad. Sci. (USA)* **75**, 2463.

Mellors, R.C., Aoki, T. and Huebner, R.J. (1969). Further implication of murine leukemia-like virus in the disorders of NZB mice. *J. Exp. Med.* **129**, 1045.

Mendlovic, S., Brocke, S., Shoenfeld, Y. *et al.* (1988). Induction of a systemic lupus erythematosus-like disease in mice by a common human anti-DNA idiotype. *Proc. Nat. Acad. Sci. (USA)* **85**, 2260.

Mendlovic, S., Fricke, H., Shoenfeld, Y. and Mozes, E. (1989). The role of anti-idiotypic antibodies in the induction of experimental systemic lupus erythematosus in mice. *Eur. J. Immunol.* **19**, 729.

Mercolino, T.J., Arnold, L.W., Hawkins, L.A. and Haughton, G. (1988). Normal mouse peritoneum contains a large population of Ly-1+ (CD5) B cells that recognize phosphatidyl choline: relationship to cells that secrete hemolytic antibody specific for autologous erythrocytes. *J. Exp. Med.* **168**, 687.

Merino, J., Schurmans, S., Duchosal, M.A., Izui, S. and Lambert, P.H. (1989). Autoimmune syndrome after induction of neonatal tolerance to alloantigens: CD4+ T cells from the tolerant host activate autoreactive F1 B cells. *J. Immunol.* **143**, 2202.

Messner, R.P., Lindstrom, F.D. and Williams, R.C., Jr (1973). Peripheral blood lymphocyte cell surface markers during the course of systemic lupus erythematosus. *J. Clin. Invest.* **52**, 3046.

Meyer, O., Hauptmann, G., Tappeiner, G., Ochs, H.D. and Mascart Lemone, F. (1985). Genetic deficiency of C4, C2 or C1q and lupus syndromes: association with anti-Ro (SS-A) antibodies. *Clin. Exp. Immunol.* **62**, 678.

Mimori, T. and Hardin, J.A. (1986). Mechanism of interaction between Ku protein and DNA. *J. Biol. Chem.* **261**, 10375.

Mimori, T., Akizuki, M., Yamagata, H. and Inada, S. (1981). Characterization of a high molecular weight acidic nuclear protein recognized by autoantibodies in sera from patients with polymyositis–scleroderma overlap. *J. Clin. Invest.* **68**, 611.

Mims, C.A. (1986). Interactions of viruses with the immune system. *Clin. Exp. Immunol.* **66**, 1.

Mimura, T., Fernsten, P., Jarjour, W. and Winfield, J.B. (1990). Autoantibodies specific for different isoforms of CD45 in systemic lupus erythematosus. *J. Exp. Med.* **172**, 653.

Minota, S. and Winfield, J.B. (1987). Identification of three major target molecules of IgM antilymphocyte autoantibodies in systemic lupus erythematosus. *J. Immunol.* **139**, 3644.

Minota, S., Cameron, B., Welch, W.J. and Winfield, J.B. (1988a). Autoantibodies to the constitutive 73-kD member of the hsp70 family of heat shock proteins in systemic lupus erythematosus. *J. Exp. Med.* **168**, 1475.

Minota, S., Koyasu, S., Yahara, I. and Winfield, J. (1988b). Autoantibodies to the heat-shock protein hsp90 in systemic lupus erythematosus. *J. Clin. Invest.* **81**, 106.

Mitchell, J.A., Batchelor, J.R., Chapel, H., Spiers, C.N. and Sim, E. (1987). Erythrocyte complement receptor type 1 (CR1) expression and circulating immune complex (CIC) levels in hydralazine-induced SLE. *Clin. Exp. Immunol.* **68**, 446.

Mittal, K.K. and Rossen, R.D. (1970). Lymphocyte cytotoxic antibodies in systemic lupus erythematosus. *Nature* **225**, 1255.

Miyachi, K., Fritzler, M.J. and Tan, E.M. (1978). Autoantibody to a nuclear antigen in proliferating cells. *J. Immunol.* **121**, 2228.

Miyakawa, Y., Yamada, A., Kosaka, K., Tsuda, F., Kosugi, E. and Mayumi, M. (1981). Defective immune-adherence (C3b) receptor on erythrocytes from patients with systemic lupus erythematosus. *Lancet* **ii**, 493.

Moldenhauer, F., David, J., Fielder, A.H., Lachmann, P.J. and Walport, M.J. (1987). Inherited deficiency of erythrocyte complement receptor type 1 does not cause susceptibility to systemic lupus erythematosus. *Arthritis Rheum.* **30**, 961.

Morimoto, C., Abe, T., Hara, M. and Homma, M. (1977). *In vitro* TNP-specific antibody formation by peripheral lymphocytes from patients with systemic lupus erythematosus. *Scand. J. Immunol.* **6**, 575.

Morimoto, C., Reinherz, E.L. and Abe, T. (1980). Characteristics of anti-T cell antibodies in systemic lupus erythematosus: evidence for selective reactivity with normal suppressor cells defined by monoclonal antibodies. *Clin. Immunol. Immunopathol.* **16**, 474.

Morimoto, C., Reinherz, E.L., Distaso, J.A., Steinberg, A.D. and Schlossman, S.F. (1984). Relationship between systemic lupus erythematosus T cell subsets, anti-T cell antibodies, and T cell functions. *J. Clin. Invest.* **73**, 689.

Morimoto, C., Steinberg, A.D., Letvin, N.L. *et al.* (1987). A defect of immunoregulatory T cell subsets in systemic lupus erythematosus patients demonstrated with anti-2H4 antibody. *J. Clin. Invest.* **79**, 762.

Morse, J.H., Muller-Eberhard, H.J. and Kunkel, H.G. (1962). Anti-nuclear factors and serum complement in systemic lupus erythematosus. *Bull. NY Acad. Med.* **38**, 641.

Mouritsen, S., Hoier-Madsen, M., Wiik, A., Orum, O. and Strandberg Pedersen, N. (1989). The specificity of anti-cardiolipin antibodies from syphilis patients and from patients with systemic lupus erythematosus. *Clin. Exp. Immunol.* **76**, 178.

Muller, S., Briand, J.P. and Van Regenmortel, M.H. (1988). Presence of antibodies to ubiquitin during the autoimmune response associated with systemic lupus erythematosus. *Proc. Nat. Acad. Sci. (USA)* **85**, 8176.

Muryoi, T., Sasaki, T., Harata, N., Takai, O., Tamate, E. and Yoshinaga, K. (1988). Heterogeneity of anti-idiotypic antibodies to anti-DNA antibodies in humans. *Clin. Exp. Immunol.* **71**, 67.

Nakamura, M., Burastero, S.E., Ueki, Y., Larrick, J.W., Notkins, A.L. and Casali, P. (1988). Probing the normal and autoimmune B cell repertoire with Epstein–Barr virus: frequency of B cells producing monoreactive high affinity autoantibodies in patients with Hashimoto's disease and systemic lupus erythematosus. *J. Immunol.* **141**, 4165.

Nakao, Y., Matsumoto, H., Miyazaki, T. *et al.* (1980). IgG heavy chain allotypes (Gm) in autoimmune diseases. *Clin. Exp. Immunol.* **42**, 20.

Naparstek, Y., Duggan, D., Schattner, A. *et al.* (1985). Immunochemical similarities between monoclonal antibacterial Waldenstrom's macroglobulins and monoclonal anti-DNA lupus autoantibodies. *J. Exp. Med.* **161**, 1525.

Naparstek, Y., Andre-Schwartz, J., Manser, T. *et al.* (1986). A single germline VH gene segment of normal A/J mice encodes autoantibodies characteristic of systemic lupus erythematosus. *J. Exp. Med.* **164**, 614.

Nasu, H., Chia, D.S., Taniguchi, O. and Barnett, E.V. (1982). Characterization of anti-F(ab')2 antibodies in SLE patients: evidence for cross-reacting auto-anti-idiotypic antibodies. *Clin. Immunol. Immunopathol.* **25**, 80.

Negoro, N., Okamura, M., Takeda, T. *et al.* (1989). The clinical significance of iC3b neoantigen expression in plasma from patients with systemic lupus erythematosus. *Arthritis Rheum.* **32**, 1233.

Ng, Y.C. and Walport, M.J. (1988). Immunogenetics of SLE and primary Sjögren's syndrome. *Baillière's Clin. Rheumatol.* **2**, 623.

Nimelstein, S.H., Brody, S., McShane, D. and Holman, H.R. (1980). Mixed connective tissue disease: a subsequent evaluation of the original 25 patients. *Medicine (Baltimore)* **59**, 239.

Nydegger, U.E., Lambert, P.H., Gerber, H. and Miescher, P.A. (1974). Circulating immune complexes in the serum in systemic lupus erythematosus and in carriers of hepatitis-B antigen. *J. Clin. Invest.* **54**, 297.

Ogata, K., Ogata, Y., Takasaki, Y. and Tan, E.M. (1987). Epitopes on proliferating cell nuclear antigen recognized by human lupus autoantibody and murine monoclonal antibody. *J. Immunol.* **139**, 2942.

Okudaira, K., Searles, R.P., Ceuppens, J.L., Goodwin, J.S. and Williams, R.C., Jr (1982a). Anti-Ia reactivity in sera from patients with systemic lupus erythematosus. *J. Clin. Invest.* **69**, 17.

Okudaira, K., Searles, R.P., Tanimoto, K., Horiuchi, Y. and Williams, R.C., Jr (1982b). T lymphocyte interaction with immunoglobulin G antibody in systemic lupus erythematosus. *J. Clin. Invest.* **69**, 1026.

Oldstone, M.B. and Dixon, F.J. (1972). Inhibition of antibodies to nuclear antigen and to DNA in New Zealand mice infected with lactate dehydrogenase virus. *Science* **175**, 784.

Padgett, R.A., Mount, S.M., Steitz, J.A. and Sharp, P.A. (1983). Splicing of messenger RNA precursors is inhibited by antisera to small nuclear ribonucleoprotein. *Cell* **35**, 101.

Parichatikanond, P., Francis, N.D., Malasit, P. *et al.* (1986). Lupus nephritis: a clinicopathological study of 162 cases in Thailand. *J. Clin. Pathol.* **39**, 160.

Pepys, M.B., Dash, A.C., Markham, R.E., Thomas, H.C., Williams, B.D. and Petrie, A. (1978). Comparative clinical study of protein SAP (amyloid P component) and C-reactive protein in serum. *Clin. Exp. Immunol.* **32**, 119.

Perrin, L.H., Lambert, P.H., Nydegger, U.E. and Miescher, P.A. (1973). Quantitation of C3PA (properdin factor B) and other complement components in diseases associated with a low C3 level. *Clin. Immunol. Immunopathol.* **2**, 16.

Perrin, L.H., Lambert, P.H. and Miescher, P.A. (1975). Complement breakdown products in plasma from patients with systemic lupus erythematosus and patients with membranoproliferative or other glomerulonephritis. *J. Clin. Invest.* **56**, 165.

Peters, M.S. and Su, W.P. (1989). Lupus erythematosus panniculitis. *Med. Clin. North Am.* **73**, 1113.

Pettersson, I., Wang, G., Smith, E.I. *et al.* (1986). The use of immunoblotting and immunoprecipitation of (U) small nuclear ribonucleoproteins in the analysis of sera of patients with mixed connective tissue disease and systemic lupus erythematosus: a cross-sectional, longitudinal study. *Arthritis Rheum.* **29**, 986.

Petz, L.D., Sharp, G.C. and Cooper, N.R. (1971). Serum and cerebrospinal fluid complement and serum autoantibodies in systemic lupus erythematosus. *Medicine (Baltimore)* **50**, 259.

Pincus, T. (1982). Studies regarding a possible function for viruses in the pathogenesis of systemic lupus erythematosus. *Arthritis Rheum.* **25**, 847.

Pincus, T., Schur, P.H., Rose, J.A., Decker, J.L. and Talal, N. (1969). Measurement of serum DNA-binding activity in systemic lupus erythematosus. *N. Engl. J. Med.* **281**, 701.

Plaué, S., Muller, S. and Van Regenmortel, M.H. (1989). A branched, synthetic octapeptide of ubiquinated histone H2A as target of autoantibodies. *J. Exp. Med.* **169**, 1607.

Plotz, P.H. (1983). Autoantibodies are anti-idiotype antibodies to antiviral antibodies. *Lancet* **ii**, 824.

Pohle, E.L. and Tuffanelli, D.L. (1968). Study of cutaneous lupus erythematosus by immunohistochemical methods. *Arch Dermatol.* **97**, 520.

Polla, B.S. (1988). A role for heat shock proteins in inflammation. *Immunol. Today* **9**, 134.

Portanova, J.P., Arndt, R.E., Tan, E.M. and Kotzin, B.L. (1987). Anti-histone antibodies in idiopathic and drug-induced lupus recognize distinct intrahistone regions. *J. Immunol.* **138**, 446.

Prelich, G., Tan, C., Kostura, M. *et al.* (1987). Functional identity of proliferating cell nuclear antigen and a DNA polymerase-δ auxiliary protein. *Nature* **326**, 517.

Provost, T.T., Watson, R., Gammon, W.R., Radowsky, M., Harley, J.B. and Reichlin, M. (1987). The neonatal lupus syndrome associated with U1RNP (nRNP) antibodies. *N. Engl. J. Med.* **316**, 1135.

Provost, T.T., Talal, N., Harley, J.B., Reichlin, M. and Alexander, E. (1988). The relationship between anti-Ro (SS-A) antibody-positive Sjögren's syndrome and anti-Ro (SS-A) antibody-positive lupus erythematosus. *Arch. Dermatol.* **124**, 63.

Query, C.C. and Keene, J.D. (1987). A human autoimmune protein associated with U1 RNA contains a region of homology that is cross-reactive with retroviral p30gag antigen. *Cell* **51**, 211.

Rader, M.D., O'Brien, C., Liu, Y.S., Harley, J.B. and Reichlin, M. (1989). Heterogeneity of the Ro/SSA antigen: different molecular forms in lymphocytes and red blood cells. *J. Clin. Invest.* **83**, 1293.

Rasmussen, E.K., Ullman, S., Hoier Madsen, M., Sorensen, S.F. and Halberg, P. (1987). Clinical implications of ribonucleoprotein antibody. *Arch. Dermatol.* **123**, 601.

Reeves, W.H. (1985). Use of monoclonal antibodies for the characterization of novel DNA-binding proteins recognized by human autoimmune sera. *J. Exp. Med.* **161**, 18.

Reeves, W.H. and Sthoeger, Z.M. (1989). Molecular cloning of cDNA encoding the p70 (Ku) lupus autoantigen. *J. Biol. Chem.* **264**, 5047.

Reeves, W.H., Sthoeger, Z.M. and Lahita, R.G. (1989). Role of antigen selectivity in autoimmune responses to the Ku (p70/p80) antigen. *J. Clin. Invest.* **84**, 562.

Rekvig, O.P. and Hannestad, K. (1980). Human autoantibodies that react with both cell nuclei and plasma membranes display specificity for the octamer of histones H2A, H2B, H3, and H4 in high salt. *J. Exp. Med.* **152**, 1720.

Reuter, R. and Luhrmann, R. (1986). Immunization of mice with purified U1 small nuclear ribonucleoprotein (RNP) induces a pattern of antibody specificities characteristic of the anti-Sm and anti-RNP autoimmune response of patients with systemic lupus erythematosus, as measured by monoclonal antibodies. *Proc. Nat. Acad. Sci. (USA)* **83**, 8689.

Reveille, J.D., Bias, W.B., Winkelstein, J.A., Provost, T.T., Dorsch, C.A. and Arnett, F.C. (1983). Familial systemic lupus erythematosus: immunogenetic studies in eight families. *Medicine (Baltimore)* **62**, 21.

Reveille, J.D., Arnett, F.C., Wilson, R.W., Bias, W.B. and McLean, R.H. (1985). Null alleles of the fourth component of complement and HLA haplotypes in familial systemic lupus erythematosus. *Immunogenetics* **21**, 299.

Revillard, J.P., Vincent, C. and Rivera, S. (1979). Anti-β2 microglobulin lymphocytotoxic autoantibodies in systemic lupus erythematosus. *J. Immunol.* **122**, 614.

Reynolds, J.T. and Panem, S. (1981). Characterization of antibody to C-type virus antigens isolated from immune complexes in kidneys of patients with systemic lupus erythematosus. *Lab. Invest.* **44**, 410.

Ridley, M.G., Maddison, P.J. and Tribe, C.R. (1984). Amyloidosis and systemic lupus erythematosus. *Ann. Rheum. Dis.* **43**, 649.

Robbins, M.L., Kornguth, S.E., Bell, C.L. *et al.* (1988). Antineurofilament antibody evaluation in neuropsychiatric systemic lupus erythematosus: combination with anticardiolipin antibody assay and magnetic resonance imaging. *Arthritis Rheum.* **31**, 623.

Robinson, M.F., Roberts, L.J., Jones, J.V. and Lewis, E.J. (1979). Circulating immune complexes in patients with lupus and membranous glomerulonephritis. *Clin. Immunol. Immunopathol.* **14**, 348.

Rordorf, C., Schnebli, H.P., Baltz, M.L., Tennent, G.A. and Pepys, M.B. (1982). The acute-phase response in (NZB × NZW)F1 and MRL/l MICE. *J. Exp. Med.* **156**, 1268.

Rosenthal, C.J. and Franklin, E.C. (1975). Depression of cellular-mediated immunity in systemic lupus erythematosus. *Arthritis Rheum.* **18**, 207.

Ross, G.D., Yount, W.J., Walport, M.J. *et al.* (1985). Disease-associated loss of erythrocyte complement receptors (CR1, C3b-receptors) in patients with systemic lupus erythematosus and other diseases involving autoantibodies and/or complement activation. *J. Immunol.* **135**, 2005.

Rothfield, N.F. and Stollar, B.D. (1967). The relation of immunoglobulin class, pattern of anti-nuclear antibody, and complement-fixing antibodies to DNA in sera from patients with systemic lupus erythematosus. *J. Clin. Invest.* **46**, 1785.

Rothfield, N.F., March, C.H., Miescher, P. *et al.* (1983). Chronic discoid lupus erythematosus. *N. Engl. J. Med.* **269**, 1155.

Roubinian, J.R., Papoian, R. and Talal, N. (1977). Androgenic hormones modulate autoantibody responses and improve survival in murine lupus. *J. Clin. Invest.* **59**, 1066.

Rowell, N.R. (1986). Lupus erythematosus, scleroderma and dermatomyositis. In *Textbook of Dermatology*, 4th edn, eds A. Rook, D.S. Wilkinson, F.J.G. Ebling and R.H. Champion, pp. 1281–1392, Blackwell Scientific Publications, Oxford.

Rubin, R.L. and Waga, S. (1987). Antihistone antibodies in systemic lupus erythematosus. *J. Rheumatol.* **14**, 118.

Rucheton, M., Graafland, H., Fanton, H., Ursule, L., Ferrier, P. and Larsen, C.J. (1985). Presence of circulating antibodies against gag-gene MuLV proteins in patients with autoimmune connective tissue disorders. *Virology*, **144**, 468.

Sagawa, A. and Abdou, N.I. (1979). Suppressor-cell antibody in systemic lupus erythematosus: possible mechanism for suppressor-cell dysfunction. *J. Clin. Invest.* **63**, 536.

Sakane, T., Steinberg, A.D. and Green, I. (1978a). Studies of immune functions of patients with systemic lupus erythematosus. I. Dysfunction of suppressor T-cell activity related to impaired generation of, rather than response to, suppressor cells. *Arthritis Rheum.* **21**, 657.

Sakane, T., Steinberg, A.D. and Green, I. (1978b). Failure of autologous mixed lymphocyte reactions between T and non-T cells in patients with systemic lupus erythematosus. *Proc. Nat. Acad. Sci. (USA)* **75**, 3464.

Sakane, T., Steinberg, A.D., Reeves, J.P. and Green, I. (1979). Studies of immune functions of patients with systemic lupus erythematosus. *J. Clin. Invest.* **63**, 954.

Sanders, M.E., Koski, C.L., Robbins, D., Shin, M.L., Frank, M.M. and Joiner, K.A. (1986). Activated terminal complement in cerebrospinal fluid in Guillain–Barré syndrome and multiple sclerosis. *J. Immunol.* **136**, 4456.

Sano, H., Kumagai, S., Namiuchi, S. *et al.* (1986). Systemic lupus erythematosus sera antilymphocyte reactivity: detection of antibodies to Tac-antigen positive T cell lines. *Clin. Exp. Immunol.* **63**, 8.

Sanz, I., Dang, H., Takei, M., Talal, N. and Capra, J.D. (1989). VH sequence of a human anti-Sm autoantibody: evidence that autoantibodies can be unmutated copies of germline genes. *J. Immunol.* **142**, 883.

Sarkany, I. (1961). Circulating antibody formation in systemic lupus erythematosus. *Arch. Dermatol.* **84**, 372.

Sasaki, T., Muryoi, T., Takai, O., Tamate, E., Saito, H. and Yoshinaga, K. (1988). Binding specificity of antiidiotypic autoantibodies to anti-DNA antibodies in humans. *J. Clin. Invest.* **82**, 748.

Scheinberg, M.A. and Cathcart, E.S. (1976). Antibody-dependent direct cytotoxicity of human lymphocytes. I. Studies on peripheral blood lymphocytes and sera of patients with systemic lupus erythematosus. *Clin. Exp. Immunol.* **24**,

317.

Schifferli, J.A., Ng, Y.C. and Peters, D.K. (1986a). The role of complement and its receptor in the elimination of immune complexes. *N. Engl. J. Med.* **315**, 488.

Schifferli, J.A., Steiger, G., Paccaud, J.P., Sjoholm, A.G. and Hauptmann, G. (1986b). Difference in the biological properties of the two forms of the fourth component of human complement (C4). *Clin. Exp. Immunol.* **63**, 473.

Schifferli, J.A., Hauptmann, G. and Paccaud, J.P. (1987). Complement-mediated adherence of immune complexes to human erythrocytes: difference in the requirements for C4A and C4B. *FEBS Lett.* **213**, 415.

Schifferli, J.A., Ng, Y.C., Estreicher, J. and Walport, M.J. (1988). The clearance of tetanus toxoid/anti-tetanus toxoid immune complexes from the circulation of humans: complement- and erythrocyte complement receptor 1-dependent mechanisms. *J. Immunol.* **140**, 899.

Schifferli, J.A., Ng, Y.C., Paccaud, J.-P. and Walport, M.J. (1989). The role of hypocomplementaemia and low erythrocyte complement receptor type 1 numbers in determining abnormal immune complex clearance in humans. *Clin. Exp. Immunol.* **75**, 329.

Schneider, J., Chin, W., Friou, G.J. *et al.* (1975). Reduced antibody-dependent cell-mediated cytotoxicity in systemic lupus erythematosus. *Clin. Exp. Immunol.* **20**, 187.

Schroeder, H.W., Jr, Hillson, J.L. and Perlmutter, R.M. (1987). Early restriction of the human antibody repertoire. *Science* **238**, 791.

Schur, P.H. and Sandson, J. (1968). Immunologic factors and clinical activity in systemic lupus erythematosus. *N. Engl. J. Med.* **278**, 533.

Schur, P.H., Pandey, J.P. and Fedrick, J.A. (1985). Gm allotypes in white patients with systemic lupus erythematosus. *Arthritis Rheum.* **28**, 828.

Schwartz, R.S. and Stollar, B.D. (1985). Origins of anti-DNA autoantibodies. *J. Clin. Invest.* **75**, 321.

Scott, A. and Rees, E.G. (1959). The relationship of systemic lupus erythematosus and discoid lupus erythematosus: a clinical and hematological study. *Arch. Dermatol.* **79**, 422.

Scott, J.S., Maddison, P.J., Taylor, P.V., Esscher, E., Scott, O. and Skinner, R.P. (1983). Connective tissue disease, antibodies to ribonucleoprotein, and congenital heart block. *N. Engl. J. Med.* **309**, 209.

Seigneurin, J.M., Guilbert, B., Bourgeat, M.J. and Avrameas, S. (1988). Polyspecific natural antibodies and autoantibodies secreted by human lymphocytes immortalized with Epstein–Barr virus. *Blood* **71**, 581.

Senecal, J.L. and Rauch, J. (1988). Hybridoma lupus autoantibodies can bind major cytoskeletal filaments in the absence of DNA-binding activity. *Arthritis Rheum.* **31**, 864.

Senecal, J.L., Oliver, J.M. and Rothfield, N. (1985). Anticytoskeletal autoantibodies in the connective tissue diseases. *Arthritis Rheum.* **28**, 889.

Serdula, M.K. and Rhoads, G.G. (1979). Frequency of systemic lupus erythematosus in different ethnic groups in Hawaii. *Arthritis Rheum.* **22**, 328.

Sharp, G.C., Irvin, W.S., Tan, E.M., Gould, R.G. and Holman, H.R. (1972). Mixed connective tissue disease — an apparently distinct rheumatic disease syndrome associated with a specific antibody to an extractable nuclear antigen (ENA). *Am. J. Med.* **52**, 148.

Shlomchik, M.J., Aucoin, A.H., Pisetsky, D.S. and Weigert, M.G. (1987). Structure and function of anti-DNA autoantibodies derived from a single autoimmune mouse. *Proc. Nat. Acad. Sci. (USA)* **84**, 9150.

Shoenfeld, Y., Isenberg, D.A., Rauch, J., Madaio, M.P., Stollar, B.D. and Schwartz, R.S. (1983). Idiotypic cross-reactions of monoclonal human lupus autoantibodies. *J. Exp. Med.* **158**, 718.

Shoenfeld, Y., Zamir, R., Joshua, H., Lavie, G. and Pinkhas, J. (1985). Human monoclonal anti-DNA antibodies react as lymphocytotoxic antibodies. *Eur. J. Immunol.* **15**, 1024.

Shores, E.W., Eisenberg, R.A. and Cohen, P.L. (1986). Role of the Sm antigen in the generation of anti-Sm autoantibodies in the SLE-prone MRL mouse. *J. Immunol.* **136**, 3662.

Shrank, A.S. and Doniach, D. (1963). Discoid lupus erythematosus: correlation of clinical factors and serum auto-antibody pattern. *Arch. Dermatol.* **87**, 677.

Siegel, M. and Lee, S.L. (1973). The epidemiology of systemic lupus erythematosus. *Semin. Arthritis/Rheum.* **3**, 1.

Sim, E., Gill, E.W. and Sim, R.B. (1984). Drugs that induce systemic lupus erythematosus inhibit complement component C4. *Lancet* **ii**, 422.

Sliwinski, A.J. and Zvaifler, N.J. (1972). Decreased synthesis of the third component of complement (C3) in hypocomplementemic systemic lupus erythematosus. *Clin. Exp. Immunol.* **11**, 21.

Smolen, J.S., Chused, T.M., Leiserson, W.M., Reeves, J.P., Alling, D. and Steinberg, A.D. (1982). Heterogeneity of immunoregulatory T-cell subsets in systemic lupus erythematosus: correlation with clinical features. *Am. J. Med.* **72**, 783.

Snyder, H.W., Jr and Fleissner, E. (1980). Specificity of human antibodies to oncovirus glycoproteins: recognition of antigen by natural antibodies directed against carbohydrate structures. *Proc. Nat. Acad. Sci. (USA)* **77**, 1622.

Solomon, G., Schiffenbauer, J., Keiser, H.D. and Diamond, B. (1983). Use of monoclonal antibodies to identify shared idiotypes on human antibodies to native DNA from patients with systemic lupus erythematosus. *Proc. Nat. Acad. Sci. (USA)* **80**, 850.

Sonnhag, C., Karlsson, E. and Hed, J. (1979). Procainamide-induced lupus erythematosus-like syndrome in relation to acetylator phenotype and plasma levels of procainamide. *Acta Med. Scand.* **206**, 245.

Sontheimer, R.D. (1989). Subacute cutaneous lupus erythematosus: a decade's perspective. *Med. Clin. North Am.* **73**, 1073.

Sontheimer, R.D. and Gilliam, J.N. (1978). DNA antibody class, subclass, and complement fixation in systemic lupus erythematosus with and without nephritis. *Clin. Immunol. Immunopathol.* **10**, 459.

Sontheimer, R.D., Thomas, J.R. and Gilliam, J.N. (1979). Subacute cutaneous lupus erythematosus: a cutaneous marker for a distinct lupus erythematosus subset. *Arch. Dermatol.* **115**, 1409.

Sontheimer, R.D., Maddison, P.J., Reichlin, M., Jordon, R.E., Stastny, P. and Gilliam, J.N. (1982). Serologic and HLA associations in subacute cutaneous lupus erythematosus, a clinical subset of lupus erythematosus. *Ann. Intern. Med.* **97**, 664.

Spies, T., Morton, C.C., Nedospasov, S.A., Fiers, W., Pious, D. and Strominger, J.L. (1986). Genes for the tumor necrosis factors alpha and beta are linked to the human major histocompatibility complex. *Proc. Nat. Acad. Sci. (USA)* **83**, 8699.

Stastny, P. and Ziff, M. (1969). Cold-insoluble complexes and complement levels in systemic lupus erythematosus. *N. Engl. J. Med.* **280**, 1376.

Steinberg, A.D., Daley, G.G. and Talal, N. (1970). Tolerance to polyinosinic-polycytidylic acid in NZB-NZW mice. *Science* **167**, 870.

Steinberg, A.D., Pincus, T. and Talal, N. (1971). The pathogenesis of autoimmunity in New Zealand mice. 3. Factors influencing the formation of anti-nucleic acid antibodies. *Immunology*, **20**, 523.

Steinberg, A.D., Raveche, E.S., Laskin, C.A. *et al.* (1984). NIH conference. Systemic lupus erythematosus: insights from animal models. *Ann. Intern. Med.* **100**, 714.

Steinman, C.R., Grishman, E., Spiera, H. and Deesomchok, U. (1977). Binding of synthetic double-stranded DNA by serum from patients with systemic lupus erythematosus: correlation with renal histology. *Am. J. Med.* **62**, 319.

Sthoeger, Z.M., Wakai, M., Tse, D.B. *et al.* (1989). Production of autoantibodies by CD5-expressing B lymphocytes from patients with chronic lymphocytic leukaemia. *J. Exp. Med.* **169**, 255.

Stollar, B.D. (1981). The antigenic potential and specificity of nucleic acids, nucleoproteins, and their modified derivatives. *Arthritis Rheum.* **24**, 1010.

Stott, D.I., McLearie, J. and Neilson, L. (1986). Analysis of the clonal origins of autoantibodies against thyroglobulin and DNA in autoimmune thyroiditis and systemic lupus erythematosus. *Clin. Exp. Immunol.* **65**, 520.

Sturfelt, G. and Sjöholm, A.G. (1984). Complement components, complement activation, and acute phase response in systemic lupus erythematosus. *Int. Arch. Allergy Appl. Immunol.* **75**, 75.

Sturfelt, G., Nived, O., Norberg, R. Thorstensson, R. and Krook, K. (1987). Anticardiolipin antibodies in patients with systemic lupus erythematosus. *Arthritis Rheum.* **30**, 382.

Takei, M., Dang, H. and Talal, N. (1987). A common idiotype expressed on a murine anti-Sm monoclonal antibody and antibodies in SLE sera. *Clin. Exp. Immunol.* **70**, 546.

Takei, M., Dang, H., Wang, R.J. and Talal, N. (1988). Characteristics of a human monoclonal anti-Sm autoantibody expressing an interspecies idiotype. *J. Immunol.* **140**, 3108.

Tan, E.M. (1989a). Antinuclear antibodies diagnostic markers for autoimmune diseases and probes for cell biology. *Adv. Immunol.* **44**, 93.

Tan, E.M. (1989b). Interactions between autoimmunity and molecular and cell biology: bridges between clinical and basic sciences. *J. Clin. Invest.* **84**, 1.

Tan, E.M. and Kunkel, H.G. (1966). An immunofluorescent study of the skin lesions in systemic lupus erythematosus. *Arthritis Rheum.* **9**, 37.

Tan, E.M., Schur, P.H., Carr, R.I. and Kunkel, H.G. (1966). Deoxyribonucleic acid (DNA) and antibodies to DNA in the serum of patients with systemic lupus erythematosus. *J. Clin. Invest.* **45**, 1732.

Tan, E.M., Cohen, A.S., Fries, J.F. *et al.* (1982). The 1982 revised criteria for the classification of systemic lupus erythematosus. *Arthritis Rheum.* **25**, 1271.

Tanaka, S., Matsuyama, T., Steinberg, A.D., Schlossman, S.F. and Morimoto, C. (1989). Antilymphocyte antibodies against CD4+2H4+ cell populations in patients with systemic lupus erythematosus. *Arthritis Rheum.* **32**, 398.

Teitelbaum, D., Rauch, J., Stollar, B.D. and Schwartz, R.S. (1984). *In vivo* effects of antibodies against a high frequency idiotype of anti-DNA antibodies in MRL mice. *J. Immunol.* **132**, 1282.

Terasaki, P.I., Mottironi, V.D. and Barnett, E.V. (1970). Cytotoxins in disease: autocytotoxins in lupus. *N. Engl. J. Med.* **283**, 724.

Theofilopoulos, A.N. and Dixon, F.J. (1979). The biology and detection of immune complexes. *Adv. Immunol.* **28**, 89.

Theofilopoulos, A.N. and Dixon, F.J. (1981). Etiopathogenesis of murine SLE. *Immunol. Rev.* **55**, 179.

Theofilopoulos, A.N. and Dixon, F.J. (1985). Murine models of systemic lupus erythematosus. *Adv. Immunol.* **37**, 269.

Theofilopoulos, A.N., Wilson, C.B. and Dixon, F.J. (1976). The Raji cell radioimmune assay for detecting immune complexes in human sera. *J. Clin. Invest.* **57**, 169.

Thomas, J.O., Wilson, C.M. and Hardin, J.A. (1984). The major core histone antigenic determinants in systemic lupus erythematosus are in the trypsin-sensitive regions. *FEBS Lett.* **169**, 90.

Thomas, T.J. and Messner, R.P. (1986). Effects of lupus-inducing drugs on the B to Z transition of synthetic DNA. *Arthritis Rheum.* **29**, 638.

Tojo, T. and Friou, G.J. (1968). Lupus nephritis: varying complement-fixing properties of immunoglobulin G antibodies to antigens of cell nuclei. *Science*, **161**, 904.

Townes, A.S., Stewart, C.R., Jr and Osler, A.G. (1963). Immunologic studies of systemic lupus erythematosus. II. Variations of nucleoprotein-reactive gamma globulin and hemolytic serum complement levels with disease activity. *Bull. Johns Hopkins Med. Sch.* **112**, 202.

Trepicchio, W., Jr, Maruya, A. and Barrett, K.J. (1987). The heavy chain genes of a lupus anti-DNA autoantibody are encoded in the germ line of a nonautoimmune strain of mouse and conserved in strains of mice polymorphic for this gene locus. *J. Immunol.* **139**, 3139.

Tron, F. and Bach, J.F. (1977). Relationships between antibodies to native DNA and glomerulonephritis in systemic lupus erythematosus. *Clin. Exp. Immunol.* **28**, 426.

Tuffanelli, D.L. (1971). Lupus erythematosus panniculitis (profundus). *Arch. Dermatol.* **103**, 231.

Tung, K.S.K., Dehoratius, R.J. and Williams, R.C. (1981). Study of circulating immune complex size in systemic lupus erythematosus. *Clin. Exp. Immunol.* **43**, 615.

Ueda, K. and Hayaishi, O. (1985). ADP-ribosylation. *Ann. Rev. Biochem.* **54**, 73.

Uwatoko, S. and Mannik, M. (1988). Low-molecular weight C1q-binding immunoglobulin G in patients with systemic lupus erythematosus consists of autoantibodies to the collagen-like region of C1q. *J. Clin. Invest.* **82**, 816.

Valentijn, R.M., Van Overhagen, H., Hazevoet, H.M. *et al.* (1985). The value of complement and immune complex determination in monitoring disease activity in patients with systemic lupus erythematosus. *Arthritis Rheum.* **28**, 904.

Van Rappard-Van der Veen, F.M., Kiesel, U., Poels, L. *et al.* (1984a). Further evidence against random polyclonal antibody formation in mice with lupus-like graft-vs-host disease. *J. Immunol.* **132**, 1814.

Van Rappard-Van der Veen, F.M., Kong, Y.M., Rose, N.R., Kimura, M. and Gleichmann, E. (1984b). Injection of mouse thyroglobulin and/or adult thymectomy do not break tolerance to thyroglobulin during the lupus like graft versus host dis. *Clin. Exp. Immunol.* **55**, 525.

Vaughan, J.H., Bayles, T.B. and Favour, C.B. (1951). Response of serum gamma globulin levels and complement titer to adrenocorticotropic hormone (ACTH) therapy in lupus erythematosus disseminatus. *J. Clin. Lab. Immunol.* **37**, 698.

Venables, P.J.W., Smith, P.R. and Maini, R.N. (1983). Purification and characterization of the Sjögren's syndrome A and B antigens. *Clin. Exp. Immunol.* **54**, 731.

Walport, M.J. and Lachmann, P.J. (1988). Erythrocyte complement receptor type 1, immune complexes, and the rheumatic diseases. *Arthritis Rheum.* **31**, 153.

Walport, M.J., Black, C.M. and Batchelor, J.R. (1982). The immunogenetics of SLE. *Clin. Rheum. Dis.* **8**, 3.

Walport, M.J., Ross, G.D., Mackworth-Young, C., Watson, J.V., Hogg, N. and Lachmann, P.J. (1985a). Family studies of erythrocyte complement receptor type 1 levels: reduced levels in patients with SLE are acquired, not inherited. *Clin. Exp. Immunol.* **59**, 547.

Walport, M.J., Peters, A.M., Elkon, K.B., Pusey, C., Lavender, J.P. and Hughes, G.R.V. (1985b). The splenic extraction ratio of antibody-coated erythrocytes and its response to plasma exchange and pulse methylprednisolone. *Clin. Exp. Immunol.* **60**, 465.

Wangel, A.G., Johansson, E. and Ranki, A. (1984). Polyclonal B cell activation and increased lymphocyte helper-suppressor ratios in discoid lupus erythematosus. *Br. J. Dermatol.* **110**, 665.

Watson, R.M., Lane, A.T., Barnett, N.K., Bias, W.B., Arnett, F.C. and Provost, T.T. (1984). Neonatal lupus erythematosus: a clinical, serological and immunogenetic study with review of the literature. *Medicine (Baltimore)* **63**, 362.

Waxman, F.J., Hebert, L.A., Cornacoff, J.B. *et al.* (1984). Complement depletion accelerates the clearance of immune complexes from the circulation of primates. *J. Clin. Invest.* **74**, 1329.

Waxman, F.J., Hebert, L.A., Cosio, F.G. *et al.* (1986). Differential binding of immunoglobulin A and immunoglobulin G immune complexes to primate erythrocytes *in vivo*: A immune complexes bind less well to erythrocytes and are preferentially deposited in glomeruli. *J. Clin. Invest.* **77**, 82.

Weinstein, A., Bordwell, B., Stone, B., Tibbetts, C. and Rothfield, N.F. (1983). Antibodies to native DNA and serum complement (C3) levels: Application to diagnosis and classification of systemic lupus erythematosus. *Am. J. Med.* **74**, 206.

Weir, D.M., Holborow, E.J. and Johnson, G.D. (1961). A clinical study of serum antinuclear factor. *Br. Med. J.* **i**, 933.

Welch, T.R., Beischel, L., Berry, A., Forristal, J. and West, C.D. (1985). The effect of null C4 alleles on complement function. *Clin. Immunol. Immunopathol.* **34**, 316.

Wener, M.H., Uwatoko, S. and Mannik, M. (1989). Antibodies to the collagen-like region of C1q in sera of patients with autoimmune rheumatic diseases. *Arthritis Rheum.* **32**, 544.

Wernet, P. and Kunkel, H.G. (1973). Antibodies to a specific surface antigen on T cells in human sera inhibiting mixed leukocyte culture reactions. *J. Exp. Med.* **138**, 1021.

Whittingham, S., Mathews, J.D., Schanfield, M.S., Tait, B.D. and Mackay, I.R. (1983). HLA and Gm genes in systemic lupus erythematosus. *Tissue Antigens* **21**, 50.

Williams, G.W., Steinberg, A.D., Reinertsen, J.L., Klassen, L.W., Decker, J.L. and Dolin, R. (1978). Influenza immunization in systemic lupus erythematosus: a double-blind trial. *Ann. Intern. Med.* **88**, 729.

Wilson, I.A., Haft, D.H., Getzoff, E.D., Tainer, J.A., Lerner, R.A. and Brenner, S. (1985). Identical short peptide sequences in unrelated proteins can have different conformations: a testing ground for theories of immune recognition. *Proc. Nat. Acad. Sci. (USA)* **82**, 5255.

Wilson, J.G., Wong, W.W., Schur, P.H. and Fearon, D.T. (1982). Mode of inheritance of decreased C3b receptors on erythrocytes of patients with systemic lupus erythematosus. *N. Engl. J. Med.* **307**, 981.

Wilson, J.G., Jack, R.M., Wong, W.W., Schur, P.H. and Fearon, D.T. (1985). Autoantibody to the C3b/C4b receptor and absence of this receptor from erythrocytes of a patient with systemic lupus erythematosus. *J. Clin. Invest.* **76**, 182.

Wilson, J.G., Murphy, E.E., Wong, W.W., Klickstein, L.B., Weis, J.H. and Fearon, D.T. (1986). Identification of a restriction fragment length polymorphism by a CR1 cDNA that correlates with the number of CR1 on erythrocytes. *J. Exp. Med.* **164**, 50.

Wilson, J.G., Wong, W.W., Murphy, E.E., III. Schur, P.H. and Fearon, D.T. (1987). Deficiency of the C3b/C4b receptor (CR1) of erythrocytes in systemic lupus erythematosus: analysis of the stability of the defect and of a restriction fragment length polymorphism of the CR1 gene. *J. Immunol.* **138**, 2708.

Wilson, R.W., Provost, T.T., Bias, W.B. *et al.* (1984). Sjögren's syndrome: influence of multiple HLA-D region alloantigens on clinical and serologic expression. *Arthritis Rheum.* **27**, 1245.

Winfield, J.B., Faiferman, I. and Koffler, D. (1977). Avidity of anti-DNA antibodies in serum and IgG glomerular eluates from patients with systemic lupus erythematosus: association of high avidity antinative DNA antibody with glomerulonephritis. *J. Clin. Invest.* **59**, 90.

Winfield, J.B., Shaw, M., Silverman, L.M., Eisenberg, R.A., Wilson, H.A., III and Koffler, D. (1983). Intrathecal IgG synthesis and blood–brain barrier impairment in patients with systemic lupus erythematosus and central nervous system dysfunction. *Am. J. Med.* **74**, 837.

Winfield, J.B., Shaw, M. and Minota, S. (1986). Modulation of IgM anti-lymphocyte antibody-reactive T cell surface antigens in systemic lupus erythematosus. *J. Immunol.* **136**, 3246.

Winfield, J.B., Shaw, M., Yamada, A. and Minota, S. (1987). Subset specificity of anti-lymphocyte antibodies in systemic lupus erythematosus. II. Preferential reactivity with T4+ cells is associated with relative depletion of autologous T4+ cells. *Arthritis Rheum.* **30**, 162.

Wolin, S.L. and Steitz, J.A. (1984). The Ro small cytoplasmic ribonucleoproteins: identification of the antigenic protein and its binding site on the Ro RNAs. *Proc. Nat. Acad. Sci. (USA)* **81**, 1996.

Yamada, A., Shaw, M. and Winfield, J.B. (1985). Surface antigen specificity of cold-reactive IgM antilymphocyte antibodies in systemic lupus erythematosus. *Arthritis Rheum.* **28**, 44.

Yamanaka, H., Penning, C.A., Willis, E.H., Wasson, D.B. and Carson, D.A. (1988). Characterization of human poly(ADP-ribose) polymerase with autoantibodies. *J. Biol. Chem.* **263**, 3879.

Yokohari, R. and Tsunematsu, T. (1985). Application, to Japanese patients, of the 1982 American Rheumatism Association revised criteria for the classification of systemic lupus erythematosus. *Arthritis Rheum.* **28**, 693.

Yoshida, H., Yoshida, M., Izui, S. and Lambert, P.H. (1985). Distinct clonotypes of anti-DNA antibodies in mice with lupus nephritis. *J. Clin. Invest.* **76**, 685.

Yu, D.T.Y., Winchester, R.J., Fu, S.M., Gibofsky, A., Ko, H.S. and Kunkel, H.G. (1980). Peripheral blood Ia-positive T cells: increases in certain diseases and after immunization. *J. Exp. Med.* **151**, 91.

Zouali, M., Stollar, B.D. and Schwartz, R.S. (1988). Origin and diversification of anti-DNA antibodies. *Immunol. Rev.* **105**, 137.

Zubler, R.H., Lange, G., Lambert, P.H. and Miescher, P.A. (1976). Detection of immune complexes in unheated sera by modified 125I−Clq binding test: effect of heating on the binding of Clq by immune complexes. *J. Immunol.* **116**, 232.

Zvaifler, N.J. and Bluestein, H.G. (1982). The pathogenesis of central nervous system manifestations of systemic lupus erythematosus. *Arthritis Rheum.* **25**, 862.

62: Systemic Vasculitides

C.O.S. Savage and C.M. Lockwood

Introduction

The term systemic vasculitis is used to delineate a group of diseases which are associated with an inflammatory reaction in or around blood-vessels. The term has clinical and pathological implications but gives no understanding of mechanisms of pathogenesis. Therefore the basic definition remains pathological, with fibrinoid necrosis of vessel walls being the salient feature of the vasculitic process. This chapter will focus on those forms of vasculitis which are considered primary and which have a particular tendency towards causing a debilitating systemic disease with multi-organ involvement, in particular the arteritis group (classical polyarteritis nodosa, microscopic polyarteritis, Henoch–Schönlein purpura) and the granulomatoses (Churg–Strauss syndrome, Wegener's granulomatosis). Other primary vasculitides (see Table 62.1) will be referred to as appropriate. This chapter will not cover vasculitis secondary to identifiable agents (drugs, infections) or other well-defined disorders (cryoglobulinaemia, systemic lupus erythematosus), most of which are discussed in other chapters.

There have been many different approaches to classification of allergic vasculitides and no attempt will be made here at a comprehensive review (Alarcon-Segovia 1977, Fauci *et al.* 1978; Fan *et al.* 1980; Cupps and Fauci 1982; McCluskey and Fienberg 1983; Savage *et al.* 1985; Croker *et al.* 1987; Lie 1988). A simple empirical system based on the type and size of vessel involvement, as originally suggested by Zeek (1953), is offered in Table 62.1. The different classification systems arose because of the scarcity of basic medical scientific data on aetiology and pathogenesis. The individual disorders are recognized by their particular pattern of clinical symptoms, signs and pathological findings, but precise diagnosis may still be difficult due to the considerable overlap between the different entities. A further difficulty is that the terminology associated with the

Table 62.1. Classification of systemic vasculitis

Primary vasculitis
1 Involving large, medium-sized and small blood-vessels:
  (a) Takayasu's arteritis
  (b) Granulomatous (giant cell) arteritis, cranial (temporal) arteritis and extracranial giant cell arteritis
2 Involving predominantly medium and small blood-vessels:
  (a) Polyarteritis (periarteritis) nodosa
  (b) Infantile polyarteritis
  (c) Kawasaki disease
  (d) Granulomatous Churg–Strauss syndrome
3 Involving predominantly small blood-vessels:
  (a) Microscopic polyarteritis (hypersensitivity vasculitis and leucocytoclastic vasculitis are terms often used when the skin is the major tissue affected)
  (b) Wegener's granulomatosis
  (c) Henoch–Schönlein purpura

Secondary vasculitis
1 Infectious:
  (a) Spirochaetal (syphilis, Lyme disease)
  (b) Mycobacterial
  (c) Pyogenic bacteria or fungal
  (d) Rickettsial
  (e) Viral
  (f) Whipple bacillus
2 Non-infectious secondary vasculitides affecting medium and small blood-vessels:
  (a) Thromboangiitis obliterans (Buerger's disease)
  (b) Sarcoidosis
  (c) Vasculitis of collagen-vascular diseases: rheumatic fever; rheumatoid arthritis; seronegative arthropathies; systemic lupus erythematosus; dermatomyositis/polymyositis; relapsing polychondritis; systemic sclerosis; Sjögren's syndrome; Behçet's syndrome; Cogan's syndrome
3 Non-infectious secondary vasculitis affecting predominantly small blood-vessels:
  (a) Serum sickness
  (b) Drug-induced vasculitis
  (c) Malignancy-associated vasculitis
  (d) Retroperitoneal fibrosis
  (e) Lymphocytic vasculitis
  (f) Essential mixed cryoglobulinaemia
  (g) Hypocomplementaemia
  (h) Inflammatory bowel disease
  (i) Primary biliary cirrhosis
  (j) Goodpasture syndrome
  (k) Transplant vasculitis

Vasculitis look-alikes
1 Coarctation–hypoplasia–dysplasia
2 Atheroembolism
3 Myxoma embolism
4 Ergotism
5 Neurofibromatosis
6 Idiopathic arterial calcification

Based on Savage *et al.* (1985) and Lie (1988).

polyarteritis group of conditions is inconsistent. The classic description of polyarteritis nodosa was given by Kussmaul and Maier in 1866, in which there was extreme vascular damage with aneurysmal formation. Then in 1948 Davson, Ball and Platt recognized that there were two patterns of polyarteritis damage, especially in the kidney; firstly a large-vessel extraglomerular arteritis compatible with classic polyarteritis nodosa, and secondly a necrotizing glomerulonephritis or microscopic polyarteritis. The association between classical polyarteritis nodosa and microscopic polyarteritis (and indeed between microscopic polyarteritis and Wegener's granulomatosis) continues to be debated, although clinical and pathological overlap undoubtedly occur (Fauci *et al.* 1978). Microscopic polyarteritis has also been termed 'hypersensitivity vasculitis' (angiitis), as proposed by Zeek in 1953 to describe the necrotizing vasculitis which was thought to be induced by drugs (sulphonamides, penicillins), heterologous sera or infection. It is likely that these agents were rarely directly causative, since systemic vasculitis can masquerade as a fever, which may be misdiagnosed as secondary to infection and for which antibiotics may be administered. Subsequently hypersensitivity vasculitis' was also applied to idiopathic small-vessel systemic vasculitis of the microscopic polyarteritis type; more recently hypersensitivity vasculitis has been equated with cutaneous leucocytoclastic vasculitis (Cupps and Fauci 1982), and indeed in our experience represents a form of microscopic polyarteritis which predominantly affects the skin, but also shows involvement of other organs. To add a further complexity to the terminology, the term idiopathic rapidly progressive glomerulonephritis appears to be a renal-limited form of microscopic polyarteritis (Serra *et al.* 1984).

Pathology

The essential lesion in the acute stage of all forms of primary vasculitis consists of fibrinoid necrosis of part or all of the vessel wall. The initial morphological changes, leading to the deposition of the fibrin-like material seen by light microscopy, have been studied using electron microscopy and scanning electron microscopy in patients with Wegener's granulomatosis (Novak *et al.* 1982). Early acute lesions showed marked alteration of the endothelial cells, with loss of cytoplasmic organelles and areas of disruption of the endothelial surface, and/or wide interendothelial cell junctions. Immediately below the endothelial surface, there was a mixture of fibrin-like strands and platelets that were partially or completely degranulated. These changes are not well appreciated by light microscopy. Other ultrastructural studies have drawn attention to lysis of cells, some with the appearance of monocytes, within capillary lumina, causing large numbers of free nuclei and cytoplasmic organelles to accumulate within capillaries where the endothelium is still intact; platelets aggregate adjacent to ruptured cells and endothelial cell necrosis, deposition of fibrin on bare basement membrane and disruption of the elastic lamina follow (Donald *et al.* 1986). These two studies suggest two early events which may contribute to vascular injury: participation of platelets, which may discharge vasoactive amines (Novak *et al.* 1982), and intravascular lysis of cells, which could at least extend tissue injury (Donald *et al.* 1986). A cellular inflammatory response generally accompanies the fibrinoid necrotic reaction with a mixed neutrophil, mononuclear and eosinophil infiltration of the vessel wall spreading out into the surrounding tissue. Such advanced changes are easily seen by light microscopy and are commonly seen in and around vessel bifurcations.

The nature of the cellular response helps to characterize certain forms of vasculitis. Granulomatous lesions develop in, for example, Wegener's granulomatosis, the Churg–Strauss syndrome and temporal (giant cell) arteritis, as well as in lymphomatoid granulomatosis. In Wegener's the granulomata may be adjacent to or distant from the vessels. The earliest recognizable lesion is an area of fibrinoid necrosis, without invading leucocytes, which then becomes surrounded by palisading histiocytes and may progress to diffuse granulomatous involvement of the affected tissue, with multinucleated giant cells (Fienberg 1981). Granulomata involving both vessels and extravascular tissue are seen also in the Churg–Strauss syndrome, accompanied by a diffuse inflammatory infiltrate composed predominantly of eosinophils (Churg and Strauss 1952; Chumbley *et al.* 1977). Lymphomatoid granulomatosis is generally considered as a granulomatous vasculitis but it differs from other forms of vasculitis under review here in that there is no leucocytoclastic vasculitis or fibrinoid necrosis; instead there is an angiotrophic and angiodestructive invasion of vessels with bizarre lymphocytoid and plasmacytoid cells (Liebow *et al.* 1972).

Immunofluorescence studies of vasculitic lesions have failed to demonstrate deposition of immunoreactants in the vessel wall beyond those deposited there through non-specific escape of plasma constituents (albumin, immunoglobulins, complement components and fibrin) into vessel walls during the acute phase of the disease (Paronetto and Strauss 1962). The presence or absence of immune complexes in vessel walls has long been debated, since immune complex generation has been proposed as a likely mechanism of injury, but electron microscopy has also failed to demonstrate ultrastructural evidence for these (Novak *et al.* 1982).

Vasculitic lesions frequently are patchily distributed along vessel walls, as has been well described in both old and new literature (Davson *et al.* 1948; Novak *et al.* 1982); this may apply particularly to the fibrinoid necrotic areas, leaving areas with only vessel wall infiltration or perivascular cuffing to suggest, but not to confirm, the underlying nature of the process. The different vasculitic syndromes also have a predilection to affect vessels of differing calibre, which has been used as a part of the basis for empirical classification of the major vasculitides (Fan *et al.* 1980; Savage *et al.* 1985). Thus, classical polyarteritis nodosa predominantly affects medium-size muscular arteries (Davson *et al.* 1948), as may the Churg–Strauss syndrome (Churg and Strauss 1952); in these disorders the segmental injury of an artery may lead to aneurysm formation, which may be a helpful diagnostic feature when radiographically demonstrated (Travers *et al.* 1979). Kawasaki disease of childhood also favours medium-sized vessels, particularly coronary arteries (Tanaka *et al.* 1976). Small arterioles and capillaries are the major target in Wegener's granulomatosis and microscopic polyarteritis, predisposing both disorders to development of a focal segmental necrotizing glomerulonephritis centred on the glomerular capillary bed (Wainwright and Davson 1950; Novak *et al.* 1982; Heptinstall 1983). The aorta and its major branches are attacked in Takayasu arteritis (Nakao *et al.* 1967) and arteries of the head and neck in temporal arteritis (Fauchald *et al.* 1972).

Differential organ involvement contributes to the characteristic patterns of clinical involvement which serve to differentiate the vasculitic syndromes. Generally there is little to distinguish the vasculitic process in the various organs, and the underlying basis for the variable involvement, as well as the patchy segmental involvement of the vessel walls themselves, is an intriguing phenomenon which is not as yet understood. However, in some organs, especially the kidney, particular pathological features do accompany each type of vasculitis. For example, hypertensive and ischaemic vascular damage is usual in classical polyarteritis nodosa. More closely associated with vasculitis is the glomerulonephritis which develops in microscopic polyarteritis and in the majority of patients with Wegener's granulomatosis. The basic lesion is focal, segmental hypercellularity of capillary loops with fibrinoid necrosis (Heptinstall 1983); platelet aggregates or microvascular thrombi may be observed at the ultrastructural level (Weiss and Crissman 1984). An increase in the number of intraglomerular neutrophils (Droz *et al*. 1979; Neild *et al*. 1983) may be seen, often associated with areas of fibrinoid necrosis or near breaks in the glomerular basement membrane (Neild *et al*. 1983; Glassock *et al*. 1986). Intraglomerular helper T cells may be distinguished using appropriate monoclonal antibody markers (ten Berge *et al*. 1985). The endocapillary lesions are usually accompanied by extracapillary proliferation, with fibrin exudation, monocyte infiltration and epithelial cell proliferation, contributing to the crescent formation (Hancock and Atkins 1984; Magil 1985), as well as infiltrating neutrophils (Neild *et al*. 1983). Silver staining, transmission electron microscopy and scanning electron microscopy after dissolution of the cellular components have revealed glomerular basement membrane perforations which may contribute to the exudation of material into Bowman's space (Serra *et al*. 1984; Bonsib 1988). Sometimes glomeruli with totally circumferential crescents show disintegration of part of Bowman's capsule, and the glomerulus is surrounded by mononuclear cells (Neild *et al*. 1983). In many cases of microscopic polyarteritis and Wegener's granulomatosis, there are endocapillary and extracapillary lesions at various stages of development, from frankly cellular to sclerosing glomerular segments or fibrous crescents, suggesting that the stimulus to tissue injury is ongoing (Balow 1985). The glomerular lesions are frequently associated with an interstitial inflammatory exudate with lymphocytes, monocytes and plasma cells; eosinophils are not prominent (Neild *et al*. 1983). In Wegener's granulomatosis large granulomas composed of histiocytes and giant cells may be present in the interstitium, or may surround necrotic glomeruli or vessels (Droz *et al*. 1979). Renal arteritis of small arteries, particularly those of interlobular size, may be seen, especially in large biopsy specimens and at autopsy (Novak *et al*. 1982; Neild *et al*. 1983; Ronco *et al*. 1983; Serra *et al*. 1984).

Clinical and therapeutic aspects of the allergic vasculitides

The allergic vasculitides together cause diverse patterns of organ involvement. They frequently present in the setting of marked constitutional upset, with specific involvement of several organ systems; the appearance of a vasculitic rash may first suggest the nature of the underlying process. The particular patterns of organ involvement which characterize the individual syndromes have been well described in other reviews (Alarcon-Segovia 1977; Fauci *et al*. 1978; Cupps and Fauci 1982) and are beyond the scope of this article; it may be useful to consider the clinical pattern in relation to the likely calibre of vessel involvement (small-vessel, medium-vessel and aortic syndromes), as has been well described by Fan (1980).

A major problem in management of allergic vasculitides lies in making a diagnosis early, before irreversible organ damage or life-threatening complications arise. In this regard, investigations have generally been supportive rather than diagnostic, reflecting the systemic nature of the diseases and the acute-phase response (raised erythrocyte sedimentation rate, normochromic normocytic anaemia, leucocytosis, thrombocytosis, reversed albumin–globulin levels, raised C-reactive protein levels, hypercomplementaemia). Involvement of individual organs, particularly kidney, liver and lung, can be confirmed by appropriate tests but do not otherwise add to the diagnosis. Arteriography of the arterial tree may be helpful in demonstrating dilatation and aneurysmal damage to medium-sized arteries in classical polyarteritis nodosa (Travers *et al*. 1979) or the arterial stenoses encountered in larger arteries in Takayasu's disease (Lande and Gross 1972). Histological confirmation of vasculitis with fibrinoid necrosis may be obtained through tissue biopsy; frequently, however, the histology only shows features consistent with vasculitis (for example, perivascular infiltrates but no fibrinoid necrosis, or a focal segmental necrotizing glomerulonephritis without evidence of vasculitis in extraglomerular vessels).

One of the most useful diagnostic tests to emerge over the last few years is the indirect immunofluorescence test for antibodies to neutrophil cytoplasm components (Davies *et al*. 1982; Van der Woude *et al*. 1985). The discovery of these antineutrophil cytoplasm antibodies (ANCA) has provided a useful tool for confirming the diagnosis in patients with Wegener's granulomatosis and microscopic polyarteritis, since ANCA, whether detected by the indirect immunofluorescence technique or using solid-phase assay systems, have a high specificity and sensitivity for these disorders (Van der Woude *et al*. 1985; Savage *et al*. 1987; Cohen Tervaert *et al*. 1989; Nolle *et al*. 1989).

Despite the potentially severe nature of the allergic vasculitides, overall patient mortality has declined dramatically in recent years following the widespread use of prednisolone and cytotoxic drugs, such as cyclophosphamide and azathioprine, both to prevent progression and to induce remission of disease. The emphasis on use of prednisolone and cyclophosphamide varies a little across the spectrum of vasculitides. Thus temporal arteritis is exquisitely sensitive to prednisolone alone (Fauchald *et al*. 1972), cyclophosphamide is the drug of choice in Wegener's granulomatosis (Fauci *et al*. 1983), and, whilst prednisolone alone is often used as first-line treatment in uncomplicated classical polyarteritis nodosa (Cohen *et al*. 1980), additional cyclophosphamide is advocated for patients with microscopic polyarteritis and renal involvement (Serra *et al*. 1984; Savage *et al*. 1985; Adu *et al*. 1987; Fuiano *et al*. 1988). Prognosis for most forms of vasculitis has thus improved markedly; for example, 80% of patients with untreated Wegener's granulomatosis were dead at 1 year (Walton 1958) but over 90% 1-year survival rates are now achievable (Reza *et al*. 1975; Fauci *et al*. 1983). The situation within the polyarteritis group is more difficult to assess, since most series do not differentiate between classical and microscopic forms of polyarteritis. However, the 5-year survival rate for patients with untreated polyarteritis nodosa was 13% in the 1967 series of Frohnert and Sheps, but use of prednisolone together with cyclophosphamide can allow 5-year actuarial survival rates of 65–80% for microscopic polyarteritis (Savage *et al*. 1985; Fuiano *et al*. 1988).

Details of recommended drug regimens are described in detail elsewhere (Savage *et al*. 1985; Balow and Fauci 1988; Fuiano *et al*. 1988). Intravenous pulse cyclophosphamide instead of oral cyclophosphamide has been used in some centres, but it is too early to recommend or discourage administration of cyclophosphamide via this route. Some caution is required since Hoffman *et al*. (1990) found that intravenous cyclophosphamide was associated with initial failure to respond to treatment and with failure both to sustain improvement and to continue treatment in 11 of 14 patients. Others have reported good results when intravenous cyclophosphamide has been substituted after 2–4 weeks of oral treatment (Ulmer *et al*. 1990). Pulse methylprednisolone or plasma exchange has been found to be effective in inducing more rapid remissions in patients with Wegener's or microscopic polyarteritis who have associated rapidly progressive glomerulonephritis (Pinching *et al*. 1983; Harrison *et al*. 1980; Hind *et al*. 1983; Pusey *et al*. 1991), particularly in those who are already dialysis-dependent at presentation (Pusey *et al*. 1991).

Finally, another therapeutic advance has been achieved of a different nature in patients with Kawasaki disease. This childhood vasculitic disease has a predilection for the coronary arteries. Improvements in outcome have been documented in children treated with intravenous immunoglobulin (Leung *et al*. 1987). The response of the allergic vasculitides to treatments which modulate the immune response suggests that immunopathogenic mechanisms may be important at least in maintaining disease activity, if not in the initiation of tissue injury, as will be discussed below.

Autoimmune responses in the systemic vasculitides

Evidence that autoimmune mechanisms are operating in the primary systemic vasculitides has emerged only within the last decade. In 1982 Davies *et al*. reported that patients with a polyarteritis-like illness and renal vasculitis at biopsy had serum autoantibodies which reacted with the cytoplasm of normal human neutrophils by indirect immunofluorescence. In 1985 a collaborative study carried out in Denmark and the Netherlands showed that sera from patients with active Wegener's granulomatosis contained ANCA (Van der Woude *et al.* 1985). Furthermore, the binding was specific since it was dependent on the $F(ab)_2$ portion of the autoantibody immunoglobulin. In 1987 we used a soluble acid extract of sonicated neutrophils as solid-phase ligand for radioimmunoassay and found that autoantibodies in sera from patients with both microscopic polyarteritis and Wegener's granulomatosis would bind specifically (Lockwood *et al.* 1987). Subsequently, two forms of ANCA have been identified that are distinguishable by their indirect immunofluorescence pattern of binding to neutrophils. The classical or cytoplasmic form of binding (C-ANCA) is identical to the pattern described by Van der Woude *et al.* (1985), with marked granular staining. The second pattern shows binding in a perinuclear distribution (P-ANCA) to ethanol-fixed neutrophils. Both C-ANCA and P-ANCA are specific for constituents of neutrophil azurophil (primary/alpha) granules and monocyte lysosomes (Falk and Jennette 1988). The P-ANCA pattern is caused by the artefactual redistribution of soluble nucleophilic proteins with high isoelectric points to a perinuclear position, while the use of formalinfixed neutrophils, which prevents the redistribution, allows C-ANCA and P-ANCA to produce granular cytoplasmic staining patterns. Wegener's granulomatosis is usually associated with C-ANCA (Falk 1990), although exceptions do occur (Gans *et al.* 1989), while microscopic polyarteritis and idiopathic rapidly progressive glomerulonephritis may be associated with either C-ANCA or P-ANCA.

Antigens recognized by anti-neutrophil cytoplasm antibodies

At least two neutrophil antigens have been identified and several others suggested. Most are enzymes, have a high pI and are associated with cellular activation. The best characterized have been myeloperoxidase (Falk and Jennette 1988) and a 29 kD serine proteinase (Goldschmeding *et al.* 1989; Niles *et al.* 1989), which has been identified as proteinase 3 (Ludemann *et al.* 1990). Sera recognizing myeloperoxidase broadly correspond to P-ANCA detected by immunofluorescence (Falk and Jennette 1988), while sera recognizing proteinase 3 broadly correspond to C-ANCA (Jennette *et al.* 1990). The different specificities could be confirmed by immunoprecipitation and Western blotting techniques. Parallel studies using monoclonal antibodies to these two antigens have been used to support the data provided by the human autoantibodies. A few P-ANCA may also react with other neutrophil constituents, such as elastase (Goldschmeding *et al.* 1989) or with the specific granule constituent lactoferrin (Lesarve *et al.* 1990). Some C-ANCA do not react with purified proteinase 3 and in these cases the azurophil granule constituent, CAP 57, may be a target antigen (Falk 1990).

Anti-neutrophil cytoplasm antibodies as diagnostic markers for primary systemic vasculitis

The value of ANCA as diagnostic markers for patients with vasculitis has been investigated in several studies. Savage *et al.* (1987) examined sera from 100 consecutive new patients referred by renal physicians in which the suspected diagnosis was renal vasculitis. Indirect immunofluorescence tests and solid-phase radioimmunoassays (with competitive inhibition tests) were used to test for ANCA. The two tests, used together, conferred both a sensitivity and a specificity of 96% for untreated Wegener's granulomatosis or microscopic polyarteritis. These findings have been confirmed by others (Ludemann and Gross 1987; Cohen Tervaert *et al.* 1989; Nolle *et al.* 1989; Falk 1990; Halma *et al.* 1990). Subsequently it became apparent that other vasculitides, including classical polyarteritis nodosa and the Churg–Strauss syndrome, and sometimes giant cell arteritis and Takayasu's disease, were also characterized by similar autoimmune responses (Cohen Tervaert *et al.* 1990a; Lai *et al.* 1990; McHugh *et al.* 1990). Thus the primary systemic vasculitides should be regarded as a spectrum of clinicopathological syndromes that have a common association with ANCA. Infrequently ANCA are associated with other diseases. For example, a few patients with systemic lupus erythematosus and renal involvement have myeloperoxidase-specific or elastase-specific P-ANCA that can be differentiated from antinuclear reactivity (Falk 1990). Children with Kawasaki disease also have P-ANCA-like autoantibody (Savage *et al.* 1989), while patients with inflammatory bowel disease have P-ANCA that may not be specific for myeloperoxidase (Falk 1990). A proportion of patients with anti-glomerular basement membrane antibody-mediated disease also have ANCA (Jayne *et al.* 1990). In general, ANCA appear to have the highest positive predictive value in groups of patients with manifestations suggestive of vasculitis or glomerulonephritis, that is, those patients where a positive diagnosis is of the greatest importance for deciding therapeutic schedules and in predicting the long-term outcome of the disease.

Value of anti-neutrophil cytoplasm antibodies in management of systemic vasculitis

The close association between clinically defined groups forming the spectrum of systemic vasculitis and the presence of ANCA suggested that autoimmune mechanisms could play some part in the development of disease. If this were the case, then autoantibody levels might reflect disease activity, and their sequential measurement might both be a guide to the efficacy of therapy and be useful in predicting disease relapse. Van der Woude *et al.* (1985) showed that, by indirect immunofluorescence assays, ANCA levels correlated with disease activity, and, more recently, Cohen Tervaert *et al.* (1990b) showed that relapses could be predicted during follow-up by rising ANCA levels, and avoided if cyclophosphamide was used when significant rises occurred. Gaskin *et al.* (1991) have found that the presence or reappearance of ANCA during follow-up may identify patients who are at risk of relapse and who are most likely to benefit from long-term immunosuppressive therapy.

Isotype, antibody class and disease expression

The immunoglobulin G (IgG) ANCA subclass distribution and its relation to disease expression have been investigated. Brouwer *et al.* (1991) found that there was a predominance of IgG-1 and IgG-4, with an increase of IgG-3 in patients with renal disease. They suggested that IgG-1 and IgG-3 might be pathogenic by virtue of their complement-fixing abilities, while they hypothesized a role for IgG-4 in binding to and activation of neutrophils. Jayne *et al.* (1991) have found increased expression of IgG-1 and IgG-3 with under-representation of IgG-2. With treatment, the normal ratio of IgG-2 to IgG-3 was restored. These findings may help to explain why some patients in remission may have raised levels of ANCA, yet little disease activity, and formal studies to examine this possibility are in progress.

In Wegener's granulomatosis and microscopic polyarteritis, ANCA were usually found to be immunoglobulins of the IgG class. Rare patients with a polyarteritis-like illness and ANCA autoantibodies of only IgM class have been identified (Jayne *et al.* 1989). These patients typically presented with severe pulmonary–renal syndromes, including pulmonary haemorrhage and renal failure. Although resembling Goodpasture's syndrome due to anti-glomerular basement membrane antibodies, these latter autoantibodies were not detected. Treatment with plasma exchange was effective when used in addition to cytotoxic drugs and steroids (which might be expected if the IgM antibody was of pathogenic important, since IgM is predominantly confined to the intravascular compartment). Interestingly, with treatment, some patients showed a late class switch of IgM to IgG, as they went into remission. In one patient, immunoglobulins of both M and G class were eluted from the kidneys at autopsy and could be shown to have specific ANCA activity. This suggested that the autoantibody (IgM) class at presentation may have determined not only the pattern of organ involvement but also the severity of disease activity. That autoantibody class may play a role in disease expression has also been suggested by Van der Wall Bake and Lobatto (1987), who showed that some patients with IgA nephritis and Henoch Schönlein purpura (in which the renal involvement may be immunohistologically identical to that in IgA nephritis) have ANCA of IgA class as well as IgG.

Pathophysiological effect of anti-neutrophil cytoplasm antibodies

Do ANCA have a central role in mediating disease? Only circumstantial evidence is available at the present time. That almost all patients with untreated active primary systemic vasculitis have detectable circulating ANCA argues that their presence is fundamental to the development of vasculitis. Furthermore, since levels correlate with disease activity, and variation in autoantibody class and subclass is associated with variety of disease expressions, these findings imply a close connection between humoral autoimmune responses and the generation of vasculitis.

Falk *et al.* (1990) have shown that ANCA can induce normal human neutrophils to undergo an oxidative burst and degranulate *in vitro*. These effects on neutrophil activation are markedly enhanced by priming neutrophils with tumour necrosis factor. These observations are complemented by *in vitro* studies which demonstrate that phorbol ester-primed neutrophils can be activated by ANCA to cause cytotoxic damage to cultured human vascular endothelial cells (Savage *et al.*, submitted).

Anti-neutrophil cytoplasm antibodies may also affect leucocyte signal transduction pathways. Using either human neutrophils or HL-60 cells (a human promyeloid cell line which grows *in vitro*), we have found that $F(ab)_2$ of ANCA +ve immunoglobulin impairs signal transduction mediated through the inositol phospholipid pathway or the translocation of protein kinase C. Stimulation of these two pathways by synthetic ligands which bind to extracellular receptors can be substantially impaired by preincubation with ANCA immunoglobulin, but not by control autoantibodies to glomerular basement membrane (Lai and Lockwood 1990). This effect is specific for neutrophils, there being no blockade of signal transduction in lymphocytes using the same ANCA antibody preparations. Signal transduction is an essential step in neutrophil activation, which occurs as part of any inflammatory stimulus. Any interference with neutrophil activation is likely to perpetuate the inflammatory state, and chronic inflammation is characteristic of systemic vasculitis.

Anti-neutrophil cytoplasm antibodies are likely to be just one of several factors that may contribute to the development of vasculitis and, as yet, the stimulus to the generation of ANCA is unknown. Genetic and environmental factors appear to influence the disease process. There is genetic linkage of Wegener's granulomatosis and microscopic polyarteritis to human leucocyte antigen (HLA) DQw7 (Spencer *et al.*, submitted). There is a seasonal incidence of vasculitis, suggesting that pathogens may contribute to the disease process, although whether as an initiator or an amplifier of injury is not clear (Falk 1990). Infection is associated with relapses of vasculitis (Pinching *et al.* 1980).

Anti-neutrophil cytoplasm antibodies and immunoregulation by the idiotypic network

If autoantibodies in patients with systemic vasculitis can mediate disease, then study of the regulation of these autoimmune responses may help guide new strategies for treatment. One type of regulatory mechanism could involve idiotypic–anti-idiotypic reactions as predicted by the network theory (Jerne 1955). Idiotypic determinants have been characterized on autoantibodies occurring in different autoimmune diseases, and heterologous anti-idiotypic antibodies to these have been shown to have a regulatory effect *in vitro* (Colvin and Olson 1985). The possibility that natural homoeostatic mechanisms operate within the network framework has been supported by the finding that 'normal' B cells possess the necessary genetic information to manufacture autoantibodies and that within the population of normal immunoglobulins there exist a range of 'natural' anti-idiotypic antibodies (Holmberg and Coutinho 1985). The therapeutic potential of pooled normal immunoglobulin has been exploited in spontaneously occurring anti-factor VIII disease (Sultan *et al.* 1987) and in Kawasaki disease, an ANCA-associated systemic vasculitis of childhood (Leung *et al.* 1987). Involvement of the idiotype–anti-idiotype network was suggested by Sultan *et al.* (1987), although other mechanisms operating via the cytokine network were suggested by Leung *et al.* (1987).

We have shown that $F(ab)_2$ of normal pooled immunoglobulin can inhibit binding of ANCA *in vitro* (Rossi *et al.* 1991). The degree of inhibition ranged from 0 to 100%, with up to 75% of a panel of 21 pretreatment ANCA +ve sera being substantially inhibited by a single $F(ab)_2$ preparation of pooled immunoglobulin. That this inhibition of binding fulfilled the criteria of idiotypic–anti-idiotypic reactions was demonstrated by showing that the $F(ab)_2$ of affinity-purified ANCA immunoglobulin reacted with, and was inhibited in its specific binding by, normal IgG. When remission sera, with no intrinsic ANCA activity, were tested with their corresponding acute (pretreatment) ANCA +ve sera, then marked inhibition was found for six of seven pairs. Such experimental data have encouraged pilot studies of the use of pooled intravenous globulin alone for certain patients with systemic vasculitis (Jayne *et al.* 1991).

Anti-endothelial cell antibodies

Antibodies to endothelial cell surface antigens (AECA) have been implicated in a number of primary systemic vasculitic disorders. In an extensive study of the role of AECA in Kawasaki disease, Leung and co-workers (1986a, b) demonstrated the presence of AECA that mediate complement-dependent cytolysis following recognition of determinants on the endothelial cell surface that are induced by the cytokines tumour necrosis factor, interleukin 1 and interferon-γ. The determinants induced by tumour necrosis factor and interleukin 1 appeared to differ from those induced by interferon-γ, suggesting recognition of multiple surface molecules.

Studies in Wegener's granulomatosis and microscopic polyarteritis have also demonstrated presence of AECA (Brasile *et al.* 1989; Ferraro *et al.* 1990; Frampton *et al.* 1990; Savage *et al.* 1991). These appear to be largely of the IgG class and recognize determinants present on cultured endothelial cells derived from human umbilical veins. The AECA are reported to mediate complement-dependent cytotoxicity in some studies (Brasile *et al.* 1989) but not others (Ferraro *et al.* 1990; Savage *et al.* 1991), but they can mediate antibody-dependent cytotoxicity in a few patients (Savage *et al.* 1991). It is possible that AECA contribute to vascular injury either directly or by promoting neutrophil adherence to the endothelium.

Conclusions

It is now evident that autoimmune mechanisms are operating in the systemic vasculitides. Study of the humoral component has not only improved their diagnosis and management, but also now offers new insights into their pathogenesis and provides new strategies for treatment.

References

Adu, D., Howie, A.J., Scott, D.G.I., Bacon, P.A., McGonigle, R.J.S. and Michael, J. (1987). Polyarteritis and the kidney. *Quart. J. Med.* **239**, 221–37.

Alarcon-Segovia, D. (1977). The necrotizing vasculitides: a new pathogenetic classification. *Med. Clin. North Am.* **61** (2), 241–60.

Alarcon-Segovia, D. (1980). Classification of the necrotising vasculitides in man. *Clin. Rheum. Dis.* **6**, 223–31.

Balow, J.E. (1985). Renal vasculitis. *Kidney Int.* **27**, 954–64.

Balow, J.E. and Fauci, A.S. (1988). Vasculitis diseases of the kidney: polyarteritis nodosa, Wegener's granulomatosis, allergic angiitis and granulomatosis, and other disorders. In *Diseases of the Kidney*, 4th edn, ed. R.W. Schrier and C.W. Gottschalk, vol. II, pp. 2335–60, Little, Brown and Co., Boston/Toronto.

Bonsib, S.M. (1988). Glomerular basement membrane necrosis and crescent organisation. *Kidney Int.* **33**, 966–74.

Brasile, L., Kremer, J.M., Clarke, J.L. and Cerilli, J. (1989). Identification of an autoantibody to vascular endothelial cell-specific antigens in patients with systemic vasculitis. *Am. J. Med.* **87**, 74–80.

Brouwer, E., Cohen Tervaert, J.W., Horst, G. *et al.* (1991). Predominance of IgG1 and IgG4 subclasses of antineutrophil cytoplasmic autoantibodies (ANCA) in patients with Wegener's granulomatosis and clinically related disorders. *Clin. Exp. Immunol.* **83**, 379–86.

Chumbley, L.C., Harrison, E.G. and DeRemee, R.A. (1977). Allergic granulomatosis and angiitis (Churg–Strauss syndrome): report and analysis of 30 cases. *Mayo Clin. Proc.* **52**, 477–84.

Churg, J. and Strauss, L. (1952). Allergic granulomatosis, allergic angiitis, and periarteritis nodosa. *Am. J. Pathol.* **27**, 277–301.

Cohen, R.D., Conn, D.L. and Ilstrup, D.M. (1980). Clinical features, prognosis, and response to treatment in polyarteritis. *Mayo Clin. Proc.* **55**, 146–55.

Cohen Tervaert, J.W., van der Woude, F.J., Fauci, A.S. *et al.* (1989). Association between active Wegener's granulomatosis and anticytoplasmic antibodies. *Arch. Intern. Med.* **149**, 2461–5.

Cohen Tervaert, J.W., Goldschmeding, R., Elema, J.D. *et al.* (1990a). Association of autoantibodies to myeloperoxidase with different forms of vasculitis. *Arthritis Rheum.* **33**, 1264–72.

Cohen Tervaert, J.W., Huitema, M.G., Hene, R.J. *et al.* (1990b). Prevention of relapses in Wegener's granulomatosis by treatment based on anti-neutrophil cytoplasm antibody titre. *Lancet* **ii**, 709–11.

Colvin, R.B. and Olson, K.A. (1985). Idiotypes in autoimmune diseases. In *Concepts in Immunopathology*, ed. J.M. Cruse and R.E. Lewis, vol. I, pp. 133–72, Karger, Basle.

Croker, B.P., Lee, T. and Gunnells, J.S. (1987). Clinical and pathologic features of polyarteritis nodosa and its renal-limited variant: primary crescentic and necrotising glomerulonephritis. *Hum. Pathol.* **18**, 38–44.

Cupps, T.R. and Fauci, A.S. (1982). The vasculitic syndromes. *Adv. Intern. Med.* **27**, 315–44.

Davies, D.J., Moran, J.E., Niall, J.F. and Ryan, G.B. (1982).

Segmental necrotising glomerulonephritis with antineutrophil antibody: possible arbovirus aetiology? *Br. Med. J.* **285**, 606.

Davson, J., Ball, J. and Platt, R. (1948). The kidney in periarteritis nodosa. *Quart. J. Med.* **17**, 175–205.

Donald, K.J., Edwards, R.L. and McEvoy, J.D.S. (1976). An ultrastructural study of the pathogenesis of tissue injury in limited Wegener's granulomatosis. *Pathology* **8**, 161–9.

Droz, D., Noel, L.H., Leibowitch, M. and Barbanel, C. (1979). Glomerulonephritis and necrotizing angiitis. *Adv. Nephrol.* **8**, 343–63.

Falk, R.J. (1990). ANCA-associated renal disease. *Kidney Int.* **38**, 998–1010.

Falk, R.J. and Jennette, J. (1988). Anti-neutrophil cytoplasmic antibodies with specificity for myeloperoxidase in patients with systemic vasculitis and idiopathic necrotising and crescentic glomerulonephritis. *N. Engl. J. Med.* **318**, 1651–7.

Falk, R.J., Terrell, R.S., Charles, L.A. and Jennette, J.C. (1990). Anti-neutrophil cytoplasmic autoantibodies induce neutrophils to degranulate and produce oxygen radicals *in vitro*. *Proc. Nat. Acad. Sci. (USA)* **87**, 4115–19.

Fan, P.T., Davis, J.A., Somer, T., Kaplan, L. and Bluestone, R. (1980). A clinical approach to systemic vasculitis. *Semin. Arthritis Rheum.* **9**, 248–304.

Fauchald, R., Rygvold, O. and Oystese, B. (1972). Temporal arteritis and polymyalgia rheumatics: clinical and biopsy findings. *Ann. Intern. Med.* **77**, 845–52.

Fauci, A.S., Haynes, B.F. and Katz, P. (1978). The spectrum of vasculitis: clinical, pathologic, immunologic, and therapeutic considerations. *Ann. Intern. Med.* **89**, 660–76.

Fauci, A.S., Haynes, B.F., Katz, P. and Wolff, S.M. (1983). Wegener's granulomatosis: prospective and clinical therapeutic experience with 85 patients for 21 years. *Ann. Intern. Med.* **98**, 76–85.

Ferraro, G., Meroni, P.L., Tincani, A. *et al.* (1990). Anti-endothelial cell antibodies in patients with Wegener's granulomatosis and micropolyarteritis. *Clin. Exp. Immunol.* **79**, 47–53.

Fienberg, R. (1981). The protracted superficial phenomenon in pathergic (Wegener's) granulomatosis. *Hum. Pathol.* **12**, 458–67.

Frampton, G., Jayne, D.R.W., Perry, G.J., Lockwood, C.M. and Cameron, J.S. (1990). Autoantibodies to endothelial cells and neutrophil cytoplasmic antigens in systemic vasculitis. *Clin. Exp. Immunol.* **82**, 227–32.

Frohnert, P.P. and Sheps, S.G. (1967). Long-term follow-up study of periarteritis nodosa. *Am. J. Med.* **43**, 8–14.

Fuiano, G., Cameron, J.S., Raftery, M., Hartley, B.H., Williams, D.G. and Ogg, C.S. (1988). Improved prognosis of renal microscopic polyarteritis in recent years. *Nephrol. Dialysis Transpl.* **3**, 383–91.

Gans, R.O.B., Goldschmeding, R., Donker, A.J.M. *et al.* (1989). Neutrophil cytoplasmic autoantibodies and Wegener's granulomatosis. *Lancet* **i**, 269–70.

Gaskin, G., Savage, C.O.S., Ryan, J.J. *et al.* (1991). Anti-neutrophil cytoplasmic antibodies and disease-activity during long-term follow-up of 70 patients with systemic vasculitis. *Nephrol. Dialysis Transpl.* **6**, 689–94.

Glassock, R.J., Cohen, A.H., Adler, S. and Ward, H. (1986). Primary glomerular diseases. In *The Kidney*, 3rd edn, ed. B.M. Brenner and F.C. Rector, Jr, vol. I, pp. 940–5, W.B. Saunders Company, Philadelphia.

Goldschmeding, R., van der Schoot, C.E., ten Bokkel Huinink, D. *et al.* (1989). Wegener's granulomatosis autoantibodies identify a novel diisopropylfluorophosphate-binding protein in the lysosomes of normal human neutrophils. *J. Clin. Invest.* **84**, 1577–87.

Halma, C., Daha, M.R., Schrama, E., Hermans, J., Van Es, L.A. and van der Woude, F.J. (1990). Anti-neutrophil cytoplasmic autoantibodies and other laboratory parameters in diagnosis and follow-up of Wegener's granulomatosis. In *Proceedings of the 2nd International ANCA Workshop*, ed. F.J. van der Woude. *Neth. J. Med.* **36**.

Hancock, W.W. and Atkins, R.C. (1984). Cellular composition of crescents in human rapidly progressive glomerulonephritis identified using monoclonal antibodies. *Am. J. Nephrol.* **4**, 177–81.

Harrison, H.L., Linshaw, M.A. and Lindsley, C.B. (1980). Bolus corticosteroids and cyclophosphamide for initial treatment of Wegener's granulomatosis. *JAMA* **244**, 1599–600.

Heptinstall, R.H. (1983). *Pathology of the Kidney*, 3rd edn, vol. II. Little, Brown and Co., Boston/Toronto.

Hind, C.R.K., Paraskevakou, H., Lockwood, C.M., Evans, D.J., Peters, D.K. and Rees, A.J. (1983). Prognosis after immunosuppression of patients with crescentic nephritis requiring dialysis. *Lancet* **i**, 263–5.

Hoffman, G.S., Leavitt, R.Y., Fleisher, T.A., Minor, J.R. and Fauci, A.S. (1990). Treament of Wegener's granulomatosis with intermittent high-dose intravenous cyclophosphamide. *Am. J. Med.* **89**, 403–10.

Holmberg, D. and Coutinho, A. (1985). Natural antibodies and autoimmunity. *Immunol. Today* **6**, 356–7.

Jayne, D.R.W., Jones, S.J., Severn, A., Shaumack, S., Murphy, J. and Lockwood, C.M. (1989). Severe pulmonary haemorrhage and systemic vasculitis in association with circulating anti-neutrophil antibodies of IgM class only. *Clin. Nephrol.* **32**, 101–6.

Jayne, D.R.W., Marshall, P.D., Jones, S.J. and Lockwood, C.M. (1990). Autoantibodies to GBM and neutrophil cytoplasm in rapidly progressive glomerulonephritis. *Kidney Int.* **37**, 965–70.

Jayne, D.R.W., Davies, M.J., Fox, C.J.V., Black, C.M. and Lockwood, C.M. (1991). Treatment of systemic vasculitis with pooled intravenous immunoglobulin. *Lancet* **337**, 1137–9.

Jayne, D.R.W., Weetman, A.P. and Lockwood, C.M. (1991). The IgG subclass distribution of autoantibodies to neutrophil cytoplasmic antigens in systemic vasculitis. *Clin. Exp. Immunol.* **84**, 476–81.

Jennette, J.C., Hoidal, J.H. and Falk, R.J. (1990). Specificity of antineutrophil cytoplasmic autoantibodies for proteinase 3. *Blood* **78**, 2263–4.

Jerne, N.K. (1955). The natural selection theory of antibody formation. *Proc. Nat. Acad. Sci. (USA)* **41**, 849–57.

Kussmaul, A. and Maier, R. (1866). Ueber eine bisher beschriebene eigenthumliche Arterienerkrankung (periarteritis nodosa), die mit morbus brightii und rapid fortschreitender allgemeiner Muskellahmung einhergeht. *Dtsch Arch. Kin. Med.* **1**, 484–517.

Lai, K.N. and Lockwood, C.M. (1990). Effect of anti-neutrophil cytoplasm autoantibodies on signal transduction in human neutrophils and HL-60 cells. *Kidney Int.* **37**, 442 (abstract).

Lai, K.N., Jayne, D.R.W., Brownlee, A. and Lockwood, C.M. (1990). The specificity of anti-neutrophil cytoplasm antibodies in systemic vasculitis. *Clin. Exp. Immunol.* **82**, 233–41.

Lande, A. and Gross, A. (1972). Total aortography in the diagnosis of Takayasu's arteritis. *Am. J. Roentgenol. Rad. Ther. Nucl. Med.* **116**, 165–78.

Lesarve, P., Chen, N., Nusbaum, P., Mecarelli, L. and Noel, L.-H. (1990). Antineutrophil cytoplasm antibodies (ANCA) with antilactoferrin activity in vasculitis. *Kidney Int.* **37**, 442 (abstract).

Leung, D.Y.M., Geha, R.S. and Newburger, J.W. (1986a). Two monokines, interleukin 1 and tumour necrosis factor, render cultured vascular endothelial cells susceptible to lysis by antibodies circulating during Kawasaki syndrome. *J. Exp. Med.* **164**, 1958–72.

Leung, D.Y.M., Collins, T., Lapierre, L.A., Geha, R.S. and Pober, J.S. (1986b). Immunoglobulin M antibodies present in the acute phase of Kawasaki syndrome lyse cultured vascular endothelial cells stimulated by gamma interferon. *J. Clin. Invest.* **77**, 1428–35.

Leung, D.Y.M., Burns, J.C., Newburger, J.W. and Geha, R.S. (1987). Reversal of lymphocyte activation *in vivo* in the Kawasaki syndrome by intravenous gamma globulin. *J. Clin. Invest.* **79**, 468–72.

Lie, J.T. (1988). Classification and immunodiagnosis of vasculitis: a new solution or promises unfulfilled? *J. Rheumatol.* **15**, 728–32.

Liebow, A.A., Carrington, C.R.B. and Friedman, P.J. (1972). Lymphomatoid granulomatosis. *Hum. Pathol.* **3**, 457–558.

Lockwood, C.M., Bakes, D., Jones, S.J., Whitaker, K.B., Moss, D.W. and Savage, C.O.S. (1987). Association of alkaline phosphatase with autoantigen recognised by circulating anti-neutrophil antibodies in systemic vasculitis. *Lancet* **i**, 716–20.

Ludemann, G. and Gross, W.L. (1987). Autoantibodies against cytoplasmic structures of neutrophil granulocytes in Wegener's granulomatosis. *Clin. Exp. Immunol.* **69**, 350–7.

Ludemann, G., Utecht, B. and Gross, W.L. (1990). Antineutrophil cytoplasm antibodies in Wegener's granulomatosis recognise an elastinolytic enzyme. *J. Exp. Med.* **171**, 357–61.

McCluskey, R.T. and Fienberg, R. (1983). Vasculitis in primary vasculitides, granulomatoses, and connective tissue disease. *Hum. Pathol.* **14**, 305–15.

McHugh, N.L., James, I.E. and Plant, G.T. (1990). Anticardiolipin and antineutrophil antibodies in giant cell arteritis. *J. Rheumatol.* **17**, 916–22.

Magil, A.B. (1985). Histogenesis of glomerular crescent. *Am. J. Pathol.* **120**, 222–9.

Nakao, K., Ikeda, M. and Kimata, S. (1967). Takayasu's arteritis: clinical report of eighty-four cases and immunological studies of seven cases. *Circulation* **35**, 1141–55.

Neild, G.H., Cameron, J.S., Ogg, C.S. *et al.* (1983). Rapidly progressive glomerulonephritis with extensive glomerular crescent formation. *Quart. J. Med.* **52**, 395–416.

Niles, J.L., McCluskey, R.T., Ahmad, M.F. and Arnaout, M.A. (1989). Wegener's granulomatosis autoantigen is a novel neutrophil serine proteinase. *Blood* **74**, 1888–93.

Nolle, B., Specks, U., Ludemann, J., Rohrbach, M.S., DeRemee, R.A. and Gross, W.L. (1989). Anticytoplasmic autoantibodies: their immunodiagnostic value in Wegener's granulomatosis. *Ann. Intern. Med.* **111**, 28–40.

Novak, R.F., Christiansen, R.G. and Sorensen, E.T. (1982). The acute vasculitis of Wegener's granulomatosis in renal biopsies. *Am. J. Pathol.* **78**, 367–71.

Paronetto, F. and Strauss, L. (1962). Immunocytochemical observations in periarteritis nodosa. *Ann. Intern. Med.* **56**, 289–96.

Pinching, A.J., Rees, A.J., Pussell, B.A., Lockwood, C.M., Mitchison, R.S. and Peters, D.K. (1980). Relapses in Wegener's granulomatosis: the role of infection. *Br. Med. J.* **281**, 836–8.

Pinching, A.J., Lockwood, C.M., Pussell, B.A. *et al.* (1983). Wegener's granulomatosis: observations on 18 patients with severe renal disease. *Quart. J. Med.* **52**, 435–60.

Pusey, C.D., Rees, A.J., Evans, D.J., Peters, D.K. and Lockwood, C.M. (1991). A randomised controlled trial of plasma exchange in rapidly progressive glomerulonephritis: evidence for benefit in dialysis dependent cases. *Kidney Int.* **40**, 757–63.

Reza, M.J., Dornfield, L., Goldberg, L.S., Bluestone, R. and Rearson, C.M. (1975). Wegener's granulomatosis: long-term follow-up of patients treated with cyclophosphamide. *Arthritis Rheum.* **18**, 501–6.

Ronco, P., Verroust, P., Mignon, F. *et al.* (1983). Immunopathological studies of polyarteritis nodosa and Wegener's granulomatosis: a report of 43 patients with 51 renal biopsies. *Quart. J. Med.* **52**, 212–23.

Rossi, F., Jayne, D.R.W., Lockwood, C.M. and Kazatchkine, M.D. (1991). Anti-idiotypes against anti-neutrophil cytoplasm antigen autoantibodies in normal human polyspecific IgG for therapeutic use and in the serum of patients with systemic vasculitis in remission. *Clin. Exp. Immunol.* **83**, 298–303.

Savage, C.O.S., Winearls, C.G., Evans, D.J., Rees, A.J. and Lockwood, C.M. (1985). Microscopic polyarteritis: presentation, pathology and prognosis. *Quart. J. Med.* **56**, 467–83.

Savage, C.O.S., Winearls, C.G., Jones, S., Marshall, P.D. and Lockwood, C.M. (1987). Prospective study of radioimmunoassay for antibodies against neutrophil cytoplasm in diagnosis of systemic vasculitis. *Lancet* **i**, 1389–93.

Savage, C.O.S., Tizard, J., Jayne, D., Lockwood, C.M. and Dillon, M.J. (1989). Antineutrophil cytoplasm antibodies in Kawasaki disease. *Arch. Dis. Child.* **64**, 360–3.

Savage, C.O.S., Pottinger, B.E., Gaskin, G., Lockwood, C.M., Pusey, C.D. and Pearson, J.D. (1991). Vascular damage in Wegener's granulomatosis and microscopic polyarteritis: presence of anti-endothelial cell antibodies and their relation to anti-neutrophil cytoplasm antibodies. *Clin. Exp. Immunol.* **85**, 14–20.

Savage, C.O.S., Pottinger, B.E., Gaskin, G., Pusey, C.D. and Pearson, J.D. (submitted). Autoantibodies developing to myeloperoxidase and proteinase 3 in systemic vasculitis stimulate neutrophil cytotoxicity towards cultured endothelial cells. (Submitted.)

Serra, A., Cameron, J.S., Turner, D.R. *et al.* (1984). Vasculitis affecting the kidney: presentation, histopathology and long-term outcome. *Quart. J. Med.* **53**, 181–207.

Spencer, S.J., Burns, A., Gaskin, G., Pusey, C.D. and Rees, A.J. (1992). HLA class II specificities in vasculitis with antibodies to neutrophil cytoplasm antigens. *Kidney Int.* **41**, 1059–63.

Sultan, Y., Rossi, F. and Kazatchkine, M.D. (1987). Recovery from anti-VIII : C (antihaemophilic factor) autoimmune disease is dependent on generation of anti-idiotypes against anti-VII : C autoantibodies. *Proc. Nat. Acad. Sci. (USA)* **84**, 828–30.

Tanaka, N., Sekimoto, K. and Nace, S. (1976). Kawasaki disease: relationship with infantile periarteritis nodosa. *Arch. Pathol. Lab. Med.* **100**, 81–6.

ten Berge, I.J., Wilmink, J.M., Meyer, C.J. *et al.* (1985). Clinical and immunological follow-up of patients with severe renal disease in Wegener's granulomatosis. *Am. J. Nephrol.* **5**, 21–9.

Travers, R.L., Allison, D.J., Brettle, R.P. and Hughes, G.R.V. (1979). Polyarteritis nodosa: a clinical and angiographic analysis of 17 cases. *Semin. Arthritis Rheum.* **8**, 184–99.

Ulmer, M., Reinhold-Keller, E. and Gross, W.L. (1990). Alternative treatment strategies in Wegener's granulomatosis: first results of a prospective study. *APMIS* **98** (suppl. 19), 51.

Van der Wall Bake, A.W.L. and Lobatto, S. (1987). IgA antibodies directed against cytoplasmic antigens of polymorphonuclear leukocytes in patients with Henoch–Schönlein purpura. *Adv. Exp. Med. Biol.* **216B**, 1593–8.

Van der Woude, F.J., Rasmussen, N., Lobatto, S. *et al.* (1985). Autoantibodies against neutrophils and monocytes: tool for diagnosis and marker of disease activity in Wegener's granulomatosis. *Lancet* **i**, 425–9.

Wainwright, J. and Davson, J. (1950). The renal appearances in the microscopic form of periarteritis nodosa. *J. Pathol. Bacteriol.* **62**, 189–96.

Walton, E.W. (1958). Giant-cell granuloma of the respiratory tract (Wegener's granulomatosis). *Br. Med. J.* **2**, 265–70.

Weiss, M.A. and Crissman, J.D. (1984). Renal biopsy findings in Wegener's granulomatosis: segmental necrotising glomerulonephritis with glomerular thrombosis. *Hum. Pathol.* **15**, 943–56.

Zeek, P.M. (1953). Periarteritis nodosa and other forms of necrotising angiitis. *N. Engl. J. Med.* **248**, 764–72.

63: Myositis: Immunological Aspects of Aetiology and Pathogenesis

R.M. Bernstein

Introduction

The inflammatory myopathies are a group of diseases characterized by proximal muscle weakness and patchy or diffuse infiltration with inflammatory cells, notably lymphocytes, around blood-vessels and between muscle fibres. When a characteristic rash is present the condition is termed dermatomyositis (DM) and without the rash polymyositis (PM). The diagnosis depends on the presence of muscle weakness, raised serum levels of muscle enzymes, characteristic electromyographic changes, the histology on muscle biopsy and the rash. Not all these features are present in every case and the diagnostic criteria suggested by Bohan and Peter (1975) are shown in Table 63.1.

Table 63.1. Diagnostic criteria for myositis

Proximal muscular weakness in a relatively symmetrical distribution, usually in both upper and lower extremities
Elevated serum enzyme levels, especially creatine kinase
The electromyogram (EMG) triad of abnormalities indicating myopathic motor unit potentials together with evidence of spontaneous activity: (a) small-amplitude, short-duration polyphasic motor unit potentials (b) insertional irritability, fibrillations, positive sharp waves; and, rarely, (c) pseudomyotonic discharges
Muscle biopsy features that typically include degeneration and regenerative changes, necrosis, phagocytosis and a mononuclear interstitial or perivascular inflammatory infiltrate
In the case of DM, the presence of characteristic skin rashes, especially a heliotrope discoloration of the upper eyelids, and Gottron's sign

Several distinct syndromes are recognized, and the myositides are almost certainly heterogeneous in aetiology as well as clinical presentation. Three classifications of increasing complexity (and the last over-embracing) are shown in Table 63.2 (Walton and Adams 1958; Bohan and Peter 1975; Dalakas 1988). In the subgroup of myositis with a connective tissue disease, correlation of various autoantibodies with clinical features suggests that there are yet more syndromes or subsets (reviewed by Bernstein and Mathews 1985). Pyogenic or tropical myositis is being reported increasingly from Europe and America, often in association with acquired immunodeficiency syndrome (AIDS) (Gaut *et al.* 1988). Retroviruses, enteroviruses, mumps virus and protozoa have been variously implicated in the cause of idiopathic myositis, and lymphocytes in the pathogenesis.

The clinical features of the myositides can be found in standard texts and recent reviews (Dalakas 1988; Strongwater 1988; Plotz *et al.* 1989). This chapter concentrates on the immunological aspects of aetiology, pathogenesis, syndrome recognition and treatment.

Table 63.2. Classification and types of myositis

Walton and Adams 1958
1 Polymyositis (PM)
2 PM with mild connective tissue disease or dermatomyositis (DM) rash
3 PM with severe connective tissue disease or DM
4 PM or DM with malignancy

Bohan and Peter 1975
Group:
I Polymyositis (PM)
II Dermatomyositis (DM)
III PM/DM with malignancy
IV Childhood PM/DM
V Myositis/connective tissue disease overlap syndromes

Dalakas 1988
Type:
1 Adult PM
2 Adult DM
3 Childhood PM
4 Childhood DM
5 PM/DM with connective tissue disease
6 PM/DM with malignancy
7 PM with monoclonal gammopathy
8 PM with AIDS
9 Focal inflammatory myopathy
10 Eosinophilic PM/DM in eosinophilic fasciitis [and eosinophilia-myalgia syndrome]
11 Putative PM/DM
12 PM/DM with other systemic illnesses
13 PM/DM induced by drugs
14 Facioscapulohumeral dystrophy simulating PM
15 Inclusion-body myositis
16 Benign acute myositis of childhood
17 Benign acute (postviral) myositis in adults
18 Postviral fatigue syndrome simulating PM
19 PM with agammaglobulinaemia
20 Fungal and mycobacterial myositis
21 Parasitic myositis
22 Tropical myositis

(1–12 amenable to steroid therapy)

Historical review

The first cases of non-infectious myositis were described by Wagner (1863), Potain (1875), Hepp (1887) and Unverricht (1887), and in a child by Batten (1912). Skin involvement was mentioned in some of these early cases, and Unverricht (1891) introduced the term 'dermatomyositis'. Oppenheim (1899) described not only cardiac involvement but also progression to scleroderma. Steiner (1903) found 28 cases in the literature, and by 1939 there were 239 cases reported (Schuermann 1951). Although DM was recognized quite readily, PM was often misdiagnosed as muscular dystrophy until Levison (1937) emphasized the round-cell infiltration in PM. Classification of myositis was attempted by Walton and Adams (1958), Bohan and Peter (1975) and Dalakas (1988). Two entities in particular were shown to be distinct from adult PM and DM: childhood DM (Banker and Victor 1966) and inclusion-body myositis (Carpenter *et al*. 1978). Pearson (1956) introduced the first animal model with experimental allergic myositis in rats, and Currie *et al*. (1971) began the study of cellular immune events in human disease. Studies of humoral autoimmunity followed, with certain aminoacyl-transfer ribonucleic acid (tRNA) synthetases the most frequent targets of myositis-specific autoantibodies (Mathews and Bernstein 1983). There are two new models of myositis induced by viruses: by a Coxsackie virus in newborn mice (Ray *et al*. 1979) and by a retrovirus in monkeys (Dalakas *et al*. 1986a). Corticosteroid therapy was introduced in the 1950s (Pearson 1962), cytotoxic agents in the 1960s, total body irradiation (Engel *et al*. 1981) and cyclosporin in the 1980s, and intravenous immunoglobulin in the 1990s.

Humoral autoimmunity

Overview

Autoantibodies recognizing intracellular antigens are found commonly in adult PM and, perhaps to a lesser extent, in DM. There are several antibody specificities, none found in more than 30% of cases. Reichlin and Arnett (1984) found antibodies by immunodiffusion against a cell extract in 55% of cases, by immunofluorescence antibodies on HEp-2 cell monolayers in 78%, and by either technique in 89%. Our own findings in a large survey of systemic rheumatic and hepatic disease were similar (Bernstein *et al*. 1984a). Both studies were rheumatology-based, so biased towards patients with myositis/connective tissue disease overlap syndromes, but they do show how autoantibodies help delineate various myositis syndromes or subsets. Several of the relevant cellular antigens are enzymes involved in tRNA charging and other aspects of protein synthesis.

Muscle antigens

Antibodies to myosin and myoglobin have been reported in myositis (Nishikai and Homma 1977; Wada *et al*. 1983; Koga *et al*. 1987), and yet antibodies to actin and 'striated muscle' are uncommon (Garlepp and Dawkins 1984). Whether this area deserves to be explored further is in doubt because antibodies to actin and myosin occur quite frequently in healthy individuals (Bijlsma *et al*. 1990).

Intracellular antigens and overlapping syndromes

Studies of serum by immunodiffusion or counter-immunoelectrophoresis against soluble tissue extracts have demonstrated the precipitating autoantibodies shown in Tables 63.3 and 63.4. The nomenclature is arcane but based on the names of patients (e.g. Jo-1, one of two precipitins in the serum of a patient called John), antigen property (RNP, ribonucleoprotein) and laboratory code (PL, precipitin line). The first report of a myositis-specific antibody, PM_1 (Wolfe *et al*. 1977), turned out to be several antibodies. The reference PM_1 is an uncommon antibody and was renamed PM-Scl because of an association with PM/scleroderma overlap syndrome (Reichlin *et al*. 1984). The second precipitin to be described in myositis, Jo-1, was found in 25–30% of cases (Nishikai and Reichlin 1980; Bernstein *et al*. 1984a; Reichlin and Arnett 1984). Anti-Jo-1 antibody is associated with other features of a connective tissue disease overlap syndrome: interstitial lung disease, Raynaud's phenomenon, arthralgias or arthritis, sicca syndrome, sometimes sclerodactyly, and occasionally glomerulonephritis, central nervous system involvement or other aspects of systemic lupus erythematosus (SLE) (Yoshida *et al*. 1983; Bernstein *et al*. 1984b). Either myositis or interstitial lung disease is seen in virtually all cases and both

Table 63.3. Antibody disease associations in the connective tissue diseases

	SLE	MCTD	Primary Sjögren's syndrome	Myositis	PSS	RA	PBC	CAH	Other
Ro	24	17	75	8	4	3	6	4	<1
La	9	3	42	1	1	—	1	—	—
Sm	4–30[a]	3	—	—	—	—	—	—	—
RNP	23	100	4	14	3	—	—	—	—
Jo-1	<1	3	—	25	1	—	—	—	—
PL-7	—	—	—	5	—	—	—	—	—
PL-12	—	—	—	3	—	—	—	—	—
PM-Scl	—	—	—	11	3	—	—	—	—
Ku	6	—	—	3	—	—	—	—	—
Scl-70	—	—	—	—	20	—	—	—	—
Centromere[b]	2	—	—	—	29	—	8	—	<1
Multiple Nuclear dots[b]	2	—	2	—	—	—	13	—	—
XR	—	—	—	—	—	—	10	24	—
SL	6	3	2	—	—	3	1	—	—
Ribosomal	3	—	2	—	1	—	—	—	—
PCNA	3	—	—	—	—	—	—	—	—
PL-4	2	—	—	—	—	—	—	—	—

a Sm in 4% of white patients and 30% of black and Chinese, 7% overall.
b Detected by immunofluorescence.
SLE = systemic lupus erythematosus; MCTD = mixed connective tissue disease; PSS = progressive systemic sclerosis; RA = rheumatoid arthritis; PBC = primary biliary cirrhosis; CAH = chronic active hepatitis. Adapted from Bernstein *et al.* (1984a).

Table 63.4. National variations in antibody frequency in myositis

Specificity	USA (%)	UK (%)	Japan (%)
Jo-1	18–25	25	21
RNP	13	14	17
Ro	7	8	19
PM-Scl	8	11	4
Ku	?	~2	14

Adapted from Mimori *et al.* 1981; Yoshida *et al.* 1983; Bernstein *et al.* 1984a; Reichlin and Arnett 1984.

together in nearly 80%. These features amount to a distinct 'Jo-1 syndrome', differing from mixed connective tissue disease (MCTD) in that myositis, lung involvement and sometimes arthralgia predominate, rather than the Raynaud's phenomenon and swollen fingers of MCTD. Two further specificities, PL-7 and PL-12, are uncommon but associated with the same clinical picture as Jo-1 antibody (Bernstein *et al.* 1984a; Marguerie *et al.* 1990), and it is striking that all three autoantibodies are directed at antigens with similar functions, the aminoacyl-tRNA synthetases for histidine, threonine and alanine (Mathews and Bernstein 1985). Targoff (1990) has, in addition, found rare examples of antibodies directed at the aminoacyl-tRNA synthetases for glycine and isoleucine. Myositis and lung disease are also sometimes associated in MCTD and in cases of PM/scleroderma overlap. In one series of myositis/pneumonitis overlap anti-Jo-1 was uncommon (Takizawa *et al.* 1987), but this differs from most series (Bernstein and Mathews 1984). Enzyme-linked immunosorbent assays (ELISA) show that anti-Jo-1 antibody is not often missed by the precipitin tests, that it is mostly of immunoglobulin G (IgG)-1 subclass, and that the level fluctuates with disease activity and may disappear during remission (Biswas *et al.* 1987; Targoff and Reichlin 1987; Miller *et al.* 1990).

PM-Scl and Ku antibodies are associated with PM/scleroderma overlap syndrome. Few patients with anti-PM-Scl have been described in detail, but their illness seems to begin with PM, going on gradually to scleroderma of the hands and face (acrosclerosis), calcinosis and pulmonary fibrosis, by which time the myositis may have disappeared. The frequency of antibody to PM-Scl in myositis is 8–12% (Bernstein *et al.* 1984a; Reichlin *et al.* 1984), but in Japanese patients another specificity, anti-Ku, is associated with scleroderma/myositis overlap (Mimori *et al.* 1981; Mimori 1987). The British experience with anti-Ku is different: of six cases seen by the author, two West Indians had a myositis overlap syndrome, but four English cases had SLE without myositis. By immunoblotting using purified Ku antigen, anti-Ku has been detected in 14–19% of patients with several connective tissue diseases (Yaneva and Arnett 1989).

Anti-RNP antibody is found with a frequency of 13–17% in myositis (Yoshida *et al.* 1983; Bernstein *et al.* 1984a; Reichlin *et al.* 1984), and in SLE muscle involvement is commoner in patients with this antibody. In MCTD (defined by high-titre RNP antibody, Raynaud's phenomenon, swollen fingers and so on), clinical or histological evidence of myositis has been reported in up to 50% of cases (Oxenhandler *et al.* 1977), but, with wider appreciation of mild and limited forms of the syndrome, the frequency of clinically significant myositis is probably much lower. Myositis may be associated with antibody to the 68 kD component rather than to the 'A' protein of the U1-(RNP) particle (Takeda *et al.* 1988).

Anti-Mi-2 is directed against an antigen in calf thymus extract. By ELISA it is found in 8% of PM/DM overall, but in pure DM the frequency is nearly 20% (Targoff and Reichlin 1985). The Mi-1 specificity, found quite commonly in myositis by a complement fixation test, was not disease-specific (Reichlin and Mattioli 1976; Targoff *et al.* 1983).

Another antibody said to be both specific and sensitive for myositis has been reported recently (Arad-Dann *et al.* 1987, 1989). The antigen is a 56 000 molecular-weight protein present in simian virus (SV)-40-transformed Syrian hamster cells. Antibody was detected by immunoblotting in 85% of 52 patients with myositis and yet was uncommon in other connective tissue disease control groups. The intensity of the protein band on immunoblots seems to vary with disease activity, disappearing during remission. Immunoblots also revealed a band of 68 000 in many cases (Arad-Dann *et al.* 1987). The 56 000 M_r antigen is said to be nuclear and part of the heterogeneous nuclear RNA processing particle, but there are no reports using other cells or tissues. It may or may not be a coincidence that the cytoplasmic signal recognition complex, involved in processing and exporting polypeptides, possesses subunits of 54 000 and 68 000 which are the target of antibodies in 4% of myositis (Kole *et al.* 1985; Reeves *et al.* 1986; Okada *et al.* 1987; Targoff *et al.* 1990).

Anti-Ro antibody is found only infrequently (about 5%) in most series of myositis, but Behan *et al.* (1987a) reported anti-Ro in 60% of cases and more often in cases with cardiac involvement; an exchange of sera is required to clarify this point.

Several of the cellular antigens related to myositis are thought to be cytoplasmic. Immunofluorescence studies of myositis sera on HEp-2 cells show cytoplasmic staining quite frequently, the pattern suggesting cytoskeletal or mitochondrial staining in different cases (Reichlin and Arnett 1984; Senecal *et al.* 1985; Gupta *et al.* 1986; Saito *et al.* 1989a). Anti-Jo-1 antibody does not stain tissues by indirect immunofluorescence but does appear to with the immunogold technique (Thiry *et al.* 1988).

Molecular characterization of myositis-related cellular antigens

In the 1970s the cellular antigens were studied by fractionation of cell extracts and susceptibility to digestion by proteases and nucleases. The results were crude and often misleading. The technique of protein A-facilitated immunoprecipitation from radiolabelled cell extracts, introduced by Lerner and Steitz (1979), led to the recognition that several antigens are complexes containing ribonucleic acids. With improved protein labelling, the polypeptide antigens themselves were demonstrated, often as parts of macromolecular complexes (Matter *et al.* 1982; Bernstein *et al.* 1984a). The Western immunoblotting technique confirmed which proteins within a complex were antigenic (Habets *et al.* 1985). Various clues then led to the precise, functional identification of several antigens (Table 63.5). In most cases these functions can be inhibited by the relevant antibody *in vitro*. The Scl-70 antigen was identified as topoisomerase I through there being two molecular-weight forms of each and by the immunofluorescence pattern (Shero *et al.* 1986). The earlier work on the function of U1(RNP) and Jo-1 antigens was based on the immunoprecipitation of an RNA–protein complex: sequencing the RNA gave a clue to the

Table 63.5. Intracellular antigens in the life of the cell

Antigen	Identity	Function
DNA	'The medium'	'The message'
Histones	Structural proteins	Packaging of DNA
Scl-70	Topoisomerase I	DNA supercoiling
PCNA	35 000 protein	Auxiliary factor for polymerase δ
Ku	60 000, 80 000 proteins	DNA binding
Nucleolar speckled	RNA polymerase I	Transcription of rRNA
RNP	(U1) ribonucleoprotein particle 68 000, A, C proteins)	RNA processing
Sm	Several (U) ribonucleoprotein particles (B/B′, D proteins)	RNA processing
Jo-1, Pl-7, PL-12	Aminoacyl-tRNA synthetases (his, thr, ala)	Protein synthesis
Ribosomal RNP	Ribosomal P proteins and rRNA	Protein synthesis
La	46 000 protein	Termination of RNA polymerase III transcription
Ro	52 000, 54 000, 60 000 proteins	RNA transport or translation control?
56KD	Component of hnRNP	RNA processing
54KD, 68KD	Signal-recognition particle	Transport of proteins into endoplasmic reticulum
PM-Scl	Nucleolar complex	Ribosomal RNA synthesis

Myositis-specific antibodies: Jo-1, PL-7, PL-12, PM-Scl, Ku, 56kD. Antibodies less closely associated with myositis: RNP (MCTD), Ro, La (Sjögren's syndrome).

cellular function of the protein. Thus, complementarity between U1–RNA and the consensus sequence at splice junctions pointed to the involvement of the U1(RNP) particle in RNA processing (Yang *et al.* 1981). In the case of Jo-1 antibody, Rosa *et al.* (1983) immunoprecipitated and sequenced the tRNA for histidine, but the pure RNA was not recognized by antibody. Mathews and Bernstein (1983) demonstrated that the antigen was a 64 000 molecular-weight polypeptide complexed with $tRNA^{his}$ and showed this to represent the enzyme histidyl-tRNA synthetase responsible for charging $tRNA^{his}$ with histidine. Using a cell extract to charge tRNA with each amino acid in turn, only the reaction of tRNA with histidine was inhibited by the presence of anti-Jo-1 or prior depletion of Jo-1 antigen. In like manner, the PL-7 and PL-12 antibodies inhibited the charging of threonine and alanine respectively. PL-12 sera differ from Jo-1 and PL-7 in containing not one but two populations of antibodies, one recognizing the enzyme (only when free of tRNA) and the other recognizing the anticodon loop of free $tRNA^{ala}$ (Bunn *et al.* 1986; Bunn and Mathews 1987). These two PL-12 antibodies may block the sites through which the enzyme and $tRNA^{ala}$ interact, in which case one autoantibody could be an anti-idiotype of the other (Bernstein and Mathews 1985, 1987; Bunn *et al.* 1986). With Jo-1 antigen the antibody does not compete with tRNA for binding (Fahoun and Young 1987), so anti-idiotypes cannot be detected in the same way. The mammalian complementary deoxyribonucleic acid (cDNA) and gene for histidyl-tRNA synthetase have been cloned (Tsui and Siminovitch 1987), but there have since been revisions to the published sequence. Epitope analysis of Jo-1 antigen by the production of a series of mutant proteins shows that autoantibodies bind to multiple sites, some of which are conformation-dependent and others not (Ramsden *et al.* 1989). Cruder analysis of Jo-1 by proteolytic cleavage indicates at least six common epitopes (Miller *et al.* 1990b).

Further tRNA-associated antigens have been studied, although not in such detail. Targoff (1988) has found individual sera inhibiting the aminoacyl-tRNA synthetases for glycine (one case) and isoleucine (two cases) and has confirmed our suggestion that another serum (Fer) recognizes elongation factor 1α (Targoff and Hanas 1989). Another antibody, anti-KJ, inhibits protein translation efficiently but not through binding to a tRNA-related protein (Targoff *et al.* 1989). An antibody named Mas reacts directly with a naked

RNA slightly larger in size than tRNA (Bernstein *et al.* 1984a; Mathews *et al.* 1985; this may be the small RNA involved in the initiation of translation. Of the other antigens, PM-Scl is a nucleolar protein complex. The Ku antigen consists of two proteins of 70 000 and 80 000 molecular weight, either or both of which are bound by separate populations of anti-Ku antibodies; the Ku proteins bind to free ends of double-stranded DNA and may have a role in DNA repair (Mimori *et al.* 1986; Mimori 1987). Antibody to the 90 kD heat-shock protein (HSP-90) has been reported in SLE and in two out of six cases of myositis (Minota *et al.* 1988; reviewed by Bernstein 1989).

General conclusions about autoantibodies to cells

Several generalizations can be drawn from the study of autoantibodies in myositis, SLE and systemic sclerosis. Autoantibodies are few in number, relatively specific for certain diseases and disease subsets, and reactive with important components of the cellular machinery for replication, transcription, processing and translation of nucleic acid and protein. In myositis the focus is mainly on the pathway from RNA processing to protein synthesis and secretion, perhaps reflecting the prominence of the cytoplasm in muscle. Autoantibodies regularly inhibit the function of their antigens, unlike most experimental antibodies: a rabbit antibody raised to threonyl-tRNA synthetase does not inhibit charging, whereas the PL-7 autoantibody does (Mathews *et al.* 1984). As well as antibody–disease associations, several autoantibodies are frequently associated together in patients' serum. These autoantibody associations are mirrored by structural associations between the relevant antigens within the cell, notably native and Z-DNA, Ro and La, Sm and RNP, the various histones, the two Ku proteins, ribosomal P proteins and ribosomal RNA, and alanyl-tRNA synthetase and $tRNA^{ala}$ (Bernstein *et al.* 1984a; Hardin 1986; Targoff and Reichlin 1988). By contrast, antibodies to Jo-1, PL-7, PL-12 and PM-Scl do not occur together in the same serum.

Autoantibodies in pathogenesis and as clues to aetiology

The pathogenesis of muscle inflammation and destruction in myositis is quite probably mediated by T lymphocytes. There is little evidence of antibody-dependent cell-mediated cytotoxicity (Behan and Behan 1985) and no report of antibody damaging the sarcolemma directly. Only anti-U1(RNP) antibody has been found within muscle cells and lymphocytes by direct immunofluorescence (Alarcon-Segovia *et al.* 1979), but autoantibodies may find their 'intracellular' antigen expressed on the cell surface. Adenovirus infection stimulates the expression of La antigen on the surface of tissue culture cells (Baboonian *et al.* 1989), and other nuclear antigens move to the surface in response to ultraviolet irradiation (LeFeber *et al.* 1984). Deoxyribonucleic acid and histones are expressed on the surface of some lymphocytes (Rekvig and Hannestad 1980).

Complement activation and immunoglobulin deposition are not prominent features in muscle biopsies of myositis (Isenberg 1983), but immunoglobulin and complement are deposited in small blood-vessels in childhood myositis (Whitaker and Engel 1972), and in adult and childhood DM the complement membrane attack complex (MAC) is deposited in the microvasculature of muscle (Kissel *et al.* 1986; Sewry *et al.* 1987). In childhood DM serum levels of C3 breakdown products may be raised (Scott and Arroyave 1987). It seems possible, therefore, that autoantibodies are involved in vascular phenomena, such as Raynaud's phenomenon in the Jo-1 syndrome, but it is then paradoxical that the known autoantibodies are less evident in childhood DM, where vasculitis is sometimes severe. Antibodies to endothelial cells occurs mainly in dermatomyositis associated with pulmonary fibrosis (Cervera *et al.* 1991).

How are antibody–disease associations to be explained? Given the paucity of evidence for antibodies mediating particular patterns of disease, it is attractive to think of them as clues to aetiology. For instance, a virus damaging muscle may generate a specific autoantibody response. Autoimmunity might arise via molecular mimicry (Query and Keene 1987), via a complex of virus and host cell components overcoming immunological tolerance (Mathews and Bernstein 1983), or through an anti-idiotype response to antiviral antibody mimicking a viral ligand for the cell (Plotz 1983). Evidence can be adduced for all three hypotheses. For molecular mimicry there are neighbouring amino acid sequences on the P30 group antigen of murine leukaemia virus, one homologous and cross-reacting with an epitope on the 70 kD U1-RNP antigen, the other homologous with an epitope of the Scl-70 antigen (Query and Keene 1987; Maul *et al.* 1989); further homologies have been suggested such as between Jo-1 (histidyl-tRNA synthetase) and encephalomyocarditis virus (Walker and Jeffrey 1988). For loss of tolerance through virus–host interaction, there are the interactions of adenovirus and Epstein–Barr virus small RNAs with the La antigen and of encephalomyocarditis virus RNA with Jo-1 (reviewed in Mathews and Bernstein 1983). For the anti-idiotype hypothesis, there are several observations, including the anti-I cold agglutinin response to *Mycoplasma* infection and the dual PL-12 specificities mentioned above (Bunn *et al.* 1986; Bunn and Mathews 1987).

The evidence is circumstantial, and there are difficulties with all three hypotheses. In the case of molecular mimicry, epitopes showing homology with a viral sequence are by no means always the dominant target for autoantibodies, which may recognize several epitopes (although this might be because mimicry just starts the ball rolling). In the case of virus–host interaction, it stretches credulity to implicate five different viruses responsible for the same syndrome but with autoantibodies induced to five different aminoacyl-tRNA synthetases. The anti-idiotype hypothesis seems contrived when it comes to intracellular antigens (Bernstein and Mathews 1984).

That autoantibodies are antigen-driven is suggested by the correlation of antibody level with disease activity, the polyclonality of autoantibodies demonstrated by spectrotype analysis (Miller *et al.* 1990) and the plurality of antigenic sites on a protein such as Jo-1 or Scl-70 and within a macromolecular complex such as the U1-RNP particle.

Cellular immune mechanisms in polymyositis and dermatomyositis

Overview

The idiopathic myositides are almost certainly a heterogeneous group of diseases. The prominent anticellular autoantibodies, such as Jo-1 referred to above, are very much linked to myositis in the context of the connective tissue diseases rather than as a purely organ-specific autoimmune disease. Studies of cellular immunity emphasize an organ-specific attack on muscle and sometimes skin. As reviewed by Ytterberg (1988), the evidence relates to alterations of lymphocyte numbers *in vivo* and function *in vitro*, distribution of mononuclear cells and membrane markers in muscle biopsies, reactivity of lymphocytes towards muscle antigens, damage to muscle by lymphocytes *in vitro*, and inhibition of muscle function by mononuclear cell products. In these studies, adult and childhood diseases are usually distinguished, and some assessment of disease activity is given, but it is often unclear whether the patients had pure PM, DM or an overlap syndrome.

Peripheral blood lymphocyte subsets and interleukins

The total lymphocyte count is usually normal in PM and DM. Iyer *et al.* (1983) found normal helper and suppressor/cytotoxic T cell numbers in seven cases, but Behan and Behan (1984, 1985) found low suppressor/cytotoxic CD8 +ve cells in five of nine patients with acute myositis and four of 14 with chronic active disease. Miller *et al.* (1990a) confirmed reduced CD8 +ve cells and found increased expression of T cell activation markers such as HLA-DR, IL-2 receptors and the late marker of cytotoxic differentiation, TLiSA1. It is more difficult to interpret modest changes in assays of overall function. For example, the autologous mixed lymphocyte reaction was suppressed compared with controls in a study of nine patients with myositis, while suppressor T cell activity induced by concanavalin A was normal (Ransohoff and Dustoor 1983). Natural killer (NK) cell activity (non-T, non-B large lymphocytes killing tumour cells independent of antibody and human leucocyte antigen (HLA) *in vitro*) was found to be suppressed in small studies of childhood and adult myositis (Miller *et al.* 1983; Behan and Behan 1984; Gonzalez-Amaro *et al.* 1987). Natural killer cells may be important in tumour surveillance, so these findings could be relevant to the increased incidence of malignancy in myositis.

Interleukins IL-1α, IL-2 and soluble IL-2 receptor (IL-2R) were studied by Wolf and Baethge (1990). Serum IL-1α was elevated in early active disease, declining rapidly with therapy; this indicates monocyte activation in myositis. Interleukin 2 was generally not detected, but soluble (and cellular) IL-2R was elevated in early active myositis, but not in inactive or late chronic disease. Serum

IL-2R correlated with weakness and the serum creatine kinase level. There are as yet no studies of cellular adhesion molecules in myositis.

Histopathology and cell membrane markers

The basis for considering the cellular immune mechanism in PM and DM is the obvious presence of cellular infiltrates, especially mononuclear cells, around small blood-vessels and surrounding and invading muscle fibres (reviewed by Bertorini 1988). The muscle fibres themselves may be necrotic, degenerate or regenerating in a patchy distribution; in DM there is also perifascicular muscle fibre atrophy. Degenerating fibres stain darkly, regenerating fibres are small with large central nuclei, and necrotic fibres may be invaded by phagocytic cells, predominantly macrophages. Chou (1968) first described myxovirus-like structures on electron microscopy in a case of chronic myositis, and Carpenter *et al.* (1978) described by light microscopy the characteristic rimmed vacuoles in frozen (but not paraffin-embedded) tissue sections and emphasized that inclusions are restricted to a distinct, relatively uncommon entity which they termed inclusion-body myositis.

The infiltrates around small blood-vessels and between living muscle fibres contain mainly lymphocytes. Muscle fibre damage (and possibly dysfunction in excess of histological change) may result from the cytotoxic effects of these lymphocytes or from small blood-vessel occlusion and ischaemia. In juvenile DM vascular damage including endothelial hyperplasia is seen in muscle, bowel and skin, and perifascicular atrophy in DM has been attributed to ischaemia.

Several studies have characterized the cellular infiltrates in muscle by using monoclonal antibodies to markers for macrophages, lymphocyte subsets, HLA Class I and II major histocompatibility complex (MHC) antigens, and immunoglobulin and complement. Rowe *et al.* (1981, 1983) showed heavy infiltrates of T lymphocytes, mostly of the helper/inducer phenotype, with fewer T cells seen in treated patients than in active myositis. Giornio *et al.* (1984) and Lemoine *et al.* (1986) confirmed that T lymphocytes predominate over B cells and are mostly of the CD4 +ve helper/inducer phenotype. They found no differences between infiltrates around blood-vessels and muscle fibres, and no differences between the myositis of PM, DM and connective tissue disease. A series of sophisticated studies using double-immunofluorescence staining and cell counting have shown some differences according to the site of infiltrate and the diagnosis (Arahata and Engel 1984, 1986, 1988; Engel and Arahata 1984; Ringel *et al.* 1986, 1987). In all biopsies Arahata and Engel found exudates of T cells, B cells and macrophages, while NK cells were rare. T lymphocytes were most frequent in perivascular infiltrates (40% of cells in DM and 16% in PM), while within endomysial and perimysial infiltrates T cells were fewer but still commoner in DM than PM (11–15% versus 1–5%). The ratio of CD4 to CD8 T lymphocytes was 1.1 to 1.7 at perivascular and perimysial sites in DM and PM but only 0.5 at endomysial (interstitial) sites in DM and 0.2 in PM. Thus there are more helper T cells around blood-vessels and more cytotoxic T cells among the muscle fibres. Endomysial helper T cells were associated closely with macrophages. About 20% of perivascular T cells bore activation markers in both PM and DM, with less frequent T cell activation at perimysial sites and more (22% in DM, 37% in PM) within endomysial infiltrates. There were relatively more B cells in the infiltrates of DM than of PM. Usually the T cells bear alpha/beta receptors, but in one case myriad cells bore gamma/delta receptors and muscle fibres expressed the 65 kD heat-shock protein (Hohlfeld *et al.* 1991).

Rowe *et al.* (1983) and Appleyard *et al.* (1985) found expression of Class I MHC antigens on muscle fibres in the inflammatory myopathies and Duchenne muscular dystrophy, and Isenberg *et al.* (1986) demonstrated interferons α, β and γ at the same sites as Class I MHC antigen expression. However, Emslie-Smith *et al.* (1989) found little interferon and rather few CD8 +ve lymphocytes at sites of copious Class I MHC antigen expression on muscle. Although Rowe *et al.* (1983) found Class I MHC HLA antigens on the membranes of damaged fibres, Class II MHC (HLA-DR) antigens were not present on muscle fibres but found around macrophages and on most T lymphocytes (indicating that these are activated). However, Zuk and Fletcher (1988) and Kalovidouris *et al.* (1991) did find evidence of Class II MHC antigen expression on myocytes in myositis, but not in muscular dystrophy or normal biopsies.

Class I MHC antigen expression on damaged fibres is consistent with attack by cytotoxic T cells, an attack presumably maintained by helper T cells. The observation of Class II MHC antigens on myocytes in myositis is of importance, because helper T cells recognize antigen presented by Class II MHC HLA-DR molecules. Class II MHC (HLA-DR) antigens are found on the surface of thyroid cells in autoimmune thyroid disease and on bile ducts in primary biliary cirrhosis, and Bottazzo *et al.* (1983) have suggested that this abnormal expression is of prime importance to the genesis of autoimmunity.

Whether aberrant Class II MHC antigen expression is a response to virus infection or to interferon-γ production, it could account for the induction of autoimmunity to neighbouring surface antigens. In myositis, helper/inducer T cells do accumulate, and we need to know whether it is HLA-DR expressed on muscle fibres, macrophages or endothelial cells that maintains the immune process. Such HLA-DR expression might be maintained by local interferon production, perhaps reflecting a virus harboured in one of these cell types.

Damage to muscle by lymphocytes *in vitro*

Several attempts have been made to demonstrate that peripheral blood lymphocytes from patients with myositis can kill muscle cells or inhibit contractility. As will be seen, the results are contradictory and there is room to question the substrates and controls. In two studies (Currie *et al.* 1971; Esiri *et al.* 1973), peripheral blood mononuclear cells proliferated in response to allogeneic muscle in 50% of cases of PM, the effect being greater during active disease. However, similar responses were seen occasionally in muscular dystrophy and polymyalgia rheumatica, and Lisak and Zweiman (1975) found no abnormality in myositis. A recent report supports the original finding: peripheral blood mononuclear cells from myositis, but not from other myopathies or SLE without myositis, show a proliferative response to homogenates of homologous and autologous muscle (Kalovidouris *et al.* 1989). In studies of leucocyte migration inhibition, lymphocytes from PM/DM responded both to crude muscle homogenates and purified myoglobin (Goust *et al.* 1974; Herrera-Esparza *et al.* 1983). In an early study of muscle damage, Johnson *et al.* (1972) incubated peripheral blood mononuclear cells with autologous muscle, and the dialysed culture supernatants were cytotoxic to human fetal muscle in 10 of 11 cases of PM (the eleventh patient being in remission on treatment); in two cases muscle biopsies containing large cellular infiltrates produced a soluble myotoxic factor without addition of peripheral blood lymphocytes.

There have been several studies of direct cytotoxicity by peripheral blood lymphocytes against muscle cells in culture. While the earlier studies appear to demonstrate cytotoxicity, two out of three more recent studies have failed to do so, including one group (Haas and Arnason 1974; Haas 1980) who were unable to confirm their earlier findings. Currie *et al.* (1971) cultured muscle explants from human and rat fetuses, assessing cell death by microscopic examination. Of 76 muscle cultures 83% were killed by mononuclear cells from 18 patients with PM, compared with 13% of 60 cultures by mononuclear cells from 15 control neurological patients. Preincubation of mononuclear cells with antilymphocyte serum inhibited the cytotoxic effect. Interestingly, myositis serum alone was cytotoxic in 19% of 36 cultures, but it is not known whether this related to the presence of autoantibodies. In a subsequent study (Dawkins and Mastaglia 1973) the cytotoxity of peripheral blood mononuclear cells was measured by ^{51}Cr released from chicken embryo muscle cells after 18 hours co-culture. Mononuclear cells from five of nine patients with active myositis were cytotoxic compared with none of four with inactive disease; serum plus complement from each of these 13 patients had no such cytotoxic effect.

Because ^{51}Cr can be taken up by fibroblasts in the myoblast cultures, more recent studies looked at the release of muscle-specific proteins. The release of creatine phosphokinase (CPK) from rat embryo muscle cultures was greater after coculture with mononuclear cells from 15 cases of myositis than with 15 controls, but in this study there was no difference between active and inactive myositis; serum alone had no effect, and these authors found no visual evidence of muscle cell killing (Haas and Arnason 1974). In a more recent study, Haas (1980) found no evidence of killing of fetal rat muscle cultures by CPK release, ^{51}Cr release or visual inspection. Cambridge and Stern (1981) were able to show killing of human fetal muscle cultures labelled with ^{3}H-carnitine, a protein taken up preferentially by muscle. After 18 hours' co-culture, mononuclear cells from nine patients with active myositis showed greater carnitine release than seven controls, and cell death was obvious on visual inspection. In childhood myositis, a study using human fetal muscle cultures showed no effect on the uptake of radio-labelled amino acids after 72 hours' co-culture with peripheral blood monocytes or lymphocytes (Iannaccone *et al.* 1982). Mononuclear cells from the blood of patients with DM can also damage human skin fibroblasts in culture (Saito *et al.* 1987, 1989b).

These are conflicting results and ultimately uninterpretable. The fetal muscle cultures employed were non-self and often non-human, ignoring both MHC restriction and surface antigens specific to fully differentiated muscle. Moreover, the abnormalities in myositis are patchy (Comola *et al.* 1987; Howel 1988), suggesting focal expression of an inciting agent or pathogenetic antigen which could well be absent from normal muscle, let alone absent from fetal muscle cultures. Peripheral blood may be deficient in the very cells attracted to muscle (Behan *et al.* 1987b). Only in two patients (Johnson *et al.* 1972) were the mononuclear cells under study already bound to muscle; in all other cases peripheral blood mononuclear cells were studied, and rarely were non-muscle targets employed as controls. Cambridge has suggested that the phenomena observed *in vitro* were mediated by NK cells, but NK cells are not prominent in blood or muscle biopsies in myositis (Arahata and Engel 1988). Recently, myocytotoxic T cell lines have been derived from inflamed muscle (Rosenschein *et al.* 1987), and these may prove a more fruitful approach to pathogenesis (Hohlfeld and Engel 1991).

Impairment of muscle contraction

Muscle weakness is sometimes out of proportion to the amount of muscle damage seen on biopsy, and the effect of peripheral blood mononuclear cells on muscle contractility has been investigated (Kalovidouris and Johnson 1980; Kalovidouris and Meiss 1984; Kalovidouris 1986). In the first study, supernatants from mitogen-stimulated normal mononuclear cells inhibited adenosine triphosphate (ATP)-dependent calcium accumulation in rat sarcoplasmic reticulum membrane preparations. Failure to accumulate and then release calcium from the sarcoplasmic reticulum would be expected to inhibit the coupling of electrical and mechanical elements in muscle, leading to weakness, and, in the second study, supernatants of mitogen-stimulated normal mononuclear cells did inhibit contraction of muscle strips *in vitro*. Inhibitory supernatants were also obtained by incubation of peripheral blood mononuclear cells with autologous muscle in eight out of 11 cases of active myositis but in none of 20 controls (Kalovidouris 1986).

In another approach to the cause of weakness, a 50% reduction of acetylcholine receptors was reported in myositis (reminiscent of myasthenia gravis), and purified myositis serum IgG increased the rate of receptor degradation on the surface of cultured mammalian muscle cells (Pestronk *et al.* 1985).

Human leucocyte antigen distribution in myositis

There are several studies associating adult and juvenile PM and DM with HLA-A1, B8 and DR3 (Pachman *et al.* 1977; Behan *et al.* 1978; Cumming *et al.* 1978; Pachman and Cooke 1980; Arnett *et al.* 1981; Hirsch *et al.* 1981; Mandel *et al.* 1982; Mellins *et al.* 1982; Friedman *et al.* 1983). In Caucasian populations these antigens are often in linkage disequilibrium within a haplotype also containing C4AQ0, a null allele of C4A. This haplotype is associated with a wide range of 'autoimmune' disease, possibly because subtle complement dysfunction impairs clearance of immune complexes (Schifferli *et al.* 1986). It may be relevant that one-third of the first-degree relatives of 33 patients with myositis had other autoimmune diseases (Walker *et al.* 1982).

Human leucocyte antigen-DR3 is increased in white patients with anti-Jo-1 antibody, being found in 54% of 11 patients with the antibody and 22% of 36 anti-Jo-1 −ve cases; HLA-DR6 was present in some DR3 +ve cases and all the DR3 −ve patients with anti-Jo-1 (Arnett *et al.* 1981). HLA-DRw52 haplotypes were found in all patients with antibodies to translation factors (Goldstein *et al.* 1990), and HLA-DQα4 is increased in myositis overall (63% versus 29% in controls), but most markedly (93%) in patients with anti-Jo-1 antibody (Gurley *et al.* 1991). C4 null alleles are increased only a little in myositis (Moulds *et al.* 1990). It is

DQ alleles that show the closest associations with autoantibodies to Sm, La and Scl-70 antigens as well as Jo-1.

Cellular immunity in animal models

Repeated injections of homogenized muscle in Freund's complete adjuvant produce myositis in rats (Pearson 1956), guinea-pigs (Dawkins 1965) and mice (Rosenberg *et al*. 1987). This experimental allergic myositis resembles PM histologically and can be transferred to naïve animals by lymphocytes but not serum. There is lymphocyte transformation in response to muscle antigens *in vitro*, and the myotoxicity of lymphocytes depends on sensitization of animals with muscle rather than other tissues. Frequent booster injections are required to maintain the myositis and in rats the picture is overshadowed by the accompanying adjuvant arthritis. In another recent model splenic cells from SJL/J mice, first activated by co-culture with syngeneic smooth muscle or striated muscle and then injected into syngeneic hosts, produced a myositis similar to human disease and with expression of Class II MHC antigens on myocytes (Hart *et al*. 1987).

Intraperitoneal injection of a strain of Coxsackie virus B1 induces persistent PM in CDI Swiss new-born mice (Ray *et al*. 1979; Strongwater *et al*. 1984). Weakness with histological evidence of myositis develops after a week and persists for 10 weeks, although virus is no longer detectable after 2 weeks, suggesting the virus has triggered a self-perpetuating immune response. New-born Swiss mice homozygous for the nude gene (*nu*/*nu*) are T-cell-deficient; their muscles recover completely within a few weeks of Coxsackie virus infection, whereas heterozygous mice with normal T cell function continue with weakness and histological degeneration, regeneration and inflammation of muscle (Ytterberg *et al*. 1987, 1989). In myocarditis the importance of T lymphocytes was first shown by Woodruff and Woodruff (1974): in Coxsackie virus B3-infected thymectomized mice, reconstitution with irradiated bone marrow led to the elimination of virus and appearance of neutralizing antibodies, but myocarditis developed only when the mice were also infused with thymocytes. Thymus-deficient *nu*/*nu* BALB/c mice infected with Coxsackie virus B3 show only mild cytopathic changes in the myocardium, whereas *nu*/*plus* mice develop myocarditis with lymphocytic infiltration (Hashimoto *et al*. 1983). In this myocarditis two populations of lymphocytes are involved: L3T4 + ve helper T cells which lyse virus-infected cells, and Lyt2 +ve cytolytic T cells autoreactive with normal cardiac myocytes (Guthrie *et al*. 1984; Estrin and Huber 1987).

Aetiology of myositis

Drugs and viruses

Apart from cases induced by drugs such as penicillamine (Takahashi *et al*. 1986; Carroll *et al*. 1987), the aetiology of PM and DM remains unknown and the different syndromes may well have different aetiopathogeneses. Myositis is uncommon; there is no evidence of epidemic onset, but a report from Greece suggests onset is commoner in the spring (Manta *et al*. 1989). There may be involvement of a rare virus strain or an unusual host response to a common virus, but conventional virological techniques have been generally disappointing, and there are no reports of consistent virus isolation.

Direct evidence for the involvement of viruses is scanty. There are isolated case reports concerning Coxsackie virus A9 (Tang *et al*. 1975), adenovirus type II (McKinlay and Mitchell 1976; Mikol *et al*. 1982), parainfluenza virus (McKinlay and Mitchell 1976), hepatitis B (Mihas *et al*. 1978) and HTLV-1 (Ishii *et al*. 1991). There are several reports concerning ultrastructural appearances interpreted as viral inclusions on light and electron microscopy (Chou 1968; Chou and Gutmann 1970; reviewed by Schiraldi and Iandolo 1978), but these observations have not been followed by virus isolation and rarely by immunological identification. Chou (1986) reviews reports of the specific immunostaining of the inclusions for mumps virus and considers that persistent mumps virus infection is the likely cause of inclusion-body myositis. However, Nishino *et al*. (1989) found no specific immunostaining or *in situ* hybridization with a cDNA probe for the mumps nucleocapsid gene. Inclusions need not represent virus directly but might be a consequence of local release of interferon-γ (H. Moutsopoulos, personal communication) or even represent glycogen particles (Katsuragi *et al*. 1981). Inclusions are seen in no more than 20% of cases, and this inclusion-body myositis is now thought to be a distinct entity (Carpenter *et al*. 1978).

Enteroviruses (Table 63.6)

Transient myositis may follow influenza, and an epidemic of acute myositis in children has been associated with influenza B virus infection (Dietzman *et al*. 1976); there was transient elevation of CPK but complete recovery in a few days. In the special situation of hypogammaglobulinaemia, myositis can occur in association with echovirus infection isolated from the cerebrospinal fluid (Webster 1984; Crennan *et al*. 1986), but the myositis is usually localized (rather than symmetrical and proximal) and muscle biopsy shows less mononuclear cell infiltration than in PM/DM. Serological surveys of myositis have been small and concerned chiefly with Coxsackie virus B following earlier studies in myocarditis (Woodruff 1980; Cambridge *et al*. 1979). Travers *et al*. (1977) showed high levels of neutralizing antibody in four of seven adults with myositis, the precise serotype varying from patient to patient, and Christensen *et al*. (1986) showed complement-fixing antibody to Coxsackie virus B in 83% of 12 children with juvenile DM, compared with 25% of 24 patients with juvenile chronic arthritis and 25% of over 2000 normal controls in the same geographical area. Serotypes B1, B2, B4 and B5 were involved in roughly equal measure, while antibodies to 14 other viruses and *Mycoplasma pneumoniae* were not increased. More detailed studies to show rising antibody titres or an IgM response at the onset of myositis are required to substantiate these observations, just as in myocarditis and juvenile diabetes mellitus, where IgM responses to Coxsackie virus B have been reported in 37% and 39% of cases respectively (El-Hagrassy *et al*. 1980; King *et al*. 1983).

Using nucleic acid hybridization techniques, Coxsackie virus B-specific sequences have been detected in myocarditis (Bowles *et al*. 1986, 1989) and myositis (Bowles *et al*. 1987; Rosenberg *et al*. 1989; Yousef *et al*. 1990). Bowles *et al*. (1986, 1987, 1989) used DNA complementary to a fragment of Coxsackie virus B genomic RNA in hydridization slot blots. They found evidence of the virus-specific sequence in nucleic acid isolated from muscle in nine of 17 cases of myocarditis and five of nine cases of myositis. In myositis the positive findings were in four of seven cases of juvenile DM and one of two adults with PM; normal muscle and four cases of Duchenne muscular dystrophy were negative (as was the one adult with myositis and anti-Jo-1 antibody).

Table 63.6. Clues to a viral aetiology of the myositis syndrome

Occasional virus isolates in acute myositis
Serological evidence of recent Coxsackie virus infection
Coxsackie virus-induced myositis and myocarditis in mice
Clues from autoantibodies
Detection of Coxsackie virus RNA in muscle biopsies

Rosenberg *et al*. (1989) carried out *in situ* hybridization using probes derived from Theiler's murine encephalomyelitis virus (TMEV), poliovirus type I and Coxsackie virus B3. The first of these probes hybridizes most avidly with TMEV and murine encephalomyocarditis virus, while the latter two are broadly cross-reactive with other human enteroviruses. The authors found evidence of TMEV-like infection of macrophages (not muscle fibres) in biopsies from three of five adults with DM, but in none of four childhood cases and none of 24 patients with other myopathies. Hybridization signals were associated with just a few of the cells staining for Mac-1 antigen (macrophages) in the biopsies. The poliovirus and Coxsackie B3 probes gave negative results.

Yousef *et al*. (1990) used a cDNA probe representing the 5′ terminal 526-base sequence in the untranslated region of Coxsackie virus B3 genome which had been shown previously to be broadly specific for enteroviruses. By *in situ* hybridization with muscle, six of 13 cases of PM were positive. The positive cases were mostly not yet on treatment, and in five of the six cases the hybridization staining was associated with areas of severe inflammation and muscle necrosis. Results were negative in muscular dystrophy (six cases) and other myopathy, myalgia or weakness (five cases).

These are exciting observations because of the epidemiological evidence of increased antibody titres to Coxsackie virus B in children with myositis and the ease with which Coxsackie virus infects myocardium and muscle in experimental animals. Unfortunately, not only are the findings of Rosenberg *et al*. (1989) and Youssef *et al*. (1990) contradictory with regard to their Coxsackie virus B3 probes, but attempts to confirm the findings of

Bowles *et al.* (1987) by the slot blot hybridization technique and the far more sensitive polymerase chain reaction have been unsuccessful (Leff *et al.* 1991; C.C. Bunn, R.M. Bernstein and M.J. Walport, unpublished observations). To explain these differences, the exact nature of the cDNA probe and the duration and type of myositis may be of importance. Furthermore, traces of virus may be scattered sparsely in muscle as happens in dilated cardiomyopathy (Bowle *et al.* 1989). The surprising question to emerge is not just whether there is an enterovirus present, but, if there is, whether muscle fibres or mononuclear cells are infected.

In the murine model, virus can be grown from muscle, and viral antigens are detectable for only 2 weeks after infection in animals with ongoing myositis; encephalomyocarditis virus nucleic acid has been detected by *in situ* hybridization a week or two longer in myositis and up to at least 12 weeks in myocarditis (Cronin *et al.* 1988). In the murine models of myocarditis and myositis induced by Coxsackie virus B3 and B1, virus was successfully detected by slot blot hybridization (Zhang *et al.* 1988). Two conclusions to be drawn from the murine models of viral myositis and myocarditis concerning a viral aetiology for human disease are, first, that very subtle differences in the viral strain (obtained through passage) dictate whether the target organ is heart or muscle, and, second, genetic differences within the MHC can dictate whether the mouse strain is susceptible or resistant to infection (Strongwater *et al.* 1984; Miller *et al.* 1987).

The case for Coxsackie virus or any other virus would be strengthened substantially by the demonstration of cellular and humoral immunity to the virus in those very patients in whom viral traces are detected. An isolated example of this combined approach is a case report in which Coxsackie virus A9 antigen was detected in muscle biopsies from an adult with PM, clinical exacerbations being accompanied by rises in the serum titre of antibody to the same virus but not to others (Kuroda *et al.* 1986).

Retroviruses

Retroviruses have long been considered in the aetiology of SLE (Schwartz 1975), and recent studies of simian and human acquired immunodeficiency syndrome (AIDS) raise the possibility of a direct involvement of retroviruses in myositis. Septic pyomyositis is now well recognized in AIDS, but myositis of idiopathic type also occurs in AIDS (Dalakas *et al.* 1986b; Bailey *et al.* 1987). In the initial report two men developed full-blown AIDS 18 months after presenting with muscle weakness. Biopsies showed the typical changes of PM, and human immunodeficiency virus (HIV) antigens were detected in CD4 +ve lymphocytes surrounding muscle fibres and invading the endomysial septa; viral antigens were not expressed in muscle fibres themselves. However, in a review of 352 patients with AIDS or generalized lymphadenopathy, clinical evidence of muscle involvement was rare: myalgia in two cases, myopathy in two cases and PM in one case (Levy *et al.* 1985). There is a marked geographical variation in prevalence of retroviruses. (Levine and Blattner 1987), and other retroviruses might be involved as well. Antibodies to human T cell lymphotrophic virus (HTLV)-1 were found in one of 49 American patients with PM, but also in seven out of seven (subsequently 11 out of 13) Jamaican cases (Mora *et al.* 1988; Morgan *et al.* 1989). Human T cell lymphotrophic virus 1 may be a secondary infection in patients with AIDS. Indeed, in one case of AIDS myopathy, HTLV-1 *tat* DNA and protein were demonstrated by *in situ* hybridization and immunochemically, but there was little lymphocytic infiltration and the HIV antigens GP41 and p24 were not detected (Wiley *et al.* 1989). In one case of myositis HTLV-1 was isolated from muscle (Ishii *et al.* 1991).

In rhesus monkeys, the type D retrovirus causing simian AIDS (SAIDS) produced myositis in 11 of 25 monkeys dying of SAIDS (Dalakas *et al.* 1986a). The histological changes were rather like human PM, but with the addition of large, vacuolated, bizarre-shaped cells of undetermined type surrounding or invading muscle fibres, and there was also extensive fibrosis. The virus isolated from inflamed muscle was able to infect muscle cells in tissue culture (Dalakas *et al.* 1987).

Sjögren's syndrome is well recognized in human AIDS, and other retroviruses may also be involved. Transgenic mice expressing the HTLV-1 *tax* gene develop epithelial proliferation and then lymphocytic infiltration of salivary glands (Green *et al.* 1989). Talal *et al.* (1990) describe antibodies to a retroviral p24 protein in about one-third of patients with various connective tissue diseases, particularly Sjögren's syndrome. If confirmed, it remains to be seen whether this reflects the presence of an aetiological agent or an enhanced immune response to an endogenous, irrelevant retrovirus, as is said to be the case with GP70 in NZB/W lupus mice.

Protozoa

Two protozoal organisms have been implicated in myositis, *Trypanosoma cruzi* and *Toxoplasma gondii*. *Trypanosoma cruzi* invades smooth muscle and myocardium in Chagas' disease, and almost 50% of patients with cardiomyopathy have high titres of antibody to the sarcolemma, compared with less than 20% in early or non-cardiac disease. Over 90% of patients with advanced cardiomyopathy have antibody to a 25 kD *T. cruzi* polypeptide, whereas the antibody is absent from non-cardiac cases (Santos-Buch *et al.* 1985). In a mouse model of PM, C3H/HeJ mice infected with *T. cruzi* developed splenic T lymphocytes responsive to *T. cruzi* antigens and cytotoxic to syngeneic skeletal muscle myoblasts; the mice developed myositis with lymphocytic infiltrates from which *T. cruzi* could not be isolated (von Kreuter and Santos-Buch 1986).

Toxoplasmosis is sometimes associated with PM in humans as well as animals, and there are several reports of PM or even DM as a major or presenting feature (Callihan *et al.* 1946; Rowland and Greer 1961; Pollock 1979). Usually the diagnosis was made on serological grounds, but in some cases muscle biopsy revealed not only mononuclear cell infiltration but also the presence of encapsulated or free organisms (Chandar *et al.* 1968; Greenlee *et al.* 1975) or specific immunofluorescence (McNicholl and Underhill 1970; Topi *et al.* 1979). In these case reports there was also clinical evidence of toxoplasmosis (fever, lymphadenopathy and so on), but could this organism cause idiopathic myositis? Three studies from Kagen and his colleagues concern the frequency of antibody to *T. gondii* in adults with typical PM and DM. In their first study (Kagen *et al.* 1974) titres of 1 : 1024 or more by the Sabin–Feldmann dye test were found in six of 10 adults with PM, two of seven adults with DM and one of 35 hospital controls. By the complement fixation test antibodies were found in 5/10 PM, 1/7 DM and 1/35 controls. *Toxoplasma* antibodies were associated chiefly with PM of less than one year's duration and not yet under corticosteroid therapy. In the second study (Phillips *et al.* 1979), complement-fixing antibodies to *T. gondii* were found in seven (35%) of 20 patients with pure PM, but infrequently in DM, myositis with a connective tissue disease or hospital controls, and in this study the Sabin–Feldmann dye test was no more often positive. Nevertheless, in 1983, Magid and Kagen reported positive dye tests in 19 (76%) of 25 patients with PM and 10 (30%) of 33 patients with DM; IgM anti-*Toxoplasma* antibodies were detected in seven patients from each group, suggesting recent infection in 24% of adults with myositis. The rarity of direct evidence of *T. gondii* infection in muscle and the frequency of subclinical toxoplasmosis in the general population signal caution in the interpretation of these results. On the other hand, in Lyme disease stage III (where the typical changes of PM can occur) the causative spirochaete can be extremely difficult to find (Duray and Steere 1988; Reimers *et al.* 1989).

Cancer

Since Stertz (1916) reported acute DM in a 55-year-old man who died shortly afterwards of gastric carcinoma and then a second report in the same year (Kankeleit 1916), there have been many case reports and series of patients suggesting an association of PM/DM with carcinoma and occasionally reticulosis. Schuermann (1951) studied the literature and found that between 1916 and 1938 7.5% of 200 cases of DM were associated with malignancy, while between 1939 and 1950 the association was reported in 15 (21%) of 75 further cases. Schuermann estimated that the incidence of malignancy in DM was about five times that of the general population, and Barnes (1976) reviewing 258 cases of DM and malignancy in the literature since 1916 came to a similar conclusion that the incidence was increased fivefold to sevenfold. In 70% of cases DM was found at the same time as the tumour or within 1 year beforehand. In most other cases the tumour preceded DM, but usually by less than a year. Intervals of up to 8 years have been reported, but until recently the whole issue was bedevilled by the absence of suitable controls. All the common cancers of lung, breast, stomach and ovary have been implicated, as well as nasopharyngeal carcinoma among the Chinese (Teo *et al*. 1989). From many series (reviewed by Masi and Hochberg 1988) it was concluded that the association with malignancy is unlikely before the age of 45 or 50 years, likelier in men than women, likelier in DM than PM, and less likely in myositis overlap syndromes like MCTD. Indeed, myositis is the only connective tissue disease in which an association with malignancy has been noted (apart from occasional cases of alveolar cell carcinoma in scleroderma with fibrosing alveolitis). No case of malignancy has been reported in a patient with myositis and anti-Jo-1 antibody, but, among eight cases with a similar overlap syndrome and the uncommon PL-12 antibodies, two patients (women aged in their 60s) had had a mastectomy about 1 year prior to the diagnosis of myositis (R.M. Bernstein and M.J. Walport, unpublished observations).

From the neurologist's point of view, myositis is just an uncommon example of malignancy-associated myopathy (Shy 1962), but is the association real? Two careful case-control studies shed doubt on the association of myositis with malignancy (Manchul *et al*. 1985; Lakhanpal *et al*. 1986). However, a critical review by Masi and Hochberg (1988) concludes that the data are sufficiently in keeping with a positive link for a further larger study to be warranted to confirm and quantify the association. In the mean time we should note that cancer is not uncommon in hospitals, that the benefits of screening tests in myositis are uncertain and limited in the literature to a few self-congratulatory anecdotes, and that aggressive investigation is expensive and uncomfortable. As several reviewers point out, the best guides are clinical history and examination, chest radiograph and pelvic ultrasound, with more extensive investigation considered only in men over 50 years of age with DM (Callen 1984; Dalakas 1988; Masi and Hochberg 1988). As to the mechanism for the association, it has been suggested that reduced NK cell function in active myositis might impair tumour surveillance (Behan and Behan 1984), but other possibilities include immunological cross-reaction between surface antigens on tumour and muscle and possibly the binding to muscle of the products of an unbridled oncogene.

Treatment of myositis

There are no controlled trials of corticosteroid therapy in myositis, but the clinical response is obvious. Prognosis appears to have improved since the introduction of steroids in the 1950s, with a mortality rate of 50% in DM (O'Leary and Waisman 1940) falling to a 5-year mortality of less than 20%, now mainly in older individuals with cardiac involvement, malignancy or other causes and not usually from the direct effects of myositis (DeVere and Bradley 1975; Carpenter *et al*. 1977; Hochberg *et al*. 1986). The need for high doses of corticosteroid was emphasized even in early studies (Pearson 1963; Rose and Walton 1966), and a recent retrospective study correlating serum CPK with muscle strength in 42 treatment periods in 30 patients concluded that a good clinical outcome depended on adequate initial corticosteroid dosage, continuation of the initial dose until or after normalization of the serum CPK, and then a slow rate of corticosteroid dose reduction (Oddis and Medsger 1988). Unfortunately, steroid myopathy (type II fibre atrophy) can be a serious problem with this aggressive approach, and a more pragmatic approach is to judge treatment according to muscle strength. For this a myometer is more helpful than the crude Medical Research Council scale of muscle power intended for the assessment of peripheral nerve injuries (Morgan *et al*. 1985; Kroll *et al*. 1986; Lane *et al*. 1989). Serial needle biopsies of muscle are also useful to assess the balance of myositis and myopathy. Adequate control of myositis probably lessens end-stage fibrosis and fatty infiltration (DeVere and Bradley 1975), but even when inflammation is well controlled some morphometric and architectural changes persist, associated with residual dynamic weakness (Lane *et al*. 1989).

Cytotoxic agents, particularly azathioprine and once-weekly methotrexate, controlled myositis effectively in several open studies, usually as adjuncts to corticosteroid therapy (Metzger *et al*. 1974; reviewed by Bunch 1988). In a prospective controlled trial, azathioprine plus prednisone was little better than prednisone alone over 3 months of treatment, but in open follow-up the combination was superior after 1 year and especially after 3 years (Bunch *et al*. 1980; Bunch 1981). Usually the recommendation is to introduce cytotoxic agents if corticosteroid therapy proves inadequate after a 2-month trial, but, since their use often allows the dose of corticosteroids to be reduced, it is now common practice to start at once with combined therapy, at least in adults with severe disease. Inclusion-body myositis is often resistant to corticosteroid and cytotoxic therapy, and a recent review supports this view (Lotz *et al*. 1989).

Myositis that is refractory or relapsing despite standard treatment has been tackled in a number of ways: combined azathioprine and methotrexate, chlorambucil, cyclophosphamide, cyclosporin A (Zabel *et al*. 1984; The *et al*. 1985; Alijotas *et al*. 1990), total body irradiation (TBI) (Engel *et al*. 1981; Morgan *et al*. 1985; Kelly *et al*. 1988), thoracic duct drainage, leucapheresis (Dau 1987), plasmapheresis (Clarke *et al*. 1988) and intravenous immunoglobulin (Gelfand 1989). Uncontrolled case reports indicate that all these treatments are beneficial sometimes but roughly in proportion to the risk of toxicity. However in a double-blind sham-controlled study of 39 patients with steroid-resistant polymyositis or dermatomyositis, neither plasmapheresis nor leucapheresis showed benefit (Miller *et al*. 1991). Intravenous immunoglobulin is being elevated in several centres. Cyclosporin A may be particularly effective in juvenile DM (B.M. Ansell, personal communication). Total body irradiation is an effective immunosuppressive therapy and more rational than total lymphoid irradiation (TLI) for killing lymphocytes in muscle. Total body irradiation (150–200 rads given as 10 treatments over 5 weeks) induced remission lasting months in most cases reported, but at the expense of fatal bone marrow depression in one patient (Morgan *et al*. 1985). It is possible that prior cytotoxic therapy increases the risk to the bone marrow and of inducing malignancy. Total body irradiation was ineffective in childhood DM (Girardin *et al*. 1988) and in inclusion body myositis (Kelly *et al*. 1986).

Epilogue

Recent years have brought greater understanding of myositis but few clear answers. Several myositis syndromes are recognized. Various autoantibody responses have been characterized and are of some use clinically, but their origin and any role in pathogenesis remain obscure. The cellular infiltrates of muscle have also been characterized with care, but how the inflammation is controlled and whether it is induced by virus infection are questions still unanswered unequivocally. Involvement of the microvasculature has been emphasized, in both idiopathic myositis and in the animal models induced by Coxsackie virus. The use of enterovirus nucleic acid probes has given conflicting results in human disease, and retroviruses are coming under closer scrutiny. Will future treatment involve immunomodulation (Cohen *et al*. 1985) or antiviral chemotherapy?

References

Alarcon-Segovia, D., Ruiz-Arguelles, A. and Fishbein, E. (1979). Antibody penetration into living cells. I. Intranuclear immunoglobulin in peripheral blood mononuclear cells in mixed connective tissue disease and systemic lupus erythematosus. *Clin. Exp. Immunol.* **35**, 364–75.

Alijotas, J., Barquinero, J., Ordi, J. and Vilardell, M. (1990). Polymyositis and cyclosporin A. *Ann. Rheum. Dis.* **49**, 66.

Appleyard, S.T., Dunn, M.J., Dubowitz, V. and Rose, M.L. (1985). Increased expression of HLA-ABC class I antigens by muscle fibres in Duchenne muscular dystrophy, inflammatory myopathy and other neuromuscular disorders . *Lancet* **i**, 361–3.

Arad-Dann, H., Isenberg, D.A., Shoenfeld, Y., Offen, D., Sperling, J. and Sperling, R. (1987). Autoantibodies against a specific nuclear RNP protein in sera of patients with autoimmune rheumatic diseases associated with myositis. *J. Immunol.* **138**, 2463–8.

Arad-Dann, H., Isenberg, D.A., Ovadia, A., Shoenfeld, Y., Sperling, J. and Sperling, R. (1989). Autoantibodies against a nuclear 56 kD protein: a marker for inflammatory muscle disease. *J. Autoimmunity* **2**, 877–88.

Arahata, K. and Engel, A.G. (1984). Monoclonal antibody analysis of mononuclear cells in myopathies. 1. Quantitation of subsets according to diagnosis and sites of accumulation and demonstration and counts of muscle fibers invaded by T cells. *Ann. Neurol.* **16**, 193–208.

Arahata, K. and Engel, A.G. (1986). Monoclonal antibody analysis of mononuclear cells in myopathies. 3. Immunoelectron microscopic aspects in cell mediated muscle fibers injury. *Ann. Neurol.* **19**, 112–25.

Arahata, K. and Engel, A.G. (1988). Monoclonal antibody analysis of mononuclear cells in myopathies. IV. Cell-mediated cytotoxicity and muscle fiber necrosis. *Ann. Neurol.* **23** (2), 168–73.

Arnett, F.C., Hirsch, T.J., Bias, W.B., Nishikai, M. and Reichlin, M. (1981). The Jo-1 antibody system in myositis: relationship to clinical features and HLA. *J. Rheumatol.* **8**, 925–30.

Baboonian, C., Venables, P.J.W., Booth, J., Williams, D.G., Roffe, L.M. and Maini, R.N. (1989). Virus infection induces redistribution and membrane localisation of the nuclear antigen La (SS-B): a possible mechanism for autoimmunity. *Clin. Exp. Immunol.* **78**, 454–9.

Bailey, R.O., Turok, D.I., Jaufmann, B.P. and Singh, J.K. (1987). Myositis and acquired immunodeficiency syndrome. *Hum. Pathol.* **18** (7), 749–51.

Banker, B.O. and Victor, M. (1966). Dermatomyositis (systemic angiopathy) of childhood. *Medicine* **45**, 261–89.

Barnes, B.E. (1976). Dermatomyositis and malignancy: a review of the literature. *Ann. Intern. Med.* **84**, 68–76.

Batten, F.E. (1912). Case of dermatomyositis in a child with pathological report. *Br. J. Child. Dis.* **9**, 247–57.

Behan, W.M.H. and Behan, P.O. (1984). Disturbance of regulatory lymphocyte subsets in polymyositis. *Ann. Neurol.* **15**, 181–2.

Behan, W.H.M. and Behan, P.O. (1985). Immunological features of polymyositis/dermatomyositis. *Semin. Immunopathol.* **8**, 267–93.

Behan, W.H.M., Behan, P.O. and Dick, H.A. (1978). HLA-B8 in polymyositis. *N. Engl. J. Med.* **298**, 1260–1.

Behan, W.H.M., Behan, P.O. and Cairns, J. (1987a). Cardiac damage in polymyositis associated with antibodies to tissue ribonucleoproteins. *Br. Heart J.* **57**, 176–80.

Behan, W.H.M., Behan, P.O., Durward, W.F. and McQueen, A. (1987b). The inflammatory process in polymyositis: monoclonal antibody analysis of muscle and peripheral blood immunoregulatory lymphocytes. *J. Neurol. Neurosurg. Psychiatry* **50**, 1468–74.

Bernstein, R.M. (1989). Heat-shock proteins and arthritis. *Br. J. Rheumatol.* **28**, 369–73.

Bernstein, R.M. and Mathews, M.B. (1984). From virus infection to autoantibody production. *Lancet* **i**, 42.

Bernstein, R.M. and Mathews, M.B. (1985). Jo-1 and other myositis autoantibodies. In *Rheumatology — 85, Excerpta Medica International Congress* Series 675, ed. P.M. Brooks and J.R. York, pp. 273–8, Elsevier Science Publishers, Amsterdam.

Bernstein, R.M. and Mathews, M.B. (1987). Autoantibodies to intracellular antigens, with particular reference to transfer RNA and related proteins in myositis. *J. Rheumatol.* **14** (suppl. 13), 83–8.

Bernstein, R.M., Bunn, C.C., Hughes, G.R.V., Francoeur, A.M. and Mathews, M.B. (1984a). Cellular protein and RNA antigens in autoimmune disease. *Mol. Biol. Med.* **2**, 105–20.

Bernstein, R.M., Morgan, S.H., Chapman, J. *et al.* (1984b). Anti-Jo-1 antibody: a marker for myositis and interstitial lung disease. *Br. Med. J.* **289**, 151–2.

Bertorini, T.E. (1988). Histopathology of the inflammatory myopathies. In *Polymyositis and Dermatomyositis*, ed. M.C. Dalakas, pp. 157–94, Butterworth, Boston.

Bijlsma, J.W.J., Plater-Zyberk, C., Mumford, P. and Maini, R.N. (1990). Lack of natural antibodies in rheumatic diseases. *Rheumatol. Int.* **10**, 107–12.

Biswas, T., Miller, F.W., Takagaki, Y. and Plotz, P.H. (1987). An enzyme-linked immunosorbent assay for the detection and quantitation of anti-Jo-1 antibody in human serum. *J. Immunol. Methods* **98** (2), 243–8.

Bohan, A. and Peter, J.B. (1975). Polymyositis and dermatomyositis. *N. Engl. J. Med.* **292**, 344–7 and 403–7.

Bottazzo, G.F., Pujol-Borrell, R., Hanafusa, T. and Feldmann, M. (1983). Role of aberrant HLA-DR expression and antigen presentation in induction of endocrine autoimmunity. *Lancet* **ii**, 1115–19.

Bowles, N.E., Richardson, P.J., Olsen, E.G.J. and Archard, L.C. (1986). Detection of coxsackie-B-virus-specific RNA sequences in myocardial biopsy samples from patients with myocarditis and dilated cardiomyopathy. *Lancet* **i**, 1120–2.

Bowles, N.E., Dubowitz, V., Sewry, C.A. and Archard, L.C. (1987). Dermatomyositis, polymyositis and coxsackie-B-virus infection. *Lancet* **i**, 1004–7.

Bowles, N.E., Rose, M.L., Taylor, P. *et al.* (1989). End stage dilated cardiomyopathy: persistence of enterovirus RNA in myocardium at cardiac transplantation and lack of immune response. *Circulation* **80**, 1128–36.

Bunch, T.W. (1981). Prednisone and azathioprine for polymyositis: long term follow-up. *Arthritis Rheum.* **24**, 45–8.

Bunch, T.W. (1988). The therapy of polymyositis. *Mt Sinai J. Med.* **55**, 483–6.

Bunch, T.W., Worthington, J.W., Combs, J.J., Ilstrup, D.M. and Engel, A.G. (1980). Azathioprine with prednisone for polymyositis a controlled clinical trial. *Ann. Intern. Med.* **92**, 365–9.

Bunn, C.C. and Mathews, M.B. (1987). Autoreactive epitope defined as the anticodon region of alancyl transfer RNA. *Science* **238**, 1116–19.

Bunn, C.C., Bernstein, R.M. and Mathews, M.B. (1986). Autoantibodies against alanyl-tRNA synthetase and tRNA^{ala} coexist and are associated with myositis. *J. Exp. Med.* **163**, 1281–91.

Callen, J.P. (1984). Myositis and malignancy. *Clin. Rheum. Dis.* **10**, 117–30.

Callihan, W.P., Russell, W.O. and Smith, M.G. (1946). Human toxoplasmosis: a clinicopathologic study with presentation of 5 cases and review of the literature. *Medicine* **25**, 343–97.

Cambridge, G. and Stern, C.M.M. (1981). The uptake of tritium-labelled carnitine by monolayer cultures of human fetal muscle and its potential as a label in cytotoxicity studies. *Clin. Exp. Immunol.* **43**, 211–19.

Cambridge, G., MacArthur, C.G.C., Waterson, A.P., Goodwin, J.F. and Oakley, C.M. (1979). Antibodies to coxsackie B viruses in congestive cardiomyopathy. *Br. Heart J.* **41**, 692–6.

Carpenter, J.R., Bunch, T.W., Engel, A.G. and O'Brien, P.C. (1977). Survival in polymyositis: corticosteroids and risk factors. *J. Rheumatol.* **4**, 207–14.

Carpenter, S., Karpati, G., Heller, I. and Eisen, A. (1978). Inclusion body myositis: a distinct variety of idiopathic inflammatory myopathy. *Neurology* **28**, 8–17.

Carroll, G.J., Will, R.K., Peter, J.B., Garlepp, M.J. and Dawkins, R.L. (1987). Penicillamine induced polymyositis and dermatomyositis. *J. Rheumatol* **14**, 995–1001.

Cervera, R., Ramirez, G., Fernández-Solà, J. *et al.* (1991). Antibodies to endothelial cells in dermatomyositis: association with interstitial lung disease. *B.M.J.* **302**, 880–1.

Chandar, K., Mair, H.J. and Mair, H.S. (1968). Case of toxoplasma polymyositis. *Br. Med. J.* **1**, 158–9.

Chou, S.M. (1968). Myxovirus-like structures and accompanying nuclear changes in chronic polymyositis. *Arch. Pathol.* **86**, 649–58.

Chou, S.M. (1986). Inclusion body myositis: a chronic persistent mumps myositis? *Hum. Pathol.* **17** (8), 765–77.

Chou, S.M. and Gutmann, L. (1970). Picornavirus-like crystals in subacute polymyositis. *Neurology* **20**, 205–13.

Christensen, M.L., Pachman, L.M., Schneiderman, R., Patel, D.C. and Friedman, J.M. (1986). Prevalence of Coxsackie B virus antibodies in patients with juvenile dermatomyositis. *Arthritis Rheum.* **29**, 1365–70.

Clarke, C.R., Dyall-Smith, D.J., Mackay, I.R., Emery, P., Jennens, I.D. and Becker, G. (1988). Plasma exchange in dermatomyositis/polymyositis: beneficial effects in three cases. *J. Clin. Lab. Immunol. (Scotland)* **27**, 149–52.

Cohen, I.R., Holoshitz, J., van Eden, W. and Frankel, A. (1985). Lymphocyte clones illuminate pathogenesis and affect therapy of experimental arthritis. *Arthritis Rheum.* **28**, 841–5.

Comola, M., Johnson, M.A., Howel, D. and Brunsdon, C. (1987). Spatial distribution of muscle necrosis in biopsies from patients with inflammatory muscle disorders. *J. Neurol. Sci.* **82**, 229–44.

Crennan, J.M., Van Scoy, R.E., McKenna, C.H. and Smith, T.F. (1986). Echovirus polymyositis in patients with hypogammaglobulinemia: failure of high-dose intravenous gammaglobulin therapy and review of the literature. *Am. J. Med.* **81**, 35–42.

Cronin, M.E., Love, L.A., Miller, F.W., McClintock, P.R. and Plotz, P.H. (1988). The natural history of encephalomyocarditis virus-linked myositis and myocarditis in mice: viral persistence demonstrated by *in situ* hybridisation. *J. Exp. Med.* **168**, 1639–48.

Cumming, W.K.J., Hudgson, P. and Wilcox, C.B. (1978). HLA antigens in adult polymyositis. (letter) *N. Engl. J. Med.* **299**, 1365.

Currie, S., Saunders, M., Knowles, M. and Brown, A.E. (1971). Immunological aspects of polymyositis in *in vitro* activity of lymphocytes on incubation with muscle antigen and muscle cultures. *Quart. J. Med.* **40**, 63–4.

Dalakas, M.C. (1988). *Polymyositis and Dermatomyositis*. Butterworths, Boston.

Dalakas, M.C., London, W.T., Gravell, M. and Sever, J.L. (1986a). Polymyositis as an immunodeficiency disease in monkeys induced by a type D retrovirus. *Neurology* **36**, 569–72.

Dalakas, M.C., Pezeshkpour, G.H., Gravell, M. and Sever, J.L. (1986b). Polymyositis associated with AIDS retrovirus. *JAMA* **256** (17), 2381–3.

Dalakas, M.C., Gravell, M., London, W.T., Cunningham, G. and Sever, J.L. (1987). Morphological changes of an inflammatory myopathy in rhesus monkeys with simian acquired immunodeficiency syndrome. *Proc. Soc. Exp. Biol. Med.* **185** (4), 368–76.

Dau, P.C. (1987). Leukocytapheresis in inclusion body myositis. *J. Clin. Apheresis* **3**, 167–70.

Dawkins, R.L. (1965). Experimental myositis associated with hypersensitivity to muscle. *J. Pathol. Bacteriol.* **90**, 619–25.

Dawkins, R.L. and Mastaglia, F.L. (1973). Cell-mediated cytotoxicity to muscle in polymyositis: effect of immunosuppression. *N. Engl. J. Med.* **288**, 434–8.

DeVere, R. and Bradley, W.G. (1975). Polymyositis: its presentations, morbidity and mortality. *Brain* **98**, 637–66.

Dietzman, D.E., Schaller, J.G., Ray, G. and Reed, M.E. (1976). Acute myositis associated with influenza B infection. *Pediatrics* **57**, 255–8.

Duray, P.H. and Steere, A.C. (1988). Clinical–pathologic correlations of Lyme disease by stage. *Ann. NY Acad. Sci.* **539**, 65–79.

El-Hagrassy, M.M.O., Banatvala, J.E. and Coltart, J.D. (1980). Coxsackie B virus specific IgM responses in patients with cardiac and other diseases. *Lancet* **ii**, 1160–2.

Emslie-Smith, A.M., Arahata, K. and Engel, A.G. (1989). Major histocompatibility complex class I antigen expression, immunolocalisation of interferon subtypes and T cell-medited cytotoxicity in myopathies. *Hum. Pathol. (US)* **20**, 224–31.

Engel, A.G. and Arahata, K. (1984). Monoclonal antibody analysis of mononuclear cells in myopathies. 2. Phenotypes of autoinvasive cells in polymyositis and inclusion body myositis. *Ann. Neurol.* **16**, 209–15.

Engel, W.K., Lichter, A.S. and Galde, A. (1981). Polymyositis: remarkable response to total body irradiation. *Lancet* **i**, 658.

Esiri, M.M., Maclennan, I.C.M. and Hazleman, B.L. (1973). Lymphocyte sensitivity to skeletal muscle in patients with polymyositis and other disorders. *Clin. Exp. Immunol.* **14**, 253–5.

Estrin, M. and Huber, S.A. (1987). Coxsackievirus B-3-induced myocarditis: autoimmunity is L3T4+ T helper cell and IL-2 independent in BALB/c mice. *Am. J. Pathol.* **127**, 335–41.

Fahoun, S.K. and Yang, D.C. (1987). Purification of mammalian histidyl-tRNA synthetase and its interaction with myositis-specific anti-Jo-1 antibodies. *Biochemistry* **26**, 5871–7.

Friedman, J.M., Pachman, L.M., Maryjowski, M.L. *et al.* (1983). Immunogenetic studies in juvenile dermatomyositis: HLA, DR antigen frequencies. *Arthritis Rheum.* **26**, 214–16.

Garlepp, M.J. and Dawkins, R.L. (1984). Immunological aspects of myositis. *Clin. Rheum. Dis.* **10**, 35–51.

Gaut, P., Wong, P.K. and Mayer, R.D., (1988). Pyomyositis in a patient with the acquired immunodeficiency syndrome. *Arch. Intern. Med.* **148**, 1608–10.

Gelfand, E.W. (1989). The use of intravenous immune globulin in collagen vascular disorders: a potentially new modality of therapy. *J. Allergy Clin. Immunol.* **84**, 613–15.

Giornio, R., Barden, M.T., Kohler, P.F. and Ringel, S.P. (1984). Histochemical characterisation of the mononuclear cells infiltrating muscle of patients with inflammatory and noninflammatory myopathies. *Clin. Immunol. Immunopathol.* **30**, 405–12.

Girardin, E., Dayer, J.M. and Paunier, L. (1988). Cyclosporine for juvenile dermatomyositis. *J. Pediatr.* **112**, 165–6.

Goldstein, R., Duvic, M., Targoff, I.N. *et al.* (1990). HLA-D region genes associated with autoantibody responses to histidyl-tRNA synthetase (Jo-1) and other translation-related factors in myositis. *Arthritis Rheum.* **33**, 1240–8.

Gonzalez-Amaro, R., Alcocer-Varela, J. and Alarcon-Segovia, D. (1987). Natural killer cell activity in dermatomyositis–polymyositis. *J. Rheumatol.* **14**, 307–10.

Goust, J.M., Castaigne, A. and Moulias, R. (1974). Delayed hypersensitivity to muscle and thymus in myasthenia gravis and polymyositis. *Clin. Exp. Immunol.* **18**, 39–47.

Green, J.E., Hinrichs, S.H., Vogel, J. and Jay, G. (1989). Exocrinopathy resembling Sjögren's syndrome in HTLV-1 *tax* transgenic mic. *Nature (London)* **341**, 72–4.

Greenlee, J.E., Johnson, N.D., Campa, J.F. *et al.* (1975). Adult toxoplasma presenting as polymyositis and cerebellar ataxia. *Ann. Intern. Med.* **82**, 367–71.

Gupta, R.C., Ringle, S., Bertorini, T. and Kaplan, S. (1986). Antibodies to cytoplasmic components in idiopathic polymyositis. *Arthritis Rheum.* **29**, S38 (abstr. 158).

Gurley, R.C., Love, L.A., Targoff, I.N., Leff, R.L., Plotz, P.H. and Miller, F.W. (1991). Associations among myositis-specific autoantibodies and HLA-DQA1 alleles. *Arthritis Rheum.* **34**, S137.

Guthrie, M., Lodge, P.A. and Huber, S.A. (1984). Cardiac injury in myocarditis induced by coxsackievirus group B, type 3 in Balb/c mice is mediated by Lyt 2+ cytologic lymphocytes. *Cell. Immunol.* **88**, 558–67.

Haas, D.C. (1980). Absence of cell-mediated cytotoxicity to muscle culture in polymyositis. *J. Rheumatol.* **7**, 671–6.

Haas, D.C. and Arnason, B.G.W. (1974). Cell-mediated immunity in polymyositis: creatine phosphokinase release from muscle cultures. *Arch. Neurol.* **31**, 192–6.

Habets, W.J., Hoet, M.H., van de Pas, J. and van Venrooij, W.J. (1985). Characterization of nuclear and cytoplasmic autoimmune antigens. In *Protides of the Biological Fluids*, vol. 33, ed. H. Peeters, pp. 199–204, Pergamon Press, Oxford.

Hardin, J.A. (1986). The lupus autoantigens and the pathogenesis of systemic lupus erythematosus. *Arthritis Rheum.* **29**, 457–60.

Hart, M.N., Linthicum, D.S., Waldschmidt, M.M., Tassell, S.K., Schelper, R.L. and Robinson, R.A. (1987). Experimental autoimmune inflammatory myopathy. *J. Neuropathol. Exp. Neurol.* **46** (5), 511–21.

Hashimoto, I., Tatsumi, M. and Nakagawa, M. (1983). The role of T lymphocytes in the pathogenesis of coxsackievirus B3 heart disease. *Br. J. Exp. Pathol.* **64**, 497–504.

Hepp, P. (1887). Ueber Pseudo-trichinose, eine besondere Form von acuter parenchymatöses Polymyositis. *Berl. Klin. Wochenschr.* **24**, 297.

Herrera-Esparza, R., Magana, L., Moreno, J., Fraga, A. and Lavalle, C. (1983). Cell-mediated immunity to myoglobin in polymyositis. *Ann. Rheum. Dis.* **42**, 182–6.

Hirsch, T.J., Enlow, R.W., Bias, W.B. and Arnett, F.C. (1981). HLA-D related (DR) antigens in various kinds of myositis. *Hum. Immunol.* **3**, 181–6.

Hochberg, M.C., Feldman, D. and Stevens, M.B. (1986). Adult onset polymyositis/dermatomyositis: an analysis of clinical and laboratory features and survival in 76 patients with a review of the literature. *Semin. Arthritis Rheum.* **15**, 168–78.

Hohlfeld, R. and Engel, A.G. (1991). Co-culture with autologous myotubes of cytotoxic T cells isolated from muscle in inflammatory myopathies. *Ann. Neurol.* **29**, 498–507.

Hohlfeld; R., Engel, A.G., Ii, K. and Harper, M.C. (1991). Polymyositis mediated by lymphocytes that express the gamma/delta receptor. *N. Engl. J. Med.* **324**, 877–81.

Howel, D. (1988). A test to detect clustering applied to muscle fibres. *Stat. Med.* **7** (11), 1157–64.

Iannaccone, S.T., Bowen, D.E. and Samaha, F.J. (1982). Cell-mediated cytotoxicity and childhood dermatomyositis. *Arch. Neurol.* **39**, 400–2.

Isenberg, D.A. (1983). Immunoglobulin deposition in skeletal muscle in primary muscle disease. *Quart. J. Med.* **207**, 297–310.

Isenberg, D.A., Rowe, D., Shearer, M., Novick, D. and Beverley, P.C.L. (1986). Localisation of interferons and interleukin 2 in polymyositis and muscular dystrophy. *Clin. Exp. Immunol.* **63**, 450–8.

Ishii, K., Yamato, K., Iwahara, Y. *et al.* (1991). Isolation of HTLV-1 from muscle of a patient with myositis. *Am. J. Med.* **90**, 267–9.

Iyer, V., Lawton, A.R. and Fenichel, G.M. (1983). T-cell subsets in polymyositis. *Ann. Neurol.* **13**, 452–3.

Johnson, R.L., Fink, C.W. and Ziff, M. (1972). Lymphotoxin formation by lymphocytes and muscle in polymyositis. *J. Clin. Invest.* **51**, 2435–49.

Kagen, L.J., Kimball, A.C. and Christian, C.L. (1974). Serologic evidence of toxoplasmosis among patients with polymyositis. *Am. J. Med.* **56**, 186–91.

Kalovidouris, A.E. (1986). Mononuclear cells from patients with polymyositis inhibit calcium binding by sarcoplasmic reticulum. *J. Lab. Clin. Med.* **107**, 23–8.

Kalovidouris, A.E. and Johnson, R.L. (1980). Mitogen-activated human mononuclear cells suppress calcium binding by sarcoplasmic reticulum. *J. Lab. Clin. Med.* **95**, 144–54.

Kalovidouris, A.E. and Meiss, R.A. (1984). Human mononuclear cells factors suppress contractility of isolated mouse soleus muscle. *J. Lab. Clin. Med.* **103**, 886–93.

Kalovidouris, A.E. and Smith, D.B. (1991). Aberrant expression of Class II and increased expression of Class I MHC antigens in muscles of patients with polymyositis-dermatomyositis. *Arthritis Rheum.* **34**, S148.

Kalovidouris, A.E., Pourmand, R., Passo, M.H. and Plotkin, Z. (1989). Proliferative response of peripheral blood mononuclear cells to autologous and allogeneic muscle in patients with polymyositis/dermatomyositis. *Arthritis Rheum. (US)* **32**, 446–53.

Kankeleit, H. (1916). Uber primare nichteitrige Polymyositis. *Dtsch. Arch. Klin. Med.* **120**, 335–49.

Katsuragi, S., Miyayama, H. and Takeuchi, T. (1981). Piconavirus-like inclusions in polymyositis: aggregation of glycogen particles of the same size. *Neurology (NY)* **31**, 1476–80.

Kelly, J.J., Jr, Madoc-Jones, H., Adelman, L.S., Andres, P.L. and Munsat, T.L. (1986). Total body irradiation not effective in inclusion body myositis. *Neurology* **36**, 1264–6.

Kelly, J.J., Madoc-Jones, H., Adelman, L.S., Andres, P.L. and Munsat, T.L. (1988). Response to total body irradiation in dermatomyositis. *Muscle Nerve* **11**, 120–3.

King, M.L., Shaikh, A., Bidwell, D., Voller, A. and Banatvala, J.E. (1983). Coxsackie-B-virus-specific IgM responses in children with insulin-dependent (juvenile-onset: type I) diabetes mellitus. *Lancet* **i**, 1397–9.

Kissel, J.T., Mendell, J.R. and Rammohan, K.W. (1986). Microvascular deposition of complement membrane attack complex in dermatomyositis. *N. Engl. J. Med.* **314**, 329–34.

Koga, K., Abe, S., Hashimoto, H. and Yamaguchi, M. (1987). Western-blotting method for detecting antibodies against human muscle contractile proteins in myositis. *J. Immunol. Methods* **105** (1), 15–21.

Kole, R., Fresco, L.D., Keene, J.D., Cohen, P.L., Eisenberg, R.A. and Andrews, P.G. (1985). Alu RNA–protein complexes formed *in vitro* react with a novel lupus autoantibody. *J. Biol. Chem.* **260**, 11781–6.

Kroll, M., Otis, J. and Kagen, L. (1986). Serum enzyme, myoglobin and muscle strength relationships in polymyositis and dermatomyositis. *J. Rheumatol.* **13**, 349–55.

Kuroda, Y., Neshige, R., Oda, K. and Shibasaki, H. (1986). Chronic polymyositis: presence of coxsackievirus A9 antigen in muscle. **25** (2), 191–4.

Lakhanpal, S., Bunch, T.W., Ilstrup, D.W. and Melton, L.J., III (1986). Polymyositis-dermatomyositis and malignant lesions: does an association exist? *Mayo Clin. Proc.* **61**, 645–53.

Lane, R.J., Emslie-Smith, A., Mosquera, I.E. and Hudgson, P. (1989). Clinical, biochemical and histological responses to treatment in polymyositis: a prospective study. *J. Roy. Soc. Med.* **82**, 333–8.

LeFeber, W.P., Norris, D.A., Ryan, S.R. *et al.* (1984). Ultraviolet light induces binding of antibodies to selected nuclear antigens on cultured human keratinocytes. *J. Clin. Invest.* **74**, 1545–51.

Leff, R.L., Love, L.A., Miller, F.W., Dalakas, M.C. and Plotz, P.H. (1991). Viral genomes from candidate viruses in myositis are absent from patient muscle biopsies by high sensitivity PCR screening. *Arthritis Rheum.* **34**, s147.

Lemoine, N.R., Ryan, J.F., Cox, E.L., Mayston, V., Revell, P.A. and Swash, M. (1986). Immunohistochemical analysis of mononuclear cell subsets in inflammatory and non-inflammatory myopathies. *J. Clin. Pathol.* **39**, 271–4.

Lerner, M.R. and Steitz, J.A. (1979). Antibodies to small nuclear RNAs complexed with proteins are produced by patients with systemic lupus erythematosus. *Proc. Nat. Acad. Sci. (USA)* **76**, 5495–9.

Levine, P.H. and Blattner, W.A. (1987). The epidemiology of diseases associated with HTLV-I and HTLV-II. *Infect. Dis. Clin. North Am.* **1** (3), 501–10.

Levison, P. (1937). Polymyositis, acute and subacute, with round-cell infiltration of muscles. *Acta Psychiatr. Neurol.* **12**, 89–96

Levy, R.M., Bredesen, D.E. and Rosenblu, M.L. (1985). Neurological manifestations of the acquired immunodeficiency syndromes (AIDS): experience of UCSF and review of the literature. *J. Neurosurg.* **62**, 475–95.

Lisak, R.P. and Zweiman, B. (1975). Mitogen and muscle extract induced *in vitro* proliferative responses in myasthenia gravis, dermatomyositis and polymyositis. *J. Neurol. Neurosurg. Psychiatry* **38**, 521–4.

Lotz, B.P., Engel, A.G., Nishino, H., Stevens, J.C. and Litchy, W.J. (1989). Inclusion body myositis: observations in 40 patients. *Brain (England)* **112**, 727–47.

McKinlay, I.A. and Mitchell, I. (1976). Transient acute myositis in childhood. *Arch. Dis. Child.* **51**, 135–7.

McNicholl, B. and Underhill, D. (1970). Toxoplasmic polymyositis. *Ir. J. Med. Sci.* **3**, 525–7.

Magid, S.K. and Kagen, L.J. (1983). Serologic evidence for acute toxoplasmosis in polymyositis-dermatomyositis: increased frequency of specific anti-*Toxoplasma* IgM antibodies. *Am. J. Med.* **75**, 313–20.

Manchul, L.A., Jin, A., Pritchard, K.I. *et al.* (1985). The frequency of malignant neoplasms in patients with polymyositis-dermatomyositis: a controlled study. *Arch. Intern. Med.* **145**, 1835–9.

Mandel, D., Segal, A., Mayes, M. *et al.* (1982). Childhood dermatomyositis: long term follow-up and new HLA findings. *Arthritis Rheum.* **25**, S151.

Manta, P., Kalfakis, N. and Vassilopoulos, D. (1989). Evidence for seasonal variation in myositis. *Neuroepidemiology* **8**, 262–5.

Marguerie, C., Bunn, C.C., Beynon, H.L. *et al.* (1990). Polymyositis, pulmonary fibrosis and autoantibodies to aminoacyl-tRNA synthetase enzymes. *Quart. J. Med.* **77**, 1019–38.

Masi, A.T. and Hochberg, M.C. (1988). Temporal association of polymyositis-dermatomyositis with malignancy: methodological and clinical considerations. *Mt Sinai J. Med.* **55**, 471–8.

Mathews, M.B. and Bernstein, R.M. (1983). Myositis autoantibody inhibits histidyl-tRNA synthetase: a model for autoimmunity. *Nature* **304**, 177–9.

Mathews, M.B., Reichlin, M., Hughes, G.R.V. and Bernstein, R.M. (1984). Anti-threonyl-tRNA synthetase, a second myositis-related autoantibody. *J. Exp. Med.* **160**, 420–34.

Mathews, M.B., Bunn, C.C. and Bernstein, R.M. (1985). Autoantibodies to Jo-1 and other t-RNA related antigens in myositis. In *Rheumatology-85, Excerpta Medica International Congress* Series 675, ed. P.M. Brooks and J.R. York, pp. 189–92, Elsevier Science Publishers, Amsterdam.

Matter, L., Schopfer, K., Wilhelm, J.A., Nyffenegger, T., Parisot, R.F. and De Robertis, E.M. (1982). Molecular characterisation of ribonucleoprotein antigens bound by antinuclear antibodies. *Arthritis Rheum.* **25**, 1278–83.

Maul, G.G., Jimenez, S.A., Riggs, E. and Ziemnicka-Kotula, D. (1989). Determination of an epitope of the diffuse systemic sclerosis marker antigen DNA topoisomerase I: sequence similarity with retroviral $p30^{gag}$ protein suggests a possible cause for autoimmunity in systemic sclerosis. *Proc. Nat. Acad. Sci. (USA)* **86**, 8492–6.

Mellins, E., Malleson, P., Schaller, J. and Hansen, J. (1982). Childhood dermatomyositis: immunogenetic and family studies. *Arthritis Rheum.* **25**; S151.

Metzger, A.L., Bohan, A., Goldberg, L.S., Bluestone, R. and Pearson, C.M. (1974). Polymyositis and dermatomyositis: combined methotrexate and corticosteroid therapy. *Ann. Intern. Med.* **81**, 182–9.

Mihas, A.A., Kirby, J.D. and Kent, S.P. (1978). Hepatitis B antigen and polymyositis. *JAMA* **239**, 221–2.

Mikol, J., Felten-Papaiconomou, A., Ferchal, F. *et al.* (1982). Inclusion-body myositis: clinicopathological studies and isolation of an adenovirus type 2 from muscle biopsy specimen. *Ann. Neurol.* **11**, 576–81.

Miller, F.W., Love, L.A., Biswas, T., McClintock, P.R., Notkin, A.L. and Plotz, P.H. (1987). Viral and host genetic factors influence encephalomyocarditis virus-induced polymyositis in adult mice. *Arthritis Rheum.* **30**(5), 549–56.

Miller, F.W., Love, L.A., Barbieri, S.A., Balow, J.E. and Plotz, P.H. (1990a). Lymphocyte activation markers in idiopathic myositis: changes with disease activity and differences among clinical and autoantibody subgroups. *Clin. Exp. Immunol.* **81**, 373–9.

Miller, F.W., Twitty, S.A., Biswas, T. and Plotz, P.H. (1990b). The origin and regulation of a disease-specific autoantibody response: antigenic epitopes, spectrotype stability and isotope restriction of anti-Jo-1 autoantibodies. *J. Clin. Invest.* **85**, 468–75.

Miller, M.L., Lantner, R. and Pachman, L.M. (1983). Natural and antibody-dependent cellular cytotoxicity in children with systemic lupus erythematosus and juvenile dermatomyositis. *J. Rheumatol.* **10**, 640–2.

Miller, F.W., Leitman, S.F., Cronin, M.E. *et al.* (1991). Failure of plasma exchange and leukaphoresis to improve polymyositis or dermatomyositis: the results of a double-blind, randomised, sham-controlled trial. *Arthritis Rheum.* **34**, S52.

Mimori, T. (1987). Scleroderma–polymyositis overlap syndrome: clinical and serologic aspects. *Int. J. Dermatol.* **26** (7), 419–25.

Mimori, T., Akizuki, M., Yamagata, H., Inada, S. and Homma, M. (1981). Characterisation of a high molecular weight acidic nuclear protein recognised by autoantibodies in sera from patients with polymyositis–scleroderma overlap. *J. Clin. Invest.* **68**, 611–20.

Mimori, T., Hardin, J.A. and Steitz, J.A. (1986). Characterisation of the DNA-binding protein antigen Ku recognised by autoantibodies from patients with rheumatic disorders. *J. Biol. Chem.* **261**, 2274–8.

Minota, S., Koyasu, S., Yahara, I. and Winfield, J. (1988). Autoantibodies to the heat-shock protein hsp90 in systemic lupus erythematosus. *J. Clin. Invest.* **81**, 106–9.

Mora, C.A., Garruto, R.M., Brown, P. *et al.* (1988). Seroprevalence of antibodies to HTLV-I in patients with chronic neurological disorders other than tropical spastic paraparesis. *Ann. Neurol.* **23** (suppl.), S192–S195.

Morgan, O.S., Rodgers-Johnson, P., Mora, C. and Char, G. (1989). HTLV-1 and polymyositis in Jamaica. *Lancet* **ii** (8673), 1184–7.

Morgan, S.H., Bernstein, R.M., Copper, J., Halnan, K.E. and Hughes, G.R.V. (1985). Total body irradiation and the course of polymyositis. *Arthritis Rheum.* **28**, 831–5.

Moulds, J.M., Rolih, C., Goldstein, R. *et al.* (1990). C4 null genes in American whites and blacks with myositis. *J. Rheumatol.* **17**, 331–4.

Nishikai, M. and Homma, M. (1977). Circulating antibody against human myoglobin in polymyositis. *JAMA* **237**, 1842–4.

Nishikai, M. and Reichlin, M. (1980). Heterogeneity of precipitating antibodies in polymyositis: characterization of the Jo-1 antibody system. *Arthritis Rheum.* **23**, 881–8.

Nishino, H., Engel, A.G. and Rima, B.K. (1989). Inclusion body myositis: the mumps virus hypothesis. *Ann. Neurol. (US)* **25**, 260–4.

Oddis, C.V. and Medsger, T.A., Jr (1988). Relationship between serum creatine kinase level and corticosteroid therapy in polymyositis-dermatomyositis. *J. Rheumatol.* **15** (5), 807–11.

Okada, N., Mimori, T., Mukai, R., Kashiwagi, H. and Hardin, J.A. (1987). Characterization of human autoantibodies that selectively precipitate 7S RNA component of the signal recognition particle. *J. Immunol.* **138**, 3219–23.

O'Leary, P.A. and Waisman, M. (1940). Dermatomyositis: a study of forty cases. *Arch. Dermatol. Syph.* **41**, 1001–19.

Oppenheim, H. (1899). Zur Dermatomyositis. *Berl. Klin. Wochenschr.* **36**, 805–7.

Oxenhandler, R., Hart, M., Corman, L., Sharp, G.E. and Adelstein, E. (1977). Pathology of skeletal muscle in mixed connective tissue disease. *Arthritis Rheum.* **50**, 985–8.

Pachman, L.M. and Cooke, N. (1980). Juvenile dermatomyositis and polymyositis. *J. Paediatr.* **96**, 226–34.

Pachman, L.M., Jonasson, O., Cannon, R.A. and Friedman, J.M. (1977). HLA-B8 in juvenile dermatomyositis. *Lancet* **ii**, 567–8.

Pearson, C.M. (1956). Development of arthritis, peri-arthritis and periostitis in rats given adjuvants. *Proc. Exp. Biol. Med.* **91**, 95–101.

Pearson, C.M. (1962). Polymyositis and dermatomyositis. *Bull. Rheum. Dis.* **12**, 269.

Pearson, C.M. (1963). Patterns of polymyositis and their responses to treatment. *Ann. Intern. Med.* **59**, 827–38.

Pestronk, A., Drachman, D.B. and Self, S.G. (1985). Measurement of junctional acetylcholine receptors in myasthenia gravis: clinical correlates. *Muscle Nerve* **8** (3), 245–51.

Phillips, P.E., Kassan, S.S. and Kagen, L.J. (1979). Increased *Toxoplasma* antibodies in idiopathic inflammatory muscle disease: a case-controlled study. *Arthritis Rheum.* **22**, 209–14.

Plotz, P.H. (1983). Autoantibodies are anti-idiotype antibodies to anti-viral antibodies. *Lancet* **ii**, 824–6.

Plotz, P.H., Dalakas, M., Leff, R.L., Love, L.A., Miller, F.W. and Cronin, M.E. (1989). Current concepts in the idiopathic inflammatory myopathies: polymyositis, dermatomyositis and related disorders. *Ann. Intern. Med. (US)* **111**, 143–57.

Pollock, J.L. (1979). Toxoplasmosis appearing to be dermatomyositis. *Arch. Dermatol.* **115**, 736–7.

Potain, C.E. (1875). Morve chronique de forme anormale. *Bull. Soc. Med. Hôp. Paris* **12**, 314.

Query, C.C. and Keene, J.D. (1987). A human autoimmune protein associated with U1 RNA contains a region of homology that is cross-reactive with retrovirus p30gag antigen. *Cell* **51**, 211–20.

Ramsden, D.A., Chen, J., Miller, F.W. *et al.* (1989). Epitome mapping of the cloned human autoantigen, histidyl-tRNA synthetase: analysis of the myositis-associated anti-Jo-1 autoimmune response. *J. Immunol. (US)* **143**, 2267–72.

Ransohoff, R.M. and Dustoor, M.M. (1983). Impaired autologous mixed lymphocyte reaction with normal concanavalin A-induced suppression in adult polymyositis. *Clin. Exp. Immunol.* **53**, 67–75.

Ray, C.G., Minnich, L.L. and Johnson, P.C. (1979). Selective polymyositis induced by coxsackievirus B1 in mice. *J. Infect. Dis.* **140**, 239–43.

Reeves, W.H., Sanjay, K.N. and Gunter, B. (1986). Human autoantibodies reactive with the signal recognition particle. *Proc. Nat. Acad. Sci. (USA)* **84**, 9507–11.

Reichlin, M. and Arnett, F.C. (1984). Multiplicity of antibodies inmyositis sera. *Arthritis Rheum.* **27**, 1150–6.

Reichlin, M. and Mattioli, M. (1976). Description of serological reaction characteristic of polymyositis. *Clin. Immunol. Immunopathol.* **5**, 12–20.

Reichlin, M., Maddison, P.J., Targoff, I. *et al.* (1984). Antibodies to a nuclear/nucleolar antigen in patients with polymyositis-overlap syndromes. *J. Clin. Immunol.* **4**, 40–4.

Reimers, C.D., Pongratz, D.E., Neubert, U. *et al.* (1989). Myositis caused by *Borrelia burgdorferi*: report of four cases. *J. Neurol.* **91**, 215–26.

Rekvig, O.P. and Hannestad, K. (1980). Human autoantibodies that react with cell nuclei and plasma membranes display specificity for the octame of histones H2A, H2B, H3 and H4 in high salt. *J. Exp. Med.* **152**, 1720–33.

Ringel, S.P., Carry, M.R., Aguilera, A.J. and Starcevich, J.M. (1986). Quantitative histopathology of the inflammatory myopathies. *Arch. Neurol.* **43** (10), 1004–9.

Ringel, S.P., Kenny, C.E., Neville, H.E., Giornio, R. and Carry, M.R. (1987). Spectrum of inclusion body myositis. *Arch. Neurol.* **44**, 1154–7.

Rosa, M.D., Hendrick, J.P., Lerner, M.R., Steitz, J.A. and Reicklin, M. (1983). A mammalian $tRNA^{His}$ containing antigen is recognised by the polymyositis-specific antibody anti-Jo-1. *Nucleic Acids Res.* **11**, 853–70.

Rose, A.L. and Walton, J.N. (1966). Polymyositis: a survey of 89 cases with particular reference to treatment and prognosis. *Brain* **89**, 747–68.

Rosenberg, N.L., Ringel, S.P. and Kotzin, B.L. (1987). Experimental autoimmune myositis in SJL/J mice. *Clin. Exp. Immunol.* **68** (1), 117–29.

Rosenberg, N.L., Ringel, S.P. and Kotzin, B.L. (1989). Evidence for a novel picornavirus in human dermatomyositis. *Ann. Neurol.* **26**, 204–9.

Rosenschein, U., Radnay, J., Shohan, D., Shainberg, A., Klajman, A. and Rozenszajn, L.A. (1987). Human muscle-derived, tissue specific, myocytotoxic T cell lines in dermatomyositis. *Clin. Exp. Immunol.* **67**, 309–18.

Rowe, D.J., Isenberg, D.A., McDougall, J. and Beverley, P.C.L. (1981). Characterisation of polymyositis infiltrates using monoclonal antibodies to human leucocyte antigens. *Clin. Exp. Immunol.* **45**, 211–19.

Rowe, D.J., Isenberg, D.A. and Beverley, P.C.L. (1983). Monoclonal antibodies to human leucocyte antigens in polymyositis and muscular dystrophy. *Clin. Exp. Immunol.* **54**, 327–36.

Rowland, L.P. and Greer, M. (1961). Toxoplasmic polymyositis. *Neurology* **11**, 367–70.

Saito, E., Kinoshita, M., Oshima, H., Wada, F. and Yoshimoto, Y. (1987). Damaging effect of peripheral mononuclear cells of dermatomyositis on cultured human skin fibroblasts. *J. Rheumatol.* **14**, 936–41.

Saito, E., Yoshimoto, Y., Oshima, H., Yohida, H. and Kinoshita, M. (1989a). Fluorescent antibodies in polymyositis using cultured human skin fibroblasts: granular perinuclear cytoplasmic staining pattern by sera from patients with polymyositis and pulmonary fibrosis. *J. Rheumatol.* **16**, 47–54.

Saito, E., Kuroda, K., Yoshimoto, Y., Oshima, H. and Kinoshita, M. (1989b). Mechanism of the damaging effect of dermatomyositis mononuclear cells on cultured human skin fibroblasts. *J. Rheumatol.* **16**, 1055–60.

Santos-Buch, C.A., Acosta, A.M., Zweerink, H.J. *et al.* (1985). Primary muscle disease: definition of a 25-kDa polypeptide myopathic specific chagas antigen. *Clin. Immunol. Immunopathol.* **37** (3), 334–50.

Schifferli, J.A., Ng, Y.C. and Peters, D.K. (1986). The role of complement and its receptor in the clearance of immune complexes. *N. Engl. J. Med.* **315**, 488–95.

Schiraldi, O. and Iandolo, E. (1978). Polymyositis accompanying Coxsackie virus B2 infection. *Infection* **6**, 32–4.

Schuermann, H. (1951). Maligne Tumoren bei Dermatomyositis und progressive Sklerodermie. *Arch. Dermatol. Syph.* **192**, 575.

Schwartz, R.S. (1975). Viruses and systemic lupus erythematosus. *N. Engl. J. Med.* **293**, 132–6.

Scott, J.P. and Arroyave, C. (1987). Activation of complement and coagulation in juvenile dermatomyositis. *Arthritis Rheum.* **30**, 572–6.

Senecal, J., Oliver, J.M. and Rothfield, N. (1985). Anticytoskeletal autoantibodies in the connective tissue diseases. *Arthritis Rheum.* **28**, 889–98.

Sewry, C.A., Dubowitz, V., Abraha, A., Luzia, J.P. and Campbell, A.K. (1987). Immunocytochemical localisation of complement components C8 and C9 in human diseased muscle: the role of complement in muscle fibre damage. *J. Neurol. Sci.* **81**, 141–53.

Shero, J.H., Bordwell, B., Rothfield, N.F. and Earnshaw, W.C. (1986). High titres of autoantibodies to topoisomerase I (Scl-70) in sera from scleroderma patients. *Science* **231**, 737–40.

Shy, G.M. (1962). The late onset myopathy — a clinicopathologic study of 131 patients. *World Neurol.* **3**, 149–60.

Steiner, W.R. (1903). Dermatomyositis, with report of a case which presented a rare muscle anomaly but once described in man. *J. Exp. Med.* **6**, 407–43.

Stertz, G. (1916). Verhandlungen arztlicher Gesellschaften. *Berl. Klin. Wochenschr.* **53**, 488–9.

Strongwater, S.L. (1988). Overview and clinical manifestations of inflammatory myositis: polymyositis and dermatomyositis. *Mt Sinai J. Med.* **55**, 435–46.

Strongwater, S.L., Dorovini-Zes, K., Ball, R.D. and Schnitzer, T.J. (1984). A murine model of polymyositis induced by coxsackie virus B1 (Tucson strain). *Arthritis Rheum.* **27**, 433–42.

Takahashi, K., Ogita, T., Okudaira, H., Yoshinoya, S., Yoshizawa, H. and Miyamoto, T. (1986). D-penicillamine-induced polymyositis in patients with rheumatoid arthritis. *Arthritis Rheum.* **29**, 560–4.

Takeda, Y., Wang, G.S., Wang, R.J. *et al.* (1989). Enzyme-linked immunoabsorbent assay using isolated (U) small nuclear ribonucleoprotein polypeptides as antigens to investigate the clinical significance of autoantibodies to these polypeptides. *Clin. Immunol. Immunopathol.* **50**, 213–30.

Takizawa, H., Shiga, J., Moroi, Y., Miyachi, S., Nishiwaki, M. and Miyamoto, T. (1987). Interstitial lung disease in dermatomyositis: clinicopathological study. *J. Rheumatol.* **14**, 102–7.

Talal, N., Dauphinée, M.J., Dang, H., Alexander, S.S., Hart, D.J. and Garry, R.F. (1990). Detection of serum antibodies to retroviral proteins in patients with primary Sjögren's syndrome (autoimmune exocrinopathy). *Arthritis Rheum.* **33**, 774–81.

Tang, T.T., Sedmar, G.V., Siegesmund, K.A. and McCreadie, S.R. (1975). Chronic myopathy associated with coxsackie virus type A9: a combined electron microscopical and viral isolation study. *N. Engl. J. Med.* **292**, 608–11.

Targoff, I.N. (1990). Autoantibodies to aminoacyl-transfer RNA synthetases for isoleucine and glycine. Two additional synthetases are antigenic in myositis. *J. Immunol.* **144**, 1737–43.

Targoff, I.N. and Hanas, J. (1989). The polymyositis-associated Fer antigen is elongation factor 1α. *Arthritis Rheum.* **32**, S81.

Targoff, I.N. and Reichlin, M. (1985). The association between Mi-2 antibodies and dermatomyositis. *Arthritis Rheum.* **28**, 796–803.

Targoff, I.N. and Reichlin, M. (1987). Measurement of antibody to Jo-1 by ELISA and comparison to enzyme inhibitory activity. *J. Immunol.* **138**, 2874–82.

Targoff, I.N. and Reichlin, M. (1988). Antibody to threonyl-transfer RNA synthetase in myositis sera. *Arthritis Rheum.* **31**, 515–24.

Targoff, I.N., Johnson, A.E. and Miller, F.W. (1990). Antibody to signal recognition particle in polymyositis. *Arthritis Rheum.* **33**, 1361–70.

Targoff, I.N., Raghu, G. and Reichlin, M. (1983). Antibodies to Mi-1 in SLE: relationship to other precipitins and reaction with bovine immunoglobulin. *Clin. Exp. Immunol.* **53**, 76–82.

Targoff, I.N., Arnett, F.C., Berman, L., O'Brien, C. and Reichlin, M. (1989). Anti-KJ: a new antibody associated with the syndrome of polymyositis and interstitial lung disease. *J. Clin. Invest. (US)* **84**, 162–72.

Teo, P., Tai, T.H. and Choy, D. (1989). Nasopharyngeal carcinoma with dermatomyositis. *Int. J. Radiation. Oncol. Biol. Phys.* **16** (2), 471–4.

The, H.S.G., Jacobs, P. and Houben, H. (1985). Cyclosporin in the treatment of intractable polymyositis. *Arthritis Rheum.* **28**, 1436–7.

Thiry, M., Humbel, R., Dicato, M., Goessens, G., Meyers, R. and Ries, F. (1988). Electron microscopy proves Jo-1 antigen to be predominantly cytoplasmic but also nuclear. *Biomed. Pharmacother.* **42** (7), 469–71.

Topi, G.C., D'Alessandro, L., Catricala, C. and Zardi, O. (1979). Dermatomyositis-like syndrome due to *Toxoplasma*. *Br. J. Dermatol.* **101**, 589–91.

Travers, R.L., Hughes, G.R.V., Cambridge, G. and Sewell, J.R. (1977). Coxsackie B neutralisation titres in polymyositis/dermatomyositis. *Lancet* **i**, 1268.

Tsui, F.W. and Siminovitch, L. (1987). Structural analysis of the 5′ region of the chromosomal gene for hamster histidyl-tRNA synthetase. *Gene* **61**, 349–61.

Unverricht, H. (1887). Polymyositis acuta progressiva. *Z. Klin. Med.* **12**, 533–49.

Unverricht, H. (1891). Dermatomyositis acuta. *Dtsch. Med. Wochenschr.* **17**, 41–4.

Von Kreuter, B.F. and Santos-Buch, C.A. (1986). Pathoimmune polymyositis induced in C3H/HeJ mice by *Trypanosoma cruzi* infection. *Clin. Exp. Rheumatol.* **4** (1), 83–9.

Wada, K., Ueno, S., Hazama, T. *et al.* (1983). Radioimmunoassay for antibodies to human skeletal muscle myosin in serum from patients with polymyositis. *Clin. Exp. Immunol.* **52**, 297–304.

Wagner, E. (1863). Fall einer seltenen Muskelkrankheit. *Arch. Heilkh.* **4**, 282.

Walker E.J. and Jeffrey, P.D. (1988). Sequence homology between encephalomyocarditis virus protein VPI and histidyl-tRNA synthetase supports a hypothesis of molecular mimicry in polymyositis. *Med. Hypotheses* **25**, 21–5.

Walker, G.L., Mastaglia, F.L. and Roberts, D.F. (1982). A search for genetic influence in idiopathic inflammatory myopathy. *Acta Neurol. Scand.* **66**, 432–3.

Walton, J.N. and Adams, R.D. (1958). *Polymyositis*. E. and S. Livingstone, London.

Webster, A.D.B. (1984). Echovirus disease in hypogammaglobulinaemic patients. *Clin. Rheum. Dis.* **10**, 189–203.

Whitaker, J.N. and Engel, W.K. (1972). Vascular deposits of immunoglobulin and complement in idiopathic inflammatory myopathy. *N. Engl. J. Med.* **286**, 333–8.

Wiley, C.A., Nerenberg, M., Cros, D. and Soto-Aguilar, M.C. (1989). HTLV-1 polymyositis in a patient also infected with the human immunodeficiency virus. *N. Engl. J. Med.* **320**, 992–5.

Wolf, R.E. and Baethge, B.A. (1990). Interleukin-1α, interleukin-2, and soluble interleukin-2 receptors in polymyositis. *Arthritis Rheum.* **33**, 1007–14.

Wolfe, J.F., Adelstein, E. and Sharp, G.C. (1977). Antinuclear antibody with distinct specificity for polymyositis. *J. Clin. Invest.* **59**, 176.

Woodruff, J.F. (1980). Viral myocarditis. *Am. J. Pathol.* **101**, 425–84.

Woodruff, J.F. and Woodruff, J.J. (1974). Involvement of T lymphocytes in the pathogenesis of coxsackie virus B3 heart disease. *J. Immunol.* **133**, 1726–34.

Yaneva, M. and Arnett, F.C. (1989). Antibodies against Ku protein in sera from patients with autoimmune diseases. *Clin. Exp. Immunol.* **76**, 366–72.

Yang, V.W., Lerner, M.R., Steitz, J.A. and Flint, S.J. (1981). A small nuclear ribonucleoprotein is required for splicing of adenoviral early RNA sequences. *Proc. Nat. Acad. Sci. (USA)* **78**, 1371–5.

Yoshida, S., Akizuki, M., Mimori, T., Yamagata, H., Inada, S. and Homma, M. (1983). The precipitating antibody to an acidic nuclear protein antigen, the Jo-1, in connective tissue diseases: a marker for a subset of polymyositis with interstitial pulmonary fibrosis. *Arthritis Rheum.* **26**, 604–11.

Yousef, G.E., Isenberg, D.A. and Mowbray, J.F. (1990). Detection of enterovirus-specific RNA sequences in muscle biopsies from patients with adult onset myositis. *Ann. Rheum. Dis.* **49**, 310–15.

Ytterberg, S.R. (1988). Cellular immunity in polymyositis-dermatomyositis. *Mt Sinai J. Med.* **55**, 494–500.

Ytterberg, S.R., Mahowald, M.L. and Messner, R.P. (1987). Coxsackievirus B1-induced polymyositis: lack of disease expression in nu/nu mice. *J. Clin. Invest.* **80**, 499–506.

Ytterberg, S.R., Mahowald, M.L. and Messner, R.P. (1988) T cells are required for coxsackievirus B1 induced murine polymyositis. *J. Rheumatol.* **15**, 475–8.

Zabel, P., Leimenstoll, A. and Gross, W.L. (1984). Cyclosporin for acute dermatomyositis. *Lancet* **i**, 343.

Zhang, H.Y., Yousef, G.E., Bowles, N.E., Archard, L.C., Mann, G.F. and Mowbray, J.F. (1988). Detection of enterovirus RNA in experimentally infected mice by molecular hybridisation: specificity of subgenomic probes in quantitative slot blot and *in situ* hybridisation. *J. Med. Virol.* **26**, 375–86.

Zuk, J.A. and Fletcher, A. (1988). Skeletal muscle expression of class II histocompatibility antigens (HLA-DR) in polymyositis and other muscle disorders with an inflammatory infiltrate. *J. Clin. Pathol.* **41**, 410–14.

64: Systemic Sclerosis (Scleroderma) and Mixed Connective Tissue Disease

G. Reimer and E.M. Tan

Systemic sclerosis (scleroderma)

Systemic sclerosis is a generalized disorder of the connective tissue clinically characterized by skin thickening, Raynaud's phenomenon and involvement of vital internal organs such as the lung, the heart, the gastrointestinal tract and the kidney (reviewed by Barnett 1974; Siegel 1977; LeRoy 1985; Medsger 1985a).

The recognition of systemic sclerosis as a distinct systemic disease entity has developed only recently. The disease has an annual mortality in the United States of between 2.1 and 2.8 per million population in two recent studies (Medsger 1985b; Hochberg *et al.* 1980). The average onset of initial scleroderma symptoms was reported between 40 and 50 years of age (Medsger and Masi 1971). Systemic sclerosis also occurs in childhood (Kass *et al.* 1966; Ansell *et al.* 1976). All ethnic groups are affected by the disease. The overall female-to-male ratio in scleroderma is 3 : 1 in Caucasians (Medsger 1985b). Several large survival studies have indicated a 5-year cumulative survival rate of between 34% and 73% (Medsger and Masi 1971) and a 10-year survival rate of between 71% and 21% (Barnett *et al.* 1988). Male sex, old age and involvement of the kidneys, heart and lungs contribute to a poorer prognosis. There appears to be no well-defined predisposing genetic background for acquiring systemic sclerosis, although there have been a number of reports of familial scleroderma (Greger 1975). Recent studies have indicated a human leucocyte antigen (HLA) association of diffuse scleroderma with A1, B8, DR5 and DR3 antigens, and the CREST (calcinosis, Raynaud's phenomenon, oesophageal dysmotility, sclerodactyly, telangiectasia) syndrome (for classification of scleroderma syndromes, see below) with DR5 and DR1 antigens (Gladman *et al.* 1981; Kallenberg *et al.* 1981; Black *et al.* 1984; Steen *et al.* 1988). However, these HLA associations with scleroderma have been questioned in other studies (Lynch *et al.* 1982; Alarcon *et al.* 1985). It is anticipated as more and more information on subgroups of patients with scleroderma is obtained that HLA associations with certain disease manifestations may evolve.

Diagnosis and classification

The term scleroderma has been applied to various cutaneous disorders characterized by hardening, tightening and inelasticity of the skin. Localized forms of scleroderma must be clearly distinguished from systemic forms. Localized scleroderma includes morphoea of the single or multiple (generalized) type and linear scleroderma with or without melorheostosis. Scleroderma *en coup de sabre*, with or without facial hemiatrophy, is the other well-recognized form of linear disease.

There are many skin diseases and systemic disorders with skin thickening as a prominent feature which must also be separated from progressive systemic sclerosis. They include diseases such as eosinophilic fasciitis (Shulman 1975; Barnes *et al.* 1979), chronic graft-versus-host disease in patients receiving bone marrow transplants, vinyl chloride disease, toxic oil syndrome (Tabuenca 1981), scleromyxoedema and Werner's syndrome. The latter diseases are not part of the spectrum of spontaneous systemic autoimmune diseases and may be differentiated by history, clinical and laboratory investigations.

Systemic sclerosis (progressive systemic sclerosis; systemic scleroderma) is a generalized, progressive, systemic, autoimmune disease, usually with Raynaud's phenomenon, skin thickening and arthritis as early clinical features. In some patients, dysphagia or intestinal motility disturbances may antedate skin thickening by years (systemic sclerosis *sine* scleroderma). The pattern of skin and internal organ involvement, however, varies in different patients, adding to the difficulties in establishing an early diagnosis. The lungs are a major internal organ target in scleroderma (Greenwald *et al.* 1987; McCarthy *et al.* 1988). Except for the occurrence of disease-specific antinuclear/antinucleolar serum autoantibodies such as anti-Scl-70 and anti-centromere antibodies (see below), there are no diagnostic laboratory tests available to separate systemic sclerosis from other chronic inflammatory diseases. The diagnosis of systemic sclerosis is traditionally based on clinical criteria, but, with the new information showing that there are auto-antibodies specific for scleroderma, this attitude is rapidly changing.

To define criteria for the diagnosis of systemic sclerosis, a prospective multicentre study was conducted by the American Rheumatism Association in 1980 (Masi *et al.* 1980). In this study, 264 patients with systemic sclerosis were compared with 413 patients suffering from other systemic autoimmune diseases or isolated Raynaud's disease. Sclerodermatous skin changes proximal to the digits were the distinguishing findings in the systemic sclerosis patient group, being present in 91% of the cases versus 1% in the control group. Sclerodactyly, digital pitting scars and bibasilar pulmonary fibrosis on chest roentgenography were established as the three minor criteria for the diagnosis of systemic sclerosis.

Systemic sclerosis is a heterogeneous disease group with a large variation of clinical manifestation and pattern of skin and internal organ involvement. It is therefore not surprising that many attempts have been made to establish a classification of the disease. These classifications distinguish between vascular–fibrotic and mesenchymal–diffuse forms of scleroderma (Winkelmann 1971, 1976), or recognize different degrees of skin involvement (Barnett 1974; Arbeitsgruppe Sklerodermie der Arbeitsgemeinschaft Dermatologische Forschung 1980; Holzmann *et al.* 1987) or distinct clinical manifestations such as the CREST syndrome and diffuse scleroderma (Winterbauer 1964; Rodnan *et al.* 1976; Giordano *et al.* 1980; Steen *et al.* 1980). Most authors distinguish between a more limited, cutaneous, stationary form of systemic sclerosis, i.e. acroscleroderma or the CREST syndrome, and the progressive, severe, diffuse, cutaneous form of scleroderma (Table 64.1) (Krieg and Meurer 1988; LeRoy *et al.* 1988).

Mixed connective tissue disease

For many years clinical rheumatologists have seen patients with concomitant clinical features of more than one defined systemic autoimmune disease and thus which did not fit the rigid classification. These patients usually display clinical findings of more than one systemic rheumatic disease, including systemic lupus erythematosus (SLE), systemic sclerosis (scleroderma) and polymyositis.

In 1972 Sharp and co-workers defined a group of patients with clinical features of polyarthritis, severe Raynaud's phenomenon, swollen hands or sclerodactyly, restrictive pulmonary disease, myositis and oesophageal dysmotility. Lymphadenopathy, alopecia, malar rash, serositis, cardiac

Table 64.1. Comparison of clinical features and cumulative survival in patients with diffuse scleroderma and the CREST syndrome

	Diffuse scleroderma (n = 305)	CREST syndrome (n = 256)
Demographic		
Age (< 40 at onset)	36.0%	51.0%
Race (non-white)	11.0%	2.0%
Sex (female)	73.0%	83.0%
Duration of symptoms (years)	4.0	11.5
Organ system involvement		
Skin (total skin score)	35.2	8.6
Telangiectasia	32.0%	82.0%
Calcinosis	7.0%	43.0%
Raynaud's phenomenon	86.0%	95.0%
Arthralgias or arthritis	80.0%	58.0%
Tendon friction rubs	67.0%	6.0%
Contractures	84.0%	45.0%
Myopathy	19.0%	8.0%
Oesophageal hypomotility	75.0%	77.0%
Pulmonary fibrosis	35.0%	37.0%
Pulmonary hypertension	< 1.0%	11.0%
Congestive heart failure	10.0%	1.0%
Renal 'crisis'	17.0%	1.0%
Cumulative survival (10 years from first diagnosis)	57.0%	75.0%

Steen *et al.* 1982.

and renal disease were less frequently observed (Table 64.2). In evaluating the sera for the presence of antinuclear antibodies, almost all these patients had a high titre (frequently >1:1 000 000 by haemagglutination) of antibodies to a ribonuclease (RNase)-sensitive antigen designated nuclear ribonucleoprotein (RNP). These serological findings have been confirmed in independent studies by other investigators (Parker 1973; Farber and Boyle 1976; Sharp *et al.* 1976; Grennan *et al.* 1977; Lemmer *et al.* 1982; Matter *et al.* 1982; Field *et al.* 1983; Williamson *et al.* 1983). The nature of this nuclear RNP antigen has been revealed in greater detail over the last 10 years and shown to be a small nuclear RNP particle complexed with U1 ribonucleic acid (RNA) (Lerner and Steitz 1979). High-titre antibodies against U1 RNP were the distinguishing feature between this disease entity, called mixed connective tissue disease (MCTD), and 'overlap syndromes', which should be reserved for patients who have overlapping features of two diseases such as combinations of SLE and scleroderma or SLE and rheumatoid arthritis or scleroderma and dermatomyositis (reviewed by Bennett 1985; Sharp and Singsen 1985).

Patients with MCTD were initially found to suffer from a disease with infrequent renal involvement, a good response to corticosteroids and a favourable prognosis (Sharp *et al.* 1972). Subsequently, it was observed that renal disease is not absent but may occur in 10–20% of cases (Mattioli and Reichlin 1973; Bennett and Spargo 1977; Nimelstein *et al.* 1980; Wiener-Kronish *et al.* 1981). Severe pulmonary involvement is also a frequent finding and may contribute to a poorer prognosis (Wiener-Kronish *et al.* 1981; Sullivan *et al.* 1984). The long-term outcome for patients with MCTD, therefore, should not *a priori* be considered to be benign.

There was debate over whether MCTD constitutes a distinct clinical entity, but this attitude is rapidly receding. In order to define MCTD clinically in a more standardized way, it would be helpful to use criteria as established in a multicentre study in Japan (Kasukawa *et al.* 1988). In this study, anti-RNP antibodies together with

Table 64.2. Characteristic features of 34 patients with mixed connective tissue disease

	Number	Percentage
Raynaud's phenomenon	31	91%
Polyarthritis	29	85%
Swollen hands or sclerodactyly	29	85%
Pulmonary disease	29	85%
Inflammatory myositis	27	79%
Oesophageal hypomotility	25	74%
Lymphadenopathy	17	50%
Alopecia	13	41%
Pleuritis	12	35%
Malar rash	10	29%
Renal disease	9	26%
Cardiac disease	9	26%
Anaemia	8	24%
Leucopenia	7	21%
Diffuse scleroderma	7	21%
Sjögren's syndrome	4	12%
Trigeminal neuropathy	2	6%
Positive antinuclear antibody	34	100%
Positive RNP antibody	34	100%
Positive rheumatoid factor	20	59%
Hypergammaglobulinaemia	18	53%
Hypocomplementaemia	11	32%
Positive lupus erythematosus (LE) cell test	6	18%

Sullivan *et al.* 1984.

either Raynaud's phenomenon or swelling of fingers or hands are required for establishing the diagnosis. In addition, other clinical findings are necessary items and they include symptoms and/or signs derived from at least two of the three diseases, SLE, scleroderma and polymyositis.

Aetiopathogenic aspects of systemic sclerosis

The aetiology of systemic sclerosis is unknown and its pathogenesis is poorly understood. From clinical, immunological and histopathological observations, three major events appear to be involved in the pathogenesis of scleroderma. These include vascular alterations, disturbances in connective tissue metabolism and its regulation and an abnormal immune response.

Vascular changes of the small arteries and microvessels in the skin and internal organs shown by histology and electron microscopy are prominent pathological findings (Norton and Nardo 1970; Fleischmajer and Perlish 1980). *In vivo*, these changes can be viewed by nail-fold capillary microscopy and consist of rarefication and dilatation of the remaining vessels (Maricq *et al.* 1982). The exact pathological events that lead to alterations of the small vessels are not known. However, serum factors cytotoxic to vascular endothelium have been detected in patients with systemic sclerosis (Kahaleh *et al.* 1979; Cohen *et al.* 1983; Drenk and Deicher 1988). However, in another study the specificity of endothelial cell cytotoxicity could not be demonstrated (Shanahan and Korn 1982). Clearly, the exact molecular nature of these cytotoxic factors needs to be revealed before their role in vascular injury can be assessed.

It is believed that damage of endothelial cells leads to release of potent factors from aggregated platelets, such as platelet-derived growth factor and transforming growth factor β. These factors, in conjunction with epidermal growth factor, are known to cause fibrosis when injected into nude mice (Roberts *et al.* 1986) and may also play a role in the events leading to fibrosis in scleroderma. An altered permeability of the vessels may also account for the penetration of mononuclear cells through the vessel wall and the formation of perivascular infiltrates. These mononuclear cells themselves may release potent mediators of inflammation, such as interleukin 1, which have a stimulating effects on the synthesis of collagen from the surrounding fibroblasts (Postlewaite *et al.* 1984). Indeed, the fibroblast in scleroderma appears to play a crucial role in the events leading to fibrosis (Peltonen *et al.* 1985). For example, enhanced production of type I and II collagens, glycoaminoglycans and fibronectin by lesional fibroblast is a characteristic finding in scleroderma (Krieg *et al.* 1977; LeRoy 1974; Fleischmajer *et al.* 1981). Elevated levels of fibronectin have been found in involved skin and bronchoalveolar lavage fluid, and their role as a growth factor for fibroblasts has been established (Rennard *et al.* 1981; Bitterman *et al.* 1983).

Evidence of an involvement of the immune system in the pathogenesis of scleroderma comes from observations such as the occurrence of an early lymphohistiocytic perivascular infiltrate in the skin (Fleischmajer *et al.* 1977; Roumm *et al.* 1984), lymphohistiocytic cells in bronchoalveolar lavage fluid (Bitterman *et al.* 1982), circulating immune complexes (Chen *et al.* 1984; Silver *et al.* 1986), decreased numbers of peripheral T lympho-

(Douvas *et al.* 1979; Tan *et al.* 1980; Bernstein *et al.* 1982). Further analysis with antigen extracted from rat liver showed that it appeared to be a protein of 70 kD by SDS gel electrophoresis and it was named Scl-70 (Douvas *et al.* 1979). In subsequent studies, the Scl-70 antigen was found to have a higher molecular weight, ranging from 86 kD (van Venrooji *et al.* 1985) to 95/100 kD (Alderuccio *et al.* 1986).

Independently, three different laboratories showed that anti-Scl-70 antibodies reacted with DNA topoisomerase I with a native molecular weight of about 100 kD (Guldner *et al.* 1986; Maul *et al.* 1986; Shero *et al.* 1986). The differences in the molecular weights of the Scl-70 antigen reported in earlier studies were shown to be due to degradation of this enzyme during extraction procedures in the absence of protease inhibitors, generating smaller immunoreactive fragments. Autoantibodies were shown to be capable of inhibiting the relaxation of supercoiled DNA induced by topoisomerase. It was also shown that topoisomerase I (Scl-70) is located within the nucleolus (Guldner *et al.* 1986), leading to subsequent observations of the nucleolus being a frequent target of scleroderma autoantibodies (Tan *et al.* 1980; Bernstein *et al.* 1982). The antigen was located in the fibrillar component of nucleoli by immunoelectromicroscopy (Rose *et al.* 1988; Raska *et al.* 1989).

This antibody was detected by immunodiffusion in 8–26% of an unselected scleroderma population (Tan *et al.* 1980; Bernstein *et al.* 1982; McCarty *et al.* 1983; Black *et al.* 1984; Meurer *et al.* 1985; Takehara *et al.* 1985; Jarzabek-Chorzelska *et al.* 1986) and in later studies, using the same assay system, it was reported to be detected in 75% of patients with diffuse scleroderma (Jarzabek-Chorzelska *et al.* 1986). Using immunoblotting techniques, anti-Scl-70 antibodies were detected in the sera from 40% (van Venrooji *et al.* 1985) and 28% of scleroderma patients (Weiner *et al.* 1988).

Antibody against Scl-70 antigen was shown in many clinical studies to be a marker antibody for scleroderma (Douvas *et al.* 1979; Tan *et al.* 1980; Cattogio *et al.* 1983; Meurer *et al.* 1985; van Venrooji *et al.* 1985; Jarzabek-Chorzelska *et al.* 1986). Of more than 300 patients with connective tissue disease other than scleroderma, <1% displayed anti-Scl-70 antibodies in their sera (Fritzler *et al.* 1980).

Anti-Scl-70 antibodies were found to be associated with diffuse scleroderma (Meurer *et al.* 1985; van Venrooji *et al.* 1985; Cattogio *et al.* 1985; Giordano *et al.* 1986; Jarzabek-Chorzelska *et al.* 1986). Clinically, diffuse scleroderma, an increased frequency of pulmonary interstitial fibrosis and peripheral vascular disease (digital pitting scars) have been observed in a recent and comprehensive clinical study of individuals with positive anti-Scl-70 antibodies. These antibodies, however, were not predictive of cardiac or renal involvement or of survival (Steen *et al.* 1988).

Convincing clinical data have emerged showing that anti-Scl-70 antibodies are marker antibodies for scleroderma. From these data it appears that the majority of patients with this antibody specificity suffer from diffuse scleroderma and rarely from the CREST syndrome, a more limited form of the disease. Anti-Scl-70 antibodies may be valuable tools not only in helping to establish the diagnosis of early scleroderma but also in predicting the natural course of the disease.

Autoantibodies against centromere (kinetochore)

Autoantibodies to centromere antigens were detected on the basis of a distinct pattern of immunofluorescent localization on tissue culture cell substrates (Fritzler *et al.* 1980; Moroi *et al.* 1981; Tan *et al.* 1980). A finite number of punctate spots in the nucleoplasm was observed to react with certain sera from scleroderma patients but the distinguishing feature was in dividing cells. The antigen segregated with and co-localized in the region of condensing metaphase chromosomes. Subsequently, immunolocalization was achieved with isolated metaphase chromosomes, which were not treated with acetic acid since the latter destroyed its antigenicity, and staining was observed in the primary constrictions of isolated chromosomes (Fig. 64.1). By immunoelectromicroscopy, centromeric antigens were localized to the inner and outer layers of the trilaminar kinetochore structure with no reaction with centromeric DNA (Brenner *et al.* 1981). Several laboratories have shown that the centromere autoantigens, which are highly conserved during evolution, consist of three proteins of 17/19 kD, 80 kD and 140 kD (Cox *et al.* 1983; Guldner *et al.* 1985; Earnshaw *et al.* 1986), and a cDNA clone which encodes about 95% of the mRNA for the 80 kD protein has been isolated (Earnshaw *et al.* 1987). Three independent antigenic epitopes have been recognized on this protein by subcloning

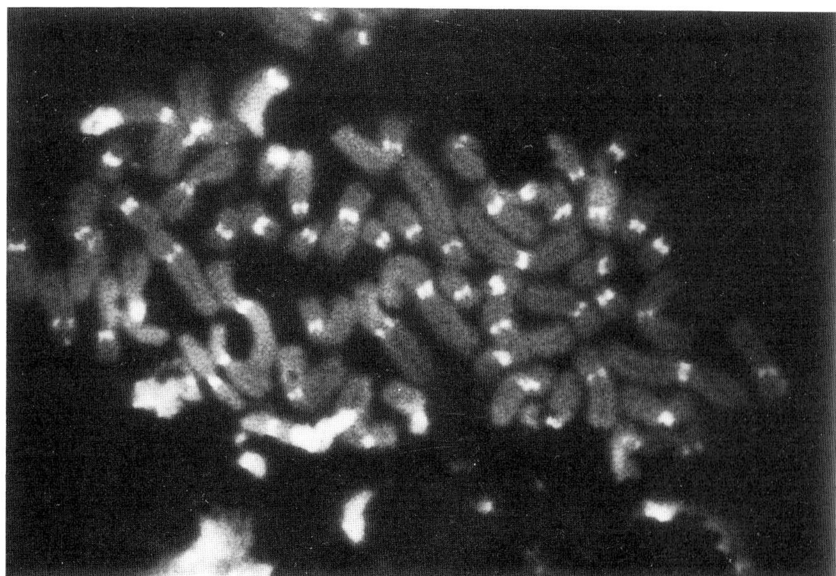

Fig. 64.1. Isolated chromosomes unfixed or fixed with acetic acid were used as substrates to localize centromere antigens. They are visible as paired structures at the centromeric regions or primary constrictions of individual chromosomes (× 2500).

of cDNA restriction fragments and analysis of expressed fusion proteins.

Autoantibodies to centromere are present in 44–98% of patients with the CREST subset of the disease (Fritzler *et al.* 1980; Tan *et al.* 1980; Catoggio *et al.* 1983; McCarty *et al.* 1983; Steen *et al.* 1988; Chorzelski *et al.* 1985; Meurer *et al.* 1985; Weiner *et al.* 1988). Anti-centromere antibodies were found to be highly specific for scleroderma in a survey on patients with connective tissue diseases (Fritzler *et al.* 1980) and the 2% of the other-category patients who were positive for anti-centromere antibodies almost always had primary Raynaud's phenomenon (Kallenberg *et al.* 1982; Tramposch *et al.* 1984; Gerbracht *et al.* 1985). In another study, approximately 25% of patients with idiopathic Raynaud's phenomenon (without other signs or symptoms of CREST) had anti-centromere antibodies (Maricq *et al.* 1982). These patients may have an early variant of CREST or a *forme fruste* and need to be followed up clinically.

Several clinical studies on the association with anti-centromere antibodies have been conducted and in almost all of these studies anti-centromere antibodies have been correlated with the more limited CREST variant of systemic sclerosis (Fritzler *et al.* 1980; Kleinsmith *et al.* 1982; McCarty *et al.* 1983; Steen *et al.* 1984, 1988; Tramposch *et al.* 1984; Meurer *et al.* 1985; Weiner *et al.* 1988). In the last study, anti-centromere antibodies were almost exclusively (96%) associated with the CREST syndrome, and the majority (57%) of the patients with a limited scleroderma subset did not have this antibody specificity. Anti-centromere antibodies were associated with more calcinosis and telangiectasia and less often had pulmonary fibrosis and restrictive lung disease (Table 64.4).

Autoantibodies against ribonucleic acid polymerase I

Autoantibodies against nucleolar antigens are a prominent serological finding in scleroderma (Beck *et al.* 1963; Fennell *et al.* 1962; Ritchie 1970; Pinnas *et al.* 1973; Tan *et al.* 1980; Bernstein *et al.* 1982). Different nucleolar staining patterns indicated a diversity in the reactive antigens (Bernstein *et al.* 1982).

In a study on the specificity of autoantibodies in scleroderma, 3% of patients were shown to produce punctate nucleolar staining by immunofluorescence in all the tissue culture cells used as substrate (Reimer *et al.* 1987b). In dividing cells, prominent staining of the nucleolar organizing regions (NOR) was observed (Fig. 64.2(a)). In 5,6-dichloro-β-D-ribofuranosyl-benzimidazole (DRB)- and actinomycin-D-segregated nucleoli, drugs which segregate nucleoli into granular and fibrillar regions (Busch and Smetana 1970), immunofluorescence staining was exclusively localized in the fibrillar regions. The granular component is known to contain the preribosomal particles whereas the fibrillar component contains nuclear proteins such as protein C23 (Ochs *et al.* 1983),

Table 64.4. Clinical features in 397 systemic sclerosis patients with antibodies to anti-Scl-70 and anti-centromere antibodies

	ACA +ve (n = 86)	ACA −ve, anti-Scl-70 −ve (n = 209)	Anti-Scl-70 +ve (n = 102)	P
Raynaud's phenomenon	97	94	97	NS
Digital pitting scars	63	56	79	< 0.05
Digital ulcers	48	33	54	NS
Mean total skin score	7	27	31	< 0.001
Telangiectasia	97	74	75	< 0.001
Calcinosis	69	24	24	< 0.001
Muscle involvement	16	28	32	< 0.05
Joint involvement	49	66	77	< 0.05
Tendon involvement	3	44	54	< 0.001
GI tract	78	64	83	NS
Lung	34	42	57	< 0.005
Heart	6	13	16	< 0.05
Kidney	0	10	6	< 0.05

Values are percentages.
ACA = anti-centromere antibodies; NS = not significant.
Steen *et al*. 1984.

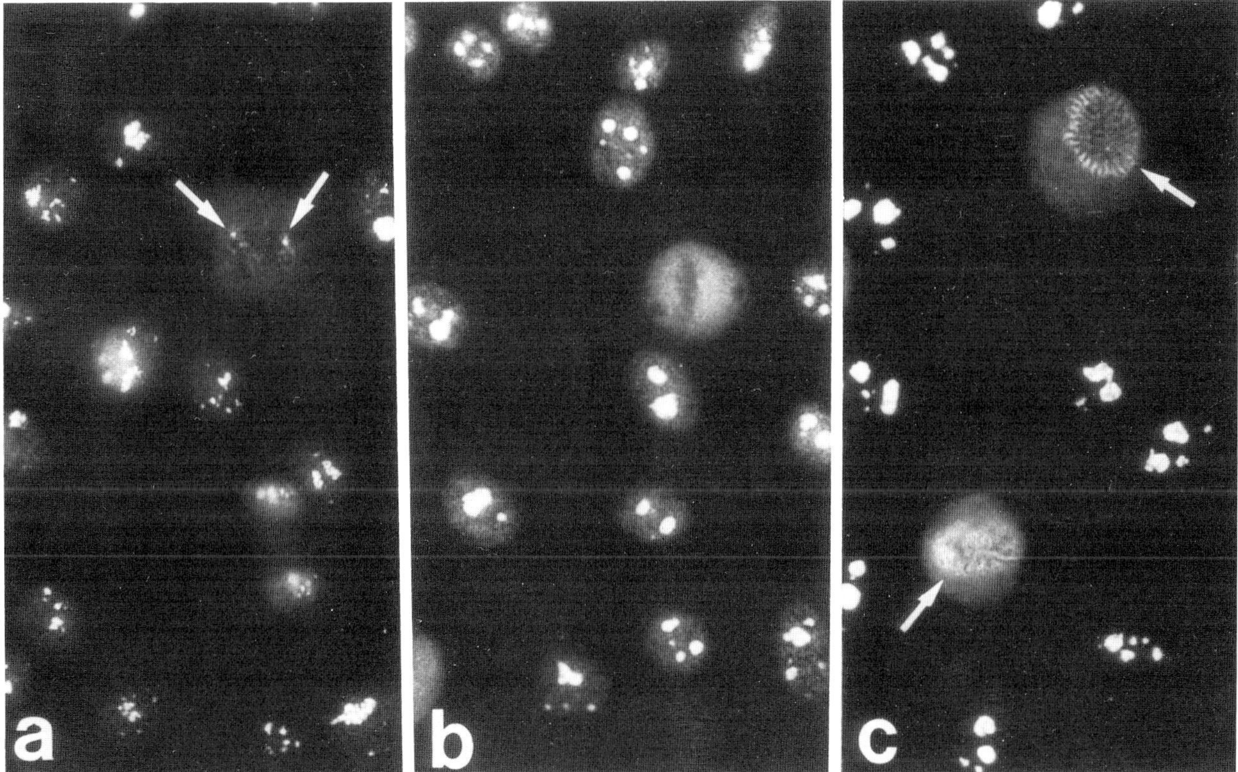

Fig. 64.2. Nucleolar staining patterns for IgG produced by scleroderma sera diluted 1 : 40 in phosphate buffered saline and processed by indirect immunofluorescence using Hep-2 cells are substrate. (a) Speckled (punctate) nucleolar staining representative of anti-RNA polymerase I serum. Arrows indicate the putative nucleolar organizing regions of a mitotic cell. (b) Homogeneous nucleolar staining with an anti-PM-Scl serum. (c) Clumpy nucleolar staining produced by a representative anti-U3-RNP serum. In metaphase cells (arrows), significant staining of the condensed chromosomes is present (magnification ×565).

fibrillarin (Ochs *et al*. 1985) and RNA polymerase I (Scheer and Rose 1984). The immunofluorescent staining properties of these scleroderma autoantibodies were identical to those described with the rabbit antibodies specific for RNA polymerase I (Scheer and Rose, 1984; Reimer *et al*. 1987b). By electron-microscopic immunocytochemistry, antibodies from certain scleroderma patients were shown to bind in the fibrillar centres but not in the granular component or dense fibrillar component of nucleoli (Reimer *et al*. 1986; Scheer and Raska 1987). The same findings were obtained with rabbit antibodies specific for RNA polymerase I (Reimer *et al*. 1987b; Scheer and Raska 1987). Ribonucleic acid polymerase I is an enzyme complex selectively transcribing the nucleolar genes which encode precursor RNA of 28S, 18S and 5.8S ribosomal RNA (rRNA) (for review see Rose *et al*. 1983).

Scleroderma antibodies against RNA polymerase I precipitated a complex particle composed of at least 13 polypeptides with molecular weights ranging from 210 kD to 12.5 kD. The complex contained phosphoproteins (180 kD, 80 kD and 18 kD) but no tightly bound RNA (Reimer *et al*. 1987b) (Fig. 64.3, lane 2). Functional evidence of the interaction between scleroderma antibodies producing punctate nucleolar staining and RNA polymerase I was obtained by demonstrating that these antibodies selectively inhibited pre-rRNA synthesis when microinjected into *Xenopus laevis* oocyte nuclei (Reimer *et al*. 1987b). These data imply that the antigenic determinants reside on or near a functionally important component of the enzyme complex, possibly the catalytic centre. In a more recent study, it was shown that microinjection of human autoantibodies to RNA polymerase I into mitotic rat kangaroo PtK2 cells inhibited reformation of nucleoli in the daughter cells. These antibodies specifically inhibited the telophasic coalescence of 'prenucleolar bodies' around the chromosomal NOR which normally leads to the reappearance of nucleoli (Benavente *et al*. 1987). Ribonucleic acid polymerase I antibodies, however, did not interfere with normal mitotic progression or early steps of nucleologenesis or the formation of 'prenucleolar bodies', which consist of structures resembling the nucleolar 'dense fibrillar component', in studies using electron microscopy. Segregation and partial disintegration of nucleolar structures by RNA polymerase I antibodies microinjected into interphase cell nuclei was also observed (Benavente *et al*. 1988). These experiments gave not only functional evidence of the interaction between human autoantibodies to RNA polymerase I and the enzyme complex in the living cells but also insights into basic mechanisms of nucleologenesis, suggesting a crucial role of RNA polymerase I and/or the transcriptional complexes for the structural organization and

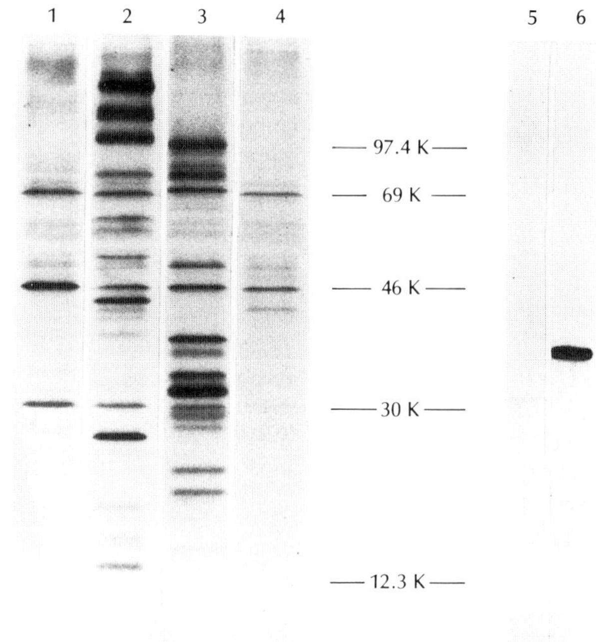

Fig. 64.3. Autoradiogram of ^{35}S-methionine-labelled HeLa cell proteins immunoprecipitated by various antinucleolar autoantibodies followed by SDS-polyacrylamide gel electrophoresis (lanes 1–3). HeLa cells were grown in monolayers and labelled *in vivo* with ^{35}S-methionine. Cell extracts were used as antigen sources for protein A-facilitated immunoprecipitation with various antibodies and controls (Reimer *et al*. 1987c). Lane 1 represents the proteins non-specifically precipitated with normal human serum IgG. Lane 2 shows the proteins precipitated by scleroderma anti-RNA polymerase I antibodies. Lane 3 shows the proteins immunoprecipitated by anti-PM-Scl antibodies from a patient with scleroderma and concomitant polymyositis. Lane 4 shows 40 kD protein of the 7–2 ribonucleoprotein complex. Immunoblots with scleroderma antibodies to fibrillarin are shown in lane 6. Proteins from isolated rat liver nucleoli were separated by SDS-polyacrylamide gel electrophoresis, electrophoretically transferred on to nitrocellulose and nitrocellulose strips incubated with normal serum and anti-fibrillarin serum (Reimer *et al*. 1987a). Lane 5 shows no binding of normal human IgG, whereas anti-fibrillarin antibodies strongly reacted with a 34 kD nucleolar protein.

integrity of transcriptionally active nucleoli in eukaryotic cells.

In a recent study, a new autoantibody in scleroderma was described that recognizes a 90 kD component of the NOR of chromatin (Rodriguez-Sanchez *et al.* 1987). This antibody specificity appears to be different from anti-RNA polymerase I and it is not clear at present whether there is any relationship to RNA polymerase I. Sera with anti-RNA polymerase I activity have also been observed in other systemic autoimmune diseases (Stettler *et al.* 1983) but their immunological specificities appear to be different from the high-titre anti-RNA polymerase I antibodies encountered in scleroderma sera (Reimer *et al.* 1987b).

Clinically, patients with anti-RNA polymerase I appear to suffer from the more severe diffuse form of scleroderma, and renal involvement may be a complicating clinical feature (Reimer *et al.* 1988). However, the number of patients in the latter study was too small for accurate statistical comparison and the result needs to be substantiated in further clinical studies.

Autoantibodies reactive with the nucleolar particle PM-Scl (polymyositis–scleroderma antigen)

A novel antigen–antibody system was described by immunodiffusion which was characteristic of certain patients with polymyositis/scleroderma overlap syndromes and hence termed the PM-Scl system (Reichlin *et al.* 1984). The PM-Scl antibody specificity was recently further investigated and the reactive antigen partially characterized on a molecular level (Reimer *et al.* 1986). Typically, anti-PM-Scl antibodies produced homogeneous nucleolar staining in cells from a variety of different species (Fig. 64.2(b)). In actinomycin-D-segregated nucleoli, anti-PM-Scl staining was mainly localized in the granular regions of segregated nucleoli. When DRB-pretreated cells were incubated with anti-PM-Scl antibodies, immunofluorescence was evenly distributed throughout the nucleoplasm without any 'necklace' staining. These 'necklace' structures, on the other hand, are known to contain RNA polymerase I (Scheer and Rose 1984) and also the nucleolar protein 'fibrillarin' (Ochs *et al.* 1985) but they lack the granular component containing the preribosomal particles (Scheer *et al.* 1984).

By electron-microscopic immunocytochemistry, anti-PM-Scl antibodies predominantly stained the granular component of nucleoli in rat liver hepatocytes. Since the granular component is the site of ribosomal assembly and packaging (reviewed by Busch and Smetana 1970), this location suggests a relationship of the PM-Scl antigen to preribosomes.

On a molecular level, anti-PM-Scl antibodies immunoprecipitated 11 polypeptides with molecular weights (M_r) ranging from 110 kD to 20 kD when incubated with ^{35}S-methionine-labelled HeLa cell proteins (Fig. 64.3, lane 3). The 80 kD and 20 kD polypeptides were phosphorylated. Unfortunately, RNA has not as yet been identified in the precipitates. Therefore a better understanding of the nature of the PM-Scl antigen is still unavailable. By immunoblotting, most anti-PM-Scl antisera reacted with the 100 kD and/or 80 kD proteins.

In the initial study by Reichlin *et al.* 1984, the PM-Scl specificity was predominately observed in patients with myositis and concomitant features of scleroderma. In a more recent study on the autoantibody specificity in scleroderma, we showed that approximately 4% of the patients with nucleolar staining displayed PM-Scl specificity (Reimer *et al.* 1988a). These patients all fulfilled the criteria for the classification of scleroderma. However, most of these patients also had serological findings or a history of myositis during the course of their disease. Thus, the anti-PM-Scl specificity may characterize a disease spectrum with myositis at one end and scleroderma at the other end.

Autoantibodies to U3-ribonucleoprotein-associated fibrillarin

Certain scleroderma sera precipitated a ribonucleoprotein particle containing U3 RNA. U3 is a highly conserved RNA species which was shown to be composed of 217 nucleotides (Suh *et al.* 1986). U3 is the only nucleolar RNA known to have a trimethylated guanosine cap at its 5′ end (Busch *et al.* 1982). The nucleolar localization (Fig. 64.2c) and its association with 28–35S RNA and partial complementarity between U3 and rRNA suggested an involvement in rRNA processing (Prestayko *et al.* 1970; Zieve and Penman 1976). It was postulated that U3 RNA mediates the cleavage separating

Table 64.5. Clinical findings in scleroderma patients with or without serum antibodies directed against defined nucleolar antigens

	With ANoA (n = 37)			
	RNA polymerase I (n = 7)	PM-Scl (n = 8)	U3-RNP (n = 22)	Without ANoA (n = 99)
Raynaud's phenomenon	85	88	95	97
Mean total skin score	29	18	21	26
Telangiectasia	86	100	95	73
Calcinosis	40	57	21	32
Arthralgias/arthritis	71*	50	14*	41
Tendon involvement	71*	75*	52	34
Muscle involvement	0	43	29	78
GI tract involvement	71	43	83	78
Lung involvement	43	67	75	59
Heart involvement	28	0	25	9
Kidney involvement	14	25	9	4

Except for total skin score, values are percentages.
*, $P < 0.05$ versus patients without ANoA.
Reimer *et al.* 1988.

5.8S from the so-called internal transcribed spacer II of pre-rRNA (Bachellerie *et al.* 1983; Crouch *et al.* 1983; Tague and Gerbi 1984).

The protein of the U3 RNA particle bearing the antigenic determinants was recently shown to be a basic (pI 8.5), 34 kD, nucleolar protein (Fig. 64.3, lane 6), rich in N^G-N^G-dimethylarginine and glycine, some of the residues clustering at the N terminus of the molecule (Lischwe *et al.* 1985). Immunolocalization of this protein by immunofluorescence and electron microscopy by scleroderma autoantibodies was exclusively in the fibrillar regions of nucleoli and hence the protein was named fibrillarin (Ochs *et al.* 1985). Scleroderma autoantibodies against fibrillarin recognize epitopes which are well conserved during evolution and occur in nucleoli not only from a variety of animal species but also from plant cells (Reimer *et al.* 1987a).

By using scleroderma anti-U3-RNP antibodies as well as a monoclonal antibody (Reimer *et al.* 1987a) in immunoprecipitation, it was shown that U3-RNP contained four non-phosphorylated proteins (36 kD, 30 kD, 13 kD and 12.5 kD) and two phosphoproteins (74 kD and 59 kD). The 36 kD protein most probably corresponds to the 34 kD nucleolar protein (fibrillarin) recognized by specific scleroderma sera in immunoblots (Parker and Steitz 1987). In this study sequencing data and structural analysis of U3 RNA showed complementarity between single-stranded regions of U3 and pre-rRNA sequences, suggesting that U3 RNA might be involved in processing events near the 3′ end of pre-rRNA.

Some interesting studies have reported that mercury chloride, when given orally to mice from susceptible strains, induces the production of autoantibodies to fibrillarin (Reuter *et al.* 1989; Hultman *et al.* 1989). This is an important observation and may allow the study of the genetics and immunopathological mechanisms leading to autoantibody production in scleroderma.

In a study on the clinical associations of antinucleolar autoantibodies in scleroderma, patients with anti-fibrillarin antibodies had less severe arthritis than patients randomly selected from a control group without antinucleolar antibodies, but otherwise they did not differ clinically from the control group (Table 64.5).

Rare antibody specificities in scleroderma include antibody against centriole antigen (Moroi *et al.* 1983) and antibody against 7–2 nucleolar RNP (Hashimoto and Steitz 1983; Reddy *et al.* 1983). The 7–2 RNP antigen contains small nucleolar 7–2 RNA and was localized in the granular component of nucleoli. A major protein component of the RNP particle was identified as a 40 kD protein (Reimer *et al.* 1987(b); Reimer *et al.* 1988b).

Autoantibodies to mitochondrial antigens in scleroderma

The association of primary biliary cirrhosis and progressive systemic sclerosis has been known for many years by gastroenterologists and rheumatologists (Murray-Lyon *et al.* 1970; Reynolds *et al.* 1971; Diaz and Schuman 1973). Antimitochondrial autoantibodies, a hallmark of primary biliary cirrhosis, have been observed by different investigators in the sera from patients with systemic sclerosis (Gupta *et al.* 1984; Alderuccio *et al.* 1986; Mouritsen *et al.* 1986). The percentage of scleroderma patients with antibodies to mitochondrial antigens as shown by immunodiffusion was reported to be 25% (Gupta *et al.* 1984) and as shown by immunoblotting approximately 15% of the patients' sera reacted with mitochondrial antigens. Only recently, it was shown that the mitochondrial antigen recognized by autoantibodies from scleroderma was directed against the M2 complex (Fregeau *et al.* 1988). The M2 complex is also the major target of autoantibodies in primary biliary cirrhosis and is located in the mitochondrial membrane in all tissues, apparently associated with the F1 subunit of the adenosine triphosphatase (ATPase) complex (Baum and Palmer 1985). The antigen is a 70 kD protein for which the cDNA has been cloned (Gershwin *et al.* 1987). Using the recombinant autoantigen, it was shown that approximately 19 of 250 scleroderma patients were reactive. Of these 19 scleroderma patients, 15 had the CREST variant of systemic sclerosis and three of the antimitochondrial antibody +ve patients also had primary biliary cirrhosis (Fregeau *et al.* 1988). Thus antimitochondrial antibodies in scleroderma appear to characterize a subgroup of patients with the CREST variant of systemic sclerosis with a high prevalence of concomitant liver disease, i.e. primary biliary cirrhosis.

Conclusion

One of the most characteristic serological features in systemic autoimmune diseases associated with fibrosis of the skin and internal organs, namely systemic sclerosis (scleroderma) and MCTD, is the occurrence of autoantibodies against nuclear and nucleolar antigens.

In recent years, a great deal of exciting information on the molecular biology of nuclear and nucleolar antigens in systemic sclerosis and MCTD has come from different laboratories and many countries. Nuclear and nucleolar autoantigens are among the best studied autoimmune targets encountered in these systemic autoimmune diseases and may advance the understanding of the aetiology of these diseases in general.

The benefit for the clinician and investigator in having molecular information on the nuclear and nucleolar target autoantigens will be in providing accurate and reproducible diagnostic and prognostic approaches for dealing with patients affected by these intractable diseases.

Acknowledgement

The research reported in this chapter was supported by NIH grants AR32063 and AI10386 (publication No. 6150-MEM from the Research Institute of Scripps Clinic).

References

Alarcon, G.S., Phillips, R.M., Wasner, C.K., Acton, R.T. and Barger, B.O. (1985). DR antigens in systemic sclerosis: lack of clinical correlations. *Tissue Antigens* **26**, 156.

Alderuccio, F., Toh, B.-H., Barnett, A.J. and Pederson, J.S. (1986). Identification and characterization of mitochondria autoantigens in progressive systemic sclerosis: identity with the 72 000 dalton autoantigen in primary biliary cirrhosis. *J. Immunol.* **137**, 1855.

Ansell, B.M., Nasseh, G.A. and Bywaters, E.G.L. (1976). Scleroderma in childhood. *Ann. Rheum. Dis.* **35**, 189.

Arbeitsgrupps Sklerodermie der Arbeitsgemeinschaft Dermatologische Forschung (ADF) (1980) Klinik der progressiven systemischen Sklerodermie (PSS). *Hautarzt* **37**, 320.

Bachellerie, J.-P., Michot, B. and Raynal, F. (1983). Recognition signals for mouse pre-rRNA processing. *Mol. Biol. Rep.* **9**, 79–86.

Barnes, E.L., Rodnan, G.P., Medsger, T.A., Jr and Short, D. (1979). Eosinophilic fasciitis: a pathologic study of twenty cases. *Am. J. Pathol.* **96**, 493.

Barnett, A.J. (1974). *Scleroderma: Progressive Systemic Sclerosis.* Charles C. Thomas, Springfield.

Barnett, A.J., Miller, M.H. and Littlejohn, G.O. (1988). A survival study of patients with scleroderma diagnosed over 30 years (1953–1983): the value of a simple cutaneous classification in the early stages of the disease. *J. Rheumatol.* **15**, 276.

Baum, H. and Palmer, C. (1985). The PBC-specific antigen. *Mol. Aspects Med.* **8**, 201–34.

Beck, J.S. (1961). Variations in the morphological patterns of 'autoimmune' nuclear immunofluorescence. *Lancet* **i**, 1203.

Beck, J.S., Anderson, J.R., Gray, K.G. and Rowell, N.R. (1963). Antinuclear and precipitating autoantibodies in progressive systemic sclerosis. *Lancet* **ii**, 1188.

Benavente, R., Rosae, K.M., Reimer, G., Hugle-Dorr, B. and Scheer, U. (1987). Inhibition of nucleolar reformation after microinjection antibodies to RNA polymerase I into mitotic cells. *J. Cell Biol.* **105**, 1483–91.

Benavente, R., Reimer, G., Roe, K.M., Hugle-Dorr, B. and Scheer, U. (1988). Nucleolar changes after microinjection of antibodies to RNA polymerase I into the nucleus of mammalian cells. *Chromosoma* **97**, 115–23.

Bennett, R.M. (1985). Mixed connective tissue disease and other overlap syndromes. In *Textbook of Rheumatology*, 2nd edn. ed. W.N. Kelly, E.D. Harris, S. Ruddy and C.B. Sledge p. 1115, W.B. Saunders Company, Philadelphia

Bennett, R.M. and Spargo, B.H. (1977). Immune complex nephropathy in MCTD. *Am. J. Med.* **63**, 534.

Bernstein, R.M., Steigerwald, J.C. and Tan, E.M. (1982). Association of antinuclear and antinucleolar antibodies in progressive systemic sclerosis. *Clin. Exp. Immunol.* **48**, 43–51.

Bitterman, P.B., Rennard, S.I., Hunninghake, G.W. and Crystal, R.G. (1982). Human alveolar macrophage growth factor for fibroblasts. *J. Clin. Invest.* **70**, 806.

Bitterman, P.B., Rennard, S.I., Adelberg, S. and Crystal, R.G. (1983). Role of fibronectin as a growth factor for fibroblasts. *J. Cell Biol.* **97**, 1925.

Black, C.M., Welsh, K.I., Maddison, P.J., Jayson, M.I.V. and Bernstein, R.M. (1984). HLA antigens, autoantibodies and clinical subsets in scleroderma. *Br. J. Rheumatol.* **23**, 267.

Bozzoni, I., Amaldi, F., Anneis, F., Beccari, E., Fragapare, P. and Pierandrei-Amaldi, P. (1984). Splicing of *Xenopus laevis* ribosomal protein RNAs is inhibited *in vivo* by antisera to snRNP. *J. Mol. Biol.* **180**, 1173.

Brenner, S., Pepper, D., Berne, M.E., Tan, E.M. and Brinkley, B.R. (1981). Kinetochore structure, duplication and distribution in mammalian cells: analysis by human autoantibodies from scleroderma patients. *J. Cell Biol.* **91**, 95.

Burnham, T.K. and Bank, P.W. (1974). Antinuclear antibodies. I. Patterns of nuclear immunofluorescence. *J. Invest. Dermatol.* **62**, 526.

Burnham, T.K., Fine, G. and Neblett, T.R. (1966). The immunofluorescent tumor imprint technique. II. The frequency of antinuclear factors in connective tissue diseases and dermatoses. *Ann. Intern. Med.* **65**, 9.

Busch, H. and Smetana, K. (1970). *The Nucleolus*. Academic Press, New York.

Busch, H., Reddy, R., Rothblum, L. and Choi, Y.C. (1982). SnRNAs, SnRNPs and RNA processing. *Ann. Rev. Biochem.* **51**, 617.

Cattogio, L.J., Bernstein, R.M., Black, C.M., Hughes, G.R.V. and Maddison, P.J. (1983). Serologic markers in progressive systemic sclerosis: clinical correlations. *Ann. Rheum. Dis.* **42**, 23.

Chen, Z., Virella, G., Tung, H.E., Ainsworth, S.K. *et al.* (1984). Immune complexes and antinuclear, antinucleolar, and anticentromere antibodies in scleroderma. *J. Am. Acad. Dermatol.* **11**, 461.

Chorzelski, T.P., Jablonska, S., Beutner, E.H. *et al.* (1985). Anticentromere antibody: an immunological marker of a subset of systemic sclerosis. *Br. J. Dermatol.* **113**, 381–9.

Cohen, S., Johnson, A.R. and Hurd, E. (1983). Cytotoxicity of sera from patients with scleroderma. *Arthritis Rheum.* **26**, 170.

Connor, G.E., Nelson, D., Wisniewolski, R., Lahita, R.G., Blobel, G. and Kunkel, H.G. (1982). Protein antigens of the RNA–protein complexes detected by anti-Sm and anti-RNP antibodies found in serum of patients with systemic lupus erythematosus and related disorders. *J. Exp. Med.* **156**, 1475.

Cox, J.V., Schenk, E.A. and Olmsted, J.B. (1983). Human anticentromere antibodies: distribution, characterization of antigens, and effect on microtubule organization. *Cell* **35**, 331–9.

Crouch, R.J., Kanaya, S. and Earl, P.L. (1983). A model for the involvement of the small nucleolar RNA (U3) in processing eukaryotic ribosomal RNA. *Mol. Biol. Rep.* **9**, 77–93.

Diaz, P.A. and Schuman, B.M. (1973). Primary biliary cirrhosis with systemic sclerosis associated with Raynaud's phenomenon and telangiectasiae. *Gastroenterology* **64**, 183–4.

Douvas, A.S., Achten, M. and Tan, E.M. (1979). Identification of a nuclear protein (Scl-70) as a unique target of human antinuclear antibodies in scleroderma. *J. Biol. Chem.* **254**, 10514–22.

Drenk, F. and Deicher, H.R.G. (1988). Pathophysiological effects of endothelial cytotoxic activity derived from sera of patients with progressive systemic sclerosis. *J. Rheumatol.* **15**, 468.

Earnshaw, E.C., Sullivan, K.F., Machlin, P.S. *et al.* (1987). Molecular cloning of cDNA for CENP-B, the major human centromere autoantigen. *J. Cell Biol.* **104**, 817.

Earnshaw, W.C., Bordwell, B., Marino, C. and Rothfield, N.F. (1986). Three human chromosomal autoantigens are recognized by sera from patients with anticentromere antibodies. *J. Clin. Invest.* **77**, 426.

Farber, S.J. and Boyle, G.G. (1976). Antibodies to components of extractable nuclear antigen. *Arch. Intern. Med.* **136**, 425.

Fennell, R.H., Jr, Rodnan, G.P. and Vazquez, J.J. (1962). Variability of tissue-localizing properties of serum from patients with different disease states. *Lab. Invest.* **11**, 24.

Field, E. Munves, E. and Schul, P.H. (1983). Antibodies to Sm and RNP prognosticators of disease involvement. *Arthritis Rheum.* **26**, 848.

Fisher, D.E., Conner, G.E., Reeves, W.H.Z., Blobel, G. and Kunkel, H.G. (1983). Synthesis and assembly of human small nuclear ribonucleoproteins generated by cell-free translation. *Proc. Nat. Acad. Sci. (USA)* **80**, 6356.

Fleischmajer, R. and Perlish, J.S. (1980). Capillary alterations in scleroderma. *J. Am. Acad. Dermatol.* **2**, 161.

Fleischmajer, R., Perlish, J.S. and Reeves, J.R.T. (1977). Cellular infiltrates in scleroderma skin. *Arthritis Rheum.* **20**, 975.

Fleischmajer, R., Perlish, J.S., Krieg, T. and Timpl, R. (1981). Variability in collagen and fibronectin synthesis by scleroderma fibroblasts in primary culture. *J. Invest. Dermatol.* **76**, 400.

Fregeau, D.R., Leung, P.S.C., Coppel, R.L., McNeilage, J., Medsger, T.A. and Gershwin, M.E. (1988). Autoantibodies to mitochondria in systemic sclerosis. *Arthritis Rheum.* **31**, 386.

Fritzler, M.J., Kinsella, T.D. and Garbutt, E. (1980). The CREST syndrome: a distinct serologic entity with anticentromere antibodies. *Am. J. Med.* **69**, 520–6.

Gerbracht, D.D., Steen, V.D., Ziegler, G.L., Medsger, T.A., Jr and Rodnan, G.P. (1985). Evolution of primary Raynaud's phenomenon (Raynaud's disease) to connective tissue diseases. *Arthritis Rheum.* **28**, 87.

Gershwin, M.E., Mackay, I.R., Sturgess, A. and Coppel, R.L. (1987). Identification and specificity of cDNA encoding the 70 kD mitochondrial antigen recognized in primary biliary cirrhosis. *J. Immunol.* **138**, 3525–31.

Giordano, M., Capelli, L., Tirri, G. and Valti, M. (1980). Vorschlag zu einer neuen Klassifizierung und Nomenklatur der progredienten generalisierten Sklerodermie (PGS). *Verh. Dtsch. Ges. Rheumatol.* **6**, 379.

Giordano, M., Valentini, G., Migliaresi, S., Picillo, U. and Vatti, M. (1986). Different antibody patterns and different prognosis in patients with scleroderma with various extent of skin sclerosis. *J. Rheumatol.* **13**, 911.

Gladman, D.D., Keystone, E.C., Baron, M., Lee, P., Cane, D. and Menest, H. (1981). Increased frequency of HLA DR5 in scleroderma. *Arthritis Rheum.* **24**, 854.

Greenwald, G.I., Tashkin, D.P., Gong, H. *et al.* (1987). Longitudinal changes in lung function and respiratory symptoms in progressive systemic sclerosis. *Am. J. Med.* **83**, 83.

Greger, R.E. (1975). Familial progressive systemic scleroderma. *Arch. Dermatol.* **111**, 81.

Grennan, D.M., Burn, C., Hughes, G.R.V., Buchanan, W.W. and Dick, W.C. (1977). Frequency and clinical significance of antibodies to ribonucleoprotein in SLE and other connective tissue disease subgroups. *Ann. Rheum. Dis.* **30**, 442.

Guldner, H.H., Lakomek, H.J. and Bautz, F.A. (1985). Human anticentromere sera recognize a 19.5 kD nonhistone chromosomal protein from HeLa cells. *Clin. Exp. Immunol.* **58**, 13.

Guldner, H.H., Szosteki, C., Vosberg, H.-P., Lakomek, H.J., Penner, E. and Bautz, F.A. (1986). Scl-70 autoantibodies from scleroderma patients recognize a 96 kDa protein identified as topoisomerase I. *Chromosoma* **94**, 132.

Gupta, R.C., Seibold, J.R., Krishnan, M.R. and Steigerwald, J.C. (1984). Precipitating autoantibodies to mitochondrial proteins in progressive systemic sclerosis. *Clin. Exp. Immunol.* **57**, 68.

Habets, W.H., Holt, M., Bingmann, P., Lechrmann, R. and Van Venrooji, W.J. (1985). Autoantibodies to ribonucleoprotein aparticles containing U2 small nuclear RNA. *EMBO J.* **4**, 1545.

Habets, W.H., DeRooji, D.H., Salden, M.H. and Van Venrooji, W.J. (1983). Antibodies against distinct nuclear matrix proteins are characteristic of mixed connective tissue disease. *Clin. Exp. Immunol.* **54**, 265.

Hashimoto, C. and Steitz, J.A. (1983). Sequential association of nucleolar 7–2 RNA with two different autoantigens. *J. Biol. Chem.* **258**, 1379–82.

Hochberg, M.C., Holt, P.M., Kane, M.G., Arnett, F.C. and Stevens, M.B. (1980). Survival in systemic sclerosis (scleroderma). *Arthritis Rheum.* **23** 689.

Holzmann, H., Sollberg, S. and Altmeyer, P. (1987). Einteilung und Klinik der progressiven systemischen Sklerodermie (PSS). In *Dermatologie und Rheuma*, ed. H. Holzmann, P. Altmeyer, W. Marsch and H.G. Vogel, p. 202, Springer, Heidelberg.

Hultman, P., Enestrom, S., Pollard, K.M. and Tan, E.M. (1989). Antifibrillarin autoantibodies in mercury-treated mice. *Exp. Cell Res. Clin. Exp. Immunol.* **78**, 470.

Inoshita, T., Whiteside, T.L., Rodnan, G.P. and Taylor, F.H. (1981). Abnormalities of T lymphocyte subsets in patients with progressive systemic sclerosis. *J. Lab. Clin. Med.* **97**, 264.

Jarzabek-Chorzelska, M., Blasczyk, M., Jablonska, S., Chorzelski, T., Kumar, V. and Beutner, E.H. (1986). Scl-70 antibody: a specific marker of systemic sclerosis. *Br. J. Dermatol.* **115**, 393.

Kahaleh, M.B., Sherer, G.K. and Leroy, E.C. (1979). Endothelial injury in scleroderma. *J. Exp. Med.* **149**, 1326.

Kallenberg, C.G.M., van der Voort-Beelen, J.M. and D'Amaro, J. (1981). Increased frequency of B8/DR3 in scleroderma and association of the haplotype with impaired cellular immune response. *Clin. Exp. Immunol.* **43**, 478.

Kallenberg, C.G.M., Pastoor, G.W., Wouda, A.A. and The, T.H. (1982). Antinuclear antibodies in patients with Raynaud's phenomenon: clinical significance of anticentromere antibodies. *Ann. Rheum. Dis.* **41**, 382.

Kass, H., Hanson, V. and Patrick, M. (1966). Scleroderma in childhood. *J. Pediatr.* **68**, 243.

Kasukawa, R., Tojo, T., Miyawaki, S. *et al.* (1988). Mixed connective tissue disease — preliminary diagnostic criteria. *Jap. J. Rheumatol.* **4**, 263.

Kleinsmith, D.M., Heinzerling, R.H. and Burnham, T.K. (1982). Antinuclear antibodies as immunologic markers for a benign subset and different clinical characteristics of scleroderma. *Arch. Dermatol.* **118**, 882.

Krieg, T. and Meurer, M. (1988). Systemic scleroderma: clinical and pathophysiologic aspects. *J. Am. Acad. Dermatol.* **18**, 457.

Krieg, T., Muller, P.K. and Goerz, G. (1977). Fibroblasts from a patient with scleroderma reveal abnormal metabolism. *Arch. Dermatol. Res.* **259**, 105.

Lemmer, J.P., Curry, N.H., Mallory, J.H. and Waller, M.V. (1982). Clinical characteristics and course in patients with high titer anti-RNP antibodies. *J. Rheumatol.* **9**, 536.

Lerner, M.R. and Steitz, J.A. (1979). Autoantibodies to small nuclear RNAs complexed with proteins are produced by patients with systemic lupus erythematosus. *Proc. Nat. Acad. Sci. (USA)* **76**, 5495–9.

LeRoy, E.C. (1974). Increased collagen synthesis by scleroderma skin fibroblast *in vitro*: a possible defect in the regulation or activation of scleroderma fibroblast. *J. Clin. Invest.* **54**, 880.

LeRoy, E.C. (1985). Systemic sclerosis (scleroderma). In *Cecil Textbook of Medicine*, 18th edn, ed. J.B. Wyngaarden and L.H. Smith, pp. 2018–24. W.B. Saunders Company, Philadelphia.

LeRoy, E.C., Black, C., Fleischmajer, R. *et al.* (1988). Scleroderma (systemic sclerosis): classification, subsets, and pathogenesis. *J. Rheumatol.* **15**, 202.

Lischwe, M.A., Ochs, R.L., Reddy, R. *et al.* (1985). Purification and partial characterization of a nucleolar scleroderma antigen (Mr = 34000; pI = 8.5) rich in N^G, N^G-dimethylarginine. *J. Biol. Chem.* **260**, 14304–10.

Lynch, C.L., Singh, G., Whiteside, T.L., Rodnan, G.P., Medsger, T.A. and Rabin, B.S. (1982). Histocompatibility antigens in progressive systemic sclerosis (PSS, scleroderma). *J. Clin. Immunol.* **2**, 314.

McCarthy, D.S., Baraggar, F.D., Dhingra, S. *et al.* (1988). The lungs in systemic sclerosis (scleroderma): a review of new information. *Semin. Arthritis Rheum.* **17**, 271.

McCarty, G.A., Rice, J.R., Bembe, M.L. and Barada, F.A., Jr (1983). Anticentromere antibody: clinical correlations and association with favorable prognosis in patients with scleroderma variants. *Arthritis Rheum.* **26**, 1.

Mackel, A.M., LeLustro, F., Harper, F.E. and LeRoy, E.C. (1982). Antibodies to collagen in scleroderma. *Arthritis Rheum.* **25**, 522.

Maricq, H.R., Weinberger, A.B. and LeRoy, E.C. (1982). Early detection of scleroderma-spectrum disorders by *in vivo* capillary microscopy: a prospective study of patients with Raynaud's phenomenon. *J. Rheumatol.* **9**, 289.

Masi, A.T., Rodnan, G.P., Medsger, T.A., Jr *et al.* (1980). Preliminary criteria for the classification of systemic sclerosis (scleroderma). *Arthritis Rheum.* **23**, 581.

Matter, L., Schopfer, K., Wilhelm, J.A., Nyffenegger, T., Parisot, R.F. and DeRobertis, E.M. (1982). Molecular characterization of ribonucleoprotein antigens bound by antinuclear antibodies: a diagnostic evaluation. *Arthritis Rheum.* **25**, 1278.

Mattioli, M. and Reichlin, M. (1973). Physical association of two nuclear antigens and mutual occurrence of their antibodies: the relationship of the Sm and the RNA-protein (Mu) systems in SLE sera. *J. Immunol.* **110**, 1318.

Maul, G.G., French, B.T., Van Venrooji, W.J. and Jiminez, S.A. (1986). Topoisomerase I identified by scleroderma 70 antisera: enrichment of topoisomerase I at the centromere in mouse mitotic cells before anaphase. *Proc. Nat. Acad. Sci. (USA)* **83**, 5145.

Medsger, T.A. (1985a). Systemic sclerosis (scleroderma), eosinophilic fasciitis, and calcinosis. In *Arthritis and Allied Conditions*, 10th edn, ed. D.J. McCarthy, p. 994, Lea Febiger, Philadelphia.

Medsger, T.A. (1985b). Epidemiology of progressive systemic sclerosis. In *Systemic Sclerosis (Scleroderma)*, ed. C. Black and A.R. Myers, p. 53, Gower, New York.

Medsger, T.A. and Masi, A.T. (1971). Epidemiology of progressive systemic sclerosis. *Ann. Intern. Med.* **74**, 714.

Meurer, M., Scharf, A., Luderschmidt, C. and Braun-Falco, O. (1984). Zentromerantikorper und Antikorper gegen Scl-70 Nucleoprotein bei progressiver Sklerodermie. *Dtsch. Med. Wochenschr.* **119**, 8.

Mimori, T., Hinterberger, M., Petterson, I. and Steitz, J.A. (1984). Autoantibodies to the U2 small nuclear ribonucleoprotein in a patient with scleroderma–polymyositis overlap syndrome. *J. Biol. Chem.* **259**, 560.

Moroi, Y., Hartmann, A.L., Nakane, P.K. and Tan. E.M. (1981). Distribution of kinetochore (centromere) antigen in mammalian cell nuclei. *J. Cell. Biol.* **90**, 254.

Moroi, Y., Murata, I., Takeuchi, A., Kamatani, N., Tanimoto, K. and Yokohari, R. (1983). Human anticentriole autoantibody in patients with scleroderma and Raynaud's phenomenon. *Clin. Immunol. Immunopathol.* **29**, 381.

Mouritsen, S., Demant, E., Permin, H. and Wilk, A. (1986). High prevalence of antimitochondrial antibodies among patients with some well-defined connective tissue diseases. *Clin. Exp. Immunol.* **60**, 68–76.

Murray-Lyon, I.M., Thompson, R.P.H., Ansell, I.D. and Williams, R. (1970). Scleroderma and primary biliary cirrhosis. *Br. Med. J.* **3**, 258–9.

Nimelstein, S.H., Brady, S., McShane, D. and Holman, H.R. (1980). Mixed connective tissue disease: a subsequent evaluation of the original 25 patients. *Medicine* **59**, 239.

Norton, W.L. and Nardo, J.M. (1970). Vascular disease in progressive systemic sclerosis (scleroderma). *Ann. Intern. Med.* **73**, 317.

Ochs, R.L., Lischwe, M.A., O'Leary, P. and Busch, H. (1983). Localization of nucleolar phosphoproteins B23 and C23 during mitosis. *Exp. Cell Res.* **146**, 139–49.

Ochs, R.L., Lischwe, M.A., Spohn, W.H. and Busch, H. (1985). Fibrillarin: a new protein of the nucleolus identified by autoimmune sera. *J. Biol. Chem.* **54**, 123–34.

Padgett, R.A., Mount, S.M., Steitz, J.A. and Sharp, P.A. (1983). Splicing of messenger RNA precursors is inhibited by antisera to small nuclear ribonucleoprotein. *Cell* **35**, 101.

Parker, K.A. and Steitz, J.A. (1987). Structural analyses of the human U3 ribonucleoprotein particle reveal a conserved sequence available for base-pairing with pre-rRNA. *Mol. Cell. Biol.* **7**, 2899–913.

Parker, M.D. (1973). Ribonucleoprotein antibodies: frequencies and clinical significance in systemic lupus erythematosus, scleroderma and mixed connective disease. *J. Lab. Clin. Med.* **82**, 769.

Peltonen, L., Palotie, A., Mylylla, R., Krieg, T. and Oikarinen, A. (1985). Collagen biosynthesis in systemic scleroderma: regulation of post-translational modifications and synthesis of procollagen in cultured fibroblasts. *J. Invest. Dermatol.* **84**. 14.

Pinnas, J.L., Northway, J.D. and Tan, E.M. (1973). Antinucleolar antibodies in human sera. *J. Immunol.* **111**, 996.

Postletwaite, A.E., Lachmann, L.B. and Kang, A.H. (1984). Induction of fibroblast proliferation by interleukin-1 derived from human monocyte leukemia cells. *Arthritis Rheum.* **27**, 995.

Prestayko, A.W., Tonato, M. and Busch, H. (1970). Low molecular weight RNA associated with 28S nucleolar RNA. *J. Mol. Biol.* **47**, 505–15.

Query, C.C. and Keene, J.P. (1987). A human autoimmune problem associated with U1 RNA contains a region of homology that is cross-reactive with viral p30 gag antigen. *Cell* **51**, 211.

Raska, I., Reimer, G., Jarnik, M., Kostrouch, Z. and Raska, K. (1989). Does the synthesis of ribosomal RNA take place within nucleolar fibrillar centers or dense fibrillar components? *Biol. Cell* **65**, 79–82.

Reddy, R., Tan., E.M., Henning, D., Nogha, K. and Busch, H. (1983). Detection of a nucleolar 7–2 ribonucleoprotein and cytoplasmic 8–2 ribonucleoprotein with autoantibodies from patients with scleroderma. *J. Biol. Chem.* **258**, 1383.

Reichlin, M., Maddison, P.J., Targoff, I. *et al.* (1984). Antibodies to a nuclear/nucleolar antigen in patients with polymyositis overlap syndromes. *J. Clin. Immunol.* **4**, 40–4.

Reimer, G., Huschka, U., Keller, J., Kammerer, R. and Hornstein, O.P. (1983). Immunofluorescence studies in progressive systemic sclerosis (scleroderma) and mixed connective tissue disease. *Br. J. Dermatol.* **109**, 27.

Reimer, G., Scheer, U., Peters, J.-M. and Tan, E.M. (1986). Immunolocalization and partial characterization of a nucleolar antigen (PM-Scl) associated with polymyositis/scleroderma overlap syndromes. *J. Immunol.* **137**; 3802–8.

Reimer, G., Pollard, K.M., Penning, C.A. *et al.* (1987a). Monoclonal autoantibody from NZB/NZW F1 mouse and some human scleroderma sera target a Mr 34 000 nucleolar protein of the U3-ribonucleoprotein particle. *Arthritis Rheum.* **30**, 793–800.

Reimer, G., Raska, I., Tan, E.M. and Scheer, U. (1987c). Human autoantibodies: probes for nucleolus structure and function. *Virchow Archiv B* **54**, 131–43.

Reimer, G., Rose, K.M., Scheer, U. and Tan, E.M. (1987b) Autoantibody to RNA polymerase I in scleroderma sera. *J. Clin. Invest.* **79**, 65–72.

Reimer, G., Raska, I., Scheer, U. and Tan, E.M. (1988b) Immunolocalization of 7–2 ribonucleoprotein in the granular component of the nucleus. *Exp. Cell Res.* **176**, 117–128.

Reimer, G., Steen, V.D., Penning, C.A., Medsger, T.A. and Tan, E.M. (1988). Correlates between autoantibodies to nucleolar antigens and clinical features in patients with systemic sclerosis (scleroderma). *Arthritis Rheum.* **31**, 525–32.

Rennard, S.I., Hunninghake, G.W., Bitterman, P.B. and Crystal, R.G. (1981). Production of fibronectin by the human alveolar macrophage: mechanism for the recruitment of fibroblasts to sites of tissue injury in interstitial lung disease. *Proc. Nat. Acad. Sci. (USA)* **73**, 7147.

Reuter, R. and Lührmann, R. (1986). Immunization of mice with purified U1 small nuclear ribonucleoprotein (RNP) induces a pattern of antibody specificities characteristic of the anti-Sm and anti-RNP autoimmune response of patients with lupus erythematosus, as measured by monoclonal antibodies. *Proc. Nat. Acad. Sci. (USA)* **83**, 8689.

Reuter, R., Tessars, G., Vohr, H.-W., Gleichmann, E. and Luhrmann, R. (1989). Mercuric chloride induces autoantibodies against U3 small nuclear ribonucleoprotein in susceptible mice. *Proc. Nat. Acad. Sci. (USA)* **86**, 237.

Reynolds, T.B., Denison, E.K., Frankl, H.D., Lieberman, F.L. and Peters, R.L. (1971). Primary biliary cirrhosis with scleroderma, Raynaud's phenomenon and telangiectasia. *Am. J. Med.* **50**, 302–12.

Ritchie, R.F. (1970). Antinucleolar antibodies: their frequency and diagnostic association. *N. Engl. J. Med.* **282**, 1174.

Roberts, A.B., Sporn, M.B., Assoian, R.K. *et al.* (1986). Transforming growth factor beta: rapid induction of fibrosis and angiogenesis *in vivo* and stimulation of collagen formation *in vitro*. *Proc. Nat. Acad. Sci. (USA)* **83**, 4167.

Rodnan, G.P., Jablonska, S. and Medsger, T.A. (1976). Classification and nomenclature of progressive systemic sclerosis (scleroderma). *Clin. Rheum. Dis.* **5**, 5.

Rodriguez-Sanchez, J.L., Gelpi, C., Juarez, C. and Hardin, J.A. (1987). A new autoantibody in scleroderma that recognizes a 90-kDA component of the nucleolus-organizing region in chromatin. *J. Immunol.* **139**, 2579.

Rose, K.M., Stettler, D.A. and Jacob, S.T. (1983). RNA polymerases from higher eukaryotes. In *Enzymes of Nucleic Acid Synthesis and Modification*, ed. S.T. Jacob, pp. 43–74, CRC Press, Boca Raton.

Rose, K.M., Szopa, J., Han, F.-S., Cheng, Y.C., Richter, A. and Scheer, U. (1988). Association of DNA topoisomerase I and RNA polymerase I: a possible role for topoisomerase I in ribosomal gene transcription. *Chromosoma* **96**, 411–16.

Rothfield, N.F. and Rodnan, G.P. (1968). Serum antinuclear antibodies in progressive systemic sclerosis (scleroderma). *Arthritis Rheum.* **11**, 607.

Roumm, A.D., Whiteside, T.L., Medsger, T.A. and Rodnan, G.P. (1984). Lymphocytes in the skin of patients with progressive systemic sclerosis: quantification, subtyping, and clinical correlations. *Arthritis Rheum.* **27**, 645.

Scheer, U. and Raska, I. (1987). Immunocytochemical localization of RNA polymerase I in the fibrillar centers of nucleoli. *Chromosomes Today* **9**, 284–94.

Scheer, U. and Rose, K.M. (1984). Localization of RNA polymerase I in interphase cells and mitotic chromosomes by light and electron microscopic immunocytochemistry. *Proc. Nat. Acad. Sci. (USA)* **81**, 1431–5.

Scheer, U., Hugle, B., Hazan, R. and Rose, K.M. (1984). Drug-induced dispersal of transcribed rRNA genes and transcriptional products: immunolocalization and silver staining of different nucleolar components in rat cells treated with 5,6-dichloro-b-D-ribofuranosylbenzimidazole. *J. Cell Biol.* **99**, 642–49.

Shanahan, W.R. and Korn, J.H. (1982). Cytotoxic activity of sera from scleroderma and other connective tissue diseases: lack of cellular and disease specificity. *Arthritis Rheum.* **25**, 1391.

Sharp, G.C. and Singsen, B.H. (1985). Mixed connective tissue disease. In *Arthritis and Allied Conditions*, ed. D.J. McCarty p. 963, Lea Febinger, Philadelphia.

Sharp, G.C., Irwin, W.S., Tan, E.M., Gould, G. and Holman, H.R. (1972). Mixed connective tissue disease — an apparently distinct rheumatic disease syndrome associated with a specific antibody to an extractable nuclear antigen (ENA). *Am. J. Med.* **52**, 148.

Sharp, G.C., Irvin, W.S., May, C.M. *et al.* (1976). Association of antibodies to ribonucleoprotein and Sm antigens with mixed connective tissue disease, systemic lupus erythematosus and other rheumatic diseases. *N. Engl. J. Med.* **295**, 1149.

Sharp, P.A. (1987). Splicing of messenger RNA precursors. *Science* **235**, 766.

Shero, J.H., Bordwell, B., Rothfield, N.F. and Earnshaw, W.C. (1986). High titers of autoantibodies to topoisomerase I (Scl-70) in sera from scleroderma patients. *Science* **231**, 737–40.

Shulman, L.E. (1975). Diffuse fasciitis with eosinophilia: a new syndrome. *Trans. Assoc. Am. Physicians* **88**, 70.

Siegel, R.C. (1977). Scleroderma. *Med. Clin. North Am.* **61**, 283.

Silver, R.M., Metcalf, J.F. and LeRoy, E.C. (1986). Interstitial lung disease in scleroderma: immune complexes in sera and bronchoalveolar lavage fluid. *Arthritis Rheum.* **29**, 525.

Steen, V.D., Medsger, T.A. and Rodnan, G.P. (1980). Clinical comparison of two variants of progressive systemic sclerosis: diffuse scleroderma and CREST syndrome (abstract). *Arthritis Rheum.* **23**, 752.

Steen, V.D., Medsger, T.A. and Rodnan, G.P. (1982). D-penicillamine therapy in progressive systemic sclerosis (scleroderma). *Ann. Intern. Med.* **97**, 652.

Steen, V.D., Ziegler, G.L., Rodnan, G.P. and Medsger, T.A., Jr (1984). Clinical and laboratory associations of anticentromere antibody in patients with progressive systemic sclerosis. *Arthritis Rheum.* **27**, 125.

Steen, V.D., Powell, D.L. and Medsger, T.A. Jr (1988). Clinical correlations and prognosis based on serum autoantibodies in patients with systemic sclerosis. *Arthritis Rheum.* **31**, 196.

Stettler, D.A., Rose, K.M., Wenger, M.E. *et al.* (1982). Antibodies to distinct polypeptides of RNA polymerase I in sera from patients with rheumatic disease. *Proc. Nat. Acad. Sci (USA)* **74**, 901.

Stupi, A.M., Steen, V.D., Owens, G.R., Barnes, E.L., Rodnan, G.P. and Medsger, T.A. (1986). Pulmonary hypertension in the CREST syndrome variant of systemic sclerosis. *Arthritis Rheum.* **29**, 515.

Suh, D., Busch, H. and Reddy, R. (1986). Isolation and characterization of a human U3 small nucleolar gene. *Biochem. Res. Comm.* **137**, 1133–40.

Sullivan, W.D., Hurst, D.J., Harman, E.E. *et al.* (1984). A prospective evaluation emphasizing pulmonary involvement in patients with mixed connective tissue disease. *Medicine (Baltimore)* **63**, 92.

Tabuenca, J.M. (1981). Toxic-allergic syndrome caused by ingestion of rapeseed oil denatured with aniline. *Lancet* **ii**, 567.

Tague, B.W. and Gerbi, S.A. (1984). Processing of the large rRNA precursor: two proposed categories of RNA–RNA interactions in eukaryotes. *J. Mol. Evol.* **20**, 362–7.

Takehara, K., Moroi, Y. and Ishibashi, Y. (1985). Antinuclear antibodies in the relatives of patients with systemic sclerosis. *Br. J. Dermatol.* **112**, 23–33.

Tan, E.M. (1989). Antinuclear antibodies: diagnostic markers for autoimmune diseases and probes for cell biology. *Adv. Immunol.* **44**, 93.

Tan, E.M. and Kunkel, H.G. (1966). Characteristics of a soluble nuclear antigen precipitating with sera of patients with systemic lupus erythematosus. *J. Immunol.* **96**, 464.

Tan, E.M., Rodnan, G.P., Garcia, I., Moroi, Y., Fritzler, M.J. and Peebles C. (1980). Diversity of antinuclear antibodies in progressive systemic sclerosis: Anti-centromere antibody and its relationship to CREST syndrome. *Arthritis Rheum.* **23**, 617.

Tan, E.M., Reimer, G. and Sullivan, K. (1989). Intracellular autoantigens: diagnostic fingerprints but aetiological dilemmas. Ciba Foundation Symposium 129. In *Autoimmunity and Autoimmune Disease*, p. 25, J. Wiley, New York.

Theissen, H., Etzerodt, M., Reuter, R. *et al.* (1987). Cloning of the human cDNA for the U1 RNA-associated 70K protein. *EMBO J.* **5**, 3209.

Tramposch, H.D., Smith, C.D., Senecal, J.-L. and Rothfield, N. (1984). A long-term longitudinal study of anticentromere antibodies. *Arthritis Rheum.* **27**, 121.

van Venrooji, W.J., Houben, S.H., Habets, W.J., Kalleenberg, C.G.M., Penner, E. and van de Putte, L.B. (1985). Scl-86, a marker antigen for diffuse scleroderma. *J. Clin. Invest.* **75**, 1053.

Verheijen, R., Kuippers, H., Vooijs, P., Van Venrooji, W. and Ramaekers, F. (1986). Distribution of the 70 K U1 RNA-associated protein during interphase and mitosis. *J. Cell Sci.* **86**, 173.

Weiner, E.S., Earnshaw, W.C., Senecal, J.-L., Bordwell, B., Johnson, P. and Rothfield, N.F. (1988). Clinical associations of anticentromere antibodies and antibodies to topoisomerase I. *Arthritis Rheum.* **31**, 378.

Wiener-Kronish, J.P., Solinger, A.M., Warnock, M.S., Churg, A., Ordernez, N. and Golden, J.A. (1981). Severe pulmonary involvement in mixed connective tissue disease. *Am. Rev. Respir. Dis.* **124**, 499.

Williams, D.G., Stocks, M.R., Smith, P.R. and Maini, R.N. (1986). Murine lupus monoclonal antibodies define five epitopes on two different Sm polypeptides. *Immunology* **58**, 495.

Williamson, G.G., Pennebaker, J. and Boyle, J.A. (1983). Clinical characteristics of patients with rheumatic disorders who possess antibodies against ribonucleoprotein particles. *Arthritis Rheum.* **26**, 509.

Winkelmann, R.K. (1971). Classification and pathogenesis of scleroderma. *Mayo Clin. Proc.* **46**, 83.

Winkelmann, R.K. (1976). Pathogenesis and staging of scleroderma. *Acta Dermatol. Venereol. (Stockholm)* **56**, 83.

Winterbauer, R.H. (1964). Multiple telangiectasia, Raynaud's phenomenon, sclerodactyly, and subcutaneous calcinosis: a syndrome mimicking hereditary hemorrhagic telangiectasia. *Bull. Johns Hopkins Hosp.* **114**, 361.

Wooley, J.C.F., Zuckerberg, L.R. and Chung, S.Y. (1983). Polypeptide components of human small nuclear ribonucleoproteins. *Proc. Nat. Acad. Sci. (USA)* **80**, 5208–12.

Yang, V.W., Lerner, M.R., Steitz, J.A. and Flint, S.J. (1981). *Proc. Nat. Acad. Sci. (USA)* **78**, 1371.

Zieve, G. and Penman, S. (1976). Small RNA species of the HeLa cell: metabolism and subcellular localization. *Cell* **8**, 19–31.

65: Juvenile Chronic Arthritis

P. Woo and B.M. Ansell

Clinical classification

It is generally agreed that juvenile chronic arthritis (JCA) is a heterogeneous group of disorders and that the majority are different from adult rheumatoid arthritis (RA). Classification of JCA is based on the different mode of onset of disease. There are three main ways in which the child presents: some 10–20% will have systemic illness with myalgia or arthralgia, and only develop arthritis later; 60–70% are pauciarticular, which describes a group with involvement of up to a maximum of four joints initially; while polyarthritis, where five or more joints are involved within the first 3 months of the illness, accounts for approximately 10–20%.

There are further clinical subgroups within the pauciarticular onset JCA, according to the initial pattern of joints involved and the association with chronic iridocyclitis. The commonest group comprises young children up to 5 or 6 years, particularly girls, who are at risk from iridocyclitis. Older boys, that is, aged 9, 10 or 11, may well have a peripheral onset of ankylosing spondylitis. Girls of 6–10 years may present with persistent monoarticular arthritis of the knee. Juvenile psoriatic arthritis frequently presents as pauciarticular disease, which later spreads. The majority of children with polyarthritis are seronegative for immunoglobulin M (IgM) rheumatoid factor (RF). Since the definition of JCA is arthritis in children up to 16 years of age, this includes the adolescent period and it is among such children that juvenile spondylitis, seropositive RA and psoriatic arthritis become more obvious.

There are no specific tests. There will be evidence of inflammation, as shown by a rise in acute-phase reactants such as C-reactive protein (CRP) or the erythrocyte sedimentation rate, and non-specific changes in immunoglobulins. Some 6–8% will be IgM RF +ve, particularly in adolescents and 25–30% antinuclear antibody (ANA) +ve, usually in young girls. Diagnosis depends on the awareness of the ways in which JCA can present and the active exclusion of a wide range of disorders varying from infections, through blood dyscrasias and orthopaedic problems to the rarer connective tissue disorders.

Systemic onset disease

Systemic onset disease is the least common form of juvenile arthritis, but the most serious. The usual age of onset is between the first and fourth birthday, but it can occur throughout childhood, and even into adult life; both sexes are equally affected. In addition to the classic triad of fever, rash and arthritis, there is frequently extensive lymphadenopathy and hepatosplenomegaly. Pericarditis is not uncommon (30–40%), but life-threatening myocarditis is seen only rarely, as is serious hepatic dysfunction and cerebral involvement. Initial differentiated diagnosis from a prolonged reaction to a viral illness is extremely difficult and the period of observation and investigation required puts a strain on both family and physician.

The course of systemic disease is unpredictable. These children are particularly susceptible to infection, which can be fatal. There are three different clinical outcomes: one episode only, or a remitting cyclic course with only minor joint residua, or recurrent systemic feature with progressive polyarthritis. Our own most recent follow-up of patients seen within 3 months of onset showed that 50% gradually went into remission over a few years, usually having had one major attack during which they could have been extremely ill. None escaped without some joint residua, the most common being loss of movement at the wrists. Patients with persistent disease, with marked stunting of growth, are extremely difficult to manage and usually require corticosteroid therapy. The majority have a widespread arthritis, often with joint destruction superimposed upon poorly or abnormally developed joints. Severe deformities can result, e.g. multiple flexion contracture or wrist and foot drop, and, in later stages, surgical corrections may be required. At 15 years from onset, radiological hip changes are present in 40% — particularly those with delay in walking due to their young age. Failure of development of the acetabulum, with overgrowth of the femoral head and persistent anteversion, is frequent.

Laboratory findings

The acute-phase response in children with systemic onset disease is characteristically high. During an acute exacerbation the erythrocyte sedimentation rate (ESR) can be over 100 mm/hr, and serum CRP and serum amyloid A (SAA) protein can both be in the region of 200–300 mg/l. There is a marked polyclonal hypergammaglobulinaemia. The white blood count can be up to $50\,000 \times 10^9$, predominantly polymorphonuclear phenotype, and platelet count too can be extremely high, frequently close to 1000×10^9. Haemoglobin is usually low at presentation, and a hypochromic microcytic anaemia of chronic disorder is seen. Patients with systemic onset disease have a negative IgM RF by latex and sheep cell agglutination tests. Very occasionally patients with persistent atypical low-grade irregular fevers and lymphadenopathy have a positive IgM RF; such patients tend to have active disease, and have persistent active polyarthritis later on which is indistinguishable from adult RA. Association with human leucocyte antigen (HLA) DR4 has been reported.

Role of infection

It is well documented that episodes of infection frequently precede exacerbation of disease activity in systemic onset JCA. Indeed the disease itself has many clinical features of an acute infection, and may be associated with increased levels of non-specific antibodies, like rubella (Cassidy *et al.* 1974). A causative infectious agent has not been positively identified so far. Many agents associated with exacerbations have been implicated on different occasions; in a prospective study of 24 episodes of disease exacerbation in 19 children suffering from systemic JCA, herpes simplex, rhinovirus and *Streptococcus* were the agents identified at the time (De-Vere Tyndall *et al.* 1984). Measurements of antibody levels to different infectious agents are, at best, only circumstantial evidence of infection, e.g. high levels of antibodies to influenza A_2N_2 were found in a cluster of children with JCA born in a Flu epidemic (Pritchard *et al.* 1988). In the study by De-Vere Tyndall *et al.* (1984), measurements of specific antibodies to a panel of microbial antigens did not reveal any significant difference from controls and a limited search for defective interferon-α (IFN-α) and IFN-γ production was not fruitful. Thus there is little evidence to implicate a specific causal infectious agent to date.

Evidence for immunoregulatory dysfunction

In the absence of an infectious agent being identified as the cause of systemic onset JCA, research has been directed to identify a possible immunoregulatory defect in these patients.

AUTOANTIBODIES, IMMUNE COMPLEXES AND COMPLEMENT

Elevated titres of classical 19S IgM RF, as detected by RAHA or latex agglutination tests, is rare in all groups of JCA. As mentioned before, a minority of patients have positive IgM RF and these patients tend to have persistent disease and also an aggressive erosive polyarthritis which is indistinguishable from adult RA (Ansell 1983; Clemens *et al*. 1983). In 1978 Moore *et al*. found 'hidden' RF in about 65% of patients with seronegative JCA. This study included all clinical forms of JCA and the presence of 'hidden' RF was independent of age, disease onset and apparently correlation with disease activity. The sera were treated initially by acid gel filtration, in order to dissociate all IgG–anti-IgG complexes. Falus *et al*. (1979) also detected 'hidden' RF, but in 25% of all JCA patients, while Wernick *et al*. (1981) failed to show 'hidden' RF in nine children and Balogh *et al*. (1980) failed to show any difference regarding 'hidden' RF between JCA patients and controls. These studies suggest that there is probably a small amount of complexed IgG–anti-IgG in normal sera as a result of normal immune response which is not detected by the latex agglutination test, and it is unlikely that these complexes are important in the pathogenesis of JCA.

Circulating immune complexes have been detected in all forms of juvenile arthritis (Miller *et al*. 1980; Moore *et al*. 1982). A review of the literature has been presented by Martini (1987) and it is clear that there is wide variation in the rate of identification of immune complexes, depending on the methods used and the disease type. None of these studies showed correlation with disease activity, except for Moore *et al*. (1982), where a correlation was also found with 'hidden' RF. However, the scoring of disease activity was crude in the study described by Moore *et al*. and the correlation can only be described as approximate.

Circulating immune complexes are cleared by several mechanisms and are fully described elsewhere in this book. Opsonization by complement activation is probably normal since complement deficiencies have not been reported in JCA. Thomsen *et al*. (1987) showed a decrease in the complement receptor CR1 on erythrocytes compared with normals in a group comprising all types of juvenile arthritis, but more so in systemics. This result may be related to clearance of immune complexes, but the decrease in CR1 level did not correlate with circulating immune complex by PEG precipitation method or C3d levels. Makela *et al*. (1983) also found decreased erythrocyte CR1 levels in severe systemic onset disease in patients with secondary amyloidosis, although the difference was not significant when compared with controls. So far, there have not been any genetic studies of complement receptors in JCA. This is unlikely to be helpful since inherited low receptor status does not appear to predispose to systemic lupus erythematosus (SLE), an immune complex disease. It is unlikely that circulating immune complexes have a major pathogenetic role.

EVIDENCE FOR DISTURBANCE IN CELLULAR IMMUNE RESPONSE

In a study of cellular immunity of 10 patients with systemic onset JCA, Tsokos *et al*. (1987) found normal numbers of the different T cell phenotypes in the circulation, but increased levels of B cells. Furthermore, a high percentage of B lymphocytes secreted Igs spontaneously. Ziegler *et al*. (1984) also demonstrated increased spontaneous Ig production in children with JCA. This *in vitro* finding is similar to that in RF +ve JCA (Tsokos *et al*. 1987), i.e. there appear to be circulating pre-activated B cells in these two groups, analogous to adult RA.

An interesting autoantibody was described by Morimoto *et al*. in 1981. Six sera from JCA patients with active systemic onset disease contained antibodies reactive with 20–50% of T lymphocytes. Using the monoclonal antibodies OKT4, OKT5 and OKT8, they were able to demonstrate the reactivity to be predominantly against the CD4 +ve subset of T cells. The authors were also able to demonstrate reactivity of the sera with T cells in JCA patients, and removal of the antibody-reactive T cells produced a marked enhancement of pokeweed mitogen (PWM)-stimulated IgG production of B cells co-cultured with the remaining JCA T cells. This *in vitro* phenomenon could represent a dysregulation of Ig production in JCA patients due to the presence of this autoantibody. Many groups have subsequently examined the T cell population in systemic onset JCA. There is no significant difference in the OKT4 : OKT8 ratios of circulating T cells compared with controls (Oen *et al.* 1985; Thoen *et al.* 1987). Moreover, Forre *et al.* (1982) used further monoclonal antibodies, Leu-2A and Leu-3A, to define the T cell population and found that the distribution of phenotypes was normal. A significant difference in the number of OKT8 +ve cells between synovial fluid and peripheral blood of patients has been found (Thoen *et al.* 1987). This is consistent with findings in other chronic joint inflammations, where there is augmentation of T8 +ve T cells in synovial fluid irrespective of the diseases aetiology or the patients' genetic constitution. There are increased DR +ve cells in the synovial fluid, a finding which is also in common with other forms of chronic active synovitis. Functional testing of helper and suppressor activity had not revealed any abnormality in T lymphocytes in patients with JCA (Oen *et al.* 1985; Thoen *et al.* 1987). Therefore there is very little evidence so far to support the hypothesis that there is immunodysregulation as a result of an anti-lymphocyte autoantibody in systemic onset JCA.

INTERLEUKIN PRODUCTION

The clinical and serological picture of systemic onset JCA could be a result of excessive cytokine production. Interleukin 1 (IL-1), IL-6, IFN-γ and also tumour necrosis factor α (TNF-α) can produce fever, malaise and hypergammaglobulinaemia. The interaction of the cytokines has been described elsewhere in this book (Chapters 14–17). It is clear that each of these cytokines can cause immune proliferative cellular responses and can potentiate further secretion of cytokines. Bacon *et al.* (1983) were unable to detect IFN-γ in 18 systemic JCA patients, and examination of IFN-γ production by mononuclear cells *in vitro* in response to a specific viral antigen (NCV) did not reveal any difference between patients and controls. More sensitive techniques are now available, including detection of messenger ribonucleic acid (RNA) production by deoxyribonucleic acid (DNA) probes, and a search for the presence of IFN-γ should be made using appropriate assays.

Preliminary examination of peripheral blood monocytes *in vitro* by Burgio and Martini (1985) showed increased IL-1 production by cells from the patients, compared with controls, and more so in active disease although the results were not significant. Prieur *et al.* (1987) showed normal to high levels of IL-1 activity in afebrile patients with arthritis. During the fever phase, however, they were not able to demonstrate high levels of IL-1. In contrast, the serum and urinary IL-1 activity was low and also they described an 'inhibitory' activity to exogenous IL-1 present in the sera. The inhibitory effect detected in the urine and serum is now attributed to the IL-1 receptor antagonist. Unfortunately, none of these measurements were performed using plasma that had been collected carefully to inhibit any enzyme activation. Therefore *in vitro* production of IL-1 during clotting and the resultant release of cytokines may cloud the true physiological picture. More careful collection of samples and sensitive enzyme-linked immunosorbent assay (ELISA) methods, using monospecific antibodies are now being applied to measure plasma IL-1, IL-6, IFN-γ and TNF-α. Raised levels of such cytokines may merely be a secondary phenomenon to an activated immune system. Alternatively, abnormal regulation of the cytokines may contribute to the pathogenesis of these diseases, and considerable work is currently being performed in this area.

Amyloidosis

There is a risk of patients developing the life-threatening complication of amyloidosis with persistent disease activity. This should be suspected in any child with systemic onset disease who has persistent proteinuria or inappropriate hepatosplenomegaly. It can occur as early as 2 years, but usually is not manifest until after several years of severe disease. The prevalence of amyloidosis in this form of arthritis is approximately 10% from our series and also from a large German series of 2000 patients (Stoeber 1981). It is interesting that amyloidosis appears to be rarer in JCA patients in the United States and Australia. The mortality rate of secondary amyloidosis is approximately 70% in the untreated group at 15 years' follow-up (Janssen *et al.* 1986; A. Howard, personal communication). The cause of death is almost invariably renal failure, with a few cases of septicaemia in patients from the Canadian Red Cross, Northwick Park and Wexham Park Hospitals. The pathogenesis of amyloidosis is described elsewhere in this book (Chapter 22). The amyloid fibre precursor is the acute-phase protein SAA, which is very high in serum of systemic JCA patients. However, previous studies in our group have shown that serum levels of SAA cannot predict amyloidosis. Susceptibility factors can include the structure of SAA itself, or a lack of appropriate synthetic or degradative control. Since there is no effective treatment of amyloidosis, it is important to prevent the onset of this complication by abolishing the acute-phase response with effective drug therapy such as chlorambucil. A marker for susceptible individuals such as the restriction fragment length polymorphism (RFLP) association described by Woo *et al.* (1987), may be useful to earmark patients for effective anti-inflammatory therapy.

Polyarthritic onset juvenile chronic arthritis

Seropositive juvenile rheumatoid arthritis

Persistent IgM RF is found in about 6–8% of all children with juvenile chronic arthritis. Seropositive polyarthritis usually occurs in girls around puberty, with involvement of hands and feet and, later, larger joints. Clinically it resembles adult RA with the early development of erosions and the later development of nodules and vasculitis, as well as other extra-articular manifestations such as pulmonary fibrosis and aortic incompetence. Active disease tends to persist into adult life. This, therefore, is a serious rheumatic disease of childhood. In Britain it is the one group that is referred to as juvenile rheumatoid arthritis (JRA) because both clinical and cellular abnormalities are similar to adult RA (Clemens *et al.* 1983; Tsokos *et al.* 1988). In addition, there is an increased association with HLA-DR4, as in adult RA (Clemens *et al.* 1983). Further RFLP and sequence analysis in DR4 +ve JRA, using complementary DNAs (cDNAs) and genomic DNAs from the DQβ region, has shown a high association with the DQ3.1 allele, analogous to the strong association between the DQ3.2 allele and insulin-dependent diabetes (Nepom *et al.* 1986). Another DR4 +ve disease is Felty's syndrome in adult RA, and this too is associated with the DQ3.1 allele (So *et al.* 1988). Such HLA associations may indicate susceptibility conferred by the Class II major histocompatibility complex (MHC) gene itself, or by another unidentified gene that is in linkage disequilibrium. The significance of HLA disease associations has already been discussed elsewhere in this book (Chapter 39). Immunogenic studies have so far contributed to the subtyping of JCA in terms of prognosis, but may contribute to the understanding of genetic susceptibility to JCA.

Seronegative polyarthritis

Seronegative polyarthritis is much more common than seropositive JCA. Girls are particularly affected and onset of disease may occur at any age throughout childhood, with a peak incidence at about 6 or 7 years. Diagnosis can be difficult at presentation, since the child (especially the younger ones) will not necessarily complain of joint pain. Deformities like flexion contractures of the knees and subluxation of the wrists can develop quickly. These children often will not develop normal hips because of their lack of mobility, even in the absence of hip involvement. Hand involvement with flexor tenosynovitis and proximal interphalangeal joint swelling are seen in severe polyarthritis, irrespective of whether it follows systemic disease or occurs *de novo*. The long-term prognosis of the seronegative disease is usually good, especially in the younger age-group. Arthritis can remit after many years of disease activity, and often without any serious residual radiological joint destruction. However, if these children are to maintain good function, deformities must be corrected as soon as they develop.

This subgroup of disease is heterogeneous both clinically and in relation to immunogenic associations. Preliminary data showed that adolescents seemed to be more at risk from the rapid development of erosive disease, particularly affecting the hips and shoulders. Immunogenetic studies have shown that there is an association with HLA-DR8 in very young children, i.e. below the age of 6. It is arguable, therefore, that the very young polyarticular onset children are at one end of the spectrum of pauciarticular disease (see below) since a proportion of these children go on to have polyarthritis 6 months to a year after pauciarticular onset, and DR8 is also strongly associated with pauciarticular onset disease. Further DNA analysis has revealed a similar association with DRβ1 0801 chain.

Active disease in the seronegative polyarthritics is usually reflected in an increased acute-phase response. Cellular abnormalities again are similar to adult RA, i.e. an increase in spontaneous Ig production and an increased number of B cells and DR +ve T-cells in the synovial fluid. 'Hidden' RFs as immune complexes have been detected in this group as well, but their significance has already been discussed in the previous section.

Pauciarticular onset

Pauciarticular onset disease is the largest group, accounting for about 60–70% of children with juvenile chronic arthritis. The most common presenting joint is the knee, which rapidly takes up a position of flexion with a valgus deformity, which is a position that minimizes pain; the ankle is the second commonest and the wrist and the hand much less common. Although approximately 10% of these children may have only one joint affected initially, the majority will develop disease in more joints. Thus the child may develop swelling of the opposite knee and/or an ankle by the second visit. Most of these children will tend to remain with two to four joints affected, usually large peripheral ones, although occasionally the hip joint is affected or a finger or toe with tenosynovitis. Seventy per cent of children with pauciarticular onset JCA are in remission some 10 years from onset (Ansell 1987). A small proportion (15%) will develop persistent polyarthritis.

Most pauciarticular onset JCA patients will be young, under the age of 5 or 6 years, with girls affected much more often than boys. These children frequently have ANAs and are at risk for the development of chronic iridocyclitis. In our prospective study, 83% of ANA +ve children developed iridocyclitis within 2 years of onset (A.M. Leak). This is often silent and can lead to blindness if their eyes are not routinely checked. Asymmetrical growth of limbs and localized deformities are common in this group. These growth anomalies can be minimized by local corticosteroid injections and the judicious use of physiotherapy combined with orthotics.

Laboratory tests

This group usually have normal or slightly raised acute-phase response with the exception of a small proportion of patients who develop persistent polyarthritis. Immune complexes have been demonstrated in this group and also 'hidden' RFs. In a study of the erythrocyte complement receptor CR1, some pauciarticular onset patients were found to have decreased levels of CR1, but this result was not significant (Thomsen *et al.* 1987).

An interesting marker of iridocyclitis in the young pauciarticular onset children is the presence of low-titre ANA. Over 90% of patients with iridocyclitis are ANA +ve. Attempts to characterize this antibody have shown this not to be anti-DNA antibody or a recognized extractable nuclear antigen (ENA) antibody. Preliminary work from Malleson *et al.* (1987) has shown in eight patients that this may be anti-histone H1. Ostensen *et al.* (1989) found predominantly anti-histone H3 in 26/28 children with ANA and uveitis and mixed anti-histone specificity in JCA with ANA but no uveitis. The presence of this ANA is not associated with hypergammaglobulinaemia or RF. It is not associated with a particular HLA-DR type or Gm type (Hall *et al.* 1985). The role of ANA in JCA children with iridocyclitis is still obscure. In common with ANA in other connective tissue diseases, ANA is probably a marker of this particular clinical presentation rather than directly responsible for the development of iridocyclitis.

Association with human leucocyte antigen Class II major histocompatibility complex antigens

Studies of different Caucasian populations in a multicentre study (Ansell and Albert 1984) in UK (Hall *et al.* 1986), USA (Glass *et al.* 1980) and Scandinavia (Morling *et al.* 1985) have shown significant association of this disease with HLA-DRw8, DR5 and A2. In the UK study (Hall *et al.* 1986), the relative risk for the heterozygote DR5/8 is very high (24), higher than the geometric sum of the risk from DR5 and DR8 alone. Restriction fragment length polymorphism studies of patients from this cohort reveal that all have a 9.5 kb RFLP band, when genomic DNA is digested with Bgl II, and probed with the cDNA of DRβ chain (A.K.L. So, A. Eberhard, B. Ansell and P. Woo, unpublished data). This band is also seen in all DR52 supertypes, to which DR5 and 8, as well as DR3 and 6, belong. These findings are consistent with those of Myers *et al.* (1987), who showed proliferation of T cell clones (raised to different DR epitopes) to peripheral blood mononuclear cells from pauciarticular onset patients. From monoclonal antibody blocking studies, as well as the known specificity of the T cell clones, the authors concluded that these T cells recognized epitopes localized on the DRβ1 and DRβ2 molecules. Thus these results strongly suggest a common epitope on the DRβ chain of pauciarticular JCA patients. Subsequent DNA sequence data confirms association with DRβ1 0801 (Nepom 1991).

A second genetic factor has been reported in this subgroup of JCA. Using alloreactive T cell clones, Hoffman and colleagues (1985, 1986) showed an association between HLA-DPw2 and pauciarticular JCA. This association was independent of DR associations and was confirmed by a population study in Denmark by Odum *et al.* (1986). Deoxyribonucleic acid analysis has located the association to DPβ1 0201 (Nepom 1991). Thus it appears that polygenic factors are implicated in the development of this disease.

Juvenile spondyloarthropathy

Pauciarticular onset disease over the age of 9 years affects boys more frequently than girls and they present with two or three lower limb joints involved, particularly knee, ankle and hip. Enthesitis, i.e. plantar fasciitis, Achilles tendonitis, or sometimes tendonitis around the hip or knee, is frequently seen in this subgroup. There is a family history of ankylosing spondylitis in some 25%. The majority are HLA-B27 +ve, but at this stage in their illness there is little evidence of sacroiliac involvement or back problems. This clinical pattern is now considered to fall into the spondyloarthropathy category. In the majority the peripheral arthropathy settles, but, unless mobility is maintained, these joints tend to stiffen. Over the following 10–15 years they may develop sacroiliitis radiologically; 60% of these ultimately develop back problems which can occur 11–33 years after the onset of arthritis (B.M. Ansell, unpublished data). The biggest problem in this group is hip disease, which can be troublesome both in adolescence and later on in life. The course of the disease may be punctuated by acute iridocyclitis (26% in the first 15 years), which is symptomatic and requires immediate attention. A few of these patients will ultimately develop inflammatory bowel disease or psoriasis. Few immunological investigations have been performed in this subgroup. Since this is associated with HLA-B27, the immunological mechanisms are assumed to be similar to adult B27 disease.

Juvenile psoriatic arthritis

Juvenile psoriatic arthritis has been regarded as part of the spondyloarthropathy group. It usually presents about the age of 8 or 9 years, affecting girls slightly more frequently than boys and, while often presenting with one or two joints, the vast majority spread to polyarthritis. Characteristically this is asymmetrical and can be locally destructive (Shore *et al.* 1982). Particular clues are the pattern of involvement with a single hand or foot digit with all three joints affected, involvement of terminal interphalanageal joints, a severe flexor tenosynovitis in a finger, a family history of psoriasis (40%) or nail pits in the child. The skin disease may follow joints by several years. Human leucocyte antigens B27 and DR1 are more prevalent in these children (Ganczarczyk *et al.* 1985), showing some difference from adult psoriatic arthritis (Gladman *et al.* 1986).

Conclusion

Immunogenic studies have helped to substantiate some of the clinical classification of JCA, suggesting that an interaction between an environmental agent (which could be infectious) and different genetic backgrounds can manifest as JCA with different clinical patterns in terms of severity and prognosis. Greater or lesser perturbation of immunological parameters have been found in the different groups of JCA, but there is as yet no evidence of dysregulation of the immune response.

References

Ansell, B.M. (1983). Juvenile chronic arthritis. *Scand. J. Rheumatol.* **66** (suppl.), 47–50.

Ansell, B.M. and Albert, E.D. (1984). Juvenile chronic arthritis: pauci-articular type. In *Histocompatibility Testing*, eds E.D. Albert, M.P. Baur and W.R. Mayr, pp. 368–74, Springer-Verlag, Berlin.

Bacon, T.H., De-Vere Tyndall, A., Tyrrell, D.A., Denman, A.M. and Ansell, B.M. (1983). Interferon system in patients with systemic juvenile chronic arthritis: *in vivo* and *in vitro* studies. *Clin. Exp. Immunol.* **54**, 23–30.

Balogh, Z., Mereley, K., Falus, A. and Bozsoky, S. (1980). Serological abnormalities in juvenile chronic arthritis: a review of 46 cases. *Ann. Rheum. Dis.* **39**, 129–39.

Burgio, G.R. and Martini, A. (1985). Interleukin production in juvenile chronic arthritis (letter). *Ann. Rheum. Dis.* **44**, 723.

Cassidy, J.T., Shillis, J.L., Brandon, F.B., Sullivan, D.B. and Brackett, R.G. (1974). Viral antibody titres to rubella and rubeola in juvenile rheumatoid arthritis. *Pediatrics* **54**, 239–44.

Clemens, L.E., Albert, E. and Ansell, B.M. (1983). HLA studies in IgM rheumatoid-factor-positive arthritis of childhood. *Ann. Rheum. Dis.* **42**, 431–4.

De-Vere Tyndall, A., Bacon, T., Parry, R., Tyrrell, D.A.J., Denman, A.M. and Ansell, B.M. (1984). Infection and interferon production in systemic juvenile chronic arthritis: a prospective study. *Ann. Rheum. Dis.* **43**, 1–7.

Falus, A., Mereley, K., Bohm, U. and Bozsoky, S. (1979). Complexed rheumatoid factor measurements in sera, synovial fluids and in immune complex fractions. *Experimentia.* **35**, 413–14.

Forre, O., Thoen, J., Dobloug, J.H. *et al.* (1982). Detection of T-lymphocyte subpopulation in the peripheral blood and the synovium of patients with rheumatoid arthritis and juvenile rheumatoid arthritis using monoclonal antibodies. *Scand. J. Immunol.* **15**, 221–6.

Ganczarczyk, M.L., Gladman, D.D. and Shore, A. (1985). Juvenile psoriatic arthritis — clinical analysis and HLA antigens. *Arthritis Rheum.* Suppl. S72, Abstr. C42.

Gladman, D.D., Anhorn, K.A.B., Schachter, R.K. and Mervart, H. (1986). HLA antigens in psoriatic arthritis. *J. Rheumatol.* **13**, 586–92.

Glass, D., Litvin, D., Wallace, K. *et al.* (1980). Early onset pauciarticular juvenile rheumatoid arthritis associated with human leukocyte antigen-DRW5, iritis, and antinuclear antibody. *J. Clin. Invest.* **66**, 426–9.

Hall, P.J., De Lange Gerd, G. and Ansell, B.M. (1985). Immunoglobulin allotypes in families with pauci-articular onset juvenile chronic arthritis. *Tissue Antigens* **25**, 212–15.

Hall, P.J., Burman, S.J., Laurent, M.R. *et al.* (1986). Genetic susceptibility to early onset pauci-articular juvenile chronic arthritis: a study of HLA and complement markers in 158 British patients. *Ann. Rheum. Dis.* **45**, 464–74.

Hall, P.J., Burman, S.J., Barash, J., Briggs, D.C. and Ansell, B.M. (1989). HLA and complement C4 antigens in polyarticular onset seronegative juvenile chronic arthritis: association of early onset with HLA-DRw8 *J. Rheumatol.* **16**, 55–9.

Hoffman, R.W., Shaw, S., Francis, L.C. *et al.* (1985). HLA-DP (SB) antigens in pauci-articular JRA with iridocyclitis (abstract). *Arthritis Rheum.* Suppl. **28**, S35.

Hoffman, R.W., Shaw, S., Francis, L.C. *et al.* (1986). HLA-DP antigens in patients with pauciarticular juvenile rheumatoid arthritis. *Arthritis Rheum.* **29**, 1057–62.

Janssen, S., Van Ruswijk, M.H., Meijer, S., Ruinen, L. and Van Der Hem, G.K. (1986). Systemic amyloidosis: a clinical survey of 144 cases. *Netherlands J. Med.* **29**, 376–85.

Makela, A.L., Erola, E., Lehtonen, O.P., Ruuska, P. and Lantto, R. (1983). Erythrocyte C3b receptors in juvenile rheumatoid arthritis. *N. Engl. J. Med.* **309**, 673.

Malleson, P.N., Fung, M. and Petty, R.E. (1987). Antigenic heterogeneity of antinuclear antibodies in juvenile rheumatoid arthritis. *Arthritis Rheum.* **30**, S126.

Martini, A. (1987). Immunological abnormalities in juvenile chronic arthritis. *Scand. J. Rheumatol.* Suppl. 66, p. 5–11.

Miller, J.J., Osborne, C.L. and Hsu, Y.P. (1980). C1q binding in serum in juvenile rheumatoid arthritis. *J. Rheumatol.* **7**, 665–70.

Moore, T.L., Zuckner, J. and Baldassare, A.R. (1978). Complement fixing hidden rheumatoid factor in juvenile rheumatoid arthritis. *Arthritis Rheum.* **21**, 935–41.

Moore, T.L., Sheridan, P.W., Traycoff, R.B., Zuckner, J. and Dorner, R.W. (1982). Immune complexes in juvenile rheumatoid arthritis: a comparison of four methods. *J. Rheumatol.* **9**, 395–401.

Morimoto, C., Reinherz, E.L., Borel, Y., Mantzouranis, E., Steinberg, A.D. and Schlossman, S.F. (1981). Autoantibodies to an immunoregulatory inducer population in patients with juvenile arthritis. *J. Clin. Invest.* **67**, 735–5.

Morling, N., Friis, J., Heilmann, C. *et al.* (1985). HLA antigen frequencies in juvenile chronic arthritis. *Scand. J. Rheumatol.* **14**, 209–16.

Myers, L.K., Ball, E.J., Nunez, G., Fink, C.W., and Stastny, P. (1987). HLA-D region epitopes associated with juvenile arthritis: recognition by alloreactive T cell clones and alloantisera. *Arthritis Rheum.* **30**, 744–51.

Nepom, B.S. (1991). Immunogenetics of juvenile rheumatoid arthritis. In *Rheumatic Disease Clinics of North America*, pp. 825–42, W.B. Saunders, Philadelphia.

Nepom, B.S., Palmer, J., Kim, S.J., Hansen, J.A., Holbeck, S.L. and Nepom, G.T. (1986). Specific genomic markers for the HLA-DQ subregion discriminate between DR4+ insulin-dependent diabetes mellitus and DR4+ seropositive juvenile rheumatoid arthritis. *J. Exp. Med.* **164**, 345–50.

Odum, N., Marlig, N., Friis, J. *et al.* (1986). Increased frequency of HLA-DPw2 in pauciarticular onset of juvenile chronic arthritis. *Tissue Antigens* **28**, 245–50.

Oen, K., Wilkins, J.A. and Krzekotowska, D. (1985) OKT4 : OKT8 ratios of circulating T cells and *in vitro* suppressor cell function of patients with juvenile rheumatoid arthritis (JRA). *J. Rheumatol.* **12**, 321–7.

Ostensen, M., Fredriksen, K., Kass, E. and Rekvig, O.P. (1989). Identification of antihistone antibodies in subsets of juvenile chronic arthritis. *Ann. Rheum. Dis.* **48**, 114–17.

Prieur, A.-M., Griscelli, C., Kaufman, M.-T. and Dayer, J.-M. (1987). Specific interleukin-1 inhibitor in serum and urine of children with systemic juvenile chronic arthritis. *Lancet* **ii**, 1240–7.

Pritchard, M.H., Matthews, N. and Munro, J. (1988). Antibodies to influenza A in a cluster of children with juvenile chronic arthritis. *Br. J. Rheumatol.* **27**, 176–80.

So, A.K.L., Warner, C.A., Sansom, D. and Walport, M.J. (1988). DQβ polymorphism and genetic susceptibility to Felty's syndrome. *Arthritis Rheum.* **31**, 990–5.

Stoeber, E. (1981). Prognosis in JCA. *Eur. J. Pediatr.* **135**, 225–8.

Thoen, J., Waalen, K. and Forre, D. (1987). Natural killer (NK) cells at inflammatory sites of patients with rheumatoid arthritis and IgM rheumatoid factor positive polyarticular juvenile rheumatoid arthritis. *Clin. Rheumatol.* **6**, 215–25.

Thomsen, B.S., Heilmann, C., Jacobsen, S.E. *et al.* (1987). Complement C3b receptors on erythrocytes in patients with juvenile rheumatoid arthritis. *Arthritis Rheum.* **30**, 967–71.

Tsokos, G.C., Mavridis, A., Inghirami, G., Pillemer, S.R., Emery, H.M. and Magilavy, D.B. (1987). Cellular immunity in patients with systemic juvenile rheumatoid arthritis. *Clin. Immunol. Immunopathol.* **42**, 86–92.

Tsokos, G.C., Inghirami, G., Pillemer, S.R., Mavridis, A. and Magilavy, D.B. (1988). Immunoregulatory aberrations in patients with polyarticular juvenile rheumatoid arthritis. *Clin. Immunol. Immunopathol.* **47**, 62–74.

Welsh, K.I., Briggs, D.C., Black, C.M. and Maddison, P.J. (1986). Positive and negative associations in the MHC with antinuclear antibodies: implications in the immunogenetics of systemic sclerosis (abstract). British Society of Rheumatology, Dublin Meeting (unpublished data).

Wernick, R., Lospalluto, J.J., Fink, C.W. and Ziff, M. (1981). Serum IgG and IgM rheumatoid factors by solid phase radioimmunoassay: a comparison between adult and juvenile rheumatoid arthritis. *Arthritis Rheum.* **24**, 1501–11.

Woo, P., Robson, M., O'Brien, J. and Ansell, B.M. (1987). A genetic marker for systemic amyloidosis in juvenile arthritis. *Lancet* **ii**, 767–9.

Ziegler, J.B., Zaunders, J.J., Cooper, D.A. *et al.* (1984). Immunoregulation in juvenile chronic arthritis. *Int. Arch. Allergy Appl. Immunol.* **75**, 196–202.

Section 8
Immunodeficiency

66: The Primary Specific Immunodeficiencies

F.S. Rosen

The primary specific immunodeficiencies are diseases that result from intrinsic defects in B and T lymphocytes. They are to be distinguished from the non-specific deficiencies such as those of the complement system or of phagocytes, which play a non-specific role in immunity. The secondary defects, as opposed to the primary defects, in the immune system are those caused by exogenous agents, such as drugs, irradiation and infections, or by environmental factors, such as malnutrition. These subjects are discussed in other chapters.

X-linked agammaglobulinaemia

In 1952, boys with recurrent pyogenic infections who had no γ-globulin in their serum were discovered by Bruton (1952). This disease has been called Bruton's disease or congenital agammaglobulinaemia but the term X-linked agammaglobulinaemia (X-LA) is preferred.

Affected male infants are usually well for the first 6–12 months of life because they are passively protected by transplacentally transmitted immunoglobulin G (IgG). Depending on environmental factors, the onset of infections may be even further delayed. Subsequently, they manifest recurrent pneumonia, otitis media, sinusitis, pyoderma and other infections due to encapsulated pyogenic bacteria. These infections are mostly due to *Haemophilus influenzae*, staphylococci, streptococci and pneumococci. Occasionally *Pseudomonas* organisms may cause infection in patients receiving many antibiotics. Although these infections are readily controlled with antibiotics, their persistent recurrence, particularly in the respiratory tract, leads to anatomical destruction and bronchiectasis (Rosen *et al.* 1984).

Genetics

X-linked agammaglobulinaemia is a monogenic defect. The gene maps to the long arm of the X chromosome at q21.2 to q22 (Kwan *et al.* 1986, 1990). The probe DXS178 is tightly linked to the X-LA locus and no crossovers have been found between this probe and X-LA in over two dozen kindred.

Obligate female heterozygous carriers are perfectly normal. However, it can be shown that there is non-random X chromosome inactivation in their B lymphocytes and that the affected X chromosome is subject to preferential inactivation (Conley *et al.* 1986; Fearon *et al.* 1987; Schwaber *et al.* 1988). No other cells of the obligate female heterozygote display this non-random X chromosome inactivation, so the disease is presumably confined to cells of B lymphocyte lineage.

Diagnosis

The diagnosis of X-LA rests on demonstrating the absence of B lymphocytes in the blood. Serum IgA and IgM levels are undetectable and serum IgG is usually less than 100 mg/dl. The bone marrow contains a normal number of pre-B cells, defined by the presence of cytoplasmic μ chains (Pearl *et al.* 1978).

T cell function in X-LA is normal. Delayed-type hypersensitivity, allograft rejection and *in vitro* responses to specific and non-specific mitogens are all normal. Biopsy of antigen-stimulated lymph nodes reveals a pattern of disorganization. There are no germinal follicles in the cortex and no plasma cells can be found in the medulla. The lymph nodes, which are small, contain only T lymphocytes.

Therapy

For the past decade, it has been possible to administer large doses of γ-globulin by the intravenous route. This advance in immunoglobulin therapy has revealed that patients were being given inadequate doses of γ-globulin by the intramuscular route, where volume limitations prevented truly prophylactic doses. The optimal dose of γ-globulin must be determined for each patient, as some require that the serum IgG concentration be kept at physiological levels to prevent the progression of obstructive lung disease. A minimal dose appears to be 400 mg/kg of body-weight at monthly intervals; in most cases, however, this dose is inadequate and more frequent administration of intravenous γ-globulin is preferable. Many of the older patients have been taught self-infusion and can administer γ-globulin to themselves at weekly intervals. Intercurrent infections should be vigorously treated with ampicillin or other appropriate antibiotics.

Complications

About one-third of boys with X-LA have swelling of the large joints, particularly of the knees, prior to diagnosis. This rheumatoid-like arthritis disappears once γ-globulin replacement therapy is started.

Patients with X-LA have been given poliovirus immunization, prior to awareness of the diagnosis, and have developed paralytic poliomyelitis. No live viral vaccines should be given to boys with X-LA, or for that matter to any immunodeficient children.

A complication resembling dermatomyositis is characterized by muscle pain and weakness, and a heliotrope rash, most prominently over the extensor surfaces of the joints. These patients also have neurological symptoms and the cerebrospinal fluid contains elevated amounts of protein and a pleocytosis. In almost all cases, this is due to echoviruses, which can be cultured from the cerebrospinal fluid (Wilfert *et al.* 1977). This complication can be readily controlled with high doses of intravenous γ-globulin that contains antibodies to the relevant echovirus (Mease *et al.* 1981). Untreated, this complication has a relentlessly downhill course and is ultimately fatal.

Pathogenesis

The basic defect in X-LA is not known. As previously mentioned, normal numbers of pre-B cells are found in the bone marrow but they mature into B cells at a markedly diminished rate so that virtually no B lymphocytes are found. When transformed with Epstein–Barr virus in culture, these X-LA pre-B cells appear not to be able to rearrange the V gene to the normally rearranged DJH segment of the μ chain (Schwaber *et al.* 1983). However, this finding has been controverted by others (Cooper *et al.* 1986). A resolution of the aetiology of X-LA awaits isolation of the gene, and that may occur in the near future.

In a few families, growth hormone deficiency has been linked to X-LA (Fleisher *et al.* 1980). It is not yet completely clear whether this is due to involvement of linked loci. Rare cases of females with a disease indistinguishable from X-LA have been reported (Hoffman *et al.* 1977).

Immunoglobulin A deficiency

One in 600 Caucasians are IgA-deficient but this deficiency is very rare in Africans and Japanese. Among Caucasians IgA deficiency is the most common immunodeficiency disease encountered. About 20% of IgA-deficient individuals have a concomitant IgG subclass deficiency and these individuals appear to be more susceptible to recurrent respiratory infections. As described elsewhere in this chapter, 50–70% of patients with hereditary ataxia telangiectasia (AT) are also IgA-deficient. An increased incidence of allergy (Burks and Steele 1986) and autoimmune disease, particularly rheumatoid arthritis (Cassidy *et al.* 1969), has been observed in IgA deficiency. There is a high incidence of antibodies to ruminant proteins of dietary source in IgA-deficient individuals and this may lead to immune complex disease when cow's milk and other bovine, ovine and caprine proteins are ingested. Patients with IgA deficiency also tend to make antibodies to immunoglobulins, particularly anti-IgA antibodies, which can give rise to anaphylactic reactions (Vyas *et al.* 1968). Some IgA-deficient patients need replacement immunoglobulin because of sinopulmonary infections despite the presence of IgA antibodies. Successful replacement has been achieved in such individuals with an IgA-depleted IgG preparation (Cunningham-Rundles *et al.* 1986).

B lymphocytes in IgA-deficient individuals bear membrane IgA and IgM but fewer mature membrane-bearing IgA cells without membrane IgM are found (Conley and Cooper 1981). These findings suggest a failure of maturation of IgA B cells in these patients. The reason for this maturation failure is unclear. In several populations IgA deficiency has been associated with human leucocyte antigen (HLA)-B8 and HLA-DR3 (Schaffer *et al.* 1991). These findings suggested that IgA deficiency might be associated with an extended HLA haplotype and this turned out to be so when it was furthermore discovered that IgA deficiency is also associated with absent C4A genes, C4B1 and the slow variant of factor B. In addition a rare C2 variant was associated with IgA deficiency (Schaffer *et al.* 1989). Multiple cases of IgA deficiency have been noted in families but the inheritance pattern has always been variable and unclear. That this deficiency may be associated with the major histocompatibility complex (MHC) locus suggests an autosomal recessive inheritance of the deficiency, which may require ill-defined environmental factors for its expression (Schaffer *et al.* 1991). In one study of 95 patients with IgA deficiency alanine and valine substitutions for aspartic acid were found at position 57 of the DQ β chain (Olerup *et al.* 1990). A similar change has been found in type I insulin-dependent diabetes mellitus.

Similar MHC extended haplotypes have been found in patients with common variable immunodeficiency (CVID) and this finding has suggested that CVID and IgA deficiency are polar ends of a spectrum of immunodeficiencies. This is further supported by the frequency of IgG subclass deficiencies in patients with IgA deficiency.

Immunoglobulin G subclass deficiency

Approximately 10% of the population have deletions of heavy chain loci on one of their chromosomes. This rarely leads to immunoglobulin deficiency of clinical consequence (Lefranc *et al.* 1991).

On the other hand, deficiencies of one or more IgG subclasses are not common and probably result from failure of isotype switching under T cell control rather than from isotype gene deletions. There are four subclasses of IgG: IgG1, IgG2, IgG3 and IgG4. Immunoglobulin G1 accounts for 67% of serum IgG and a deficiency of this subclass would be indistinguishable from CVID, since it comprises the bulk of serum IgG. Immunoglobulin G2 constitutes 20–25% of serum IgG and IgG3 5–10%. As IgG4 comprises less than 5% of serum IgG, its deficiency appears to have no clinical consequences except in those cases where it is accompanied by IgG2 deficiency. Thus isolated deficiency of IgG2, and to a lesser extent of IgG3, is clinically important. Almost all human antibody to the polysaccharide capsules of pyogenic bacteria, such as pneumococci and *Haemophilus influenzae,* is found in the IgG2 fraction. Isolated IgG2 deficiency can thus lead to recurrent pyogenic infections such as are seen in males with X-LA. The diagnosis of IgG2 subclass deficiency should be suspected when there is a relevant clinical history and the total serum IgG level is at the lower limits of normal. However, an inability to respond to capsular polysaccharides has been observed in children with normal IgG levels and this incapacity results in clinical findings indistinguishable from IgG2 subclass deficiency (Ambrosino *et al*. 1988; Preud'Homme and Hanson 1990).

Isolated IgG3 deficiency can also lead to recurrent bacterial infections but the pathophysiology of this isolated defect is less well understood. In any case, patients with selective IgG subclass deficiency benefit from immunoglobulin replacement therapy.

Immunodeficiency with increased immunoglobulin M

A clinical syndrome resembling X-LA has been found in patients who have no IgA, very little IgG but increased concentrations of IgM. In addition to increased susceptibility to pyogenic infections, these patients tend to make IgM autoantibodies to neutrophils and platelets, and even rarely to T lymphocytes and erythrocytes. Thus neutropenia and thrombocytopenia tend to complicate the immunodeficiency. This defect is commonly inherited as an X-linked recessive character but autosomal recessive inheritance has also been reported. The deficiency was acquired in several cases during the rubella pandemic of the early 1960s. Increased numbers of plasmacytoid cells that secrete IgM are found in the blood of these patients (Geha *et al*. 1979) as well as in tissue infiltrates, particularly in the gastrointestinal tract. These infiltrates can become malignant in their tissue invasiveness and can prove fatal in many cases.

There appears to be a defect in isotype switching from IgM to IgA and IgG in these patients. In some the defect appears to be intrinsic to the immature μ-bearing B cells. In most a T cell defect appears to be present in that isotype switching of the patients' B cells can be forced by lymphoma cells of T cell lineage (Mayer *et al*. 1986).

Common variable immunodeficiency

A heterogeneous group of disorders that do not readily lend themselves to classification have been lumped together under the designation CVID; this was formerly referred to as acquired or late-onset agammaglobulinaemia. Cases of CVID are equally divided between males and females; surprisingly most cases have their onset before the age of 25. They have recurrent pyogenic infections of the respiratory tract, resulting in severe obstructive pulmonary disease if untreated. Indeed, the diagnosis should be suspected in any adolescent or adult with chronic progressive bronchiectasis. Patients with CVID frequently develop gastrointestinal disease with chronic diarrhoea, steatorrhoea and malabsorption with protein-losing enteropathy. In many cases, this is due to infestation of the gastrointestinal tract with *Giardia lamblia*; they can be rapidly eliminated with atabrine or metronidazole. In some cases, intolerance to milk proteins or gluten is encountered. Giant lymphoid hyperplasia of the gastrointestinal tract in CVID patients imparts a moth-eaten appearance to a barium study of the gastrointestinal tract. More than half of the patients with CVID develop achlorhydria and pernicious anaemia. The consequent megaloblastic changes in the bone marrow and vitamin B_{12} deprivation lead to faulty phagocytic function that compounds susceptibility to infection. Frequently patients with CVID whose infections appear not to respond to adequate antibiotic therapy have become B_{12}-deficient.

Splenomegaly is present in many patients with CVID, and lymph nodes may be palpable in the cervical, axillary and inguinal regions. As with the intestinal giant lymphoid hyperplasia, the lymphoid exuberance is usually benign in these patients. Sometimes non-caseating, sarcoid-like granulomas are found in the skin, spleen, liver, gut, lung and other viscera. The cause of these granulomas is not known and they are controlled with steroid therapy. Some patients with CVID have contracted acquired immune deficiency syndrome (AIDS) and, curiously, this cures their agammaglobulinaemia (Wright *et al*. 1987).

The serum of patients with CVID contains less than 500 mg/dl of IgG. Depression of IgA and IgM concentration is variable and usually less than 50 mg/dl. Cooper and Lawton (1972) observed that most of these patients have circulating B lymphocytes, and a heterogeneity of defects was found in the circulating B cells of CVID patients (Geha *et al.* 1974). About 20% of these patients have no circulating B lymphocytes. The precise defects in the B cells of the remaining 80% of the patients are obscure. The various B cell phenotypes and the accompanying functional abnormalities found in CVID patients has recently been reviewed by Spickett *et al.* (1990). T cell function in CVID may be normal, and many patients exhibit a progressive decline in their capacity to respond to non-specific mitogens and antigens.

As previously discussed, there appears to be a spectrum of disease between isolated IgA deficiency at one extreme and CVID at the other. Like IgA deficiency, CVID has been associated with certain HLA haplotypes but the interpretation of these findings is as yet unclear.

Patients with CVID should be treated with immunoglobulin replacement therapy as described for X-LA. Those patients who are vitamin B_{12}-deficient should receive 1000 μg of vitamin B_{12} at monthly intervals by subcutaneous injection. Appropriate antibiotics should be used to treat intercurrent infections.

Transient hypogammaglobulinaemia of infancy

The serum of normal human new-borns contains an amount of IgG that is roughly equilibrated with the maternal IgG concentration. As this dowry of IgG is slowly consumed by the new-born, the onset of endogenous immunoglobulin synthesis begins in the 3rd month of life. This physiological event may be abnormally delayed and leaves the infant with depressed serum concentrations of IgG up to 36 months of age. The phenomenon does not appear to be genetically determined, although a familial incidence has been noted. Many of these infants have milk intolerance and a tendency to develop mild obstructive pulmonary disease. However, the prognosis is generally favourable and only a few of these children require immunoglobulin replacement therapy. The cause of the delay in IgG synthesis is not entirely clear. T and B cell numbers are normal in peripheral blood. CD4 T cells in these infants appear to provide inadequate help for IgG synthesis (Siegel *et al.* 1981).

Severe combined immunodeficiency

Severe combined immunodeficiency (SCID) is a phenotypic description of a fatal illness of infancy, which has many genotypic causes. Infants with SCID have no cell-mediated immunity and no humoral immunity. The disease is incompatible with survival. By 3 months of age affected infants manifest opportunistic infections. Most commonly the first infection is widespread moniliasis of the mouth and the nappy area. Persistent pertussis-like cough usually betrays the presence of interstitial pneumonitis, most commonly due to *Pneumocystis carinii* or to giant-cell pneumonia from respiratory syncytial virus. Persistent diarrhoea is usually due to rotavirus infection or enteropathic *Escherichia coli* or *Salmonella* infection. Immunization with bacillus Calmette–Guérin or vaccinia virus results in progressive disease with a fatal outcome.

The diagnosis of SCID must always be suspected in the face of thrush, intractable diarrhoea and persistent pneumonitis, because it presents a medical emergency; unless such infants are rescued, usually by transplants of bone marrow, the outcome is invariably fatal. Failure to gain weight is an important feature of the disease. On chest X-ray, the thymus shadow is absent.

Diagnosis

Infants with SCID are lymphopenic and contain less than 3000 lymphocytes/mm^3 of blood. The number of natural killer cells may be normal or elevated, but CD3+ve T lymphocytes are absolutely depressed in number and may even be of maternal origin when they are found. As mentioned, the thymus is not visible in the chest film, but it is sometimes required to have a skilled thoracic surgeon obtain a biopsy of the thymic remnant, which can be located with fibre optics; the pathognomonic feature of the disease lies in the histopathology of the thymus gland, which appears fetal in that the endodermal anlage is present but has failed to become lymphoid. Peripheral blood mononuclear cells from SCID patients are unresponsive to non-specific mitogens, such as phytohaemagglutinin or pokeweed or concanavalin A, as well as to specific antigens and to allogeneic stimuli.

The ratio of affected males to females is three to one. The most common form of SCID is X-linked, and affected males usually have normal numbers of B lymphocytes in their peripheral blood, in contrast to the autosomal recessive forms of the disease where B lymphocytes are absent from the blood. All lymphoid tissue is poorly developed and lymph node biopsies to establish the diagnosis are ill-advised as the biopsy site frequently becomes a portal of entry for infection.

Therapy

All forms of SCID can be corrected with transplants of bone marrow (Gatti *et al*. 1968). When a histoidentical donor (usually a sibling) is available, a successful transplant can be achieved with as few as 50×10^6 donor marrow cells. Complete lymphoid chimerism becomes manifest in 10–14 days and the transplanted lymphoid cells mature to reconstitute the entire immune system of the recipient. As these infants are extemely susceptible to graft-versus-host disease (Kretschmer *et al*. 1969), it has been difficult to achieve lymphoid reconstitution with haploidentical marrow, a desirable goal in view of the fact that 40% of SCID patients do not have a histoidentical sibling. This has been achieved by depleting donor marrow of T lymphocytes with monoclonal antibodies (Reinherz *et al*. 1982) or with lectin columns (Reisner *et al*. 1983). O'Reilly *et al*. (1989) has recently reviewed the world-wide experience with haplo-identical marrow transplants. Recent attempts at gene therapy will be discussed below.

Genetics

Severe combined immunodeficiency may have many genetic causes. As mentioned, there are three times as many affected males as females and the X-linked form of the disease is the most common form. The defect has been mapped to the proximal portion of the long arm at Xq13.1 to Xq13.3 because of its tight linkage to the deoxyribonucleic acid (DNA) probes for PGK1 and DXS72 (Goodship *et al*. 1989; Puck *et al*. 1989). Obligate female heterozygous carriers exhibit non-random X chromosome inactivation in their T cells and in mature B cells (but not in immature μ-bearing B cells) (Conley *et al*. 1988).

The autosomal recessive form of the disease appears to have several genetic bases; about half of these patients have a defect in one of the purine degradation enzymes, adenosine deaminase (ADA) or purine nucleoside phosphorylase (PNP). Adenosine deaminase has been mapped to chromosome 20q13.11 and PNP to chromosome 14q13.1. Point mutations and exon deletions in ADA and PNP have been found in many affected kindred, and these have recently been reviewed by Hirschhorn (1990) and Markert (1991). Rare ADA mutants have also been found that do not result in SCID (Hirschhorn 1990).

Pathogenesis

The discovery of defects in purine degradation enzymes in SCID was fortuitous and led to a flurry of research to explain the pathogenic relationship between the biochemical defects and immunodeficiency. Adenosine deaminase and PNP are ubiquitously distributed in mammalian cells, and the connection between the lymphoid pathology and the biochemical defect was not immediately apparent. Adenose deaminase catalyses the deamination of adenosine and 2′-deoxyadenosine to inosine with the production of ammonia. Purine nucleoside phosphorylase catalyses the conversion of guanosine to guanine and of inosine to hypoxanthine. As a consequence of these enzyme defects, adenosine triphosphate (ATP) and deoxyadenosine triphosphate (dATP) accumulate in ADA-deficient lymphoid cells and guanosine triphosphate (GTP) and deoxyguanosine triphosphate (dGTP) in PNP-deficient lymphoid cells. Deoxyadenosine triphosphate and dGTP are toxic to the enzyme ribonucleotide reductase, which is needed for DNA synthesis. The reasons for the preferential accumulation of these toxic metabolites in lymphoid cells are not entirely clear (Carson *et al*. 1977). None the less, bone marrow transplants clear these metabolites (Hirschhorn *et al*. 1981). This led to the idea that benefit might be obtained from pure enzyme replacement. Adenosine deaminase was conjugated to polyethylene glycol and administered to ADA-deficient patients, with improvement in immunological function (Hershfield *et al*. 1987). More recently the

ADA gene inserted into a retroviral vector has been transfected into lymphoid cells of an ADA-deficient child. Early results from this labour-intensive experiment appear promising (R.M. Blaese, pers. comm.).

Rare SCID phenotypes have been traced to defects in well-defined molecules of the immune system. In one child with SCID, CD7 was absent from T cells (Jung *et al.* 1986). Children in two Mennonite kindred have had a deficiency of CD8 +ve cells and SCID; at least two affected children were successfully transplanted with bone marrow (Roifman *et al.* 1989). In a Spanish kindred, CD3 was defective in a child affected with SCID; this was traced to defective biosynthesis of the γ chain of CD3 (Alarcon *et al.* 1988). In a French child CD3 was absent from T cells, also due to a defect in the γ chain (Thoenes *et al.* 1990).

Signal transduction defects and cytokine defects have also been associated with SCID. Chatila *et al.* (1989) described a boy who was unable to transduce signals when stimulated with mitogens or antigens; the defect could be circumvented *in vitro* with phorbol esters. Severe combined immunodeficiency has been associated with a defect in the interleukin 2 gene (Weinberg and Parkman 1990); failure of transcription of multiple lymphokine genes (Chatila *et al.* 1990); and defective interleukin 1 receptors (Chu *et al.* 1984).

Reticular dysgenesis is a form of SCID in which granulocytes are also absent. These infants die very rapidly unless rescued with bone marrow transplants (Levinsky and Tiedman 1983).

Another variant of SCID is called Omenn's syndrome. It is inherited as an autosomal recessive, and affected infants have erythroderma, hepatosplenomegaly, histiocytosis, eosinophilia and elevated serum concentrations of IgE. The number of circulating T cells may be normal but they have poor function (Businco *et al.* 1987).

Another SCID variant is found in children with cartilage–hair hypoplasia. The defect is common in Amish children and apparently in Finland. Metaphyseal dysostosis results in short-limbed dwarfism and hair is sparse and depigmented. The defect in cell-mediated immunity is variable, from frank SCID to much milder forms of immunodeficiency. Fatal varicella has been frequently observed in affected children (Lux *et al.* 1970; Ranki *et al.* 1978; Pierce and Polmar 1982).

Class II major histocompatibility complex deficiency

Defective expression of Class II MHC molecules has been observed in almost two dozen kindred, mostly North African immigrants in Western Europe. The defect is inherited as an autosomal recessive phenomenon. Antigen-presenting cells and B lymphocytes of affected children do not express DP, DQ or DR molecules. The I invariant chain is normally expressed. Interferon-γ does not induce Class II MHC expression in affected infants (de Preval *et al.* 1988). Because of the Class II MHC deficiency, CD4 +ve cells are also deficient, presumably due to the failure of positive selection for these cells in the thymus by Class II MHC molecules. Delayed-type hypersensitivity cannot be elicited in affected children, but, in contrast to SCID, their T cells respond *in vitro* to non-specific mitogens and allogeneic stimuli. Because they lack CD4 +ve T cell helper function, antibody formation is poor and these infants tend to be hypogammaglobulinaemic. Clinically they resemble the SCID phenotype and have many opportunistic infections. Affected infants have been noted to have protracted diarrhoea and malabsorption (Griscelli *et al.* 1989). Several affected infants have been successfully treated with bone marrow transplants.

Class II MHC deficiency is not linked to the genes for Class II MHC molecules, which are encoded on the short arm of chromosome 6. The defect lies in the failure of proteins that bind to the promoter boxes, upstream from the Class II MHC genes (Reith *et al.* 1988; Kara and Glimcher 1991). There may be different defects in different kindred that can complement each other but the number of complementation groups is not yet precisely known. There is a diminished level of Class I MHC expression in affected infants. The prior description of the so-called bare lymphocyte syndrome, in which Class I MHC expression was defective, probably concerned the same disease.

Wiskott–Aldrich syndrome

In 1937 Wiskott described four unrelated male infants with bloody diarrhoea and eczema. They had marked thrombocytopenia and the remaining platelets were abnormally small in diameter. Subsequently Aldrich *et al.* (1954) described the same defect in five generations of males of a single kindred and demonstrated that the defect is inherited as an X-linked phenomenon.

Affected male infants do indeed tend to bleed easily from birth, for instance, following circumcision. They develop petechiae and have bloody diarrhoea. The eczema has its onset in the first 6 months of life; it becomes readily infected, usually with staphylococci, and is aggravated by pruritus and excessive scratching. In addition to increased susceptibility to pyogenic infections, which leads to frequent otitis media and pyoderma, boys with Wiskott–Aldrich syndrome (WAS) may have very severe varicella and other childhood exanthems.

In the past these male children did not survive beyond the first decade of life. Almost half of them died from haemorrhage, usually into the brain, and the remainder from overwhelming infections. There is a high incidence of lymphoid malignancies in these males, and B cell lymphomas are emerging with great frequency in those who now survive into adulthood.

Several kindred have been described with a mild form of WAS, in which there is thrombocytopenia but the immunological defect is not found (Canales and Mauer 1967).

Genetics

Wiskott–Aldrich syndrome, in all its phenotypic forms, is a monogenic disease that maps to the short arm of the X chromosome at Xp11.23 to Xp11.3. Two flanking DNA probes, TIMP and DXS255, are each within 2 centiMorgans of the gene and make prenatal diagnosis possible (Peacocke and Siminovitch 1987; Kwan *et al.* 1988, 1991).

Obligate female heterozygous carriers of WAS exhibit non-random inactivation of the X chromosome in all cells of blood lineage but in no other cells (Fearon *et al.* 1988; Greer *et al.* 1989). This clearly implies that the defect involves not only platelets and T lymphocytes, the cells that appear defective in WAS, but also granulocytes, cells of monocyte–macrophage lineage and B lymphocytes. In any case, these obligate female carriers are clinically normal.

Diagnosis

The diagnosis of WAS may prove difficult in some cases. The platelet size is invariably small (effective average diameter 1.82 μm compared with the normal of 2.23 μm). Because of their small size, the platelet count is invariably greater than the numbers reported by electronic counting. Patients may have platelet counts of less than 20 000 and show no signs of haemorrhage; in fact, their platelet count is underestimated by 25–50%. The platelets and the T lymphocytes have a characteristic morphology on scanning electron microscopy; the T lymphocytes appear bald and lack villous projections (Kenney *et al.* 1986). Although cumbersome to perform, this appears to be the most reliable manner in which to ascertain the diagnosis. Tests of lymphocyte function *in vitro* are very variable in WAS and no characteristic pattern emerges that clarifies the diagnosis. A peculiarity of WAS is the inability of affected males to make antibodies to polysaccharide antigens such as blood group substance or the capsular polysaccharides of pneumococci and *Haemophilus influenzae* (Blaese *et al.* 1968; Cooper *et al.* 1968). Serum IgG is normal in concentration but the IgA and IgE are elevated and the IgM decreased.

Therapy

The most favourable therapy for WAS is a bone marrow transplant (Parkman *et al.* 1978). Since 1978 dozens of affected males have been readily rendered into complete bone marrow chimeras, with transplants from histoidentical donors (usually siblings) following total body irradiation or preparation with busulphan. On the other hand, it has been very difficult to transplant the children with bone marrow from haploidentical donors; some recent success has been reported (Rumelhard *et al.* 1990).

Splenectomy is often a useful stopgap measure and may have prolonged benefits. It variably increases the platelet count and size (Lum *et al.* 1980; Corash *et al.* 1985). Intravenous γ-globulin helps prevent pyogenic infections and is particularly useful in preventing sepsis in boys who have been splenectomized.

Pathogenesis

The cause of WAS is not known. The first unsuccessful transplants of WAS patients led to the establishment of only partial T cell chimerism.

Thereupon the eczema disappeared, normal responses to polysaccharide antigens were measured and immunoglobulin levels became normal (Parkman *et al.* 1978).

It subsequently became apparent that the major sialoglycoproteins of platelets (GPIb) and nucleated blood cells (CD43) were defective (Parkman *et al.* 1981; Remold-O'Donnell *et al.* 1984). The biosynthesis of CD43, also known as sialophorin or leucosialin, is normal in WAS T lymphocytes (Remold-O'Donnell and Rosen 1990) but CD43 is rapidly degraded from WAS T cells. When the gene for CD43 was cloned (Pallant *et al.* 1989; Shelley *et al.* 1989), it was found to map to the short arm of chromosome 16, thereby ruling out the defect in this protein as the basic defect in WAS. CD43 is important in signal transduction (Silverman *et al.* 1989) and in T cell activation (Mentzer *et al.* 1987). The ligand for CD43 appears to be ICAM-1 (Park *et al.* 1991; Rosenstein *et al.* 1991). The central enigma of WAS is to explain the cause of the abnormal degradation of sialoglycoproteins on the surfaces of blood cells.

Boys with WAS respond variably to stimulation with mitogens and antigens (Oppenheim *et al.* 1970). As they grow older, their lymphocyte count declines, particularly after the age of 6 (Ochs *et al.* 1980), and their immunological performance *in vitro* gets worse. Their blood cells appear to have a rapid turnover and poor survival in the circulation. The explanation for these various and sundry observations awaits the isolation of the WAS gene.

Hereditary ataxia telangiectasia

Boder and Sedgwick (1958) described the syndrome of hereditary AT. It is inherited as an autosomal recessive. Affected children develop ataxia at about 18–20 months of age, shortly after they start to walk. During the 5th year of life telangiectasia develops, first in the conjuctivae of the eyes and then on exposed areas of skin, most prominently in the elbow creases and necklace area. Boder and Sedgwick (1958) also noted undue susceptibility to sinopulmonary infections, and Peterson *et al.* (1964) demonstrated a defect in cell-mediated immunity and in thymic morphology. Patients with AT are prone to develop lymphoid malignancies and leukaemia and other tumours in the second decade of life and later (Swift 1990).

A wide variety of immunological defects have been described in AT. Perhaps half the patients have a deficiency of IgA. The IgA deficiency may be associated with deficiencies of IgG2 and IgG4; in these patients sinopulmonary disease and bronchiectasis are prominent (Oxelius *et al.* 1982). The lymphoid tissue is sparse and disorganized. However, circulating T cell number is normal, although a large number of $\gamma\delta$ T cells are present in peripheral blood (Carbonari *et al.* 1990). Karyotype examination reveals many chromosomal breaks and they are usually at the sites of immunoglobulin heavy-chain genes or T cell receptor genes on chromosome 7 and 14. T cell responses to mitogens, antigens and allogeneic stimuli are poor. Almost all patients with AT have an elevated serum level of α-1-fetoprotein (Waldmann and McIntire 1972). This observation provides a useful test for early diagnosis.

Gotoff *et al.* (1967) noted an unusual sensitivity to ionizing irradiation in a patient with AT. This was subsequently shown to pertain to their cells in culture; they have difficulty repairing chromosomal breaks following γ irradiation. At least five complementation groups are known in AT. Thus, when heterokaryons are produced between cells in two different complementation groups, they cross-correct sensitivity to ionizing irradiation (Jaspers *et al.* 1988). The most common complementation groups have been mapped to chromosome 11q22–23 (Gatti *et al.* 1985). It has been estimated that approximately 1.4% of the population in the United States is heterozygous for AT, and the age-specific cancer rate in relatives of AT patients is significantly higher than expected (Swift 1990).

The DiGeorge anomaly

In 1968, DiGeorge described four infants with congenital hypoparathyroidism and congenital thymic aplasia with faulty cell-mediated immunity. The parathyroid and the thymus glands are derived from the third and fourth pharyngeal pouches. In experiments with avian neural crest development, it has been shown that extirpation of cephalic neural crest cells results in abnormalities of these glands and the lower parts of the face, the tongue, etc. (Bockman and Kirby 1984; Le Douarin 1986). Recently, elimination of a homoeobox gene in mice has led to an experimental model of the DiGeorge anomaly (Chisaka and Capecchi 1991). In addition to these abnormalities, almost all infants with the DiGeorge anomaly have congenital malformation of the heart, most commonly interrupted aortic arch, right-sided aortic arch, truncus arteriosus and tetralogy of Fallot.

The diagnosis of the DiGeorge anomaly can usually be made by the bizarre facial features of affected infants, with hypertelorism, micrognathia, low-set ears and shortened filtrum of the upper lip. The thymus shadow is absent from the chest X-ray and the aforementioned cardiac abnormalities are observed. The infants are hypocalcaemic. Their T lymphocytes are usually decreased in number, and they respond poorly to non-specific mitogens. Various chromosomal abnormalities are present, particularly monosomy 10p and 22q11. The ossification centre of the hyoid bone is absent (Hong 1991). The transmission of the DiGeorge anomaly does not appear to be Mendelian and almost all cases are sporadic. However, multiple cases in families have been reported (Rohn *et al.* 1984).

In most cases of DiGeorge anomaly, cell-mediated immunity is sufficient to spare the infant serious opportunistic infections. Thymus transplants have corrected the cell-mediated immune defect (August *et al.* 1968; Cleveland *et al.* 1968). The cardiac malformation is the most serious threat to these infants and leads to surgical intervention. Graft-versus-host disease ensues when fresh blood is given or used to prime the pump for extracorporeal circulation during surgery. Only oxygenated, irradiated blood should be used in such circumstances, to prevent graft-versus-host disease.

Immunodeficiency secondary to other diseases

A variety of diseases have been associated with immunodeficiency. They include chromosomal abnormalities such as Bloom's syndrome, Fanconi anaemia and Down's syndrome; in addition, multiple organ system abnormalities and hereditary metabolic defects may have associated immunodeficiency. Hypercatabolism of immunoglobulin may lead to a deficiency of IgG; in addition, in intestinal lymphangiectasia there may be loss of significant numbers of lymphocytes into the gut. Immunodeficiency may be secondary to infection such as occurs in leprosy or mucocutaneous candidiasis. An X-linked syndrome of aplastic anaemia, lymphoma and agammaglobulinaemia follows a primary exposure to Epstein–Barr virus; this has been variously called the X-linked lymphoproliferative syndrome or Duncan's syndrome (Sullivan and Woda 1989). The major conditions associated with immunodeficiency are given in Table 66.1 (WHO Sponsored Meeting 1989).

Table 66.1. Other syndromes associated with immunodeficiency

Chromosome abnormalities
Bloom's syndrome
Fanconi's anaemia
Down's syndrome
Multiple organ system abnormalities
Partial albinism
Short-limbed dwarfism
Cartilage–hair hypoplasia
Agenesis of the corpus callosum
Hereditary metabolic defects
Transcobalamin-2 deficiency
Acrodermatitis enteropathica
Type I orotic aciduria
Biotin-dependent carboxylase deficiency
Hypercatabolism of immunoglobulin
Familial hypercatabolism immunoglobulin
Myotonic dystrophy
Intestinal lymphangiectasia
Other
Hyper IgE syndrome
Chronic mucocutaneous candidiasis
Thymoma
Immunodeficiency following hereditarily determined susceptibility to Epstein–Barr virus

References

Alarcon, B., Regueiro, J.R., Arnaiz-Villena, A. and Terhorst, C. (1988). Familial defect in the surface expression of the T cell receptor–CD3 complex. *N. Engl. J. Med.* **319**, 1203–8.

Aldrich, R.A., Steinberg, A.G. and Campbell, D.C. (1954). Pedigree demonstrating a sex-linked recessive condition characterized by draining ears, eczematoid dermatitis and bloody diarrhea. *Pediatrics* **13**, 133–9.

Ambrosino, D.M., Umetsu, D.T., Siber, G.R. *et al.* (1988). Selective defect in the antibody response to *Haemophilus influenzae* type B in children with recurrent infections and normal serum IgG subclass levels. *J. Allergy Clin. Immunol.* **81**, 1175–9.

August, C.S., Rosen, F.S., Filler, R.M., Janeway, C.A., Markowski, B. and Kay, H.E.M. (1968). Implantation of a foetal thymus, restoring immunological competence in a patient with thymic aplasia (DiGeorge's syndrome). *Lancet* **ii**, 1210–11.

Blaese, R.M., Strober, W., Brown, R.S. and Waldmann, T.A. (1968). The Wiskott–Aldrich syndrome: a disorder with a possible defect in antigen processing or recognition. *Lancet* **i**, 1056–61.

Bockman, D.E. and Kirby, M.L. (1984). Dependence of thymus development on derivatives of the neural crest. *Science* **223**, 498–500.

Boder, E. and Sedgwick, R.P. (1958). Ataxia-telangiectasia: a familial syndrome of progressive cerebellar ataxia, oculocutaneous telangiectasia and frequent pulmonary infection. *Pediatrics* **21**, 526–54.

Bruton, O.C. (1952). Agammaglobulinemia. *Pediatrics* **9**, 722–8.

Burks, A.W., Jr and Steele, R.W. (1986). Selective IgA deficiency. *Ann. Allergy* **57**, 3–8.

Businco, L., DiFazio, A., Ziruolo, M.G. *et al.* (1987). Clinical and immunological findings in four infants with Omenn's syndrome: a form of severe combined immunodeficiency with phenotypically normal T cells, elevated IgE, and eosinophilia. *Clin. Immunol. Immunopathol.* **44**, 123–33.

Canales, L. and Mauer, A.M. (1967). Sex-linked hereditary thrombocytopenia as a variant of Wiskott–Aldrich syndrome. *N. Engl. J. Med.* **277**, 899–901.

Carbonari, M., Cherchi, M., Paganelli, R. *et al.* (1990). Relative increase of T cells expressing the gamma/delta rather than the alpha/beta receptor in ataxia-telangiectasia. *N. Engl. J. Med.* **322**, 73–6.

Carson, D.A., Kaye, J. and Seegmiller, J.E. (1977). Lymphospecific toxicity in adenosine deaminase deficiency and purine nucleoside phosphorylase deficiency: possible role of nucleoside kinase(s). *Proc. Nat. Acad. Sci. (USA)* **74**, 5677–81.

Cassidy, J.T., Burt, A., Petty, R. and Sullivan, D. (1969). Selective IgA deficiency in connective tissue diseases. *N. Engl. J. Med.* **280**, 275.

Chatila, T., Wong, R., Young, M., Miller, R., Terhorst, C. and Geha, R.S. (1989). An immunodeficiency characterized by defective signal transduction in T lymphocytes. *N. Engl. J. Med.* **320**, 696–702.

Chatila, T., Castigli, E., Pahwa, R. *et al.* (1990). Primary combined immunodeficiency resulting from defective transcription of multiple T-cell lymphokine genes. *Proc. Nat. Acad. Sci. (USA)* **87**, 10033–7.

Chisaka, O. and Capecchi, M.R. (1991). Regionally restricted developmental defects resulting from targeted disruption of the mouse homeobox gene hox-1.5. *Nature* **350**, 473–9.

Chu, E.T., Roserwasser, L.J., Dinarello, C.A., Rosen, F.S. and Geha, R.S. (1984). Immunodeficiency with defective T cell response to interleukin 1. *Proc. Nat. Acad. Sci. (USA)* **81**, 4945–9.

Cleveland, W.W., Fogel, B.J., Brown, W.T. and Kay, H.E. (1968). Foetal thymic transplant in a case of DiGeorge's syndrome. *Lancet* **ii**, 1211–14.

Conley, M.E. and Cooper, M.D. (1981). Immature IgA B cells in IgA-deficient patients. *N. Engl. J. Med.* **305**, 495–7.

Conley, M.E., Brown, P., Pickard, A.R. *et al.* (1986). Expression of the gene defect in X-linked agammaglobulinemia. *N. Engl. J. Med.* **315**, 564–7.

Conley, M.E., Lavoie, A., Briggs, C., Brown, P., Guerra, C. and Puck, J.M. (1988). Nonrandom X chromosome inactivation in B cells from carriers of X chromosome linked severe combined immunodeficiency. *Proc. Nat. Acad. Sci. (USA)* **85**, 3090–4.

Cooper, M.D. and Lawton, A.R. (1972). Circulating B-cells in patients with immunodeficiency. *Am. J. Pathol.* **69**, 513–28.

Cooper, M.D., Chase, H.P., Lowman, J.T., Krivit, W. and Good, R.A. (1968). Wiskott–Aldrich syndrome: an immunologic deficiency disease involving the afferent limb of immunity. *Am. J. Med.* **44**, 499–513.

Cooper, M.D., Burrows, P.D. and Kubagawa, H. (1986). Ontogeny of B cells and their abnormal development in immunodeficiency disease. In *Recent Advances in Immunodeficiences*, ed. F. Aiuti, F. Rosen and M.D. Cooper, pp. 19–29, Raven Press, New York.

Corash, L., Shafer, B. and Blaese, R.M. (1985) Platelet-associated immunoglobulin, platelet size, and the effect of splenectomy in the Wiskott–Aldrich syndrome. *Blood* **65**, 1439–43.

Cunningham-Rundles, C. Wong, S., Bjorkander, J. and Hanson, L.A. (1986). Use of an IgA-depleted intravenous immunoglobulin in a patient with an anti-IgA antibody. *Clin. Immunol. Immunopathol.* **38**, 141–9.

de Preval, C., Hadam, M.R. and Mach, B. (1988). Regulation of genes for HLA class II antigens in cell lines from patients with severe combined immunodeficiency. *N. Engl. J. Med.* **318**, 1295–300.

DiGeorge, A.M. (1968). Congenital absence of the thymus and its immunologic consequences: concurrence with congenital hypoparathyroidism. In *Birth Defects*, ed. D. Bergsma, pp. 116–21, Original Articles Series, IV, The National Foundation, New York.

Fearon, E.R., Winkelstein, J.A., Civin, C.I., Pardoll, D.M. and Vogelstein, B. (1987). Carrier detection in X-linked agammaglobulinemia by analysis of X-chromosome inactivation. *N. Engl. J. Med.* **316**, 427–31.

Fearon, E.R., Kohn, D.B., Winkelstein, J.A., Vogelstein, B. and Blaese, R.M. (1988). Carrier detection in the Wiskott–Aldrich syndrome. *Blood* **72**, 1735–9.

Fleisher, T.A., White, R.M., Broder, S. *et al.* (1980). X-linked hypogammaglobulinemia and isolated growth hormone deficiency. *N. Engl. J. Med.* **302**, 1429–33.

Gatti, R.A., Meeuwissen, H.J., Allen, H.D., Hong, R. and Good, R.A. (1968). Immunological reconstitution of sex-linked lymphopenic immunological deficiency. *Lancet* **ii**, 1366–9.

Gatti, R.A., Boehnke, M., Crist, M. and Sparkes, R.S. (1985). Genetic linkage studies in ataxia-telangiectasia: Gm markers. *Kroc. Found. Ser.* **19**, 163–72.

Geha, R.S., Schneeberger, E., Merler, E. and Rosen, F.S. (1974). Heterogeneity of 'acquired' or common variable agammaglobulinemia. *N. Engl. J. Med.* **291**, 1–6.

Geha, R.S., Hyslop, N., Alami, S., Farah, F., Schneeberger, E.E. and Rosen, F.S. (1979). Hyper immunoglobulin M immunodeficiency (dysgammaglobulinemia): presence of immunoglobulin M-secreting plasmacytoid cells in peripheral blood and failure of immunoglobulin M–immunoglobulin G switch in B-cell differentiation. *J. Clin. Invest.* **64**, 385–91.

Goodship, J., Levinsky, R. and Malcolm, S. (1989). Linkage of PGK-1 to X-linked severe combined immunodeficiency (IMD4) allows predictive testing in families with no surviving male. *Hum. Genet.* **84**, 11–14.

Gotoff, S.P., Amirmokri, E. and Liebner, E.J. (1967). Ataxia telangiectasia: neoplasia, untoward response to X-irradiation and tuberous sclerosis. *Am. J. Dis. Child.* **114**, 617–25.

Greer, W.L., Kwong, P., Peacocke, M., Ip, P., Rubin, L.A. and Siminovitch, K.A. (1989). X-chromosome inactivation in the Wiskott–Aldrich syndrome: a marker for detection of the carrier state and identification of cell lineages expressing the gene defect. *Genomics* **4**, 60–7.

Griscelli, C., Lisowska-Grospierre, B. and Mach, B. (1989). Combined immunodeficiency with defective expression in MHC class II genes. *Immunodeficiency Rev.* **1**, 135–53.

Hershfield, M.D., Buckley, R.H., Greenberg, M.L. *et al.* (1987). Treatment of adenosine deaminase deficiency with polyethylene glycol-modified adenosine deaminase. *N. Engl. J. Med.* **316**, 589–96.

Hirschhorn, R. (1990). Adenosine deaminase deficiency. *Immunodeficiency Rev.* **2**, 175–98.

Hirschhorn, R., Roegner-Maniscalco, V., Kuritsky, L. and Rosen, F.S. (1981). Bone marrow transplantation only partially restores purine metabolites to normal in adenosine deaminase-deficiency patients. *J. Clin. Invest.* **68**, 1387–93.

Hoffman, T., Winchester, R., Schulkind, M., Frias, J.L., Ayoub, E.M. and Good, R.A. (1977). Hypogammaglobulinemia with normal T cell function in female siblings. *Clin. Immunol. Immunopathol.* **7**, 364–71.

Hong, R. (1991). The DiGeorge anomaly. *Immunodeficiency Rev.* **3**, 1–14.

Jaspers, N.G., Gatti, R.A., Baan, C., Linssen, P.C. and Bootsma, D. (1988). Genetic complementation analysis of ataxia telangiectasia and Nijmegen breakage syndrome: a survey of 50 patients. *Cytogenet. Cell Genet.* **49**, 259–63.

Jung, L.K.L., Fu, S.M., Hara, T., Kapoor, N. and Good, R.A. (1986). Defective expression of T cell-associated glycoprotein in severe combined immunodeficiency. *J. Clin. Invest.* **77**, 940–6.

Kara, C.J. and Glimcher, L.H. (1991). *In vivo* footprinting of MHC class II genes: bare promoters in the bare lymphocyte syndrome. *Science* **252**, 709–12.

Kenney, D.M., Cairns, L., Remold-O'Donnell, E., Peterson, J., Rosen, F.S. and Parkman, R. (1986). Morphological abnormalities in the lymphocytes of patients with Wiskott–Aldrich syndrome. *Blood* **68**, 1329–32.

Kretschmer, R., Jeannet, M., Mereu, T.R., Kretschmer, K., Winn, H. and Rosen, F.S. (1969). Hereditary thymic dysplasia: a graft-versus-host reaction induced by bone marrow cells with a partial 4a series histoincompatibility. *Pediatr. Res.* **3**, 34–40.

Kwan, S.-P., Kunkel, L., Bruns, G., Wedgwood, R.J., Latt, S. and Rosen, F.S. (1986). Mapping of the X-linked agammaglobulinemia locus by use of restriction fragment length polymorphism. *J. Clin. Invest.* **77**, 649–52.

Kwan, S.-P., Sandkuyl, L.A., Blaese, M. *et al.* (1988). Precise gene mapping of the Wiskott–Aldrich syndrome. *Genomics* **3**, 39–43.

Kwan, S.-P., Terwilliger, J., Parmley, R. *et al.* (1990). Identification of a closely linked DNA marker, DXS178, to further refine the X-linked agammaglobulinemia locus. *Genomics* **6**, 238–42.

Kwan, S.-P., Lehner, T., Hagemann, T. *et al.* (1991). Localization of the gene for the Wiskott–Aldrich syndrome between two flanking markers TIMP and DXS255 on Xp11.2–11.3. *Genomics* **10**, 29–33.

Le Douarin, N.M. (1986). Investigations on the neural crest: methodological aspects and recent advances. *Ann. NY Acad. Sci.* **486**, 66–86.

Lefranc, M.-P., Hammarstrom, L., Smith, C.I.E. and Lefranc, G. (1991). Gene deletions in the human immunoglobulin heavy chain constant region locus: molecular and immunological analysis. *Immunodeficiency Rev.* **2**, 265–81.

Levinsky, R.J. and Tiedman, K. (1983). Successful bone-marrow transplantation for reticular dysgenesis. *Lancet* **i**, 671–3.

Lum, L.G., Tubergen, D.G., Corash, L. and Blaese, R.M. (1980). Splenectomy in the management of the thrombocytopenia of the Wiskott–Aldrich syndrome. *N. Engl. J. Med.* **302**, 892–6.

Lux, S.E., Johnston, R.B., Jr, August, C.S. *et al.* (1970). Chronic neutropenia and abnormal cellular immunity in cartilage–hair hypoplasia. *N. Engl. J. Med.* **282**, 231–6.

Markert, M.L. (1991). Purine nucleoside phosphorylase deficiency. *Immunodeficiency Rev.* **3**, 45–81.

Mayer, L., Kwan, S.-P., Thompson, C. *et al.* (1986). Evidence for a defect in 'switch' T cells in patients with immunodeficiency and hyperimmunoglobulinemia M. *N. Engl. J. Med.* **314**, 409–13.

Mease, P.J., Ochs, H.D. and Wedgwood, R.J. (1981). Successful treatment of echovirus meningoencephalitis and myositis-fasciitis with intravenous immune globulin therapy in a patient with X-linked agammaglobulinemia. *N. Engl. J. Med.* **304**, 1278–81.

Mentzer, S.J., Remold-O'Donnell, E., Crimmins, M.A.V., Bierer, B.E., Rosen, F.S. and Burakoff, S.J. (1987). Sialophorin, a surface sialoglycoprotein defective in the Wiskott–Aldrich syndrome, is involved in human T lymphocyte proliferation. *J. Exp. Med.* **165**, 1383–92.

Ochs, H.D., Slichter, S.J., Harker, L.A., Von Behrens, W.E., Clark, R.A. and Wedgwood, R.J. (1980). The Wiskott–Aldrich syndrome: studies of lymphocytes, granulocytes and platelets. *Blood* **55**, 243–52.

Olerup, O., Smith, C.I.E. and Hammarstrom, L. (1990). Different amino acids at position 57 of the HLA-DO β chain associated with susceptibility and resistance to IgA deficiency. *Nature* **347**, 289–90.

Oppenheim, J.J., Blaese, R.M. and Waldmann, T.A. (1970). Defective lymphocyte transformation and delayed hypersensitivity in Wiskott–Aldrich syndrome. *J. Immunol.* **104**, 835–44.

O'Reilly, R.J., Keever, C.A., Small, T.N. and Brochstein, J. (1989). The use of HLA-non-identical T-cell-depleted marrow transplants for correction of severe combined immunodeficiency disease. *Immunodeficiency Rev.* **1**, 273–309.

Oxelius, V.A., Berkel, A.I. and Hanson, L.A. (1982). IgG2 deficiency in ataxia-telangiectasia. *N. Engl. J. Med.* **306**, 515–17.

Pallant, A., Eskenazi, A., Mattei, M.-G. *et al.* (1989). Characterization of cDNAs encoding human leukosialin and localization of the leukosialin gene to chromosome 16. *Proc. Nat. Acad. Sci. (USA)* **86**, 1328–32.

Park, J.K., Rosenstein, Y.J., Remold-O'Donnell, E., Bierer, B.E., Rosen, F.S. and Burakoff, S.J. (1991). Enhancement of T-cell activation by the CD43 molecule whose expression is defective in Wiskott–Aldrich syndrome. *Nature* **350**, 706–9.

Parkman, R., Rappeport, J., Geha, R. *et al.* (1978). Complete correction of the Wiskott–Aldrich syndrome by allogeneic bone-marrow transplantation. *N. Engl. J. Med.* **298**, 921–7.

Parkman, R., Remold-O'Donnell, E., Kennev, D.M., Perrine, S. and Rosen, F.S. (1981). Surface protein abnormalities in the lymphocytes and platelets from patients with Wiskott–Aldrich syndrome. *Lancet* **ii**, 1387–90.

Peacocke, M. and Siminovitch, K.A. (1987). Linkage of the Wiskott–Aldrich syndrome with polymorphic DNA sequences from the human X chromosome. *Proc. Nat. Acad. Sci. (USA)* **84**, 3430–3.

Pearl, E.R., Vogler, L.B., Okos, A.J., Crist, W.H., Lawton, A.R. III and Cooper, M.D. (1978). B lymphocyte precursors in human bone marrow: an analysis of normal individuals and patients with antibody-deficient states. *J. Immunol.* **120**, 1169–75.

Peterson, R.D.A., Kelly, W.D. and Good, R.A. (1964). Ataxia-telangiectasia: its association with a defective thymus, immunological-deficiency disease, and malignancy. *Lancet* **i**, 1189–93.

Pierce, G.F. and Polmar, S.H. (1982). Lymphocyte dysfunction in cartilage–hair hypoplasia: evidence for an intrinsic defect in cellular proliferation. *J. Immunol.* **129**, 570–5.

Preud'Homme, J.-L. and Hanson, L.A. (1990). IgG subclass deficiency. *Immunodeficiency Rev.* **2**, 129–49.

Puck, J., Nussbaum, R., Smead, D. and Conley, M.E. (1989). X-linked severe combined immunodeficiency: localization within the region Xq13.1–q21.1 by linkage and deletion analysis. *Am. J. Hum. Genet.* **44**, 724–30.

Ranki, A., Perheentupa, J., Anderson, L.C. and Hayry, P. (1978). *In vitro* T- and B-cell reactivity in cartilage hair hypoplasia. *Clin. Exp. Immunol.* **32**, 352–60.

Reinherz, E.L., Geha, R., Rappeport, J.M. *et al.* (1982). Reconstitution after transplantation with T lymphocyte-depleted HLA haplotype-mismatched bone marrow for severe combined immunodeficiency. *Proc. Nat. Acad. Sci. (USA)* **79**, 6047–51.

Reisner, Y., Kapoor, N., Kirkpatrick, D. *et al.* (1983). Transplantation for severe combined immunodeficiency with HLA-A,B,D,DR incompatible parental marrow cells fractionated by soybean agglutinin and sheep red blood cells. *Blood* **61**, 341–8.

Reith, W., Satola, S., Sanchez, C.H. *et al.* (1988). Congenital immunodeficiency with a regulatory defect in MHC class II gene expression lacks a specific HLA-DR promoter binding protein, RF-X. *Cell* **53**, 897–906.

Remold-O'Donnell, E. and Rosen F.S. (1990). Sialophorin (CD43) and the Wiskott–Aldrich syndrome. *Immunodeficiency Rev.* **2**, 151–74.

Remold-O'Donnell, E., Kenney, D.M., Parkman, R., Cairns, L., Savage, B. and Rosen, F.S. (1984). Characterization of a human lymphocyte surface sialoglycoprotein that is defective in Wiskott–Aldrich syndrome. *J. Exp. Med.* **159**, 1705–23.

Rohn, R.D., Leffell, M.S., Leadem, P., Johnson, D., Rubio, T. and Emanuel, B.S. (1984). Familial third-fourth pharyngeal pouch syndrome with apparent autosomal dominant transmission. *J. Pediatr.* **105**, 47–51.

Roifman, C.M., Hummel, D., Martinez-Valdez, H. *et al.* (1989). Depletion of CD8+ cells in human thymic medulla results in selective immune deficiency. *J. Exp. Med.* **170**, 2177–82.

Rosen, F.S., Cooper, M.D. and Wedgwood, R.J.P. (1984). The primary immunodeficiencies. I. *N. Engl. J. Med.* **311**, 235–42.

Rosenstein, Y., Park, J.K., Hahn, W.C., Rosen, F.S., Bierer, B.E. and Burakoff, S.J. (1991). CD43, a molecule defective in Wiskott–Aldrich syndrome, binds ICAM-1. *Nature* **354**, 233–5.

Rumelhard, S.L., Trigg, M., Horowitz, S.D. and Hong, R. (1990). Monoclonal antibody T-cell-depleted HLA-haploidentical bone marrow transplantation for Wiskott–Aldrich syndrome. *Blood* **75**, 1031–5.

Schaffer, F.M., Palermos, J., Zhu, Z.B., Barger, B.O., Cooper, M.D. and Volanakis, J.E. (1989). Individuals with IgA deficiency and common variable immunodeficiency share polymorphisms of major histocompatibility complex class III genes. *Proc. Nat. Acad. Sci. (USA)* **86**, 8005–19.

Schaffer, F.M., Monteiro, R.C., Volanakis, J.E. and Cooper, M.D. (1991). IgA deficiency. *Immunodeficiency Rev.* **3**, 15–44.

Schwaber, J., Molgaard, H., Orkin, S.H., Gould, H.J. and Rosen, F.S. (1983). Early pre-B cells from normal and X-linked agammaglobulinemia produce C-mu without an attached V-H region. *Nature* **304**, 355–8.

Schwaber, J., Payne, J. and Chen, R. (1988). B lymphocytes from X-linked agammaglobulinemia: delayed expression of light chain and demonstration of lyonization in carriers. *J. Clin. Invest.* **81**, 514–22.

Shelley, C.S., Remold-O'Donnell, E., Davis, A.E., III *et al.* (1989). Molecular characterization of sialophorin (CD43), the lymphocyte surface sialoglycoprotein defective in Wiskott–Aldrich syndrome. *Proc. Nat. Acad. Sci. (USA)* **86**, 2819–23.

Siegel, R.L., Issekutz, T., Schwaber, J., Rosen, F.S. and Geha, R.S. (1981). Deficiency of T helper cells in transient hypogammaglobulinemia of infancy. *N. Engl. J. Med.* **305**, 1307–13.

Silverman, L.B., Wong, R.C.K., Remold-O'Donnell, E. *et al.* (1989). Mechanism of mononuclear cell activation by an anti-CD43 (sialophorin) agonistic antibody. *J. Immunol.* **142**, 4194–200.

Spickett, G.P., Webster, A.D.B. and Farrant, J. (1990). Cellular abnormalities in common variable immunodeficiency. *Immunodeficiency Rev.* **2**, 199–219.

Sullivan, J.L. and Woda, B.A. (1989). X-linked lymphoproliferative syndrome. *Immunodeficiency Rev.* **1**, 325–47.

Swift, M. (1990). Genetic aspects of ataxia-telangiectasia. *Immunodeficiency Rev.* **2**, 67–81.

Thoenes, G., Le Deist, F., Fischer, A., Griscelli, C. and Lisowska-Grospierre, B. (1990). Immunodeficiency associated with defective expression of the T-cell receptor-CD3 complex. *N. Engl. J. Med.* **322**, 1399 (letter).

Vyas, G.N., Perkins, H.A. and Fudenberg, H.H. (1968). Anaphylactoid transfusion reactions associated with anti-IgA. *Lancet* **ii**, 312–15.

Waldmann, T.A. and McIntire, K.R. (1972). Serum alpha-fetoprotein levels in patients with ataxia-telangiectasia. *Lancet* **ii**, 1112–15.

Weinberg, K. and Parkman, R. (1990). Severe combined immunodeficiency due to a specific defect in the production of interleukin-2. *N. Engl. J. Med.* **322**, 1741–3.

WHO Sponsored Meeting (1989). Primary immunodeficiency diseases. *Immunodeficiency Rev.* **1**, 173–205.

Wilfert, C.M., Buckley, R.H., Mohanakumar, T. *et al.* (1977). Persistent and fatal central-nervous-system echovirus infections in patients with agammaglobulinemia. *N. Engl. J. Med.*

296, 1485–9.

Wiskott, A. (1937). Familiarer, angeborenor morbus Werlhofii. *Monatsch. Kinderheil* **68**, 212–18.

Wright, J.J., Birx, D.L., Wagner, D.K., Waldmann, T.A., Blaese, R.M. and Fleisher, T.A. (1987). Normalization of antibody responsiveness in a patient with common variable hypogammaglobulinemia and HIV infection. *N. Engl. J. Med.* **317**, 1516–20.

Primary Non-specific Immunodeficiency

67: Complement Deficiencies — Genetic and Acquired

P.J. Lachmann

Introduction

The complement system differs from, for example, the coagulation system in that the study of deficiencies of individual components played a relatively small part in the original delineation of the reaction mechanisms. Although a strain of complement-deficient guinea-pigs was described at the end of World War I (Moore 1919), they died out and were not extensively studied. It was not until the 1960s that other complement deficiency states were described both in other laboratory animals and in man. A remarkable feature of all the early discoveries of complement deficiency (with the exception of C1 inhibitor deficiency) was that they were ascertained in normal animals and not infrequently in humans with no disease that could be obviously attributed to their complement deficiency. This was in striking contrast to the increasing knowledge of the activities of the complement system as an enhancer of inflammation and phagocytosis as well as its well-known actions as a cytolytic and bactericidal agent. This gave rise to doubts about the role of the complement system *in vivo*. It was only with the analysis of more substantial numbers of complement-deficient subjects that their association with disease became clearer. In most instances the association of complement deficiency with diseases was not directly causal but the complement deficiency produced an increased susceptibility to certain disease processes, notably infection. This is what is known as a 'diathesis' — a genetically determined predisposition to react in particular, harmful ways to environmental stimuli. It is because there is a considerable degree of 'belt and braces' in the mechanisms that resist infection, and indeed in those that enhance inflammation and phagocytosis, that the failure of one mechanism does not unfailingly lead to a severe immunity deficiency.

Only absence of polymorphonuclear leucocytes rapidly — and absence of the whole immunological apparatus (as in severe combined immunodeficiency) more slowly — inevitably lead to lethal infections. Deficiencies of individual components of the immune response, particularly of the humoral effector mechanism, are more subtle in their effects.

It is perhaps particularly puzzling that patients with identical complement deficiencies whose complement profiles are indistinguishable should nevertheless vary most strikingly in their clinical presentation and lifetime experience of complications. The most plausible explanation lies in the recognition that we are the product not only of our genes but also of our immunological history. The circumstances under which we first encounter antigens affect critically the consequences of subsequent exposure to them. In the context of complement deficiency, it is clearly important in what circumstances an infectious agent is first encountered. If the primary exposure is to a small dose of organism or occurs at a time when the host still has some immunoglobulin G (IgG) antibody passively acquired from the mother, then the absence of an intact complement system may be much less important than if the organism is first encountered in a larger dose or when no IgG antibody is present. A high level of IgG antibody can substitute for many of the actions of the complement system in the enhancement of phagocytosis and even in the induction of inflammation via the IgG Fc (Fc_{γ}) receptors. On the other hand, the IgM antibodies made in the primary immune responses are very dependent upon complement fixation for their biological effects.

However, it is now clear that complement deficiency does predispose to infections and, as will be shown, to immune complex diseases; and, since the clinical manifestations are very variable from person to person, the problem arises whether and in what circumstances one should consider replacement therapy for complement-deficient children. This problem has been relatively little discussed and no proper trials on the subject are known to the author. A particular difficulty arises from the parodoxical relationship that complement has, for example, to immune complex disease where its deficiency is indubitably a powerful predisposing cause to developing the diseases but, once developed, there are also compelling reasons for believing that the complement system plays a role in their pathogenesis. Nevertheless, particularly in those deficiencies, for example of C1 and C4, where the risk of developing immune complex disease is high, the *a priori* case for treating clinically normal children is hard to deny and the time would certainly seem to be ripe for some properly constructed controlled studies.

Table 67.1 gives a summary of the known complement deficiencies. It shows that isolated component deficiencies have been described in all the four commonest laboratory animals as well as in man. All these deficiencies are described in some detail in the volume of *Progress in Allergy* devoted to complement deficiencies (Rother and Rother 1986) and only a brief account is given here.

Complement deficiency in animals

Complement deficiency in guinea-pigs (see Bitter-Suermann and Burger 1986)

It may not be a coincidence that the earliest complement deficiency was described in the guinea-pig since it was the blood from this species that was normally used as a source of complement. Early in the twentieth century animals deficient in haemolytic complement were described (Moore 1919; Hyde 1923). The component analysis available at that time showed the deficiency to be in what was then called C′3 and would now be regarded as comprising any of the terminal components, C3 to C9. The animals were apparently healthy but were more susceptible to experimental challenge with bacteria. The strain died out after a number of years. While this may be related to complement deficiency, this should not readily be assumed since the inbreeding of laboratory animals is notoriously difficult.

A distinct strain of animals deficient in C4 was discovered and bred at the National Institute of Health (NIH) (Ellman *et al.* 1971). These guinea-pigs have been established in many parts of the world, are healthy under laboratory conditions and breed well. They are usually bred in closed colonies and not inbred. In striking contrast to human C4 deficiency, C4-deficient guinea-pigs do not obviously suffer from autoimmune immune complex disease. The reason for this difference does not seem to lie in the completeness of C4 deficiency since the C4-deficient guinea-pigs do

Table 67.1. Complement deficiencies

Complement component	Total patients	Pedigrees (if, reported)	Clinical associations	Comments	Reference
C1q	11	7	Skin and renal lesions — SLE or SLE-like syndrome; infections		Orihara *et al.* 1987
C1q	7	3	Skin and renal lesions — SLE or SLE-like syndrome: infections		
C1r/C1s	10	6	Skin and renal lesions — SLE or SLE-like syndrome; infections		Loos and Heinz 1986; Garty *et al.* 1987
C4	17	11	SLE +/− infections; two normal		Hauptmann *et al.* 1986, 1988
C2	>77		SLE; other immune complex disease; some infections; about 30% healthy	Caucasians only; ? incidence 1/10 000 of population	Ruddy 1986
C3	18		Pyogenic infections; glomerulonephritis		Day 1986b; Borzy *et al.* 1988; Grumach *et al.* 1988; Roord *et al.* 1989; Botto *et al.* 1990
Factor I	12	0	Pyogenic infections; neisserial infection; immune complex disease; healthy		Day 1986; Porteu *et al.* 1986; Moller- Rasmussen *et al.* 1988
Factor H	5	2	Haemolytic uraemic syndrome; SLE; healthy		Day 1986a; Brai *et al.* 1988;
Properdin	25	16	Infections, particularly neisserial		Wyatt 1986; Fijen *et al.* 1989; Schlesinger *et al.* 1990
Factor D	1	1	Neisserial infection (N.B. Patient is thin)	Factor D = adipsin	Hiemstra *et al.* 1989
C5	18	10	Neisserial + some other infections; SLE (rare); can be healthy		McCarty and Snyderman 1986; Nielsen and Koch 1987; Rosen *et al.* 1988
C6	56	12	Neisserial infections predominate; often healthy		Rother 1986; Orren *et al.* 1987
C7	28	11	Neisserial infections predominate; often healthy		Zeitz *et al.* 1986; Zimran *et al.* 1987; Fijen *et al.* 1989; Schlesinger *et al.* 1990
C6 + C7	2	2	Candidiasis; healthy		Lachmann *et al.* 1978; Morgan *et al.* 1989
C8αγ	6		Predominantly neisserial infection; occasional SLE; some healthy	Gene found so far only in US Blacks	Tedesco 1986
C8β	25		Predominantly neisserial infection occasional SLE; some healthy		
C9	Many		Predominantly healthy; occasional neisserial infection but rare in Caucasians; affects *c.* 1/1000 Japanese		Lint and Gewurz 1986
DAF	Rare		INAB phenotype of Cromer blood group; healthy		Telen and Green 1989
C1-ina	Many		Hereditary angio-oedema; 5% have immune complex disease (N.B. Patients are heterozygotes)		Cullmann and Opferkuch 1986

not seem to have any C4. Although the exact nature of the mutation producing the deficiency is unknown, it gives rise to the production of a primary ribonucleic acid (RNA) transcript that is not properly processed into messenger RNA (mRNA).

C2-deficient guinea-pigs were encountered in Germany in 1981 (Bitter-Suermann *et al.* 1981) and a colony has been bred from them. These animals appear to make small amounts of a dysfunctional C2 protein and the defect is therefore presumably in the structural gene. The animals are also healthy.

A further component deficiency was discovered in Germany in 1983, namely a true C3 deficiency (Burger *et al.* 1986). The deficiency is subtotal, the homozygous deficient animals having low but detectable quantities of C3 in their blood. It has been suggested that the defect is due to unstable C3 being produced but the molecular basis is still incompletely known. Again these animals are healthy under laboratory conditions and differ from human C3-deficient subjects in not suffering from infections.

Complement-deficient guinea-pigs respond poorly to low doses of antigen, particularly when these are given without adjuvants. Conversion of the antibody response to IgG is impaired. The defect is more marked in the C3-deficient animals than in those deficient in C4 or C2 (Bottger *et al.* 1986). However, the animals are not hypogammaglobulinaemic, so that, under the normal *in vivo* conditions of immunization, they seem to make adequate antibody responses, and their failure to suffer from infections under laboratory circumstances suggests that their failure in raising antibodies is not sufficient to reduce the immunity to the pathogens among which they live.

Complement deficiency in rabbits

C6 DEFICIENCY IN THE RABBIT

C6 deficiency in rabbits was first discovered by Klaus and Ursula Rother in laboratory rabbits in Heidelberg (Rother and Rother 1961) and within a few years C6-deficient rabbits were also encountered in laboratory-bred animals in Cambridge (Lachmann 1970) and among rabbits offered for sale in Mexico City (Biro and Garcia 1965). It is therefore clear that C6 deficiency in rabbits is not a very rare mutation found only as a result of extensive screening of normal animals but that it is probably a fairly common rabbit gene which is widely distributed. This raises the possibility that the gene either in homozygous or in heterozygous form may carry some selective advantage. Although there is no evidence on this point in rabbits, this possibility will be discussed in more detail with regard to C6 deficiency in man.

Under laboratory conditions the C6-deficient rabbits are entirely healthy. It can be demonstrated that they have increased susceptibility to experimental neisserial infection and that in contrast they show an increased resistance to endotoxin shock. The nature of the molecular defect is not known since C6 has proved difficult to clone and probes are only just becoming available. However, they have no C6 protein in their blood and make anti-C6 antibodies with remarkably wide cross-reactivity among C6s of different species, suggesting that they have a fairly complete lack of tolerance to the whole molecule.

C8$\alpha\gamma$ DEFICIENCY IN THE RABBIT

Two rabbits deficient in C8$\alpha\gamma$ were discovered in 1985 in Japan (Komatsu *et al.* 1985). They have bred a colony from these rabbits and shown that the deficiency is inherited as a single autosomal recessive. The nature of the molecular defect is not so far known. The homozygous deficient rabbits are said to be smaller than their normal or heterozygous littermates and it was further observed that the average litter size for deficient does was significantly smaller, mean 2.7, than that in normals or heterozygotes, mean 6.2. The authors also demonstrated a reduced survival in the deficient animals compared with the normals and heterozygotes in the first 3 months of life. Although this may demonstrate that C8$\alpha\gamma$ deficiency causes reduced lifespan, this is by no means certain since the inbreeding of rabbits causes considerable problems with reduction in litter size and premature mortality; one would need to have much more detailed information about the degree of inbreeding in the homozygotes compared with the heterozygotes and normals.

C3 DEFICIENCY IN THE RABBIT

Examples of C3 deficiency have been described in

the same Japanese colony of rabbits in which C8αγ deficiency was identified (Komatsu *et al.* 1988). The C3 deficiency is not total, the affected animals having approximately 10% of the normal C3 concentration. The C3 is apparently normal in haemolytic activity and there is no evidence of excess C3 destroying activity in the serum and no information on the C3 gene in these rabbits or on the level of mRNA has been reported. The deficiency seems to be somewhat similar to that described in guinea-pigs by Burger *et al.* (1986) and it is therefore possible that it is due, as Burger and his colleagues have suggested, to the production of an unstable C3 molecule that is susceptible to intracellular proteolysis. The rabbit serum with reduced C3 levels shows a reduced bactericidal activity and the affected rabbits are again said to have an increased mortality in the first 3 months although, unlike the C8αγ-deficient rabbits, they are not of smaller size.

Complement deficiency in mice

C5 DEFICIENCY IN MICE

C5-deficient mice were first described by Rosenberg and Tachibana in 1962, though it was not until 1967 (Nelson and Muller-Eberhard 1967) that it was established that it was indeed C5 that was the missing component. Before this time Cinader (Cinader *et al.* 1964) had shown that the deficiency of complement described by Rosenberg and Tachibana (1962) went along with a serum protein antigen that they had called MUB1. C5 deficiency is remarkably common among inbred strains of mice and a list of C5-deficient inbred strains is given in Table 67.2. The genetic defect has been suspected for some time not to be the structural gene itself since fusion of the spleen cells of deficient mice with chicken erythrocytes gave rise to the formation of mouse C5 in the heterokaryon (Ooi and Colten 1979). Biologically, C5 deficiency is an interesting model since C5 deficiency not only interferes with the formation of the membrane attack complex (MAC) but also prevents the formation of the most powerful anaphylatoxin. The biological consequences of C5 deficiency have been extensively studied and reviewed by Rosenberg and Tachibana (1986). The findings are on the whole not striking. There are some reports of reduced immunity to certain bacterial infections but not to virus infections or parasitic infections. C5-deficient mice certainly survive normally under laboratory conditions.

Table 67.2. Incidence of C5 deficiency in inbred strains of mice

Sufficient	Deficient
B10D2 — new line	B10D2 — old line
BALB/c	A
BDP	A/He
BRVR/Sr	AKR
BSVS/Sr	AU
BUB/Bn	BUA/Wi
BUB/Bn-C	BUC/Wi
BUB/Wi	BUE/Wi
CBA	CE
C3H	DBA/2
CHI/St	DDK
C57BL/6	DM/Ms
C57BL/10	FAKI
C57BR/cdJ	GFF
C57L	IF/Bcr
C58	I/FnLn
DBA/1	JU/Fa
F/St	KK
FU	MaS/A
HR/De	NBL/N
MA/J	NC
MO/Ko	NS/Fr
NZO/B1	NXB/B1
PHL	NZB
P	PHH
PL	RF
PS	SMA/Ms
RIII/An	ST/J
RIII/Wy	SWR
SEA/Gn-se	YBR/HeWiHa
SEC/1Gn	
SJL	
SL/R1	
SM	
STOLI/Lw	
T6	
WH/Ht	
129	
2BC3H	
2C3H	

From Cinader *et al.* (1964) and Olac Manual (1976).

C6 DEFICIENCY IN MICE

Very recently C6 deficiency has been discovered among certain animals in the so-called Peruvian strain of mice, which are known to be somewhat genetically unstable (A. Orren, pers. comm.). This deficiency is currently being bred into an inbred strain of mice. Little else is so far known about it.

It is disappointing that a wider range of complement deficiencies is not available among mice since these are such convenient experimental animals. It is also unfortunate that the only complement-deficient rats ever described (C. Arroyave, pers. comm.), a strain deficient in C4, have apparently died out.

Genetic complement deficiencies in man

The first complement component deficiency in human subjects was not described until 1960 but in the three decades that have elapsed since then the deficiencies of all the complement components, except factor B, have been described. Even factor B deficiency is known in heterozygous form. This undoubtedly reflects the growing extent to which complement estimations have been done in clinical laboratories. That deficiency of the components of the classical pathway and the membrane attack complex were described earlier than those of the alternative pathway is because the former causes the CH50 to be absent (or severely reduced) whereas this is not the case in the latter.

It is probably no longer possible, and almost certainly no longer profitable, to try to give a complete account of every case of human complement component deficiency that has been described. Furthermore there is a recent detailed compilation in book form (Rother and Rother 1986) which reviews the literature as far as 1986. What is to be attempted here is to give an account of the deficiencies and their molecular basis where this is known and in particular to discuss what the study of complement-deficient subjects has contributed to our knowledge of the functions of the complement system *in vivo*.

Deficiencies of the early components of the classical pathway

THE DEFICIENCIES OF C1Q (see Loos and Heinz 1986)

There are two distinct varieties of C1q deficiency: one with a total deficiency and no dysfunctional protein and the other where there is a highly abnormal C1q molecule, which can readily be distinguished by fractionating as a pseudoglobulin. This abnormal protein has been studied by Reid and Thompson (1983) and the defect appears to be in the α chain, causing failure to assemble the molecule properly. The consequences of the two deficiencies are rather similar: both types of pedigree have both immune complex disease and, in particular, rather nasty skin infections.

C1r and C1s are closely linked genes and it may be for this reason that the deficiencies of these two components are not clearly distinguished. Though distinctly uncommon, they are again associated largely with immune complex disease as well as infections. It is interesting that the presence of free C1q in these patients does not seem to give rise to any recognizable biological effects. It is known that isolated C1q is a powerful precipitator of immune complexes and that it can react with the C1q receptor much better than can C1q in whole C1. It might therefore be anticipated either that the C1r and C1s deficiencies would have a lesser biological effect on immune complex disease than C1q deficiency, or (more probably) that they would make it worse. However, neither appears to be the case and this must throw some doubt about the importance of C1q–C1q receptor reactions *in vivo*.

C4 DEFICIENCY (see Hauptmann *et al.* 1986)

C4 deficiency is of great interest, partly because the gene is duplicated and the resulting two isotypes have different functions. C4A has a preference for making amide bonds and binds well to immune complexes, while having a lower haemolytic activity than C4B. In contrast, C4B prefers to make ester bonds and has a high haemolytic activity but binds less well to immune complexes.

Null alleles, both at the C4A and at the C4B locus, are surprisingly common. On the other hand, double deficiency haplotypes are extremely rare, probably because they are harmful and have a short half-life.

The reported cases of total C4 deficiency occur on quite different human leucocyte antigen (HLA) backgrounds, suggesting that they have arisen separately from each other, and this is quite different from what is seen in the case of C2 deficiency.

Total C4 deficiency is a more or less sufficient cause for developing systemic lupus erythematosus (SLE) or a related autoimmune immune complex disease. Heterozygous deficiency of C4A also shows a significant rise in the risk of developing SLE and more than 50% of patients with this disease carry a C4AQ0 allele. In Caucasian populations the bulk of C4AQ0 is carried in a single haplotype (A1, B8, C4AQ0 C4B3, C2S, BfS, DR3). This haplotype carries susceptibility genes not only for SLE but, separately, for coeliac disease and autoimmune endocrinopathies. It is fairly clear that the susceptibility gene for these latter diseases is not the same as that which predisposes to SLE since homozygous C4-deficient subjects do not appear to be at an increased risk of getting coeliac disease or autoimmune endocrinopathy. Presumably this haplotype, which is the commonest of all Caucasian haplotypes, survives not because of all its disease associations but because it provides protection against some infectious diseases. However, it is a nuisance in analysing the relative contributions of individual genes such as C4AQ0 to the disease susceptibility and, for this reason, these studies have also been carried out in non-Caucasian populations where this haplotype does not occur. It is interesting that, among orientals (Dunckley *et al.* 1987) and among American Blacks (Wilson *et al.* 1988), the same association of C4AQ0 and SLE have been found. The C4BQ0 allele does not appear to share this disease association, though its association with schizophrenia (Rudduck *et al.* 1985) and IgA nephropathy (Welch *et al.* 1989) have been reported. The mechanism involved in the association of autoimmune immune complex disease with complement deficiency is discussed in a later section of this chapter.

C2 DEFICIENCY

C2 deficiency is the commonest isolated complement component deficiency among Caucasians but has not been encountered at all in the extensive surveys done in Japan. In Israel too it seems to be found only among the Ashkenazi and not the Sephardi population.

C2 deficiency, in more than 90% of cases, is found on a single HLA haplotype, A10, B18, C4A4B2, BfS, C2Q0, DR2. This haplotype must also have had a survival value in the past among the Caucasian population and it has not so far been discovered what it may have been.

C2 deficiency is relatively less harmful than C4 or C1 deficiency and this must presumably be due to the fact that bound C4 shares many of the activities of bound C3, although it performs them less well. For this reason, a subject is less compromised in regard to immune complex binding to CR1, in particular, by being C2-deficient, than by being C4- or C1-deficient.

The published figures in Rother and Rother (1986) probably overestimate the percentage of C2-deficient subjects who are sick, since in recent years the reporting of healthy C2-deficient subjects has probably decreased. It is likely that the older view that about one-third of patients with C2 deficiency were entirely healthy, while a third had SLE and probably one-third had other immune complex disease and/or minor infections, is nearer the truth.

C1 INHIBITOR DEFICIENCY AND HEREDITARY ANGIO-OEDEMA

Hereditary angio-oedema (HAE) as a disease has been known for over a century but it is only in the last 30 years that it has become clear that the disease is due to deficiency of C1 inhibitor (Donaldson and Evans 1963). It was the first deficiency of a complement factor to be associated with a particular disease.

Hereditary angio-oedema remains an unusual deficiency disease. It is transmitted as an autosomal dominant with high penetrance. This means that the patients are heterozygotes and have one normal gene. While this would be most unusual for enzyme deficiencies, it is not unknown for enzyme inhibitors. At least one related enzyme inhibitor deficiency, that of antithrombin III, has similar dominant inheritance. It would appear that such inhibitors are not made in large excess of physiological requirement and one functioning gene is not enough.

The disease itself is episodic and for most of the time patients are free of symptoms. Attacks of HAE are fairly characteristic. They occur at one subcutaneous site (the face or one limb) and last characteristically between 48 and 72 hours. Hereditary angio-oedema does not itch and is not associated with urticaria. Whether or not the lesions hurt presumably depends on the depth of the lesion and the degree of stretching of the tissues involved. In addition the subcutaneous angio-oedema attacks may involve either the upper respiratory tract or the bowel. Attacks in the bowel are usually very painful and may be mistaken for appendicitis. If a barium meal is done during the acute phase, the characteristic X-ray appearances of bowel oedema are seen. It is, however, the respiratory attacks that give the disease its slightly sinister reputation. Oedema may extend from the upper airways right down into the larger bronchi and cause respiratory obstruction which is difficult to reverse.

Pathogenesis of the individual attack is not known with certainty. The commonest predisposing factor is trauma, for example dental extraction or a blow, but many attacks have no obvious predisposing cause. However, what appears to happen is that, at an extravascular site, there is exhaustion of the limited amount of C1 inhibitor available due to its consumption by one of the enzymes with which it can react. These are C1r and C1s, kallikrein, plasmin, and factors XIIa and XIa of the coagulation system (see Fig. 67.1). The association with trauma suggests that plasmin activation is important in bringing about the local exhaustion of inhibitor. The absence of C1 inhibitor permits the autoactivation of C1 (Ziccardi and Cooper 1978) and the generation of free C1s and of the other locally available serine proteases which C1 inhibitor regulates, notably kallikrein and plasmin. This disregulation of the serine proteases produces the mediators giving rise to the angio-oedema. There is still some dispute about the relative importance of bradykinin on the one hand (produced by kallikrein from plasma kininogen) and a kinin-like peptide generated from C2 in the presence of C1, C4 and plasmin (Strang *et al.* 1988). The evidence in favour of bradykinin includes its detection in HAE blister fluid (Curd *et al.* 1980) and the inhibition of its production by C1 inhibitor. On the other hand injected bradykinin gives rise to a sharply painful inflammatory reaction which does not resemble clinical HAE attacks. Evidence that the complement system is itself involved in the attacks comes from some early work showing that the injection of purified C1s produces no inflammatory reaction in patients who are C2-deficient; produces a wheal and flare in normal subjects; and produces an attack of HAE in C1 inhibitor-deficient subjects. A kinin-like fragment has also been produced from C2 and sequenced (Lopez-Trascasa *et al.* 1982) although some doubt has been expressed whether enough of this material could be produced to account for the clinical effects. It is, of course, possible that

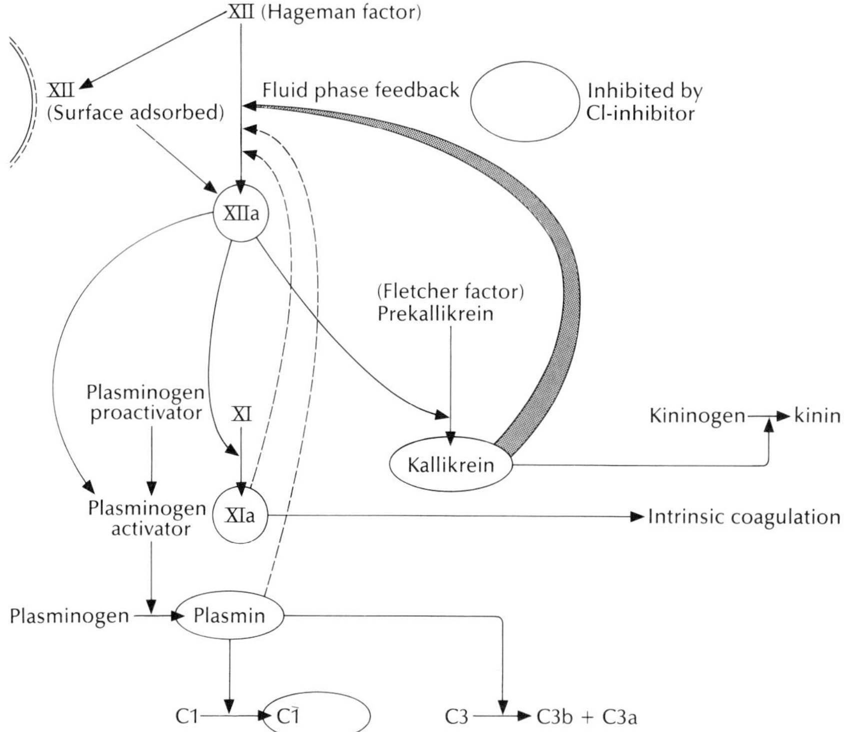

Fig. 67.1. The functions of C1 inhibitor.

both types of mediator are involved synergistically.

What is perhaps more mysterious is what causes the attack to go away after 48–72 hours. If there is an autocatalytic activation of C1 and of plasmin, kallikrein and factor XII over a large local area, it is difficult to see how homoeostasis would be restored by the introduction of further C1 inhibitor from the circulation. It used to be believed that there was activated C1 present in the circulation during attacks of HAE, which would make it even more difficult to restore homoeostasis, but it is likely that the detection of C1 in freshly taken blood during attacks may be artefactual and result from activation in the drawn blood following the venepuncture. In plasma, α-2-macroglobulin inhibits plasmin but this is largely absent from the normal extravascular space. However, once capillary permeability is much increased, α-2-macroglobulin will enter the extracellular fluid and by inhibiting plasmin may help to bring an attack to an end.

The diagnosis of hereditary angio-oedema

The disease can frequently be diagnosed clinically from the characteristic history but biochemical diagnosis requires the demonstration of low levels of C1 inhibitor activity. In several series (Hadjiyannaki and Lachmann 1971; Rosen *et al.* 1971; Agostoni 1989) 10–15% of pedigrees of HAE have normal antigenic levels in the presence of low functional levels. This is due to the presence of dysfunctional proteins rather than failure to make protein. It is customary to call those where both antigenic and functional level are low 'type 1 HAE' and those with dysfunctional proteins 'type 2 HAE'.

A good deal of effort has gone into identifying the abnormalities of the dysfunctional proteins. It has been found that approximately half have mutations at the P1 residue, i.e. the reactive centre of the inhibitor. In C1 inhibitor this P1 'bait' residue is an arginine. The codon contains a CpG dinucleotide. There are two common products of mutation from this codon, one giving a histidine and one giving a cysteine. Both of these have been identified in multiple pedigrees (Aulak *et al.* 1988, 1989). Recently one serine at the P1 site has also been found (Aulak *et al.* 1990).

It is curious that although the patients are heterozygotes the normal inhibitor level in type 1 HAE is 15–30% protein; and that in type 2 patients usually more than 90% of the protein is of the dysfunctional type and very little is normal. This strange state of affairs has been explained by Lachmann and Rosen (1984) on the basis that catabolism of C1 inhibitor is in part effected by the increased catabolism of the inhibitor–enzyme complex, which is faster than the catabolism of the inhibitor alone. This enhanced catabolism occurs only with functional proteins. This leads to relative hypercatabolism of normal inhibitor, particularly when there is increased enzyme activation (as occurs in HAE). Since the enzyme–inhibitor complex-dependent metabolism is essentially independent of the concentration of inhibitor, this route of metabolism leads to a greater consumption of normal inhibitor than expected from the synthetic rate alone.

The treatment of hereditary angio-oedema

Since the pathogenesis of HAE is essentially understood, rational lines of treatment are available.

Prophylactic treatment Since the patients have one normal C1 inhibitor gene, it is possible to raise the levels of the normal protein by treatments that enhance the gene transcription and translation. It was originally found by Spaulding (1960) that treatment with testosterone improved the disease. Although this was, at the time, an entirely empirical treatment, it gave rise to the recognition that the C1 inhibitor gene is androgen-responsive and to the treatment of the disease with modified androgens such as danazol and stanazol (Gadek *et al.* 1979). These compounds when given in sufficient dosage normalize the C1 inhibitor level. However, they have undesirable side-effects, delaying puberty in children, preventing the establishment of pregnancy, increasing muscle bulk and producing some degree of virilization. Most importantly, they produce changes in liver histology that give rise to suspicion of malignancy although actual tumours are very rare. For this reason they are used in the lowest possible dose to prevent attacks rather than a dose to normalize the biochemistry.

An alternative method of prophylaxis is to inhibit the activation of the enzymes with which C1 inhibitor reacts. For this purpose inhibitors of plasmin activation such as epsilon aminocaproic acid or tranexamic acid can be used. Epsilon aminocaproic acid has to be given in rather large doses and because it is nauseating it is unpopular with patients. Tranexamic acid is free from this problem and is thus more acceptable. Patients on tranexamic acid should have their eyes regularly examined, since it produces retinal damage though so far only in dogs. It has occasionally been reported to cause muscle necrosis.

Whereas both the androgenic hormones and the plasmin inhibitors are effective, they act in quite different ways and it is logical, though not always necessary, to give them together, since one causes an increase in the amount of inhibitor synthesized and the other a diminution in the amount of inhibitant needed to maintain homoeostasis.

Treatment of attacks Attacks can be treated by replacing inhibitor. For this purpose purified inhibitor preparations are available from Immuno AG and the Netherlands Red Cross, and they generally terminate attacks rapidly. It is also possible to use fresh frozen plasma. This is generally highly effective but carries the potential disadvantage that giving further C4 and C2 may cause a temporary aggravation of symptoms before the attack is brought to an end. This is potentially dangerous in patients with severe respiratory attacks, and it makes the point that if an attack is to be treated in this way it should be treated early rather than waiting until the patient already has a considerable degree of respiratory obstruction.

The great majority of C1 inhibitor-deficient subjects have no disease other than HAE, but a minority — some 2–5% — do show manifestations of autoimmune immune complex disease — similar to that seen in C2 and C4 deficiency, which these patients have, albeit in incomplete form.

C3 deficiency

C3 deficiency is expected to be the severest complement deficiency clinically, and in general this is true, a high proportion of C3-deficient subjects suffering severe bacterial immunodeficiency of the same sort as seen in antibody deficiency syndromes. Occasional C3-deficient subjects, however, have much milder infectious manifestations. Thus, if they first encounter a pathogen when they still have maternal antibody and they encounter it in relatively small amounts, then they may form a good IgG antibody response, without having severe clinical problems. If they first encounter a pathogen at a subsequent stage, they may develop more severe clinical complications. Furthermore, it must be remembered that the generation of good IgG responses may be impaired in the presence of a severe complement deficiency (see later).

Abnormality of antibody formation in conjunction with complement deficiencies

The observation that complement depletion impaired antibody responses was first made by Pepys (1972) to show that cobra venom-treated mice failed to make good IgG responses to sheep cells.

It was subsequently observed (Ellman *et al.* 1971; Ochs *et al.* 1983) that C4-deficient guinea-pigs also had an impaired capacity to make IgG antibodies, especially to small doses of antigens given without adjuvant, and similar work has been done by Burger and his colleagues (1986), on C2-deficient and C3-deficient guinea-pigs. The latter are the most seriously disadvantaged and, in these animals, antibody responses cannot be normalized entirely either by giving adjuvant or by raising the dose of antigen given.

The most convincing explanation of this phenomenon was given by Klaus and Humphrey (1977), who demonstrated that it required both complement and IgM antibody for antigen to be localized on the follicular dendritic cells in the germinal follicles of lymph nodes and that antigen so localized is required for the development of B cell memory. This is the site where antigen is presented for the secondary antibody response.

In humans it has been difficult to demonstrate deficiency of specific antibodies in complement-deficient subjects. They appear to have normal levels of antibodies to the organisms with which they become infected and have normal overall levels of immunoglobulin. An exception to this is the finding by Bird and Lachmann (1988) that patients with genetic deficiencies of C1, C4, C2 and C3 have reduced levels of IgG4. This is at first sight a slightly surprising finding since IgG4 does not fix complement by the classical pathway and it seems a perverse consequence of complement deficiency to fail to make a non-complement-fixing antibody. However, it is more likely that the explanation lies in the fact that IgG4 is the last IgG subclass to be made during the generation of the B cell memory and this defect of IgG4 may be the extent of the defect in memory generation that is shown in complement-deficient humans.

Deficiencies of factor I and factor H

Factor I deficiency has clinical manifestations rather similar to C3 deficiency, and, indeed, factor I deficiency causes a severe secondary C3 deficiency as well as a secondary deficiency of factor B, both due to hypercatabolism. It is nevertheless interesting that some of the patients suffer only from neisserial infections and one or two have been reported as healthy, in spite of having the same complement profile.

Factor H deficiency appears to be very rare. Although such patients cannot make complexes of C3b at complement fixation sites, this does not apparently make their clinical status any different from that of factor I-deficient patients. Thus, while factor H receptors do indeed exist, these deficiencies give little clue to their functions. It is also interesting that complement receptor type 1 (CR1), which shares the factor I cofactor activity of factor H, can clearly not substitute for factor H in controlling the C3b feedback cycle in solution.

Deficiencies of the membrane attack complex

Deficiencies of the MAC may be treated as a group since their biological effects are closely similar. They are associated almost exclusively with neisserial infections, predominantly with an increased incidence of meningococcal meningitis. It is curious that C5 deficiency does not show separate manifestations in view of the known *in vitro* importance of the C5 anaphylatoxin.

All the terminal complement components of deficiency seem to be relatively rare among Caucasian populations in the developed world. It is, however, clear that that is not the case elsewhere. There is a striking incidence of C6 deficiency among the Cape Coloured population in South Africa (Orren *et al*. 1987). In this population the interesting observation has been made that there is a marked excess of homozygous C6-deficient subjects over statistical expectation, approximately half the children in the affected families being homozygous for C6 deficiency. The most plausible explanation for this is that C6 deficiency has a compensating protective advantage in early or fetal life. This population suffers a high infant mortality from gastroenteritis and associated shock states. This disease must be a good candidate for that which C6 deficiencies protects against — and it was shown by Brown and Lachmann (1973) that C6 deficiency does indeed protect rabbits from endotoxin shock.

Similarly, Schlesinger *et al*. (1990) have described a high frequency of C7 and C8 deficiency among North African Arabs and Sephardic Jews suffering from meningococcal meningitis. It seems not unlikely, therefore, that terminal deficiencies under Third World conditions do have some selective advantage and that this is balanced by the tendency of the affected subjects to be more prone to develop meningococcal meningitis.

The meningococcal meningitis seen in complement-deficient subjects shows some characteristic features. Firstly, it occurs later in life than it does in the complement-sufficient population, i.e. the increased susceptibility does not appear to show until adolescence. Secondly, although subsequent attacks appear to get less severe, the chance of having a further attack increases after the first. This has led A. Orren (pers. comm.) to question whether the antibodies formed are, in the absence of complement, protective rather than the reverse. This is a matter that needs clarification since it has important practical implications on whether complement-deficient children should be immunized against meningococci or whether they should be treated with chemoprophylaxis. At the present time, the latter course may seem the more prudent.

C9 DEFICIENCY

C9 deficiency is strikingly common among Japanese (Inai *et al*. 1979) and there are detailed studies demonstrating that, both in Japanese blood donors and in Japanese hospital patients, about 1 in 1000 is homozygous for C9 deficiency, giving an allele frequency of about 1 in 16. The reason for this high incidence is unknown and C9 deficiency produces only a minor increase in susceptibility to meningococcal disease (if any) so that the 'down' side of the deficiency is small. If there is any compensating advantage, it has yet to be discovered.

It is surprising how slight the effects of C9 deficiency are on the total haemolytic titre. Some of the deficient subjects have been shown to have normal haemolytic titres when they have an acute-phase response. This has led to suspicions that the deficiency may be subtotal, but recent claims have denied this (Takata *et al.* 1989).

Suggestions have been made that the MAC of complement may be involved in the pathogenesis of multiple sclerosis (MS), (Morgan *et al.* 1984), and that the high incidence of C9 deficiency may contribute to the surprisingly low incidence of MS in Japan (considering its latitude) is an intriguing but entirely unproved possibility.

Deficiencies of alternative pathway factors

There is no known homozygous deficiency of factor B, although a heterozygous form has been described by Mauff *et al.* (1980) and Bertrams and Mauff (1985). C3 deficiency can be regarded as an alternative pathway deficiency but has been described separately. This leaves only factor D and properdin.

One pedigree of factor D deficiency is known from Holland (Hiemstra *et al.* 1989). This pedigree is perhaps of particular interest now it has been established that factor D is identical to adipsin, a serum proteinase found in fat cells and low levels of which are associated with genetic forms of obesity in animals (Rosen *et al.* 1989). It is interesting that the factor D-deficient propositus is lean and seems to have no obvious problems with his fat metabolism (M. Daha, pers. comm.). Since the function of adipsin in adiposites is unknown, no further explanation for this can so far be given. However, it is again perhaps interesting how relatively benign this deficiency is, in view of the widespread belief that the alternative pathway plays a major role in non-specific immunity.

On the other hand, properdin deficiency is not benign and, in the original pedigrees described in Sweden, it was associated with severe bacterial immunodeficiencies and high mortality. Schlesinger and his colleagues (1990) have recently described properdin deficiency in Israel among patients who only have meningococcal meningitis, and, to this extent, properdin deficiency is beginning to resemble factor I deficiency, which may show severe manifestations of general immunodeficiency, on the one hand, or only neisserial deficiencies, on the other.

MANNAN-BINDING PROTEIN

A common immunodeficiency syndrome characterized by recurrent pyogenic infections in infancy, chronic diarrhoea and failure to thrive was described in association with the failure of serum to opsonize *Saccharomyces cerevisiae* for phagocytosis by normal polymorphs (Miller *et al.* 1968). This same opsonic defect is present in up to 5% of a Caucasoid population (Soothill and Harvey 1976) and the strength of its association with increased infectious disease in adult life has not been established. The defect of opsonization was correlated with reduced deposition of C3 on to the yeast cells and the basis of this remained a mystery for a number of years because no abnormality in the complement system was found which could explain the decreased uptake of C3. The discovery that a lectin which bound mannan, mannan-binding protein (MBP), could opsonize *Saccharomyces cerevisiae* with C3 by a C1q-independent route led to the elucidation of the mechanism of the immunodeficiency. It was found that there was polymorphism of expression of the level of major basic protein (MBP) in the population and that reduced levels of MBP, which showed dominant inheritance within families, correlated with the opsonic defect (Super *et al.* 1989). The molecular basis of this polymorphism has recently been shown to be due to an asp to gly substitution within the collagen-like chain of the MBP monomer. The presence of this substitution may disrupt the formation of the normal triple helix, accounting for the dominant expression of the lesion (Sumiya *et al.* 1991).

Acquired complement deficiencies

Acquired complement deficiencies of the classical complement pathway as exemplified by cold haemolytic antibody disease

Cold haemolytic antibody disease (CHAD) is due to the formation of antibodies to the I antigen on erythrocytes. Such antibodies are often found for a time following *Mycoplasma pneumoniae* infection or chronically as a result of a monoclonal immunoglobulin proliferation. The antibodies are of low affinity and bind sufficiently to produce either agglutination or complement fixation only at reduced temperature. It is therefore in cold weather and in parts of the body, e.g. hands and feet, that have a lower body temperature that symptoms — Raynaud's phenomenon and in more severe cases persistent anoxia — are seen. The patients tend to have very low complement levels due to the persistent activation of the classical complement pathway, and levels of C1, C4, C2 and C3 are all much reduced. Indeed, the low levels of serum complement play a role in limiting the complement activation and it is recorded that blood transfusion containing fresh plasma may make the patients worse. Studies on their red cells show that they circulate as microspherocytes, carrying increased numbers of C3dg and reduced numbers of CR1 on their membranes. Indeed, red cells in this disease have the highest levels of C3dg and some of the lowest levels of CR1 that have been observed *in vivo*; and in this disease it is quite clear that these anomalies result from the complement activation.

The microspherocytes are resistant to complement lysis by further anti-I antibody and they have a normal (or supranormal) survival time *in vivo*. The resistance to further lysis presumably means that all the membrane sites adjacent to the I antigen sites where the antibody can combine are already occupied by C3dg and/or C4d fragments, so that further productive complement fixation is not possible. The normal survival time demonstrates that the reaction of C3dg with the complement receptors with which this fragment reacts (CR2 and CR4) does not lead to clearance, which is in strong contrast to the reaction of iC3b with CR3 and CR1. The chronic haemolytic anaemia accentuated by cold is the major clinical problem for these patients with anti-I antibody and they do not have problems either with infections or with immune complex diseases such as SLE.

Systemic lupus erythematosus, reduced numbers of complement receptor type 1 on erythrocytes and the pathogenesis of autoimmune immune complex disease

Low CR1 levels on erythrocytes were first found in SLE, where it was postulated that this might reflect a genetic predisposition to the disease (Wilson *et al.* 1982). Although genetic variation in CR1 numbers does occur, it has since been shown by allotyping both normal patients and patients with SLE that they are not obviously a risk factor for SLE, and it has been demonstrated in a variety of ways that the low CR1 numbers are the result of the disease rather than its cause. Thus low CR1 numbers and raised C3dg levels are found in a variety of diseases associated with complement activation, either by anti-red cell antibodies or by immune complexes, and C3dg levels go down and CR1 levels go up when diseases remit. The reduction in CR1 is an *in vivo* phenomenon and cannot be replicated by incubating red cells with anti-red cell antibodies and complement *in vitro*. It is believed that during passage through the liver, where complement-coated red cells are temporarily held on the Kupffer cells before being released

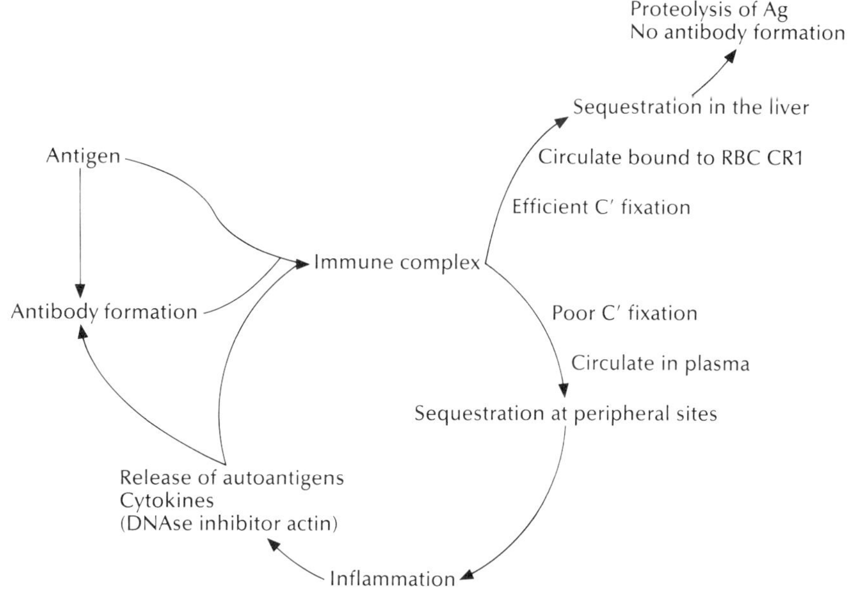

Fig. 67.2. Schema for the handling of immune complexes.

again, the cleavage of iC3b to C3dg takes place and the proteolytic removal of CR1. It has been demonstrated by the transfusion of compatible cells (Walport *et al.* 1987) that loss of CR1 and acquisition of C3dg can be monitored *in vivo* on such cells. The reason that these changes in red cells are believed to be important is that, *in vivo*, immune complexes are believed to be carried bound to red cell CR1 and that this carriage transport by red cells keeps immune complexes away from endothelial surfaces and allows them to be sequestered in the liver without feedback antibody formation. If this mechanism fails, immune complexes sequester elsewhere and give rise to inflammation and subsequent feedback antibody formation where the antigens concerned are autoantigens (as is the case in SLE). This scheme is shown in Fig. 67.2 and is discussed in more detail by Lachmann and Walport (1987) and Lachmann (1990).

This mechanism fails *in vivo* where there is a deficiency of the early components of the classical pathway rather than when there are genetically reduced CR1 numbers. The failure of this pathway is believed to explain the association of C4AQ0 with SLE and other autoimmune immune complex diseases.

Complement depletion by the alternative pathway as seen in sickle-cell disease

Complement depletion by the alternative pathway is not particularly severe since total haemolytic complement is often not significantly expressed. Patients with sickle-cell anaemia do have a defective alternative complement pathway, particularly demonstrated by low levels of factor B. This has been shown by turnover studies to be due to hypercatabolism and not to hyposynthesis. It seems that the sickled red cells activate the alternative pathway *in vivo*. The importance of this example of acquired complement deficiency is that these patients do suffer from an increased incidence of infection and this is a not uncommon cause of death.

Nephritic factor

Nephritic factor provides a rare but dramatic example of an acquired complement deficiency. The name 'Nef' is an abbreviation of nephritic factor and describes the factor in the plasma of patients with the dense deposit form of mesangiocapillary glomerulonephritis (MCGN) that is capable of giving rise to C3 cleavage in normal serum. After a period of dispute it was established that Nef is an autoantibody to the alternative pathway C3 convertase which has the property of stabilizing the convertase against dissociation by factor H and thus causes the alternative pathway to cycle to exhaustion. Patients with Nef have very low C3 levels but do not usually have great depletion of factor B. The reason for this appears to be that there is a feedback reduction in the synthesis of C3 and the C3 levels become so low that the cycling of the alternative pathway is greatly reduced. Although Nef was described in relation to MCGN, it is not found only in this disease. There is indeed a stronger association with the strange condition known as partial lipodystrophy. In this condition the fat is lost from the subcutaneous tissues, usually only in part of a body, and not infrequently above a horizontal level. The loss of fat in the face with a consequent hollowing of the cheeks gives such patients a characteristic appearance. Partial lipodystrophy is not a genetic disease and tends to come on after virus infections, sometimes measles. The recognition that factor D is the same as adipsin and is made in adipose tissue has reawakened interest in the mechanism of this particular disease association.

About 85% of children with partial lipodystrophy have Nef and it is interesting that some of these later go on to develop MCGN. This provides evidence that the association is likely to be in the direction that the hypercomplementaemia consequent upon having Nef predisposes to the nephritis rather than vice versa. Nef is rarely seen in SLE and there is at least one reported case of it being encountered in someone who is clinically normal (Tedesco *et al.* 1985). Association with excessive infection has not been a feature of most patients with Nef. The stimulus for forming this strange autoantibody remains completely unknown but it is possible that patients who carry the C3F allele are more likely to develop it. The C3F allele is limited to Caucasians and interestingly MCGN is an entirely Caucasian disease. Another disease association that has been described for C3F (but where there is no Nef) is with Indian childhood cirrhosis, which again seems to be restricted to the Caucasian parts of northern India.

'Critical time' complement deficiencies

'Critical time' complement deficiency is the term proposed to describe situations where complement depletion at a critical time when a host is encountering an infectious agent may establish sequestered infections which it is subsequently difficult or impossible to eliminate, even though the complement level has long returned to normal when the subsequent disease is recognized. Thus, subacute sclerosing panencephalitis (SSPE) is a late consequence of measles virus infection and before measles vaccination was initiated it occurred in western countries in approximately one in a million cases of measles. In some parts of the world, however, particularly where early measles virus infection (i.e. before the age of 2) is common, the incidence of SSPE is appreciably greater. The phenomenon which is believed to underlie the pathogenesis of this disease was described by Joseph and Oldstone (1975) and Joseph *et al*. (1976). They showed that, if cells infected with the measles virus were cultured in the presence of antibody but in the absence of complement, the surface viral glycoproteins would be 'capped off' and extruded from the cells as a large immune complex and these surface antigens would not be re-expressed while the cells were grown in the presence of antibody. Such cells then became resistant to immune attack — at least by antibody, complement and antibody-dependent cell-mediated cytotoxicity (ADCC). At the time it was not realized that cytotoxic T cells do not recognize the intact viral glycoproteins but rather see processed peptides; and the capacity of these modulated measles virus-infected cells to be killed by measles-specific cytotoxic T lymphocytes (CTL) was not assessed. However, it was shown that mRNA production for the haemagglutinin and fusion protein was much decreased, so that it is likely that even the peptides are not adequately made. When the amounts of antibody and complement required to produce modulation were investigated (Gorman and Lachmann 1982) it was found that in the presence of high levels of antibody very substantial complement depletion is needed to produce a living modulated cell. However, there is a 'window' of antibody formation round about 50 μg of antibody per ml when quite moderate degrees of complement depletion can give rise to modulation. It had previously been shown that complement depletion does occur in acute measles infection. It therefore seems entirely plausible that in rare cases the conditions required for successful modulation of the central nervous infection of measles occur. In this way an infection is set up which can subsequently not be eliminated and which persists for long periods of time, gradually causing the hypoimmunization of the host and eventually leading to sufficient destruction of neurones to give rise to the clinical features. A final twist was added to this story when it was shown by Rittner *et al*. (1984) that, of the children who develop SSPE in Europe, a substantial number show partial genetic C4 deficiency, so that it may be that starting with a somewhat impaired complement system it is easier to achieve the conditions that predispose to SSPE.

Acquired C1 inhibitor deficiency

C1 inhibitor deficiency has long been known in its genetic form, giving rise to the disease of hereditary angio-oedema as discussed in an earlier section. In more recent years, an acquired disease has been encountered, generally in elderly people, who have similar attacks of angio-oedema without a family history and whose complement profile, low C1 inhibitor level, low C2 and low C4, is similar except that in this acquired form they also show a low level of C1. This disease is frequently associated with a covert B cell lymphoma and it has been proposed that its pathogenesis is due to an unusual complement-fixing reaction produced by the interaction of the immunoglobulin idiotype on the abnormal B cells and auto-anti-idiotypic antibody (Geha *et al*. 1985). It remains to be explained why this particular reaction should fix so much C1 as to produce C1 inhibitor deficiency while producing relatively little fixation of C3. Even more recently a further form of this disease has been encountered and this is associated with autoantibodies to C1 inhibitor in the circulation (Jackson *et al*. 1986; Alsenz and Loos 1989). In at least the case of the Irish patient whose serum the author's laboratory have studied, the level of C1 inhibitor is relatively normal antigenically while highly defective functionally, i.e. he resembles an acquired form of type II hereditary angio-oedema. However, the abnormal protein is not dysfunctional in the same way. The protein that is circulating in the plasma of this patient is in the cleaved form, i.e. it has reacted with an enzyme, giving rise to cleavage, but without forming a firm complex. This cleaved form is not only inactive but is remarkably heat-stable and can be detected antigenically after heating to 90 °C (Pemberton *et al.* 1989). We have also demonstrated that his autoantibody fails to react with this cleaved form of the inhibitor, i.e. it reacts only with normal functional inhibitor and therefore must be directed to somewhere in the region of the binding site. It is interesting that no mouse monoclonal of this specificity has so far been raised. This reactivity also accounts for the fact that he can have at the same time an antibody to C1 inhibitor and a normal level of C1 inhibitor without any evidence of immune complex formation between them.

The pathogenesis of this disease is unclear. The antibody present in the patient does not itself cleave C1 inhibitor. On the other hand, it produces some inhibition of the activity of the inhibitor and this can be pictured as giving rise to auto C1 activation. Alsenz and Loos (1989) have shown that C1 cleavage in the presence of antibody can give rise to the abnormal cleaved inhibitor, and it is possible that a process of this kind is going on *in vivo*. As is the case in hereditary angio-oedema the process would have to occur intermittently and presumably at extravascular sites as a result of abnormal enzyme activation or inhibitor consumption of some kind. Whether the formation of the antibody is the primary cause of the disease or is a secondary phenomenon still remains to be elucidated.

References

Agostoni, A. (1989). Inherited C1 inhibitor deficiency. *Complement Inflamm.* **6**, 112–18.

Alsenz, J. and Loos, M. (1989). The acquired C1-INH deficiencies with autoantibodies (AAE type II). *Behring Inst. Mitt.* **84**, 165–72.

Aulak, K.S., Pemberton, P.A., Rosen, F.S., Carrell, R.W., Lachmann, P.J. and Harrison, R.A. (1988). Dysfunctional C1-inhibitor (At), isolated from a type II hereditary angio-oedema plasma, contains a P1 'reactive centre' (Arg 444 → His) mutation. *Biochem. J.* **253**, 615–18.

Aulak, K.S., Rosen, F.S., Lachmann, P.J. and Harrison, R.A. (1989). Are the dysfunctional 1-inhibitor proteins expressed in Type II hereditary angio-oedema of limited structural heterogeneity? *Behring Inst. Mitt.* **84**, 198 (abstract).

Aulak, K.S., Cicardi, M. and Harrison, R.A. (1990). Identification of a new P1 residue mutation (444 Arg → Ser) in a dysfunctional C1-inhibitor protein contained in a type II hereditary angioedema plasma. *FEBS Lett.* **266**, 13–16.

Bertrams, J. and Mauff, G. (1985). Another family with a silent allele of properdin factor B polymorphism (BF QO). *Hum. Genet.* **70**, 321–3.

Bird, P. and Lachmann, P.J. (1988). The regulation of IgG subclass production in man: low serum IgG4 in inherited deficiencies of the classical pathway of C3 activation. *Eur. J. Immunol.* **18**, 1217–22.

Biro, C.E. and Garcia, G. (1965). The antigenicity of aggregated and aggregate-free human gamma-globulin for rabbits. *Immunology* **8**, 411–19.

Bitter-Suermann, D. and Burger, R. (1986). Hereditary deficiencies in animals. 1. Guinea pigs deficient in C2, C4, C3 or the C3a receptor. *Prog. Allergy* **39**, 134–58.

Bitter-Suermann, D., Hoffmann, T., Burger, R. and Hadding, U. (1981). Linkage of total deficiency of the second component (C2) of the complement system and of genetic C2-polymorphism to the major histocompatibility complex of the guinea pig. *J. Immunol.* **127**, 608–12.

Borzy, M.S., Gewurz, A., Wolff, L., Houghton, D. and Lovrien, E. (1988). Inherited C3 deficiency with recurrent infections and glomerulonephritis. *Am. J. Dis. Child.* **142**, 79–83.

Bottger, E.C., Metzger, S., Bitter-Suemann, D., Stevenson, G., Kleindienst, S. and Burger, R. (1986). Impaired humoral immune response in complement C3-deficient guinea pigs: absence of secondary antibody response. *Eur. J. Immunol.* **16**, 1231–5.

Botto, M., Fong, K.Y., So, A.K., Rudge, A. and Walport, M.J. (1990). Molecular basis of hereditary C3 deficiency *J. Clin. Invest.* **86**, 1158–63.

Brai, M., Misiano, G., Maringhini, S., Cutaja, I. and Hauptmann, G. (1988). Combined homozygous factor H and heterozygous C2 deficiency in an Italian family. *J. Clin. Immunol.* **8**, 50–6.

Brown, D.L. and Lachmann, P.J. (1973). The behaviour of complement and platelets in lethal endotoxin shock in rabbits. *Int. Arch. Allergy Appl. Immunol.* **45**, 193–205.

Burger, R., Gordon, J., Stevenson, G. *et al.* (1986). An inherited deficiency of the third component of complement, C3, in guinea pigs. *Eur. J. Immunol.* **16**, 7–11.

Cinader, B., Dubiski, S. and Wardlaw, A.C. (1964). Distribution, inheritance and properties of an antigen, MUB1 and its relation to hemolytic complement. *J. Exp. Med.* **120**, 897–924.

Cullmann, W. and Opferkuch, W. (1986). Deficiencies in regulator proteins. 1. C1 inhibitor. *Prog. Allergy* **39**, 311–34.

Curd, J.G., Prograis, L.J. and Cochrane, C.G. (1980). Detection of active kallikrein in induced blister fluids of hereditary angioedema patients. *J. Exp. Med.* **152**, 742–7.

Day, N.K. (1986a). Deficiencies in regulator proteins. 2. Factor I and H. *Prog. Allergy* **39**, 311–34.

Day, N.K. (1986b). Complement deficiencies. 2. The third component. *Prog. Allergy* **39**, 335–8.

Donaldson, V.H. and Evans, R.R. (1963). A biochemical abnormality in hereditary angioneurotic edema: absence of serum inhibitor of C1 esterase. *Am. J. Med.* **35**, 37–44.

Dunckley, H., Gatenby, P.A., Hawkins, B., Naito, S. and Serjeantson, S.W. (1987). Deficiency of C4A is a genetic determinant of systemic lupus erythematosus in three ethnic groups. *J. Immunogenet.* **14**, 209–18.

Ellman, L., Green, I., Judge, F. and Frank, M.M. (1971). *In vivo* studies in C4-deficient guinea pigs. *J. Exp. Med.* **134**, 162–87.

Fijen, C.A.P., Kuijper, E.J., Hannema, A.J., Sjoholm, A.G. and van Putten, J.P.M. (1989). Complement deficiencies in patients over ten years old with meningococcal disease due to uncommon serogroups. *Lancet* **ii**, 585–8.

Gadek, J.E., Hosea, S.W., Gelfand, J.A. and Frank, M.M. (1979). Response of variant hereditary angioedema phenotypes. *J. Clin. Invest.* **64**, 280–6.

Garty, B.Z., Conley, M.E., Douglas, S.D. and Kolski, G.B. (1987). Recurrent infections and staphylococcal liver abscess in a child with C1r deficiency. *J. Allergy Clin. Immunol.* **80**, 631–5.

Geha, R.S., Quinti, I., Austen, K.F., Cicardi, M., Sheffer, A. and Rosen, F.S. (1985). Acquired C1-inhibitor deficiency associated with antiidiotypic antibody to monoclonal immunoglobulins. *N. Engl. J. Med.* **312**, 534–40.

Gorman, N.T. and Lachmann, P.J. (1982). *In vitro* modulation of viral cell surface glycoproteins by anti-viral antibody in the presence of complement. *Clin. Exp. Immunol.* **50**, 507–14.

Grumach, A.S., Vilela, M.M., Gonzales, C.H. *et al.* (1988). Inherited C3 deficiency of the complement system. *Braz. J. Med. Biol. Res.* **21**, 247–57.

Hadjiyannaki, K. and Lachmann, P.J. (1971). Hereditary angiooedema: a review with particular reference to pathogenesis and treatment. *Clin. Allergy* **1**, 221–33.

Hauptmann, G., Goetz, J., Uring-Lambert, B. and Grosshans, E. (1986). Complement deficiences. 2. The fourth component. *Prog. Allergy* **39**, 232–49.

Hauptmann, G., Tappeiner, G. and Schifferli, J.A. (1988). Inherited deficiency of the fourth component of human complement. *Immunodeficiency Rev.* **1**, 3–32.

Hiemstra, P.S., Langeler, E., Compier, B. *et al.* (1989). Complete and partial deficiencies of complement factor D in a Dutch family. *J. Clin. Invest.* **84**, 1957–61.

Hyde, R.R. (1923). Complement-deficient guinea-pig serum. *J. Immunol.* **8**, 267–86.

Inai, S., Kitamura, H., Hiramatsu, S. and Nagaki, K. (1979). Deficiency of the ninth component of complement in man. *J. Clin. Lab. Immunol.* **2**, 85–7.

Jackson, J., Sim, R.B., Whelan, A. and Feighery, C. (1986). An IgG autoantibody which inactivates C1-inhibitor. *Nature* **323**, 722–4.

Joseph, B.S. and Oldstone, M.B.A. (1975). Immunologic injury in measles virus infection. II. Suppression of immune injury through antigenic modulation. *J. Exp. Med.* **142**, 864–76.

Joseph, B.S., Cooper, N.R. and Oldstone, M.B.A. (1976). Immunologic injury of cultured cells infected with measles virus. I. Role of IgG antibody and the alternative complement pathway. *J. Exp. Med.* **141**, 761–74.

Klaus, G.G.B. and Humphrey, J.H. (1977). The generation of memory cells. I. The role of C3 in the generation of B memory cells. *Immunology* **33**, 31–40.

Komatsu, M., Yamamoto, K.I., Kawashima, T. and Magita, S. (1985). Genetic deficiency of the $\alpha\gamma$ subunit of the eighth complement component in the rabbit. *J. Immunol.* **134**, 2607–9.

Komatsu, M., Yamamoto, K.I., Nakanu, Y. *et al.* (1988). Hereditary C3 hypocomplementaemia in the rabbit. *Immunology* **64**, 363–8.

Lachmann, P.J. (1970). C6-deficiency in rabbits. In *XVII Colloquium of Protides of the Biological Fluids, Bruges 1969*, ed. H. Peeters, pp. 301–9, Pergamon Press.

Lachmann, P.J. (1990). Complement deficiency and the pathogenesis of autoimmune immune complex disease. *Chem. Immunol.* **49**, 245–63.

Lachmann, P.J. and Rosen, F.S. (1984). The catabolism of C1-inhibitor and the pathogenesis of hereditary angio-edema. *Acta Pathol. Microbiol. Immunol. Scand. Sect. C* (Suppl. 284), **92**, 35–9.

Lachmann, P.J. and Walport, M.J. (1987). Deficiency of the effector mechanisms of the immune response and autoimmunity. *Ciba Found. Symp.* **129**, 149–65.

Lachmann, P.J., Hobart, M.J. and Woo, P. (1978). Combined genetic deficiency of C6 and C7 in man. *Clin. Exp. Immunol.* **33**, 193–203.

Lint, T.F. and Gewurz, H. (1986). Complement deficiencies. 9. The ninth component. *Prog. Allergy* **39**, 307–10.

Loos, M. and Heinz, H.-P. (1986). Complement deficiencies. 1. The first component C1q, C1r and C1s. *Prog. Allergy* **39**, 212–31.

Lopez-Trascasa, M., Moisy, M., Pirotzky, E., Blouquit, Y., Blanc, C. and Sobel, A.T. (1982). Isolation and characterization of a biologically active C2 derived oligopeptide. *Mol. Immunol.* **19**, 1403 (abstract).

McCarty, G.A. and Snyderman, R. (1986). Complement deficiencies. 5. The fifth component. *Prog. Allergy* **39**, 271–82.

Mauff, G., Federmann, G. and Hauptmann, G. (1980). A hemolytically inactive gene product of Factor B. *Immunobiology* **158**, 96–100.

Miller, M.E., Seals, J., Kaye, R. and Levitsky, L.C. (1968). A familial, plasma-associated defect of phagocytosis: a new cause of recurrent bacterial infections. *Lancet* **ii**, 60–3.

Moller-Rasmussen, J., Teisner, B., Jepsen, H.H. *et al.* (1988). Three cases of factor I deficiency: the effect of treatment with plasma. *Clin. Exp. Immunol.* **74**, 131–6.

Moore, H.D. (1919). Complement and opsonic functions in their relation to immunity: a study of the serum of guinea-pigs naturally deficient in complement. *J. Immunol.* **4**, 425–41.

Morgan, B.P., Campbell, A.K. and Compston, D.A.S. (1984). Terminal component of complement (C9) in cerebrospinal fluid of patients with multiple sclerosis. *Lancet* **ii**, 251–5.

Morgan, B.P., Vora, J.P., Bennett, A.J., Thomas, J.P. and Matthews, N. (1989). A case of hereditary combined deficiency of complement components C6 and C7 in man. *Clin. Exp. Immunol.* **75**, 396–401.

Nelson, U.R. and Muller-Eberhard, H.J. (1967). Deficiency of the fifth component of complement in mice with an inherited complement defect. *J. Exp. Med.* **125**, 1–16.

Nielsen, H.E. and Koch, C. (1987). Meningococcal disease in congenital absence of the fifth component of complement. *Scand. J. Infect. Dis.* **19**, 635–9.

Ochs, H.D., Wedgewood, R.J., Frank, M.M., Heller, S.R. and Hosea, S.W. (1983). The role of complement in the induction of antibody responses. *Clin. Exp. Immunol.* **53**, 208–16.

OLAC Manual, 2nd edn (1976). Compiled by C. Hetherington. OLAC, Bicester.

Ooi, Y.M. and Colten, H.R. (1979). Genetic defect in secretion of complement C5 in mice. *Nature* **282**, 207–8.

Orihara, T., Tsuchiya, K., Yamasaki, S. and Furuya, T. (1987). Selective C1q deficiency in a patient with systemic lupus erythematosis. *Br. J. Dermatol.* **117**, 247–54.

Orren, A., Potter, P.C., Cooper, R.C. and du Toit, E. (1987). Deficiency of the sixth component of complement and susceptibility to *N. meningitidis* infections: studies in ten families and five isolated cases. *Immunology* **62**, 249–53.

Pemberton, P.A., Harrison, R.A., Lachmann, P.J. and Carrell, R.W. (1989). The structural basis for neutrophil inactivation of C1 inhibitor. *Biochem. J.* **258**, 193–8.

Pepys, M.B. (1972). Role of complement in the induction of the allergic response. *Nature N. Biol.* **237**, 157–9.

Porteu, F., Fischer, A., Descamps-Latscha, B. and Halbwachs-Mecarelli, L. (1986). Defective complement receptors (CR1 and CR3) on erythrocytes and leukocytes of factor I (C3b-inactivator) deficient patients. *Clin. Exp. Immunol.* **66**, 463–71.

Reid, K.B.M. and Thompson, R.A. (1983). Characterization of a nonfunctional form of C1q found in patients with a genetically linked deficiency of C1q activity. *Mol. Immunol.* **20**, 1117–25.

Rittner, C., Meier, E.M., Stradmann, B. *et al.* (1984). Partial C4 deficiency in subacute sclerosing panencephalitis. *Immunogenetics* **20**, 407–15.

Roord, J.J., van Diemen-van Steenvoorde, R.A., Shuurman, H.-J. *et al.* (1989). Membranoproliferative glomerulonephritis in a patient with congenital deficiency of the third component of complement; effect of treatment with plasma. *Am. J. Kidney Dis.* **13**, 413–17.

Rosen, B.S., Cook, K.S., Yaglom, J. *et al.* (1989). Adipsin and complement factor D activity: an immune-related defect in obesity. *Science* **244**, 1483–7.

Rosen, F.S., Alper, C.A , Pensky, J., Klemperer, M.R. and Donaldson, V.H. (1971). Genetically determined heterogeneity of the C1 esterase inhibitor in patients with hereditary angioneurotic edema. *J. Clin. Invest.* **50**, 2143–9.

Rosen, M.S., Lorber, B. and Myers, A.R. (1988). Chronic meningococcal meningitis: an association with C5 deficiency. *Arch. Intern. Med.* **148**, 1441–2.

Rosenberg, L.T. and Tachibana, D.K. (1962). Activity of mouse complement. *J. Immunol.* **89**, 861–7.

Rosenberg, L.T. and Tachibana, D.K. (1986). Hereditary deficiencies in animals: mice deficient in C5. *Prog. Allergy* **39**, 169–91.

Rother, K. and Rother, U. (eds.) (1986). Hereditary and acquired complement deficiencies in animals and man. *Prog. Allergy* **39** (whole volume).

Rother, U. (1986). Component deficiencies. 6. The sixth component. *Prog. Allergy* **39**, 283–8.

Rother, U. and Rother, K. (1961). Uber einen angeborenen Komplement-Defekt bei Kaninchen. *Z. Immun. Forsch. Exp. Ther.* **121**, 224.

Rudduck, C., Beckman, L., Franzen, G., Jacobsson, L. and Lindstrom, L. (1985). Complement factor C4 in schizophrenia. *Hum. Hered.* **35**, 223–6.

Ruddy, S. (1986). Component deficiencies. 3. The second component. *Prog. Allergy* **39**, 250–6.

Schlesinger, M., Nave, Z., Levy, Y., Slater, P.E. and Fishelson, Z. (1990). Prevalence of hereditary properdin, C7 and C8 deficiencies in patients with meningococcal infections. *Clin. Exp. Immunol.* **81**, 423–7.

Soothill, J.F. and Harvey, B.A.M. (1976). Defective opsonisation: a common immunity deficiency. *Arch. Dis. Child.* **51**, 91–9.

Spaulding, W.B. (1960). Methyltestosterone therapy for hereditary episodic edema (hereditary angioneurotic edema). *Ann. Intern. Med.* **53**, 739–45.

Strang, C.J., Cholin, S., Spragg, J. *et al.* (1988). Angioedema induced by a peptide derived from complement component C2. *J. Exp. Med.* **168**, 1685–98.

Sumiya, M., Super, M., Tabona, P. *et al.* (1991). Molecular basis of opsonic defect in immunodeficient children. *Lancet* **337**, 1569–70.

Super, M., Lu, J., Thiel, S., Levinsky, R.J. and Turner, M.W. (1989). Association of low levels of mannan-binding protein with a common defect of opsonisation. *Lancet* **ii**, 1236–9.

Takata, Y., Moriyama, T., Fukumori, Y., Yoden, A., Shima, M. and Inai, S. (1989). A biotin–avidin sandwich ELISA for quantification of intact complement component C9: the sera from hereditary C9 deficient individuals completely lack C9. *J. Immunol. Methods* **117**, 107–13.

Tedesco, F. (1986). Complement deficiencies. 8. The eighth component. *Prog. Allergy* **39**, 295–306.

Tedesco, F., Tovo, P.A., Tamaro, G., Basaglia, M., Perticarari, S. and Villa, M.A. (1985). Selective C3 deficiency due to C3 nephritic factor in an apparently healthy girl *Ric. Clin. Lab.* **15**, 323–9.

Telen, M.J. and Green, A.M. (1989). The Inab phenotype: characterization of the membrane protein and complement regulatory defect. *Blood* **74**, 437–41.

Walport, M.J., Ng, Y.C. and Lachmann, P.J. (1987). Erythrocytes transfused into patients with SLE and haemolytic anaemia lose complement receptor type 1 from their cell surface. *Clin. Exp. Immunol.* **69**, 501–7.

Welch, T.R., Beischel, L.S. and Choi, E.M. (1989). Molecular genetics of C4B deficiency in IgA nephropathy. *Hum. Immunol.* **26**, 353–63.

Wilson, J.G., Wong, W.W., Schur, P.H. and Fearon, D.T. (1982). Mode of inheritance of decreased C3b receptors on erythrocytes of patients with systemic lupus erythematosus. *N. Engl. J. Med.* **307**, 981–6.

Wilson, W.A., Perez, M.C. and Armatis, P.E. (1988). Partial C4A deficiency is associated with susceptibility to systemic lupus erythematosus in black Americans. *Arthritis Rheum.* **31**, 1171–5.

Wyatt, R.J. (1986). Deficiencies in regulator proteins. 3. Properdin. *Prog. Allergy* **39**, 339–43.

Zeitz, H.J., Lint, T.F., Gewurz, A. and Gewurz, H. (1986). Complement deficiencies. 7. The seventh component. *Prog. Allergy* **39**, 289–94.

Ziccardi, R.J. and Cooper, N.R. (1978). Modulation of the antigenicity of C1r and C1s by C1-inactivator. *J. Immunol.* **121**, 2148–52.

Zimran, A., Rudensky, B., Kramer, M.R. *et al.* (1987). Hereditary complement deficiency in survivors of meningococcal disease: high prevalence of C7/C8 deficiency in Sephardic (Moroccan) Jews. *Quart. J. Med.* **63**, 349–58.

68: Leucocyte Adhesion Molecule Deficiency and Chronic Granulomatous Disease

M.A. Arnaout and P.E. Newburger

Introduction

Over the past few years significant progress has been made in elucidating the molecular basis of leucocyte adhesion deficiency (LAD) and chronic granulomatous disease (CGD), two inherited disorders of leucocyte function. Classical genetics and reverse genetics were used respectively in understanding the pathogenesis of these two disorders. In this chapter we review the clinical and pathogenetic aspects of these two disease processes and the impact such an understanding had in identifying new treatment modalities and possible chemotherapeutic interventions in controlling phagocyte-mediated tissue injury.

Leucocyte adhesion deficiency

Leucocyte adhesion deficiency is a rare inherited disease characterized by recurrent and often fatal bacterial infections and presenting in the first 2 years of life (Dana and Arnaout 1988). Phagocytes from affected individuals have defects in adhesion-related functions such as chemotaxis, aggregation, phagocytosis, endothelial cell- and complement iC3b-binding and antibody-dependent cellular toxicity. Less severe defects in lymphocyte functions are also present. The disease results from partial or total lack in surface membrane expression of three leucocyte surface glycoprotein heterodimers which constitute an integrin receptor subfamily (β_2 integrins). In the majority of cases the disease is inherited on an autosomal recessive basis.

Historical perspective

In the late 1970s and early 1980s, several patients with severe and recurrent bacterial infections were described whose leucocytes displayed a constellation of defects spanning such diverse functions as binding to complement iC3b, phagocytosis, particle-induced superoxide generation, chemotaxis, homotypic cell adhesion, binding to endothelial cell monolayers and cell-mediated cytotoxicity (van der Meer *et al.* 1975; Weening *et al.* 1976; Gallin *et al.* 1978; Hayward *et al.* 1979; Crowley *et al.* 1980; Abramson *et al.* 1981; Bissenden *et al.* 1981; Arnaout *et al.* 1982; Bowen *et al.* 1982; Buchanan *et al.* 1982; Davies *et al.* 1982; Fischer *et al.* 1983). Between 1980 and 1982, three groups independently found that neutrophils from such patients are missing a protein of 110–180 kD (Crowley *et al.* 1980; Arnaout *et al.* 1982; Bowen *et al.* 1982) which is glycosylated and expressed on the cell surface (Arnaout *et al.* 1982). A year later, it was shown that this missing glycoprotein is identical to Mo1 (also known as CR3, OKM1, Mac-1) and that these patients are deficient in the alpha (155 kD) and beta (94 kD) subunits of this heterodimer (Dana *et al.* 1983, 1984; Arnaout *et al.* 1984). Similar findings were independently shown in another patient (Beatty *et al.* 1984). Mo1(Mac-1) antigen was defined a few years earlier (Springer *et al.* 1979; Breard *et al.* 1980; Todd *et al.* 1981), using monoclonal antibodies raised against whole monocytes or macrophages. An identical structure was also identified in guinea-pig macrophages (named GP160), based on its high sensitivity to proteolytic enzymes (Remold-O'Donnell 1980, Remold-O'Donnell and Savage, 1988). Work by several investigators also showed that the beta subunit of Mo1 is shared by lymphocyte function-associated antigen 1 (LFA-1) (also known as TA1) and p150,95 (also known as Leu-M5), two additional surface glycoprotein heterodimers with distinct alpha subunits of 180 kD and 150 kD respectively (LeBien and Kersey 1980; Davignon *et al.* 1981; Pierres *et al.* 1982; Trowbridge and Omary 1981; Sanchez-Madrid *et al.* 1983; Lanier *et al.* 1985). This family of leucocyte adhesion molecules is also referred to as the CD11/CD18 glycoprotein complex with the individual alpha subunits of LFA-1, Mo1 and p150,95 named CD11a, b and c respectively and the beta subunit named CD18. Subsequently many of the previously described patients with similar clinical and laboratory findings were found to have a complete or partial deficiency of leucocyte adhesion molecules (Anderson *et al.* 1984, 1985; Kobayashi *et al.* 1984; Thompson *et al.* 1984; Buescher *et al.* 1985; Fischer *et al.* 1985; Miedema *et al.* 1985; Fujita *et al.* 1986) and the disease is now commonly referred to as leucocyte adhesion deficiency (LAD), CR3 deficiency, β_2 integrin deficiency or CD11/CD18 deficiency.

Incidence

Leucocyte adhesion deficiency is a rare disease. Approximately 60 patients have so far been described world-wide. Despite its rarity, this experiment of nature established the biological role of cell adhesion in mediating such diverse and seemingly unrelated leucocyte functions as chemotaxis, phagocytosis and cell-mediated killing. It also opened the possibility for new chemotherapeutic agents which could control leucocyte-mediated tissue injury through inhibition of cell adhesion. Leucocyte adhesion deficiency is commonly seen in the paediatric age group and affects males and females equally (Dana and Arnaout 1988; Fischer *et al.* 1988). In the majority of cases, the mode of inheritance is autosomal recessive. The bulk of the patients described are Caucasians (with different ethnic backgrounds). Two Japanese patients have been reported (Fujita *et al.* 1986).

Clinical manifestations

The clinical manifestations of LAD are summarized in Table 68.1. The most common presentation is recurrent and often life-threatening pyogenic infections of the skin, mucous membranes or deep tissues, similar to what is often observed in patients with neutropenias. Recurrent otitis media, severe gingivitis, pharyngitis, stomatitis and perirectal abscesses are common. Deep-seated infections of the lungs, gastrointestinal tract or nervous system may progress despite aggressive therapy. Increased susceptibility to infections is directly related to the inability of granulocytes and monocytes from these patients to migrate to sites of tissue infection and to exhibit other normal functions essential to mount a host defence against pathogens. Infected areas (e.g. skin and gut) are thus often devoid of phagocytic cells, resulting in impaired clearance of bacteria and poor wound healing. Increased susceptibility to viral infections is unusual. The severity of the clinical disease is directly related to the degree of the deficiency (Anderson *et al.* 1985). Patients totally lacking in surface expression of CD11/CD18 often die at an early age with overwhelming sepsis. Patients with

Table 68.1. Clinical manifestations of leucocyte adhesion deficiency

Recurrent pyogenic infections
Persistent neutrophilia
Poor leucocyte mobilization
Impaired wound healing
Delayed umbilical cord separation

partial deficiency (10–20% of normal levels of CD11/CD18 expressed on the leucocyte surface) have a milder form of the disease and usually survive into adulthood. Heterozygous individuals are usually asymptomatic.

Laboratory findings and their structural basis

The diagnostic laboratory finding is the complete (0–2%) or partial (10–20%) absence of CD11/CD18 glycoproteins on the cell surface of circulating leucocytes. Another characteristic finding is persistent neutrophilia, which is invariably seen even during infection-free periods (Arnaout *et al.* 1982; Anderson *et al.* 1984, 1985; Kobayashi *et al.* 1984; Thompson *et al.* 1984; Buescher *et al.* 1985; Fischer *et al.* 1985). Serum immunoglobulins and complement levels are normal. Skin testing with antigens is normal as is delayed hypersensitivity (Dana and Arnaout 1988). Other laboratory findings are summarized in Table 68.2. These findings reveal the profound defects in adhesion-related leucocyte functions. Adhesion-independent functions such as superoxide generation and degranulation in response to soluble stimuli are normal. In one family, a defect in actin polymerization has been shown (Boxer *et al.* 1974; Southwick *et al.* 1989). This defect is not present in 11 other patients with complete or partial deficiency, suggesting the presence of a unique mutation affecting cytoskeletal assembly or the coexistence of two unrelated defects in this family. The variable degree (0–20%) of cell surface expression of CD11/CD18 in different patients (a reflection of the heterogeneous mutations affecting the CD18 gene (see below)) may explain the somewhat variable leucocyte functions described in various reports. Quantification of CD11/CD18 expressed on the leucocyte surface has been useful in prenatal diagnosis (Weisman *et al.* 1985).

Table 68.2. Leucocyte defects in leucocyte adhesion deficiency and their structural basis

Impaired function	Deficient heterodimer
Myeloid series	
Binding to iC3b	CD11b,c/CD18
Aggregation	CD11a,b/CD18
Phagocytosis	CD11b/CD18
Particle-induced oxidative burst and degranulation	CD11b/CD18
Spreading/random migration/ chemotaxis	Cd11a–c/CD18
Adhesion to endothelium	CD11a–c/CD18
ADCC	CD11a
Persistent leucocytosis	CD11a–c/CD18
Lymphoid series	
Antigen-, mitogen- or alloantigen-induced proliferation	CD11a
NK, K and CTL	CD11a–c/CD18
T and B cell aggregation	CD11a/CD18
Baseline adhesion to endothelium	CD11a/CD18
Helper activity for *in vitro* immunoglobulin production	CD11a/CD18

ADCC = antibody-dependent cell-mediated cytotoxicity; NK = natural killer; K = killer; CTL = cytotoxic T lymphocyte.

The various inherited defects in leucocyte functions observed in these patients can be reproduced *in vitro* and *in vivo* using monoclonal antibodies directed against the various subunits of CD11/CD18 (Arnaout *et al.* 1983, 1984, 1985; Beatty *et al.* 1984; Dana *et al.* 1984; Buescher *et al.* 1985; Fischer *et al.* 1985; Miedema *et al.* 1985; Anderson *et al.* 1986; Dana and Arnaout 1988; Timonin *et al.* 1988). Through this approach, the contributions of each subunit to various aspects of leucocyte adhesion were defined (Table 68.2). *In vivo*, monoclonal antibodies directed against CD11b/CD18 blocked neutrophil migration into many organs, including skin, myocardium, gastrointestinal tract and liver (Arfors *et al.* 1987; Hernandez *et al.* 1987; Ismail *et al.* 1987; Price *et al.* 1987; Simpson *et al.* 1988; Vedder *et al.* 1988), suggesting that one reason for increased susceptibility to infections results from impaired phagocyte emigration into infected tissues.

Defects in B and T lymphocyte functions such as antigen-, mitogen- or alloantigen-induced proliferation, natural killing, antibody-dependent killing and T-cell-dependent antibody production are usually demonstrable in these patients *in vitro* (Arnaout *et al.* 1984; Fischer *et al.* 1985; Ross *et al.* 1985; Weisman *et al.* 1985; Kohl *et al.* 1986; Mentzer *et al.* 1986; Miedema *et al.* 1986). These defects are more profound at low concentrations of the stimulus or during primary stimulation (Arnaout *et al.* 1984; Mentzer *et al.* 1986; Brown *et al.* 1988). At higher concentrations of the stimulus or during secondary stimulation, many of these functions become normal, especially in patients with the partial deficiency. In natural killer (NK) cells which express all three antigens, anti-CD11/CD18 monoclonal antibodies produce partial inhibition of effector–target cell binding and cytotoxicity (Timonin *et al.* 1988). These data suggest that alternative mechanisms are utilized by deficient lymphocytes (for example, use of other cell adhesion pathways) that compensate for deficiency of CD11/CD18 antigens. This may explain the variable response seen in NK activity (Arnaout *et al.* 1984; Ross *et al.* 1985) and the lack of unusual susceptibility to viral infections.

Each member of the CD11/CD18 family mediates specific and/or overlapping adhesion-promoting functions of leucocytes (Table 68.2). These functions are affected through interaction of each member with several ligands, some of which have been identified. CD11a/CD18 binds to at least two different ligands, named intercellular adhesion molecules (ICAM-1 and ICAM-2) (Dustin *et al.* 1986; Patarroyo *et al.* 1987; Simmons *et al.* 1988; Staunton *et al.* 1989). These two ligands are members of the immunoglobulin supergene family. Both CD11b/CD18 and CD11c/CD18 bind to a complement C3 fragment named iC3b (Beller *et al.* 1982; Arnaout *et al.* 1983; Wright *et al.* 1983). In activated cells, CD11b/CD18 also binds to coagulation factor X and to fibrinogen (Altieri and Edgington 1988; Altieri *et al.* 1988; Wright *et al.* 1988). All three glycoprotein heterodimers may bind to lipopolysaccharides (Wright and Jong 1986). In B and T lymphocytes, all CD11/CD18-dependent functions are mediated by CD11a/CD18 since this is the only heterodimer normally expressed on these cells. On the other hand, granulocytes, monocytes and NK cells express all three heterodimers, accounting for the wider range of CD11/CD18-dependent functions mediated by these cells. All functions mediated by CD11/CD18 are dependent on divalent cations. Metal chelators such as ethylenediamine tetra-acetic acid (EDTA) abolish CD11/CD18 adhesion functions in leucocytes.

Using subunit-specific monoclonal antibodies, it was further shown that selective domains within the alpha subunits mediate distinct functions. Certain monoclonal antibodies directed against CD11b, for example, only inhibit binding to iC3b-coated surfaces, while others inhibit neutrophil aggregation and binding to endothelium without affecting binding to iC3b (Dana *et al.* 1986; Arnaout *et al.* 1988a). The ability of anti-CD11/CD18 monoclonal antibodies to produce an acquired form of immune deficiency was exploited in controlling tissue injury mediated by neutrophils *in vivo*. Certain anti-CD11b antibodies significantly reduced the size of myocardial infarcts in dogs (Simpson *et al.* 1988). Other monoclonal antibodies directed against CD18-inhibited hepatic and intestinal ischaemia–reperfusion tissue injury (Hernandez *et al.* 1987; Vedder *et al.* 1988). Anti-CD11a antibodies were also found to reduce rejection in recipients of haplotype-matched bone marrows (Fischer *et al.* 1986).

Quantitative as well as qualitative changes in CD11/CD18 occur upon cell activation and may be required for enhanced adhesion mediated by these receptors. Resting granulocytes and monocytes both contain intracellular pools of CD11b/CD18 and CD11c/CD18 (located in secondary and tertiary secretory granules) (Arnaout *et al.* 1984; Lanier *et al.* 1985; O'Shea *et al.* 1985; Yancey *et al.* 1985; Bainton *et al.* 1987; Freyer *et al.* 1988; Singer *et al.* 1989). Activation of these cells by several inflammatory stimuli, both *in vitro* and *in vivo*, results in a rapid translocation of CD11b,c/CD18 receptors from these intracellular pools to the cell surface, leading to a 3–10-fold increase in surface expression of these two antigens (Dana and Arnaout 1988). This quantitative up-regulation is associated with increased ability of these cells to undergo homotypic or heterotypic cell adhesion. These findings led to the hypothesis that a quantitative increase in surface expression of these heterodimers is responsible for the enhanced adhesion observed in activated phagocytes (Arnaout *et al.* 1984; Todd *et al.* 1984; Anderson *et al.* 1986). Two additional observations support this hypothesis. Granulocytes from patients with inherited deficiency of specific granules (a major intracellular storage site for CD11b/CD18) are defective in their ability to undergo enhanced adhesion and chemotaxis in response to inflammatory stimuli (Gallin *et al.* 1982). Granulocytes from neonates are relatively deficient in specific granules and exhibit similar defects in enhanced cell adhesion upon activation (Anderson *et al.* 1987).

Evidence for qualitative changes in these receptors as a prerequisite for optimal functional activity has been more recently shown. Kinetic analysis of F-Met-Leu-Phe-induced neutrophil aggregation revealed that aggregation precedes a detectable increase in CD11b/CD18 on the cell surface and is reversed despite persistent up-regulation of this antigen (Buyon *et al.* 1988). Stimulated adhesion of granulocytes to endothelial cell monolayers was unaffected by the presence of inhibitors of degranulation (and therefore of increased CD11b/CD18 surface expression), suggesting that no detectable quantitative rise in CD11b/CD18 surface expression is required for leucocyte–endothelial interactions (Vedder and Harlan 1988). Homotypic and heterotypic adhesion mediated by CD11a/CD18 on activated T or B lymphocytes occurs despite the lack of an intracellular pool for this receptor (Arnaout *et al.* 1984; Mentzer *et al.* 1985, 1986; Patarroyo *et al.* 1985).

Among the qualitative changes that occur in CD11/CD18 is phosphorylation. All three alpha subunits are intrinsically phosphorylated in isolated human mononuclear cells. Phorbol myristate acetate (PMA) rapidly induces phosphorylation of the CD18 subunit in leucocytes (within one-half minute) (Chatila *et al.* 1989). This CD18-induced phosphorylation correlates with the increased adhesion induced by PMA. The chemotactic peptide F-Met-Leu-Phe also produces a rapid and reversible phosphorylation of CD18 with kinetics similar to FMLP-induced homotypic adhesion (aggregation) in phagocytes (Chatila *et al.* 1989). Stimulus-induced phosphorylation may be a mechanism for enhancing CD11/CD18 functions through altering CD11/CD18–cytoskeleton or CD11/CD18–ligand interactions. Taken together these data show that CD11/CD18 functions are regulated quantitatively as well as qualitatively. The relative functional importance of these receptor modifications may vary depending on the specific adhesion receptor involved, the functions mediated (e.g. adherence vs. translocation across endothelium) and the availability of ligands.

Molecular cloning studies revealed that CD11/CD18 are members of a large gene family involved in cell–cell/cell–matrix adhesion (integrins) (Tamkun *et al.* 1986; Argraves *et al.* 1987a; Bogaert *et al.* 1987; Corbi *et al.* 1987, 1988a; Fitzgerald *et al.* 1987; Hemler *et al.* 1987; Kishimoto *et al.* 1987a; Law *et al.* 1987; Poncz *et al.* 1987; Suzuki *et al.* 1987; Arnaout *et al.* 1988b, c; Pytela 1988; Takada *et al.* 1988; Staunton *et al.* 1989). Three subfamilies of integrins have been described, each with a unique beta subunit (β_1, β_2 and β_3) that is shared by several distinct alpha subunits (Hynes 1987). The β_1 subfamily includes the fibronectin receptor and other very late activation (VLA) antigens; the β_2 subfamily consists of leucocyte CD11/CD18; and the β_3 subfamily includes platelet IIb/IIIa and the vitronectin receptor. The beta subunits of integrins are highly conserved (an overall homology of 40–48%) and contain a characteristic extracellular region which is rich in cysteines (20% of the residues are cysteines within a 256 amino acid stretch). These cysteines are arranged in four repeating units of 60–70 amino acids each (Fig. 68.1). The alpha subunits of integrins are also homologous to each other but to a lesser degree (18–35% overall homology) than the beta subunits.

The genes for all three alpha subunits of CD11/CD18 (β_2 integrins) are located on chromosome 16 and might have arisen through duplication of a primordial gene (Arnaout *et al.* 1988c; Corbi *et al.* 1988b). The common beta subunit is located on chromosome 21 (Corbi *et al.* 1988b). The large N-terminal extracellular region of the alpha subunits of CD11/CD18 contains several interesting features (Fig. 68.1). First, it contains seven homologous tandem repeats, each ~60 amino acids long, which could have arisen by a series of duplication events. These repeats are also conserved in the alpha subunits of other integrin subfamilies. (Arnaout *et al.* 1988b; Pytela 1988; Larson *et al.* 1989). In the CD11/CD18 subfamily, repeats 5–7 each contain the metal-binding consensus non-

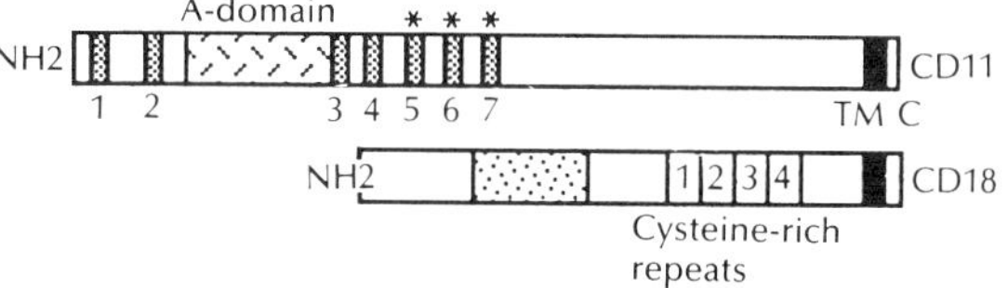

Fig. 68.1. Structure of CD11/CD18. Each heterodimer consists of a distinct alpha subunit (CD11) non-covalently associated with an identical beta subunit (CD18). The N-terminal portion of the alpha subunit contains seven repeats, three of which (*) contain a putative metal-binding site, each in the 'lock-washer' configuration. Inserted between the second and third repeats is a 200 amino acid peptide (A domain) with homology to the collagen/heparin/platelet GPIb binding A domains of von Willebrand's factor and of cartilage matrix protein, VLA-2 and complement factors B and C2. The dark areas are the membrane-spanning portions (TM). C represents the cytoplasmic portion. A striking feature of CD18 is a highly conserved cysteine-rich motif repeated four times. Another region in CD18 which is also conserved among the beta subunits of integrins is outlined (hatched box). This region as well as the cysteine-rich repeats appear to be essential for heterodimer assembly and surface membrane expression.

apeptide, DXXDXGXXD. The latter sequence is not immediately followed by the invariant glutamic acid at position 12 as is the case in other EF-loop structures. For metal-binding to occur, a non-contiguous glutamic acid residue is necessary to provide the sixth and seventh oxygen atoms for approximating the divalent cation. In the case of galactose-binding protein, a chemotactic receptor of bacteria, the required glutamic acid is provided by a non-contiguous segment of the protein, thus generating a 'lock-washer' configuration for the metal-binding site (Vyas *et al.* 1987). By analogy, in integrins, the glutamic acid residue could be provided by another segment in the alpha chain, in the beta chain or in the ligand recognized by these receptors. In integrins such a lock-washer structure may underlie the dependence of heterodimer formation and stabilization on the presence of divalent cations and may also promote a reversible interaction between these receptors and various ligands.

A second feature of CD11/CD18 is the presence of a large insertion, of ~200 amino acids (Fig. 68.1) in the extracellular region between the second and third homologous repeats which is not present in the fibronectin, vitronectin or platelet IIb/IIIa receptors. This additional domain (A domain) is homologous to a conserved domain repeated one or more times in several proteins involved in adhesive interactions, such as von Willebrand factor (Girma *et al.* 1987), cartilage matrix protein (a collagen-binding protein) (Argraves *et al.* 1987b), VLA-2 (platelet Ia/IIa, a collagen receptor) (M.E. Hemler 1989, pers. comm.) and complement proteins C2 and factor B (Shelton-Inoloes *et al.* 1986). In von Willebrand factor, three homologous repeats are involved in binding to collagen/heparin/platelet Ib (Girma *et al.* 1987). These data suggest that, in CD11/CD18, this domain may be involved in some of the cell–cell/cell–matrix adhesion-promoting functions.

A third feature which differentiates CD11/CD18 from other integrin subfamilies is the lack of a proteolytic cleavage site within the alpha subunits. This is due to a small deletion in the CD11 molecules in the region corresponding to the one containing the proteolytic cleavage sites in other integrins (Corbi *et al.* 1987; Arnaout *et al.* 1988b).

The short cytoplasmic regions of the alpha subunits are non-homologous. In CD11b, one serine residue serves as a potential phosphorylation site. Multiple threonines and/or serines are present in CD11c and CD11a respectively, which could account for phosphorylation of these subunits (Chatila *et al.* 1989). The single tyrosine residues present in the cytoplasmic region of CD11b,c are not phosphorylated by phorbol esters (Chatila *et al.* 1989). The cytoplasmic domain of CD18 contains tyrosine, serine and threonine residues that could serve as potential phosphorylation sites.

Molecular basis for leucocyte adhesion deficiency

The basic defect in LAD is abnormal synthesis of the common CD18 precursor. This leads to the failure to form αβ complexes, a step which is required for normal processing and membrane expression of these heterodimers (Marlin *et al.* 1986; Dana *et al.* 1987; Dimanche *et al.* 1987; Kishimoto *et al.* 1987b). Different sizes and quantities of CD18 protein precursor are detected in non-related patients (Table 68.3). Depending on the nature of the CD18 defect, none or small amounts of αβ complexes are processed and expressed on the cell surface, accounting for the observed phenotypes (Dana *et al.* 1987; Dimanche *et al.* 1987; Kishimoto *et al.* 1987b). Expression of other integrins is unaffected, reflecting the specificity of αβ interactions within integrin subfamilies.

Molecular cloning studies have revealed different mutations in the CD18 gene. In the first patient in which the diagnosis was made, two amino acid substitutions, presumably reflecting two mutant alleles, were observed in the extracellular region of CD18 (Arnaout *et al.* 1989). One substitution (a lysine-to-threonine change) occurs within a 248 amino acid domain which is highly conserved among integrins (overall homology of 50–60%) (Fig. 68.1). These data suggest that mutations within this region could impair αβ assembly and subsequent surface membrane expression. The other point mutation results in replacement of an arginine residue with a cysteine. This occurs in the fourth cysteine-rich repeat (Fig. 68.1). The replaced arginine is conserved in an identical site in all mammalian integrins, suggesting that mutations affecting this residue will impair expression of various members of this supergene family. In a second patient (Kishimoto *et al.* 1989), a mutation at a splice site results in deletion of 30 amino acids (one exon) from the coding region. It is interesting to note that this deletion also occurred

Table 68.3. Heterogeneity leucocyte adhesion deficiency

Cell phenotype	Disease phenotype	CD18 precursor	CD18 mRNA levels	Molecular defects
Partial deficiency	Moderate	nl size and quantity (10–15% of nl surface expression)	Normal (10–15% maturation)	Point-mutations
		Trace, nl size	Low	
		Trace, small size	Normal	Splice mutation
Complete deficiency	Severe	nl size and quantity	Normal	
		Large size, nl quantity	Normal	Aberrant additional glycosylation site
		Trace, multiple small-size forms	Normal	
		Absent	Normal	
		Absent	Absent	

Modified from Dana and Arnaout (1988) and Fischer *et al.* (1988).

within the highly conserved 248 amino acid domain, further supporting a role for this domain in heterodimer formation. Additional studies in other patients may be very helpful in further elucidation of the structure–function relationships of these adhesion receptors.

Prognosis and therapy

Complete LAD is invariably fatal, often within the first few years of life (Dana and Arnaout 1988; Fischer *et al.* 1988). Patients with the partial form of the disease have a milder course and may survive into adulthood with appropriate therapy. The mainstay of treatment is antibiotic therapy, both as prophylaxis and during infections. Two patients with partial deficiency followed for 8 years have done well with prophylactic antibiotics. Prolonged courses of treatment are often needed during established infections. Granulocyte transfusions may be used in some cases unresponsive to antibiotics, although their use is limited because of development of alloantibodies.

Bone marrow transplantation has been curative (Fischer *et al.* 1986) and is probably the best hope for patients with the complete deficiency. Successful bone marrow transplantation has been reported in two out of three patients with human leucocyte antigen (HLA)-matched transplants and three out of three mismatched transplants (Fischer *et al.* 1988). In all six patients, a stable chimerism was achieved, allowing adequate leucocyte adhesion functions. One patient subsequently died from graft vs. host disease and another died accidentally. The remaining four patients are still alive 1–6 years after bone marrow transplantation.

Since the basic defect involves only the common beta subunit, somatic gene therapy through introduction of the normal beta subunit gene into leucocyte precursors would seem to be a suitable curative approach. Recombinant retroviruses could be used to transfer the complementary deoxyribonucleic acid (cDNA) into haemopoietic stem cells. Despite difficulties in expression of cDNA in stem cells, a minimum of 5–10% expression may be sufficient to change the phenotype from the invariably fatal form of the disease to the milder form, which could then be managed clinically. Much remains to be done, however, before gene therapy could be used clinically for treatment of this and other genetic disorders (Williams and Orkin 1986).

Chronic granulomatous disease

Chronic granulomatous disease is an uncommon hereditary disorder, characterized by recurrent pyogenic infections which usually present early in life and may lead to death in childhood (Tauber *et al.* 1983; Forrest *et al.* 1988). Phagocytes from CGD patients display normal chemotaxis, ingestion and degranulation; but microbial killing is deficient, due to the failure of a membrane-associated nicotinamide adenine dinucleotide phosphate (NADPH) oxidase to produce superoxide and related toxic oxygen metabolites (Babior 1987). The disease is inherited in both X-linked and autosomal recessive forms (Mills and Quie 1983).

Historical perspective

Janeway and his colleagues provided the first, nearly inadvertent, description of CGD (Janeway *et al.* 1954). In the course of investigating hypogammaglobulinaemia, they noted a group of patients with increased infections, yet elevated serum immunoglobulins; several were later found to have CGD. Good's group provided the first definitive clinical recognition of the disease in 1957 (Berendes *et al.* 1957). They described four male children with recurrent pyogenic infections, hypergammaglobulinaemia and leucocytosis; all died in the first decade of life, leading the authors to name the syndrome 'fatal granulomatous disease of childhood'. In 1959, the Minnesota group demonstrated that CGD granulocytes ingested bacteria normally but failed to kill them (Quie *et al.* 1959). Biochemical studies shortly thereafter localized the defect to the respiratory burst pathway of oxygen metabolism (Baehner and Nathan 1967; Holmes *et al.* 1967), and later narrowed the basis of the disease to a deficiency of phagocyte superoxide generation (Curnutte *et al.* 1974). The use of nitroblue tetrazolium (NBT) dye reduction for the diagnosis of CGD was developed in 1968 (Baehner and Nathan 1968) and remains the standard test to this date (see below). In 1975, an enzymatic defect in phagocyte NADPH oxidase activity was reported from two laboratories (Curnutte *et al.* 1975; Hohn and Lehrer 1975). The next major step in the molecular basis of CGD came from Segal's demonstration of the absence of a unique, low midpoint potential, cytochrome b from phagocytes of many patients with CGD (Segal *et al.* 1978). Further studies showed that, in this genetically heterogeneous disease, phagocytes lacked the cytochrome in virtually all kindreds with X-linked CGD and a subset of those with autosomal recessive disease (Segal *et al.* 1983). In a classic exercise in 'reverse genetics', Orkin's group cloned the gene responsible for the X-linked form of CGD (Royer-Pokora *et al.* 1986) on the basis of its chromosomal localization and transcript biology, rather than the traditional route starting from a known protein. The gene product turned out to be the heavy chain of the cytochrome b, which was found nearly simultaneously to be a heterodimer of 90 kD heavily glycosylated and 22 kD non-glycosylated subunits (Dinauer *et al.* 1987; Teahan *et al.* 1987). The Orkin and Jesaitis laboratories soon cloned and characterized the cytochrome b light (22 kD) chain gene (Parkos *et al.* 1988) as well. Most recently, autosomal recessive CGD with normal cytochrome b has been shown to derive from defects in cytosolic proteins necessary for *in vitro* activation of the NADPH oxidase (Curnutte 1985; McPhail *et al.* 1985). Two forms of this subset of CGD complement each other in the *in vitro* assay (Nunoi *et al.* 1988; Curnutte *et al.* 1989) and appear related to the absence of either a 47- or a 67-kD cytosolic protein (Nunoi *et al.* 1988; Volpp *et al.* 1988).

Incidence

Over 400 cases of CGD have been reported (Forrest *et al.* 1988) and the incidence estimated at approximately 1 in 1 000 000 persons (Gallin *et al.* 1983). Thus, this 'most common' phagocytic disorder is a very rare disease. However, CGD constitutes one of the best examples of the principle that inherited diseases represent experiments of nature that lead to profound insights into normal processes. In fact, as discussed above, the disease provided the basis for the first 'reverse genetic' approach to the cloning of a gene without prior identification of its protein product. Male predominance, with reported ratios of 6 : 1 to 3 : 1 (Forrest *et al.* 1988), reflects the mixed X-linked and autosomal recessive inheritance patterns in CGD. More recent reviews have tended to report lower male : female ratios, perhaps reflecting increased awareness of autosomal disease.

Clinical manifestations

The chronic and recurrent pyogenic infections characteristic of CGD usually present in the first years of life, but may not become evident until adulthood, particularly in milder cases. Because clinical suspicion of CGD usually rests upon recurrence or chronicity of infection, the diagnosis usually follows the presentation by months or years. Exceptions to this rule include patients with infections by unusual pathogens (see below) or with known family histories of the disease. A recent review combined the published literature with the clinical experiences of the Children's

Table 68.4. Sites of infection in 441 cases of chronic granulomatous disease

Infection	Patient number	%
Pneumonitis	331	75
Dermatitis	297	67
Lymphadenitis	263	60
Hepatic/perihepatic abscess	171	39
Osteomyelitis	135	31
Persistent diarrhoea	82	19
Septicaemia/meningitis	74	17
Conjunctivitis	70	16
Perianal abscess	64	15
Stomatitis	64	15

Each patient number represents the occurrence of that finding in a single patient on at least one occasion. Adapted from Forrest *et al.* (1988).

Hospital of Philadelphia, University of California at Los Angeles (UCLA) Medical Center and University of Michigan's Mott Children's Hospital (Forrest *et al.* 1988). In the group of 19 patients from the three institutions, the mean age at diagnosis was 3.6 years, with 10 diagnosed in the first year of life, including one prenatal and two neonatal diagnoses. The sites of infection and their relative frequencies in the entire group of 441 patients reviewed are shown in Table 68.4. Infections of the lung, skin and lymph nodes predominate. Pneumonitis may appear patchy, lobar or nodular (with or without cavitation). Scarring is frequent and often leads to chronic lung disease in older patients. Overwhelming acute pneumonia or pneumonitis in the setting of chronic lung disease are frequent causes of death in CGD patients. Manifestations of dermatitis include both acute pyoderma or subcutaneous abscesses and chronic rashes that may appear eczematous in infants and acneiform in older patients. Suppurative, often draining, lymphadenitis is common, as indicated, and chronic reactive lymphadenopathy nearly universal. Hepatic and other intra-abdominal abscesses are less common, but occur so infrequently in patients with intact host defence that any such infection should raise the suspicion of CGD.

As the name of the disease implies, granuloma formation is common and chronic. Reactive granulomata containing plasma cells, lymphocytes, macrophages and occasionally multinucleated giant cells can occur in any organ (Tauber *et al.* 1983). Pigmented lipid histiocytes (Landing and Shirkey 1957) are frequently present, but may be rare. These large macrophages, containing finely granular yellow or brown pigment in a foamy cytoplasm, are highly characteristic of CGD but may also occur in lymph nodes draining necrotizing malignant tumours (Hotchi *et al.* 1980). The pigment appears to be a complex mixture of fatty acids, phospholipids and glycoproteins, probably representing degradation products of leucocytes (Hotchi *et al.* 1980; Tauber *et al.* 1983). The granulomata may produce severe obstructive lesions, particularly in the gastric antrum and urinary tract (Griscom *et al.* 1974; Forrest *et al.* 1988). Both small and large bowel may be affected by lesions indistinguishable from Crohn's disease or granulomatous colitis (Donowitz and Mandell 1983).

Aetiological agents of infection in CGD include a wide range of bacteria and fungi. Table 68.5 lists organisms identified in a study of 119 major febrile episodes (defined as requiring intravenous antibiotics) in 14 CGD patients followed for 150 patient-years at the US National Institutes of Health (Gallin *et al.* 1983). As in a major survey a decade earlier (Johnston and Baehner 1971), *Staphylococcus aureus* was the most common organism, but many of the others are microbes that rarely, if ever, infect the immunocompetent. Several, including *Chromobacterium violaceum* (Macher *et al.* 1982), *Pseudomonas cepacia* (Bottone *et al.* 1975) and non-nosocomial *Serratia marcescens*, are particularly indicators of CGD. Although *S. aureus* is consistently the most frequent isolate,

Table 68.5. Organisms causing infection in chronic granulomatous disease (in order of frequency of occurrence)

Staphylococcus aureus
Aspergillus species
Chromobacterium violaceum
Pseudomonas cepacia
Nocardia species
Salmonella typhimurium
Serratia marcescens
Mycobacterium fortuitum
Klebsiella species
Escherichia coli
Actinomyces species
Legionella bosmanii
Clostridium difficile
Streptococcus pneumoniae

Adapted from Gallin *et al.* (1983).

a review in 1975 (Lazarus and Neu 1975) noted that it accounted for only 9% of fatal infections, whereas Gram-negative bacilli caused 80% of infectious deaths in that series.

As expected for a phagocyte defect, there is no reported increase in frequency or severity of viral, protozoal or helminthic disease. *Pneumocystis carinii* pneumonia has been reported in only two patients with CGD (Tauber *et al.* 1983), but one had disease refractory to both trimethoprim/sulphamethoxazole and pentamidine.

The list of pathogenic organisms is also notable for the low frequency of infection by bacteria such as *Streptococcus* and *Haemophilus* species, which do not contain catalase. Granulocytes from CGD patients are capable of killing these organisms *in vitro* (Kaplan *et al.* 1968), and presumably *in vivo*, most probably by utilization of the peroxide produced and released by the microbes in the absence of endogenous catalase. Alternatively, these organisms may be highly susceptible to oxygen-independent killing mechanisms.

In addition to the patients with the classic clinical features of severe, recurrent infections beginning early in life, a heterogeneous group of 'variant' CGD patients have been described whose phagocytes possess markedly decreased but still detectable NADPH oxidase activity (Lew *et al.* 1981; Seger *et al.* 1983; Shurin *et al.* 1983). These individuals tend to present later (in the second or third decade of life) and to have less frequent or less severe infections; but severe infections may down-regulate their residual respiratory burst function (Newburger *et al.* 1986) and hence initiate a 'vicious circle' resulting in life-threatening or fatal illness. The clinical suspicion of CGD usually derives from the identification of an unusual pathogen.

Laboratory findings

Standard laboratory tests in CGD patients reveal only non-specific signs of acute inflammation during periods of infection. Leucocytosis, anaemia and elevation of the erythrocyte sedimentation rate usually resolve during infection-free intervals (Forrest *et al.* 1988). The erythrocyte sedimentation rate has proved to be the most reliable blood test for the detection of infection in these patients (Gallin *et al.* 1983). Signs of chronic inflammation, such as hypergammaglobulinaemia and anaemia with increased transferrin saturation, are less common now with modern antibiotic management than at the time of the original descriptions of CGD.

The first, and still standard, test for the diagnosis of CGD (Baehner and Nathan 1968) measures the superoxide-mediated reduction of NBT from a water-soluble yellow dye to insoluble blue formazan particles (Baehner *et al.* 1976). Activated CGD phagocytes fail to produce superoxide and hence do not reduce NBT. The test may be performed quantitatively (Baehner and Nathan 1968), by spectrophotometric measurement of formazan dissolved in an organic solvent, or histochemically (Gifford and Malawista 1970), by examination of cells adherent to glass slides or cover-slips (Fig. 68.2). The latter method is generally preferable, even though qualitative, because it permits determination of the distribution of cells capable of NBT reduction in CGD carriers or in patients with partial activity of the superoxide-generating oxidase.

Other methods for measurement of phagocyte oxidase activity include a spectrophotometric assay of superoxide dismutase-inhibitable cytochrome c reduction (Newburger *et al.* 1980), which is more specific for superoxide than the NBT test, and luminol-enhanced chemiluminescence (Trush *et al.* 1978), which is more sensitive.

Prenatal diagnosis of CGD is possible by application of these assays to fetal granulocytes obtained by fetoscopic or ultrasound-guided placental venepuncture (Newburger *et al.* 1979; Matthay *et al.* 1984). More recently, prenatal diagnosis has been performed by analysis of amniotic cell DNA for restriction fragment length polymorphisms linked to the X chromosome CGD locus (Lindlöf *et al.* 1987). However, the high rate of genetic recombination in the region of the CGD locus limits the accuracy of this method until probes are developed either within or more closely linked to the gene.

Patients with X-linked CGD should also be tested for determination of the red blood cell Kell phenotype. In several kindreds with X-linked CGD, the disease has been associated with the McLeod phenotype (Densen *et al.* 1981), a rare disorder in which red blood cells lack the Kell-related surface antigen Kx. The locus encoding Kx, termed Xk, is very closely linked to that for X-linked CGD, as demonstrated by several patients with both syndromes due to small interstitial de-

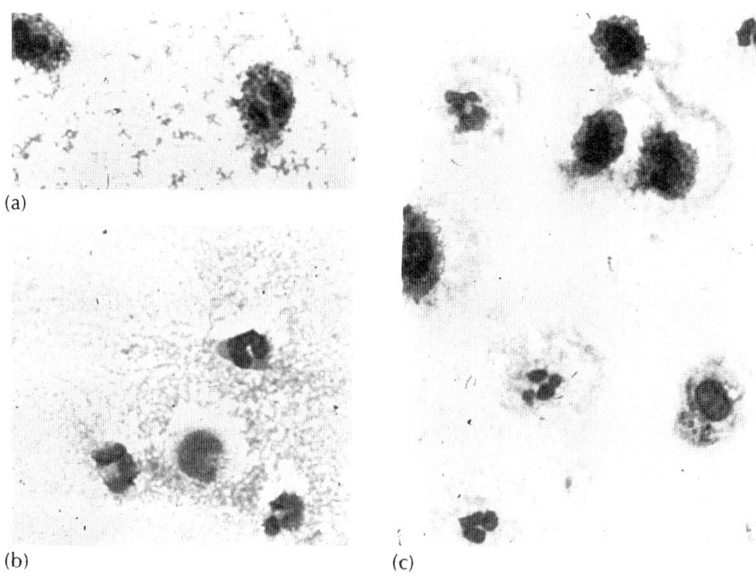

Fig. 68.2. Nitroblue tetrazolium slide test. Dark formazan deposits are evident in granulocytes and monocytes of a normal subject (panel a) but not in phagocytes from a CGD patient (panel b). Phagocytes from a carrier of X-linked CGD (panel c) show a distribution of normal and CGD phenotypes, in accordance with random X chromosome inactivation. Incubations of phorbol ester-stimulated phagocytes with nitroblue tetrazolium were performed as previously described (Newburger *et al*. 1979).

letions in the X chromosome (Francke *et al*. 1985; De Saint-Basile *et al*. 1988). Although the McLeod phenotype produces only a mild haemolytic disorder, the weak and unusual presentation of Kell antigens in the red cells presents a risk of sensitization to transfusions.

Molecular defects

Several recent commentaries (Dinauer and Orkin 1988; Ezekowitz and Newburger 1988) have reviewed the important and still evolving story of the molecular genetics of CGD.

The first major step was the identification and cloning of the gene mutated in X-linked CGD. The strategy of the 'reverse genetic' approach was based upon the fine mapping of the gene by a combination of deletion analysis and formal linkage studies. The X chromosome map position was first approximated on the basis of individuals with cytogenetically visible interstitial deletions in the region Xp21 and resulting combined syndromes of CGD, Duchenne muscular dystrophy, retinitis pigmentosa and McLeod phenotype in one patient (Francke *et al*. 1985) and of CGD and Duchenne muscular dystrophy in another (Baehner *et al*. 1986). The locus was then mapped to Xp21.1 by formal genetic linkage analysis of recombination frequencies between the CGD locus and a collection of cloned cDNA probes that recognize restriction fragment length polymorphisms in Xp21 (Baehner *et al*. 1986).

The assignment of the X-linked CGD gene to Xp21.1 confined the locus to approximately 0.1% of the human genome, within about 3000 kilobases of DNA. Transcripts relevant to phagocytic function were then isolated from cDNA prepared from HL-60 myeloid leukaemia cells (Collins *et al*. 1978) induced to differentiate *in vitro* and hence in the process of acquiring NADPH oxidase activity (Newburger *et al*. 1984). To enrich for transcripts relevant to the oxidase and derived from the Xp21 region, the cDNA underwent subtractive hybridization to an excess of messenger ribonucleic acid (mRNA) from an Epstein–Barr virus-transformed B cell line from the patient with CGD and Duchenne muscular dystrophy due to a deletion in Xp21 (Royer-Pokora *et al*. 1986). The subtracted pool of cDNA still contained an estimated 500 transcripts. Rather than analyse each for Xp21.1 localization, the entire pool was radiolabelled and used as a hybridization probe against a panel of genomic clones from Xp21. These clones represented only about 5–10% of the region, but fortuitously two overlapping clones hybridized with the subtracted pool and were shown to encode a transcript up-regulated in differentiating HL-60 cells and abnormal in expression or structure in phagocytes from patients with X-linked CGD (Royer-Pokora *et al*. 1986).

The protein predicted from the 'X-CGD' gene did not bear any significant sequence homology to any cytochromes or other polypeptides known at the time. However, soon thereafter two groups purified the phagocyte cytochrome b and reported its structure as a heterodimer of a 90-kD glycoprotein (termed the 'heavy chain') and a non-glycosylated 22-kD polypeptide ('light chain') (Parkos *et al.* 1987; Segal 1987). Antisera to synthetic and fusion peptides from the X-CGD gene reacted with the cytochrome b heavy chain (Dinauer *et al.* 1987) and the N-terminal amino acid sequence matched that predicted from the cDNA sequence (Teahan *et al.* 1987). These findings not only established the protein product mutated or missing in X-linked CGD, but also demonstrated the essential role of the cytochrome b in the phagocyte oxidase.

Using polyclonal antisera against the light chain to probe an expression library from induced HL-60 cells, cDNA encoding the 22-kD subunit was isolated and cloned (Parkos *et al.* 1988). Like the heavy chain, this polypeptide shares no sequence homology with known proteins. Phagocytes of patients with either X-linked or autosomal cytochrome b −ve CGD lack both protein components (Segal 1987; Parkos *et al.* 1989), even though only one subunit is genetically altered — the heavy chain in X-linked and the light chain in autosomal CGD (Royer-Pokora *et al.* 1986; M.C. Dinauer and S.H. Orkin, pers. comm.). This finding explains the lack of spectrophotometrically detectable cytochrome b in both X-linked and some autosomal recessive CGD phagocytes and further suggests that each subunit of the cytochrome is unstable in the monomeric form.

Most recently, autosomal recessive CGD with normal cytochrome b has been shown to derive from defects in cytosolic proteins necessary for *in vitro* activation of the NADPH oxidase (Nunoi *et al.* 1988; Volpp *et al.* 1988; Bolscher *et al.* 1989; Curnutte *et al.* 1989). Two forms of this subset of CGD complement each other in the *in vitro* assay and appear related to the absence of either a 47- or a 67-kD cytosolic protein.

On the basis of this current knowledge of the molecular pathology of CGD, a working classification of the disease has been proposed (Curnutte 1988). Table 68.6 presents an updated (J.T. Curnutte, pers. comm.) classification scheme. Type I CGD is the most common form, representing approximately 65% of cases (Curnutte 1988); inheritance is X-linked and phagocytes contain no cytochrome b. Type II represents about 30% of cases; this autosomal recessive, cytochrome b +ve form derives from abnormalities in the cytosolic 47-kD protein. Type V, which accounts for approximately 5% of cases, results from abnormality or absence of the other, 67-kD, cytosolic protein. The other categories are rare, each representing one to eight reported cases. Type III is autosomal recessive, cytochrome b −ve due to defects in the cytochrome b light chain gene. Type IV is X-linked, but cytochrome b +ve (that is, the protein is detectable immunogenically and spectrophotometrically); one case appears to be due to a point mutation in the heavy chain gene that renders the cytochrome b non-functional but stable (Dinauer *et al.* 1989).

Subcategories of IA, IIA, etc. (not shown) indicate the 'variant', less severe forms of each grouping. However, as the molecular basis of each category is elucidated, a spectrum of defects will probably emerge that will blur the distinction between 'classic' and 'variant' forms of CGD.

In addition, one CGD kindred with autosomal dominant inheritance has been reported (Gallin *et al.* 1983), but not included in the classification because of a lack of current information on their biochemical or molecular characterization.

Table 68.6. Classification and molecular characteristics of chronic granulomatous disease

		Cytochrome b					
		Protein		Gene		Cytosolic proteins	
Scripps 1 classification	Inheritance	91 kD	22 kD	91 kD	22 kD	47 kD	67 kD
I	X-linked	Absent	Absent	Abnormal	Normal	Normal	Normal
II	Autosomal recessive	Present	Present	Normal	Normal	Abnormal	Normal
III	Autosomal recessive	Absent	Absent	Normal	Abnormal	Normal	Normal
IV	X-linked	Present	Present	Abnormal	Present	Normal	Normal
V	Autosomal recessive	Present	Present	Present	Present	Normal	Abnormal

Prognosis and therapy

Since the first descriptions of the syndrome, the commonly used name has evolved from 'fatal granulomatous disease of childhood' to the current term 'chronic granulomatous disease'. This change in nomenclature reflects the impact of early recognition of the disease and aggressive antibiotic management on its clinical course.

A 1971 review (Johnston and Baehner 1971) reported 40% mortality in patients under 7 years of age. A more recent retrospective analysis (Forrest *et al*. 1988) found a 5% mortality. Both series were small; no large natural history study has been performed for CGD. It is still possible to conclude that the prognosis has improved in successive decades, but that fatal infections remain a risk. Previously undiagnosed patients may also present *in extremis*, in which case documentation of the disease is still essential for genetic counselling of the family.

Antibiotic therapy, both prophylactic and infection-related, remains the mainstay of treatment for CGD. Because CGD phagocytes ingest micro-organisms but do not kill them, antibiotics that achieve high intracellular levels are preferred and prolonged courses of treatment are necessary for established infections. Trimethoprim–sulphamethoxazole (TMP–SMZ) is particularly useful because of its broad spectrum of activity, low toxicity and demonstrated bactericidal function in CGD granulocytes (Johnston *et al*. 1975; Gmünder and Seger 1981). Rifampin may also be useful, in combination with other antibiotics (Ezer and Soothill 1974).

Although never subjected to a randomized trial, the use of prophylactic TMP–SMZ is generally accepted. In a review of 16 patients followed before and after institution of TMP–SMZ prophylaxis (Forrest *et al*. 1988), the incidence of infection decreased as did the number of microbial isolates, particularly of *Staphylococcus aureus*. In patients unable to tolerate TMP–SMZ, most clinicians substitute a beta-lactamase-resistant semi-synthetic penicillin such as dicloxacillin.

Prolonged use of antibiotics is appropriate not only for documented infection, but also for obstructive lesions due to granulomata in the gastrointestinal or urinary tracts (Forrest *et al*. 1988). These lesions may also respond to judicious use of corticosteroids (Chin *et al*. 1987), but these drugs need to be used with extreme caution because of the risk of increasing susceptibility to other, especially fungal, infections.

Incision and drainage of abscesses is generally necessary, but often leads to scarring due to poor wound healing. Surgical treatment of obstructive lesions should probably be considered only for emergency decompression or in case of failure of prolonged attempts at medical management.

Granulocyte transfusions have been used in some cases of infection unresponsive to antibiotics, but the balance of efficacy and toxicity is uncertain (Johnston 1983). The limitations of number and persistence of transfused granulocytes ensures a very high ratio of ineffective CGD cells relative to the effective transfused leucocytes.

Recently, recombinant human interferon gamma (rhIFN-γ) has emerged as a promising potential treatment for infection or prophylactic drug in patients with CGD. The physiological functions of the cytokine include activation of macrophages and enhancement of granulocyte superoxide production (Nathan and Tsunawaki 1986). Studies of CGD phagocytes have demonstrated improved respiratory burst and bactericidal activity after rhIFN-γ treatment both *in vitro* (Ezekowitz *et al*. 1987) and *in vivo* (Ezekowitz *et al*. 1988; Sechler *et al*. 1988). Part of the action of the drug appears to be due to up-regulation of cytochrome b heavy chain gene expression (Newburger *et al*. 1988), but other mechanisms probably contribute as well. The effect occurs in phagocytes from both X-linked and autosomal recessive CGD patients, but to varying degrees and not in all patients in any one disease category. Although all patients whose phagocytes have responded to rhIFN-γ *in vitro* have also shown *in vivo* responses (usually greater in magnitude), the lack of an *in vitro* effect of rhIFN-γ does not necessarily predict the absence of *in vivo* activity. At least two patients have responded to rhIFN-γ *in vivo* despite no detectable enhancement of phagocyte function *in vitro* (Ezekowitz *et al*. 1988).

The only definitive, curative treatment for CGD is bone marrow transplantation. One patient showed sustained clinical improvement after partial engraftment of marrow from an unrelated, histocompatible donor (Westminster Hospital's bone-marrow transplant team 1977). Of three allogeneic transplants, all showed biochemical correction after engraftment, but only one has had continued clinical improvement, with mixed chimeric engraftment (Kamani *et al.* 1988). The other two resulted in graft rejection with return of the CGD phenotype at 3 months post-transplant (Goudemand *et al.* 1976) and in death from graft-versus-host disease and infection at day 112 post-transplant (Rappeport *et al.* 1982). Bone marrow transplantation is not advisable in most cases in view of the improving prognosis for CGD with medical management and the present morbidity and mortality of the procedure. Furthermore, transplantation presents the highest risk to older patients with chronic infection and tissue damage; yet younger, uninfected patients are clearly better off with conventional therapy.

With the cloning of the genes for CGD, treatment with somatic gene therapy has become a topic for hopeful discussion. However, the practical application of recombinant DNA technology to clinical uses will require much further research before it can be considered for patient treatment (Williams and Orkin 1986).

Acknowledgements

We thank Ms Lisa Firicano for assistance in preparing this manuscript. This work was supported by National Institute of Health grants, Established Investigatorship grants and a March of Dimes grant.

References

Abramson, J.S., Mills, E.L., Sawyer, M.K., Regelmann, W.R., Nelson, J.D. and Quie P.G. (1981). Recurrent infections and delayed separation of the umbilical cord in an infant with abnormal phagocytic cell locomotion and oxidative response during partial phagocytosis. *J. Pediatr.* **99**, 887–94.

Altieri, D.C. and Edgington, T.S. (1988). The saturable high affinity association of factor X to ADP stimulated monocytes defines a novel function of the MAC-1 receptor. *J. Biol. Chem.* **263**, 7007–15.

Altieri, D.C., Bader, R., Mannucci, P.M. and Edgington, T.S. (1988). Oligospecificity of the cellular adhesion receptor MAC-1 encompasses an inducible recognition specificity for fibrinogen. *J. Cell Biol.* **107**, 1893–900.

Anderson, D.C., Schmalsteig, F.C., Arnaout, M.A. *et al.* (1984). Abnormalities in polymorphonuclear function associated with a heritable deficiency of a high molecular weight surface glycoprotein (GP 138): common relationship to diminished cell adherence. *J. Clin. Invest.* **74**, 536–51.

Anderson, D.C., Schmalsteig, F.C., Finegold, M.J. *et al.* (1985). The severe and moderate phenotypes of heritable Mac-1, LFA-1 deficiency: their quantitative definition and relation to leukocyte dysfunction and clinical features. *J. Infect. Dis.* **152**, 668–89.

Anderson, D.C., Miller, L.J., Schmalsteig, F.C., Rothlein, R. and Springer, T.A. (1986). Contributions of the Mac-1 glycoprotein family to adherence-dependent granulocyte functions: structure–function assessments employing subunit-specific monoclonal antibodies. *J. Immunol.* **137**, 15–27.

Anderson, D.C., Becker-Freeman, K.L., Heerdt, B., Hughes, B.J., Jack, R.M. and Smith, C.W. (1987). Abnormal stimulated adherence of neonatal granulocytes: impaired induction of surface Mac-1 by chemotactic factors or secretagogues. *Blood* **70**, 740–50.

Arfors, K.-E., Lundberg, C., Lindbom, L., Lundberg, K., Beatty, P.G. and Harlan, J.M. (1987). A monoclonal antibody to the membrane glycoprotein complex CD18 inhibits polymorphonuclear leukocyte accumulation and plasma leakage *in vivo*. *Blood* **69**, 338–40.

Argraves, W.S., Suzuki, S., Arai, H., Thompson, K., Pierschbacher, M.D. and Ruoslahti, E. (1987a). Amino acid sequence of the human fibronectin receptor. *J. Cell Biol.* **105**, 1183–90.

Argraves, W.S., Deak, F., Sparks, K.J., Kiss, I. and Goetinck, P.F. (1987b). Structural features of cartilage matrix protein deduced from cDNA. *Proc. Nat. Acad. Sci. (USA)* **84**, 464–8.

Arnaout, M.A., Pitt, J., Cohen, H.J., Melamed, J., Rosen, F.S. and Colten, H.R. (1982). Deficiency of a granulocyte-membrane glycoprotein (gp 150) in a boy with recurrent bacterial infections. *N. Engl. J Med.* **306**, 693–9.

Arnaout, M.A., Todd, R.F., III, Dana, N., Melamed, J., Schlossman, S.F. and Colten, H.R. (1983). Inhibition of phagocytosis of complement C3- or immunoglobulin-G-coated particles and of C3bi binding by monoclonal antibodies to a monocyte–granulocyte membrane glycoprotein (Mo1). *J. Clin. Invest.* **72**, 171–9.

Arnaout, M.A., Spits, H., Terhorst, C., Pitt, J. and Todd R.F., III (1984). Deficiency of a leukocyte surface glycoprotein (LFA-1) in two patients with Mo1 deficiency: effects of cell activation on Mo1/LFA-1 surface expression in normal and deficient leukocytes. *J. Clin. Invest.* **74**, 1291–300.

Arnaout, M.A., Hakim, R.M., Todd, R.F., III, Dana, N. and Colten, H.R. (1985). Increased expression of an adhesion-promoting surface glycoprotein in the granulocytopenia of hemodialysis. *N. Engl. J. Med.* **312**, 457–62.

Arnaout, M.A., Lanier, L.L. and Faller, D.V. (1988a). The relative contribution of the leukocyte molecules Mo1, LFA-1, p150,95 (LeuM5) in adhesion of granulocytes and monocytes to vascular endothelium is tissue- and stimulus-specific. *J. Cell. Physiol.* **137**, 305–9.

Arnaout, M.A., Remold-O'Donnell, E., Pierce, M.W., Harris, P., & Tenen, D.G. (1988b) Molecular cloning of the alpha subunit of human and guinea pig leukocyte adhesion glycoprotein Mo1: chromosomal localization and homology to the alpha subunits of integrins. *Proc. Nat. Acad. Sci. (USA)* **85**, 2776–80.

Arnaout, M.A., Gupta, S.K., Pierce, M.W. and Tenen, D.G. (1988c). Amino acid sequence of the alpha subunit of human leukocyte adhesion receptor Mo1 (complement receptor type 3). *J. Cell Biol.* **106**, 2153–8.

Arnaout, M.A., Dana, N., Simmons, D., Gupta, S.K., Tenen, D. and Fathallah, D. (1989). Two point mutations in the leukocyte CD18 gene in a patient with CD11/CD18 deficiency. *Fed. Proc.* **3**, A802.

Babior, B.M. (1987). The respiratory burst oxidase. *Trends*

Biochem. Sci. **12**, 241–5.

Baehner, R.L. and Nathan, D.G. (1967). Leukocyte oxidase: defective activity in chronic granulomatous disease. *Science* **155**, 835–6.

Baehner, R.L. and Nathan, D.G. (1968). Quantitative nitrobule tetrazolium test in chronic granulomatous disease. *N. Engl. J. Med.* **278**, 971–6.

Baehner, R.L., Boxer, L.A. and Davis, J. (1976). The biochemical basis of nitroblue tetrazolium reduction by normal human and chronic granulomatous disease polymorphonuclear leukocytes. *Blood* **48**, 309–13.

Baehner, R.L., Kunkel, L.M., Monaco, A.P. *et al.* (1986). DNA linkage analysis of X chromosome-linked chronic granulomatous disease. *Proc. Nat. Acad. Sci. (USA)* **83**, 3398–401.

Bainton, D.F., Miller, L.J., Kishimoto, T.K. and Springer, T.A. (1987). Leukocyte adhesion receptors are stored in peroxidase-negative granules of human neutrophils. *J. Exp. Med.* **166**, 1641–53.

Beatty, P.G., Harlan, J.M., Rosen, H. *et al.* (1984). Absence of monoclonal-antibody defined protein complex in a boy with abnormal leukocyte function. *Lancet* **i**, 535–7.

Beller, D.I., Springer, T.A. and Schreiber, R.D. (1982). Anti-Mac-1 selectively inhibits the mouse and human type three complement receptor. *J. Exp. Med.* **156**, 1000–9.

Berendes, H., Bridges, R.A. and Good, R.A. (1957). A fatal granulomatosus of childhood: the clinical study of a new syndrome. *Minnesota Med.* **40**, 309–12.

Bissenden, J.G., Haeney, M.R., Tarlow, M.J. and Thompson, R.A. (1981). Delayed separation of the umbilical cord, severe widespread infections and immunodeficiency. *Arch. Dis. Child.* **56**, 397–9.

Bogaert, T., Brown, N. and Wilcox, M. (1987). The *Drosophila* PS2 antigen is an invertebrate integrin that, like the fibronectin receptor, becomes localized to muscle attachments. *Cell* **61**, 929–40.

Bolscher, B.G.J.M., Van Zwieten, R., Kramer, I.M., Weening, R.S., Verhoeven, A.J. and Roos, D. (1989). A phosphoprotein of Mr 47 000, defective in autosomal chronic granulomatous disease, copurifies with one of two soluble components required for NADPH : O_2 oxidoreductase activity in human neutrophils. *J. Clin. Invest.* **83**, 757–63.

Bottone, E.J., Douglas, S.D., Rausen, A.R. and Keusch, G.T. (1975). Association of *Pseudomonas cepacia* with chronic granulomatous disease. *J. Clin. Microbiol.* **1**, 425–8.

Bowen, T.J., Ochs, H.D., Altman, L.C. *et al.* (1982). Severe recurrent bacterial infections associated with defective adherence and chemotaxis in two patients with neutrophils deficient in a cell-associated glycoprotein. *J. Pediatr.* **101**, 932–40.

Boxer, L.A., Hedley-Whyte, E.T. and Stossel, T.P. (1974). Neutrophil actin dysfunction and abnormal neutrophil behavior. *N. Engl. J. Med.* **291**, 1093–9.

Breard, J., Reinhertz, E.L., Kung, P.C., Goldstein, G. and Schlossman, S.F. (1980). A monoclonal antibody reactive with peripheral blood monocytes. *J. Immunol.* **124**, 1943–8.

Brown, E.J., Bohnsack, J.F. and Gresham, H.D. (1988). Mechanism of inhibition of immunoglobulin G-mediated phagocytosis by monoclonal antibodies that recognize the Mac-1 antigen. *J. Clin. Invest.* **81**, 365–75.

Buchanan, M.R., Crowley, C.A., Rosin, R.E., Gimbrone, M.A. and Babior, B.M. (1982). Studies on the interaction between gp-180-deficient neutrophils and vascular endothelium. *Blood* **60**, 160–5.

Buescher, E.S., Gaither, T., Nath, J. and Gallin, J.I. (1985). Abnormal adherence-related functions of neutrophils, monocytes and Epstein–Barr virus-transformed B cells in a patient with C3bi receptor deficiency. *Blood* **65**, 1382–90.

Buyon, J.P., Abramson, S.B., Philips, M.R. *et al.* (1988). Dissociation between increased surface expression of Gp165/95 and homotypic neutrophil aggregation. *J. Immunol.* **140**, 3156–60.

Chatila, T., Geha, R.S. and Arnaout, M.A. (1989). Phosphorylation of leukocyte adhesion molecules (CD11/CD18) in human monocytes. *Fed. Proc.* **3**, A963.

Chin, T.W., Stiehm, E.R., Falloon, J. and Gallin, J.I. (1987). Corticosteroids in the treatment of obstructive lesions of chronic granulomatous disease. *J. Pediatr.* **111**, 349–52.

Collins, S.J., Ruscetti, F.W., Gallagher, R.E. and Gallo, R.C. (1978). Terminal differentiation of human promyelocytic leukemia cells induced by dimethyl sulfoxide and other polar solvents. *Proc. Nat. Acad. Sci. (USA)* **75**, 2458–62.

Corbi, A.L., Miller, L.J., O'Connor, K., Larson, R.S. and Springer, T.A. (1987). cDNA cloning and complete primary structure of the subunit of a leukocyte adhesion glycoprotein, p150,95. *EMBO J.* **6**, 4023–8.

Corbi, A.L., Kishimoto, T.K., Miller, L.J. and Springer, T.A. (1988a). The human leukocyte adhesion glycoprotein Mac-1 (complement receptor type 3, CD11b) α subunit. *J. Biol. Chem.* **263**, 12403–11.

Corbi, A.L., Larson, R.S., Kishimoto, T.K., Springer, T.A. and Morton, C.C. (1988b). Chromosomal location of the genes encoding the leukocyte adhesion receptors LFA-1, Mac-1 and p150,95: identification of a gene cluster involved in cell adhesion. *J. Exp. Med.* **167**, 1597–607.

Crowley, C.A., Cunnette, J.T., Rosin, R.E. *et al.* (1980). An inherited abnormality of neutrophil adhesion: its genetic transmission and its association with a missing protein. *N. Engl. J. Med.* **302**, 1163–8.

Curnette, J.T. (1985). Activation of human neutrophil nicotinamide adenine dinucleotide phosphate, reduced oxidase by arachidonic acid in a cell-free system. *J. Clin. Invest.* **75**, 1740–3.

Curnutte, J.T. (1988). The classification of chronic granulomatous disease. *Hematol. Oncol. Clin. North Am.* **2**, 241–52.

Curnutte, J.T., Whitten, D.M. and Babior, B.M. (1974). Defective superoxide production by granulocytes from patients with chronic granulomatous disease. *N. Engl. J. Med.* **290**, 593–7.

Curnutte, J.T., Kipnes, R.S. and Babior, B.M. (1975). Defect in pyridine nucleotide dependent superoxide production by a particulate fraction from the granulocytes of patients with chronic granulomatous disease. *N. Engl. J. Med.* **293**, 628–32.

Curnutte, J.T., Scott, P.J. and Mayo, L.A. (1989). Cytosolic components of the respiratory burst oxidase: resolution of four components, two of which are missing in complementing types of chronic granulomatous disease. *Proc. Nat. Acad. Sci. (USA)* **86**, 825–9.

Dana, N. and Arnaout, M.A. (1988). Leukocyte adhesion molecular (CD11/CD18) deficiency. In *Baillière's Clinical Immunology and Allergy*, ed. M. Kazatchine, vol. II, pp. 453–76, W.B. Saunders, London.

Dana, N., Pitt, J., Todd, R.F., Melamed, J., Colten, H.R. and Arnaout, M.A. (1983). Deficiency of a monocyte–granulocyte surface glycoprotein (Mo1) in man. *Clin. Res.* **31**, 489.

Dana, N., Todd, R.F., III, Pitt, J., Springer, T.A. and Arnaout, M.A. (1984). Deficiency of a monocyte–granulocyte surface glycoprotein Mo1 in man. *J. Clin. Invest.* **73**, 153–9.

Dana, N., Styrt, B., Griffin, J.D., Todd, R.F., III, Klempner, M.S. and Arnaout, M.A. (1986). Two functional domains in the phagocyte membrane glycoprotein Mo1 identified with monoclonal antibodies. *J. Immunol.* **137**, 3259–63.

Dana, N., Clayton, L.K., Tenen, D.G. *et al.* (1987). Leukocytes from four patients with complete or partial Leu-CAM deficiency contain the common-subunit precursor and -subunit messenger RNA. *J. Clin. Invest.* **79**, 1010–15.

Davies, E.G., Isaacs, D. and Levinsky, R.J. (1982). Defective immune interferon production and natural killer activity associated with poor neutrophil mobility and delayed umbilical cord separation. *Clin. Exp. Immunol.* **50**, 454–60.

Davignon, D., Martz, E., Reynolds, T., Kurzinger, K. and Springer, T.A. (1981). Lymphocyte function-associated antigen-1 (LFA-1): a surface antigen distinct from Lyt-2,3 that participates in T lymphocyte-mediated killing. *Proc. Nat. Acad. Sci. (USA)* **78**, 4535–9.

Densen, P., Wilkinson-Kroovand, S., Mandell, G.L., Sullivan, G., Oyen R. and Marsh, W.L. (1981). Kx: its relationship to chronic granulomatous disease and genetic linkage with Xg. *Blood* **58**, 34–7.

De Saint-Basile, G., Bohler, M.C., Fischer, A. *et al.* (1988). Xp21 DNA micro-deletion in a patient with chronic granulomatous disease, retinitis pigmentosa, and McLeod phenotype. *Hum. Genet.* **80**, 85–9.

Dimanche, M.T., LeDeist, F., Fisher, A., Arnaout, M.A., Griscellis, C. and Lisowska-Grospierre, B. (1987). LFA-1 beta-chain synthesis and degradation in patients with leukocyte adhesive-proteins deficiency. *Eur. J. Immunol.* **17**, 417–20.

Dinauer, M.C. and Orkin, S.H. (1988). Molecular genetics of chronic granulomatous disease. *Immunodeficiency Rev.* **1**, 55–69.

Dinauer, M.C., Orkin, S.H., Brown, R., Jesaitis, A.J. and Parkos, C.A. (1987). The glycoprotein encoded by the X-linked chronic granulomatous disease locus is a component of the neutrophil cytochrome b complex. *Nature* **327**, 717–20.

Dinauer, M.C., Curnutte, J.T., Rosen, H. and Orkin, S.H. (1989). A missense mutation in the neutrophil cytochrome b heavy chain in cytochrome-positive X-linked chronic granulomatous disease. *J. Clin. Invest.* **84**, 2012–6.

Donowitz, G.R. and Mandell, G.L. (1983). Clinical presentation and unusual infections in chronic granulomatous disease. In *Chronic Granulomatous Disease*, ed J.I. Gallin and A.S. Fauci, pp. 55–75, Raven Press, New York.

Dustin, M.L., Rothlein, R., Bhan, A.K., Dinarello, C.A. and Springer, T.A. (1986). A natural adherence molecule (ICAM-1): induction by IL1 and interferon-gamma, tissue distribution, biochemistry and function. *J. Immunol.* **137**, 245–54.

Ezekowitz, R.A.B. and Newburger, P.E. (1988). New perspectives in chronic granulomatous disease. *J. Clin. Immunol.* **8**, 419–25.

Ezekowitz, R.A.B., Orkin, S.H. and Newburger, P.E. (1987). Recombinant interferon gamma augments phagocyte superoxide production and X-chronic granulomatous disease gene expression in X-linked variant chronic granulomatous disease. *J. Clin. Invest.* **80**, 1009–16.

Ezekowitz, R.A.B., Dinauer, M.C., Jaffe, H.S., Orkin, S.H. and Newburger, P.E. (1988). Partial correction of the phagocyte defect in patients with X-linked chronic granulomatous disease by subcutaneous interferon gamma. *N. Engl. J. Med.* **319**, 146–51.

Ezer, G. and Soothill, J.F. (1974). Intracellular bactericidal effects of rifampicin in both normal and chronic granulomatous disease polymorphs. *Arch. Dis. Child.* **49**, 463–6.

Fischer, A., Trung, P.H., Deschamps-Latscha, B. *et al.* (1983). Bone-marrow transplantation for inborn error of phagocytic cells associated with defective adherence, chemotaxis, and oxidative response during opsonized particle phagocytosis. *Lancet* **ii**, 473–6.

Fischer, A., Seger, R., Durandy, A. *et al.* (1985). Deficiency of the adhesion protein complex lymphocyte function antigen 1, complement receptor type 3, glycoprotein p150,95 in a girl with recurrent bacterial infections. *J. Clin. Invest.* **76**, 2385–92.

Fischer, A., Griscelli, C., Blanche, S. *et al.* (1986). Prevention of graft failure by anti-HLFA-1 monoclonal antibody in HLA-mismatched bone marrow transplantation. *Lancet* **ii**, 1058–61.

Fischer, A., Lisowska-Grospierre, B., Anderson, D.C. and Springer, T.A. (1988). Leukocyte adhesion deficiency: molecular basis and functional consequences. *Immunodeficiency Rev.* **1**, 39–54.

Fitzgerald, L.A., Steiner, B., Rall, S.C., Lo, S.S. and Philips, D.R. (1987). Protein sequence of endothelial glycoprotein IIIa derived from a cDNA clone. *J. Biol. Chem.* **262**, 3936–9.

Forrest, C.B., Forehand, J.R., Axtell, R.A., Roberts, R.L. and Johnston, R.B., Jr (1988). Clinical features and current management of chronic granulomatous disease. *Hematol. Oncol. Clin. North Am.* **2**, 253–66.

Francke, U., Ochs, H.D., DeMartinville, B. *et al.* (1985). Minor Xp21 chromosome deletion in a male associated with expression of Duchenne muscular dystrophy, chronic granulomatous disease, retinitis pigmentosa, and McLeod syndrome. *Am. J. Hum. Genet.* **37**, 250–67.

Freyer, D.R., Morganroth, M.L., Rogers, C.E., Arnaout, M.A. and Todd, R.F., III (1988). Regulation of surface glycoproteins CD11/CD18 (Mo1, LFA-1, p150,95) by human mononuclear phagocytes. *J. Clin. Immunol. Immunopathol.* **46**, 272–83.

Fujita, K., Kobayashi, K., Uchida, M. and Kajii, T. (1986). Neutrophil adhesion abnormality with deficient surface membrane proteins (gp110 and p98): the effect of their antibodies on the function of normal neutrophils. *Pediatr. Res.* **20**, 361–6.

Gallin, J.I., Malech, H.L., Wright, D.G., Whisnant, J.K. and Kirkpatrick, C.H. (1978). Recurrent severe infections in a child with abnormal leukocyte function: possible relationship to increased microtubule assembly. *Blood* **51**, 919–33.

Gallin, J.I., Fletcher, M.P., Seligman, B.E., Hoffstein, S., Cehrs, K. and Mounessa, N. (1982). Human neutrophil specific granule deficiency: a model to assess the role of neutrophil-specific granules in the evolution of the inflammatory response. *Blood* **59**, 1317–29.

Gallin, J.I., Buescher E.S., Seligmann, B.E., Nath, J., Gaither, T. and Katz, P. (1983). Recent advances in chronic granulomatous disease. *Ann. Intern. Med.* **99**, 657–74.

Gifford, R.H. and Malawista, S.E. (1970). A simple rapid micromethod of detecting chronic granulomatous disease of childhood. *J. Lab. Clin. Med.* **75**, 511–19.

Girma, J.-P., Myer, D., Verweij, C.L., Pannekock, H. and Sixma, J.J. (1987). Structure–function relationship of human von Willebrand factor. *Blood* **70**, 605–11.

Gmünder, F.K. and Seger, R.A. (1981). Chronic granulomatous disease: mode of action of sulfamethoxazole/trimethoprim. *Pediatr. Res.* **15**, 1533–7.

Goudemand, J., Anssens, R., Delmas-Marsalet, Y., Farriaux, J.P. and Fontaine, G. (1976). Attempt to treat a case of chronic familial granulomatous disease by allogeneic bone marrow transplantation. *Arch. Fr. Pediatr.* **33**, 121–9.

Griscom, N.T., Kirkpatrick, J.A., Jr, Girdany, B.R., Berdon, W.E., Grand, R.J. and Mackie, G.G. (1974). Gastric antral narrowing in chronic granulomatous disease of childhood. *Pediatrics* **54**, 456–60.

Hayward, A.R., Leonard, J., Wood, C.B.S., Harvey, B.A.M., Greenwood, M.C. and Soothill, J.F. (1979). Delayed separation of the umbilical cord, widespread infections and defective neutrophil mobility. *Lancet* **i**, 1099–101.

Hemler, M.E., Huang, C. and Schwarz, L. (1987). The VLA protein family: characterization of five distinct cell surface heterodimers each with a common 130,000 molecular weight beta subunit. *J. Biol. Chem.* **262**, 7660–5.

Hernandez, L.A., Grisham, M.B., Twohig, B., Arfors, K.E., Harlan, J.M. and Granger, D.N. (1987). Role of neutrophils in ischemia–reperfusion-induced microvascular injury. *Am. J. Physiol.* **253**, H699–703.

Hohn, D.C. and Lehrer, R.I. (1975). NADPH oxidase deficiency in X-linked chronic granulomatous disease. *J. Clin. Invest.* **55**, 707–13.

Holmes, B., Page, A.R. and Good, R.A. (1967). Studies of the metabolic activity of leukocytes from patients with a genetic abnormality of phagocyte function. *J. Clin. Invest.* **46**, 1422–32.

Hotchi, M., Fujiwara, M., Hata, S. and Nasu, T. (1980). Chronic granulomatous disease associated with peculiar *Aspergillus* lesions: patho-anatomical report based on two autopsy cases and a brief review of all autopsy cases reported in Japan. *Virchows Arch. (Pathol. Anat.)* **387**, 1–15.

Hynes, R.O. (1987). Integrins: a family of cell surface receptors. *Cell* **48**, 549–54.

Ismail, G., Morganroth, M.L., Todd, R.F., III and Boxer, L.A. (1987). Prevention of pulmonary injury in isolated perfused rat lungs by activated human neutrophils preincubated with anti-Mo1 monoclonal antibodies. *Blood* **69**, 1167–74.

Janeway, C.A., Craig, J., Davidson, M., Downey, W., Gitlin, D. and Sullivan, J.C. (1954). Hypergammaglobulinemia associated with severe recurrent and chronic nonspecific infection. *Am. J. Dis. Child.* **88**, 388–92.

Johnston, R.B., Jr (1983). Management of patients with chronic granulomatous disease. In *Chronic Granulomatous Disease*, ed. J.I. Gallin and A.S. Fauci, pp. 77–88, Raven Press, New York.

Johnston, R.B., Jr and Baehner, R.L. (1971). Chronic granulomatous disease: correlation between pathogenesis and clinical findings. *Pediatrics* **48**, 730–9.

Johnston, R.B., Jr, Wilfert, C.M., Buckley, R.H., Webb, L.S., Dechatelet, L.R. and McCall, C.E. (1975). Enhanced bactericidal activity of phagocytes from patients with chronic granulomatous disease in the presence of sulphisoxazole. *Lancet* **i**, 824–7.

Kamani, N., August, C.S., Campbell, D.E., Hassan, N.F. and Douglas, S.D. (1988). Marrow transplantation in chronic granulomatous disease: an update, with 6-year follow-up. *Pediatrics* **113**, 697–700.

Kaplan, E.L., Laxdal, T. and Quie, P.G. (1968). Studies of plymorphonuclear leukocytes from patients with chronic granulomatous disease of childhood: bactericidal capacity for streptococci. *Pediatrics* **41**, 591–9.

Kishimoto, T.K., O'Connor, K., Lee, A., Roberts, T.M. and Springer, T.A. (1987a). Cloning of the beta subunit of the leukocyte adhesion proteins: homology to an extracellular matrix receptor defines a novel supergene family. *Cell* **48**, 681–90.

Kishimoto, T.K., Hollander, N., Roberts, T.M., Anderson, D.C. and Springer, T.A. (1987b). Heterogeneous mutations in the beta subunit common to the LFA-1, Mac-1 and p150,95 glycoproteins cause leukocyte adhesion deficiency. *Cell* **50**, 193–202.

Kishimoto, T.K., O'Connor, K. and Springer, T.A. (1989). Leukocyte adhesion deficiency: aberrant splicing of a conserved integrin sequence causes a moderate deficiency phenotype. *J. Biol. Chem.* **264**, 3588–95.

Kobayashi, K., Fujita, K., Okino, F. and Kajii, T. (1984). An abnormality of neutrophil adhesion: autosomal recessive inheritance associated with missing neutrophil glycoproteins. *Pediatrics* **73**, 606–10.

Kohl, S., Loo, L.S., Schmalsteig, F.C. and Anderson, D.C. (1986). The genetic deficiency of leukocyte surface glycoprotein Mac-1, LFA-1, p150,95 in humans is associated with defective antibody-dependent cellular cytotoxicity *in vitro* and defective antibody-dependent cellular cytotoxicity *in vitro* and defective protection against herpes simplex virus infection *in vivo*. *J. Immunol.* **137**, 1688–94.

Landing, B.H. and Shirkey, H.S. (1957). A syndrome of recurrent infection and infiltration of the viscera by pigmented lipid histiocytes. *Pediatrics* **20**, 431–42.

Lanier, L.L., Arnaout, M.A., Schwarting, R., Warner, N.L. and Ross, G.D. (1985). p150,95, third member of the LFA-1/CR3 polypeptide family identified by anti-LeuM5 monoclonal antibody. *Eur. J. Immunol.* **15**, 713–18.

Larson, R.S., Corbi, A.L., Berman, L. and Springer, T.A. (1989). Primary structure of the leukocyte function-associated molecule-1 α subunit: an integrin with an embedded domain defining a protein superfamily. *J. Cell Biol.* **108**, 703–12.

Law, S.K.A., Gagnon, J., Hildreth, J.E.K., Wells, C.E., Willis, A.C. and Wong, A.J. (1987). The primary structure of the beta-subunit of the cell surface adhesion glycoproteins LFA-1, CR3 and p150,95 and its relationship to the fibronectin receptor. *EMBO J.* **6**, 915–19.

Lazarus, G.M. and Neu, H.C. (1975). Agents responsible for infection in chronic granulomatous disease of childhood. *Pediatrics* **86**, 415–17.

LeBien, T.W. and Kersey, J.H. (1980). A monoclonal antibody (TA-1) reactive with human lymphocytes and monocytes. *J. Immunol.* **125**, 2208–14.

Lew, P.D., Southwick, F.S., Stossel, T.P., Whitin, J.C., Simons, E.R. and Cohen, H.J. (1981). A variant of chronic granulomatous disease: deficient oxidative metabolism due to a low-affinity NADPH oxidase. *N. Engl. J. Med.* **305**, 1329–33.

Lindlöf, M., Kere, J., Ristola, M. *et al.* (1987). Prenatal diagnosis of X-linked chronic granulomatous disease using restriction fragment length polymorphism analysis. *Genomics* **1**, 87–92.

Macher, A.M., Casale, T.B. and Fauci, A.S. (1982). Chronic granulomatous disease of childhood and *Chromobacterium violaceum* infections in the southeastern United States. *Ann. Intern. Med.* **97**, 51–5.

McPhail, L.C., Shirley, P.S., Clayton, C.C. and Snyderman, R. (1985). Activation of the respiratory burst enzyme from human neutrophils in a cell-free system: evidence for a soluble cofactor. *J. Clin. Invest.* **75**, 1735–9.

Marlin, S.D., Morton, C.C., Anderson, D.C. and Springer, T.A. (1986). LFA-1 immunodeficiency disease: definition of the genetic defect and chromosomal mapping of the alpha and beta subunits of the lymphocyte function-associated antigen (LFA-1) by complementation in hybrid cells. *J. Exp. Med.* **164**, 855–67.

Matthay, K.K., Golbus, M.S., Wara, D.W. and Mentzer, W.C. (1984). Prenatal diagnosis of chronic granulomatous disease. *Am. J. Med. Genet.* **17**, 731–9.

Mentzer, S.J., Gromkowski, S.H., Krensky, A.M., Burakoff, S.J. and Martz, E. (1985). LFA-1 membrane molecule in the regulation of homotypic adhesion of human B lymphocytes. *J. Immunol.* **135**, 9–11.

Mentzer, S.J., Bierer, B.E., Anderson, D.C., Springer, T.A. and Burakoff, S.J. (1986). Abnormal cytolytic activity of lymphocyte function associated antigen 1 deficient human cytolytic T lymphocyte clones. *J. Clin. Invest.* **78**, 1387–91.

Miedema, F., Tetteroo, P.A.T., Terpstra, F.G. *et al.* (1985). Immunologic studies with LFA-1 and Mo1-deficient lymphocytes from a patient with recurrent bacterial infections. *J. Immunol.* **134**, 3075–81.

Miedema, F., Terpstra, F.G. and Melief, C.J.M. (1986). Functional studies with monoclonal antibodies against function-associated leukocyte antigens. In *Leukocyte Typing II*, vol. III, *Human Myeloid and Hematopoietic Cells*, ed. E.L. Reinherz, B.F. Haynes, L.M. Nadler and I.D. Bernstein, pp. 55–68, Springer-Verlag, New York.

Mills, E.L. and Quie, P.G. (1983). Inheritance of chronic granulomatous disease. In *Chronic Granulomatous Disease*, ed. J.I. Gallin and A.S. Fauci, pp. 25–53, Raven, Press, New York.

Nathan, C.F. and Tsunawaki, S. (1986). Secretion of toxic oxygen products by macrophages: regulatory cytokines and their effects on the oxidase. *Ciba Found. Symp.* **118**, 211–30.

Newburger, P.E., Cohen, H.J., Rothchild, S.E., Hobbins, J.C., Malawista, S.E. and Mahoney, M.J. (1979). The prenatal diagnosis of chronic granulomatous disease. *N. Engl. J. Med.* **300**, 178–81.

Newburger, P.E., Chovaniec, M.E. and Cohen, H.J. (1980). Activity and activation of the granulocyte superoxide generating system. *Blood* **55**, 85–92.

Newburger, P.E., Speier, C., Borregaard, N., Walsh, C.E., Whitin, J.C. and Simons, E.R. (1984). Development of the superoxide-generating system during differentiation of the HL-60 promyelocytic leukemia cell line. *J. Biol. Chem.* **259**, 3771–6.

Newburger, P.E., Luscinskas, F.W., Ryan, T. *et al.* (1986). Variant chronic granulomatous disease: modulation of the neutrophil defect by severe infection. *Blood* **68**, 914–19.

Newburger, P.E., Ezekowitz, R.A.B., Whitney, C., Wright J. and Orkin, S.H. (1988). Induction of phagocyte cytochrome b heavy chain gene expression by interferon gamma. *Proc. Nat. Acad. Sci. (USA)* **85**, 5215–19.

Nunoi, H., Rotrosen, D., Gallin, J.I. and Malech, H.L. (1988). Two forms of autosomal chronic granulomatous disease lack distinct neutrophil cytosol factors. *Science* **242**, 1298–301.

O'Shea, J.J., Brown, E.J., Seligmann, B.E., Metcalf, J.A., Frank, M.M. and Gallin, J.I. (1985). Evidence for distinct intracellular pools of receptors for C3b and C3bi in human neutrophils. *J. Immunol.* **134**, 2580–7.

Parkos, C.A., Allen, R.A., Cochrane, C.G. and Jesaitis, A.J. (1987). Purified cytochrome b from human granulocyte plasma membrane is comprised of two polypeptides of 91 000 and 22 000 relative molecular weights. *J. Clin. Invest.* **80**, 732–42.

Parkos, C.A., Dinauer, M.C., Walker, L.E., Allen, R.A., Jesaitis, A.J. and Orkin, S.H. (1988). The primary structure and unique expression of the 22 kilodalton light chain of human neutrophil cytochrome b. *Proc. Nat. Acad. Sci. (USA)* **85**, 3319–23.

Parkos, C.A., Dinauer, M.C., Jesaitis, A.J., Orkin, S.H. and Curnutte, J.T. (1989). Absence of both the 91K and 22K subunits of the human neutrophil cytochrome b in two genetic forms of chronic granulomatous disease. *Blood* **73**, 1416–20.

Patarroyo, M., Beatty, P.G., Fabre, J.W. and Gahmberg, C.G. (1985). Identification of a cell surface protein complex mediating phorbol ester-induced adhesion (binding) among mononuclear leukocytes. *Scand. J. Immunol.* **22**, 171–82.

Patarroyo, M., Clark, E.A., Prieto, J., Kantor, C. and Gahmberg, C.G. (1987). Identification of a novel adhesion molecule in human leukocytes by monoclonal antibody LB-2. *FEBS Lett.* **210**, 217–31.

Pierres, M., Goridis, C. and Golstein, P. (1982). Inhibition of murine T cell-mediated cytolysis and T cell proliferation by a rat monoclonal antibody immunoprecipitating two lymphoid cell surface polypeptides of 94 000 and 180 000 molecular weight. *Eur. J. Immunol.* **12**, 60–9.

Poncz, M.R., Eisman, R., Heidenreich, R. *et al.* (1987). Structure of the platelet glycoprotein IIb. *J. Biol. Chem.* **262**, 8476–82.

Price, T.H., Beatty, P.G. and Corpuz, S.R. (1987). *In vivo* inhibition of neutrophil function in rabbit using monoclonal antibody to CD18. *J. Immunol.* **139**, 4174–7.

Pytela, R. (1988). Amino acid sequence of the murein Mac-1 a chain reveals homology with the integrin family and an additional domain related to von Willebrand factor. *EMBO J.* **7**, 1371–8.

Quie, P.G., White, J.G., Holmes, B. and Good, R.A. (1959). *In vitro* bactericidal capacity of human polymorphonuclear leukocytes: diminished activity in chronic granulomatous disease of childhood. *J. Clin. Invest.* **46**, 668–79.

Rappeport, J.M., Newburger, P.E., Goldblum, R.M., Goldman, A.S., Nathan, D.G. and Parkman, R. (1982). Allogeneic bone marrow transplantation for chronic granulomatous disease. *Pediatrics* **101**, 952–5.

Remold-O'Donnell, E. (1980). A macrophage component gp160, a major trypsin-sensitive surface glycoprotein. *J. Exp. Med.* **152**, 1699–708.

Remold-O'Donnell, E. and Savage, B. (1988). Characterization of macrophage adhesion molecule (MAM). *Biochemistry* **27**, 39–41.

Ross, G.D., Thompson, R.A., Walport, M.J. *et al.* (1985). Characterization of patients with increased susceptibility to bacterial infections and genetic deficiency of leukocyte membrane complement receptor type 3 and the related membrane antigen LFA-1. *Blood* **66**, 882–90.

Royer-Pokora, B., Kunkel, L.M., Monaco, A.P. *et al.* (1986). Cloning the gene for an inherited disorder — chronic granulomatous disease — on the basis of its chromosomal location. *Nature* **322**, 32–8.

Sanchez-Madrid, F., Nagy, J.A., Robbins, E., Simon, P. and Springer, T.A. (1983). A human leukocyte differentiation antigen family with distinct alpha subunits and a common beta subunit: the lymphocyte function associated antigen (LFA-1), the C3bi complement receptor (OKM1/Mac-1), and the p150,95 molecule. *J. Exp. Med.* **158**, 1785–803.

Sechler, J.M.G., Malech, H.L., White, C.J. and Gallin, J.I. (1988). Recombinant human interferon-gamma reconstitutes defective phagocyte function in patients with chronic granulomatous disease of childhood. *Proc. Nat. Acad. Sci. (USA)* **85**, 4874–8.

Segal, A.W. (1987). Absence of both cytochrome b-245 subunits from neutrophils in X-linked chronic granulomatous disease. *Nature* **326**, 88–91.

Segal, A.W., Jones, O.T.G., Webster, D. and Allison, A.C. (1978). Absence of a newly described cytochrome b from neutrophils of patients with chronic granulomatous disease. *Lancet* **ii**, 446–9.

Segal, A.W., Cross, A.R., Garcia, R.C. *et al.* (1983). Absence of cytochrome b-245 in chronic granulomatous disease: a multicenter European evaluation of its incidence and relevance. *N. Engl. J. Med.* **308**, 245–51.

Seger, R.A., Tiefenauer, L., Matsunage, T., Wildfeuer, A. and Newburger, P.E. (1983). Chronic granulomatous disease due to granulocytes with abnormal NADPH oxidase activity and deficient cytochrome b. *Blood* **61**, 423–8.

Shelton-Inoloes, B.B., Titani, K. and Sadler, J.E. (1986). cDNA sequences for human von Willebrand factor reveal five types of repeated domains and five possible protein sequence polymorphisms. *Biochemistry* **25**, 3164–71.

Shurin, S.B., Cohen, H.J., Whitin, J.C. and Newburger, P.E. (1983). Impaired granulocyte superoxide production and prolongation of the respiratory burst due to a low-affinity NADPH-dependent oxidase. *Blood* **62**, 564–71.

Simmons, D., Makgoba, M.W. and Seed, B. (1988). ICAM, an adhesion ligand of LFA-1 is homologous to the neutral adhesion molecule NCAM. *Nature* **331**, 625–7.

Simpson, P.J., Todd, R.F., III, Fantone, J.C. *et al.* (1988). Reduction of experimental canine myocardial reperfusion injury by a monoclonal antibody (anti-Mo1, anti-CD11b) that inhibits leukocyte adhesion. *J. Clin. Invest.* **81**, 624–9.

Singer, I.I., Scott, S., Kawka, D.W., Kazazis, D.M. and Segui-Real, B. (1989). Laminin receptors are localized in the specific granules of human leukocytes. *J. Cell Biol.* **107**, 801a.

Southwick, F.S., Howard, T.H., Holbrook, T., Anderson, D.C., Stossel, T.P. and Arnaout, M.A. (1989). The relationship between CR3 deficiency and neutrophil actin dysfunction. *Blood* **73**, 1973–9.

Springer, T.A., Galtre, G., Secher, D.S. and Milstein, C. (1979). Mac-1: a macrophage differentiation antigen identified by monoclonal antibody. *Eur. J. Immunol.* **9**, 301–6.

Staunton, D.E., Dustin, M.L. and Springer, T.A. (1989). Molecular characterization of ICAM-1 and ICAM-2: alternate ligands for LFA-1. *Fed. Proc.* **3**, a446.

Suzuki, S., Argraves, W.S., Arai, H., Languino, L.R., Pierschbacher, M.D. and Ruoslahti, E. (1987). Amino acid sequence of the vitronectin receptor α subunit and comparative expressing of receptor mRNAs. *J. Biol. Chem.* **83**, 8614–18.

Takada, Y., Wayner, E.A., Carter, W.G. and Hemler, M.E. (1988). Extracellular matrix receptors, ECMR II and ECMR I, for collagen and fibronectin correspond to VLA-2 and VLA-3 in the VLA family of heterodimers. *J. Cell. Biochem.* **37**, 385–93.

Tamkun, J.W., DeSimone, D.W., Fonda, D. *et al.* (1986). Structure of integrin, a glycoprotein involved in the transmembrane linkage between fibronectin and actin. *Cell* **46**, 271–82.

Tauber, A.I., Borregaard, N., Simons, E.R. and Wright, J. (1983). Chronic granulomatous disease: a syndrome of phagocyte oxidase deficiencies. *Medicine* **62**, 286–309.

Teahan, C., Rowe, P., Parker, P., Totty, N. and Segal, A.W. (1987). The X-linked chronic granulomatous disease gene codes for the beta-chain of cytochrome b-245. *Nature* **237**, 720–1.

Thompson, R.A., Candy, D.C.A. and McNeish, A.S. (1984). Familial defect of polymorph neutrophil phagocytosis associated with absence of a surface glycoprotein (OKM1). *Clin. Exp. Immunol.* **58**, 229–36.

Timonin, T., Patarroyo, M. and Gahmberg, C.G. (1988). CD11a–c/D18 and GP84 (LB-2) adhesion molecules on large granular lymphocytes and their participation in natural killing. *J. Immunol.* **141**, 1041–6.

Todd, R.F., Nadler, L.M. and Schlossman, S.F. (1981). Antigens on human monocytes identified by monoclonal antibodies. *J. Immunol.* **126**, 1435–42.

Todd, R.F., III, Arnaout, M.A., Rosin, R.E. *et al.* (1984). Subcellular localization of the subunit of Mo1 (Mo1 alpha; formerly gp 110), a surface glycoprotein associated with neutrophil adhesion. *J. Clin. Invest.* **74**, 1280–90.

Trowbridge, I.S. and Omary, M.B. (1981). Molecular complexity of surface glycoproteins related to the macrophage differentiation antigen Mac-1. *J. Exp. Med.* **154**, 1517–24.

Trush, M.A., Wilson, M.E. and Van Dyke, K. (1978). The generation of chemiluminescence by phagocytic cells. *Methods Enzymol.* **57**, 462–75.

van der Meer, J., Zwet, T.L. and van Furth, R. (1975). New familial defect in microcidal function of polymorphonuclear leucocytes. *Lancet* **ii**, 630–2.

Vedder, N.B. and Harlan, J.M. (1988). Increased surface expression of CD11b/CD18 (Mac-1) is not required for stimulated neutrophil adherence to cultured endothelium. *J. Clin. Invest.* **81**, 676–82.

Vedder, N.B., Winn, R.K., Rice, C.L., Chi, E.Y., Arfors, K.E. and Harlan, J.M. (1988). A monoclonal antibody to the adherence-promoting leukocyte glycoprotein, CD18, reduces organ injury and improves survival from hemorrhagic shock and resuscitation in rabbits. *J. Clin. Invest.* **81**, 939–44.

Volpp, B.D., Nauseef, W.M. and Clark, R.A. (1988). Two cytosolic neutrophil oxidase components absent in autosomal chronic granulomatous disease. *Science* **242**, 1295–7.

Vyas, N.K., Vyas, M.N. and Quiocho, F.A. (1987). A novel calcium-binding site in galactose-binding protein of bacterial transport and chemotaxis. *Nature (London)* **327**, 635–8.

Weening, R.S., Roos, D., Weemaes, C.M.R., Homan-Muller, J.W.T. and van Schaik, M.L.J. (1976). Defective initiation of the metabolic stimulation in phagocytizing granulocytes: a new congenital defect. *J. Lab. Clin. Med.* **88**, 757–68.

Weisman, S.J., Berkow, R.L., Plautz, G. *et al*. (1985). Glycoprotein-180 deficiency: genetics and abnormal neutrophil activation. *Blood* **65**, 696–704.

Westminster Hospital's Bone-Marrow Transplant Team (1977). Bone-marrow transplant from an unrelated donor for chronic granulomatous disease. *Lancet* **i**, 210–13.

Williams, D.A. and Orkin, S.H. (1986). Somatic gene therapy: current status and future prospects. *J. Clin. Invest.* **77**, 1053–6.

Wright, S.D. and Jong, M.T.C. (1986). Adhesion-promoting receptors on human macrophages recognize *E. coli* by binding to lipopolysaccharides. *J. Exp. Med.* **164**, 1876–88.

Wright, S.D., Rao, P.E. and van Voorhis, W.C. (1983). Identification of the C3bi receptor of human monocytes and macrophages by using monoclonal antibodies. *Proc. Nat. Acad. Sci. (USA)* **80**, 5699–703.

Wright, S.D., Weitz, J.I., Huang, A.J., Levin, S.M., Silverstein, S.C. and Loike, J.D. (1988). Complement receptor type 3 (CD11b/CD18) of human polymorphonuclear leukocytes recognizes fibrinogen. *Proc. Nat. Acad. Sci. (USA)* **85**, 7734–8.

Yancey, K.B., O'Shea, J., Chused T. *et al*. (1985). Human C5a modulates monocyte Fc and C3 receptor expression. *J. Immunol.* **135**, 465–70.

69: Nutrition and Immunity

R.K. Chandra

Introduction

Malnutrition is the commonest cause of immunodeficiency world-wide. The frequent presence of nutritional deficiencies in developing countries is well known. It has been estimated that more than 300 million individuals suffer from protein–energy malnutrition (PEM) and another 250 million from deficiencies of iron, vitamin A and iodine. It has now been revealed that mild to moderate undernutrition is not uncommon even in industrialized countries. For example, iron deficiency is seen in about 10% of North American and European populations. The incidence of nutritional deficiencies is higher in certain at-risk groups, such as the elderly. In hospitalized patients, obvious malnutrition is frequent. The major causes of malnutrition can be divided into primary and secondary factors. Included in the former are poverty, illiteracy and lack of nutrition education, and certain age-groups, e.g. low-birth-weight (LBW) infants, adolescents, pregnant and nursing mothers, and the elderly. Secondary causes include a variety of systemic diseases that lead to nutritional problems, e.g. cancer, inflammatory bowel disease, chronic renal failure, diabetes, etc.

The combination of malnutrition and infection is responsible for much of the morbidity and mortality in all age-groups. In patients with a variety of primary diseases, such as cancer and Crohn's disease, nutritional deficiencies further complicate the picture and increase the risk of infectious illnesses. Although much of the initial work on nutrition and immunity was done on young children in developing countries (Chandra 1972), the general principle that nutrition is a critical determinant of immunocompetence is applicable universally.

The initial studies showed that, in malnourished patients, impaired delayed cutaneous hypersensitivity, lymphocyte proliferation response to mitogens, complement activity and secondary antibody response to certain antigens were frequently found. Subsequent work has demonstrated that PEM results in a reduced number of rosetting T lymphocytes, increased deoxynucleotidyl transferase activity, decreased serum thymic factor, fewer helper T cells, impaired production of interferon gamma and interleukin 2, reduced antibody affinity, impaired secretory immunoglobulin A (IgA) antibody response and phagocyte dysfunction. Malnutrition, however, is not a single entity but rather a broad syndrome. We now know that deficiencies of trace elements and vitamins impair immunity. Both in humans and laboratory animals, intrauterine malnutrition causes prolonged, even permanent, depression of immunity in the offspring. Furthermore, nutrition is an important determinant of waning immunity in old age.

The pathogenesis of immunological changes in undernutrition has been studied extensively. The severity and extent of dysfunction caused by malnutrition in various organ systems depends on several factors, including the rate of cell proliferation, the amount and rate of protein synthesis and the role of individual nutrients in metabolic pathways. Lymphoid tissues are very vulnerable to this damaging effect. Many cells of the immune system are known to depend for their function on metabolic pathways that employ various nutrients as critical co-factors. Numerous enzymes require the presence of zinc, iron, vitamin B_6 and other micronutrients. Any discussion of the effects of nutritional deficiencies on immune responses must be prefaced by emphasizing the complexities and heterogeneity of immunocompetent cells, their subpopulations and products such as interleukins and interferons, and other inducer/regulator systems, e.g. complement, involved in immune responses. Also, malnutrition is a complex syndrome where several deficiencies exist simultaneously. Even in laboratory animals deprived of a single nutrient, the functional effects may be the consequence of changes in the absorption or body stores of other substances. Thus what is observed in an undernourished individual or a deprived animal is the sum of contributions and responses of many components of the immune system that have been altered by one or more nutrient deficiencies.

Epidemiology

Population data and clinical observations indicate that infection and malnutrition are invariably linked together, each aggravating the other. Factors such as lack of health education, illiteracy, poor sanitation, contaminated food and water and overcrowding are important in worsening the situation. In addition, the consistent impairment of immunity in PEM and the recognized increase in infections in patients with primary immunodeficiencies are compatible with the hypothesis that a depressed immune system in malnutrition enhances the risk and severity of infection.

Longitudinal studies of infants in underprivileged communities demonstrate the interaction between nutritional status as judged by anthropometric measurements, immune responses and infection. In the infant illustrated in Fig. 69.1, reduction in two parameters of immunocompetence preceded clinical infection and growth faltering. Findings such as these suggest, firstly, that altered immune responses are early functional indices of growth failure secondary to latent nutritional deficiency and, secondly, that episodes of infection worsen the child's nutritional state.

Several epidemiological studies have documented the adverse effect of PEM on morbidity and mortality (Scrimshaw *et al.* 1968). In rural India, there was a significant correlation between weight-for-height as an index of protein–energy status and risk of death from infectious disease (Chandra 1983a). Pathological examination of tissues from children dying of PEM showed the frequent presence of several opportunistic microorganisms, including *Pneumocystis carinii* (Purtilo and Connor 1975). Morbidity due to diarrhoeal disease is increased (Tomkins 1981; Chandra 1983b), particularly among those children whose weight-for-height is less than 70% of standard (Fig. 69.2). Incidence of diarrhoea is increased slightly but this is not a consistent observation. On the other hand, there is a more profound and universally observed effect on the duration of each episode. This in turn would be expected to worsen malnutrition. Similar observations have been made with respect to respiratory infection and fever (Scrimshaw *et al.* 1968; Chandra and Newberne 1977). In a recent report, Victora and colleagues (1990) studied the synergism between nutritional status and hospital admissions due to diarrhoea and pneumonia in a cohort of 5914 live births in southern Brazil and found that malnutrition was a more important risk factor for pneumonia than for diarrhoea whereas diarrhoea was a stronger predictor of malnutrition than was pneumonia, the association being strongest in the first 2 years of life.

Lymphoid tissues

Lymphoid atrophy is a prominent feature of

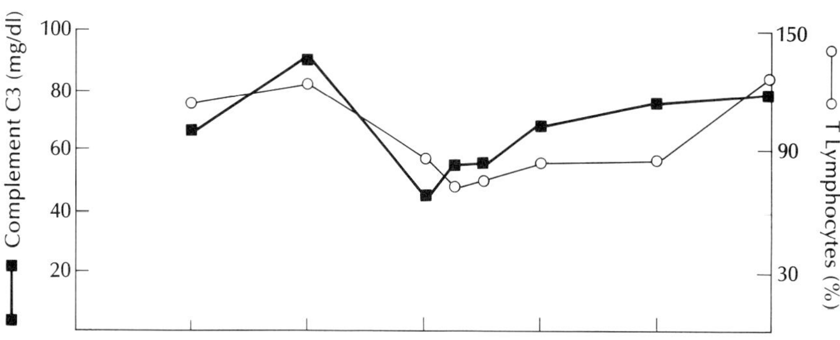

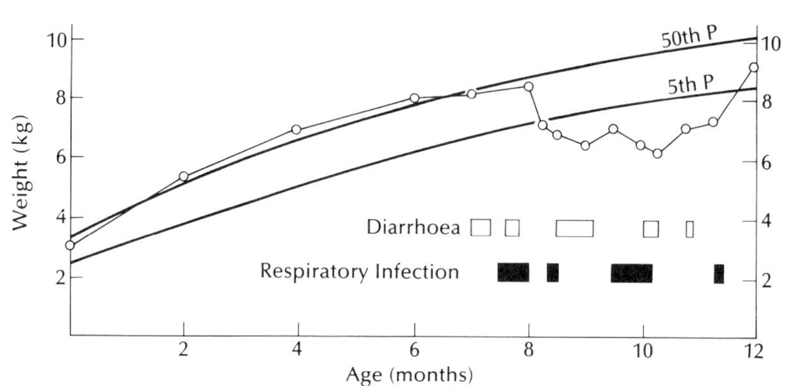

Fig. 69.1. Course of events in an infant in a village near New Delhi, India, followed from birth until 12 months of age. Soon after weaning at the age of 5 months, there is a reduction in the number of T lymphocytes and the concentration of C3 (bottom panel). These immunological changes precede the occurrence of clinical manifestations (diarrhoea, respiratory infection) and the obvious growth faltering seen at about 8 months (upper panel). The findings suggest that immunological changes are sensitive and functional indices that serve as prognostic indicators of future clinical events.

nutritional deprivation. Anatomical changes in lymphoid tissues in malnutrition have been described for well over 144 years. The thymus was noted to be 'a barometer of malnutrition, and a very sensitive one' (Simon 1845). The term 'nutritional thymectomy' illustrates the profound changes that occur in the thymus in malnutrition. The size and weight of the thymus are reduced. Histologically, there is a loss of corticomedullary differentiation, there are fewer lymphoid cells, and the Hassall bodies are enlarged, degenerated and, occasionally, calcified. These changes are easily differentiated from findings in primary immunity deficiency, such as DiGeorge's syndrome. In the spleen, there is a loss of lymphoid cells around small blood-vessels. In the lymph node, the thymus-dependent paracortical areas show depletion of lymphocytes.

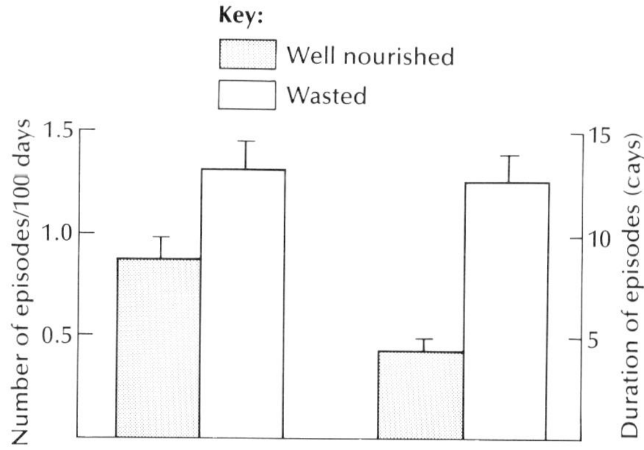

Fig. 69.2. Differences in morbidity due to diarrhoea in well-nourished and wasted (decreased weight-for-height below 70% of National Centre for Health Statistics reference standard) infants in rural India. There is a slight increase in the number of episodes suffered and a more profound increase in the average duration of each episode. Based on data from Chandra (1983b).

Immunocompetence in protein–energy malnutrition

Beisel (1991) and Chandra (1991a) have reviewed the history of early immunological studies in malnutrition, and several monographs and reviews (Chandra and Newberne 1977; Suskind 1977; Chandra 1980a, 1988a; Gershwin *et al.* 1984; Watson 1984; Chandra and Chandra 1986) have provided comprehensive listing of work in this field. In PEM, most of the host defence mechanisms are

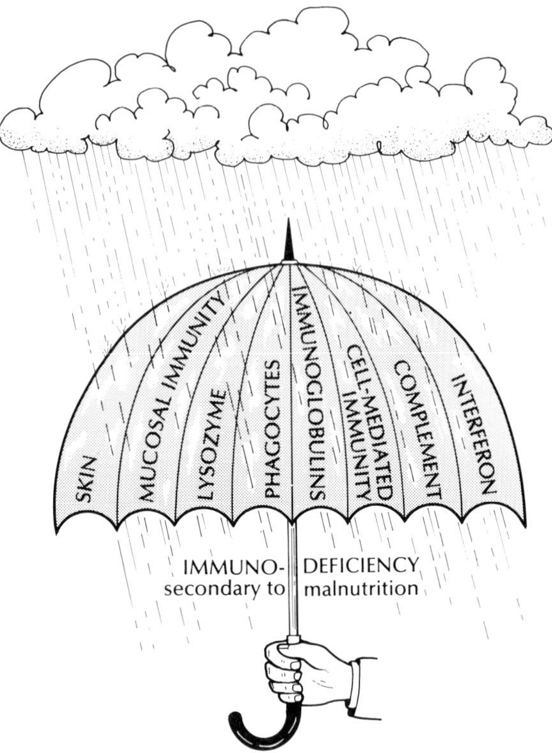

Fig. 69.3. In protein–energy malnutrition, most of the host defence mechanisms are breached, allowing microbes to invade and produce clinical infection which is more severe and prolonged. Copyright ARTS Biomedical Publishers, 1981.

breached (Fig. 69.3). Delayed cutaneous hypersensitivity responses to both recall and new antigens are markedly depressed (Fig. 69.4). It is not uncommon to have complete anergy to a battery of different antigens (Smythe *et al.* 1971; Chandra 1972). These changes are observed in moderate deficiencies as well. Findings in patients with kwashiorkor are more striking compared with those in marasmus. The skin reactions are restored after appropriate nutritional therapy for several weeks or months.

One obvious reason for reduced cell-mediated immunity in PEM is the reduction in mature fully differentiated T lymphocytes that can be recognized by the classical technique of rosette formation or by the newer method of fluorescent labelling with monoclonal antibodies (Chandra 1983c). The reduction in serum thymic factor activity observed in primary PEM (Chandra 1979; Wade *et al.* 1985) may underlie the impaired maturation of T lymphocytes. There is an increase in the amount of deoxynucleotidyl transferase activity in leucocytes (Chandra 1983b), a feature of immaturity. The proportion of helper/inducer T lymphocytes recognized by the presence of CD4 +ve antigen on the cell surface is markedly decreased (Fig. 69.5). There is a moderate reduction in the number suppressor/cytotoxic CD8 +ve cells. Thus the ratio CD4 +ve/CD8 +ve is significantly decreased compared with that in well-nourished controls (Chandra 1983c). Moreover, co-culture experiments have shown a reduction in the number of antibody-producing cells and in the amount of immunoglobulin secreted. This may largely be due to decreased 'help' provided by T lymphocytes (Fig. 69.6). Lymphocyte proliferation and synthesis

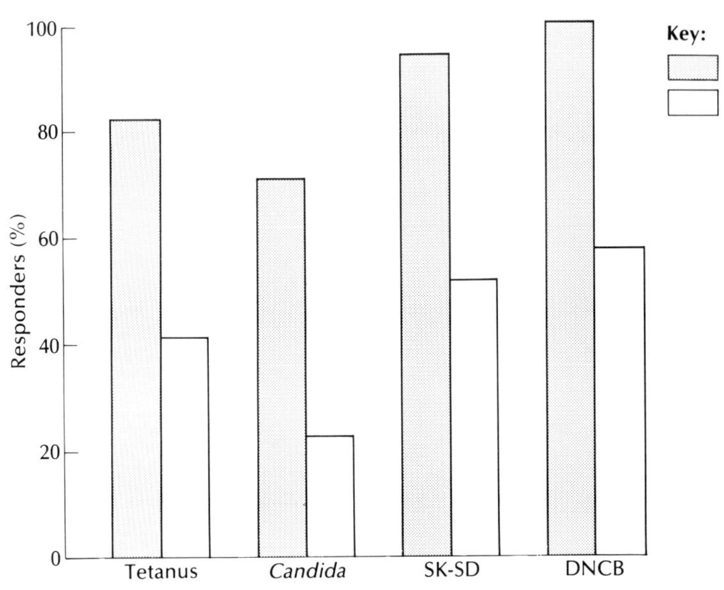

Fig. 69.4. Delayed hypersensitivity skin responses. The percentage of young children who showed a positive response to various antigens is shown. SK-SD, streptokinase-streptodornase; DNCB, 2,4-dinitrochlorobenzene. There is marked reduction in the proportion of wasted children who respond to these recall antigens and chemical sensitization.

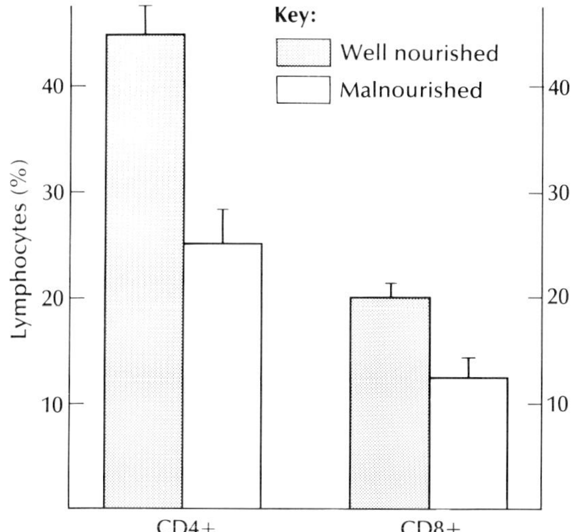

Fig. 69.5. The proportion of two subsets of T lymphocytes. There is a marked reduction in the proportion of CD4 +ve helper/inducer cells in malnourished children ($p < 0.001$). Differences between the two groups for CD8 +ve cytotoxic/suppressor cells are less but are statistically significant ($p < 0.05$).

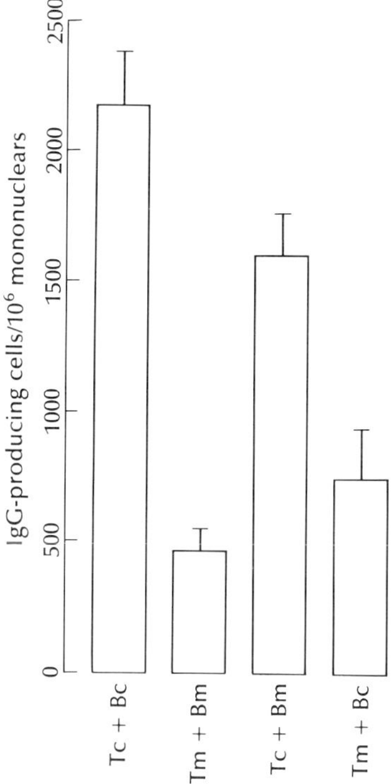

Fig. 69.6. Immunoglobulin production in co-culture experiments where T and B lymphocytes are mixed and are stimulated with pokeweed mitogen for 7 days. Immunoglobulin-producing cells are recognized by lytic areas in a reverse haemolytic plaque assay. Compared with well-nourished controls (first column), there is a marked reduction in the number of antibody-producing cells in malnourished children (second column). When T cells of healthy controls (Tc) are mixed with B cells of malnourished patients (Bm), there is a significant improvement in response (third column), whereas the opposite combination (Tm + Bc) results in a moderate increase (fourth column).

of deoxyribonucleic acid (DNA) are reduced, especially when autologous patient's plasma is used in cell cultures. This may be the result of inhibitory factors as well as deficiency of essential nutrients lacking in the patient's plasma (Beatty and Dowdle 1978). Another aspect of lymphocyte function that changes in PEM is the traffic and 'homing' pattern. For example, lymphocytes derived from mesenteric lymph nodes of immunized rodents revert back to the intestine in large numbers, whereas in malnutrition this homing is reduced (Fig. 69.7).

A critical analysis of the published literature suggests that serum antibody responses are generally intact in PEM, particularly when antigens in adjuvant are administered or in the case of those materials that do not evoke T cell response. Rarely, the antibody response to organisms such as *Salmonella typhi* may be decreased. However, before impaired antibody response can be attributed to nutritional deficiency, one must carefully rule out infection as a confounding factor. Recently, antibody affinity was found to be decreased in patients who are malnourished. This may provide an explanation for a higher frequency of antigen–antibody complexes found in such patients. As opposed to serum antibody responses, secretory IgA antibody levels after deliberate immunization with viral vaccines are decreased (Chandra 1975a); there is a selective reduction in secretory IgA levels (Watson *et al.* 1985). This may have several clinical implications, including an increased frequency of septicaemia commonly observed in undernourished children.

The process of phagocytosis is also affected in PEM. Complement is an essential opsonin and the levels and activity of most complement components are decreased (Chandra 1975b; Haller *et al.* 1978). The best-documented is a reduction in C3, C5, factor B and total haemolytic activity (Table 69.1). There is a slight reduction in opsonic activity of plasma when tests are run using plasma diluted 1:10 or more (Smythe *et al.* 1971). Although the ingestion of particles by phagocytes is intact, subsequent metabolic activation and destruction of bacteria are reduced. Finally, recent work in man and animals has demonstrated that the

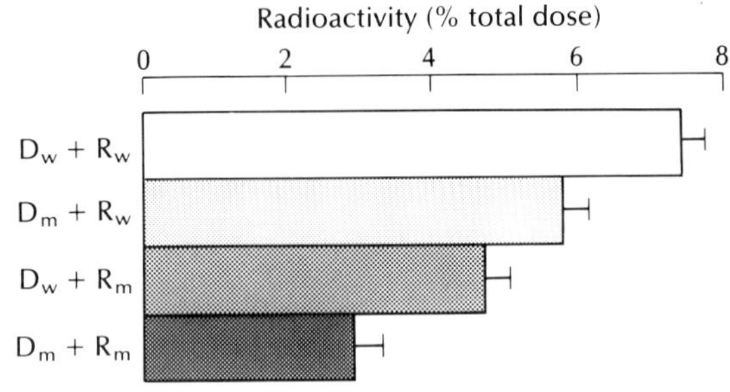

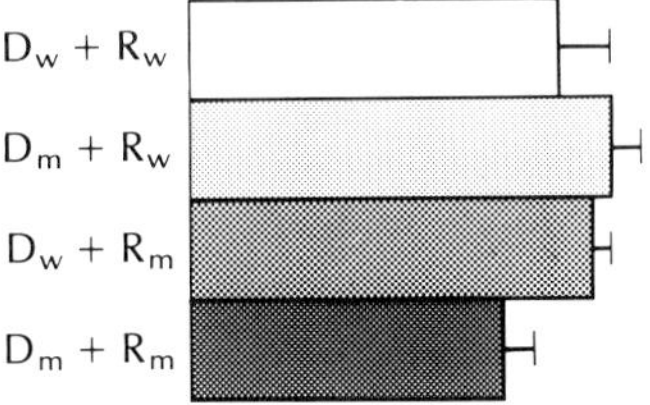

Fig. 69.7. Lymphocyte traffic. Lymphoblasts recovered from mesenteric lymph nodes of well-nourished (D_w) or malnourished (D_m) donor rats immunized with sheep red blood cells intraperitoneally were isolated, radiolabelled and injected back into syngeneic well-nourished (R_w) or malnourished (R_m) recipient animals. The amount of radioactivity seen in the intestine (upper panels) and in the spleen (lower panels) was estimated. Malnutrition either in the donor or in the recipient reduced the homing of lymphocytes to the intestine. The effect was more pronounced when both the donor and the recipient were malnourished. There was no significant effect of malnutrition on the homing of cells to the spleen.

Table 69.1. Complement system[a]

	Healthy	Protein-energy malnutrition
Total hemolytic complement activity, CH_{50} (kU/l)	116 ± 19	67 ± 12
C3 (g/l)	1.43 ± 0.15	0.61 ± 0.09
C5 (g/l)	0.081 ± 0.003	0.049 ± 0.002
Factor B (g/l)	2.29 ± 0.17	1.21 ± 0.11

a $\bar{x}$ ± SEM.
From Chandra 1991d.

production of several cytokines including interleukins 1 and 2 and interferon gamma is decreased in PEM. Moreover, malnutrition alters the ability of T lymphocytes to respond appropriately to cytokines (Hoffman-Goetz *et al.* 1984).

There is very little work on the effect of malnutrition on the integrity of physical barriers, quality of mucus and several other innate immune defences. For example, lysozyme levels are decreased, largely the result of reduced production by monocytes and neutrophils and also increased excretion in the urine. Adherence of bacteria to epithelial cells is a first step before invasion and infection can occur. The number of bacteria adhering to respiratory epithelial cells is increased in PEM (Chandra and Gupta 1991).

Individual nutrients and immune responses

Several investigations have pointed to the crucial role of some nutrients in key metabolic pathways and immunological cell functions (Beisel 1982; Chandra and Dayton 1982; Bendich and Chandra 1990; Chandra 1991b). Isolated deficiencies of micronutrients are rare with the exception of iron, vitamin A and zinc. However, they frequently complicate PEM and many systemic diseases. Moreover, human malnutrition is usually a composite syndrome of multiple nutrient deficiencies. Observations in laboratory animals deprived of one dietary element and findings in the rare patient with a single nutrient deficiency have confirmed the crucial role of several vitamins and trace elements in immunocompetence.

Five general concepts have been advanced (Chandra 1990):

1 Alterations in immune responses occur early in the course of reduction in micronutrient intake.

2 The extent of immunological impairment depends upon the type of nutrient involved, its interactions with other essential nutrients, severity of deficiency, presence of concomitant infection and age of the subject.

3 Immunological abnormalities predict outcome, particulary the risk of infection and mortality.

4 In the case of many micronutrients, excessive intake is associated with impaired immune responses.

5 Tests of immunocompetence are useful in titration of physiological needs and in assessment of safe lower and upper limits of intake of micronutrients.

Vitamin A deficiency results in a slight reduction in the weight of the thymus, decreased lymphocyte proliferation in response to mitogens, antigen-specific antibody production and T lymphocyte proliferation *in vitro*, and increased bacterial adherence to respiratory epithelial cells (Chandra and Au 1981; Nauss *et al.* 1985; Friedman and

Sklan 1989). Vitamin A has been known as an 'anti-infective vitamin' and its deficiency is believed to have an impact on both morbidity and mortality but the precise quantitative relationships for these interactions have to be worked out. Carotenoids have important immunoregulatory functions involving T and B lymphocytes, natural killer cells and macrophages.

Vitamin B_6 deficiency causes profound changes in immune responses in animals (Robson and Schwartz 1980; Sudhakaran and Chandra 1990). The thymus is smaller and thymic hormone activity is decreased. Impaired cell-mediated immunity is shown by failure of delayed cutaneous hypersensitivity reactions, reduced T lymphocyte cytotoxicity and delayed rejection of allografts. Lymphocyte responses to mitogens and antigens are decreased. There is decreased antibody formation after both primary and secondary immunization. Isolated vitamin B_6 deficiency is rare in humans.

The role of vitamin C in phagocyte function is recognized. Moderately severe deficiency is associated with retarded locomotion and decreased bactericidal capacity of neutrophils and macrophages; cell-mediated immunity and antibody production are relatively unaffected (Anderson *et al.* 1990). Severe vitamin E deficiency results in impaired cell-mediated immunity and decreased antibody synthesis.

Zinc deficiency, both acquired and inherited, is associated with lymphoid atrophy, decreased cutaneous delayed hypersensitivity responses and homograft rejection, and lower thymic hormone activity (Chandra 1980b; Chandra and Au 1980a; Prasad *et al.* 1988). This is best illustrated in patients with acrodermatitis enteropathica (Table 69.2), who have impaired lymphocyte response to phytohaemagglutinin, decreased thymulin activity and reduced delayed hypersensitivity skin reactions (Chandra 1980b). In laboratory animal models these findings can be confirmed and in addition one can demonstrate a reduced number of antibody-forming cells in the spleen and impaired T killer cell activity. There is much recent interest in the role of zinc in macrophage function. Zinc deficiency results in decreased ingestion and phagocytosis. The nutrient is probably involved in stimulation of nicotinamide adenine dinucleotide phosphate (NADPH) oxidase through its role as a co-factor for phospholipase A2 and/or phospholipase C. Zinc may stabilize 20:4 arachidonic acid against oxidation by iron complexes. Zinc complexes may react with oxygen, generating products highly toxic to ingested pathogens. Wound healing is impaired. Zinc deficiency increases morbidity and mortality of animals challenged with various organisms, including coxsackie B virus and *Listeria monocytogenes*. Zinc deficiency promotes the establishment of nematodes and alters the characteristics of their expulsion from the intestine, although spontaneous cure was unaffected (Fenwick *et al.* 1990). Important questions that remain unanswered in the zinc-immunity field include: Is leucopenia the main reason for the immunodeficiency observed in zinc deficiency? Are antibody responses to T-cell-independent antigens normal in zinc deficiency? Are there significant shifts in the distribution of cells bearing different surface markers? What is the molecular basis of impaired lymphocyte and phagocyte functions in zinc deficiency?

Table 69.2. Immunological findings in acrodermatitis enteropathica[a]

Index	Before therapy (n = 8)	After therapy (n = 8)
Serum zinc (μmol/l)	7.40 ± 1.72[b]	13.61 ± 1.33
Delayed cutaneous hypersensitivity reactions	3 of 8	8 of 8
Serum thymulin activity (median titre)	1:2	1:32
Lymphocyte stimulation index[c]	23.4 ± 7.6[b]	79.5 ± 12.4

a Patients were treated orally with 150 mg Zn/day for 6 weeks.
b $\bar{x}$ ± SEM.
c Lymphocyte response to phytohaemagglutinin, expressed as cpm of the culture containing phytohaemagglutinin divided by cpm of the culture containing saline.
From Chandra 1991d.

Copper deficiency may occur rarely in association with PEM. In the Menkes' kinky-hair disease with altered copper metabolism and in animals deprived of dietary copper, there is an increased susceptibility to infection, particularly *Salmonella*. Copper deficiency results in altered immune responses (Vyas and Chandra 1983). These changes are organ-specific and are influenced by the type of carbohydrate in the diet (Babu and Failla 1989). The function of the reticuloendothelial system is depressed and the microbicidal activity of phagocytes is decreased. This has been attributed to the role of copper in the superoxide dismutase and cytochrome c oxidase enzyme systems. There is a reduction in antibody response to T-cell-dependent antigens.

Deficiency of iron is the commonest nutritional problem world-wide, even in industrialized countries. On the one hand, free iron is necessary for bacterial growth: removal of iron with the help of lactoferrin or other chelating agents reduces bacterial multiplication, particularly in the presence of specific antibody. On the other hand, iron is needed by natural killer cells, neutrophils and lymphocytes for optimal function. Thus, bactericidal capacity is reduced in iron deficiency (Fig. 69.8). This may be due to the deficiency of iron-dependent myeloperoxidase and cytochrome enzymes. Also, the lymphocyte proliferation response to mitogens and antigens is impaired: response to tetanus toxoid and herpes simplex antigens is low in iron-deficiency subjects and iron therapy results in a significant improvement in their response. It is interesting to note that persons with a history of recurrent herpes labialis are more often iron-deficient than controls matched for age and sex. The molecular explanation for impaired lymphocyte proliferation in iron deficiency may lie in part in the deficiency of the ribonucleotidyl reductase that is needed for cell proliferation.

Does the amount of dietary iron influence the risk of infection? In the case of no other trace element is the discussion of deficiency and risk of infection so biased and controversial as it is in the case of iron (Vyas and Chandra 1984; Hershko *et al.* 1988). The concept of 'iron nutritional immunity' emphasizing the effect of iron deprivation in limiting the multiplication of bacteria is an attractive hypothesis with considerable *in vitro* evidence, but clinical data do not support the suggestion that iron deficiency protects against infection or that correction of iron deficiency, particularly if it is achieved gradually by oral iron therapy, increases the incidence or severity of infectious disease in man.

The role of other micronutrients and of toxic heavy metals has been reviewed elsewhere (Beisel 1982; Chandra and Dayton 1982; Chowdhury and Chandra 1987; Bendich and Chandra 1990; Chandra 1991b).

Amino acids modulate immune responses in many different ways. Dietary deficiencies of selected amino acids decrease antibody responses; in other states of amino acid imbalance, the overall response may be enhanced, indicating that changes in suppressor cells may occur. The phagocytic clearance of macromolecules from the blood is reduced, as is antibody affinity in inbred animals (Coovadia and Soothill 1976). There is recent evidence for the immunostimulatory and anti-infective role of glutamine and arginine.

There is much evidence to indicate that dietary lipids have an immunoregulatory role (Erickson *et al.* 1983; Gogos *et al.* 1990). The postulated pathogenetic mechanisms include modulation of eicosanoid synthesis, changes in the cell membrane, altered number and density of receptors, changes in the number and function of selected subsets of cells, and altered production and action

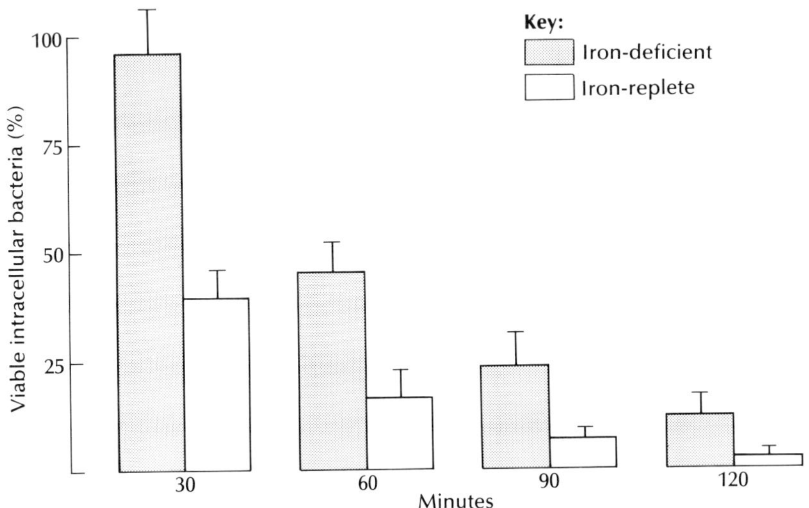

Fig. 69.8. Bactericidal capacity of neutrophils in iron-deficient and iron-replete individuals. Percentage of viable intracellular bacteria at various time intervals after the start of cell–bacteria cultures is shown.

of cytokines. Essential fatty acid deficiency reduces a variety of immune responses. However, the main focus of work has been on the effect of excess intake of lipids (see below).

Immunocompetence of low-birth-weight infants

There is good clinical evidence that neonates have suboptimal immune responses and are susceptible to infection. When growth retardation and nutritional deficiency complicate the picture, as in LBW infants, impairment of immunocompetence is more marked and longer-lasting (Chandra 1975c, 1991c).

The world-wide incidence of low birth weight, defined as weight less than 2500 g, varies considerably from one population group to another, from 8% in some industrialized countries to a high of 41% in some developing countries of Africa. The aetiology of fetal growth retardation includes maternal malnutrition and infection, hypertension, toxaemia, smoking, substance abuse and 'placental insufficiency'. More than one factor is often at work.

Low birth weight is associated with a higher mortality. Whereas the total proportion of infants who die or are handicapped is similar in appropriate for gestational age (AGA) and small-for-gestational-age (SGA) groups, the former are at higher risk of death in the immediate post-natal period whereas the latter are at higher risk of morbidity in the 1st year of life. Infection is one of the recognized causes of increased illness in SGA infants. Upper and lower respiratory tract infections are three times more frequent in SGA infants compared with AGA infants. The SGA group is also at risk of developing infection with opportunistic micro-organisms, such as *Pneumocystis carinii*, as observed also in postnatal malnutrition.

Small-for-gestational-age infants show atrophy of the thymus and prolonged impairment of cell-mediated immunity (Fig. 69.9). Delayed cutaneous hypersensitivity to a variety of microbial recall antigens as well as to the strong chemical sensitizer 2,4-dinitrochlorobenzene is impaired. Serum thymic factor activity is lower in SGA infants tested at 1 month of age or later. In contrast to AGA LBW infants, who recover immunologically by about 2–3 months of age, SGA infants continue to exhibit impaired cell-mediated immune responses for several months or even years. This is particularly true of those infants whose weight-for-height is less than 80% of standard. The prolonged immunosuppression in some SGA infants correlates with clinical experience of infectious illness, and thus may have considerable biological significance. In animal models of intrauterine nutritional deficiency, protein–energy malnutrition (Fig. 69.10; Chandra 1975d) as well as deprivation of selected nutrients (Robson and Schwartz 1975; Beach *et al.* 1982) results in reduced immune responses in the offspring.

Phagocyte function is deranged in LBW infants.

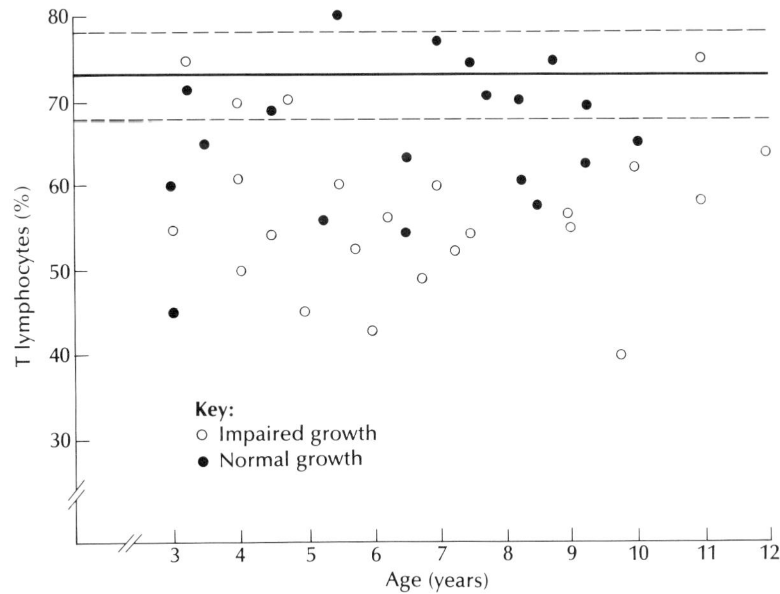

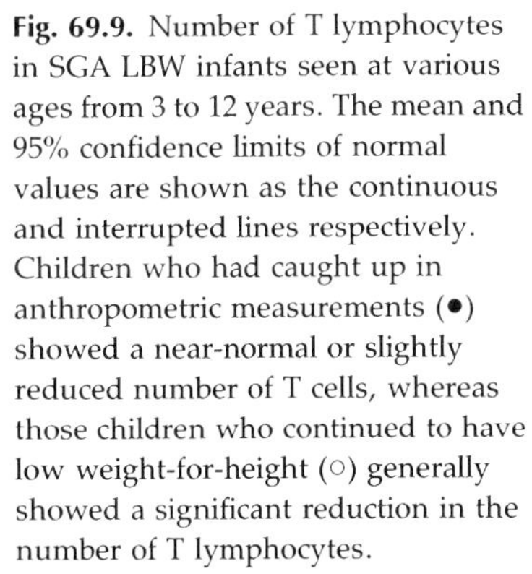
Fig. 69.9. Number of T lymphocytes in SGA LBW infants seen at various ages from 3 to 12 years. The mean and 95% confidence limits of normal values are shown as the continuous and interrupted lines respectively. Children who had caught up in anthropometric measurements (●) showed a near-normal or slightly reduced number of T cells, whereas those children who continued to have low weight-for-height (○) generally showed a significant reduction in the number of T lymphocytes.

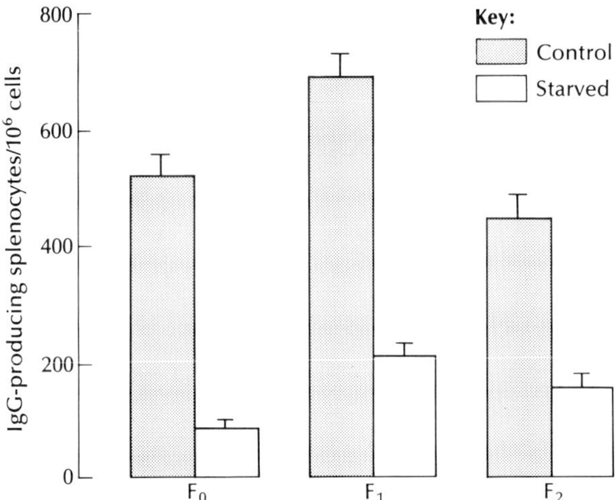

Fig. 69.10. Intergenerational effects of nutritional deficiency. Immunoglobulin G antibody-producing spleen cells were estimated in mice subjected to partial starvation (65% of energy intake in controls). The offspring were given *ad libitum* access to food. The F_1- and F_2-generation offspring of starved female dams mated with healthy well-nourished males showed a significant reduction in antibody response. F_0 and F_1 animals were tested at age 9 weeks and F_2 at age 6 weeks. Data from Chandra (1975d). Copyright American Association for Advancement of Science, 1975.

There is a slight reduction in ingestion of particulate matter and a significant reduction in both metabolic activity and bactericidal capacity.

Immunoglobulin G from the mother, acquired through placental transfer, is the principal immunoglobulin in cord blood. Physiological hypoimmunoglobulinaemia seen between 3 and 5 months of age is pronounced and prolonged in LBW infants (Chandra 1975c) since their level of IgG at birth is significantly lower compared with full-term infants. There is a progressive rise in IgG concentration with gestational age and birth weight, especially in infants below 2500 g. All four subclasses of IgG are detected in fetal sera as early as 16 weeks of gestation, the bulk being formed by IgG1. In SGA LBW infants, the cord blood levels of IgG1 are reduced much more than those of other subclasses. Thus the infant : maternal ratio is significantly low for IgG1 but not for IgG2. The number of immunoglobulin-producing cells and the amount of immunoglobulin secreted is decreased in SGA infants who are symptomatic, i.e. those who have recurrent infections. In the 2nd year of life, SGA infants show a marked reduction in IgG2 levels and often show infections with organisms that have a polysaccharide capsule.

Table 69.3. Zinc supplementation of preterm low-birthweight infants[a]

	Supplemented (n = 18)	Control (n = 16)
T lymphocytes (%)	56 ± 4[b]	38 ± 6
Lymphocyte stimulation index	62 ± 12	21 ± 7
Serum thymulin activity (median titre)	1 : 32	1 : 8

a Infants received orally 1 mg Zn/kg body wt/day. The infants were tested at age 4 weeks.
b $\bar{x}$ ± SEM.
From Chandra 1991d.

In preterm infants with birth weight between 1800 and 2200 g, moderate amounts of oral zinc supplements accelerate immunological recovery (Table 69.3).

Nutritional regulation of immunity in old age

Four questions have been posed (Chandra 1989):
1 Is immunological decline an inevitable part of aging?
2 How common are nutritional deficiencies in the elderly?
3 Would correction of nutritional deficiencies improve immune responses?
4 If nutritional therapy improves immunity, will this result in reduced illness?

A critical review of published work related to nutrition, immunity and morbidity in old age has been presented (Chandra 1989). It has been observed that the average of immune responses in the elderly is significantly lower than that seen in the young. However, there is a much wider range of responses found in the former, so that there are some among the very old whose immune responses are as vigorous as those observed in younger subjects. Several surveys have shown that almost one-third of apparently healthy elderly people have a reduction in the intake of several nutrients; this is reflected to some extent in reduced blood concentrations. The most common deficiencies are those of iron, zinc and vitamin C. Correction of these deficiencies by nutritional advice and dietary or medicinal supplements results in a significant improvement in immunocompetence (Fig. 69.11). There is recent evidence to

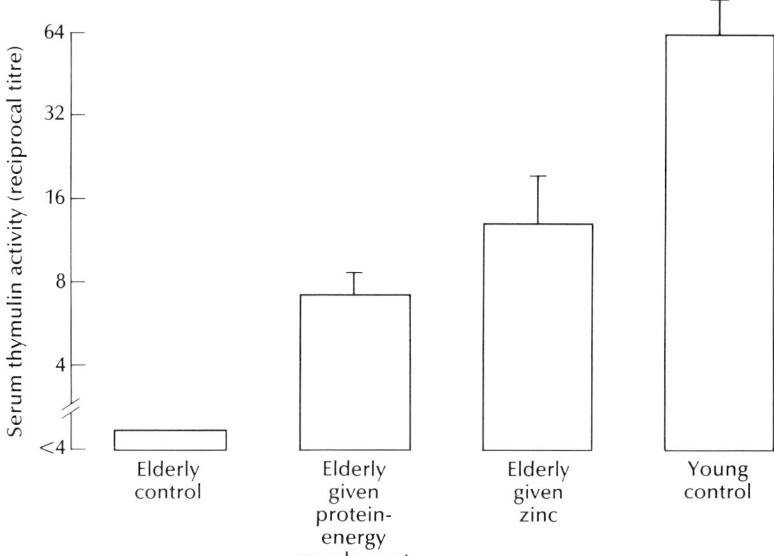

Fig. 69.11. Serum thymulin activity in elderly subjects who were given appropriate nutritional advice and supplements for 3 months.

indicate that improved immune responses are associated with decreased morbidity due to common respiratory infections.

Immune responses in obesity and excessive intake of nutrients

Genetically obese animals show alterations in a variety of immune responses (Chandra and Au 1980b). The weight of the thymus expressed as a proportion of body-weight is decreased and there are fewer lymphocytes present. Natural killer cell activity is decreased. The generation of cytotoxic T lymphocytes following stimulation *in vivo* is decreased but is normal if sensitization is carried out *in vitro*. This suggests that the microenvironment of the obese animal, including hyperlipidaemia, hyperglycaemia and altered levels of insulin, glucagon, cortisol and adrenocorticotrophic hormones, may be responsible for impaired cellular responses.

Human obesity is a heterogeneous syndrome. Nevertheless, obese adolescents and adults show a higher risk of infection, including postoperative sepsis, than lean controls (Pasulka *et al*. 1986). In the obese, there is a slight impairment of delayed cutaneous hypersensitivity responses, decreased lymphocyte response to mitogens and reduced bactericidal capacity of neutrophils (Chandra and Kutty 1980). Some of the abnormalities may be due to associated deficiencies of selected micronutrients such as iron and zinc, which are encountered more frequently in the obese compared with lean controls.

There are considerable data implicating excess lipid intake in impaired immune responses (Gurr 1983; Johnston and Marshall 1984; Chandra 1988b). An increase in either saturated fat or polyunsaturated fatty acids to more than 16% of calories results in decreased cell-mediated immunity, including cytotoxic function, delayed cutaneous hypersensitivity, lymphocyte response to mitogen stimulation and natural killer cell activity. In autoimmune disease-prone mice, reduction in fat intake protects against immune complex pathology. A marine-oil diet decreased the lymphoid hyperplasia induced by the *lpr* gene, prevented an increase in macrophage Ia expression and the formation of circulating retroviral sp70 immune complexes and delayed the onset of disease, thereby prolonging survival (Kelley *et al*. 1985).

A slight excess intake of certain nutrients may be associated with enhanced immune responses. These include beta-carotene, vitamin A, vitamin E, zinc and selenium. Increased amounts of selected amino acids, such as arginine, and other compounds, such as nucleotides, are reported to enhance immune responses, particularly in the face of stress such as burns, trauma or sepsis.

At the same time, it must be emphasized that all nutrients given in quantities beyond a certain threshold will reduced immune responses. This has been shown for zinc (Fig. 69.12; Chandra 1984), selenium and vitamins A and E. Iron overload

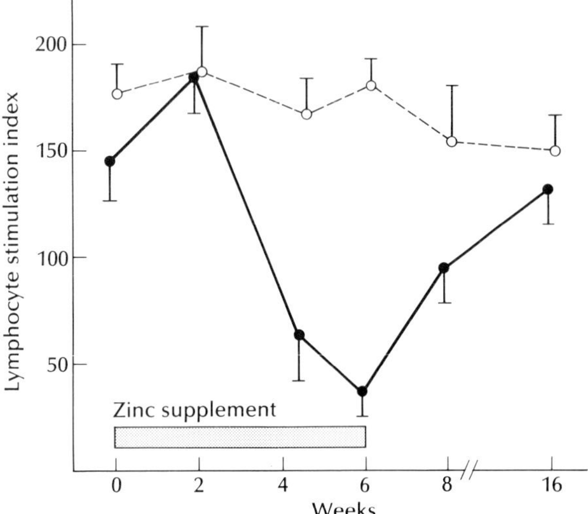

Fig. 69.12. Lymphocyte stimulation response to phytohaemagglutinin in young adults given zinc supplements 150 mg twice a day for 6 weeks (●) or placebo (○). Data shown were optimal results obtained on dose–response curves. Based on Chandra (1984). Copyright American Medical Association, 1984.

may promote bacterial septicaemia and increase the frequency of symptomatic malaria in endemic areas. The mechanisms of these immunotoxic effects are not clear, but, in the case of zinc overdose, alterations in serum and cell-bound low-density lipoproteins, reduced levels of other nutrients and changes in membrane structure and receptor expression are some possibilities.

Clinical and applied significance

Nutritional regulation of immunity and risk of illness have several practical applications. First, changes in immune responses occur early in the course of nutritional deficiency. Thus, we can employ immunocompetence as a sensitive functional indicator of nutritional status. In patients with obvious primary or secondary malnutrition, the number of T lymphocytes is a useful measure of response to supplementation therapy. Secondly, anergy and other immunological changes correlate with poor outcome both in medical and surgical patients in terms of complications, duration of hospital stay and mortality (Table 69.4). This is particularly useful when impaired immunity is considered in association with hypoalbuminaemia. In field surveys, impaired cell-mediated immunity and reduced levels of complement

Table 69.4. Reliability of preoperative anergy (absence of delayed cutaneous hypersensitivity) to predict postoperative malnutrition and associated complications[a]

Outcome	Sensitivity	Specificity	Positive predictive value	Negative predictive value
Sepsis	61 (50–80)	74 (62–90)	28 (14–39)	92 (84–97)
Mortality	49 (37–60)	74 (60–88)	25 (21–29)	91 (90–92)

a $\bar{x}$ (and range) of values obtained from several reported studies, largely based on adults undergoing major surgery for a variety of primary diagnoses.
From Chandra 1991d.

components precede and predict the occurrence of infection. Thirdly, opportunistic infections occur more frequently among those patients with cancer who are also malnourished. The incidence of complicating infections can be reduced if appropriate preventative and therapeutic nutritional management is carried out in patients with leukaemia. Fourthly, there is an uncanny similarity between the immunological findings in nutritional deficiencies and those seen in acquired immune deficiency syndrome (AIDS) (Jain and Chandra 1984). It has been postulated that nutritional deficiency may influence the biological gradient and natural history of this infection. Recent surveys indicate that attention to the nutritional needs of the human immunodeficiency virus (HIV)-infected individual is an important part of the overall management of this life-threatening infection (Winick *et al.* 1989). Fifthly, response to immunization is modulated by the nutritional status of the host and protective efficacy of vaccines may be suboptimal in the undernourished individual. Finally, immune responses can be used to define safe upper and lower limits of nutrient intake (Chandra 1991d). The era of nutritional immunology has finally arrived.

References

Anderson, R., Smit, M.J., Joone, G.K. and van Staden, A.M. (1990). Vitamin C and cellular immune functions. In *Micronutrients and Immune Functions*, ed. A. Bendich and R.K. Chandra, pp. 34–48, New York Academy of Sciences, New York.

Babu, U. and Failla, M.L. (1989). Superoxide dismutase activity and blastogenic response of lymphocytes from copper-deficient rats fed diets containing fructose or corn starch. *Nutr. Res.* **9**, 273–82.

Beach, R.S., Gershwin, M.E. and Hurley, L.S. (1982). Gestational zinc deprivation in mice: persistence of immunodeficiency for three generations. *Science* **218**, 469–72.

Beatty, D.W. and Dowdle, E.B. (1978). The effects of kwashiorkor serum on lymphocyte transformation *in vitro*. *Clin. Exp. Immunol.* **32**, 134–43.

Beisel, W.R. (1982). Single nutrients and immunity. *Am. J. Clin. Nutr.* **35**, 417–68.

Beisel, W.R. (1991). The history of nutritional immunology. *J. Nutr. Immunol.* **1**, 62–78.

Bendich, A. and Chandra, R.K. (eds) (1990). *Micronutrients and Immune Functions*. New York Academy of Sciences, New York.

Chandra, R.K. (1972). Immunocompetence in undernutrition. *J. Pediatr.* **81**, 1194–200.

Chandra, R.K. (1975a). Reduced secretory antibody response to live attenuated measles and poliovirus vaccines in malnourished children. *Br. Med. J.* **2**, 583–5.

Chandra, R.K. (1975b). Serum complement and immunoconglutinin in malnutrition. *Arch. Dis. Child.* **50**, 225–9.

Chandra, R.K. (1975c). Fetal malnutrition and postnatal immunocompetence. *Am. J. Dis. Child.* **125**, 450–5.

Chandra, R.K. (1975d). Antibody formation in first and second generation offspring of nutritionally deprived rats. *Science* **190**, 289–90.

Chandra, R.K. (1979). Serum thymic hormone activity in protein–energy malnutrition. *Clin. Exp. Immunol.* **38**, 228–30.

Chandra, R.K. (1980a). *Immunology of Nutritional Disorders*. Edward Arnold, London.

Chandra, R.K. (1980b). Acrodermatitis enteropathica: zinc levels and cell-mediated immunity. *Pediatrics* **66**, 789–91.

Chandra, R.K. (1983a). Nutrition, immunity and infection: present knowledge and future directions. *Lancet* **i**, 688–91.

Chandra, R.K. (1983b). The nutrition–immunity–infection nexus: the enumeration and functional assessment of lymphocyte subsets in nutritional deficiency. *Nutr. Res.* **3**, 605–15.

Chandra, R.K. (1983c). Numerical and functional deficiency in T helper cells in protein–energy malnutrition. *Clin. Exp. Immunol.* **51**, 126–32.

Chandra, R.K. (1984) Excessive intake of zinc impairs immune responses. *JAMA* **252**, 1443–6.

Chandra, R.K. (ed.) (1988a). *Nutrition and Immunology*. Alan R. Liss, New York.

Chandra, R.K. (1988b). Dietary factors in immune responsiveness. In *Dietary Fat Requirements in Health and Disease*, ed. J. Beare-Rogers, pp. 143–9, American Oil Chemists Society, Champaign, Illinois.

Chandra, R.K. (1989). Nutritional regulation of immunity and risk of infection in old age. *Immunology* **67**, 141–7.

Chandra, R.K. (1990). Micronutrients and immune functions, an overview. *Ann. NY Acad. Sci.* **587**, 9–16.

Chandra, R.K. (1991a). Immunocompetence in protein–energy malnutrition, a historical perspective. *J. Nutr.* **122**, 597–600.

Chandra, R.K. (1991b). Trace elements and immune responses. In *Trace Elements in the Nutrition of Children*, ed. R.K. Chandra, vol. II, pp. 201–14, Raven Press, New York.

Chandra, R.K. (1991c). Interactions between early nutrition and the immune system. In *The Childhood Environment and Adult Disease*, ed. D.J.P. Barker and J. Whelan, Ciba Foundation Symposium 156, pp. 77–88, Wiley, London.

Chandra, R.K. (1991d). Nutrition and immunity: lessons from the past and new insights into the future. *Am. J. Clin. Nutr.* **53**, 1087–101.

Chandra, R.K. and Au, B. (1980a). Single nutrient deficiency and cell-mediated immune responses. I. Zinc. *Am. J. Clin. Nutr.* **33**, 736–8.

Chandra, R.K. and Au, B. (1980b). Spleen hemolytic plaque forming cell response and generation of cytotoxic cells in genetically obese (C57Bl/6J *ob/ob*) mice. *Int. Arch. Allergy Appl. Immunol.* **62**, 94–8.

Chandra, R.K. and Au, B. (1981). Single nutrient deficiency and cell-mediated immune responses. III. Vitamin A. *Nutr. Res.* **1**, 181–5.

Chandra, R.K. and Dayton, D.H. (1982). Trace element regulation of immunity and infection. *Nutr. Res.* **2**, 721–33.

Chandra, R.K. and Gupta, S.P. (1990). Increased bacterial adherence to respiratory epithelial cells in protein–energy malnutrition. *Immunol. Infect. Dis.* **1**, 55–7.

Chandra, R.K. and Kutty, K.M. (1980). Immunocompetence in obesity. *Acta Paediatr. Scand.* **69**, 25–30.

Chandra, R.K. and Newberne, P.M. (1977). *Nutrition, Immunity and Infection: Mechanisms of Interactions*. Plenum, New York.

Chandra, S. and Chandra, R.K. (1986). Nutrition, immune responses, and outcome. *Prog. Food Nutr. Sci.* **10**, 1–65.

Chowdhury, B.A. and Chandra, R.K. (1987). Biological and health implications of toxic heavy metal and essential trace element interactions. *Prog. Food Nutr. Sci.* **11**, 55–113.

Coovadia, H.M. and Soothill, J.F. (1976). The effect of amino acid restricted diets on the clearance of ^{125}I-labelled polyvinyl pyrrolidone in mice. *Clin. Exp. Immunol.* **23**, 562–7.

Erickson, K.L., Adams, D.A. and McNeill, C.J. (1983). Dietary lipid modulation of immune responsiveness. *Lipids* **18**, 468–74.

Fenwick, P.K., Aggett, P.J., Macdonald, D.C., Huber, C. and Wakelin, D. (1990). Zinc deprivation and zinc repletion: effect on the response of rats to infection with *Strongyloides ratti*. *Am. J. Clin. Nutr.* **52**, 173–7.

Friedman, A. and Sklan, D. (1989). Antigen-specific immune response impairment in the chick as influenced by dietary vitamin A. *J. Nutr.* **119**, 790–5.

Gershwin, M.E., Beach, R.S. and Hurley, L.S. (1984). *Nutrition and Immunity*. Academic Press, New York.

Gogos, C.A., Kalfarentzos, F.E. and Zoumbos, N.C. (1990). Effect of different types of total parenteral nutrition on T-lymphocyte subpopulations and NK cells. *Am. J. Clin. Nutr.* **51**, 119–22.

Gurr, M.I. (1983). The role of lipids in the regulation of the immune system. *Prog. Lipid Res.* **22**, 257–87.

Haller, L., Zubler, R.H. and Lambert, P.H. (1978). Plasma levels of complement components and complement hemolytic activity in protein–energy malnutrition. *Clin. Exp. Immunol.* **34**, 248–54.

Hershko, C., Peto, T.E.A. and Weatherall, D.J. (1988). Iron and infection. *Br. Med. J.* **296**, 660–4.

Hoffman-Goetz, L., Bell, R.C. and Deir, R. (1984). Effect of protein malnutrition and interleukin-1 on *in vitro* rabbit lymphocyte mitogenesis. *Nutr. Res.* **4**, 769–80.

Jain, V.K. and Chandra, R.K. (1984). Does nutritional deficiency predispose to acquired immunodeficiency syndrome? *Nutr. Res.* **4**, 537–42.

Johnston, P.V. and Marshall, L.A. (1984). Dietary fat, prostaglandins and the immune response. *Prog. Food Nutr. Sci.* **8**, 3–35.

Kelley, V.E., Feretti, A., Izui, S. and Strom, T.B. (1985). A fish oil diet rich in eicosopentaenoic acid reduces cycloxygenase metabolites and suppresses lupus in MRL-lpr mice. *J. Immunol.* **134**, 1914–19.

Nauss, K.M., Phua, C.-C., Ambrogi, L. and Newberne, P.M. (1985). Immunological changes during progressive stages of vitamin A deficiency in the rat. *J. Nutr.* **115**, 109–18.

Pasulka, P.S., Bistrian, B.R., Benotti, P.N. and Blackburn, G.L. (1986). The risks of surgery in obese patients. *Ann. Intern. Med.* **104**, 540–6.

Prasad, A.S., Meftah, S., Abdallah, J. *et al.* (1988). Serum thymulin in human zinc deficiency. *J. Clin. Invest.* **82**, 1202–10.

Purtilo, D.T. and Connor, D.H. (1975). Fatal infections in protein–calorie malnourished children with thymolymphatic atrophy. *Arch. Dis. Child.* **50**, 149–52.

Robson, L.C. and Schwartz, M.R. (1975). Vitamin B6 deficiency and the lymphoid system: effects of vitamin B6 deficiency *in utero* on the immunological competence of the offspring. *Cell. Immunol.* **16**, 145–56.

Robson, L.C. and Schwartz, M.R. (1980). The effects of vitamin B6 deficiency on the lymphoid system and immune responses. In *Vitamin B6 Metabolism and Role in Growth*, ed. G.P. Tryfiates, pp. 205–22, Food Nutrition Press, Westport, Connecticut.

Scrimshaw, N.S., Taylor, C.E. and Gordon, J.E. (1968). *Interactions of Nutrition and Infection*. World Health Organization, Geneva.

Simon, J. (1845). *A Physiological Essay on the Thymus Gland.* Renshaw, London, pp. 1–100.

Smythe, P.M., Brerton-Stiles, G.G., Grace, H.J. *et al.* (1971). Thymolymphatic deficiency and depression of cell-mediated immunity in protein–calorie malnutrition. *Lancet* **ii**, 939–43.

Sudhakaran, L. and Chandra, R.K. (1990). Vitamin B6 and immune regulation. *Ann. NY Acad. Sci.* 404–23.

Suskind, R. (ed.) (1977). *Malnutrition and the Immune Response.* Raven Press, New York.

Tomkins, A. (1981). Nutritional status and severity of diarrhoea among pre-school children in rural Nigeria. *Lancet* **i**: 860–2.

Victora, C.G., Barros, F.C., Kirkwood, B.R. and Vaughan, J.P. (1990). Pneumonia, diarrhoea, and growth in the first 4 y of life: a longitudinal study of 5914 urban Brazilian children. *Am. J. Clin. Nutr.* **52**, 391–6.

Vyas, D. and Chandra, R.K. (1983). Thymic factor activity, lymphocyte stimulation response and antibody-forming cells in copper deficiency. *Nutr. Res.* **3**, 343–50.

Vyas, D. and Chandra, R.K. (1984). Functional implications of iron deficiency. In *Iron Nutrition in Infancy and Childhood*, ed. A. Stekel, pp. 45–59, Raven Press, New York.

Wade, S., Bleiberg, F.K., Moose, A. *et al.* (1985). Thymulin (Zn-facteur thymique sérique) activity in anorexia nervosa patients. *Am. J. Clin. Nutr.* **41**, 275–80.

Watson, R.R. (ed.) (1984). *Nutrition, Disease Resistance, and Immune Function*. Marcel Dekker, New York.

Watson, R.R., McMurray, D.N., Martin, P. and Reyes, M.A. (1985). Effect of age, malnutrition and renutrition on free secretory components and IgA in secretions. *Am. J. Clin. Nutr.* **41**, 281–8.

Winick, M., Andrassy, R.J., Armstrong, D. *et al.* (1989). Guidelines for nutrition support in AIDS. *Nutrition* **5**, 39–46.

Acquired Immune Deficiency Syndrome

70: Paediatric Acquired Immune Deficiency Syndrome

T.A. Calvelli, M.J. Sicklick and A. Rubinstein

History

At about the same time that Kaposi's sarcoma and *Pneumocystis carinii* pneumonia (PCP) were seen in homosexual males, increasing numbers of children were referred to our immunology service for an apparent congenital immune deficiency. These children had recurrent bacterial infections, an interstitial pneumonitis, diarrhoea and failure to thrive. Immune evaluation showed decreased mitogenic responses (primarily to pokeweed mitogen), as well as a remarkable hypergammaglobulinaemia. There was no evidence of an immune deficiency linked to previously described *in utero* infections, and the immunological profile of these children did not fit any of the known congenital immunodeficiencies. These turned out to be the first cases of paediatric acquired immune deficiency syndrome (AIDS) (Gupta *et al.* 1982; Rubinstein *et al.* 1983). The number of children infected with the AIDS virus (human immunodeficiency virus — HIV) has increased dramatically since that time.

Definition

Paediatric AIDS has been defined by the Centers for Disease Control (CDC), Atlanta, Georgia, for epidemiological surveys. Because of limited clinical and laboratory data, the initial definition was narrow and required documentation of certain opportunistic infections (e.g. PCP) or malignancies (e.g. Kaposi's sarcoma). With time, the definition has been broadened to include an increased roster of diagnostic infections, malignancies and intercurrent syndromes. The most current CDC case definition encompasses almost the entire spectrum of HIV infection in children, ranging from the asymptomatic stage, to full-blown AIDS with opportunistic infection leading to severe debilitation and death (Table 70.1).

Table 70.1. Classification of human immunodeficiency virus infection in children

Class P-0. Indeterminate infection
Class P-1. Asymptomatic infection
Subclass A. Normal immune function
Subclass B. Abnormal immune function
Subclass C. Immune function not tested
Class P-2. Symptomatic infection
Subclass A. Non-specific findings
Subclass B. Progressive neurological disease
Subclass C. Lymphoid interstitial pneumonitis
Subclass D. Secondary infectious diseases
Category D-1. Specified secondary infectious diseases listed in the CDC surveillance definition for AIDS
Category D-2. Recurrent serious bacterial infections
Category D-3. Other specified secondary infectious diseases
Subclass E. Secondary cancers
Category E-1. Specified secondary cancers listed in the CDC definition for AIDS
Category E-2. Other cancers possibly secondary to HIV infection
Subclass F. Other diseases possibly due to HIV infection

Virology

Human immunodeficiency virus (HIV-1) is the third human retrovirus to be identified. Retroviruses have been studied throughout the twentieth century in conjunction with animal and human cancers. The retrovirus family, formerly known as ribonucleic acid (RNA) tumour viruses and oncornaviruses, is comprised of oncogenic and non-oncogenic subgroups.

In the 1970s, Essex (1975) showed that feline leukaemia virus (FeLV), which caused malignant transformation of feline leucocytes, aplasias and an immune deficiency (Hardy 1982), could be transmitted horizontally among unrelated cats in a household. In 1970, Temin and Mizutani (1970) and Baltimore (1970) simultaneously reported the discovery of reverse transcriptase, the retroviral enzyme capable of synthesizing a deoxyribonucleic acid (DNA) molecule from the virus genomic RNA template. This discovery was substantially facilitated by the development of efficient culture methods, making possible the long-term *in vitro* growth of animal cells, particularly those of haemotological origin. Human cells, however, remained notoriously refractory to extended growth in culture. The identification of a factor capable of stimulating growth of human T lymphocytes *in vitro* (T cell growth factor, now known at interleukin 2) (Poiesz *et al.* 1980a) made possible the first isolation of retrovirus from human cells. Human T cell lymphotrophic virus type 1 (HTLV-1), isolated from cells of a patient with a malignancy of mature CD4 +ve T lymphocytes (Poiesz *et al.* 1980b), has since been unequivocally associated with related strains of adult T cell leukaemia (ATL) (Catovsky *et al.* 1984; Gallo *et al.* 1982, 1983; Hanaoka *et al.* 1982; Popovic *et al.* 1983). A second human retrovirus, HTLV-2, was isolated in 1982 from a patient with hairy cell leukaemia (Kalyanaraman *et al.* 1982). These two human retroviruses shared a tropism for human T lymphocytes, particularly those expressing the CD4 antigen on their surface.

In 1983, Robert C. Gallo, National Cancer Institute (NCI), National Institutes of Health (NIH) (Gallo *et al.* 1983) and Luc Montagnier (the Pasteur Institute) (Barre-Sinoussi *et al.* 1983) independently reported the isolation of a human retrovirus associated with leucocytes from patients with AIDS. The Gallo isolate was initially named HTLV-3, as next in the sequence of isolates from his laboratory, and the Paris isolate was designated LAV (lymphadenopathy-associated virus). The most troubling aspects of assignment of the AIDS-associated retrovirus to the HTLV family were absence of evidence for a capacity to induce malignant transformation and differing morphology of extracellular virions. Infection of cells with the AIDS-associated virus caused death and/or pathology rather than cancerous transformation (Gallo and Wong-Staal 1985; Ho *et al.* 1987; Fauci 1988), and virions resembled lentiviruses (e.g. visna; equine infectious anaemia virus) (Gonda *et al.* 1985) rather than type C (e.g. murine leukaemia virus; FeLV; HTLV-1) retroviruses.

As more sequence data emerged, it became clear that these AIDS-associated retroviruses did in fact share greater genomic homology with the lentiviruses, or 'slow' viruses, than with HTLV-1 and HTLV-2 (Chiu *et al.* 1985; Gonda *et al.* 1985, 1986; Sonigo *et al.* 1985). The lentiviruses, associated with slowly developing, progressive multi-system disease occurring primarily in sheep, horses and goats, are characterized by restricted viral expression and latency of disease (Haase 1986). Human immunodeficiency virus is now, by international agreement, the accepted nomenclature for human AIDS-associated retroviruses. As a member of the lentivirus subfamily. HIV shares a number of properties with other members of this group: (i) latency of disease (Haase 1975); (ii) virion morphology; (iii) similar genome size (9–10 kb); (iv) significant homologies in nucleotide and amino acid sequences (particularly in conserved gag–pol regions) (Gonda *et al.* 1985; Stephens *et al.* 1986); (v) similar size of envelope glycoproteins; (vi) cytopathic effects in culture (Haase *et al.* 1982; Gendelman *et al.* 1986; Lairmore *et al.* 1987); (vii) high incidence of neurological complications *in vivo* (Haase *et al.* 1982; Levy and Bredesen 1988); (viii) restriction of number of infected cells *in vivo*; (ix) a *trans*-activating regulatory element (Arya *et al.* 1985; Hess *et al.* 1985); (x) a complex pattern of transcription (Davis *et al.* 1987); (xi) an Mg^{2+} rather than an Mn^{2+} cation requirement for its reverse transcriptase (Hoffman *et al.* 1985); and (xii) high genetic variability (Clements *et al.* 1980; Shaw *et al.* 1984; Wong-Staal *et al.* 1985a; Alizon *et al.* 1986; Hahn *et al.* 1986; Payne *et al.* 1987; Stanley *et al.* 1987).

The two human immunodeficiency lentiviruses identified to date, HIV-1 and HIV-2, probably diverged from a common retrovirus ancestor (Smith *et al.* 1988). Human immunodeficiency virus 2, originally isolated from individuals in west Africa (Clavel *et al.* 1987), is more closely related to a simian T lymphotrophic retrovirus (simian immunodeficiency virus (SIV)) which induces an AIDS-like syndrome in non-human primates (Daniel *et al.* 1985; Letvin *et al.* 1985; Henderson *et al.* 1988). Although HIV-2 infection is most prevalent in West Africa, it has recently spread to Western Europe. Since only HIV-1 is currently clearly associated with AIDS in the paediatric population, discussion will be limited to that virus.

Morphologically, HIV-1 resembles the ungulate lentiviruses: a 100 nm diameter spheroid comprised of a proteolipid bilayer 'envelope' containing a central electron-dense bar-shaped core comprised of the virion RNA, reverse transcriptase and core proteins. Human immunodeficiency virus structural proteins are encoded by the three genes shared with other members of the retrovirus family: gag, env and pol. The major envelope component (gp120) makes up knob-like projections on the external virion surface (Takahashi *et al.* 1989), and is responsible for the T cell tropism of HIV (Dalgleish *et al.* 1984; Klatzmann *et al.* 1984; McDougal *et al.* 1985, 1986). High-avidity binding of gp120 to the CD4 molecule on the surface of helper T lymphocytes (and other cells expressing surface CD4) is the first step in the HIV infection cycle. Internalization appears to be mediated by the envelope transmembrane glycoprotein gp41, which provides an anchor for gp120 and effects membrane fusion via its hydrophobic N terminus (Veronese *et al.* 1985; Brasseur *et al.* 1988). The internal components of HIV virions are cleavage products of a precursor (p55) coded for by the gag gene (Robey *et al.* 1985). Adjacent to the inner surface of the envelope is p17, which has partial amino acid sequence homology with human thymosine-α-l (Sarin *et al.* 1986; Naylor *et al.* 1987). The major gag protein, p24, as well as p7 and p9, is found in the cylindrical core of mature virions. Multiple molecules of the pol gene product, an RNA-dependent DNA-polymerase (reverse transcriptase) (Hoffman *et al.* 1985; Veronese *et al.* 1986), are associated with two identical single-stranded molecules of genomic RNA within the core.

The infectious cycle of HIV involves a series of complex interactions between virus and cell. The first phase of infection occurs when gp120 binds to CD4 on the cell surface and the virus envelope fuses with the cell membrane. This 'uncoating' process results in emptying of the viral RNA and proteins into the cytoplasm. The second phase of the cycle is initiated when reverse transcriptase makes a DNA copy (complementary DNA (cDNA)) of the viral RNA. A second DNA copy is transcribed, yielding circularized double-stranded DNA (the 'provirus') capable of entering the nucleus of the cell. A third viral enzyme, an integrase, splices HIV proviral DNA into the cellular genomic DNA, where it remains for the life of the cell. The fate of the integrated viral genome is controlled by a complex network of at least six regulatory genes, some of which appear to be unique to HIV: tat, rev, nef, vif, vpr and vpu (Fig. 70.1) (Gallo *et al.* 1988). Each regulatory gene codes for a protein which can interact with a specific sequence of HIV cDNA nucleotides to up-regulate (Arya *et al.* 1985) or down-regulate (Luciw *et al.* 1987; Ahmad and Venkatesan 1988) virus replication and generation of new HIV particles.

Human immunodeficiency virus-infected cells can harbour the integrated provirus cryptically without producing new virions (latent infection),

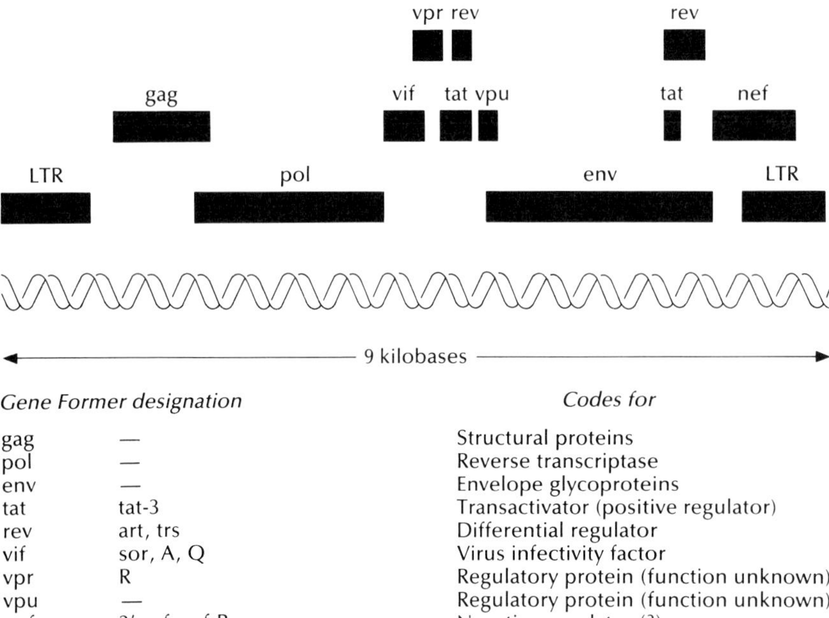

Gene	*Former designation*	*Codes for*
gag	—	Structural proteins
pol	—	Reverse transcriptase
env	—	Envelope glycoproteins
tat	tat-3	Transactivator (positive regulator)
rev	art, trs	Differential regulator
vif	sor, A, Q	Virus infectivity factor
vpr	R	Regulatory protein (function unknown)
vpu	—	Regulatory protein (function unknown)
nef	3′ orf, orf-B	Negative regulator (?)

Fig. 70.1. Structure of the HIV-1 genome.

due at least in part to feedback repression of viral replication by nef and/or rev proteins. Activation of the infected cell (e.g. stimulation of T lymphocytes by antigen), with consequent transcription of the cellular DNA, initiates the third phase of the infectious cycle: replication of the HIV genome and active production of virions. The most potent positive regulator operative in this phase is the tat gene or *trans*-activator (Arya *et al.* 1985; Dayton *et al.* 1986; Rosen *et al.* 1986; Wright *et al.* 1986), which is essential for HIV replication and amplifies virus expression up to 500-fold. The rev gene product acts in concert with tat, differentially influencing regulatory and structural genes, and selectively controlling whether regulatory proteins or virion components are produced (Feinberg *et al.* 1986; Knight *et al.* 1987; Hammarskjold *et al.* 1989). The positive effect of rev on production of virus components, combined with negative feedback of rev to suppress nef action, may modulate HIV disease clinically by controlling the switch from latent to active infection. In addition, interactions of the tat–rev–nef regulatory network could determine whether and when HIV-infected individuals present with low-level symptomatology or with rapidly progressive fulminant disease. The majority of infants infected with HIV pre- or perinatally, present with symptoms in the first year of life, rather than exhibiting the lengthy latent phase of disease seen in adults. Whether this is due to the timing of infection during gestation, to the immunological immaturity of the new-born or to differences in tat–rev–nef interactions in congenitally infected infants is unknown.

Following activation of an infected cell, HIV proviral DNA is transcribed into RNA and the viral RNA is translated into virion proteins. Some HIV proteins undergo post-translational modification (e.g. myristylation of p17, glycosylation of gp160) mediated by cellular enzymes (Sarngadharan *et al.* 1987; Kozarsky *et al.* 1989; Pal *et al.* 1989). Viral RNA, reverse transcriptase and precursor polyproteins migrate to cell surface for assembly of new virions. Structural components aggregate at points where the gp120/gp41 HIV envelope complex has been inserted into the cell membrane. As proteases cleave the gag and env precursors to yield the final core and envelope proteins, two molecules of viral RNA associate with the nascent virion. During this process, the cell membrane gradually bulges outward at the site of virus assembly and formation for free virus particles is completed by 'budding' of completed virions from the cell surface. The ability of free virus to infect cells is influenced by the product of another regulatory gene, vif (Fisher *et al.* 1987; Strebel *et al.* 1987), prior to budding. Although the mechanism by which the vif protein enhances virus infectivity is unknown, deletion of the vif gene results in formation of particles capable of binding to, but not infecting, target cells (Strebel *et al.* 1987). Thus, the virulence of free HIV particles from infected individuals, and undoubtedly cell-free transmission of the virus, could be influenced by mutations in vif. This point is of potential importance for pre- and perinatal HIV infection, since therapeutic modalities directed against vif would only be applicable if cell-free transmission from an infected mother were the primary mechanism of infection.

Epidemiology

Human immunodeficiency virus has been cultured from blood and other body fluids, including saliva, semen, breast milk, tears, urine and stool. To date, the vast majority of adult AIDS cases in the United States have been transmitted through blood, blood products and semen.

Current estimates for paediatric HIV disease indicate that approximately 77% were infected by maternal–fetal transmission; 13% via transfusion of blood products; and 5% during the treatment of haemophilia or other bleeding disorders. In a small number, the risk factors have not been satisfactorily determined (Wiznia and Rubinstein 1988). As screening of blood for HIV antibody became more effective, the percentage of children newly infected via blood and blood products decreased, while an increasing role was ascribed to materno-fetal transmission. Preventing HIV infection in women of childbearing age is therefore of paramount importance to the control of paediatric AIDS. In order to achieve this goal, it is important to understand more clearly the risk factors for infection in women. These factors vary geographically.

In Africa, most women are infected through heterosexual contact (Melbye *et al.* 1986). In Europe and the United States, however, the vast majority of seropositive women were infected through drug use (Rogers *et al.* 1987; European Collaborative Study 1988; Italian Multicenter Study 1988). A recent report showed that an increasing number of women are being infected with HIV through heterosexual contact with high-risk partners (Wiznia *et al.* 1988). As a result, these women frequently do not consider themselves at high risk for HIV infection, let alone for delivering an HIV +ve infant. The overall incidence of HIV +ve babies is increasing rapidly. In November 1987, the incidence of cord blood positivity in New York City was 1 in 61, and in the Bronx, a borough of New York City, 1 in 43 (Novick *et al.* 1988). More recent surveys in the Bronx demonstrated the seropositivity of cord bloods to range from 4 to 8%.

The rate of transmission from a positive mother to her offspring has been estimated to range from 12.5 to 35% (Rubinstein and Bernstein 1986; Mok *et al.* 1987). It appears that after a mother delivers one HIV-infected child, the odds shift toward the higher transmission rate. A variety of postulated, though unconfirmed, factors could affect the rate of maternal–fetal transmission. These may include maternal viral load, overall maternal health, intercurrent infections, maternal nutrition, maternal drug use and possibly genetic predisposition. A potential association between maternal antibody responses to HIV-1 gp120, and materno-fetal transmission of HIV has been suggested by several studies. Broliden *et al.* (1989) and Rossi *et al.* (1989) reported that 31% and 46%, respectively, of healthy uninfected neonates born to HIV-infected mothers, had circulating maternal IgG reactive with HIV-1 gp120 'hypervariable loop' sequences which include the 'principal neutralizing domain' (PND) of the virus (Javaherian *et al.* 1989). Another investigation found that the absence of high titre maternal antibodies to HIV-1 gp120 positively correlated with increased risk of HIV infection in infants (Goedert *et al.* 1989b). We have demonstrated a positive correlation between the presence of high affinity/avidity maternal IgG reactive with the hypervariable gp120 'loop' PND of the HTLV-IIIMN strain of HIV-1, and absence of pre-/perinatal transmission (Devash *et al.* 1990). There continues however, to be debate regarding a global correlation between the presence or absence of maternal anti-gp120 antibody and maternal–fetal transmission of HIV. Another study failed to confirm a statistically significant correlation between the presence of maternal anti-gp120 MN-PND and maternal–fetal transmission (Parekh *et al.* 1991). Yet, in more recent investigations, we and others have extended these findings, confirming correlation between absence of maternal–fetal HIV-1 transmission and presence of maternal high affinity IgG reactive with the MN-PND in *some* but *not all* populations (unpublished observations; Rossi, pers. comm.). It is becoming apparent that fetal infection by an 'escape mutant' of HIV-1, against which the mother does not have high affinity antibodies, can occur. Recently, Wolinsky *et al.* (1992) demonstrated that a woman may be infected with several MN strains of HIV-1 during pregnancy, with only selective transplacental transfer of the strain infecting the fetus. Absence of a protective maternal antibody response to this particular strain would theoretically increase the potential for fetal infection. It is hoped that extension of these findings will lead to identification of reliable predictors of *in utero* transmission and avenues for potential therapeutic intervention. Most puzzling to the understanding of maternofetal transmission are the reports of discordant HIV infection in twins with/without identical genetic background (Rubinstein 1986). While data indicate that HIV does, in fact, cross the placental barrier during pregnancy, the mechanism by which intact infectious virions are transferred to the fetus occurs has not yet been delineated. The placental architecture in higher mammals prevents direct mixing of maternal and fetal blood. Exchange of both soluble and cellular elements between mother and fetus has, however, been demonstrated (Adinolfi and Gorvette 1974; Olding 1979; Zilliacus *et al.* 1975; Lala *et al.* 1983), indicating that the placental 'barrier' is permeable to some extent. The trophoblastic tissue of human placental chorionic villi has the closest contact with the maternal blood saturating the intervillous space. Several cell populations comprising the trophoblastic tissue are potential targets for HIV. The CD4 antigen has been shown to be expressed on a subpopulation of trophoblastic cells (Maury *et al.* 1989). This study also suggested that these CD4-bearing cells might be cytotrophoblasts, which are morphologically and antigenically similar to Langerhans' cells, which are susceptible to HIV infection. Located in the connective tissue stroma adjacent to the placental trophoblastic tissue, Hofbauer cells represent an additional potential HIV target. These large macrophages express both the CD4 antigen cell surface Fc receptors (McNabb *et al.* 1975; Matre and Johnson 1977; Down *et al.* 1989). While Fc receptor expression by trophoblastic cells is believed to play a role in transplacental transfer of maternal IgG to the fetus (Matre and Johnson 1977), it could potentially facilitate Fc-receptor-mediated uptake of HIV (Gendelman *et al.* 1985; Ho *et al.* 1986; Bender *et al.* 1988; Jouault *et al.* 1989) by placental cells.

Evidence that HIV is transmitted *in utero* includes: (i) identification of HIV genomic DNA in abortuses (Lyman *et al.* 1987, 1988); (ii) lack of decreased infection rate in babies delivered by caesarean section (Cowan *et al.* 1984); (iii) AIDS embryopathy in the neonatal period (Marion *et al.* 1986); and (iv) culture of HIV from cord blood (Rubinstein and Bernstein 1986) or fetal tissues (Di Maria *et al.* 1986). In addition, the time to diagnosis of perinatally acquired AIDS has a median of 9 months, whereas the mean time to diagnosis in transfusion-related AIDS is 17 months (Rogers *et al.* 1987). This implies early infection with likely *in utero* acquisition of HIV, or an unusually short incubation period.

A study of 100 sets of twins and one set of triplets born to HIV-1 infected women suggested that the first-born of dizygotic twins may be at higher risk for HIV infection than the second-born twin (Goedert *et al.* 1991). This study appeared to indicate that a considerable proportion of HIV transmission may occur at delivery. No correlation, however, was found between infection and invasive medical/surgical procedures such as use of scalp electrodes. Moreover, a substantial proportion of both the first- and second-born twins delivered by caesarian section, were found to be infected with HIV.

Recent data also suggests that HIV transmission occurs perinatally. Ehrnst *et al.* (1991) have, for example, shown that despite the fact that HIV was cultured from peripheral blood mononuclear cells or from plasma of 83% of HIV-infected women, it could not be cultured from their newborn's blood at birth. Human immunodeficiency virus could be recovered from the blood of all infected infants within the first 6 months of life, however. Based on this finding, the authors suggest that there is no consistent spread of HIV across the placenta during maternal viraemic episodes, and that in most cases, transmission occurs close to, or at, delivery. Similar temporal observations were made using the polymerase chain reaction (PCR) technique, or HIV p24 antigen capture assay, as a measure of viraemia. Of all HIV-infected infants born to infected mothers, about 50% tested positive at birth with these techniques. Moreover, in some infants, an acute viraemic syndrome could be documented at a few months of age, also suggesting infection at or near delivery. However, the delayed detection of HIV in the peripheral blood of neonates may also be explained by preferential homing of the virus to lymphoid organs rather than to the periphery. The European Collaborative Study has also shown that transmission was somewhat higher with vaginal deliveries in which episiotomy, scalp electrodes, forceps or vacuum extractors were used, but only in centres where these procedures were not routine. So far no study has shown a statistically significant benefit of Caesarian sections. Taken together, it appears that transmission may occur throughout pregnancy, including the time of delivery; the predominant time of transmission has however, yet to be determined. The development of successful strategies to prevent transmission rests largely on defining when and how perinatal HIV transmission occurs (Pizzo and Butler 1991).

Several cases of breast-milk-transmitted AIDS have been reported. All occurred in circumstances wherein the mother was transfused with an infected unit of blood during the post-partum period (Ziegler *et al.* 1985). Infectious HIV has been isolated by culture from breast milk. Recently, Van de Perre *et al.* (1988; 1991) demonstrated the presence of HIV-specific immunoglobulin G (IgG), IgA and IgM antibodies in the breast milk of infected mothers. It is not clear, however, whether these antibodies have any protective role.

Although the risk of transmission from saliva has not been established, one case of seroconversion has been reported following a human bite (Wahn *et al.* 1986).

Finally, at least one case of transmission through child abuse has been confirmed (Rubinstein 1986): a 5-year-old male was sodomized by his HIV-infected father and subsequently developed AIDS. More recently, a 10-year-old child of an HIV-negative mother died of HIV disease with no history of transfusion of blood or blood products. Sexual abuse is a suspected mode of transmission in this case.

There is no evidence that normal day-to-day intra-household contact of uninfected children with HIV-infected children constitutes a risk factor. Human immunodeficiency virus −ve children who shared table food, utensils, toothbrushes and beds with HIV +ve siblings did not seroconvert (Rubinstein *et al.* 1984a; Sicklick *et al.* 1985).

Immunopathology

Human immunodeficiency virus preferentially infects cells expressing the CD4 antigen, due to high-avidity binding of gp120 to the CD4 molecule. The CD4 molecule is expressed on the surface of a variety of cells, including helper T lymphocytes and cells of macrophage−monocyte lineage (the Langerhans cells of the skin, dendritic cells in lymph nodes, Kuppfer cells in the liver, pulmonary alveolar cells and glial cells in the central nervous system). In the peripheral circulation, the primary target of HIV is the helper (T4 or CD4 +ve) lymphocyte. The devastating effects of HIV infection on the immune system result from the central position of the CD4 +ve lymphocyte in the immunoregulatory network. The absolute lymphopenia, which occurs frequently in infected adults, is the result of CD4 +ve lymphocyte depletion. A variety of mechanisms for the cytocidal effects of HIV have been proposed: (i) lysis of infected cells by 'explosive' virus budding accompanying cellular proliferation (Zagury *et al.* 1986); (ii) fusion of an infected cell with surface HIV gp120 with uninfected CD +ve cells, resulting in syncytium formation and cell death (Lifson *et al.* 1986); (iii) accumulation of unintegrated HIV cDNA in the cytoplasm of infected cells (Wong-Staal *et al.* 1985): (iv) antibody-dependent cell-mediated cytotoxicity (ADCC) mediated by binding of anti-gp120 to the surface of infected cells (Lyerly *et al.* 1987a, 1987b; Weinhold *et al.* 1989); (v) ADCC caused by reaction of autoantibody directed against a modified 'self' antigen on the surface of infected cells (Rubinstein *et al.* 1985; Kowalski *et al.* 1989); (vi) direct ADCC mediated by CD16 +ve natural killer/killer (NK/K) cells having surface-bound anti-gp120 (Tyler *et al.* 1989); and (vii) cytotoxic T-cell-mediated cytolysis of infected cells (Siliciano *et al.* 1988; Weinhold *et al.* 1988). Paradoxical effects on the immune system *in vitro* can be caused by HIV gp120 alone. Incubation with purified gp120 can cause activation of resting T cells (Kornfeld *et al.* 1988), and yet suppression of mitogen- (Mann *et al.* 1987), antigen- and anti-CD3-driven T cell proliferation (Weinhold *et al.* 1989).

Depletion of CD4 +ve lymphocytes, sometimes coupled with an increase in circulating suppressor (T8) T cells, results in an imbalance in the helper/

suppressor cell ratio (T4/T8 ratio) in HIV-infected children (Oleske *et al.* 1983, Rubinstein *et al.* 1983; Scott *et al.* 1984; Thomas *et al.* 1984; Pahwa *et al.* 1986a; Rubinstein 1986; see Table 70.2). A decreased or reversed T4/T8 ratio is common in both adult and paediatric AIDS, although most infants pre- or perinatally infected with HIV typically do not show markedly reversed ratios in the first year of life. Other manifestations of deficits in T cell function in congenitally infected children include decreased production of thymulin (Incefy *et al.* 1986; Pahwa *et al.* 1986a; Rubinstein *et al.* 1986a), interleukin 2 and interferon (Rubinstein 1986). Decreased thymulin may be the result of infection of the fetal thymus. Human immunodeficiency virus has been detected in some fetal tissues, as early as the 12th–15th week of gestation (Rubinstein 1986; Sprecher *et al.* 1986), and HIV antigen has been detected in thymuses of infected children (Lapointe *et al.* 1985; Joshi *et al.* 1986). Infectious HIV, demonstrated by co-cultivation, has been isolated from both fetal and infant thymus glands (Jovaisas *et al.* 1985; Rubinstein 1986; Calvelli and Rubinstein 1990). Histopathological evaluation of biopsy and autopsy thymic tissues from HIV-infected children has shown that the gland, frequently small in size, often exhibits depletion of lymphocytic elements, and cortico-medullary differentiation may be obscured by infiltrates of mononuclear leucocytes or plasmacytes (Joshi and Oleske 1985; Joshi *et al.* 1986; Rubinstein *et al.* 1986a; Savino *et al.* 1986). In one study, serum thymosine-α-1, measured by radioimmunoassay, was found to be elevated in 16 of 24 HIV-infected children studied (Rubinstein *et al.* 1986a). This detected elevation was, however, later found to be due to cross-reactivity of thymosine-α-1 with HIV p17, rather than to over-production of the hormone (Sarin *et al.* 1986; Naylor *et al.* 1987).

Table 70.2. Immunological defects in human immunodeficiency virus-infected children

B cell abnormalities
Defective antibody production (hypergammaglobulinaemia or hypogammaglobulinaemia)
Decreased *in vitro* lymphoproliferative responses to B cell mitogens (pokeweed mitogen (PWM); *Staphylococcus aureus*) and antigens (e.g. tetanus; *Candida*; streptokinase)
Defective *in vivo* primary and secondary B cell responses (e.g. ΦX 174; Pneumovax; tetanus toxoid)
Defective IgM–IgG class switching
Elevated circulating immune complexes
Increased peripheral B lymphocytes

Other abnormalities
Reversed CD4/CD8 ratio
Autoimmune phenomena (e.g. antinuclear antibodies, Coombs antibodies)
Decreased *in vitro* lymphoproliferative responses to T cell mitogens (e.g. phytohaemagglutin (PHA); Concanavalin A typically occurs later than decreased responsiveness to B cell mitogens)
Decreased thymulin

While the hallmark of HIV infection in adults is depletion of CD4 +ve lymphocytes, congenitally infected infants more commonly exhibit defective humoral (B-cell-mediated) immunity (Lane *et al.* 1983; Bernstein *et al.* 1985a, b; Pahwa *et al.* 1986b, 1987). Maturation of B-cell-mediated immunity, accompanied by development of the capacity to produce antibodies, occurs after birth and is reliant upon lymphokine signals produced by functionally intact helper T cells. In addition to direct cytocidal effects of HIV on infected CD4 +ve lymphocytes, functional abnormalities in helper activity also occur (Hoxie *et al.* 1986; Diamond *et al.* 1988), indirectly affecting B cell, suppressor T cell and NK cell functions. Linette *et al.* (1988) recently demonstrated that HIV-1-infected T cells exhibit selective impairment of membrane signalling. Stimulation of the T cells by antibody to the CD3 surface antigen failed to elicit a proliferative response, suggesting that HIV-infected T cells are unable to respond to antigen signalling mediated by the CD3/antigen receptor. Such indirect effects are particularly evident in infants congenitally infected with HIV, with B cell defects able to be identified earlier than T cell defects (Bernstein *et al.* 1985a,b; Pahwa *et al.* 1986b, 1987; Rubinstein 1986). Their consequent compromised ability to produce specific antibody results in a high frequency of serious or recurrent bacterial infection. Such deficits in B cell function are reflected in depressed *in vitro* lymphoproliferative responses to T-cell-dependent (pokeweed mitogen (PWM)) and T-cell-independent (*Staphylococcus aureus* Cowan A (SAC)) mitogens, as well as to panels of common specific antigens (e.g. tetanus, *Candida*, streptokinase) (Bernstein *et al.* 1985a, b; Pahwa *et al.* 1986b; Borokowsky *et al.* 1987a). In addition, suppression of *in vivo* primary and secondary B cell responses in congenitally infected children has been demonstrated by immunization with ΦX 174, a T-cell-dependent neo-antigen, pneumococcal polysaccharide antigen (Pneumovax) and tetanus toxoid (Bernstein *et al.* 1985b). Primary responses were blunted, secondary responses were decreased and IgM–IgG class switch was absent in most cases.

Despite defective ability to mount specific antibody responses *in vivo*, infants and children with HIV infection frequently exhibit abnormally elevated levels of serum immunoglobulin (IgG, IgA, IgM, IgD) (Lane *et al.* 1983; Bernstein *et al.* 1985b). Hypergammaglobulinaemia resulting from polyclonal B cell activation frequently occurs prior to other identifiable immunological abnormalities (Bernstein *et al.* 1985b; Rubinstein 1986; Cavelli and Rubinstein 1990). Both HIV particles and gp120 alone in the absence of infectious HIV particles have been reported to induce B cell activation *in vitro* (Schnittman *et al.* 1986). Polyclonal B cell activation may also be caused by HIV gp120-induced over-production of B cell stimulatory factor (BSF), as demonstrated by a recent study (Nakajima *et al.* 1989). Whether gp120 contributes to the *in vivo* over-production of immunoglobulin observed so frequently in paediatric patients is not known. In our experience with over 300 HIV-infected infants, up to 3% exhibit hypogammaglobulinaemia in the first months of life; later, these infants may later become hypergammaglobulinaemic.

HIV-infected infants with elevated serum immunoglobulin levels also frequently exhibit high elevated levels of circulating immune complexes (CIC), although infants with normal or decreased serum immunoglobulin concentration can also have increased CIC (Rubinstein *et al.* 1983; Scott *et al.* 1984; Bernstein *et al.* 1985a; Rubinstein 1986; Ellaurie *et al.* 1988; Falloon 1989; Calvelli and Rubinstein 1990; Ellaurie *et al.* 1990a). The Raji cell assay has shown far greater sensitivity in detecting CIC in HIV-infected children, than the C1q assay, presumably because CIC in these children form in antigen excess and therefore bind complement poorly (Rubinstein 1986; Ellaurie *et al.* 1988; Calvelli and Rubinstein 1990; Ellaurie *et al.* 1990b). The Raji cell assay, which is capable of binding CIC by both complement and Fc receptors, is not reliant only on the presence of complement in CIC, and can therefore detect complexes formed in antigen excess.

Studying 55 congenitally HIV-infected children (ages 3 months to 9 years), we found that 60% had HIV protein(s) (p17; p24; gp120) associated with their CIC (HIV-Ag-CIC) (Ellaurie *et al.* 1990b). The concentration of CIC-associated HIV protein showed positive correlation with disease stage, and was predictive of disease course.

Other manifestations of defective humoral immunity include: (i) IgG subclass deficiencies, predominantly IgG2 and IgG4 (Rubinstein *et al.* 1983; Church *et al.* 1984; Rubinstein 1986; Honda *et al.* 1987); (ii) isohaemagglutinin deficiency (Blanche *et al.* 1986); and (iii) autoimmune phenomena (e.g. antinuclear antibodies, Coombs antibodies, anti-T-cell antibodies) (Scott *et al.* 1984; Rubinstein *et al.* 1985; Rubinstein 1986; Blanche *et al.* 1986).

Immune system activation has been described for both paediatric and adult patients with HIV-1 disease (Grieco *et al.* 1984; Amadori *et al.* 1989; Fahey *et al.* 1990; Prince *et al.* 1990; Calvelli *et al.* 1991). Recent studies have implicated cellular activation in disease progression (Bogner *et al.* 1988; Chan *et al.* 1990; Fahey *et al.* 1990). Using flow cytometric analysis, we have shown that cell surface markers of cellular activation in infants and children congenitally infected with HIV, show positive correlation with both serum immunoglobulin status (Calvelli *et al.* 1990), and disease stage (Calvelli *et al.* 1991). Human immunodeficiency virus infected infants and children with elevated serum immunoglobulin levels, and in advanced disease state, consistently exhibit increased expression of phenotypic markers of cellular activation (e.g. CD38; HLA-DR) on both T and B lymphocytes. We have found that elevated expression of CD45RO on CD8+ve lymphocytes is a sensitive indicator of advancing disease stage in congenitally HIV-infected children (Calvelli *et al.* 1991).

Elevated serum concentration of soluble markers of cellular activation, has been reported for both HIV-infected adults (Grieco *et al.* 1984; Fuchs *et al.* 1988; Bogner *et al.* 1988; Reddy *et al.* 1989; Fahey *et al.* 1990), and children (Ellaurie and Rubinstein 1990; Chan *et al.* 1990). Beta-2-microglobulin (B2M) and neopterin (Npt) are the most-studied soluble activation markers in serum and urine. These markers may be potentially useful prognostic indicators of disease progression in HIV-infected children (Ellaurie and Rubinstein 1990). We have found that children with persistent serum B2M concentrations greater than 3.0 mg/l showed disease progression; on the other hand, those whose serum B2M levels decreased with time exhibited a stable disease course (Ellaurie and Rubinstein 1990). The concentration of B2M and Npt in serum can overlap significantly at different stages of HIV disease stage in infected children (Chan *et al.* 1990), perhaps due to cellular activation in response to infection with other pathogens secondary to infection with HIV.

The immunopathology resultant from direct and indirect effects of HIV infection of helper T lymphocytes is the most highly noted consequences of infection. The consequence of infection of monocyte–macrophage lineage cells with HIV may be more insidious and ultimately more devastating, since it has the potential of causing pathology in multiple organ systems (Bender *et al.* 1988). Expression of surface CD4 antigen by monocyte–macrophage lineage cells renders them susceptible to HIV infection mediated by gp120–CD4 binding. Alternatively, HIV may enter monocytes/macrophages by Fc-receptor-mediated uptake due to binding of anti-gp120 complexed to whole virus (Takeda *et al.* 1988; Jouault *et al.* 1989). Unlike T cells, monocytes and macrophages only rarely divide, increasing the likelihood of chronic latent infection. Recently, however, expression and replication of HIV in spinal cord macrophages of three adults with AIDS was demonstrated by *in situ* hybridization and immunohistochemistry (Eilbott *et al.* 1989). Macrophages are resident elements of a variety of tissues, including skin, brain, lymph nodes, lung, liver and bone marrow. As such, they may provide a reservoir for HIV within critical tissue compartments (Gendelman *et al.* 1985; Ho *et al.* 1986; Klatzmann and Gluckman 1986; Pauza 1988). For instance, Langerhan cells, the macrophage lineage population found within the epidermis and in certain lymph nodes, have the capacity to present antigen to T cells *in vitro* (Streilen and Bergstresser 1980). They may also be important components in mediating dermatological lesions having immunological aetiology, and can harbour the AIDS virus. No specific pathological condition in children has as yet been associated with HIV infection of Langerhans cells. It is conceivable, however, that compromised ability of these cells to process antigen could contribute to the high incidence of infection with common pathogens in perinatally infected infants. In a similar manner, HIV infection of alveolar macrophages (Gartner *et al.* 1986a) could contribute directly or indirectly to the frequent development of lymphocytic interstitial pneumonitis in these children. Human immunodeficiency virus RNA, as well as the DNA of Epstein–Barr virus (EBV), has been detected in lung tissue from HIV-infected children with lymphoid interstitial pneumonitis, (LIP) (Andiman *et al.* 1985; Fackler *et al.* 1985; Chayt *et al.* 1986; Rubinstein *et al.* 1986; Joshi *et al.* 1987), and production of anti-HIV antibody within the lung has been demonstrated (Resnick *et al.* 1987).

Macrophages also have the ability to traverse blood-vessels and tissue barriers. Infected cells could therefore act as 'Trojan horses', carrying cryptic HIV into tissue compartments, such as the brain, unlikely to be infected by free virions. In fact, children congenitally infected with HIV have a high incidence of neurological complications (Belman *et al.* 1985, 1988; Ultmann *et al.* 1985, 1987; Epstein *et al.* 1987, Pahwa *et al.* 1986a; Rubinstein 1986). The precise mechanism by which HIV infects the central nervous system (CNS) has not yet been elucidated, but at least three possible routes can be hypothesized: (i) HIV-infected macrophages transport the virus from the peripheral circulation across the blood–brain barrier; (ii) CD4 +ve cells may be infected with HIV during fetal life prior to the formation of an intact blood–brain barrier; and (iii) free HIV may infect neuronal cells by entering the brain during fetal life. Human immunodeficiency virus antigens, DNA and RNA have been detected in brain and cerebrospinal fluid (CSF) from infected adults and children (Sharer *et al.* 1986); and infectious HIV has been cultivated from CNS-derived cells. In adults, the primary infected cell populations in the brain appear to be macrophages and glial cells (Epstein *et al.* 1985; Shaw *et al.* 1985; Gartner *et al.* 1986b; Koenig *et al.* 1986). In addition, it has recently been demonstrated that HIV replicates in, and is expressed by, macrophages in the spinal cords of adult AIDS patients with myelopathy (Eilbott *et al.* 1989). There is some evidence for infection of neuronal cells in fetal brain tissue by HIV as early as 14 weeks' gestation (Lyman *et al.* 1988).

Whether the CNS pathology observed in HIV-infected children and adults is caused directly by infection of CNS cells with the virus, or by as yet unidentified secondary mechanisms, is not currently known. However, one postulated mechanism involves the potential action of HIV gp120 on neurons. The gp120 molecule from numerous HIV isolates has partial homology to vasoactive intestinal peptide (VIP) (Ruff *et al.* 1987; Lee *et al.* 1988). Brenneman *et al.* (1988) demonstrated that gp120 could induce neuropathology by blocking the action of VIP, a factor important for the survival of neurones in culture, causing neuronal cell death.

Case definition and disease classification

The original surveillance definition for acquired immune deficiency syndrome (AIDS) formulated by the Centers for Disease Control (CDC) was developed prior to identification of the human immunodeficiency virus (HIV), and delineation of the differences in disease presentation in adults and children. The original CDC definition of AIDS was based on the disease in adults, defined by the spectrum of opportunistic infections (OIs) and malignancies observed in that population. As increasing numbers of infants and children presented with symptoms of an immunodeficiency apparently related to parental or blood-/blood-product-associated risk factors for AIDS, it became clear that the clinical manifestations of this syndrome differed from those of adult AIDS. In 1985 and 1987, the CDC released an additionally revised surveillance definition for HIV infection in children under 13 years of age, which includes an amalgam of virologic and immunologic laboratory criteria (Centers for Disease Control, 1987c), in addition to broader clinical criteria. The clinical criteria have been categorized using a classification system (Table 70.3) comprised of three principal groups based on symptomatology: (1) indefinite infection in young infants under the age of 15 months; (2) asymptomatic infection; and (3) symptomatic infection. While the CDC is considering a surveillance definition and classification system for adults based on CD4 T cell count, development of a CD4 cell count-based system for children would be complicated by the age-dependent variability in CD4 cell percentages and white blood cell count, during the first years of life.

Clinical picture

Approximately half of infected children identified to date have become symptomatic in the first year of life, with 90% diagnosed by the age of 4 (New York State Department of Health 1988). That study also suggested that up to 10% may go undiagnosed until the age of 10. An increasing number of children first presenting with symptoms of HIV infection over 4 years of age, yet apparently pre-perinatally infected, are being seen by our immunology service. It has yet to be determined how many of these 'later-onset disease' are actually related to perinatal infection. Ongoing prospective studies using more sophisticated serological and virological tests will determine the rate of long-term asymptomatic infection in children. In our experience the rate of asymptomatic infection by 6 years of age has been less than 3%.

Table 70.3. Classification of human immunodeficiency virus infection in children

Class P-O. Indeterminate infection

Class P-1. Asymptomatic infection
Subclass A. Normal immune function
Subclass B. Abnormal immune function
Subclass C. Immune function not tested

Class P-2. Symptomatic infection
Subclass A. Non-specific findings
Subclass B. Progressive neurologic disease
Subclass C. Lymphoid interstitial pneumonitis
Subclass D. Secondary infectious diseases
- Category D-1. Specified secondary infectious diseases listed in the CDC surveillance definition for AIDS
- Category D-2. Recurrent serious bacterial infections
- Category D-3. Other specified secondary infectious diseases

Subclass E. Secondary Cancers
- Category E-1. Specified secondary cancers listed in the CDC definition for AIDS
- Category E-2. Other cancers possibly secondary to HIV infection

Subclass F. Other diseases possibly due to HIV infection

Infections

As previously mentioned, HIV-infected children have abnormalities of both cell-mediated and humoral immune systems (Bernstein *et al.* 1985a, b; Pahwa *et al.* 1987). As such, they are susceptible to a variety of pathogens, including common organisms. Organisms frequently causing infections in these children include *Streptococcus pneumoniae*, *Haemophilus influenzae*, *Neisseria meningitidis* and *Salmonella enteritidis* (Bernstein *et al.* 1985a). Of HIV +ve children, 20–76% have had significant bacterial infections (Calvelli and

Rubinstein 1986; New York State Department of Health 1988), often with an atypical disease course. Following successful treatment of an acute bacteraemia or enteritis, carrier states have been noted to develop, especially with non-typhoid *Salmonella* (Wiznia and Rubinstein 1988). In addition, drug-resistant superinfections may occur following a course of antibiotics.

Human immunodeficiency virus +ve children frequently develop either acute or chronic diarrhoea. Aside from the common causes of diarrhoea in children, other agents that must be considered include *Salmonella*, *Mycobacterium avium intracellulare* (MAI), *Cryptosporidium*, cytomegalovirus and *Candida*. *Mycobacterium avium intracellulare* was documented in 11% of paediatric AIDS patients (Rogers *et al*. 1987). Typical symptoms of disseminated MAI include night sweats, fevers, weight loss, diarrhoea and abdominal pain. Examination may reveal hepatosplenomegaly and lymphadenopathy. Suggestive laboratory findings include anaemia and elevated serum alkaline phosphatase. Appropriate diagnostic tests for suspected MAI include blood cultures, liver biopsy and/or bone marrow biopsy.

The clinical presentation of pulmonary pneumocystosis can be quite variable. Usually, an acute respiratory decompensation is noted. The patient presents with tachypnoea, flaring of nostrils, chest wall retractions and fever. Physical examination reveals wheezes and rales. Chest X-ray is either normal or shows a diffuse interstitial pattern. Arterial blood gases reveal marked hypoxia (Rubinstein *et al*. 1986). Isomorphic elevation of serum lactate dehydrogenase may precede or accompany the disease. Rarely, patients present with a subacute or chronic course. Definitive diagnosis usually requires identification of the organism, and should be undertaken whenever the diagnosis is in doubt or when the patient's clinical condition warrants it. In children, bronchoalveolar lavage appears to be safer than an open lung biopsy, without loss of diagnostic sensitivity (Bye *et al*. 1987).

Usual viral childhood illnesses can be devastating in HIV-infected children. Failure to form crusts and prolonged vesiculation during a course of varicella is often an ominous sign. Exposed children should be treated immediately with zoster immune globulin, and with acyclovir at the onset of symptoms. Disseminated herpes zoster can occur, as is well described in other immune deficiencies. There are also reports of fatal rubeola in these children (MMWR 1988b).

Pulmonary lymphoid hyperplasia/lymphoid interstitial pneumonitis complex

Pulmonary lymphoid hyperplasia/lymphoid interstitial pneumonitis (PLH/LIP) occurs in 48% of cases of paediatric AIDS. Associated with hepatosplenomegaly and lymphadenopathy, the usual course of PLH/LIP is subacute or chronic, leading eventually to hypoxia and respiratory failure. These children frequently show clubbing of their fingers similar to that observed in cystic fibrosis. On chest X-ray, multiple nodules (1–5 mm) are visible throughout the lung. The mediastinum is widened with hilar prominence (Rubinstein *et al*. 1986a). Unlike patients with PCP, children with PLH/LIP have a normal or mildly elevated serum LDH. On biopsy, the lung tissue pattern is quite characteristic. In LIP, the lymphoid infiltrates are diffuse in the lung parenchyma. Conversely, in PLH, the nodularity is conspicuous, and the lesions are somewhat localized to the mucosa and wall of the bronchi and bronchioles (Rubinstein *et al*. 1988). The EBV genome has been found in most lung specimens of these patients (Andiman *et al*. 1985; Rubinstein *et al*. 1986a), and it has been postulated that EBV stimulation of intrapulmonary B cells may cause the hyperplasia lymphoid elements.

Neurodevelopmental abnormalities

Developmental delay and microcephaly were noted in the first description of cases of paediatric AIDS (Rubinstein *et al*. 1983). Further longitudinal studies have shown that neurological problems are a major part of HIV disease in both adults and children. In fact, up to 93% of infected children have neurodevelopmental abnormalities. Almost all exhibit some degree of developmental delay, and half have microcephaly. Cognitive defects and spasticity related to bilateral pyramidal tract involvement are also fairly common (Belman *et al*. 1985). In fact, corticospinal tract (CST) signs represent the most frequent manifestation of HIV-associated encephalopathy in children. In contrast to the vacuolar myelopathy of the spinal cord commonly seen in HIV-infected adults, children with AIDS most frequently have CST degeneration (Dickson *et al*. 1989).

There are three major courses of HIV-related neurological complications. Twenty per cent of children develop a progressive encephalopathy resulting in loss of previously attained milestones, pyramidal tract involvement and desocialization. Fifty per cent exhibit a less fulminant course. They may retain previously acquired milestones, but either fail to gain new ones or do so at a slower rate than normal. Their spasticity due to pyramidal tract involvement is less severe, and they may have neurologically stable periods. Eventually, as their overall disease progresses, their neurological deterioration accelerates. The third group, comprising approximately 7% of involved children, shows periods of neurological plateauing, and, at times, some degree of spontaneous improvement (Belman *et al*. 1988).

Computerized tomography scans of the brain reveal cortical atrophy, ventricular enlargement and white matter abnormalities in almost all cases. A significant number have bilateral basal ganglial calcifications that may be detectable at birth. Cerebrospinal fluid examination may be normal, or show elevated protein and/or cell count. Human immunodeficiency virus particles, as well as the p24 core antigen, have been demonstrated in the brains of some of these children (Epstein *et al*. 1987).

Embryopathy

The features of AIDS embryopathy are consistent with fetal infection in the first half of gestation. Microcephaly, a prominent box-like forehead, a flattened nasal bridge and columella, increased intercanthal distance, blue sclerae and long palpebral fissures are characteristic (Marion *et al*. 1986). The embryopathy is not present in all infected children. In those with more pronounced dysmorphic features, clinical symptoms of AIDS typically occur in the first year of life (Marion *et al*. 1987).

Malignancies

Kaposi's sarcoma, well described in adult HIV patients, is extremely rare in paediatric AIDS (Rogers *et al*. 1987). There have been a few reports of Kaposi lesions found in lymph nodes at autopsy (Buck *et al*. 1983). Prelymphomatous conditions involving B cell proliferation have been described by Joshi *et al*. (1987), characterized by pulmonary involvement. B and T cell lymphomas represent the most common malignancy in HIV-infected children; these often spread rapidly to a variety of organs (e.g. lymph nodes, liver, spleen, kidney and bone marrow) (Wiznia and Rubinstein 1988). Central nervous system lymphomas have been observed in a few patients. Despite chemotherapy and radiotherapy, CNS lymphomas tend to progress and are generally fatal within 1 year of diagnosis. In one of our patients, Burkitt's lymphoma of the tongue was noted. In general, malignancies in HIV-infected children are less frequent than in HIV-infected adults.

Other complications

LIVER

It is common to find elevated serum transaminases in children with AIDS, and biopsy reports have shown nodular lymphoid aggregates in the portal triads, cellular damage, and changes suggesting chronic, active hepatitis (Duffy *et al*. 1986).

KIDNEY

Renal involvement has been well described in adult AIDS. Proteinuria and proximal tubular acidosis are common early findings in HIV-infected children. Progression to renal failure is often noted. Nephrotic syndrome with focal glomerular sclerosis has also been described (Pardo *et al*. 1987). It has recently been suggested that the renal pathology seen in HIV-infected patients may occur as a result of direct infection of glomerular cells expressing the CD4 antigen (Karlsson-Parra *et al*. 1989).

HEART

Cardiomyopathy in HIV-infected children has also been described (Joshi *et al*. 1988; Lipshultz *et al*. 1989). Cardiomegaly is a prominent feature, with congestive heart failure as a common finding. Other HIV-associated cardiac abnormalities include tachycardia and arrhythmias; tachypnoea; and cardiomegaly associated with conductive defects. In addition to primary cardiac involvement in HIV disease, it has been suggested that some degree of cor pulmonale may develop in those patients with chronic pulmonary disease (Joshi *et al*. 1988; Rubinstein 1989). One of our patients first presented at the age of 10 years with a rapidly fatal cardiomyopathy.

Recently, a prospective study of cardiovascular function in 31 HIV-infected infants/children suggested that cardiac abnormalities are common in this population (Lipshultz *et al*. 1989). Cardiac dysfunction often may not, however, be clinically apparent.

AUTOIMMUNE COMPLICATIONS

Autoimmune thrombocytopenia, anaemia, neutropenia and lymphopenia have also been described in infected children. Autoimmune anaemia, seen in most patients, is frequently superimposed on a baseline underlying anaemia due to chronic infection and poor nutrition. Thrombocytopenia is seen in 13% of a paediatric AIDS patients, and usually presents in the first 18 months of life. A high percentage of infants have circulating IgG anti-platelet antibodies (82%) and circulating immune complexes (74%) Ellaurie *et al*. 1988).

HAEMATOLOGIC COMPLICATIONS

Virtually all congenitally HIV-infected children develop anaemia (Rubinstein 1986); blood transfusion is however, rarely necessary. Erythrocyte autoantibodies have not been detected. Frequently, the anaemia occurs secondary to chronic conditions such as inadequate nutrition and lymphoma. Progressive anaemia is prognostic of advancing disease, and shows better correlation with poor outcome than decreasing CD4/CD8 ratios (Ellaurie *et al*. 1990b).

Children congenitally infected with HIV-1 frequently develop neutropenia as a frequent haematologic complication in paediatric HIV infection (Rubinstein 1986; Falloon 1989). Neutrophil autoantibodies may play a role in HIV-associated neutropenia. Although lymphopenia has been reported in infected children, it is rarely severe, at least in early disease stage.

Thrombocytopenia is a frequent haematologic complication in HIV-infected children. It occurs in children with both asymptomatic and symptomatic disease; greater than 10% of symptomatic children develop thrombocytopenia (Rubinstein 1986; Ellaurie 1988; Falloon 1989; Calvelli and Rubinstein 1990). Circulating anti-platelet IgG, and circulating immune complexes (CIC) are found in 82% and 74% respectively, of HIV-infected infants (Rubinstein 1986; Ellaurie *et al*. 1988; Calvelli and Rubinstein 1990; Rigaud *et al*. 1992). HIV-1 infected children may present with thrombocytopenia as the first and only symptom, or it may develop in association with advancing disease. The megakaryocyte number in these children's bone marrows may be normal, or elevated. When thrombocytopenia occurs early in the disease course, it may spontaneously resolve; it has also been seen to resolve or improve with zidovudine (AZT) therapy. High dose intravenous gammaglobulin and corticosteroid treatment usually have only a transient effect. Insomuch as CNS bleeding in thrombocytopenic children is much higher than adults, these treatments should at least be attempted. In a recent study, corticosteroid treatment was administered to six children who had failed to improve with intravenous gammaglobulin infusions (Rigaud *et al*. 1992). Sustained remission occurred however, only in one case.

Laboratory diagnosis

In adults, HIV infection is diagnosed by means of serological testing for antibody reactive with the viral antigens, and is staged by clinical symptomatology (Centers for Disease Control 1987b). Serodiagnosis is carried out using an enzyme-linked immunosorbent assay (ELISA), which depends upon reactivity of patient IgG with HIV lysate adsorbed to a solid phase. Reactivity is confirmed by Western blot assay, in which IgGs directed against specific HIV proteins separated by electrophoresis are identified using defined criteria (Table 70.4) (Consortium for Retrovirus Serology Standardization 1989). Antibodies to some HIV proteins may be present without these criteria being met, yielding an indeterminate result (i.e. the sample is neither truly negative nor confirmed positive).

Serological diagnosis of infants with congenital HIV infection is complicated by a number of factors (Table 70.5; Goedert 1986; Calvelli *et al*. 1990). Although the rate of transmission of HIV from an infected mother to her infant pre-/perinatally ranges from 35% to 60% (Rubinstein 1986; Rogers

Table 70.4. Defined criteria for interpretation of human immunodeficiency virus antibody Western blots

US Public Health Service criteria	
Positive (I)	p24, p31 *and* gp41 or gp120/gp160
Probably Positive (II)	
IIa	p24 *and* gp41 or gp120/gp160
IIb	p31 *and* gp41 or gp120/gp160
IIc	gp41 *and* gp120/gp160
IId	Any other combination of HIV-specific bands: one from each gene product (gag; env; pol)
Indeterminate (III)	
IIIa	One band only: p24, p31, gp41, or gp120/160
IIIb	Other non-HIV-specific bands
Negative (IV)	No bands present
Consortium for Retrovirus Serology Standardization	
Positive	p24 or p31 *and* gp41 or gp120/gp160
Indeterminate	Any bands present, but pattern does not meet the criteria for positive
Negative	No bands present

Table 70.5. Problems with serodiagnosis of human immunodeficiency virus infection in infants

Presence of maternal anti-IgG in the infant circulation (for up to 18 months)
Delayed or absent antibody responses in infected infants
Symptomatology similar to congenital immunodeficiencies
Inability of p24 antigen capture assays to detect low-level or latent HIV infection
Absence of free p24 due to binding by passively transferred maternal antibodies
Inability of negative co-cultures to rule out infection
Unreliability of IgM anti-HIV assays due to short or absent IgM responses in infected infants

et al. 1987; Wiznia and Rubinstein 1988; Falloon *et al.* 1989; Calvelli and Rubinstein 1990), newborns of infected mothers invariably test positive using serological assays, whether or not they are actually infected (Amman and Levy 1986). Transplacentally transferred maternal antibody (IgG anti-HIV), detectable by ELISA and Western blot, may persist in the infant circulation for as long as 23 months, complicating serodiagnosis (MMWR 1987a; Pyun *et al.* 1987b; Calvelli and Rubinstein 1990). Testing of serial serum samples by ELISA can be used to assess disappearance of maternal antibody (Rubinstein 1986; Pyun *et al.* 1987a). Also, evaluation of changes in Western blot patterns, reflecting specific HIV protein reactivities or IgG subclass reactivities not present in the maternal serum, can suggest *de novo* production of anti-HIV antibody by the infant (Johnson *et al.* 1987; Krilov *et al.* 1987).

An additional problem in serodiagnosis arises from the frequency of defective humoral immunity in infected infants. Up to 5% of pre- or perinatally infected children are unable to mount antibody responses to common immunogens (e.g. tetanus toxoid, Pneumovax), and remain negative for antibody to HIV even though they are infected (Pahwa *et al.* 1986a; Rubinstein 1986; Borokowsky *et al.* 1987b; Hu *et al.* 1987; Maloney *et al.* 1987; Pyun *et al.* 1987b; Falloon *et al.* 1989). Also, even infants who are hypergammaglobulinaemic as a result of polyclonal B cell activation may not be able to form specific antibody responses.

One approach to diagnosis of HIV infection in infancy has been evaluation of the presence of IgM anti-HIV in the neonatal/infant circulation (Landesman *et al.* 1987). Since maternal IgM anti-HIV does not normally cross the placenta, any IgM anti-HIV present in infant sera would be undeniably of infant origin, indicating current HIV infection. To date, detection of IgM anti-HIV has proved to be of limited value in diagnosis, since it has been shown that production of IgM anti-HIV by infected infants may be transient or absent (Gaetano *et al.* 1987; Johnson *et al.* 1987; Pyun *et al.* 1987a).

Interpretation of concentration differences between IgG subclass anti-HIV antibodies in maternal versus neonatal sera should however, be approached with care since particular IgG subclasses, specifically IgG1, cross the placenta preferentially (Einhorn *et al.* 1987) and may be present in the neonatal circulation at higher concentration than maternal blood.

In addition, several investigators have demonstrated IgA specifically reactive with HIV-1 in the serum of HIV-infected children in the first months of life (Landesman *et al.* 1991; Martin *et al.* 1991).

Another experimental strategy for serological diagnosis of congenital paediatric HIV infection is *in vitro* production of HIV-specific antibody by cultured peripheral blood B cells. The rationale for this approach focuses on the fact that circulating B lymphocytes of an infant infected with HIV would form 'memory' responses of HIV antigens, even if the immaturity of the humoral immune system prevented secretion of specific antibody. Stimulation with polyclonal activators (e.g. PWM, EBV) should push these cells through maturation, resulting in secretion of anti-HIV antibody, if the infant is infected. This method is currently being standardized for potential clinical use (Amadori *et al.* 1988).

An alternative approach to early diagnosis is directed toward detection of the virus itself. The search for HIV in an infected individual is complicated by (i) scarcity of cells in the peripheral circulation actually infected (as few as 1 in 100 000); (ii) sequestering of the virus in a cryptic or latent state within cells or tissues; and (iii) low proviral copy number in cells harbouring HIV cDNA. The first method employed to detect the AIDS-associated virus in infected individuals was expansion of HIV *in vitro* by co-cultivation of patient peripheral blood leucocytes with target cells susceptible to infection with HIV (Popovic *et al.* 1983). Infected target cells can be examined by immunofluorescence for HIV proteins, and cell-free culture fluids assayed for the presence of HIV reverse transcriptase or for HIV p24 antigen (Foerino *et al.* 1987). This methodology is, however, a labour- and cost-intensive undertaking. Improvements in the sensitivity of antigen capture assays now make possible the detection of 5 pg/ml HIV p24. Another caveat regarding this technique is the possibility of false negative results due to removal of p24 from the infant's circulation as a result of complexing with passively transferred maternal anti-p24.

Detection of HIV proviral DNA (see Table 70.6) in biopsy/autopsy material, either directly or following expansion of HIV signals by co-cultivation, has been attempted by some investigators using *in situ* hybridization. In one study, HIV cDNA was detected in co-cultures of peripheral blood, obtained 24 hours after birth from the new-born of an HIV-infected mother (Harnish *et al.* 1987). This methodology is, however, highly subject to sampling error, tedious to perform and relatively insensitive, and a negative result does not rule out infection. A revolutionary method for amplification of nanogram to microgram quantities of cellular DNA and RNA has recently been developed (Cetus Corp., Emeryville, CA). This technique, the polymerase chain reaction (PCR) (Chien *et al.* 1976; Saiki *et al.* 1985; Scharf *et al.* 1986; Abbot *et al.* 1988), employs repeated cycles of template denaturation, oligonucleotide primer annealing and polymerase-mediated chain extension. Coupled with HIV-specific nucleotide primers and probes, this methodology will facilitate highly specific and sensitive detection of HIV genomic sequences in patient blood and tissue samples, present in quantities below the limits of sensitivity of currently used techniques. The polymerase chain reaction holds the additional promise of estimating proviral copy number in latent infections, as well as detecting HIV in productive infections and in cultures at levels below the limit of sensitivity of other methods (Ou *et al.* 1988). At the present time, PCR for HIV detection is in a nascent phase of implementation. Although additional HIV-specific primers and probes continue to be developed, they are being evaluated by a limited number of laboratories and it is too early to assess the significance of either positive or negative results. Although these methods do sometimes enable identification of infants infected with HIV in cases where serological testing is not useful (e.g. prior to disappearance of maternal anti-HIV antibody; compromised infant ability to mount specific antibody responses), a negative result does not exclude the presence of HIV infection. Conversely, a positive result using new-born peripheral blood may be due to HIV within residual maternal cells. Such cells could be cleared by the infant's immune system without causing active neonatal infection (Calvelli and Rubinstein 1990).

A recent report describes two attempts at prenatal diagnosis of HIV infection employing sampling of fetal blood during the second trimester (Daffos *et al.* 1989). Although maternally transferred HIV antibody was present in both fetuses, no evidence of HIV infection was found, with total lymphocytes, CD4 lymphocytes and CD4/CD8 ratios within the normal range. Since only about half of infants born to infected mothers will prove to be infected, further investigation of this approach may be appropriate.

In addition to laboratory methods directed toward identification of serological or virological indices of HIV infection, several non-specific *in vitro* tests of immununological parameters can be useful adjuncts in the differential diagnosis of infants born to infected mothers. Elevated levels of serum immunoglobulins, particularly IgG and IgD, are frequently the first indication of HIV infection in these infants (Rubinstein 1986; Falloon *et al.* 1989; Wiznia and Rubinstein 1988). Defective B

Table 70.6. Laboratory evaluation of paediatric human immunodeficiency virus infection

Test	Detects	Comments
Virologic		
HIV antibody ELISA	IgG anti-HIV	Maternal IgG anti-HIV preferentially detected over infant IgM anti-HIV
Western blot	IgG against specific HIV proteins	Maternal IgG anti-HIV preferentially detected over infant IgM anti-HIV
HIV p24 antigen capture ELISA	p24	Specific for presence of HIV, but patient must be antigenaemic for positive result; negative result does not exclude infection
HIV IgM or IgA ELISA/ Western blot	IgM or IgA anti-HIV	No kits commercially available; infant IgM or IgA not reliably produced; IgG anti-HIV out-competes IgM or IgA due to affinity/avidity binding
Co-culture	Infectious HIV in cells and/or body fluids	Expensive, time-consuming; negative result does not exclude infection
Polymerase chain reaction	HIV DNA or RNA	Requires dedicated lab space and set-up of DNA technology; expensive; negative result does not exclude infection
Immunologic		
Serum immunoglobulins	Serum IgG, IgA, IgM, IgD	Detects elevated or deficient Ig production (hyper/ hypogammaglobulinaemia) suggestive of HIV infection
Circulating immune complexes	CIC in serum	Detects CIC in peripheral blood; elevated CIC is suggestive of HIV infection
Immunization with ΦX 174, diphtheria, tetanus toxoid	Deficits in primary and secondary responses to antigens	Infected infants frequently have abnormal primary and secondary responses *in vivo*
Mitogen-induced lymphoproliferation	Functional B or T cell deficits	Infected infants frequently show reduced responses to PWM and *Staphylococcus aureus*
Circulating thymulin	Serum thymulin level	Decreased in many perinatally infected infants

cell function may also be reflected in decreased proliferative responsiveness of peripheral blood mononuclear cells to PWM and *Staphylococcus aureus*. Depressed lymphoproliferative responses of infected infants to T cell mitogens frequently precede impaired responses to T cell mitogens (phytohaemagglutinin (PHA) and concanavalin A (Con A)) (Bernstein *et al*. 1985b; Pahwa *et al*. 1986b). Human immunodeficiency virus-infected adults typically show decreased responses to the T cell mitogens before the B cell mitogens. Assays to detect circulating immune complexes (CIC) (C1q assay, Raji cell assay) may also provide circumstantial evidence of HIV infection: infants and children infected with HIV frequently exhibit elevated CIC, particularly when measured by the

Raji cell assay (Bernstein *et al.* 1985b; Rubinstein 1986; Ellaurie *et al.* 1988). The presence of HIV antigens associated with CIC by complexing with either maternal or infant antibodies, can also be used to identify HIV-infected infants (Calvelli *et al.* 1988; Ellaurie *et al.* 1990a). Diagnosis of HIV infection in the paediatric population may also be aided by *in vivo* assessment of B-cell-mediated immune function: abnormal primary and secondary responses to immunization with diphtheria, tetanus toxoid or pneumococcal polysaccharide vaccine may be indicative of HIV-associated B cell deficiency (Bernstein *et al.* 1985a,b). Although abnormal results for any of the above tests alone may be indicative of a congenital non-HIV immunodeficiency, the pattern of abnormalities in combination with clinical signs and symptoms, and serological and virological testing, should determine the extent of follow-up as well as the need for repeated HIV testing.

Therapeutic intervention

Antiretroviral therapy

In addition to specific pharmaceuticals directed toward eradication, prevention or control of the infectious (bacterial, non-HIV viral and fungal infections) and non-infectious (e.g. immunological, pulmonary) complications of HIV infection, therapeutic modalities directed against the virus itself are being developed. Specific steps in the HIV infectious cycle which are potential targets of antiretroviral therapy include binding of gp120 to cell surface CD4; viral uncoating; reverse transcription, including digestion of the RNA template by viral ribonuclease (RNase); integration of proviral DNA into the host genome; transcription of integrated viral DNA to RNA; translation of viral RNA; post-translational modifications of HIV proteins necessary for production and assembly of virion components; and viral budding. The step in the viral replication cycle which is the target of all of the antiretroviral agents developed to the point of use in HIV-infected patients is reverse transcription (Yarchoan and Broder 1987). A number of these are currently in phase I and II clinical trials in HIV-infected adults. Trials of antiretroviral agents in infants and children have only recently been initiated. The most extensively evaluated antiretroviral therapy at present is 3′-azido-2′,3′-dideoxythymidine (azidothymidine (AZT), zidovudine) (Fig. 70.2), a thymidine nucleoside analogue in which the 3′-hydroxy group is modified so that the phosphodiester linkages necessary for formation of nucleic acid chains cannot be formed (Furman *et al.* 1986). *In vitro*, AZT has been shown to be a potent inhibitor of HIV replication, causing termination of DNA chains during reverse transcription of viral RNA (Fig. 70.3). Results from the blind placebo-armed trials have not yet been analysed, and the long-term sequelae associated with AZT are not known. However, data from adults receiving the drug outside the trials suggest that increased survival, immunological improvements and decreased circulating HIV antigen may be achieved. In addition, some studies have reported significant decrease in the serum concentration of p24 as a result of treatment with AZT (Chaisson *et al.* 1986; Surbone *et al.* 1988). Phase II clinical trials to assess the potential efficacy of AZT alone, and in combination with either intravenous gamma globulin or 2′,3′-dideoxycytidine (ddC), have been initiated in congenitally infected children. The fact that AZT has shown excellent penetration of the blood–brain barrier (Yarchoan *et al.* 1987; Klecker *et al.* 1987) may be of particular importance in the paediatric population, since infected infants

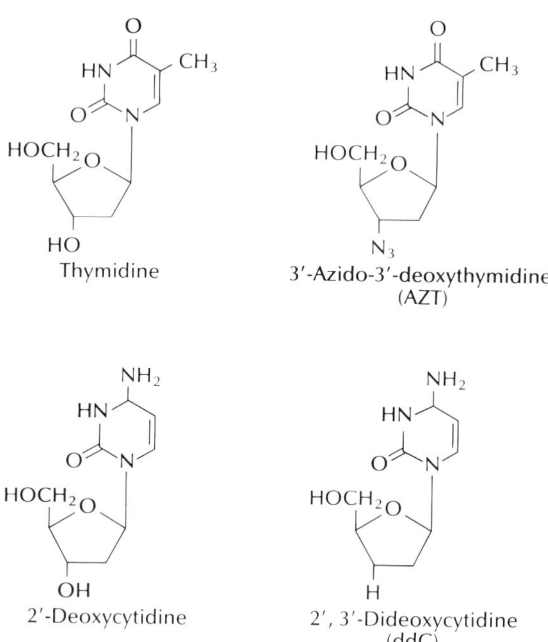

Fig. 70.2. Structure of dideoxynucleosides.

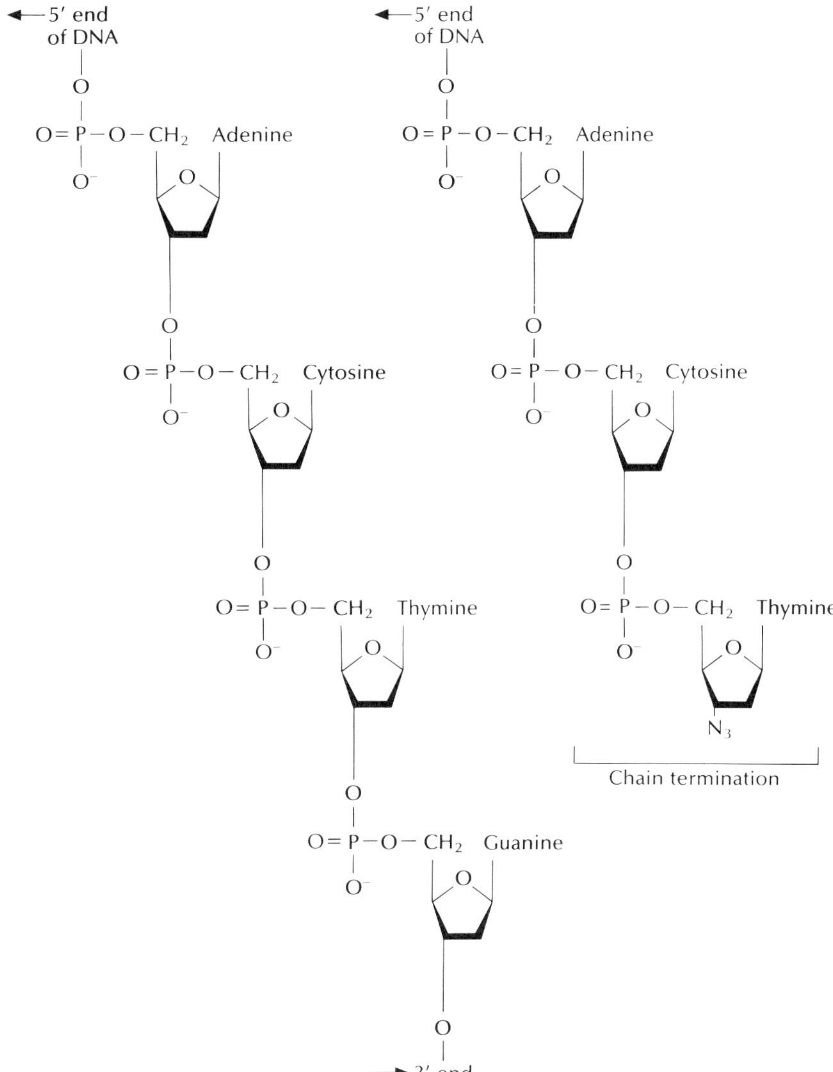

Fig. 70.3. DNA chain termination by AZT. Formation of DNA molecules proceeds by addition of nucleoside triphosphate bases from the 5′ to the 3′ end by the action of cellular DNA polymerase. When AZT triphosphate is incorporated into the 3′ end of a DNA chain, no further phosphodiester linkages can form to couple additional nucleoside triphosphates, resulting in premature chain termination.

present with a high incidence of neurological complications. Another pyrimidine analogue, ddC (Fig. 70.2), is phosphorylated by cellular kinases to its active form (Mitsuya and Broder 1986). Phase I trials to assess the toxic side effects of ddC in both adults and children are currently under way. Although this drug has shown extremely potent inhibition of HIV replication *in vitro*, toxic side-effects have been reported *in vivo* (Hagler and Frame 1986; Richman *et al.* 1987a). While both of these agents inhibit reverse transcription of HIV RNA, neither has effects on the integrated provirus in latent infection. In addition, Richman *et al.* (1987b) demonstrated that the dideoxynucleosides fail to inhibit HIV replication in human macrophages *in vitro*. As a consequence of this, neither agent has the ability to eliminate HIV from an infected individual, and both are limited to holding spread of the virus in check by interfering with formation of proviral DNA in newly infected cells. It has, in fact, been shown that the concentration of HIV p24 in the peripheral circulation increases if AZT treatment is stopped (Chaisson *et al.* 1986). Another study demonstrated *in vitro* that, although AZT controlled infection of uninfected cells, cell-to-cell spread of HIV took place in the presence of the drug (Gupta *et al.* 1989). Other treatment modalities directed toward the control or elimination of HIV in infected patients, or toward stimulation of the immune system, are currently in development in trials in adults, but will not be discussed here.

Early treatment of neonates and infants with antiretroviral drugs has been limited in part by the difficulties inherent in diagnosis of HIV infection in preperinatally infected children, discussed above. The ultimate goal of therapeutic intervention for congenitally acquired paediatric HIV infection is prevention of transmission of the virus from an infected mother to the developing fetus during gestation. Development of potential treatment modalities which could be used safely in pregnant HIV-infected women without compromising efficacy is a critical area for investigation.

The AIDS Clinical Trial Group (ACTG), under the auspices of the National Institute of Allergy & Infectious Diseases (NIAID) Division of AIDS (DAIDS), is currently conducting a Phase I trial to evaluate the effects of AZT treatment of HIV-infected pregnant women during the last trimester of pregnancy, on both the incidence of HIV transmission and time to symptomatic disease in infants who do become infected. In so much as fetal studies (Rubinstein 1986; Calvelli and Rubinstein 1990) indicate that transmission of HIV can occur in the first trimester of pregnancy, therapeutic antiretroviral intervention may be necessary for prevention of materno-fetal infection, despite the inherent embryopathic risks.

The ultimate goal of therapeutic intervention in congenital HIV infection is prevention of transmission during fetal life. In addition to use of antiretroviral therapy to inhibit transmission of HIV from an infected to the developing fetus during pregnancy, the use of hyperimmune serum during pregnancy to provide passive immunotherapy to prevent *in utero* transmission deserves consideration. Data indicating that materno-fetal transmission correlates with the absence of maternal antibodies to gp120, specifically to peptides of the V3 PND hypervariable loop (Goedert *et al.* 1989a,b; Devash *et al.* 1990) may ultimately find application in this context.

Intravenous gamma globulin

Intravenous gamma globulin (intravenous immunoglobulin (IVIG)) has been used in the treatment of HIV-infected children for the past 10 years (Rubinstein *et al.* 1984b). It has been our experience that IVIG treatment reduces the frequency of febrile illnesses, as well as the frequency of episodes of sepsis in children. In some patients, increased helper:suppressor (T4/T8) ratios and improvement of mitogenic responses were observed (Calvelli and Rubinstein 1986). In addition, IVIG treatment restored T cell suppressor activity in these children (Gupta *et al.* 1986). For children with recurrent bacterial infections or B cell defects, IVIG at a dosage of 300 mg/kg every other week is recommended (Rubinstein 1986). Gamma globulin has also been used for treatment of thrombocytopenia, starting with an infusion of 500 mg/kg/day for 5 consecutive days, and doubling the dose if the response is insufficient. Haemmorhagic episodes decreased in all patients who responded with elevation of their platelet count. In treatment failures, corticosteroids were only rarely effective over long periods of time.

Antibacterial agents

Children presenting with fever and/or elevated white count must always be evaluated for sepsis and treated with broad-spectrum antibiotics. Trimethoprim–sulphamethoxazole is the first line treatment for PCP, but, as in adults, fever, rash, leucopenia, thrombocytopenia or rising liver transaminases may develop. Children who have had one episode of PCP, or who have less than 200 helper (T4) cells, are routinely placed on trimethoprim–sulphamethoxazole prophylaxis. The alternative drug for treatment of PCP is pentamidine, which has the same side-effects in children as in adults. Prophylactic aerosolized pentamidine in children is currently under investigation.

Mycobacterial infections are extremely difficult to treat, and their presence is a poor prognostic sign. The response to currently available antituberculosis drug regimens is minimal. Cryptosporidium, a cause of chronic diarrhoea in HIV-infected children, is also not typically responsive to specific treatment. Care is essentially symptomatic and supportive.

Non-human-immunodeficiency-virus antiviral agents

Herpes zoster and herpes simplex infections should be treated with acyclovir, since these viral infections may disseminate rapidly. Cytomegalovirus (CMV) can be cultured from stool, urine and blood, and may also disseminate. Ophthalmological CMV involvement is, however, surprisingly infrequent in HIV-infected children compared with adult AIDS patients. Gancyclovir has been used with some success for disseminated CMV infection.

Corticosteroids

Lymphoid interstitial pneumonitis/pulmonary lymphoid hyperplasia responds well to oral steroids. After initial treatment with 1–2 mg/kg/day of prednisone, the dosage should be quickly tapered to an alternate-day regimen designed to maintain a Po_2 over 70 mmHg (Rubinstein *et al.* 1988).

Routine health care

It is well known that immune deficient patients are at risk for complications from live vaccines. Both bacillus Calmette–Guérin and varicella immunization have been linked to childhood death in immunocompromised patients. The question of risk versus benefit in regard to immunization of HIV-infected children is still unresolved. In addition, evidence clearly shows that HIV-infected infants do not effectively form antibody in response to vaccinations (Bernstein *et al.* 1985a,b). Experience to date does, however, suggest that non-live vaccines, such as diphtheria–pertussis–tetanus and Haemophilus influenza B, can be administered safely. Regarding live vaccines, it is preferable to administer killed polio vaccine, since it is available, rather than the live oral vaccine. Policies concerning measles, mumps and rubella vaccines are controversial. It is currently recommended that HIV-infected asymptomatic, as well as symptomatic, children be vaccinated (Centers for Disease Control 1987b). However, it must be kept in mind that the immune response to the vaccine may be insufficient to offer protection, and passive immunization with gamma globulin is recommended at the time of exposure to an infectious agent.

In general, care for paediatric AIDS patients involves care for families, since the parent(s) are also, more often than not, HIV-infected (Rubinstein 1987).

References

Abbot, M.A., Poiesz, B.J., Byrne, B.C., Kwok, S., Sninsky, J.J. and Ehrlich, G.D. (1988). Enzymatic gene amplification: qualitative and quantitative methods for detecting proviral DNA amplified *in vitro*. *J. Infect. Dis.* **158**, 1158–63.

Adinolfi, M. and Gorvette, D.P. (1974). The transfer of lymphocytes through the human placenta. In *Proceedings First International Congress Immunology, Obstetrics and Gynaecology* (Padua), Excerpta Medica International Congress Series No. **327**, 177–82.

Ahmad, N. and Venkatesan, S. (1988). Nef protein of HIV-1 is a transcriptional repressor of HIV-1 LTR. *Science* **241**, 1481–5.

Alizon, M., Wain-Hobson, S., Montagnier, L. and Sonigo, P. (1986). Genetic variability of the AIDS virus: nucleotide sequence analysis of two isolates from African patients. *Cell* **46**, 63–74.

Amadori, A., de Rossi, A., Giaquinto, C., Faulkner-Valle, G., Zacchello, F. and Chieco-Bianchi, L. (1988). *In-vitro* production of HIV-specific antibody in children at risk of AIDS. *Lancet* **i**, 852–4.

Amadori, A., Zamarchi, R., Ciminale, V. *et al.* (1989). HIV-1-specific B cell activation. A major constituent of spontaneous B cell activation during HIV-1 infection. *J. Immunol.* **143**, 2146–52.

Amman, A.J. and Levy, J. (1986). Laboratory investigation of pediatric acquired immunodeficiency syndrome. *Clin. Immunol. Immunopathol.* **40**, 122–7.

Andiman, W.A., Eastman, R., Martin, K. *et al.* (1985). Opportunistic lymphoproliferations associated with Epstein–Barr viral DNA in infants and children with AIDS. *Lancet* **ii**, 1390–3.

Arya, S.K., Guo, C., Josephs, S.F. and Wong-Staal, F. (1985). *Trans*-activator gene of human T-lymphotropic virus type III (HTLV-III). *Science* **229**, 69–73.

Baltimore, D. (1970). RNA-dependent-DNA-polymerase in virions of RNA tumor viruses. *Nature* **226**, 1209–11.

Barre-Sinoussi, F., Chermann, J.C., Rey, R. *et al.* (1983). Isolation of a T-lymphotropic retrovirus from a patient at risk for acquired immune deficiency syndrome (AIDS). *Science* **220**, 868–71.

Belman, A.L., Ultmann, M.H., Horoupian, D. *et al.* (1985). Neurological complications in infants and children with acquired immune deficiency syndrome. *Ann. Neurol.* **18**, 560–6.

Belman, A.L., Diamond, G., Dickson, D., Horoupian, D., Llena, J. and Rubinstein, A. (1989). Pediatric acquired immunodeficiency syndrome: neurological syndromes. *Am. J. Dis. Child.* **142**, 29–35.

Bender, B.S., Davidson, B.L., Kline, R., Brown, C. and Quinn, T.C. (1988). Role of the mononuclear phagocyte system in the immunopathogenesis of human immunodeficiency virus infection and the acquired immunodeficiency syndrome. *Rev. Infect. Dis.* **10**, 1142–54.

Bernstein, L.J., Krieger, B.Z., Novick, B, Sicklick, M.J. and Rubinstein, A. (1985a). Bacterial infection in the acquired immunodeficiency syndrome of children. *Pediatr. Infect. Dis.* **4**, 472–5.

Bernstein, L.J., Ochs, H.D., Wedgwood, R.J. and Rubinstein, A.

(1985b). Defective humoral immunity in pediatric acquired immunodeficiency syndrome. *J. Pediatr.* **107**, 352–7.

Blanche, S., Le Deist, F., Fischer, A., Veber, F., Debre, M., Chamaret, S., Montagnier, L. and Griscelli, C. (1986). Longitudinal study of 18 children with perinatal LAV/HTLV III infection: attempt at prognostic evaluation. *J. Pediatr.* **109**, 965–70.

Bogner, J.R., Matuschke, A., Heinrich, B., Eberle, E. and Goebel, F.D. (1988). Serum neopterin levels as predictor of AIDS. *Klin. Wschr.* **66**, 1015–18.

Borkowsky, W., Steele, C.J., Grubman, S., Moore, T., La-Russa, P. and Krasinski, K. (1987a). Antibody responses to bacterial toxoids in children infected with human immunodeficiency virus. *J. Pediatr.* **110**, 563–6.

Borkowsky, W., Krasinski, K., Paul, D., Moore, T., Bebenroth, D. and Chadwani, S. (1987b). Human-immunodeficiency-virus infections in infants negative for anti-HIV by enzyme-linked immunoassay. *Lancet* **i**, 1168–71.

Brasseur, R., Cornet, B., Burny, A., Vandenbranden, M. and Ruysschaert, J.M. (1988). Mode of insertion into a lipid membrane of the N-terminal HIV gp41 peptide segment. *AIDS Res. Hum. Retroviruses* **4**, 83–90.

Brenneman, D.E., Westbrook, G.L., Fitzgerald, S.P., Ennist, D.L., Elkins, K.L., Ruff, M.R. and Pert, C.B. (1988). Neuronal cell killing by the envelope protein of HIV and its prevention by vasoactive intestinal peptide. *Nature* **335**, 639–42.

Broliden, P.A., Moschese, V., Lounggren, K. *et al.* (1989). Diagnostic implication of specific immunoglobulin G patterns born to HIV-infected mothers. *AIDS* **9**, 577–82.

Buck, B.E., Scott, G., Valdes-Dapena, M., Parks, W. *et al.* (1983). Kaposi sarcoma in two infants with acquired immune deficiency syndrome. *J. Pediatr* **103**, 911–13.

Bye, M., Bernstein, L., Shah, K., Ellaurie, M. and Rubinstein, A. (1987). Diagnostic broncho-alveolar lavage in children with AIDS. *Pediatr Pulm.* **3**, 425–8.

Calvelli, T.A. (1991). Flow cytometry and the evaluation of HIV-infected children. 6th Annual Meeting, *Clinical Applications of Cytometry*, [Plenary session] September 1991, Charleston, SC.

Calvelli, T.A. and Rubinstein, A. (1986). Intravenous gammaglobulin in infant acquired immunodeficiency syndrome. *Pediatr. Infect. Dis.* **5**, S207–S210.

Calvelli, T.A. and Rubinstein, A. (1990). Pediatric HIV infection: a review. *Immunodeficiency Rev.* **2**, 83–127.

Calvelli, T.A., Ellaurie, M. and Rubinstein, A. (1988). HIV protein associated with circulating immune complexes (CIC) in pediatric AIDS/ARC. in *IV International Conference on AIDS* (abstr.).

Calvelli, T.A., Golodner, M., Shliozberg, J., Keswani A. and Rubinstein, A. (1990). Expression of cell-surface activation markers by congenitally HIV-infected children. *6th Internat. AIDS Conf.* F.B. 456, Vol 2: 192.

Calvelli, T.A., Dubrovsky, L., Freyman, B., Lyman, W.D., Soeiro, R. and Rubinstein, A. (1991). IgA and IgM in amniotic fluid in HIV-positive pregnancies: anti-HIV reactivity and association with immune complexes. *7th Internat. AIDS Conf.*, June 1991, W.C. 1326.

Centers for Disease Control (1987a). Immunization of children infected with HTLV-III/LAV: recommendations of the immunizations advisory committee. *Ann. Intern. Med.* **106**, 75–8.

Centers for Disease Control (1987b). Revision of the CDC surveillance: case definition for acquired immunodeficiency syndrome. *Morb. Mort. Weekly Rep.* **36**, 1S–15S.

Centers for Disease Control (1987c). Classification system for human immunodeficiency virus (HIV) infection in children under 13 years of age. *MMWR* **36**, 1–6.

Chaisson, R.E., Allain, J.P., Leuther, M. and Volberding, P.A. (1986). Significant changes in HIV antigen level in the serum of patients treated with azidothymidine (letter). *N. Engl. J. Med.* **315**, 1610–11.

Chan, M.M., Campos, J.M., Josephs, S. and Rifai, N. (1990). β_2-microglobulin and neopterin: predictive markers for human immunodeficiency virus type 1 infection in children? *J. Clin. Microbiol.* **28**, 2215–19.

Chayt, K.S., Harper, M.E., Marselle, L.M., Lewin, E.B., Rose, R.M., Oleske, J.M., Epstein, L.G., Wong-Staal, F. and Gallo, R.C. (1986). Detection of HTLV-III RNA in lungs of patients with AIDS and pulmonary involvement. *JAMA* **256**, 2356–9.

Chien, A., Edgar, D.B. and Trela, J.M. (1976). Deoxyribonucleic acid polymerase from the extreme thermophile thermus aquaticus. *J. Bacteriol.* **127**, 1550–7.

Chiu, I.-M., Yaniv, A., Dahlberg, J.E., Gazit, A., Skuntz, S.F., Tronick, S.R. and Aaronson, S.A. (1985). Nucleotide sequence evidence for relationship of AIDS retrovirus to lentiviruses. *Nature* **317**, 366–8.

Church, J.A., Lewis, J. and Spotkov, J.M. (1984). IgG subclass deficiencies in children with suspected AIDS. *Lancet* **i**, 279.

Clavel, F., Mansinho, K., Chamaret, S., Guetard, D., Favier, V., Nina, J., Santos-Ferreira, M.-O., Champalimaud, J.-L. and Montagnier, L. (1987). Human immunodeficiency virus type 2 infection associated with AIDS in West Africa. *N. Engl. J. Med.* **316**, 1180–5.

Clements, J.E., Narayan, O., Griffin, D.E. and Johnson, R.T. (1980). Genomic changes associated with antigenic variation of visna virus during persistent infection *Proc. Nat. Acad. Sci. (USA)* **77**, 4454–8.

Consortium for Retrovirus Serology Standardization (1988). Serological diagnosis of human immunodeficiency virus infection by Western blot testing. *JAMA* **260**, 674–9.

Cowan, M.J., Hellman, D., Chudwin, D., Wara, D., Chang, R.S. and Ammann, A.J. (1984). Maternal transmission of acquired immune deficiency syndrome. *Pediatrics* **73**, 382–6.

Daffos, F., Forestier, F., Mandelbrot, L., Pialoux, G., Rey, M.A. and Brun-Vezinet, F. (1989). Prenatal diagnosis of HIV infection: two attempts using fetal blood sampling. *J. Acquired Immune Deficiency Syndr.* **2**, 205–7.

Dalgleish, A.G., Beverly, P.C.L., Clapham, P.R. Crawford, D.H., Greaves, M.F. and Weiss, R.A. (1984). The CD4 (T4) antigen is an essential component of the receptor for the AIDS retrovirus. *Nature* **312**, 763–7.

Daniel, M.D., Letvin, N.L., King, N.W., Kannagi, M., Sehgal, P.K., Hunt, R.D., Kanki, P.J., Essex, M. and Desrosiers, R.C. (1985). Isolation of T-cell tropic HTLV-III-like retrovirus from macaques. *Science* **228**, 1201–4.

Davis, J.L., Molineaux, S. and Clements, J.E. (1987). Visna virus exhibits a complex transcriptional pattern: one aspect of gene expression shared with the acquired immunodeficiency syndrome retrovirus. *J. Virol.* **61**, 1325–31.

Dayton, A.I., Sodroski, J.G., Rosen, C.A., Goh, W.C. and Haseltine, W.A. (1986). The *trans*-activator gene of the human T cell lymphotropic virus type III is required for replication.

Cell **44**, 941–7.

Devash, Y., Calvelli, T.A., Wood, D.G., Reagan, K.J. and Rubinstein, A. (1990). Vertical transmission of HIV correlated with the absence of high affinity/avidity maternal antibodies to the gp120 principal neutralizing domain. *Proc. Nat. Acad. Sci. (USA)* **87**, 3445–9.

Diamond, D.C., Sleckman, B.P., Gregory, T., Lasky, L.A., Greenstein, J.L. and Burakoff, S.J. (1988). Inhibition of CD4+ T cell function by the HIV envelope protein, gp120. *J. Immunol.* **141**, 3715–17.

Dickson, D.W., Belman, A.L., Kim, T.S., Horoupian, D.S. and Rubinstein, A. (1989). Spinal cord pathology in pediatric acquired immunodeficiency syndrome. *Neurology* **39**, 227–35.

Di Maria, H., Courpotin, C., Rouzioux, C., Cohen, D., Rio, D. and Boussin, F. (1986). Transplacental transmission of human immunodeficiency virus. *Lancet* **ii**, 215–16.

Down, J.A., Kawakami, M., Klein, M.H. and Dorrington, K.J. (1989). Proteins associated with activity of Fc receptors on isolated human placental syncytiotrophoblast microvillous plasma membranes. *Placenta* **10**, 227–46.

Duffy, L.F., Daum, F., Kahn, E., *et al.* (1986). Hepatitis in children with acquired immune deficiency syndrome: histopathologic and immunocytologic features. *Gastroenterology* **90**, 173–81.

Ehrnst, A., Londgren, S., Dictor, M. *et al.* (1991). HIV in pregnant women and their offspring: evidence for late transmission. *Lancet* **337**, 253–60.

Eilbott, D.J., Peress, N., LaNeve, D., Orenstein, J., Gendelman, H.E., Seidman, R. and Weiser, B. (1989). Human immunodeficiency virus type 1 in spinal cords of acquired immunodeficiency syndrome patients with myelopathy: expression and replication in macrophages. *Proc. Nat. Acad. Sci. (USA)* **86**, 3337–41.

Einhorn, M.S., Granoff, D.M., Nahm, M.H., Quinn, A. and Shackelford, P.G. (1987). Concentration of antibodies in paired maternal and infant sera: Relationship to IgG subclass. *J. Pediatr.* **111**, 783–8.

Ellaurie, M. and Rubinstein, A. (1990). Beta-2-microglobulin concentrations in pediatric human immunodeficiency virus infection. *Pediatr Infect. Dis. J.* **9**, 807–9.

Ellaurie, M., Burns, E., Bernstein, L., Shah, K. and Rubinstein, A. (1988). Thrombocytopenia and human immunodeficiency virus in children. *Pediatrics* **82**, 905–8.

Ellaurie, M., Calvelli, T.A. and Rubinstein, A. (1990a). Human immunodeficiency virus (HIV) circulating immune complexes in infected children. *AIDS Res. Human Retrovir.* **6**, 1437–41.

Ellaurie, M., Burns, E.R. and Rubinstein, A. (1990b) Hematologic manifestations in pediatric HIV infection: severe anemia as a prognostic factor. *Am. J. Pediatr. Hematol./Oncol.* **12**, 449–53.

Epstein, L.G., Sharer, L.R., Cho, E.S., Myenhofer, M., Navia, B. and Price R.W. (1985). HTLV-III/LAV-like retrovirus particles in the brains of patients with AIDS encephalopathy. *AIDS Res* **1**, 447–54.

Epstein, L.G., Goudsmit, J., Paul, D.A., Morrison, S.H., Connor, E.M., Oleske, J.M. and Holland, B. (1987). Expression of human immunodeficiency virus in cerebrospinal fluid of children with progressive encephalopathy. *Ann. Neurol.* **21**, 397–401.

Essex, M. (1975). Horizontally and vertically transmitted oncornaviruses of cats. *Adv. Cancer Res.* **21**, 175–248.

European Collaborative Study (1988). Mother-to-child transmission of HIV infection. *Lancet* **ii**, 1039.

Fackler, J.C., Nagel, J.E., Adler, W.H., Mildvan, P.T. and Ambinder, R.F. (1985). Epstein–Barr virus infection in a child with acquired immune deficiency syndrome. *Am. J. Dis. Child.* **139**, 1000–4.

Fahey, J.L., Taylor, R., Detels, R. *et al.* (1990). The prognostic value of cellular and serologic markers in infection with human immunodeficiency virus type 1. *N. Engl. J. Med.* **322**, 166–72.

Falloon, J., Eddy, J., Wiener, L. and Pizzo, P. (1989). Human immunodeficiency virus in children. *J. Pediatr.* **114**, (1), 1–30.

Fauci, A.S. (1988). The human immunodeficiency virus: infectivity and mechanisms of pathogenesis. *Science* **239**, 617–22.

Feinberg, M.B., Jarrett, R.F., Aldovini, A., Gallo, R.C. and Wong-Staal, F. (1986). HTLV-III expression and production involve complex regulation at the levels of splicing and translation of viral RNA. *Cell* **46**, 807–17.

Fisher, A.G., Ensoli, B., Ivanoff, L., Chamberlain, M., Peetway, S., Ratner, L., Gallo, R.C. and Wong-Staal, F. (1987). The sor gene of HIV-1 is required for efficiency virus transmission *in vitro*. *Science* **237**, 888–93.

Feorino, P., Forrester, B., Schable, C., Warfield, D. and Schochetman, G. (1987). Comparison of antigen capture assay and reverse transcriptase assay for detecting human immunodeficiency virus in culture. *J. Clin. Microbiol.* **25**, 2344–96.

Fuchs, D.A., Hausen, A., Reibnegger, G., Werner, E.R., Dierich, M.P. and Wachter, H. (1988). Neopterin as a marker for activated cell-mediated immunity: application in HIV infection. *Immunol. Today* **9**, 150–5.

Furman, P.A., Fyfe, J.A., St Clair, M.H., *et al.* (1986). Phosphorylation of 3′-azido-3′-deoxythymidine and selective interaction of the 5′-triphosphate with human immunodeficiency virus reverse transcriptase. *Proc. Nat. Acad. Sci. (USA)* **83**, 8333–7.

Gaetano, C., Scano, G., Carbonari, M., Giannini, G., Mezzaroma, I., Aiuti, F., Marolla, L., Casadei, A.M. and Carapella, E. (1987). Delayed and defective anti-HIV IgM response in infants. *Lancet* **i**, 631.

Gallo, R.C. and Wong-Staal, F. (1985). A human T-lymphotropic retrovirus (HTLV-III) as the cause of the acquired immune deficiency syndrome. *Ann. Intern. Med.* **103**, 679–89.

Gallo, R.C., Mann, D., Broder, S., Ruscetti, F.W., Maeda, M., Kalyanaraman, V.S., Robert-Guroff, M. and Reitz, M.S. (1982). Human T-cell leukemia-lymphoma virus (HTLV) is in T but not B lymphocytes from a patient with cutaneous T-cell lymphoma. *Proc. Nat. Acad. Sci. (USA)* **79**, 5680–3.

Gallo, R.C., Kalyanaraman, V.S., Sarngadharan, M.G., *et al.* (1983). Association of the human type C retrovirus with a subset of adult T-cell cancers. *Cancer Res.* **43**, 3892–9.

Gallo, R., Wong-Staal, F., Montagnier, L., Haseltine, W.A. and Yoshida, M. (1988). HIV/HTLV gene nomenclature. *Nature* **333**, 504.

Gartner, S., Markovits, P., Markovitz, D.M., Kaplan, M.H., Gallo, R.C. and Popovic, M. (1986a). The role of mononuclear phagocytes in HTLV-III/LAV infection. *Science* **233**, 215–19.

Gartner, S., Markovits, P., Markovitz, D.M., Betts, R.F. and Popovic, M. (1986b). Virus isolation from and identification of HTLV-III/LAV-producing cells in brain tissue from a patient with AIDS. *JAMA* **256**, 2365–71.

Gendelman, H.E., Narayan, O., Kennedy-Stoskopf, S., Clements, J.E. and Ghotbi, A. (1985). Slow persistant replication of lentiviruses: role of macrophages and macrophage-precursors in bone marrow. *Proc. Nat. Acad. Sci. (USA)* **82**, 7086–90.

Gendelman, H.E., Narayan, O., Kennedy-Stoskopf, S., Kennedy, P.G.E., Ghotbi, Z., Clements, J.E., Stanley, J. and Pezeshkpour, G. (1986). Tropism of sheep lentiviruses for monocytes: susceptibility to infection and virus gene expression increases during maturation of monocytes to macrophages. *J. Virol.* **58**, 67–74.

Goedert, J.J. (1986). Testing for human immunodeficiency virus. *Ann. Intern. Med.* **105**, 609–10.

Goedert, J.J., Mendez, H., Willoughby, A. and Landesman, S.H. (1989). High perinatal HIV rates with prematurity or low anti-gp120. *5th International Conference on AIDS, Montreal, Canada.* [abstr] Th.A.0.6. p. 71.

Goedert, J.J., Mendez, H., Willoughby, A. and Landesman, S.H. (1989a). High perinatal HIV rates with prematurity or low anti-gp120. *5th International Conference on AIDS, Montreal, Canada.* [abstr] Th.A.0.6. p. 71.

Goedert, J.J., Mendez, H., Drummond, J.E. *et al.* (1989b). Mother-to-infant transmission of human immunodeficiency virus type 1: association with prematurity or low anti-gp120. *Lancet* **ii**, 1351–4.

Goedert, J.J., Duliege, A.-M., Amos, C.J. *et al.* (1991). High risk of HIV-1 infection for first-born twins. *Lancet* **338**, 1471–5.

Gonda, M.A., Wong-Staal, F., Gallo, R.C., Clements, J.E., Narayan, O. and Gilden, R.V. (1985). Sequence homology and morphologic similarity of HTLV-III and visna virus, a pathogenic lentivirus. *Science* **227**, 173–7.

Gonda, M.A., Braun, M.J., Clements, J.E. *et al.* (1986). HTLV-III shares sequence homology with a family of pathogenic lentiviruses. *Proc. Nat. Acad. Sci. (USA)* **83**, 4007–11.

Grieco, M.H., Reddy, M.M., Kothari, H.B., Lange, M., Buimovici-Klein, E. and William, D. (1984). Elevated β_2-microglobulin and lysozyme levels in patients with acquired immune deficiency syndrome. *Immunol. Immunopathol.* **32**, 174–84.

Gupta, A., Sicklick, M., Bernstein, L.B., Rubinstein, E., Silverman, B. and Rubinstein, A. (1982). Recurrent infections, interstitial pneumonia, hypergammaglobulinemia and reversed T4/T8 ratio in children with high antibody titer to Epstein-Barr virus. *Proc. Am. Acad. Pediatr.* (abstr.).

Gupta, A., Novick, B., Rubinstein, A. *et al.* (1986). Restoration of suppressor T-cell functions in children with AIDS following intravenous gamma globulin treatment. *Am. J. Dis. Child.* **140**, 143–6.

Gupta, P., Balachandran, R., Ho, M., Enrico, A. and Rinaldo, C. (1989). Cell-to-cell transmission of human immunodeficiency virus type 1 in the presence of azidothymidine and neutralizing antibody. *J. Virol.* **63**, 2361–5.

Haase, A.T. (1975). The slow infection caused by visna virus. *Curr. Topics Microbiol. Immunol.* **72**, 101–56.

Haase, A.T. (1986). Pathogenesis of lentivirus infections. *Nature* **322**, 130–6.

Hȧase, A.T., Stowring, L., Pelus, R. *et al.* (1982). Visna virus DNA and the tempo of infection *in vitro*. *Virology* **119**, 399–410.

Hagler, D.N. and Frame, P.T. (1986). Azidothymidine neurotoxicity. *Lancet* **ii**, 1392–3.

Hahn, B.H., Shaw, G.M., Taylor, M.E. *et al.* (1986). Genetics variation in HTLV-III/LAV over time in patients with AIDS or at risk for AIDS. *Science* **232**, 1548–53.

Hammarskjold, M.-L., Heimer, J., Hammarskjold, B., Sangwan, I., Albert, L. and Rekosh, D. (1989). Regulation of human immunodeficiency virus env expression by the rev gene product. *J. Virol.* **63**, 1959–66.

Hanaoka, M., Takatsuki, K. *et al.* (eds) (1982). Adult T-cell leukemia and related disease. *Gann Monogr. Cancer Res.* **28**, 1–237.

Hardy, W.D. (1982). Immunopathology induced by the feline leukemia virus. *Springer Semin. Immunopathol.* **5**, 75–106.

Harnish, D.G., Hammerberg, O. and Rosenthal, K.L. (1987). Early detection of HIV infection in a newborn. *N. Engl. J. Med.* **316**, 272–3.

Henderson, L.E., Benveniste, R.E., Sowder, R., Copeland, T.D., Schultz, A.M. and Oroszlan, S. (1988). Molecular characterization of gag proteins from simian immunodeficiency virus (SIV_{Mne}). *J. Virol.* **62**, 2587–95.

Hess, J.L., Clements, J.E. and Narayan, O. (1985). *Cis* and *trans*-acting transcriptional regulation of visna virus. *Science* **229**, 482–5.

Ho, D.D., Rota, T.R. and Hirsch, M.S. (1986). Infection of human monocyte/macrophage by human T lymphotropic virus type III. *J. Clin. Invest.* **77**, 1712–15.

Ho, D.D., Pomerantz, R.J. and Kaplan, J.C. (1987). Pathogenesis of infection with human immunodeficiency virus. *N. Engl. J. Med.* **317**, 278–86.

Hoffman, A.D., Banapour, B., Levy, J.A. (1985). Characterization of the AIDS-associated retrovirus reverse transcriptase and optimal conditions for its detection in virions. *Virology* **147**, 326–35.

Honda, N.S., Sun, N.C.J. and Heiner, D.C. (1987). Isolated IgG4 subclass deficiency and malignant lymphoma in a child with acquired immunodeficiency syndrome. *Am. J. Dis. Child.* **141**, 398–9.

Hoxie, J.A., Alpers, J.D., Rackowski, J.L. *et al.* (1986). Alterations in T4 (CD4) protein and mRNA synthesis in cells infected with HIV. *Science* **234**, 1123–7.

Hu, P.K., Ochs, H.D. and Wedgwood, R.J. (1987) Seronegativity and paediatric AIDS. *Lancet* **i**, 1152–3.

Incefy, G.S., Pahwa, S., Pahwa, R., Sarngadharan, M.G., Menez, R. and Fikrig, S. (1986). Low circulating thymulin-like activity in children with AIDS and AIDS-related complex. *AIDS Res.* **2**, 109–16.

Italian Multicenter Study (1988). Epidemiology, clinical features and prognostic factors of pediatric HIV infection. *Lancet* **ii**, 1043.

Javaherian, K., Langlois, A.J., McDanal, C. *et al.* (1989). Principal neutralizing domain of the human immunodeficiency virus type 1 envelope protein. *Proc. Nat. Acad. Sci. (USA)* **86**, 6768–72.

Johnson, J.P., Nair, P. and Alexander, S. (1987). Early diagnosis of HIV infection in the neonate. *N. Engl. J. Med.* **316**, 273–4.

Joshi, V.V. and Oleske, J.M. (1985). Pathologic appraisal of the thymus glands in acquired immunodeficiency syndrome in children: a study of four cases and a review of the literature. *Arch. Pathol. Lab. Med.* **109**, 142–6.

Joshi, V.V., Oleske, J.M., Saad, S. *et al.* (1986). Thymus biopsy in children with acquired immunodeficiency syndrome. *Arch. Pathol. Lab. Med.* **110**, 837–42.

Joshi, V.V., Kauffman, S., Oleske, J.M. *et al.* (1987). Polyclonal polymorphic B-cell lymphoproliferative disorder with prominent pulmonary involvement in children with acquired immune deficiency syndrome. *Cancer* **59**, 1455–62.

Joshi, V.V., Gadol, C., Connor, C., Oleske, J.M., Mendelson, J. and Marin-Garcia, J. (1988). Dilated cardiomyopathy in children with acquired immunodeficiency syndrome: a pathologic study of five cases. *Hum. Pathol.* **19**, 69–73.

Jouault, T., Chapuis, F., Olivier, R., Parravicini, C., Bahraoui, E. and Gluckman, J.-C. (1989). HIV infection of monocytic cells: role of antibody-mediated virus binding to Fc-gamma receptors. *AIDS* **3**, 125–33.

Jovaisas, E., Koch, M.A., Schafer, A., Stauber, M. and Lowenthal, D. (1985). LAV/HTLV-III in 20-week fetus. *Lancet* **ii**, 1129.

Kalyanaraman, V.S., Sarngadharan, M., Robert-Guroff, M. *et al.* (1982). A new subtype of human T-cell leukemia virus (HTLV-II) associated with a T-cell variant of hairy cell leukemia. *Science* **218**, 321–3.

Karlsson-Parra, A., Dimeny, E., Fellstrom, B. and Klareskog, L. (1989). HIV receptors (CD4 antigen) in normal human glomerular cells. *N. Engl. J. Med.* **320**, 741.

Klatzmann, D. and Gluckman, J.C. (1986). HIV infection: facts and hypotheses. *Immunol. Today* **7**, 291–6.

Klatzmann, D., Champagne, E., Chamaret, S. *et al.* (1984). T-lymphocyte T4 molecule behaves as the receptor for human retrovirus LAV. *Nature* **312**, 767–8.

Klecker, R.W., Collins, J.M., Yarchoan, R. *et al.* (1987). Plasma and cerebrospinal fluid pharmacokinetics of 3′-azido-3′-deoxythymidine: a novel pyrimidine analog with potential application for the treatment of AIDS and related disorders. *Clin. Pharmacol. Ther.* **41**, 407–12.

Knight, D.M., Flomerfelt, F.A. and Ghrayeb, J. (1987). Expression of the art/trs protein of HIV and study of its role in viral envelope synthesis. *Science* **236**, 837–40.

Koenig, S., Gendelman, H.E., Orenstein, J.M. *et al.* (1986). Detection of AIDS virus in macrophages in brain tissue from AIDS patients with encephalopathy. *Science* **233**, 1089–93.

Kornfeld, H., Cruikshank, W.W., Pyle, S.W., Berman, J.S. and Center, D.M. (1988). Lymphocyte activation by HIV-1 envelope glycoprotein. *Nature* **335**, 445–8.

Kowalski, M., Ardman, B., Basiripour, L. *et al.* (1989). Antibodies to CD4 in individuals infected with human immunodeficiency virus type 1. *Proc. Nat. Acad. Sci. (USA)* **86**, 3346–50.

Kozarsky, K., Penman, M., Basiripour, L., Haseltine, W., Sodroski, J. and Krieger, M. (1989). Glycosylation and processing of the human immunodeficiency virus type 1 envelope protein. *J. Acquired Immune Deficiency Syndr.* **2**, 163–9.

Krilov, L.R., Kamani, N., Hendry, R.M., Wittek, A.E. and Quinnan, G.V. (1987). Longitudinal serologic evaluation of an infant with acquired immunodeficiency syndrome. *Pediatr. Infect. Dis. J.* **6**, 1066–7.

Lairmore, M.D., Akita, G.Y., Russell, H.I. and DeMartini, J.C. (1987). Replication and cytopathic effects of ovine lentivirus strains in alveolar macrophages correlate with *in vivo* pathogenicity. *J. Virol.* **61**, 4038–42.

Lala, P.K., Cahtterjee-Hasrouni, S., Kearns, M., Montgomery, B. and Colavincenzo, V. (1983). Immunobiology of the maternal–fetal interface. *Immunol. Rev.* **75**, 87–116.

Landesman, S., Mendez, H., Pluda, J.M. *et al.* (1987). Evaluation of HIV IgM and antigen assays for determination of perinatal infection with HIV. In: *III International Conference on Acquired Immunodeficiency Syndrome (AIDS)*, June 1–5, abstract THP. 71, Paris.

Landesman, S., Weiblen, B., Mendez, H. *et al.* (1991). Clinical utility of HIV-IgA immunoblot assay in the early diagnosis of perinatal HIV infection. *JAMA* **266**, 3443–46.

Lane, H.C., Masur, H. *et al.* (1983). Abnormalities of B-cell activation and immunoregulation in patients with the acquired immunodeficiency syndrome. *N. Engl. J. Med.* **309**, 453–8.

Lapointe, N., Michaud, J., Pekovic, D., Chausseau, J.P. and Dupuy, J.-M. (1985). Transplacental transmission of HTLV-III virus. *N. Engl. J. Med.* **312**, 1325–6.

Lee, M.R., Ho, D.D. and Gurney, M.E. (1988). Functional interaction and partial homology between human immunodeficiency virus and neuroleukin. *Science* **237**, 1047–51.

Letvin, N.L., Daniel, M.D., Sehgal, P.K. *et al.* (1985). Induction of AIDS-like disease in macaque monkeys with T-cell tropic retrovirus STLV-III. *Science* **230**, 71–3.

Levy, J.A., Hoffman, A.D., Kramer, S.M., Landis, J.A., Shimabukuro, J.M. and Oshino, J.M. (1984). Isolation of lymphocytopathic retroviruses from San Francisco patients with AIDS. *Science* **225**, 840–2.

Levy, R.M. and Bredesen, D.E. (1988). Central nervous system dysfunction in acquired immunodeficiency syndrome. *J. Acquired Immune Deficiency Syndr.* **1**, 41–64.

Lifson, J.D., Reyes, G.R., McGrath, M.S., Stein, B.S. and Engleman, E.G. (1986). AIDS retrovirus induced cytopathology: giant cell formation and involvement of CD4 antigen. *Science* **323**, 1123–7.

Linette, G.P., Hartzman, R.J., Ledbetter, J.A. and June, C.H. (1988). HIV-1-infected T cells show a selective signaling defect after perturbation of CD3/antigen receptor. *Science* **241**, 573–5.

Lipshultz, S.E., Chaock, S., Sanders, S.P., Colan, S.D., Perez-Atayde, A. and McIntosh, K. (1989). Cardiovascular manifestations of human immunodeficiency virus infection in infants and children. *Am. J. Cardiol.* **63**, 1489–97.

Luciw, P.A., Cheng-Mayer, C. and Levy, J.A. (1987). Mutational analysis of the human immunodeficiency virus: The orf-B region down-regulates virus replication. *Proc. Nat. Acad. Sci. (USA)* **84**, 1434–8.

Lyerly, H.K., Matthews, T.J., Langlois, A.J., Bolognesi, D.P. and Weinhold, K.J. (1987a). Anti-gp120 antibodies from HIV seropositive individuals mediate broadly reactive anti-HIV ADCC. *AIDS Res. Hum. Retroviruses* **3**, 409–22.

Lyerly, H.K., Matthews, T.J., Langlois, A.J., Bolognesi, D.P. and Weinhold, K.J. (1987b). Human T-cell lymphotropic virus III B glycoprotein (gp120) bound to CD4 determinants on normal lymphocytes and expressed by infected cells serves as target for immune attack. *Proc. Nat. Acad. Sci. (USA)* **84**, 4601–5.

Lyman, W.D., Kress, Y., Rashbaum, W.K. *et al.* (1987). An AIDS-virus associated antigen localized in human fetal brain. *J. Neuroimmunol.* **16**, 11 (abstr.).

Lyman, W.D., Kress, Y., Rashbaum, W.K. *et al.* (1988). Evidence of human immunodeficiency virus infection in human fetal tissues. *Ann. N. York Acad. Sci.* **549**, 258–9.

McDougal, J.S., Mawle, A., Cort, S.P. *et al.* (1985). Cellular tropism of the human retrovirus HTLV-III/LAV. I. Role of T cell activation and expression of the T4 antigen. *J. Immunol.* **135**, 3151–62.

McDougal, J.S., Kennedy, M.S., Sligh, J.M., Cort, S.P., Mawle, A. and Nicholson, J.K.A. (1986). Binding of HTLV-III/LAV to T4+ T cells by a complex of the 110K viral protein and the T4 molecule. *Science* **231**, 382–5.

McNabb, T., Kuh, T.Y., Dorrington, K.J. and Painter, R.H. (1975). Structure and function of immunoglobulin domains. V. Binding of immunoglobulin G and fragments to placental membrane preparations. *J. Immunol.* **117**, 882–8.

Maloney, M.J., Guill, M.F., Wray, B.B., Lobel, S.A. and Ebbeling, W. (1987). Pediatric acquired immune deficiency syndrome with pan-hypogammaglobulinemia. *J. Pediatr.* **110**, 266–7.

Mann, D.L., Lasane, F., Popovic, M. *et al.* (1987). HTLV-III large envelope protein (gp120) suppresses PHA-induced lymphocyte blastogenesis. *J. Immunol.* **138**, 2640–4.

Marion, R.W., Wiznia, A.A., Hutcheon, R., Rubinstein, A. (1986). Human T-cell lymphotrophic virus type III (HTLV-III) embryopathy: A new dysmorphic syndrome associated with intrauterine HTLV-III infection. *Am. J. Dis. Child.* **140**, 638–45.

Marion, R.W., Wiznia, A.A., Hutcheon, R.G. and Rubinstein, A. (1987). Fetal AIDS syndrome score: correlation between severity of dysmorphism and age at diagnosis of immunodeficiency. *Am. J. Dis. Child.* **141**, 429–31.

Martin, N.L., Levy, J.A., Legg, H., Weintraub, P.S., Cowan, M.J. and Wara, D.W. (1991). Detection of infection with human immunodeficiency virus (HIV) type 1 in infants by an anti-HIV immunoglobulin A assay using recombinant proteins. *J. Pediatr.* **118**, 354–8.

Matre, R. and Johnson, P.M. (1977). Multiple Fc receptors in the human placenta. *Acta Pathol. et Microbiol. Scand.* **85**, Section C, 314–16.

Maury, W., Potts, B.J. and Rabson, A.B. (1989). HIV-1 infection of first-trimester and term human placental tissue: a possible mode of maternal–fetal transmission. *J. Inf. Dis.* **160**, 583–8.

Melbye, M., Njelesani, E.K., Bayley, A. *et al.* (1986). Evidence for heterosexual transmission and clinical manifestations of human immunodeficiency virus infection and related conditions in Lusaka, Zambia. *Lancet* **ii**, 1113–15.

Mitsuya, H. and Broder, S. (1986). Inhibition of the *in vitro* infectivity and cytopathic effect of human T-lymphotropic virus type III/lymphadenopathy-associated virus (HTLV-III/LAV) by 2',3'-dideoxynucleosides. *Proc. Nat. Acad. Sci. (USA)* **83**, 1911–15.

MMWR (1988a). Update: serologic testing for antibody to human immunodeficiency virus. *Morb. Mort. Weekly Rep.* **36**, 833–45.

MMWR (1988b). Measles in HIV-infected children. *Morb. Mort. Weekly Rep.* **37**, 183–6.

Mok, J.Q., Giaquinto, C., De Rossi, A., Grosh-Warner, I., Ades, A.E. and Peckham, C.S. (1987). Infants born to mothers seropositive for human immunodeficiency virus: preliminary findings from a European multicentre study. *Lancet* **i**, 1164–8.

Nakajima, K., Martinez-Maza, O., Hirano, T. *et al.* (1989). Induction of IL-6 (B cell stimulatory factor-2/IFN- beta 2) production by HIV. *J. Immunol.* **142**, 531–6.

Naylor, P.H., Naylor, C.W., Badamchian, M. *et al.* (1987). Human immunodeficiency virus contains an epitope immunoreactive with thymosin alpha$_1$ and the 30-amino acid synthetic p17 group-specific antigen peptide HGP-30. *Proc. Nat. Acad. Sci. (USA)* **84**, 2951–5.

New York State Department of Health (1988). AIDS among New York State children. *Epidemiol. Notes* **10**, 1–2.

Novick, L.F., Berns, D., Strickoff, R. and Stevens, R. (1988). HIV seroprevalence in newborn infants in New York State. In *4th International Conference on AIDS*, abstr. 7221.

Olding, L.B. (1979). Interactions between maternal and fetal/neonatal lymphocytes. In *Current Topics in Pathology*, ed. E. Grundmann, No. **66**, *Perinatal Pathology*, 83–104.

Oleske, J., Minnefor, A., Cooper, R. *et al.* (1983). Immune deficiency syndrome in children. *JAMA* **249**, 2345–9.

Ou, C.-Y., Kwok, S., Mitchell, W. *et al.* (1988). DNA amplification for direct detection of HIV-1 in DNA of peripheral blood mononuclear cells. Science **239**, 295–7.

Pahwa, R., Good, R.A. and Pahwa, S. (1987). Prematurity, hypogammaglobulinemia, and neuropathology with human immunodeficiency virus (HIV) infection. *Proc. Nat. Acad. Sci. (USA)* **84**, 3826–30.

Pahwa, S., Kaplan, M., Fikrig, S. *et al.* (1986a). Spectrum of human T-cell lymphotropic virus type III infection in children: recognition of symptomatic, asymptomatic, and seronegative patients. *JAMA* **255**, 2299–305.

Pahwa, S., Fikrig, S., Menez, R. and Pahwa, R. (1986b). Pediatric acquired immunodeficiency syndrome: demonstration of B lymphocyte defects *in vitro*. *Diagn. Immunol.* **4**, 24–30.

Pahwa, S., Pahwa, R., Good, R.A., Gallo, R.C. and Saxinger, C. (1986c). Stimulatory and inhibitory influences of human immunodeficiency virus on normal B lymphocytes. *Proc. Nat. Acad. Sci. (USA)* **83**, 9124–8.

Pal, R., Hoke, G.M. and Sarngadharan, M.G. (1989). Role of oligosaccharides in the processing and maturation of envelope glycoproteins of human immunodeficiency virus type 1. *Proc. Nat. Acad. Sci. (USA)* **86**, 3384–8.

Pardo, V., Meneses, R., Ossa, L. *et al.* (1987). AIDS-related glomerulopathy: occurrence in specific risk groups. *Kidney Int.* **31**, 1167–73.

Parekh, B.S., Shaffer, N., Chou-Pong, P. *et al.* (1991). Lack of correlation between maternal antibodies to V3 loop peptides of gp120 and perinatal transmission. *AIDS* **5**, 1179–84.

Pauza, C.D. (1988). HIV persistence in monocytes leads to pathogenesis and AIDS. *Cell. Immunol.* **112**, 414–24.

Payne, S.L., Fang, F.-D., Liu, C.-P. *et al.* (1987). Antigenic variation and lentivirus persistence: variations in envelope gene sequences during EIAV infection resemble changes reported for sequential isolates of HIV. *Virology* **161**, 321–31.

Pizzo, P.A. and Butler, K.M. (1991). In the vertical transmission of HIV, timing may be everything. *N. Engl. J. Med.* **325**, 652–4.

Poiesz, B.J., Ruscetti, F.W., Mier, J.W., Woods, A.M. and Gallo, R.C. (1980a). T-cell lines established from human T-lymphocytic neoplasias by direct response to T-cell growth factor. *Proc. Nat. Acad. Sci. (USA)* **77**, 6815–19.

Poiesz, B.J., Ruscetti, F.W., Gazdar, A.F., Bunn, P.A., Minna, J.D. and Gallo, R.C. (1980b). Detection and isolation of type C retrovirus particles from fresh and cultured lymphocytes of a patient with cutaneous T-cell lymphoma. *Proc. Nat. Acad. Sci. (USA)* **77**, 7415–19.

Popovic, M., Reitz, M.S. *et al.* (1983). Isolation and transmission of human retrovirus (human T-cell leukemia virus). *Science* **219**, 856–9.

Prince, H.E., Kleinman, S., Czaplicki, C., John, J. and Williams, A.E. (1990). Interrelationships between serologic markers of immune activation of T lymphocyte subsets in HIV infection. *J. Acq. Imm. Def. Syndr.* **3**, 525–30.

Pyun, K.H., Ochs, H.D., Dufford, M.T.W. and Wedgwood, R.J. (1987a). Perinatal infection with human immunodeficiency virus: specific antibody responses by the neonate. *N. Engl. J. Med.* **317**, 611–14.

Pyun, K.H., Ochs, H.D., Wedgwood, R.J., Marshall, G.S., Barbour, S.D. and Plotkin, S.A. (1987b). Seronegativity and paediatric AIDS. *Lancet* **i**, 1152–3.

Reddy, M.M., Lange, M. and Grieco, M.H. (1989). Elevated soluble CD8 levels in sera of human immunodeficiency virus infected populations. *J. Clin. Microbiol.* **27**, 257–60.

Resnick, L., Pitchenik, A.E., Fisher, E. and Croney, R. (1987). Detection of HTLV-III/LAV-specific IgG and antigen in bronchoalveolar lavage fluid from two patients with lymphocytic interstitial pneumonitis associated with AIDS-related complex. *Am. J. Med.* **82**, 553–6.

Richman, D.D., Kornbluth, R.S. and Carson, D.A. (1987a). Failure of dideoxynucleosides to inhibit human immunodeficiency virus replication in cultured human macrophages. *J. Exp. Med.* **166**, 1144–9.

Richman, D.D., Fischl, M.A., Grieco, M.H. *et al.* (1987b). The toxicity of 3′-azido-3′-deoxythymidine (azidothymidine) in the treatment of patients with AIDS and AIDS-related complex: a double-blind, placebo-controlled trial. *N. Engl. J. Med.* **317**, 192–7.

Rigaud, M., Leubovitz, E., Quee, C.S. *et al.* (1992). Thrombocytopenia in children infected with human immunodeficiency virus: long-term follow-up and therapeutic considerations. *J. Acq. Imm. Def. Syndr.* **5**, 450–5.

Robey, W.G., Safai, B., Oroszlan, S. *et al.* (1985). Characterization of envelope and core structural gene products of HTLV-III with sera from AIDS patients. *Science* **228**, 593–5.

Rogers, M.F., Thomas, P.A., Starcher, E.T., Noa, M.C., Bush, T.J. and Jaffe, H.W. (1987). Acquired immunodeficiency syndrome in children: report of the Centers for Disease Control national surveillance, 1982 to 1985. *Pediatrics* **79**, 1008–14.

Rosen, C.A., Sodroski, J.G., Goh, W.C., Dayton, A.I., Lippke, J. and Haseltine, W.A. (1986). Post-transcriptional regulation accounts for the *trans*-activation of the human T-lymphotropic virus type III. *Nature* **319**, 555–9.

Rossi, P., Moschese, V., Broliden, P.A. *et al.* (1989). Presence of maternal antibodies to human immunodeficiency virus 1 envelope glycoprotein gp120 epitopes correlates with the uninfected status of children born to seropositive mothers. *Proc. Nat. Acad. Sci. (USA)* **86**, 3055–8.

Rubinstein, A. (1986). Pediatric AIDS. *Curr. Prob. Pediatr.* **16**, 361–409.

Rubinstein, A. (1987). Supportive care and treatment of pediatric AIDS: United States Department of Health and Human Services report of the surgeon general's workshop on children with HIV infection and their families. DHHS publication HRS-D-MC 87-i, 29–31.

Rubinstein, A. and Bernstein, L.J. (1986). The epidemiology of pediatric acquired immunodeficiency syndrome. *Clin. Immunol. Immunopathol.* **40**, 115–21.

Rubinstein, A., Sicklick, M.J., Gupta, A. *et al.* (1983). Acquired immunodeficiency with reversed T4/T8 ratio in infants born to promiscuous and drug-addicted mothers. *JAMA* **249**, 2350–6.

Rubinstein, A., Sicklick, M.J., Bernstein, L.J., Mayers, M., Lee, H. and Hollander, M. (1984a). The spectrum of AIDS in infants: lack of evidence for intrafamilial spread. *Pediatr. Res.* **18**, 264A (abstr.).

Rubinstein, A., Sicklick, M.J., Bernstein, L.J. *et al.* (1984b). Treatment of AIDS with intravenous gamma globulin. *Pediatr. Res.* **18**, 264A (abstr.).

Rubinstein, A., Small, C.B. and Bernstein, L.J. (1985). Autoantibodies to T cells in adult and pediatric AIDS. *Ann. N. York Acad. Sci.* **437**, 508–12.

Rubinstein, A., Morecki, R., Silverman, B. *et al.* (1986a). Pulmonary disease in children with acquired immune deficiency syndrome and AIDS-related complex. *J. Pediatr.* **108**, 498–503.

Rubinstein, A., Novick, B.E., Sicklick, M.J. *et al.* (1986b). Circulating thymulin and thymosin-alpha-1 activity in pediatric acquired immune deficiency syndrome: *in vivo* and *in vitro* studies. *J. Pediatr.* **109**, 422–7.

Rubinstein, A., Bernstein, L.J., Charytan, M., Krieger, B.Z. and Ziprowski, M. (1988). Corticosteroid treatment for pulmonary lymphoid hyperplasia in children with the acquired immune deficiency syndrome. *Pediatr. Pulm.* **4**, 13–17.

Ruff, M.R., Martin, B.M., Ginns, E.I., Farrar, W.L. and Pert, C.B. (1987). CD4 receptor binding peptides that block HIV infectivity cause human monocyte chemotaxis. *FEBS Lett.* **211**, 17–22.

Saiki, R.K., Scharf. S.J., Faloona, F. *et al.* (1985). Enzymatic amplification of B-globin genomic sequences and restriction site analysis for diagnosis of sickle cell anemia. *Science* **230**, 1350–4.

Sarin, P.S., Sun, D.K., Thornton, A.H., Naylor, P.H. and Goldstein, A.L. (1986). Neutralization of HTLV-III/LAV replication by antiserum to thymosin $alpha_1$. *Science* **232**, 1135–7.

Sarngadharan, M.G., Veronese, F.D., Oroszlan, S., Arya, S. and Gallo, R.C. (1987). Structural proteins of HTLV-/LAV. In *Acquired Immunodeficiency Syndrome*, ed. J.C. Gluckman and E. Vilmer, pp. 43–6, Elsevier, North-Holland, Paris.

Savino, W., Dardenne, M., Marche, C. *et al.* (1986). Thymic epithelium in AIDS: an immunohistologic study. *Am. J. Pathol.* **122**, 302–7.

Scharf, S.J., Horn, G.T. and Erlich, H.A. (1986). Direct cloning and sequence analysis of enzymatically amplified genomic sequences. *Science* **233**, 1976.

Schnittman, S.M., Lane, H.C., Higgins, S.E., Folks, T. and Fauci, A.S. (1986). Direct polyclonal activation of human B lymphocytes by the acquired immune deficiency syndrome virus. *Science* **233**, 1084–6.

Scott, G.B., Buck, B.E., Leterman, J.G., Bloom, F.L. and Parls, W.P. (1984). Acquired immunodeficiency syndrome in infants. *N. Engl. J. Med.* **310**, 76–81.

Sharer, L.R., Epstein, L.G., Cho, E.-S. *et al.* (1986). Pathologic features of AIDS encephalopathy in children: evidence for LAV/HTLV-III infection of brain. *Hum. Pathol.* **17**, 271–84.

Shaw, G.M., Hahn, B.H., Arya, S.K., Groopman, J.E., Gallo, R.C. and Wong-Staal, F. (1984). Molecular characterization of human T-cell leukemia (lymphotropic) virus type III in the acquired immune deficiency syndrome. *Science* **226**, 1165–71.

Shaw, G.M., Harper, M.E., Hahn, B.H. *et al.* (1985). HTLV-III infection in brains of children adults with AIDS encephalopathy. *Science* **227**, 177–82.

Sicklick, M.J., Novick, B. and Rubinstein, A. (1985). Is AIDS transmitted horizontally? *Pediatr. Res.* **19**, 209A (abstr.).

Siliciano, R.F., Lawton, T., Knall, C. *et al.* (1988). Analysis of host–virus interactions in AIDS with anti-gp120 T cell clones: effect of HIV sequence variation and a mechanism for $CD4^+$ cell depletion. *Cell* **54**, 561–75.

Silverman, B. and Rubinstein, A. (1985). Serum lactate dehydrogenase levels in adults and children with AIDS and ARC: possible indicator of B-cell lymphoproliferation and disease activity: effect of intravenous gammaglobulin on enzyme levels. *Am. J. Med.* **78**, 728–36.

Smith, T.F., Srinivasan, A., Schochetman, G., Marcus, M. and Myers, G. (1988). The phylogenetic history of immunodeficiency viruses. *Nature* **333**, 573–5.

Sonigo, P., Alizon, M., Staskus, K. *et al.* (1985). Nucleotide sequence of the visna lentivirus: relationship to the AIDS virus. *Cell* **42**, 369–82.

Sprecher, A., Soumenkoff, G., Puissant, F. and Degueldre, M. (1986). Vertical transmission of HIV in 15-week fetus. *Lancet* **ii**, 288–9.

Stanley, J., Bhaduri, L.M., Narayan, O. and Clements, J.E. (1987). Topographical rearrangements of visna virus envelope glycoprotein during antigenic drift. *J. Virol.* **61**, 1019–28.

Stephens, R.M., Casey, J.W. and Rice, N.R. (1986). Equine infectious anemia virus gag and pol genes: relatedness to visna and AIDS virus. *Science* **231**, 589–94.

Strebel, K., Daugherty, D., Clouse, K., Cohen, D., Folks, T. and Martin, M.A. (1987). The HIV 'A' (sor) gene product is essential for virus infectivity. *Nature* **328**, 728–30.

Streilein, J.W. and Bergstresser, P.R. (1980). Ia antigen and epidermal Langerhans cells. *Transplantations* **30**, 319–23.

Surbone, A., Yarchoan, R., McAtee, N. *et al.* (1988). Treatment of acquired immunodeficiency syndrome (AIDS) and AIDS-related complex with a regimen of 3'-azido-2',3'-dideoxythymidine (azidothymidine or zidovudine) and acyclovir: a pilot study. *Ann. Intern. Med.* **108**, 534–40.

Takahashi, I., Takama, M., Ladhoff, A.-M. and Scholz, D. (1989). Envelope structure model of human immunodeficiency virus type 1. *J. Acquired Immune Deficiency Syndr.* **1**, 136–40.

Takeda, A., Tuazon, C.U. and Ennis, F.A. (1988). Antibody-enhanced infection by HIV-1 via Fc receptor-mediated entry. *Science* **242**, 580–3.

Temin, H.M. and Mizutani, S. (1970). RNA-dependent-DNA polymerase in virions of Rous sarcoma virus. *Nature* **226**, 1211–13.

Thomas, P.A., Jaffe, H.W., Spira, T.J., Reiss, R., Guerro, I.C. and Auerbach, D. (1984). Unexplained immunodeficiency in children: a surveillance report. *JAMA* **252**, 639–44.

Tyler, D.S., Nastala, C.L., Stanley, S.D. *et al.* (1989). gp120 specific cellular cytotoxicity in HIV-1 seropositive individuals: evidence for circulating $CD16^+$ effector cells armed *in vivo* with cytophilic antibody. *J. Immunol.* **142**, 1177–82.

Ultmann, M.H., Belman, A.L. and Ruff, H.A. (1985). Developmental abnormalities in infants and children with acquired immunodeficiency syndrome (AIDS) and AIDS-related complex. *Dev. Med. Child. Neurol.* **27**, 563–71.

Ultmann, M.H., Diamond, G.W., Ruff, H.A. *et al.* (1987). Developmental abnormalities in children with acquired immunodeficiency syndrome (AIDS): a follow-up study. *Int. J. Neurosci.* **32**, 661–7.

Van de Perre, P., Hitimana, D.G. and Lepage, P. (1988). Human immunodeficiency virus antibodies of IgG, IgA, and IgM subclasses in milk of seropositive mothers. *J. Pediatr.* **113**, 1039–41.

Veronese, F.D., DeVico, A.L., Copeland, T.D., Oroszlan, S., Gallo, R.C. and Sarangadharan, M.G. (1985). Characterization of gp41 as the transmembrane protein coded by HTLV-III/LAV envelope gene. *Science* **229**, 1402–5.

Veronese, F.D., Copeland, T.D., DeVico, A.L. *et al.* (1986). Characterization of highly immunogenic p66/p51 as the reverse transcriptase of HTLV-III/LAV. *Science* **231**, 1289–91.

Wahn, V., Kramer, H., Voit, T., Bruster, H., Scrampical, B. and Scheid, A. (1986). Horizontal transmission of HIV infection between two siblings. *Lancet* **ii**, 694.

Weinhold, K.J., Lyerly, H.K., Matthews, T.J. *et al.* (1988). Cellular anti-gp120 cytolytic reactivities in HIV-1 seropositive individuals. *Lancet* **i**, 902–5.

Weinhold, K.J., Lyerly, H.K., Stanley, S.D., Austin, A.A., Matthews, T.J. and Bolognesi, D.P. (1989). HIV-1 gp120-mediated immune suppression and lympohocyte destruction in the absence of viral infection. *J. Immunol.* **142**, 3091–7.

Wiznia, A. and Rubinstein, A. (1988). Acquired immunodeficiency syndrome in infants and children. *Ann. Nestlé* **46**, 154–75.

Wiznia, A., Kashkin, J., Patterson, S. and Rubinstein, A. (1988). Increase in heterosexual contact as a risk factor in mothers of HIV infected children. In *4th International Conference on AIDS*, Stockholm, abstr. 4023.

Wolinsky, S.M., Wike, C.M., Korber, B.T.M. *et al.* (1992). Selective transmission of human immunodeficiency virus type-1 variants from mothers to infants. *Science* **255**, 1134–7.

Wong-Staal, F., Shaw, G.M., Hahn, B.H. *et al.* (1985). Genomic diversity of human T-lymphotropic virus type III (HTLV-III). *Science* **229**, 759–62.

Wright, C.M., Felber, B.K., Paskalis, H. and Pavlakis, G.N. (1986). Expression and characterization of the *trans*-activator of HTLV-III/LAV virus. *Science* **234**, 988–92.

Yarchoan, R. and Broder, S. (1987). Development of antiretroviral therapy for the acquired immunodeficiency syndrome and related disorders. *N. Engl. J. Med.* **316**, 557–64.

Yarchoan, R., Grafman, J., Brouwers, P. *et al.* (1987). Response of human immunodeficiency-virus-associated neurological disease to 3'-azido-3'deoxythymidine. *Lancet* **i**, 132–5.

Zagury, D., Bernhard, J., Leonard, R. *et al.* (1986). Long-term culture of HTLV-III-infected T cells: a model of cytopathology of T-cell depletion in AIDS. *Science* **231**, 850–3.

Ziegler, J.B., Cooper, D.A., Johnson, R.O. and Gold, J. (1985). Post-natal transmission of AIDS-associated retrovirus from mother to infant. *Lancet* **i**, 896–8.

Zilliacus, R., dela Chapelle, A., Schroder, J., Tilikainen, A., Kohne, E. and Kleihauer, E. (1975). Transplacental passage of foetal blood cells. *Scand. J. Haematol.* **15**, 333–8.

71: Immunological Abnormalities in Human Immunodeficiency Virus Infection

M. Seligmann

Introduction

Infection with the human immunodeficiency virus (HIV) results in a profound immunosuppression responsible for most of the clinical features of the acquired immune deficiency syndrome (AIDS). The virus devastates the immune system because its main target is the T4 lymphocyte, which is the key component for generating and regulating the immune response. The cellular receptor for HIV, the membrane glycoprotein CD4, is found mainly on the surface of this major subpopulation of T lymphocytes and also on other cell types such as the monocyte/macrophage series. The human immunodeficiency virus can destroy CD4 cells and causes functional impairment in T cells, B cells and monocytes. Host factors that may affect clinical outcome and immunological markers that may predict progression of HIV disease are currently being delineated. Protective humoral and cell-mediated immune responses to HIV are either poor or not sustained. A central question regarding immunity to HIV is its beneficial versus deleterious effects. The development of an AIDS vaccine faces many difficulties and still unanswered questions.

The crucial role of the CD4 molecule in human immunodeficiency virus infection

Since the observation that CD4 (T4) T lymphocytes

can be selectively infected by HIV, it has been demonstrated that the very molecule defining that subset, the CD4 glycoprotein, serves as the cellular receptor for the virus.

The interaction of CD4 with the human immunodeficiency virus envelope glycoprotein

A number of experimental data are now available which, taken together, demonstrate that the human CD4 molecule specifically binds the envelope glycoprotein gp120 of the HIV. Some monoclonal antibodies directed to the CD4 glycoprotein were shown to inhibit HIV binding, penetration and activity (Dalgleish *et al.* 1984; Klatzmann *et al.* 1984). A physical interaction between CD4 and HIV gp120 was further demonstrated by immunoprecipitation of these two antigens as a complex from infected cells (McDougal *et al.* 1986a). Maddon *et al.* (1986) showed that human cells that were CD4 −ve and refractory to infection with HIV acquired the ability to bind virus and became susceptible to HIV infection following transfection with cloned CD4 complementary deoxyribonucleic acid (cDNA). However, transfected murine cell lines expressing human CD4 efficiently bound HIV but were not susceptible to infection and could not fuse with HIV-infected human cells, suggesting that additional factors found in human cells but not in mouse cells are required for infection. A number of investigators (Smith *et al.* 1987; Berger *et al.* 1988; Deen *et al.* 1988; Fisher *et al.* 1988; Hussey *et al.* 1988; Traunecker *et al.* 1988) have described efficient expression systems in which a recombinant soluble form of CD4 (sCD4) is secreted into tissue culture medium supernatants. This sCD4 binds to gp120 with high affinity (K_D 10^{-9}M) (Lasky *et al.* 1987) and blocks HIV binding to CD4 +ve lymphocytes, resulting in a striking inhibition of syncytium formation and virus infectivity.

Much effort has been aimed at mapping the HIV gp120-binding site on CD4 and inversely at mapping the CD4-binding site on HIV gp120. An essential epitope for HIV binding had been defined by mapping with monoclonal antibodies (Sattentau *et al.* 1986). This epitope is located within the first of four immunoglobulin (Ig)-like domains of CD4, designated V1, as shown by cross-inhibition and peptide inhibition studies. Anti-idiotypic antibodies to CD4 monoclonals reactive with that epitope do recognize a conserved region on gp120 of HIV (Dalgleish *et al.* 1987). The sCD4 molecules have allowed a more precise delineation of the HIV-binding site. Studies of truncated or chimeric CD4 molecules, as well as elegant mutational analyses (Clayton *et al.* 1988; Mizukami *et al.* 1988; Peterson and Seed 1988) have identified stretches of sequence critical for recognition and binding of gp120 which are located in a relatively short region of the V1 domain, homologous to the complementarity-determining region 2 (CDR2) of Ig light chains. Mapping with site-directed mutants and anti-idiotypes (Sattentau *et al.* 1989) showed that the location of the epitopes is consistent with a folded Vκ-like structure of V1, most of the epitopes lying within regions of predicted exposed loops. Arthos *et al.* (1989) have quantitated the affinities for gp120 of several truncated derivatives of sCD4, as well as their ability to inhibit HIV infection *in vitro*. In addition, they have analysed a series of 26 amino acid substitutions within the V1 domain for gp120 binding and inhibition of HIV infection. These quantitative analyses demonstrated that there is a single binding site within this domain from residue 42 to 55. The crystal structure reveals that this region protrudes, is exposed on one face of the first domain and is structurally analogous to the second complementarity determining region (CDR2) of immunoglobulin light chains (Ryu *et al.* 1990). The recognition by gp120 of such a small loop on CD4 may forbid the recognition of the receptor-binding site by antibodies and thus allow the virus to evade the immune response. It should, however, be emphasized that the binding of gp120 is dependent on the stabilized tertiary structure of this small-sized binding region (Richardson *et al.* 1988; Ibegbu *et al.* 1989). CD4 +ve T lymphocytes interact with antigen-bearing target cells that express Class II major histocompatibility complex (MHC) molecules which associate specifically with CD4. The CD4 residues important in Class II MHC interaction involve a broader region than those involved in gp120 binding and appear to overlap with them, aminoacids Phe 43 and Gly 47 comprising an intimate part of both binding sites (Bowman *et al.* 1990). Clayton *et al.* (1989) have shown that mutations in CDR2 that destroy gp120 binding affect CD4-Class II MHC binding similarly. In addition, binding of soluble gp120 to CD4-transfected cells abrogates their ability to interact with Class II MHC-bearing B lymphocytes. However, the MHC-binding and gp120-binding functions of CD4 are separable (Lamarre *et al.* 1989a). Indeed Fleury *et al.* (1991) showed, in the context of the CD4 crystal structure, that mutations affecting the interaction with Class II MHC molecules are located on three exposed loops from CD4 domains 1 and 2 and specifically implicate residues 19, 89 and 165 situated on a surface opposite to the gp120-binding site.

Several studies using *in vitro* mutagenesis or monoclonal antibodies capable of blocking the gp120–CD4 interaction have indicated that the conserved carboxyterminal region of gp120 within amino acid residues 425–437 is critical for interaction with CD4 (Kowalski *et al.* 1987; Lasky *et al.* 1987; Sun *et al.* 1989). Further studies showed the conformation-dependent and discontinuous nature of the receptor-binding region and have identified carboxyterminal, as well as aminoterminal, regions of gp120 that affect its interaction with CD4 (Syu *et al.* 1990; Olshevsky *et al.* 1990) and could be closely positioned in the tertiary structure of the native envelope. Conservation of the tertiary structure of gp120 had indeed been shown to be necessary to retain binding activity for CD4 (McDougal *et al.* 1986b). Carbohydrates of CD4 and of gp120 do not appear to play a significant role in the *in vitro* interaction between these two molecules (Fenouillet *et al.* 1989).

Ivey-Hoyle *et al.* (1991) measured the affinity of envelope from diverse HIV strains and found a large variation. Human immunodeficiency virus 2 has been reported to require higher doses of sCD4 for neutralization than does HIV-1, a property attributed to lower affinity for CD4 (Moore 1990) or greater retention of envelope by HIV-2 (Looney *et al.* 1990).

Target cells

The CD4 molecule expression is not restricted to cells of the T lymphocyte lineage. Monocytes/macrophages, as well as monocyte lines, express CD4 to a variable degree and can be infected *in vitro* with HIV (Ho *et al.* 1986; Nicholson *et al.* 1986). In addition to attachment to the CD4 receptor, HIV can infect monocytes via phagocytic engulfment, and antibodies present in sera from HIV-infected individuals may enhance the infectivity of such Fc receptor-bearing cells (Homsy *et al.* 1988). However, CD4 is a dominant entry pathway for HIV-1 infection of macrophage (Collman *et al.* 1990) and interaction with CD4 is required for infectivity even under conditions of antibody-mediated binding of HIV-1 to Fc receptors for IgG (Connor *et al.* 1991). The monocyte may serve as a reservoir for HIV in the body and play an important role in the initiation and propagation of HIV infection. There is a biological variation in the tropism of HIV *in vitro* for lymphocytes or monocytes. Monocytotropic and lymphocytotropic strains of HIV-1 show distinctive patterns of replication (Collmann *et al.* 1989; Schwartz *et al.* 1989). Determinants responsible for HIV-1 tropism for mononuclear phagocytes have been identified in regions of gp120 outside the CD4-binding domain (O'Brien *et al.* 1990) and more precisely in the third variable domain (Westervelt *et al.* 1991) where a 20-amino acids sequence in the V3 loop is sufficient to confer macrophage tropism (Hwang *et al.* 1991). Hattori *et al.* (1990) showed that the *vpr* gene is essential for productive infection of human macrophages.

Follicular dendritic cells of germinal centres (Tenner-Racz *et al.* 1986) and Langerhans cells in the skin (Tschachler *et al.* 1987) also express CD4 and replicate virus. Dendritic cells support the active replication of all strains of HIV-1, including T cell tropic and monocytotropic isolates, suggesting that this antigen-presenting cell population may play a central role in HIV pathogenesis (Langhoff *et al.* 1991). Some B cell lines transformed by Epstein–Barr virus (EBV) are infectible in culture and may express surface CD4 or CD4 messenger ribonucleic acid (mRNA) (Montagnier *et al.* 1984; Malkovsky *et al.* 1988); the infection of normal B cells, however, has not been demonstrated. Neurological manifestations imply cells of the central nervous system as another target for HIV. The predominant cell type in the brain that is infected is the macrophage and the related microglial cell (Koenig *et al.* 1986; Vazeux *et al.* 1987). The implication of endothelial cells in the brain (Wiley *et al.* 1986) is still a matter of controversy. There is very little evidence of *in vivo* infection in neurons, oligodendrocytes or astrocytes (Price *et al.* 1988). However, neurons and glial cells, as well as other CD4 –ve cells such as fibroblastic cells or rhabdomyosarcoma cell lines, can be infected *in vitro* at low efficiency (Clapham *et al.* 1989; Harouse *et al.* 1989; Tateno *et al.* 1989), even in the presence of sCD4 and monoclonal antibodies to CD4. Infection of immature bone marrow cells (Folks *et al.* 1988) and detection of productive infection of CD8 +ve CD4 −ve lymphocyte lines (Tsubota *et al.* 1989a) have also been described. It cannot be however ruled out that infection of these cells occurred at a stage during which CD4 was expressed. All these findings suggest the possibility of an alternative, less efficient, route of virus entry. Antibodies to galactosyl ceramide inhibit uptake and infection of HIV-1 in neural cell lines (Harouse *et al.* 1991) and recombinant gp120 specifically binds to galactosyl ceramide (Bhat *et al.* 1991), suggesting that this molecule may serve as an alternative receptor for HIV in the nervous system. On the other hand, Boyer *et al.* (1991) showed that complement in the absence of antibody may enhance infection of C3 receptor-bearing T cells with HIV-1 and that the interaction of opsonized virus with the CR2 receptor may result by itself in the infection of target T cells in a CD4 −ve and antibody-independent fashion.

Virus entry and cytopathic effects of human immunodeficiency virus infection

The precise mechanism of virus entry into the target cell is not yet fully understood. Internalization of CD4 molecules is observed after exposure of CD4 +ve T cells to either phorbol ester or appropriate antigen-bearing target cells. This and other observations have suggested that the complex of HIV and CD4 on the cell surface could be internalized via endocytosis, leading to virus entry. However, the pH-independent entry of HIV into cells (Stein *et al.* 1987) suggests that receptor-mediated endocytosis is not essential for internalization. Bedinger *et al.* (1988) have shown that internalization of HIV does not require the cytoplasmic domains of CD4. Indeed, Maddon *et al.* (1988) introduced a series of mutations in the cytoplasmic domain of the CD4 cDNA that block internalization of the CD4 molecule and showed that cells expressing the mutant CD4 molecules remain susceptible to HIV infection. These studies indicate that HIV entry proceeds via direct fusion of the viral envelope with the cell membrane. A hydrophobic aminoterminal region of gp41 provides at least one fusion site (Kowalski *et al.* 1987) which has recently been more precisely characterized (Freed *et al.* 1990). In addition, Ho *et al.* (1988) have shown that the second conserved domain of gp120 is important in post-binding events during virus penetration; within this region, there exists a site (residue 269) that appears critical for infectivity (Willey *et al.* 1988). Gowda *et al.* (1989) provided evidence that HIV entry and HIV envelope-dependent cell-to-cell fusion require T cell activation. The study by Pantaleo *et al.* (1991) of CD4 +ve T lymphocytes genetically deficient in LFA-1 has demonstrated that LFA-1 is required for HIV-mediated cell fusion but not for viral transmission.

The CD4 molecule itself may play an important role in the fusion process. CD4 +ve cells from the chimpanzee bind HIV and support viral infection but do not fuse with HIV-infected cells. A recent study by Camerini and Seed (1990) suggests that the inability of CD4 +ve cells from the chimpanzee to support syncytium formation is inherent in the CD4 molecule itself and can be traced to a single amino acid change at position 87, well outside the virus-binding site. Interestingly, benzylated derivatives corresponding to the 81−92 sequence were shown to block fusion and also binding (Kalyanaraman *et al.* 1990). The presence of a glutamic acid at position 87 in this sequence is more critical for the CD4/gp120 interaction leading to syncytium formation than for the CD4/gp120 interaction leading to primary infection of CD4 +ve cells (Lifson *et al.* 1991). Nevertheless, it is possible that other regions of CD4 are required after binding for successful fusion and infection. Celada *et al.* (1990) detected a conformational change in CD4 as a consequence of gp120 binding and antibodies that recognized the conformational change inhibited HIV fusion with CD4 cells. Healey *et al.* (1990) and Truneh *et al.* (1991) identified several anti-CD4 monoclonal antibodies that do not block gp120 binding but inhibit virus fusion and infectivity.

Moore *et al.* (1990) reported that sCD4 causes the release of gp120 from virions resulting in irreversible inactivation of HIV infectivity. This gp120 dissociation occurs at 37°C but not 4°C and requires occupancy by CD4 of multiple binding sites on a gp120−gp41 oligomer (Moore *et al.* 1991). Recent experiments with short synthetic CD4 peptide derivatives provided evidence for the significance of gp120 release for membrane fusion and suggest the involvement of the specific region corresponding to residues 81−92 (Berger *et al.* 1991). The engagement of cellular CD4 by the virion might induce a secondary change in the virion that is required for penetration, such as exposition of gp120 to a protease, allowing a fusion domain in gp41 to contact the cell membrane.

After penetrating the target cell, the virus remains latent and increased viral replication is only observed upon activation of the host CD4 +ve cell. HIV-1 can persist in a non-productive extra chromosomal state in resting T cells (Stevenson *et al*. 1990) and initiate synthesis of only incomplete viral DNA species (Zack *et al*. 1990). Activation of these T cells by antigens, mitogens, select cytokines or various gene products of different viruses creates a permissive cellular environment that promotes a high level of HIV replication. Many of these activating agents induce the expression of host transcription factors such as the NF-κB family of enhancer binding proteins. When active replication of virus occurs, the host cell is usually killed. Of note is the fact that the monocyte and dendritic cell are resistant to the cytopathic effect of HIV. The precise mechanisms of direct cell-killing by HIV remain unknown. The accumulation of large amounts of unintegrated viral DNA in the infected cells has been suggested as an important factor (Shaw *et al*. 1984). It is also possible that formation of intracellular complexes of CD4 and viral envelope proteins may trigger the fusogenic activity of gp41 and play a role in the cytopathic effect (Hoxie *et al*. 1986). The susceptibility to cytopathic effects has been correlated with the density of CD4 expressed on the cell surface (Hoxie *et al*. 1986). Salmon *et al*. (1988) have shown that the initial diminution in surface CD4 observed after infection results from the interaction of CD4 with surface gp120 and that, late in infection, levels of CD4 mRNA decrease significantly. However, Schnittman *et al*. (1989) have shown that the CD4 +ve T cell in AIDS patients maintains expression of its surface CD4 molecule despite actively expressing HIV-1.

Mechanisms of CD4-positive cell depletion in human-immunodeficiency-virus-infected individuals

Low numbers of T cells appear to be actively engaged in virus replication *in vivo* at any one time (Harper *et al*. 1986). The precursor frequency of CD4 +ve T cells that are actively expressing HIV-1 (as determined by *in situ* hybridization, immunofluorescence to detect viral antigens and limiting dilution analysis of co-cultures) in patients with AIDS is approximately 1/1000 cells (Schnittman *et al*. 1989). The same authors found, with polymerase chain reaction (PCR) technique, that the frequency of CD4 +ve T cells that contain proviral DNA is at least 1/100 in patients with AIDS and in the order of 1/10 000 cells in asymptomatic seropositive individuals. The relatively high viral burden may thus be an important cause for the accelerated decline in T4 cell number in patients with AIDS.

In addition to this direct cytopathic effect of HIV, several other mechanisms may account for the profound depletion of CD4 +ve cells. One such mechanism is cell fusion. A single infected cell can fuse with many CD4 +ve uninfected lymphocytes, form syncytia and then lyse (Lifson *et al*. 1986; Sodroski *et al*. 1986). Another potential mechanism of T4 cell depletion involves autoimmune phenomena (Klatzmann and Montagnier 1986; Ziegler and Stites 1986). The molecular mimicry between HIV and human leucocyte antigen (HLA) Class II MHC antigens may lead to the generation of autoantibodies reacting with both the carboxyl terminus of gp160 and Class II MHC molecules, contributing to immune dysfunction in HIV-infected individuals (Golding *et al*. 1989). Allo-immune and autoimmune mice were shown to make anti-HIV antibodies, without being exposed to HIV, as well as anti-anti-MHC antibodies (Kion and Hoffmann 1991). Autoantibodies to sCD4 have been found in a significant portion of HIV-infected patients (Chams *et al*. 1988; Thiriart *et al*. 1988; Kowalski *et al*. 1989). Most of these antibodies are directed against a region of CD4 distinct from the virus-binding domain. Their pathogenic significance and clinical relevance remain to be defined. More importantly, uninfected cells that have bound with high affinity shed gp120 to the CD4 molecule could be recognized as non-self. It is evident that host defence mechanisms such as antibody-dependent cellular toxicity or HLA-restricted cytotoxicity might contribute to pathogenesis by eliminating, in addition to HIV-infected lymphocytes, such uninfected cells targeted by the attachment of free gp120 to CD4. These bystander cells become targets for anti-gp120 antibodies and can be killed via antibody-dependent cell-mediated cytotoxicity (ADCC) (Lyerly *et al*. 1987a).

Also, such bystander uninfected cells can internalize gp120 bound tightly to CD4 on their surface, process it and present peptides derived from it on their Class II MHC molecules, thus becoming sensitive, even at low gp120 concentrations, to lysis by gp120-specific cytotoxic T cells (Lanzavecchia *et al.* 1988; Siliciano *et al.* 1988). Finally, it is most intriguing that destroyed CD4 +ve T cells are not regenerated by bone marrow precursors. The possibility exists that HIV infects an intrathymic T4 cell precursor or that HIV induces secretion of soluble factors which are toxic to T4 cells (Fauci 1988).

Recent findings suggest the possibility that activation-induced death by apoptosis might account for the progressive depletion of CD4 +ve T cells. Ameisen and Capron (1991) have proposed that inappropriate induction of apoptosis could account for both early qualitative and late quantitative CD4 +ve T lymphocyte defects in HIV-infected individuals; this group has shown (Groux *et al.* 1992) that the failure of CD4 +ve T cells from asymptomatic HIV-infected patients to proliferate *in vitro* to TCR mobilization by Class-II-dependent superantigens and to pokeweed mitogen is indeed due to this active cell death process. The mechanisms by which T cells in HIV-infected individuals are programmed for death upon further activation by various stimuli such as antigens and superantigens is unknown. Systemic effects of HIV-proteins or disturbances of cytokine networks (IFNγ, TGFβ) may well be involved. Janeway (1991) has proposed that, like the mammary tumour virus, HIV might encode a superantigen responsible for CD4 +ve T cell depletion, possibly by both priming for and inducing apoptosis. Imberti *et al.* (1991) have examined the repertoire of TCR V regions in persons infected with HIV and claimed the absence of a common set of Vβ regions, possibly indicating the presence of HIV-encoded superantigens since the lack of these Vβ segments was not correlated with the existence of opportunistic infections. This finding has not been confirmed by B. Autran and F. Sigau (pers. comm.). On the other hand, Terai *et al.* (1991) and Laurent-Crawford *et al.* (1991) recently showed that the cytopathic effect induced by acute HIV infection of T-cell lines or of normal activated mononuclear cells is associated with apoptosis.

Therapeutic approaches

The understanding of the interaction between CD4 and gp120 has allowed the design of new therapeutic strategies to inhibit HIV infection and spread *in vivo*. Dextran sulphate was found to block the binding of virions to target T lymphocytes and to inhibit syncytium formation. However no efficiency has been demonstrated in patients. Aurin tricarboxylic acid selectively binds to the CD4 receptor for HIV and also interferes with the staining of membrane-associated gp120 by a specific monoclonal antibody (Schols *et al.* 1989). The use of anti-CD4 monoclonal antibodies in humans is limited by the development of an immune response against murine Ig. In addition, in view of the partial overlap of the Class II MHC-binding site on CD4 with the gp120-binding site, some anti-CD4 antibodies may have immunosuppressive effects *in vivo*.

The ability of soluble CD4 to bind gp120 and inhibit viral infection *in vitro* immediately suggested the potential use of sCD4 as an antiviral agent in patients. The CD4-binding domain of gp120 is the only part that the virus cannot afford to change. Thus, sCD4 is likely to be a universal inhibitor of HIV infection. *In vitro* quantitative assays showed that sCD4 reduces the infectivity of HIV-1 by at least 4 logs when used at concentrations approaching 10 μg/ml (Deen *et al.* 1988). The optimal inhibition of HIV infection is obtained when sCD4 is maintained throughout the culture, even with low sCD4 doses (Byrn *et al.* 1989). It should, however, be noted that sCD4 blocks HIV-2 infectivity less effectively and does not inhibit infection of glioma and rhabdomyosarcoma cell lines (Clapham *et al.* 1989). Moreover, there is recent evidence from Daar *et al.* (1991) that isolates of HIV freshly obtained from patients are substantially less sensitive to the inhibitory effects of soluble CD4 than the laboratory strains initially used to define this activity. This phenomenon, which is not due to lower binding affinity between sCD4 and free gp120 from primary isolates (Ashkenazi *et al.* 1991), may pose an important problem for sCD4-based treatment of HIV-infected patients.

The use of sCD4 in man will depend upon its pharmacokinetics, its immunogenicity, its effect upon the cellular immune response and its ability to display important antiviral activities *in vivo*.

Watanabe *et al.* (1989) have shown that sCD4 was able to protect two macaques from simian immunodeficiency virus (SIV) and that isolation of the virus became very difficult in two others that were already SIV-infected. More recently the same group (Watanabe *et al.* 1991) demonstrated that human sCD4 elicits in immunized Rhesus monkeys an IgG antibody response that inhibits SIV replication. Soluble CD4 has been used in phase I–II clinical trials (Schooley *et al.* 1990; Kahn *et al.* 1990). Its half-life is short. The molecule appears to be well tolerated at doses up to 30 mg/day and to exert minimal immunosuppressive effects, thus corroborating *in vitro* data showing that sCD4 does not significantly inhibit the activation of human peripheral blood lymphocytes by mitogens, tetanus toxoid or allogeneic cells (Liu and Liu 1988). Serum concentrations of sCD4 were achieved that were comparable to concentrations shown to have antiviral activity *in vitro*. A decline in p24 antigen was seen in some patients receiving 30 mg of sCD4 daily. However, no significant decrease in viral titres was found during therapy (Daar *et al.* 1990).

A number of groups have developed a second generation of agents by modifying the sCD4 molecule in order to enhance its antiviral capabilities. Till *et al.* (1988) conjugated sCD4 to the active subunit of the toxin ricin. This conjugate killed HIV-infected H-9 cells but was 1/1000 as toxic to uninfected H-9 cells and was not toxic to Daudi cells (which express Class II MHC antigens). A second elegant CD4 chimera has been constructed by Chaudary *et al.* (1988). This hybrid molecule consists of the first 178 amino acids of CD4 fused to domains II and III of the *Pseudomonas* exotoxin protein. The major problems of these chimeras lie in their potential toxicity for non-infected cells, their potential immunogenicity and the possible destruction of HLA Class II MHC-expressing cells. Moreover Tsubota *et al.* (1990) recently demonstrated that CD4 −ve *Pseudomonas* exotoxin conjugates do not fully inhibit HIV replication in lymphocytes *in vitro*.

Antibody-like molecules containing the gp120-binding domain of CD4 have been constructed. These chimeric molecules (CD4 immunoadhesin) may overcome the half-life problem of sCD4 and confer upon the sCD4 molecules some of the important effector functions of Ig, thus making them good candidates for therapeutic use. Capon *et al.* (1989) have designed hybrid CD4 molecules in which the variable domain of a human γ-1 heavy-chain Ig gene is replaced with either the two N-terminal domains or the four domains of sCD4. This hybrid is efficiently secreted as a stable dimer. It binds gp120 with high affinity and inhibits viral infection *in vitro* as efficiently as the intact sCD4. The chimeric molecule exhibits a longer half-life than CD4 and binds well to Fc receptors (but not to C1q). It is transferred across the placenta of rhesus monkeys and can mediate ADCC towards HIV-infected cells, although it does not allow ADCC towards uninfected CD4 +ve cells that have bound gp120 (Byrn *et al.* 1990). No evidence was found for enhancement of infection by the hybrid in cells which express high-affinity Fc receptors. CD4 derivatives which intrinsically lack the ability to bind Class II MHC molecules are currently being developed. In contrast to recombinant sCD4, CD4-IgG immunoadhesin does block syncytium formation by HIV-2-infected lymphoid cells (Serigawa *et al.* 1990). Ward *et al.* (1991) recently demonstrated that pretreatment with CD4-IgG immunoadhesin can prevent the infection of chimpanzees with HIV-1. Since this molecule efficiently crosses the placenta, this finding points to possible prevention of materno-fetal transfer of HIV infection. Traunecker *et al.* (1989) generated molecules where the V_H and C_H1 domains of mouse γ-2a or μ heavy chains are replaced with the first two N-terminal domains of CD4. These molecules are secreted in the absence of any Ig light chain. The pentameric CD4–IgM chimera is at least 1000-fold more active than the dimeric CD4–IgG in syncytium inhibition assays. Effector functions, such as the binding of Fc receptors and of C1q, are retained. No negative effects on humoral and cellular immune responses were observed in transgenic mice expressing constitutively high serum levels of these soluble CD4–Ig molecules. Human clinical trials will assess efficacy of these second-generation CD4-based molecules *in vivo*.

Main immunological abnormalities in human immunodeficiency virus disease

There is a trend towards more severe immunological abnormalities with clinical progression from an asymptomatic state to AIDS-related complex (ARC) and to AIDS (Lane *et al.* 1985a).

Furthermore, within AIDS patients, those with Kaposi's sarcoma alone usually have fewer abnormalities than those with opportunistic infections.

T cells

The hallmark of the immune defect in AIDS is a quantitative and qualitative defect of CD4 +ve cells. Since this T cell subset has a central role in the immune response, loss of its activity will compromise the function of other cell types. For example, the induction of T cytotoxic responses requires CD4 +ve cells, as does antibody production by B cells. The defects of CD4 +ve cells result in reduced elaboration of lymphokines.

A profound decline in the number of circulating CD4 T cells and the occurrence of impaired delayed-type hypersensitivity reactions are relatively late events in the course of HIV disease. Since the number of CD8 T cells is usually increased, the total T cell level remains often near normal, and profound lymphopenia is rarely observed. There is no major imbalance in the number of T lymphocytes bearing the $\gamma\delta$ receptor, or their subsets (Autran *et al.* 1989). A selective loss of CD29 +ve T4 memory cells has been consistently observed in asymptomatic HIV-infected individuals with still normal numbers of CD4 +ve T cells (Giorgi and Detels 1989; van Noesel *et al.* 1990). These CD4 +ve memory T cells are preferentially infected by HIV-1 (Schnittman *et al.* 1990). Early depletion of memory T cells may partly explain functional defects.

Human immunodeficiency virus causes a number of functional abnormalities in the remaining CD4 T cells, even in the absence of any CD4 cell depletion. The earlier abnormality that occurs in HIV +ve asymptomatic individuals is a selective defect in lymphocyte proliferative responses to HIV antigens (Gurley *et al.* 1989), even in the presence of recombinant interleukin 2 (IL-2) (Krowka *et al.* 1989). An impairment of proliferative responses to soluble recall antigens (Shearer *et al.* 1984), such as tetanus toxoid (Lane *et al.* 1985b; Gurley *et al.* 1989), other microbial antigens (Ballet *et al.* 1988) or influenza A virus (Clerici *et al.* 1989a), indicating a selective defect in CD4 +ve MHC-restricted T helper function, usually occurs a little later in the course of HIV infection, and is found in most patients with few symptoms. An impairment of the proliferative response of highly purified T cells to anti-CD3 antibodies and to a lesser degree to anti-CD2 antibodies, is also observed at a relatively early stage (Miedema *et al.* 1988; Bentin *et al.* 1989; Gruters *et al.* 1990). Helper activity induced by pokeweed mitogen is low (Terpstra *et al.* 1989; Hofmann *et al.* 1989). Although the selective inhibition of the proliferative response of clonal CD4 +ve T lymphocytes to alloantigen is an early consequence of *in vitro* HIV infection (Laurence *et al.* 1989), the loss of response of the patient's lymphocytes to HLA alloantigens occurs later than the previous defects (Clerici *et al.* 1989a). Those mitogen responses such as phytohaemagglutinin, which are not critically dependent on the CD4–Class II MHC interaction, remain normal in many patients with a selective defect in antigen responses. Langhoff *et al.* (1989) have shown that T cells from seropositive individuals, even those with markedly reduced CD4 cell counts, exhibit a normal cloning efficiency and proliferative capacity.

Several groups have shown that the HIV envelope protein gp120 can specifically inhibit *in vitro*, in a dose-dependent way, the Class II MHC-restricted antigen-driven proliferative responses of peripheral blood T cells, human CD4-transfected murine T cell hybridoma and tetanus toxoid-specific T cell clones (Shalaby *et al.* 1987; Diamond *et al.* 1988; Gurley *et al.* 1989; Weinhold *et al.* 1989; Chirmule *et al.* 1990), as well as OKT3-driven proliferation of cloned CD4 +ve lymphocytes (Weinhold *et al.* 1989). The precise mechanism of this gp120-mediated immune suppression, which is based on its unique interaction with CD4, is still unclear. Immunosuppression by gp120 can be inhibited by soluble CD4 *in vitro* (Lamarre *et al.* 1989b). Oyaizu *et al.* (1990) have shown that the inhibitory effect of gp120 occurred concomitantly with decreased IL-2 production, reduced expression of the gene encoding IL-2 and reduced surface IL-2 receptor. Glycoprotein 120 appears to interfere with an essential role of the CD4 molecule in signal transduction through the CD3–antigen receptor complex. Indeed, such signal transduction mechanisms appear to be modified in HIV-infected T cells (Gupta and Vayuvegula 1987; Linette *et al.* 1988). Nye and Pinching (1990) showed that HIV-1 infection alters key parameters of the inositol polyphosphate pathway. Cefai *et al.* (1990) demonstrated that HIV-1 envelope glycoproteins specifically inhibit this CD3/TcR phosphoinositide transduction pathway. Mittler and Hoffmann (1989) have shown that CD4-bound gp120 attracts gp120-specific antibodies to form a trimolecular complex with itself and CD4. The gp120-specific antibody thus functions as an antibody to CD4 and there is a synergism between gp120 and anti-gp120 in blocking T cell activation.

CD8 +ve T lymphocytes also show profound functional defects in persons infected with HIV. They contain increased percentages of cells with phenotypes associated with activation, expressing MHC Class II markers during the asymptomatic stage and abundant CD38 and CD57 markers at later stages. These activated CD8 +ve cells are apparently refractory to further *in vitro* signals for proliferation (Pantaleo *et al.* 1990) and are reported to die in culture (Prince and Jensen 1991).

Thus chronic activation, with defective signal transduction, leading to impaired responses to further stimulation is observed in CD4 +ve, as well as CD8 +ve T cells (and also B cells) (Pinching and Nye 1990). Impaired T cell signal transduction mediated by HIV proteins may prime CD4 +ve T cells (and possibly other cells such as neurons) from HIV-infected individuals for apoptosis in response to antigens and superantigens (see above: Mechanisms of CD4 cell depletion). This hypothesis provides a possible explanation not only for CD4 +ve T cell dysfunction but also for CD8 +ve T cell and B cell hyperactivation since apoptosis is associated with early lymphokine secretion and with release of nucleosomes that can activate B cells (Ameisen 1992).

B cells

Infection with HIV leads to significant abnormalities of B cell function. Polyclonal activation of B cells and hypergammaglobulinaemia are usual from early stages of infection. This polyclonal hyperactivity of B cells is probably due to multiple factors. The high incidence of infection with EBV and cytomegalovirus (CMV), both of which are polyclonal B cell activators, may contribute to this phenomenon. Human immunodeficiency virus itself or subunits of the virus can polyclonally activate B cells *in vitro*, either by direct stimulation or through the induction of B cell growth factors in T cells (Pahwa *et al.* 1986; Schnittman *et al.* 1986; Yarchoan *et al.* 1986). IL-6 expression is upregulated (Nakajima *et al.* 1989) and IL-6 serum levels in individuals infected with monocytotropic HIV correlates directly with serum IgG levels (Birx *et al.* 1990). Delfraissy *et al.* (1991) showed that HIV or its recombinant *env* gp160 protein can render B cells responsive to the growth-promoting effect of several T cell-derived interleukins. This competence signal is provided in the absence of monocytes and the CD4 molecule is not involved. *In vitro* spontaneous immunoglobulin synthesis is a prominent feature of seropositive subjects (Yarchoan *et al.* 1986; Teeuwsen *et al.* 1987; Mizuma *et al.* 1988). Amadori *et al.* (1989) showed that B cell activation is mainly orientated towards a specific response to HIV determinants.

Oligoclonal Ig components are frequently detected by sensitive techniques in the serum of HIV-infected patients or asymptomatic individuals (Papadopoulos *et al.* 1985; Crapper *et al.* 1987). Many of these sera contain several detectable monoclonal Ig, with predominance of IgG3 and IgG4 subclasses and of λ light chains (Briault *et al.* 1988). Ng *et al.* (1989) have shown that IgG1κ paraproteins found in five HIV-1-infected individuals displayed at least two light chain species and were reactive with multiple HIV-1 viral antigens. They showed in addition that subsequent clinical evaluation of the patients failed to correlate the presence of oligoclonal Ig with the development of lymphoma over a 2–3-year period.

Despite hypergammaglobulinaemia, there is a deficient antibody response to new antigens (Lane *et al.* 1983). B cell functional defects represent probably one of the first immunological abnormalities in the course of HIV infection (reviewed in Pinching 1991). Ballet *et al.* (1987) found that antibody responses to polysaccharide antigens were impaired in most asymptomatic patients, including those with normal humoral response to protein antigens and normal CD4 T cell numbers. Miedema *et al.* (1988) showed that in such individuals B cell differentiation in a pokeweed mitogen-driven system was completely absent. A recent longitudinal study by the same group (Terpstra *et al.* 1989) showed that this defect occurred shortly after seroconversion and was not restored by addition of normal CD4 +ve T cells. The addition of envelope peptides to a pokeweed mitogen-induced B cell activation system results in suppression of Ig synthesis by normal lymphocytes (Nair *et al.* 1988). Delfraissy *et al.* (1991)

showed that HIV is able to render B cells susceptible to suppression by tumour necrosis factor (TNF)-α, which down-regulates the B cell response to various interleukins.

These B cell defects explain why frequent and severe pyogenic infections, particularly with encapsulated bacteria, are encountered in patients with AIDS (Polsky *et al.* 1986); they are especially frequent in HIV-infected children. The occurrence of pyogenic infections is significantly associated with deficiency in IgG2 subclass (Parkin *et al.* 1989). Natural antibacterial activity against *Salmonella* is significantly decreased in AIDS patients as well as in asymptomatic HIV-infected individuals (Tagliabue *et al.* 1988).

Antigen-presenting cells

Evidence is accumulating to support the theory that monocytes and macrophages are involved in the pathogenesis of HIV infection. The virus can be isolated from or identified in monocytes obtained from the blood and mainly from cells of monocytic lineage in the brain and alveolar macrophages in the lung (Gartner *et al.* 1986; Ho *et al.* 1986; Nicholson *et al.* 1986). Normal, nonproliferating monocytes differ from T lymphocytes in that a productive HIV-1 infection can occur independently of cellular DNA synthesis (Weinberg *et al.* 1991). These results suggest that mononuclear phagocytes which are resistant to the destructive effects of the virus, may serve as persistent and productive reservoirs for HIV-1 *in vivo*. However, monocytes are neither a primary nor an exclusive reservoir of HIV infection in the blood and bone marrow (McElrath *et al.* 1989; Schnittman *et al.* 1989). Efficient transmission of virus from macrophages to activated T cells during antigen presentation has been demonstrated (Mann *et al.* 1990; Massari *et al.* 1990), supporting the notion that tissue macrophages are the main producers of HIV. Macrophages and monocytes show reduced HLA Class II MHC expression and a number of functional defects that can impair both antigen-presenting and effector functions (Smith *et al.* 1984; Poli *et al.* 1985; Eales *et al.* 1987; Rich *et al.* 1988). Normal monocytes infected with HIV-1 or exposed to purified gp120 demonstrate a down-regulation of chemotactic ligand receptors and migratory function (Wahl *et al.* 1989) and a deficiency in intracellular killing ability (Baldwin *et al.* 1990). Longitudinal studies showed that antigen-presenting cell functions are not significantly affected in early infection (Clerici *et al.* 1990). Monocyte defects are found in approximately 50% of ill patients, but not in asymptomatic HIV-infected individuals (Clerici *et al.* 1991a).

Monocytes treated with recombinant IFN-α at the time of HIV challenge show no evidence of virus infection 3 weeks later and the IFN-α induced antiviral activity is equally dramatic when monocytes were infected prior to treatment (Gendelman *et al.* 1990). Glutathione and N-acetyl cysteine suppress in a dose-dependent fashion the induction of HIV expression mediated by PMA, TNF-α and IL-6 in chronically infected monocytic cells (Kalbic *et al.* 1991). It should also be noted that HIV-infected macrophages produce soluble factors that cause histological and neurochemical alterations in cultured human brains (Pullian *et al.* 1991).

Dendritic cells and Langerhans cells, which have a major antigen-presenting role, are extensively infected by HIV at an early stage. Decreased expression of HLA Class II antigens and severe functional impairment has been noted in these cells (Eales *et al.* 1988; Macatonia *et al.* 1990). Circulating dendritic cells are depleted in asymptomatic and symptomatic HIV infection (Macatonia *et al.* 1990). Dendritic cells, which travel from mucosa to the lymph node via the circulation, may be a site of primary infection. They can readily be infected by a variety of HIV-1 lymphocytotropic and monocytotropic strains. They produce large amounts of virus in the absence of detectable cytopathic effects (Langhoff *et al.* 1991) and may play an important role in CD4 +ve T cell infection.

Interleukins

There is general agreement that IL-2 and interferon-γ production are impaired by HIV infection (Murray *et al.* 1984, 1988). The loss of such lymphokine activities may affect multiple components of the immune system. For instance, natural killer cell function is usually impaired in AIDS patients and may be reconstituted by the addition of IL-2 (Rook *et al.* 1983).

Conversely HIV infection results in increased production of IL-6 (Nakajima *et al.* 1989), IL-1α (Weiss *et al.* 1989) and TNF-α (Roux-Lombard *et al.* 1989) by monocytes. Patients with AIDS have elevated levels of circulating TNF-α (Lahdevirta *et al.* 1988). It should be noted that stimulation by

Candida albicans (Djeu *et al.* 1988) or by some herpes group viruses such as CMV and EBV (Clouse *et al.* 1989) induce the production of this monokine. Tumour necrosis factor α, in turn, induces HIV replication and expression in chronically infected cells (Folks *et al.* 1989). This stimulation of the HIV enhancer is mediated by the cellular transcription factor NF(nuclear factor)-κB (Osborn *et al.* 1989). IL-6 and GM-CSF are also able to induce HIV expression in infected monocytic cells, alone or in synergy with TNF-α, by post-transcriptional mechanisms (Poli *et al.* 1990a). Activated B cells from HIV-infected persons are capable of inducing HIV expression by virtue of secretion of cytokines such as TNF-α and IL-6 (Rieckmann *et al.* 1991). Human immunodeficiency virus 1 can thus augment its own expression by inducing the secretion of monokines which upregulate HIV expression in the infected cells and function in an autocrine manner (Poli *et al.* 1990b; Rosenburg and Fauci 1990).

In contrast, to the induction of HIV expression, certain interleukins can actually downregulate the expression of HIV. Interferon alpha has such properties and blocks the budding of HIV from chronically infected cell lines (Poli *et al.* 1989). Tumour necrosis factor beta suppresses HIV expression induced by PMA or by IL-6 (Fauci 1991).

Autoimmune phenomena and haematological disorders

A number of autoimmune phenomena, usually not associated with clinical expression, have been described in HIV-infected patients (Kopelman and Zolla-Pazner 1988). Anti-cardiolipin antibodies are frequently observed in these patients (Stimmler *et al.* 1989), as well as autoantibodies directed to CD4 +ve T lymphocytes, whose significance has been discussed in the previous section. Human immunodeficiency virus 1 infection was recently shown to be specifically associated with the production of autoantibodies that bind to CD43 on normal T lymphocytes. Several researchers believe that autoimmune phenomena, host immunoregulatory mechanisms and allogeneic stimuli may play an important role in the pathogenesis of AIDS (Via *et al.* 1990; Hoffmann *et al.* 1991).

The issue of HIV infection of hematopoietic precursor cells is still a matter of controversy (Folks 1991). Among the HIV-associated haematological disorders (Scadden *et al.* 1989), immune thrombocytopenia deserves special consideration. This condition occurs in 5–10% of HIV-infected individuals, in all risk groups and at any stage of the natural history of HIV disease, mainly in CDC (Center for Disease Control) groups II and III. Patients with thrombocytopenia are not at greater risk for development of AIDS than seropositive non-thrombocytopenic individuals (Oksenhendler and Seligmann 1990). The precise mechanism(s) leading to immune thrombocytopenia remain unclear; the respective role of autoantibodies or immune complexes in the peripheral platelet destruction is still debated, as well as the direct or indirect responsibility of HIV itself. Van der Lelie *et al.* (1987) and Bettaieb *et al.* (1989) found in the serum and platelet eluates of such patients autoantibodies to normal platelets with, sometimes, a specificity similar to that observed in classic autoimmune thrombocytopenic purpura. The responsibility of non-specific immune complexes was first suggested by Walsh *et al.* (1984). Karpatkin *et al.* (1988) have claimed that 50% of eluted platelet IgG contain anti-HIV-1 antibodies complexed with anti-idiotypic antibodies, in the absence of detectable HIV-1 antigens or proviral DNA. Human immunodeficiency virus may directly affect megakaryocytes: HIV transcripts have been detected by *in situ* hybridization in megakaryocytes from patients with AIDS (Zucker-Franklin and Cao 1989) and from AIDS-free seropositive thrombocytopenic patients (Louache *et al.* 1991). Human immunodeficiency virus infection of megakaryocytes could thus favour thrombocytopenia through the expression of low amounts of HIV antigens on platelets. Indeed, a direct or indirect role of HIV in the process of platelet destruction is suggested by the effectiveness of Zidovudine therapy (Swiss Group 1988; Oksenhendler *et al.* 1989). In our present experience, with a median follow-up of 24 months, Zidovudine provides a sustained response in about 60% of the patients, while on therapy (Oksenhendler and Seligmann 1990).

Immunological aspects of the natural history of human immunodeficiency virus disease

Cohort studies of people with HIV infection have helped to define those factors which can influence the clinical outcome. These studies represent the natural history of HIV infection at the earliest stage of the pandemic and in those patients who have acquired HIV most readily. They may therefore not be truly representative of the wider natural history in the longer term (Pinching 1988). The follow-up study of the San Francisco cohort leads to an estimate that 13% of cohort members will have developed AIDS within 5 years of seroconversion and 51% within 10 years (Rutherford *et al.* 1990). Lui *et al.* (1988) estimate that the mean incubation period for AIDS in homosexual men is 7.8 years, which is close to the estimate of 8.2 years for adults developing transfusion-associated AIDS. They estimate from their model that the probability of infected homosexual men likely to develop AIDS is 0.99.

Immunological signs of primary infection

Primary infection is associated with extremely high titres of HIV in plasma and high numbers of productively infected peripheral blood T cells. This high virus load rapidly declines with increasing titres of anti-HIV antibodies (Clark *et al.* 1991; Daar *et al.* 1991). Viraemia is accompanied by a transient, sometimes dramatic, lymphocytopenia of both CD4+ve and CD8+ve T cells which recovers following seroconversion. A subsequent selective increase of activated CD8 cells, expressing CD38 and HLA Class II, may be observed for at least 2 months after seroconversion (Miedema 1992). Patients infected with syncytium-inducing, fast replicating, HIV variants have severe immunological and clinical abnormalities, indicators for rapid progression to AIDS (Miedema 1992).

Serological latency

Human immunodeficiency virus seropositivity, as routinely defined by the presence of antibodies directed against the virion structural proteins, occurs 1–2 months after direct bloodstream infections. The duration of the silent period that follows sexual exposure to HIV is poorly defined since the precise date of contamination is often unknown. The existence of prolonged latency in sexually transmitted HIV infection has been the subject of a controversy. Ranki *et al.* (1987a) reported a substantial number of high-risk individuals and of sexual partners of AIDS or ARC patients with fluctuating HIV antigenaemia contrasting with no or low-titre antibodies to structural proteins for 6–34 months before conventional seroconversion. Imagawa *et al.* 1989 have claimed that a very long period of latency can indeed occur. Their study deals with a cohort of 133 seronegative homosexual men who continued to be involved in high-risk sexual activity. Human immunodeficiency virus 1 was isolated in at least some of the sequential blood samples in 31 (23%) of these individuals, 27 of whom remained seronegative for up to 36 months after the first positive culture; the other four men seroconverted 11–17 months after the isolation of HIV-1. Proviral DNA was detected by gene amplification (PCR) in cryopreserved lymphocytes obtained from three of these four men 23–35 months before seroconversion. The same group (Wolinsky *et al.* 1989) subsequently detected, by PCR, HIV-1 nucleic acid sequences in the peripheral blood mononuclear cells from 20 of 24 homosexual men 6–42 months before seroconversion (median 18 months). Identification of HIV proviral DNA sequences by PCR had indeed been previously reported in five seronegative individuals at risk for HIV infection (Loche and Mach 1988) and in five children of HIV-infected mothers who had lost maternal antibodies to HIV at the age of 1 year (Laure *et al.* 1988). Ameisen *et al.* (1989) have also detected HIV-1 proviral DNA in eight individuals at risk for HIV infection and seronegative by conventional methods.

Jehuda-Cohen *et al.* (1990) showed that 30 of 165 seronegative individuals who were at high risk for HIV infection had circulating B cells which, upon *in vitro* polyclonal activation with pokeweed mitogen, produced antibodies reactive with HIV. The presence of HIV-specific DNA sequences was demonstrated by PCR in a significant number of samples from these individuals.

In contrast, Groopman *et al.* (1988) concluded, from a longitudinal study of high-risk individuals, to lack of evidence of prolonged HIV infection before antibody seroconversion, since they found neither circulating viral antigen nor positive direct virus culture. Pan *et al.* (1991) found evidence of virus by culture and PCR in only one of 59 seronegative men who practised high-risk sexual behaviour. Horsburgh *et al.* (1989) detected HIV DNA before seroconversion in only 4 of 39 men, PCR being positive only in the seronegative sample taken closest to the time of seroconversion. They consider that HIV infection for longer than 6 months without detectable antibody seems uncommon. Imagawa and Detels (1991) recently provided additional information about their initial report (Imagawa *et al.* 1989) and subsequent studies. They found no evidence of contamination leading to false-positive results in PCR testing. However, when studying fresh samples recently obtained from the previously HIV virus-positive 27 men who never seroconverted, virus was isolated from only one man. They conclude that these results are more consistent with the hypothesis of incomplete infection than with latent, persistent infection.

Detection of antibodies to regulatory gene products was reported by Ranki *et al.* (1987a) in some individuals several months before full seroconversion. Using purified recombinant protein and synthetic peptides, Ameisen *et al.* (1989) demonstrated antibodies to the product of the *nef* regulatory gene by Western blot and radioimmunoassay in 9 of 22 high-risk seronegative individuals who were prospectively studied. They also found such antibodies, as well as HIV-1 proviral DNA, in a case of spontaneous complete HIV seronegativation, with negative antigenaemia and negative virus culture. Farzadegan *et al.* (1988) had previously observed such a loss of HIV-1 antibody in three homosexual men in whom the Western blot assay for antibodies, antigenaemia and viral culture remained negative after a 6–12 months follow-up, whereas the detection of HIV-1 proviral DNA by PCR was positive.

Whatever the mechanism(s) responsible for these observations, the implications of these probably very rare states of serological latency are of obvious importance. Whether such individuals harbour sufficient numbers of infectious virions to allow transmission of HIV infection through sexual contact or blood transfusion is a currently unanswered question.

Co-factors for progression

Cohort studies have provided evidence that cofactors for progression exist. The spectrum of clinical outcomes of HIV infection may reflect different *host factors*, including protective immune response against HIV. It has been possible to identify some intercurrent events that affect the risk of progression to ARC or AIDS. Some cohort studies on seropositive homosexual men showed that sexually transmitted diseases clearly increase the risk of progression (Weber *et al.* 1986; Quinn *et al.* 1987). It is not yet clear whether any major systemic infection could exert such an effect. Some studies have suggested that co-infection with human T cell lymphotrophic virus 1 (HTLV-1) is associated with increased risk of progression to AIDS (Bartholomew *et al.* 1987), in accordance with *in vitro* evidence that HTLV-1 can increase HIV replication (Siekevitz *et al.* 1987) and stimulate HIV-1-infected blood T cells to produce large quantities of virus (Zack *et al.* 1988). The herpesvirus HHV-6 and HIV-1 can also productively co-infect human CD4 +ve T lymphocytes, resulting in accelerated HIV-1 expression and cellular death (Lusso *et al.* 1989). HHV-6 might thus contribute to progression towards AIDS. Viruses such as CMV and EBV could operate through the production of TNF-α, leading to HIV replication in chronically infected T4 cells or macrophages.

Evidence concerning *genetic factors* affecting susceptibility to HIV infection remains rather scanty. Human leucocyte antigen associations with specific manifestations of HIV disease such as Kaposi's sarcoma are not consistent. An association of HLA-DR5 with HIV-related thrombocytopenia has been noted in a series of French Caucasian patients (Raffoux *et al.* 1987). The prevalence of HLA-DR5 was also increased in a series of patients with sicca syndrome (Itescu *et al.* 1989). Cameron *et al.* (1988) found a very high incidence of C4b null alleles in patients with persistent generalized lymphadenopathy. We failed to find such a significant association between C4 null allele frequency and HIV-related thrombocytopenia. Various HLA phenotypes have been claimed to represent a risk factor in progression to full-blown HIV disease. The most consistent findings are those of Steel *et al.* (1988) and Kaslow *et al.* (1990), who showed that the A1, B8, DR3 haplotype was strongly associated with a rapid decline in T4 cells and early development of AIDS.

The biological properties of HIV-1 may correlate with its virulence in the host and carry prognostic significance. Cheng-Mayer *et al.* (1988) and Tersmette et al (1989) showed, in sequential studies of isolates obtained at intervals during infection, that the development of severe disease corresponded to the emergence of HIV-1 variants that were more cytopathic *in vitro* and had increased replicative capacity.

Markers for progression

Immunological markers are useful in predicting clinical outcome of HIV infection. Numerous studies on groups of subjects showed that serial measurements of circulating CD4 +ve cell numbers provide an important index of progression of HIV infection (Fahey *et al.* 1987; Goedert *et al.* 1987; Polk *et al.* 1987; De Wolf *et al.* 1988; Moss *et al.* 1988). Asymptomatic subjects with the most extensive and/or rapid fall in CD4 +ve lymphocyte absolute numbers and percentages are the most likely to develop AIDS within 2 years (Giorgi and Detels 1989). Burcham *et al.* (1991) found that baseline CD4% had greater prognostic value than baseline CD4 cell count for AIDS-free survival time. Phillips, A.N. *et al.* (1991) concluded that differences in the duration of the asymptomatic period can largely be explained by differences in rates of decline of CD4 lymphocyte counts. The Dutch study (Miedema 1992), over a 5-year follow-up, shows that non-progressors display a continuous and steady decline of the mean number of CD4 +ve cells whereas in more than 90% of the progressors, the decline is 3–5 times faster during the last 18 months preceding diagnosis of AIDS. Rapid declining CD4 cell numbers is an independent predictive marker for development of disease that may be used in addition to baseline CD4 cell counts. The earlier depletion of CD29 +ve CD4 +ve T memory cells and impairment of T cell reactivity precedes the decline in T4 cell numbers (Gruters *et al.* 1991a).

Clerici *et al.* (1989a) obtained evidence for sequential patterns of T cell dysfunction that correlated with distinct phases of infection. Hofmann *et al.* (1987) showed that low responsiveness to PWM has independent predictive value. Anti-CD3 induced T cell proliferation is decreased in non-progressing stable asymptomatics but remains at a level of 40–50% of normal controls, whereas it declines to very low levels 2–3 years before development of symptoms (Schellekens *et al.* 1990; Gruters *et al.* 1991b). Low CD4 +ve lymphocyte numbers and anti-CD3 reactivity are good independent prognostic markers for development of AIDS (Miedema 1992).

Some studies have shown that elevated CD8 +ve T cell counts independently predict the development of AIDS whereas other studies have failed to show such an association; the findings suggest a complex relationship between CD8 +ve cell counts and progression to AIDS, with the possibility that various subsets of CD8 +ve lymphocytes play different roles (Anderson *et al.* 1991). Outgrowth of CD8 cells has been interpreted as immune activation (Fahey *et al.* 1990). Stites *et al.* (1989) found that increased numbers or percentages of DR +ve CD8 cells were an independent predictor of progression. Nishanian *et al.* (1991) have shown that serum soluble CD8 level, a marker of CD8 T cell activation, predicts CD4 +ve T cell fall relatively early in infection and subsequent occurrence of AIDS.

In the study of the San Francisco cohort (Moss *et al.* 1988), the level of serum β2 microglobulin, which may reflect activation in target cell populations of HIV infection, was a better single predictor of progression than p24 antigenaemia or T4 cell number. Although β2M is not a marker specific for HIV infection, the predictive value of elevated levels has been confirmed in numerous reports and appears to be independent of the CD4 lymphocyte count (Anderson *et al.* 1990), but has not always been found to be a better predictor than p24 antigenaemia or CD4 +ve cell depletion. Neopterin concentrations in urine, and more recently serum, have also been proposed as predictors of progression (Fuchs *et al.* 1988; Krämer *et al.* 1989). The combination of serum β2 microglobulin, p24 antigenaemia and CD4 +ve lymphocyte counts identifies larger groups at high risk than T4 cell counts alone (Moss *et al.* 1988). A subsequent study from the same group (Osmond *et al.* 1991) showed that β2M, neopterin and soluble CD8 predicted AIDS independently of both CD4 count and p24 antigen in multivaried analysis and that, within the range of CD4 counts of 200–500, these immune activation markers, used in combination with p24 antigen level, identify individuals at high risk of AIDS.

The patterns of antibody responses against specific HIV components change over time in infected subjects who progress to ARC or AIDS. Declining levels of antibodies to gp160, its conserved domain or its main neutralization epitope are inconstant and not significantly associated with disease progression. In contrast, several longitudinal studies have shown that antibody to core protein, mainly anti-p24, progressively declines before the onset of symptoms (Allain *et al.* 1987;

Goudsmit *et al.* 1987; McDougal *et al.* 1987; Weber *et al.* 1987). Measurement of specific HIV antigenaemia is also an important marker of progression, as shown in cohorts of both seropositive haemophiliacs (Allain *et al.* 1987) and seropositive homosexual men (Moss *et al.* 1988). The p24 core antigen is usually first detectable at infection and then disappears. The asymptomatic individuals who continue to be positive for the antigen or in whom antigenaemia reappears are at risk of progressing to AIDS. Although p24 antigen bound in immune complexes is not detected by the standard assays, p24 antigenaemia has been found to be a good predictor of AIDS.

The magnitude of plasma viraemia was recently found to be a much better correlate of the clinical stage of disease and of disease progression than the results of tests for p24 antigenaemia or for antibody to this antigen (Coombs *et al.* 1989). Low HIV-1 proviral DNA burden detected by negative PCR correlates with slower disease progression (Schechter *et al.* 1991).

The emergence and overt replication of syncytiuminducing, highly virulent HIV variants occurs in about half of infected individuals who progress to AIDS (Tersmette *et al.* 1989). This phenotypic switch occurs 18–24 months before AIDS, concomitantly with increase in the rate of CD4 +ve T cell decline, and there is a significant correlation between the fast decline of CD4 +ve cells and the presence of more virulent HIV-1 variants (Miedema 1992). Among zidovudine-treated asymptomatic individuals, the majority of those who progressed to AIDS had detectable syncytiuminducing isolates and an extremely low responsiveness to anti-CD3 1 year before the start of treatment (Gruters *et al.* 1991b). Moreover, the lag time between phenotype switch and AIDS was not prolonged by zidovudine and CD4 +ve cell decline was not inhibited in treated individuals with virulent isolates (C. Boucher, pers. comm.). Zidovudine treatment resulted in transient improvement of T cell function in progressors while no significant improvement was noted in non-progressors (Miedema 1992). Immunological, as well as virological, surrogate markers in the evaluation of treatment for HIV infection (Valentine and Jacobson 1990; Machado *et al.* 1990) should clearly be validated in therapy protocols that use true clinical end-points in parallel.

Immunological markers used in Europe and America for the study of HIV infection have yet to be validated in various areas of Africa, where environmental factors such as fungal or parasitic infections and malnutrition induce additional polyclonal B cell activation signals and a different range of immunological values (Seligmann *et al.* 1987).

Paediatric acquired immune deficiency syndrome

Human immunodeficiency virus infection of the fetus or new-born infant results in an immunodeficiency disease which is distinct from AIDS in the adult (Falloon *et al.* 1989; Calvelli and Rubinstein 1990). There is evidence for a bimodal evolution in HIV-1-infected infants (Auger *et al.* 1988; Scott *et al.* 1989). Ten to 20% of patients have a rapid downhill course with early opportunistic infections and often severe encephalopathy. In contrast, the other HIV-infected children have a probability of survival at 3 years of 97%, whether or not bacterial infections, which are prevented by the administration of intravenous γ-globulins (The National Institute of Child Health and Human Development Intravenous Immunoglobulin Study Group 1991), or lymphoid interstitial pneumopathy occur (Blanche *et al.* 1990). Immunological parameters obtained during the first year of life have a good predictive value: poor proliferative responses to soluble antigens *in vitro*, absent delayed-type hypersensitivity, CD4 cell counts below 500/mm^3 and/or absence of serum antibodies to core HIV proteins correlate with poor subsequent clinical evolution (Blanche *et al.* 1990).

Humoral and cell-mediated immune responses to human immunodeficiency virus

It remains to be clearly established whether humoral and cell-mediated immune responses may prevent HIV primary infection and/or protect against disease progression. In contrast, host defence mechanisms can contribute to pathogenesis.

Neutralizing antibodies

Human immunodeficiency virus-infected individuals develop antibodies to many viral proteins. Molecular characterization of such antibodies showed that they use different germ-line V_H gene segments and display extensive somatic mutations typical of an antigen-driven immune response

(Andris *et al.* 1991). The first studies showed that comparably low titres of neutralizing antibodies were detected in the sera of both asymptomatic seropositive individuals and patients with AIDS (Robert-Guroff *et al.* 1985; Weiss *et al.* 1986), suggesting that naturally developing neutralizing antibodies offer little protection. This notion is supported by the study of a cohort in which, despite higher titres of anti-p24 antibodies in individuals who remained asymptomatic, neuralizing activity in their sera was not significantly different from that in patients whose disease progressed (Weber *et al.* 1987). However, in the study of Ranki *et al.* (1987b), dealing with sequential serum samples of 28 HIV-infected individuals followed for 2–3 years, an increase in neutralization titre was associated with a stable clinical course. Robert-Guroff *et al.* (1988) followed for 6 years the spectrum of HIV-1 neutralizing antibodies in a cohort of homosexual men and found that decreasing titres signalled poor prognosis. Similar observations prompted two groups to attempt passive immunoneutralization. Jackson *et al.* (1988) infused 50–500 ml plasma from donors selected for high anti-p24 and neutralizing antibodies to six patients with AIDS. Antigenaemia cleared immediately for up to 11 weeks and the authors claim that infusions were followed by clinical improvement. Karpas *et al.* (1988; 1990) treated 10 patients with ARC or AIDS and also observed sustained clearance of p24 antigen, as well as of cell-free virus in plasma which became undetectable by PCR; they claimed clinical improvement with stable CD4+ve cell counts in ARC patients. All these early studies were performed before identification of the various epitopes involved in antibody neutralization.

The best candidates for possibly efficient neutralizing activity are antibodies reactive with the envelope. In experimental animals immunized with gp160 or fragments thereof, a large fraction of the neutralizing antibody activity appears to be directed against linear epitopes of an immunodominant portion of gp120 located in the V3 region between residues 307 and 330 (Rusche *et al.* 1988). Palker *et al.* (1988) have identified synthetic peptides representative of this segment of gp120 which induce neutralizing antibodies. Neutralizing monoclonal antibodies have been found to bind the same region of gp120 (Skinner *et al.* 1988; Thomas *et al.* 1988). This dominant neutralization epitope, consisting of a loop between two disulphide-linked cysteine residues, induces, in HIV-1-infected chimpanzees, antibodies restricted to the homologous viral strain (Goudsmit *et al.* 1988). Although the amino acid sequence within this V3 loop is variable, the loop itself is present in gp120 from different strains of the virus. The principal neutralizing determinant (PND) has been mapped to eight amino acids, this sequence containing a central Gly–Pro–Gly–Arg which is generally conserved between different HIV-1 isolates (Javaherian *et al.* 1989). LaRosa *et al.* (1990) found a consensus sequence that is relatively preserved in 245 HIV European and North American isolates. Also Devash *et al.* (1990a) reported that a majority of infected individuals in North America and Europe have antibodies reactive with a MN-like variant of the V3 loop. Contrasting with the usual isolate-specificity of neutralizing antibodies to the PND of the V3 loop, Ohno *et al.* (1991) recently described a broadly neutralizing monoclonal antibody that reacts with diverse HIV-1 isolates through the Gly–Pro–Gly–Arg sequence of the V3 loop. Antibodies to this region neutralize virus infectivity by interfering with the post-binding step, probably linked to the fusion process (Skinner *et al.* 1988). At least two hypervariable regions other than the V3 domain are capable of eliciting neutralizing antibodies to gp120 (Haigwood *et al.* 1990). Peptides mimicking selected disulphide loops of gp120, other than V3, elicit relatively high levels of anti-gp120 antibodies which, however, fail to neutralize the infectivity of HIV-1 (Neurath *et al.* 1991).

Several groups have recently identified a second category of anti-gp120 neutralizing antibodies induced in HIV-1-infected humans (Ho *et al.* 1991a; Steimer *et al.* 1991; Kang *et al.* 1991). These antibodies react with conformational discontinuous epitopes of gp120, interfere with gp120–CD4 binding and neutralize a broader spectrum of HIV-1 isolates than V3-specific antibodies. These antibodies are less potent than V3 region-specific antibodies in neutralizing a specific isolate (Kang *et al.* 1991).

Longitudinal examination of the humoral response which arose after accidental inoculation of a laboratory worker showed (Gallo *et al.* 1989) that isolate-restricted neutralizing antibodies against the V3 region of gp120 occurred relatively early after seroconversion, following the emergence of

ADCC antibodies. Broad neutralizing activity, directed to more conserved structural regions and blocking gp120 binding to CD4, occurred 18 months later. A role for these broadly neutralizing conformation-dependent antibodies to gp120 in protection against disease progression has not been established. Contradictory results for such a protective role of V3-specific neutralizing antibodies have been published. The findings of Boucher *et al.* (1989), who tested for the presence of antibodies to the dominant V3 neutralization epitope sequential sera of a cohort of seropositive men, argue against a protective role. On the other hand, Neurath *et al.* (1990) concluded that it was possible to predict the unfavourable outcome of disease by comparative measurements of levels of antibodies to a peptide corresponding to the V3 hypervariable loop of gp120, providing evidence for declining levels of these antibodies during the course of infection. Since efficient neutralizing activity of V3 specific antibodies is mainly type-specific, accurate assessment of how neutralizing antibody may affect disease progression would require examining serial serum samples of a given patient against his own particular virus isolate. Moreover, Albert *et al.* (1990) have shown that escape variants arise during the course of infection since the patient's serum antibodies can neutralize the virus that was isolated from that patient early in the course of infection, but not a virus that was isolated after 118 weeks of infection.

Some, but not all, infants born to mothers infected with HIV are infected *in utero*. Some studies suggest that maternal antibodies directed against gp120 may be associated with a lower rate of vertical transmission. Rossi *et al.* (1989) found that neutralizing antibodies against select hypervariable epitopes of gp120 may play a role in preventing mother-to-child transmission of HIV-1 infection. Devash *et al.* (1990b) found a lower transmission rate among women with high-affinity antibodies to the gp120 PND measured by ELISA. However, Goedert *et al.* (1989) found that prevention of mother-to-infant transmission was not associated with anti-V3 antibodies and that protection was conferred by antibodies to another gp120 epitope. Pareka *et al.* (1991) stated that there was a lack of correlation between perinatal HIV-1 transmission and the presence of maternal antibodies to V3 loop peptides, without any differences in their affinity. In this respect, it should be emphasized that Prince *et al.* (1988) had been unable to block HIV infection in chimpanzees who had received, before challenge, immunoglobulins prepared from plasma of seropositive donors selected for high neutralizing antibody titres. However, they reported recently (Prince *et al.* 1991) that such immunoglobulins protected against a challenge dose 10-fold lower than that used previously.

Other regions of the envelope located in gp41 (Banapour *et al.* 1987) may also represent targets of neutralizing human antibodies. Klasse *et al.* (1988) claimed that the presence of antibodies directed against a discrete region of gp41 is strongly associated with the absence of progression to AIDS. Various studies point to a conserved site on gp41 (735–752) as a region which can induce neutralizing antibodies and block fusion in a broad fashion (Dalgleish *et al.* 1988; Thomas *et al.* 1988). Evans, D.J. *et al.* (1989) reported that up to 80% of cross-neutralizing activity in human HIV +ve sera could be abolished by previous incubation with this gp41 epitope.

Neutralization epitopes have been mapped by monoclonal antibodies to the aminoterminal region of the p17 core protein (Papsidero *et al.* 1989). Antibodies to HIV reverse transcriptase, which appear to inhibit the catalytic activity of this enzyme in some HIV-treated subjects (Laurence *et al.* 1987), are detected in 79% of HIV-infected individuals (DeVico *et al.* 1988), with only slight variations of their level according to the clinical stages of HIV disease.

Khalife *et al.* (1988) have investigated the isotypic profile of the antibody response to HIV structural proteins. Whereas the response to *gag* products was polyisotypic, that to envelope proteins was strikingly restricted to the IgG1 isotype, suggesting different regulatory mechanisms.

The antigenic sites recognized by the neutralizing antibodies of HIV-1-infected humans are distinct from those recognized by cloned, type-specific, T helper cells (Walker, C.M. *et al.* 1988). Conversely, Ahearne *et al.* (1988) showed, with several recombinant and native peptides, that the immunodominant neutralizing epitope of gp120 does not produce significant lymphocyte proliferation.

Antibody-dependent cellular cytotoxicity and enhancing antibodies

Sera from a wide spectrum of HIV-infected patients, ranging from asymptomatic to overt AIDS, were shown to contain high titres of antibodies that mediate ADCC. Such antibodies are among the earliest to appear. They were detected in serum samples from a laboratory worker who had been exposed to HIV-1 prior to the appearance of any other functionally active antibodies, and these ADCC antibodies were broadly reactive from the start (Tyler *et al*. 1989b). The study of Ljunggren *et al*. (1987) suggests that a slight decline in anti-HIV ADCC may occur with disease progression. The predominant isotype of these antibodies appears to be IgG1 (Ljunggren *et al*. 1988).

Another manifestation of ADCC, which may provide a primary cytotoxic host defence, is a gp120-specific, MHC-unrestricted cellular toxicity directed by cytophilic antibodies which arm circulating CD16 +ve natural killer/killer (NK/K) cells (Tyler *et al*. 1989a). Weinhold *et al*. (1988) found that such cellular cytotoxicity against autologous or heterologous gp120-bearing target cells is present at higher levels in symptomless individuals than in patients with ARC or AIDS. The loss of ADCC-directing antibodies, combined with poorly defined cellular defects, can contribute to the observed decline (Tyler *et al*. 1990).

In contrast to a report showing some correlation of ADCC activity with the presence of anti-p24 (Rook *et al*. 1987), subsequent studies showed that gp120 is the major target (Lyerly *et al*. 1987a). These anti-gp120 antibodies mediate broadly reactive, group-specific anti-HIV ADCC (Lyerly *et al*. 1987b). Antibodies that mediate ADCC can also be directed against gp41 (Evans, L.A. *et al*. 1989). As discussed in the first section, ADCC antibodies can kill uninfected cells targeted by the attachment of free gp120 to CD4 (Lyerly *et al*. 1987a).

An additional deleterious effect of ADCC antibodies could potentially facilitate HIV infection: Fc receptor-mediated antibody-dependent enhancement. Antibodies that enhance HIV infection via Fc receptors were first described by Homsy *et al*. (1988) and Takeda *et al*. (1988). Several subsequent reports supported the findings that subneutralizing amounts of patient's serum could significantly enhance virus replication. Two mechanisms have been suggested: one implicates Fc receptors and CD4 while the second involves only Fc receptor on target cells. Several authors have demonstrated that CD4 is required since enhanced infection of monocytes and of the human monocytic cell line U937 is blocked by inhibitors of CD4-gp120 binding (Jouault *et al*. 1989; Zeira *et al*. 1990; Perno *et al*. 1990). Other authors believe that Fc receptors alone can enhance HIV-1 infection in primary monocyte cultures (Homsy *et al*. 1989). This mechanism of enhancement has also been demonstrated using fibroblasts infected with cytomegalovirus and therefore expressing Fc receptors (McKeating *et al*. 1990).

Another mechanism for *in vitro* enhancement involves antibody to HIV in combination with complement proteins (Robinson *et al*. 1988). This complement-mediated, antibody-dependent enhancement requires both CD4 and complement receptor type II (CR_2) (Robinson *et al*. 1990a).

Some epitopes serving as targets for enhancing antibodies appear to be distinct from neutralizing epitopes. Robinson *et al*. (1990b) showed that several human monoclonal antibodies against the HIV-1 envelope glycoproteins could enhance infection but did not neutralize HIV-1 *in vitro*. The ability of these monoclonals to enhance infection was not determined by their IgG subclass or their ability to activate complement (Robinson *et al*. 1990c). These monoclonal antibodies were mainly directed against two linear, conserved immunodominant domains of gp41 (Robinson *et al*. 1990c, 1991). Jiang *et al*. (1991) found that, in addition to these domains of gp41, many other regions in gp120/41 elicit enhancing antibodies and that V3 hypervariable loop from one isolate may elicit antibodies enhancing infection by another HIV-1 isolate.

Although it has been difficult to demonstrate the *in vivo* relevance of enhancing antibodies, they may play a part in the pathogenesis of HIV infection. Homsy *et al*. (1990) showed that Fc receptor-mediated enhancement correlates with disease progression and that homotypic viral isolates were enhanced and not neutralized by patient's sera. The occurrence of complement-dependent enhancing antibodies correlated also with severity of disease in man (Toth *et al*. 1991) and SIV-infected macaques (Montefiori *et al*. 1990).

It should also be noted that some sera from healthy subjects immunized with gp160 contained enhancing antibodies (Dolin *et al.* 1991).

Helper T cell immunity

Helper T cell immunity is likely to be an important component of the immune defence against HIV. We have outlined in a previous section the compromised helper T cell function in infected individuals, who often fail to respond to HIV proteins early in the course of infection. The ability to generate and maintain a vigorous helper T cell response to HIV may be important in preventing progression to AIDS. Human immunodeficiency virus-infected non-human primates who do not develop HIV-related disease, have sustained proliferative responses to HIV antigens (Lusso *et al.* 1988). Schrier *et al.* (1988) have shown that the synthetic peptide corresponding to amino acids 598–609 of gp41, which includes a T cell epitope and an immunodominant B cell epitope, was capable of generating IgG antibodies in normal mice but not in athymic mice.

The specificity of helper T cells required for a protective antibody immune response against HIV has not been established. Recombinant or native *env* proteins have been used to induce helper T cell responses in man and experimental animals. Attempts to induce helper T cells specific for HIV core proteins have met with varying degrees of success. Some epitopes recognized by HIV-specific helper T cells have been identified by Wahren *et al.* (1989), by Schrier *et al.* (1989) through the use of synthetic peptides and by Clerici *et al.* (1989b), who used IL-2 secretion as an index of T cell activation. Helper T cell epitopes have also recently been defined by Mills *et al.* (1990) on the *gag* protein p24. The mapping of epitopes which can be presented to helper T cells by several Class II MHC molecules is of special importance. Such epitopes have been identified in conserved regions of the HIV envelope protein which contain several overlapping or adjacent antigenic sites (reviewed in Berzofsky 1991). Peptides encompassing such multideterminant clusters of HIV envelope have been constructed and shown to induce *in vitro* T cell responses in mice and humans of multiple MHC types (Berzovsfy *et al.* 1991).

Human-immunodeficiency-virus-specific cytotoxicity

Human immunodeficiency virus-specific, HLA-restricted cytotoxic T lymphocytes (CTL) were first reported in the peripheral blood (Walker *et al.* 1987) and bronchoalveolar lavages (Plata *et al.* 1987) from HIV-infected persons. Most such HIV-specific CTL are CD8 +ve T cells and Class I-restricted. They may play a critical role in limiting viral spread. Human immunodeficiency virus-specific CTL kill autologous HIV-infected target cells and heterologous infected targets that share at least one HLA-1 antigen. The simplest approach is to use targets and CTL from the same donor. Autologous macrophages and EBV-transformed B lymphocytes infected by HIV have been used as target cells. Another approach for the production of target cells is the infection of HLA-matched EBV lymphoblasts with recombinant vaccinia viruses. Plata *et al.* (1987) chose a third approach involving the double transfection of mouse cells with a human HLA gene and an HIV gene. The cells were selected for expression of the transfected gene products and were cloned. The use of small antigenic peptides which can be absorbed and efficiently presented in the groove of MHC antigens circumvents the need for antigen processing or endogenous synthesis.

Human immunodeficiency virus-specific HLA-restricted CTL are present in sufficient numbers in seropositive donors to be detected directly by the incubation of fresh blood leucocytes with ^{51}Cr-labelled target cells (Koenig *et al.* 1988). Quantitative analyses by limiting dilution (Hoffenbach *et al.* 1989) indicate that there is a surprisingly high number of circulating virus-specific CTL (0.7–4.0 per 10 000 leucocytes). These CTL numbers can be amplified by *in vitro* restimulation with HIV antigens. Most circulating cells with anti-*env* cytotoxic activity present in seropositive subjects are CD16 +ve cells mediating ADCC (Rivière *et al.* 1989b). They coexist with primary MHC-restricted CTL (McChesney *et al.* 1990). Bronchoalveolar washes of patients with lymphocytic interstitial pneumonitis are a source of both CTL and infected macrophages (Langlade-Demoyen *et al.* 1988; Hoffenbach *et al.* 1989).

An unexpected finding by Hoffenbach *et al.* (1989) was that seronegative donors have circulating

HIV-specific CTL precursor cells and can generate virus-specific CTL upon stimulation with HIV proteins. This highly unusual situation may indicate that humans are naturally primed to HIV in the absence of infection, presumably by cross-reactive antigens that have yet to be identified. Several other groups have not been able to confirm these findings. However, S.E. Macatonia and S.C. Knight (pers. comm.) have generated HIV-specific CTL in seronegative individuals by using dendritic cells in microculture.

Virus-immune CTL consist in general of multiple lymphocyte subpopulations that recognize different virus proteins and HIV-specific CTL appear to follow this pattern. The HIV glycoproteins coded by the *env* gene are recognized by MHC-restricted CTL, as shown by Plata *et al.* (1987), Walker *et al.* (1987), Koenig *et al.* (1988) and Sethi *et al.* (1988). Internal *gag* and *pol* structural proteins of HIV are also detected by CTL (Koenig *et al.* 1988; Nixon *et al.* 1988; Walker, B.D. *et al.* 1988; Rivière *et al.* 1989b). Finally, regulatory *nef* and *vif* proteins are recognized by CTL on HIV-infected cells (Rivière *et al.* 1989a; Chenciner *et al.* 1989; Culmann *et al.* 1989). HIV-infected humans carry coexisting CTL subpopulations of different specificities, each appearing to vary in intensity among different individuals. Cytotoxic T lymphocytes specific for *nef* protein appear to be a major constituent of the human immune response to HIV.

Occasional CD4 +ve, Class II-restricted CTL have been isolated from infected donors. They seem to require *in vitro* expansion for detection (Koenig *et al.* 1988). Sethi *et al.* (1988) have described a few cytotoxic CD4 +ve T lymphocyte clones from cerebrospinal fluid. The use of CD4 +ve activated helper T lymphocytes as presenting cells permitted the generation from seronegative donors of CD4 +ve CTL specific for gp120 and Class II-restricted (Siliciano *et al.* 1988; Lanzavecchia *et al.* 1988). It should also be noted that CD4 +ve CTL have been generated in vaccinated individuals (Orentas *et al.* 1990; Hammond *et al.* 1991). In contrast, naturally elicited CTL responses in infected persons consist predominantly of CD8 +ve, HLA-I-restricted cells. Plata *et al.* (1989) suggested that a hierarchy of HLA molecules could eventually be established for the presentation of diverse HIV proteins.

Synthetic peptides have been used in order to identify the fine specificity of human HIV-immune CTL, which seem often to recognize conserved epitopes (reviewed in Nixon and McMichael 1991). More than 40 CTL epitopes have currently been identified in the *gag* protein (Nixon *et al.* 1988; Claverie *et al.* 1988; Johnson *et al.* 1991), reverse-transcriptase (Walker *et al.* 1989; Hosmalin *et al.* 1990), *nef* protein (Koenig *et al.* 1990; Culmann *et al.* 1991) and the envelope protein (Clerici *et al.* 1991b; Dadaglio *et al.* 1991). An immunodominant epitope of a variable segment of gp160, recognized by CD8 +ve CTL, which overlaps the major B cell epitope, had been defined in mice by Takahashi *et al.* (1988) and is recognized by HLA-A2 restricted CTL in HIV-infected patients (Clerici *et al.* 1991b; Dadaglio *et al.* 1991). The study of HIV CTL epitopes has demonstrated that a single peptide can be recognized in association with two or more different HLA molecules and that a single HLA molecule can act as restricting element for multiple peptides, even from the same protein.

Purified envelope proteins in ISCOMs (Takahashi *et al.* 1990) and carrier-free, non-derivatized HIV synthetic peptides (Hart *et al.* 1991) can be used *in vivo* to induce anti-HIV CD8 +ve CTL responses.

The *in vivo* relevance of HIV-specific CTL raises a number of important and yet poorly solved issues. Sequential studies have clearly shown that circulating (Hoffenbach *et al.* 1989), as well as bronchoalveolar (Autran *et al.* 1989), CTL numbers decrease gradually with time in HIV-infected individuals and become undetectable when major clinical deterioration occurs. Similarly, CTL precursor cell frequencies progressively drop to undetectable levels. A striking point is that this phenomenon is observed for all kinds of HIV-specific CTL, in spite of their phenotypic and functional heterogeneity. This generalized 'paralysis' of cytotoxic cells could be related (Plata *et al.* 1989) to an impairment of precursor cells in the bone marrow and other lymphoid tissues. Moreover, suppressor T cells have been found in the lungs of patients with advanced HIV disease in whom a considerable decline of alveolar anti-HIV CTL activity had been demonstrated (Joly *et al.* 1989). These suppressor cells displayed the CD3, CD8 and CD57 markers, where CD4 −ve and CD16 −ve and lacked NK activity. Their function was not restricted by HLA Class I MHC antigens. These suppressor T cells could partly explain the inefficiency of host defence against HIV at rather late stages of HIV disease. Their inhibitory activity is mediated by a non-antigen specific soluble factor (Sadat-Sowti *et al.* 1991).

Phillips *et al.* (1991) have recently demonstrated, in a longitudinal study of HIV seropositive haemophiliacs, fluctuations in the specificity of cytotoxic T cells matched by genetic variation in *gag* CTL epitopes leading to loss of CTL recognition. Accumulation of unseen viral epitopes could thus be one way by which HIV escapes immune surveillance.

On the other hand, important data suggest that CD8 +ve T lymphocytes can block *in vitro* the replication of both HIV and SIV. A controversy persists about the mechanism involved in such protection. Walker (1989) has shown the generation in HIV-infected individuals of inhibitory CD8 +ve T lymphocytes which appear to suppress virus replication, without destruction by a cytotoxic mechanism of the virus-containing cells. Tsubota *et al.* (1989b) have demonstrated control of HIV and SIV replication by CD8 +ve T cells. They showed that MHC restriction was necessary and there was contact through the lymphocyte function-associated antigen (LFA)-1 adhesion molecule. The extent of antiviral activity exhibited *in vitro* by CD8 +ve lymphocytes from individuals infected by HIV-1 correlates significantly with their clinical status: decreased activity is related to progression to disease (Mackewicz *et al.* 1991).

Michel *et al.* (1988) have in fact shown that mice immunized against the HIV envelope glycoproteins developed both CD4 and CD8 T lymphocyte HIV-specific immunity, and were protected from challenge with a syngeneic transfected tumour expressing HIV envelope gp160. Elimination of cells expressing HIV antigens can thus be induced by vaccination in this murine model.

On the other hand, there is suggestive evidence that HIV-specific CTL might be deleterious to the infected host by inducing destruction of immunocompetent target cells with surface-bound gp120 (Lanzavecchia *et al.* 1988; Siliciano *et al.* 1988) and/or by producing local inflammatory reactions. Human immunodeficiency virus-specific CTL have indeed been detected in the lungs of seropositive patients with lymphocytic aleveolitis and lymphocytic interstitial pneumonitis (Plata *et al.* 1987; Autran *et al.* 1988) and in cerebrospinal fluid of patients with neurological disorders (Sethi *et al.* 1988), suggesting a role for CTL-mediated lysis of HIV-infected macrophages. The eventual attack of host tissues by CTL becomes a rather alarming possibility when one considers the large number of cell types that can be infected by HIV. For these reasons, immunotherapies or vaccines aimed at exacerbating the HIV-specific CTL response, particularly to gp120, should perhaps be considered with caution.

Prospects for vaccine development

Since it is widely agreed that vaccine development is crucial to the containment of the HIV epidemic, the effort devoted by the international scientific community to this challenge is unprecedented for any infectious agent. Early disappointments in the quest for an AIDS vaccine are now tempered by some signs of optimism. A number of important issues still need to be resolved since several properties of HIV complicate the development of an effective and safe vaccine (Ada 1988; Fauci 1989; Sonigo *et al.* 1989; Berzofsky 1991).

Obstacles to vaccine efficacy

Virological and immunological obstacles impede the development of an AIDS vaccine. Immunization against a virus whose target is an important component of the immune system and which establishes persistent infection in cells of the immune system presents particular difficulties. The constitution of reservoirs of viral genetic material invisible to the immune system in cells such as macrophages has been described as a 'Trojan horse strategy' for persistence of the lentivirus (Haase 1986). The importance of this obstacle might be tempered by recent findings establishing that, although cells of the monocyte–macrophage lineage may provide important reservoirs of HIV infection elsewhere in the body, most of the cell-associated virus in the blood is contained within the CD4 +ve T cells (Schnittman *et al.* 1989) and that many patients have circulating infectious HIV present in their plasma throughout most of the course of HIV disease (Coombs *et al.* 1989; Ho *et al.* 1989), implying that there is some viral replication. However both of these assumptions have been recently challenged: most groups did not confirm the positivity of plasma viraemia in asymptomatic individuals. McElrath *et al.* (1991), using a PCR method, found that a fraction of both T cells and monocytes in blood carry a latent infection in all stages of HIV disease.

Another strategy by which the virus may escape immune elimination is the development of structural changes within immunodominant regions. Different strains of HIV-1 show considerable diversity of nucleotide sequence as well as amino acid sequences in envelope proteins which have hypervariable domains. Efficient neutralizing activity is mainly directed towards these domains and isolate-restricted. It is therefore essential to determine the prevalence of different serotypes in the population of the relevant geographic area in order to design rational antigen mixtures for multivalent vaccines.

Longitudinal studies of HIV-infected subjects show an increasing spectrum of sequence variation with time. The nucleotide sequences of virus recovered from infected persons continually vary throughout HIV disease (Saag *et al*. 1988; Meyerhans *et al*. 1989). The virus may change not only its antigenic properties but also other main features that influence its relationship with the infected host, such as cellular tropism, syncitium-inducing capacities and replication kinetics (Cheng-Mayer *et al*. 1988; Tersmette and Miedema 1990). Furthermore, several strains of HIV may infect a given individual and recurrent selection may occur since *in vitro* experiments using neutralizing antibodies support the principle of strain selection (Robert-Guroff *et al*. 1986). Reitz *et al*. (1988) demonstrated that the generation of a neutralization-resistant variant of HIV-1 is due to selection for a point mutation in the envelope gene. Neutralization-escape mutants have been selected using monoclonal antibodies mapping to the type-specific V3 loop of gp120 containing the immunodominant epitope (McKeating and Willey 1989). The evolution of V3 sequences is host dependent, rapid, continuous and independent of the level of antigenic expression (Wolfs 1990). However, recent studies have provided evidence that there is considerable pressure to conserve a critical portion of the central part of this loop (Goudsmit *et al*. 1989; LaRosa *et al*. 1990). Moreover, Ohno *et al*. (1991) have recently studied a broadly neutralizing monoclonal antibody that reacts with diverse HIV-1 isolates through this central sequence of the V3 loop. Berkower *et al*. (1989) showed the predominance of a group-specific neutralizing epitope that persists despite genetic variation. Several groups have recently demonstrated the presence in the serum of HIV-1 infected humans of group-specific neutralizing antibodies that react with conformation-dependent discontinuous epitopes and prevent gp120 binding to CD4 (Steimer *et al*. 1991; Ho *et al*. 1991a; Posner *et al*. 1991; Kang *et al*. 1991). It has unfortunately not been possible so far to elicit this type of broadly neutralizing antibodies by active immunization in chimpanzees nor in human volunteers. Ho *et al*. (1991b) have recently identified, with a monoclonal antibody generated by immunizing mice with purified gp120, another discontinuous epitope involved in neutralization of HIV-1.

Takahashi *et al*. (1989a) showed that the V3 region encompasses also a Class I-restricted isolate-specific determinant for cytotoxic T lymphocytes and that a single amino acid exchange can lead to a complete reversal of the CTL specificity (Takahashi *et al*. 1989b). Such spontaneously occurring variations could contribute to escape of HIV from CTL immunity, as recently shown by R.E. Phillips *et al*. (1991). Human immunodeficiency virus may also escape from immune elimination by molecular masking or sequestration of some important B or T cell epitopes, and carbohydrates of the *env* glycoproteins may play a role in this mechanism.

Despite the enormous amount of research on the characterization of the immune response to the virus, the definition of protective immunity against initial infection with HIV remains uncertain. Since infection can be transmitted as either a free or a cell-associated virus, a protective response should deal not only with the virus itself but also with the infected cells. To be effective against the various modes of natural HIV transmission, a clearance mechanism for the infection must be established through vaccination. Studies by Emini *et al*. (1990) have shown that, when given with the virus, neutralizing antibodies to the principal neutralizing epitope of the V3 loop of gp120 can protect chimpanzees against HIV infection. Putkonen *et al*. (1991) showed that passively transferred antibodies can protect cynomolgus monkeys against a low-dose challenge by HIV-2 or SIV. Moreover vaccine protection of chimpanzees has been associated with induction of high levels of neutralizing antibodies (Girard *et al*. 1991).

Since enhancement of helper T cell activity could give higher-titre antibody responses, identification of HIV epitopes that can be presented to helper T cells by several Class II MHC molecules is certainly of importance. Indeed Vahlne *et al.* (1991) recently showed that some gp120 synthetic peptides are able to induce in immunized monkeys both cross-neutralizing antibodies and IL-2 production as well as lymphocyte proliferation in culture, and that the corresponding domains accommodate T-cell recognition sites. Since most HIV infections occur transmucosally, the possibility that secretory IgA may be an initial important local defence must also be considered (Archibald *et al.* 1987). Prophylactic vaccination should probably also elicit CTL immunity so that the virus that evades neutralization can be rapidly eliminated in order to provide sustained protection.

When infection is established, the possible benefits of vaccination are less clear. The best hope to limit viral replication and spread during the chronic phase probably lies in the virus-specific CTL. Cell killing by CTL may, however, induce deleterious effects in such patients. The possibility that the host cellular immune response to HIV contributes to the development of AIDS has been suggested by Zinkernagel (1988), in analogy with the situation observed in the lymphocytic choriomeningitis virus model in mice or in aggressive hepatitis B virus infection. In addition, antigenic stimulation in such patients could induce viral replication and apoptosis.

Indeed, another central question which is critical to the rational design of a safe AIDS vaccine is whether the immune response to HIV can be detrimental to the host. We have discussed a number of potential deleterious effects: elimination by ADCC or CTL of uninfected cells targeted by gp120 bound to CD4 or peptides derived from gp120; enhanced infection of monocytes by anti-HIV antibodies, through the ADCC mechanism; involvement of HIV-specific CTL in severe inflammatory reactions; autoimmune phenomena. Jiang *et al.* (1991) recently showed that antisera to peptides encompassing the V3 loop of several HIV-1 isolates contained enhancing antibodies. It should also be outlined that certain HIV peptides, encompassing regions suggested as vaccine candidates, have the potential to inhibit immune reactivity (reviewed in Bolognesi 1989). Deleterious effects of anti-idiotypic or anti-gp120 antibodies with anti-CD4 activity must also be considered (Martinez *et al.* 1988).

The lack of an adequate animal model limits the development of an HIV vaccine. The chimpanzee is currently the only animal that can be readily infected by HIV. A state of chronic infection is established in these animals, with immune responses similar to those in humans. To date, however, no disease has occurred in chimpanzees and testing a vaccine in this species may not be relevant to vaccination in humans. Additional difficulties arise from the logistic constraints of the chimpanzee model, including availability of animals and cost. The SCID-hu mouse chimeras in which components of the human immune system are able to survive for several months can be infected by HIV (Namikawa *et al.* 1988). However, a clear demonstration that these animals can mount an immune response to virus is lacking and this model may prove more useful for testing the effect of antiviral drugs than for vaccine development. Macaques are susceptible to infection by SIV, which results in an AIDS-like disease. Since SIV is closely related to HIV-2, this animal model is important for providing concepts and strategies for vaccine development. However, in view of recent data (Stott 1991) all protection data in the SIV model need to be reassessed (see below).

Vaccine strategies

Since we still miss guidelines for the development of long term protection against HIV infection in humans, the ideal vaccine should contain epitopes able to induce neutralizing antibodies, antibodies involved in complement-mediated virus and/or cell lysis, as well as helper and cytotoxic T lymphocytes. Vaccine preparations should be able to confer protection against all strains and preferably all HIV types, to protect against infection by cell-associated virus and probably to induce mucosal immunity. On the other hand, one should avoid the induction of enhancing antibodies, the induction of CTL directed against some envelope epitopes which could lead to destruction of non-infected bystander cells, the administration of immunosuppressive components of the virus and the induction of autoimmune response to sequences showing homology with normal self components.

Attenuated live vaccines mimic natural infection.

Although it is now possible to introduce irreversible deletions in some viral genomes, the risk exists, in the case of HIV, of reverse mutations that would restore virulence. In addition, recombination with or promotion of adjacent cellular oncogenes may occur through viral enhancers. This approach therefore has major potential drawbacks. Viruses with a deletion in *nef* sequences might be used for making live-attenuated strains since Kestler *et al.* (1991) have recently demonstrated that *nef* is required for maintaining high virus loads and for full pathogenic potential.

The use of an *inactivated HIV vaccine* in noninfected humans may also raise major objections since the risk exists of imperfect inactivation, which could escape quality controls. Such preparations are not strongly immunogenic and require multiple injections and strong adjuvants. Salk (1987) has designed the use of an inactivated, γ-irradiated, envelope-depleted preparation for active immunotherapy in already infected people.

Live recombinant vaccines are built by genetic recombination between HIV genes and nonvirulent vectors. Different viruses can be used as live vectors, such as adenoviruses, vaccinia virus or other poxviruses. The use of bacteria has also been advocated: Bacillus Calmette–Guérin (BCG) might be an advantageous vector. These recombinant vaccines elicit a strong cellular immune response and a rather weak humoral response, only after several boosts. Vaccinia virus has been the most often used live vector. The cellular immunity against vaccinia considerably limits the efficiency of boosting. To avoid this problem, Zagury *et al.* (1988) used as boost formalin-fixed autologous cells infected *in vitro* with the vaccinia recombinant, followed by further boosts of intramuscular gp160. This problem should not be met in the case of recombinant avian poxviruses (canary-pox) since they do not multiply in mammalian hosts. Vaccination by a live recombinant vaccine followed by boost with an envelope-based subunit vaccine is an appealing strategy, leading to both cell-mediated and humoral immune responses. The use of recombinant vaccines containing genes coding for selected interleukins, in addition to those coding for HIV proteins, has also been advocated.

Subunit vaccines are made of antigens purified from virions or produced by genetic engineering. In the case of HIV proteins, many expression systems have been used such as bacteria, yeast and animal or insect cell lines. These vaccines are safe. The main problems are their low immunogenicity and the choice of the viral antigens to be included. Immunization of chimpanzees by gp120, gp160 and V3 peptides has resulted in protection against intravenous challenge with homologous HIV. The presentation of both linear and conformational epitopes of gp120 might induce protective humoral immunity to a broader spectrum of virus isolates.

Chimeric vaccines allow the use of conserved poorly immunogenic HIV epitopes in a different structural and immunological context, which enhances their immunogenicity. Different presentation vectors have been chosen. For instance, Evans, D.J. *et al.* (1989) have inserted a highly conserved epitope of gp41, considered to be a neutralization target, in the VP1 domain of polio virus. The major disadvantage of this approach is the maximal acceptable size of the inserted epitopes, which becomes a problem if immunity against a large number of epitopes is necessary for protection.

One of the approaches currently devised by several groups is to construct complex *synthetic vaccines* capable of engaging both T and B cells. The choice of the synthetic peptides to be included in such a vaccine relies on epitope mapping of HIV. Just as selection of the epitopes that induce the desired immune responses is essential, the identification of sites that promote immunosuppression, autoimmunity and enhancement of viral infectivity is critical in order to delete these from vaccine regimens. Currently, rapid progress has been made in the identification of peptide epitopes recognized by HIV-specific B (Bolognesi 1989) and T (Mills *et al.* 1989) cells. A possible solution to the low immunogenicity of synthetic peptides resides in the coupling of peptides to strong T immunogens, according to the intermolecular–intrastructural T cell help concept developed by Milich (1988), who showed that priming with a peptide of the hepatitis B virus nucleocapsid corresponding to a T epitope, followed by injection of complete viral particles, elicited a secondary response not only against the nucleocapsid antigen but also against the viral envelope B epitopes (HBs). This approach has led to the design by Palker *et al.* (1989) of a polyvalent

HIV synthetic immunogen comprised of gp120 T helper cell sites and B cell neutralization epitopes which elicited high-titre neutralizing antibodies as well as T cell responses to more than one HIV isolate. Hart *et al.* (1990) have reported good immunogenicity of V3 peptides coupled to peptides with a sequence of T helper-cell epitopes. It will also be necessary to fuse such neutralizing B epitopes with T epitopes of broad CTL reactivity in diverse HLA haplotypes.

A challenge in HIV vaccine design which lies outside the selection of target epitopes is the mode of antigen presentation necessary to induce the desired response and immunological memory. The use of effective safe adjuvants is necessary to induce a response of sufficient magnitude. At present, the only adjuvants approved for human use are aluminium phosphate and aluminium hydroxide. Muramyl dipeptide-based adjuvants are currently in development. Other promising adjuvants could be the immunostimulating complexes (ISCOMs) derived from a detergent that forms complexes with viral glycoproteins, and liposomes that reproduce artificially the external envelope structure of the virus.

First trials

The very first AIDS vaccine trials were done in chimpanzees (reviewed in Girard and Eichberg 1990). They have used recombinant gp120, vaccinia recombinants expressing the *gag* and/or *env* gene products or purified proteins in adjuvant, as immunization agents. In all cases, high levels of antibodies, with a moderate titre of neutralizing antibodies, and T cell responses were obtained. They were, however, insufficient to confer protection against the infectious viral challenge, even when anti-gp120 antibodies were able to neutralize HIV-1 infectivity *in vitro* (Berman *et al.* 1988; Arthur *et al.* 1989). However, recent studies have shown that such protective immunity may, in fact, be attainable in chimpanzees. After the pilot study of Emini *et al.* (1990) demonstrating that neutralizing antibody specific for the V3 loop can indeed protect chimpanzees from HIV infection, Berman *et al.* (1990) showed that recombinant gp120, but not gp160, can elicite in chimpanzees protective immunity against a homologous strain of HIV-1. Girard *et al.* (1991) elicited sustained high titres of neutralizing antibodies in three chimpanzees after sequential injections of different HIV-1 antigen preparations that included recombinant gp160 and V3 synthetic peptide. The three chimpanzees appeared uninfected by serologic and virologic criteria including PCR, for 6 months following intravenous HIV-1 challenge. However, one of the animals became virus isolation positive at 32 weeks; the two other chimpanzees remained uninfected during longer follow up.

Evidence for protective immunity in macaques was also recently obtained in prophylactic vaccine studies using inactivated whole SIV with adjuvant. Desrosiers *et al.* (1989) obtained complete protection against challenge with live SIV in two out of six animals immunized with purified, disrupted, non-infectious virus. The four other animals became infected but viral load appeared much lower and disease onset significantly slower than in the non-immunized controls. Using a smaller inoculum for challenge, Murphey-Corb *et al.* (1989) obtained complete protection in eight of nine monkeys immunized with a formalin-inactivated whole SIV vaccine potentiated with adjuvant. Gardner (1990) reported that betapropiolactone-inactivated whole virus vaccination protected 3 of 3 monkeys when given in MDP adjuvant, 1 of 2 monkeys when given in complete Freund's adjuvant and 1 of 3 monkeys when given without adjuvant. He has also recently shown that both inactivated and live attenuated SIV vaccines provide some degree of protective immunity against cell-free intravenous challenge, but not when the virus was delivered intravaginally. Recent data suggest that subunit vaccines containing sufficient quantities of viral glycoproteins (Murphey-Corb *et al.* 1991) or envelope-peptide vaccines (Shafferman *et al.* 1991) can protect macaques against SIV infection. Johnson *et al.* (1992) recently demonstrated that inactivated whole SIV vaccine confered protection against homologous and heterologous challenge. Shen *et al.* (1991) have demonstrated that SIV gag peptide-specific CTL can be generated by vaccination with a recombinant SIV-vaccinia virus construct.

A provocative study recently reported by Stoot (1991) casts some doubt on the validity of some of these vaccine data in macaques. These investigators had previously found that vaccination with inactivated SIV-infected allogeneic cells in quil-A adjuvant protected macaques against live virus challenge (Stoot *et al.* 1990). They also saw protection of some control animals vaccinated with uninfected allogeneic cells in quil-A (Stoot 1991). Moreover, protection appeared to correlate with the development of anti-cell antibodies in these monkeys. These results are therefore most probably due to an immune response to a cellular component of the viruses used for the preparation of the vaccine and for the challenge of the vaccinated animals, and not to a viral antigen. The antigen responsible for the unexpected protection artefact might be one of the major histocompatibility antigens. All protection data in the SIV model therefore need to be reassessed. This does not however apply to the successful protection experiment reported by Hu *et al.* (1992) using vaccinia virus- SIV-gp140 recombinant followed by purified recombinant SIV-gp140 antigen which elicited high titres of neutralizing antibodies.

The SIV system in macaques has also been used to investigate post-exposure immunotherapy. A single inoculation of inactivated whole SIV immunogen in adjuvant, given to healthy seropositive macaques 4 months after infection, did not alter antigenaemia, recovery of cell-associated virus or disease course (Gardner *et al.* 1989). Stoot *et al.* (1990) also found that when the vaccine was given after infection, it had no effect on virus recovery.

Whether efficacy should be established in an animal model before testing in humans has been debated for some time. Since some researchers believe that much can be learned about the safety of a product and the development of an immune response in humans before successful efficacy trials in monkeys, phase I trials of an HIV vaccine have begun in seronegative healthy human volunteers, as well as some trials of post-infection immunization.

Zagury *et al.* (1988) have performed the first human immunizations with a candidate AIDS vaccine, using a recombinant vaccinia virus expressing the gp160 protein of HIV. Boosting with paraformaldehyde-fixed autologous cells previously infected with the vaccinia recombinant, followed by subsequent boost with purified recombinant gp160, induced an anamnestic humoral and cellular immune response. Such a vaccine strategy is too complex to be utilized on a large scale. Several phase I trials of safety and immunogenicity in human volunteers are currently in progress in the USA (Koff and Schultz 1990). They use recombinant vaccinia expressing HIV genes, recombinant subunit proteins such as gp160 produced in a baculovirus expression system or gp120 produced in yeast, and synthetic peptides. All these products have been determined to be safe. Cooney *et al.* (1991) showed that a recombinant vaccinia virus vaccine expressing gp160 elicited in vaccinia-naive subjects strong and sustained T cell responses to homologous and heterologous HIV and some antibodies to HIV envelope, whereas in vaccinia-primed subjects T-cell responses were transient and antibodies not detectable. A baculovirus-expressed recombinant gp120 candidate vaccine was used at a 40 or 80 μg dose on days 0, 30 and 180 with a boost on day 540 in a randomized trial with hepatitis B vaccine or placebo as controls (Dolin *et al.* 1991). Antibody responses (Western blot) markedly increased in rate after the third dose and the fourth dose resulted in homologous neutralizing activity in sera from 20% of subjects, as well as in complement-mediated antibody-dependent enhancement in sera from 6 of 24 subjects. Some of these vaccinees had gp160-specific CTLs that were shown by cloning to be CD4 +ve. Certain clones recognized gp160 from diverse HIV isolates and did not kill uninfected CD4 +ve T cells that had bound gp120 (Orentas *et al.* 1990). The most encouraging results were observed after priming with recombinant vaccinia virus-gp160 followed by boosting with purified gp160 (Corey 1992) since over 50% of vaccinia-naive individuals developed antibodies to the V3 loop, fusion inhibition antibodies and neutralizing antibodies.

On the other hand, Salk (1987) hypothesized that, by boosting the protective host immune responses against HIV during the asymptomatic period, it might be possible to reduce the viral burden and thereby prevent the clinical progression to AIDS. Thus, a post-infection immunization strategy is currently undergoing preliminary evaluation, using the Salk irradiated, envelope-depleted HIV immunogen emulsified in Freund's incomplete adjuvant. Preliminary data have indicated that this preparation is safe (Levine 1991). Active immunotherapy with recombinant gp160 in asymptomatic HIV-infected individuals resulted, in subjects with more than 600 CD4 cell counts at entry, in seroconversion to selected envelope epitopes and new T cell proliferative responses to gp160. There were no obvious systemic or immunologic adverse reactions (Redfield *et al*. 1991). Active immunotherapy using vaccinia recombinant should be avoided in potentially immunodeficient individuals.

The development of a vaccine for a virus such as HIV presents a formidable challenge. Despite the many obstacles, the recent advances leading to new strategies as well as recent evidence of protective responses by candidate vaccine in monkeys, raise hope for eventual production of an effective AIDS vaccine. However, the evaluation of efficacy of a vaccine candidate in humans will be a very difficult task in view of the low transmission rate of HIV infection in the population and the long and variable interval between infection and disease. In anticipation of future efficacy trials in the field, WHO has selected four developing countries, Brazil, Rwanda, Uganda and Thailand, as locations to prepare cohorts, train personnel and gather logistical support. Such trials may begin within the next few years.

Acknowledgements

I thank Mrs M.T. Miglierina and M. Bargis-Touchard for invaluable secretarial assistance.

References

Ada, G.I. (1988). Prospects for HIV vaccines. *J. Acquired Immune Deficiency Syndr.* **1**, 295–303.

Ahearne, P.M., Matthews, T.J., Lyerly, H.K., White, G.C., Bolognesi, D.P. and Weinhold, K.J. (1988). Cellular immune response to viral peptides in patients exposed to HIV. *AIDS Res. Hum. Retroviruses* **4**, 259–67.

Allain, J.P., Laurian, Y., Paul, D.A. *et al.* (1987). 'Long-term evaluation of HIV antigen and antibodies to p24 and gp41 in patients with hemophilia: potential clinical importance. *N. Engl. J. Med.* **317**, 1114–21.

Albert, J., Abrahamsson, B., Nagy, K. *et al.* (1990). Rapid development of isolate-specific neutralizing antibodies after primary HIV-1 infection and consequent emergence of virus variants which resist neutralization by autologous sera. *AIDS* **4**, 107–12.

Amadori, A., Zamarchi, R., Ciminale, V. *et al.* (1989). HIV-1 specific B cell activation: a major constituent of spontaneous B cell activation during HIV-1 infection. *J. Immunol.* **143**, 2146–52.

Ameisen, J.C. (1992). The programmed cell death theory of AIDS pathogenesis: implications, testable predictions, and confrontation with experimental findings. *Immunodeficiency Rev.* **3**, 237–46.

Ameisen, J.C. and Capron, A. (1991). T-cell dysfunction and depletion in AIDS: the programmed cell death hypothesis. *Immunol. Today* **7**, 102–5.

Ameisen, J.C., Guy, B., Chamaret, S. *et al.* (1989). Antibodies to the *nef* protein and to nef peptides in HIV-1-infected seronegative individuals. *AIDS Res. Hum. Retroviruses* **5**, 279–91.

Anderson, R.E., Lang, W., Shiboski, S.C., Royce, R., Jewell, N. and Winkelstein, W. Jr. (1990) Use of β2-microglobulin level and CD4 lymphocyte count to predict development of acquired immunodeficiency syndrome in persons with human immunodeficiency virus infection. *Arch. Intern. Med.* **150**, 73–7.

Anderson, R.E., Shiboski, S.C., Royce, R., Jewell, N.P., Lang, W. and Winkelstein, W. Jr. (1991). CD8+ T lymphocytes and progression to AIDS in HIV-infected men: some observations. *AIDS* **5**, 213–5.

Andris, J.S., Johnson, S., Zolla-Pazner, S. and Capra, J.D. (1991). Molecular characterization of five human anti-human immunodeficiency virus type 1 antibody heavy chains reveals extensive somatic mutation typical of an antigen-driven immune response. *Proc. Nat. Acad. Sci. (USA)* **88**, 7783–7.

Archibald, D.W., Barr, C.E., Torosian, J.P., McLane, M.F. and Essex, M. (1987). Secretory IgA antibodies to human immunodeficiency virus in the parotid saliva of patients with AIDS and AIDS-related complex. *J. Infect. Dis.* **155**, 793–6.

Ardman, B., Sikorski, M.A., Settles, M. and Staunton, D.E. (1990). Human immunodeficiency virus type-1 infected individuals make autoantibodies that bind to CD43 on normal thymic lymphocytes. *J. Exp. Med.* **172**, 1151–8.

Arthos, J., Deen, K.C., Chaikin, M.A. *et al.* (1989). Identification of the residues in human CD4 critical for the binding of HIV. *Cell* **57**, 469–81.

Arthur, L.O., Bess, J.W., Waters, D.J. *et al.* (1989). Challenge of chimpanzees (Pan troglodytes) immunized with human immunodeficiency virus envelope glycoprotein gp120. *J. Virology* **63**, 5046–53.

Ashkenazi, A., Smith, D.H., Marsters, S.A. *et al.* (1991). Resistance of primary isolates of human immunodeficiency virus type 1 to soluble CD4 is independent of CD4-rgp120 binding affinity. *Proc. Nat. Acad. Sci. (USA)* **88**, 7056–60.

Auger, I., Thomas, P., De Gruttola, V. *et al.* (1988). Incubation periods for paediatric AIDS patients. *Nature* **336**, 575–7.

Autran, B., Mayaud, C., Raphael, M. *et al.* (1988). Evidence for a cytotoxic T-lymphocyte alveolitis in human immunodeficiency virus-infected patients. *AIDS* **2**, 179–83.

Autran, B., Triebel, F., Katlama, C., Rozenbaum, W., Hercend, T. and Debre, P. (1989). T cell receptor γ/δ^+ lymphocyte subsets during HIV infection. *Clin. Exp. Immunol.* **75**, 206–10.

Baldwin, G.C., Fleischmann, J., Chung, Y., Koyanagi, Y., Chen, I.S. and Golde, D.W. (1990). Human immunodeficiency virus causes mononuclear phagocyte dysfunction. *Proc. Nat. Acad. Sci. (USA)* **87**, 3933–7.

Ballet, J.J., Sulcebe, G., Couderc, L.J. *et al.* (1987). Impaired antipneumococcal antibody response in patients with AIDS-related persistent generalized lymphadenopathy. *Clin. Exp. Immunol.* **68**, 479–87.

Ballet, J.J., Couderc, L.J., Rabian-Herzog, C. *et al.* (1988). Impaired T lymphocyte dependent immune responses to microbial antigens in patients with HIV-I associated persistent generalized lymphadenopathy. *AIDS* **2**, 291–7.

Banapour, B., Rosenthal, K., Rabin, L. *et al.* (1987). Characterization and epitope mapping of a human monoclonal antibody reactive with the envelope glycoprotein of human immunodeficiency virus. *J. Immunol.* **139**, 4027–33.

Bartholomew, C., Blattner, W. and Cleghorn, F. (1987). Progression to AIDS in homosexual men coinfected with HIV and HTLV-I in Trinidad. *Lancet* **ii**, 1469.

Bedinger, P., Moriarty, A., Von Borstel, R.C., Donovan, N.J., Steimer, K.S. and Littman, D.R. (1988). Internationalization of the human deficiency virus does not require the cytoplasmic domain of CD4. *Nature* **334**, 162–5.

Bentin, J., Tsoukas, C.D., McCutchan, J.A., Spector, S.A., Richman, D.D. and Vaughan, J. (1989). Impairment in T-lymphocyte responses during early infection with the human immunodeficiency virus. *J. Clin. Immunol.* **9**, 159–68.

Berger, E.A., Fuerst, T.R. and Moss, B. (1988). A soluble recombinant polypeptide comprising the amino-terminal half of the extracellular region of the CD4 molecule contains an active binding site for human immunodeficiency virus. *Proc. Nat. Acad. Sci. (USA)* **85**, 2357–61.

Berger, E.A., Lifson, J.D. and Eiden, L.E. (1991). Stimulation of glycoprotein gp120 dissociation from the envelope glycoprotein complex of human immunodeficiency virus type 1 by soluble CD4 and CD4 peptide derivatives: implications for the role of the complementarity-determining region 3-like region in membrane fusion. *Proc. Nat. Acad. Sci. (USA)* **88**, 8082–6.

Berkower, I., Smith, G.E., Giri, C. and Murphy, D. (1989). Human immunodeficiency virus 1: predominance of a group-specific neutralizing epitope that persists despite genetic variation. *J. Exp. Med.* **170**, 1681–95.

Berman, P.W., Groopman, J.E., Gregory, T.J. *et al.* (1988). Human immunodeficiency virus type 1 challenge of chimpanzees immunized with recombinant envelope glycoprotein GP120. *Proc. Nat. Acad. Sci. (USA)* **85**, 5200–4.

Berman, P.W., Gregory, T.J., Riddle, L. *et al.* (1990). Protection of chimpanzees from infection by HIV-1 after vaccination with recombinant glycoprotein GP120 but not GP160. *Nature* **345**, 622–5.

Berzofsky, J.A. (1991). Approaches and issues in the development of vaccines against HIV. *J. Acquired Immune Deficiency Syndr.* **4**, 451–9.

Berzofsky, J.A., Pendleton, C.D., Clerici, M. *et al.* (1991). Construction of peptides encompassing multideterminant clusters of human immunodeficiency virus envelope to induce *in vitro* T cell responses in mice and humans of multiple MHC types. *J. Clin. Invest.* **88**, 876–84.

Bettaieb, A., Oksenhendler, E., Fromont, P., Duedari, N. and Bierling, P. (1989). Immunochemical analysis of platelet autoantibodies in HIV-related thrombocytopenic purpura: a study of 68 patients. *Br. J. Haematol.* **73**, 241–7.

Bhat, S., Spitalnik, S.L., Gonzalez-Scarano, F. and Silberberg, D.H. (1991). Galactosyl ceramide or a derivative is an essential component of the neural receptor for human immunodeficiency virus type 1 envelope glycoprotein gp120. *Proc. Nat. Acad. Sci. (USA)* **88**, 7131–4.

Birx, D.L., Redfield, R.R., Tencer, K., Fowler, A., Burke, D.S. and Tosato, G. (1990). Induction of interleukin-6 during human immunodeficiency virus infection. *Blood* **76**, 2303–10.

Blanche, S., Tardieu, M., Duliege, A.M. *et al.* (1990). Longitudinal study of 94 symptomatic infants with perinataly acquired HIV infection: evidence for a bimodal expression of clinical and biological symptoms. *Am. J. Dis. Child.* **144**, 1210–5.

Bolognesi, D.P. (1989). HIV antibodies and vaccine design. *AIDS* **3** (suppl. 1), S111–S118.

Boucher, C.A.B., de Wolf, F., Houweling, J.T.M. *et al.* (1989). Antibody response to a synthetic peptide covering a LAV-1/HTLV-IIIB neutralization epitope and disease progression. *AIDS* **3**, 71–6.

Bowman, M.R., MacFerrin, K.D., Schreiber, S.L. and Burakoff, S.J. (1990). Identification and structural analysis of residues in the V1 region of CD4 involved in interaction with human immunodeficiency virus envelope glycoprotein gp120 and class II major histocompatibility complex molecules. *Proc. Nat. Acad. Sci. (USA)* **87**, 9052–6.

Boyer, V., Desgranges, C., Trabaud, M.A., Fischer, E. and Kazatchkine, M.D. (1991). Complement mediates human immunodeficiency virus type 1 infection of a human T cell line in a CD4- and antibody-independent fashion. *J. Exp. Med.* **173**, 1151–8.

Briault, S., Courtois-Capella, M., Duarte, F., Aucouturier, P. and Preud'homme, J.L. (1988). Isotypy of serum monoclonal immunoglobulins in human immunodeficiency virus-infected adults. *Clin. Exp. Immunol.* **74**, 182–4.

Burcham, J., Marmor, M., Dubin, N. *et al.* (1991). CD4% is the best predictor of development of AIDS in a cohort of HIV-infected homosexual men. *AIDS* **5**, 365–72.

Byrn, R.A., Sekigawa, I., Chamow, S.M. *et al.* (1989). Characterization of *in vitro* inhibition of human immunodeficiency virus by purified recombinant CD4. *J. Virol.* **63**, 4370–5.

Byrn, R.A., Mordenti, J., Lucas, C. *et al.* (1990). Biological properties of a CD4 immunoadhesin. *Nature* **344**, 667–70.

Calvelli, T.A. and Rubinstein, A. (1990). Pediatric HIV infection: a review. *Immunodeficiency Rev.* **2**, 83–127.

Camerini, D. and Seed, B. (1990). A CD4 domain important for HIV-mediated syncytium formation lies outside the virus binding site. *Cell* **60**, 747–54.

Cameron, P.U., Cobain, T.J., Zhang, W.J., Kay, P.H. and Dawkins, R.L. (1988). Influence of C4 null genes on infection with human immunodeficiency virus. *Br. Med. J.* **296**, 1627–8.

Capon, D.J., Chamow, S.M., Mordenti, J. *et al.* (1989). Designing CD4 immunoadhesins for AIDS therapy. *Nature* **337**, 525–31.

Cefai, D., Debre, P., Kaczorek, M., Idziorek, T., Autran, B. and Bismuth, G. (1990). Human immunodeficiency virus-1 glycoproteins gp120 and gp160 specifically inhibit the CD3/T cell-antigen receptor phosphoinositide transduction pathway. *J. Clin. Invest.* **86**, 2117–24.

Celada, F., Cambiaggi, C., Maccari, J. *et al.* (1990). Antibody raised against soluble CD4-gp120 complex recognizes the CD4 moiety and blocks membrane fusion without inhibiting CD4-gp120 binding. *J. Exp. Med.* **172**, 1143–50.

Chams, V., Jouault, T., Fenouillet, E., Gluckman, J.C. and Klatzmann, D. (1988). Detection of anti-CD4 autoantibodies in the sera of HIV-infected patients using recombinant soluble CD4 molecules. *AIDS* **2**, 353–61.

Chaudary, V.K., Mizukami, T., Fuerst, T.R. *et al.* (1988). Selective killing of HIV-infected cells by recombinant human CD4-pseudomonas exotoxin hybrid protein. *Nature* **335**, 369–72.

Chenciner, N., Michel, F., Dadaglio, G. *et al.* (1989). Multiple subsets of HIV-specific cytotoxic T lymphocytes in humans and in mice. *Eur. J. Immunol.* **19**, 1537–44.

Cheng-Mayer, C., Seto, D., Tateno, M. and Levy, J.A. (1988). Biologic features of HIV-1 that correlate with virulence in the host. *Science* **240**, 80–2.

Chirmule, N., Kalayanaraman, V.S., Oyaizu, N. *et al.* (1990). Inhibition of functional properties of tetanus antigen-specific T-cell clones by envelope glycoprotein gp120 of human immunodeficiency virus. *Blood* **75**, 152–9.

Clapham, P.R., Weber, J.N., Whitby, D. *et al.* (1989). Soluble CD4 blocks the infectivity of diverse strains of HIV and SIV for T cells and monocytes but not for brain and muscle cells. *Nature* **337**, 368–70.

Clark, S.J., Saag, M.S., Don Decker, W. *et al.* (1991). High titres of cytopathic virus in plasma of patients with symptomatic primary HIV-1 infection. *New Engl. J. Med.* **324**, 954–60.

Claverie, J.M., Kourilsky, P., Langlade-Demoyen, P. *et al.* (1988). T-immunogenic peptides are constituted of rare sequence patterns. Use in the identification of T epitopes in the human immunodeficiency virus *gag* protein. *Eur. J. Immunol.* **18**, 1547–53.

Clayton, L.K., Hussey, R.E., Streinbrich, R., Ramachandran, H., Husain, Y. and Reinherz, E.L. (1988). Substitution of murine for human CD4 residues identifies amino acids critical for HIV-gp120 binding. *Nature* **335**, 363–6.

Clayton, L.K., Sieh, M., Pious, D.A. and Reinherz, E.L. (1989). Identification of human CD4 residues affecting class II MHC versus HIV-1 gp120 binding. *Nature* **339**, 548–51.

Clerici, M., Stocks, N.I., Zajac, R.A. *et al.* (1989a). Detection of three distinct patterns of T helper cell dysfunction in asymptomatic, human immunodeficiency virus-seropositive patients. Independence of $CD4^+$ cell numbers and clinical staging. *J. Clin. Invest.* **84**, 1892–9.

Clerici, M., Stocks, N.I., Zajac, R.A. *et al.* (1989b). Interleukin-2 production used to detect antigenic peptide recognition by T-helper lymphocytes from asymptomatic HIV-seropositive individuals. *Nature* **339**, 383–5.

Clerici, M., Stocks, N.I., Zajac, R.A., Boswell, R.N. and Shearer, G.M. (1990). Accessory cell function in asymptomatic human immunodeficiency virus-infected patients. *Clin. Immunol. Immunopathol.* **54**, 168–73.

Clerici, M., Landay, A.L., Kessler, H.A. *et al.* (1991a). Multiple patterns of alloantigen presenting/stimulating cell dysfunction in patients with AIDS. *J. Immunol.* **146**, 2207–13.

Clerici, M., Lucey, D.R., Zajac, R.A. *et al.* (1991b). Detection of cytotoxic T lymphocytes specific for synthetic peptides of gp160 in HIV-seropositive individuals. *J. Immunol.* **146**, 2214–9.

Clouse, K.A., Robbins, P.B., Fernie, B., Ostrove, J.M. and Fauci, A.S. (1989). Viral antigen stimulation of the production of human monokines capable of regulating HIV1 expression. *J. Immunol.* **143**, 470–5.

Collman, R., Hassan, N.F., Walker, R. *et al.* (1989). Infection of monocyte-derived macrophages with human immunodeficiency virus type 1 (HIV-1). Monocyte-tropic and lymphocyte-tropic strains of HIV-1 show distinctive patterns of replication in a panel of cell types. *J. Exp. Med.* **170**, 1149–63.

Collman, R., Godfrey, B., Cutilli, J. *et al.* (1990). Macrophage-tropic strains of human immunodeficiency virus type 1 utilize the CD4 receptor. *J. Virol.* **64**, 4468–76.

Connor, R.I., Dinces, N.B., Howell, A.L., Romet-Lemonne, J.L., Pasquali, J.L. and Fanger, M.W. (1991). Fc receptors for IgG (FcγRs) on human monocytes and macrophages are not infectivity receptors for human immunodeficiency virus type 1 (HIV-1): studies using bispecific antibodies to target HIV-1 to various myeloid cell surface molecules, including the FcγR. *Proc. Nat. Acad. Sci. (USA)* **88**, 9593–7.

Coombs, R.W., Collier, A.C., Allain, J.P. *et al.* (1989). Plasma viremia in human immunodeficiency virus infection. *N. Engl. J. Med.* **321**, 1626–31.

Cooney, E.I., Collier, A.C., Greenberg, P.D. *et al.* (1991). Safety and immunological response to a recombinant vaccinia virus vaccine expressing HIV envelope glycoprotein. *Lancet* **337**, 567–72.

Corey, L. (1992). Phase I trials of subunit gp160 vaccines: a current summary. In: *Sixième Colloque des Cent Gardes: Retroviruses of Human AIDS and Related Animal Diseases*, ed. M. Girard and L. Valette, pp. 287–92.

Crapper, R.M., Deam, D.R. and MacKay, I.R. (1987). Paraproteinemias in homosexual men with HIV infection. Lack of association with abnormal clinical or immunologic findings. *Am. J. Clin. Pathol.* **88**, 348–51.

Culmann, B., Gomard, E., Kieny, M.P. *et al.* (1989). An antigenic peptide of the HIV-1 Nef protein recognized by cytotoxic T lymphocytes of seropositive individuals in association with different HLA-B molecules. *Eur. J. Immunol.* **12**, 2383–6.

Culmann, B., Gomard, E., Kieny, M.P. *et al.* (1991). Six epitopes reacting with human cytotoxic CD8+ T cells in the central region of the HIV-1 Nef protein. *J. Immunol.* **146**, 1560–5.

Daar, E.S., Li, X.L., Moudgil, T. and Ho, D.D. (1990). High concentrations of recombinant soluble CD4 are required to neutralize primary human immunodeficiency virus type 1 isolates. *Proc Nat. Acad. Sci. (USA)* **87**, 6574–8.

Daar, E.S., Moudgil, T., Meyer, R.D. and Ho, D.D. (1991). Transient high levels of viremia in patients with primary human immunodeficiency virus type 1 infection. *New Engl. J. Med.* **324**, 961–4.

Dadaglio, G., Leroux, A., Langlade-Demoyen, P. *et al.* (1991). Epitope recognition of conserved HIV envelope sequences by human cytotoxic T lymphocytes. *J. Immunol.* **147**, 2302–9.

Dalgleish, A.G., Beverley, P.C., Clapham, P.R., Crawford, D.H., Greaves, M.F. and Weiss, R.A. (1984). The CD4 (T4) antigen is an essential component of the receptor for the AIDS retrovirus. *Nature* **312**, 763–7.

Dalgleish, A.G., Thomson, B.J., Chanh, T.C., Malkovsky, M. and Kennedy, R.C. (1987). Neutralization of HIV isolates by anti-idiotypic antibodies which mimic the T4 (CD4) epitope: a potential AIDS vaccine. *Lancet* **ii**, 1047–50.

Dalgleish, A.G., Chanh, T.C., Kennedy, R.C., Kanda, P., Clapham, P.R. and Weiss, R.A. (1988). Neutralization of diverse HIV1 strains by monoclonal antibodies raised against a gp41 synthetic peptide. *Virology* **165**, 209–15.

Deen, K.C., McDougal, J.S., Inacker, R., *et al.* (1988). A soluble form of CD4 (T4) protein inhibits AIDS virus infection. *Nature* **331**, 82–4.

Delfraissy, J.F., Wallon, C., Boué, F., Barre-Sinoussi, F. and Galanaud, P. (1991). Tumor necrosis factor α inhibits the competence signal delivered by HIV to normal B cells. *J. Immunol.* **146**, 1516–21.

Desrosiers, R.C., Wyand, M.S., Kodama, T. *et al.* (1989). Vaccine protection against simian immunodeficiency virus infection. *Proc. Nat. Acad. Sci. (USA)* **86**, 6353–7.

Devash, Y., Matthews, T.J., Drummond, J.E. *et al.* (1990a). C-terminal fragments of gp120 and synthetic peptides from five HTLV-III strains: prevalence of antibodies to the HTLV-III-MN isolate in infected individuals. *AIDS Res. Hum. Retrov.*

6, 307–16.

Devash, Y., Calvelli, T.A., Wood, D.G., Reagan, K.J. and Rubinstein, A. (1990b). Vertical transmission of human immunodeficiency virus is correlated with the absence of high-affinity/avidity maternal antibodies to the gp120 principal neutralizing domain. *Proc. Nat. Acad. Sci. (USA)* **87**, 3445–9.

DeVico, A.L., Veronese, F.D., Lee, S.L., Gallo, R.C. and Sarngadharan, M.G. (1988). High prevalence of serum antibodies to reverse transcriptase in HIV-1-infected individuals. *AIDS Res. Hum. Retroviruses* **4**, 17–22.

De Wolf, F., Lange, J.M., Houweling, J.T. *et al.* (1988). Numbers of CD4+ cells and the levels of core antigens of and antibodies to the human immunodeficiency virus as predictors of AIDS among seropositive homosexual men. *J. Infect. Dis.* **158**, 615–22.

Diamond, D.C., Sleckman, B.P., Gregory, T., Lasky, L.A., Greenstein, J.L. and Burakoff, S.J. (1988). Inhibition of $CD4^+$ T cell function by the HIV envelope protein, gp120. *J. Immunol.* **141**, 3715–17.

Djeu, J.Y., Blanchard, D.K., Richards, A.L. and Friedman, H. (1988). Tumor necrosis factor induction by *Candida albicans* from human natural killer cells and monocytes. *J. Immunol.* **141**, 4047–52.

Dolin, R., Graham, B.S., Greenberg, S.B. *et al.* (1991). The safety and immunogenicity of a human immunodeficiency virus type 1 (HIV-1) recombinant gp160 candidate vaccine in humans. *Ann. Intern. Med.* **114**, 119–27.

Eales, L.J., Moshtael, D. and Pinching, A.J. (1987). Microbicidal activity of monocyte derived macrophages in AIDS and related disorders. *Clin. Exp. Immunol.* **67**, 227–35.

Eales, L.J., Farrant, J., Helbert, M. and Pinching, A.J. (1988). Peripheral blood dendritic cells in persons with AIDS and AIDS related complex: loss of high intensity class II antigen expression and function. *Clin. Exp. Immunol.* **71**, 423–7.

Emini, E.A., Nara, P.I., Schlief, W.A. *et al.* (1990). Antibody mediated *in vitro* neutralization of human immunodeficiency virus type 1 abolishes infectivity for chimpanzees. *J. Virol.* **64**, 3674–8.

Evans, D.J., McKeating, J., Meredith, J.M. *et al.* (1989). An engineered poliovirus chimera elicits broadly reactive HIV-1 neutralizing antibodies. *Nature* **339**, 385–8.

Evans, L.A., Thomson-Honnebier, G., Steimer, K. *et al.* (1989). Antibody-dependent cellular cytotoxicity is directed against both the gp120 and gp41 envelope proteins of HIV. *AIDS* **3**, 273–6.

Fahey, J.L., Giorgi, J., Martinez-Maza, O., Detels, R., Mitsuyasu, T.R. and Taylor, J.M. (1987). Immunopathogenesis AIDS and related syndromes. *Ann. Immunol. (Inst. Pasteur)* **138**, 245–52.

Fahey, J.L., Taylor, J.M., Detels, R. *et al.* (1990). The prognostic value of cellular and serologic markers in infection with human immunodeficiency virus type 1. *N. Engl. J. Med.* **322**, 166–72.

Falloon, J., Eddy, J., Wiener, L. and Pizzo, P.A. (1989). Human immunodeficiency virus infection in children. *J. Pediatr* **114**, 1–30.

Farzadegan, H., Polis, M.A., Wolinsky, S.M. *et al.* (1988). Loss of human immunodeficiency virus type 1 (HIV-1) antibodies with evidence of viral infection in asymptomatic homosexual men. A report from the multicenter AIDS cohort study. *Ann. Intern. Med.* **108**, 785–90.

Fauci, A.S. (1988). The human immunodeficiency virus infectivity and mechanisms of pathogenesis. *Science* **239**, 617–22.

Fauci, A.S. (moderator) (1989). NIH conference. Development and evaluation of a vaccine for human immunodeficiency virus (HIV) infection. *Ann. Intern. Med* **110**, 373–85.

Fauci, A.S. (1991). The relation between HIV and the human immune system. In: Immunopathogenic mechanisms in human immunodeficiency virus (HIV) infection. *Ann. Intern. Med.* **114**, 678–93.

Fenouillet, E., Clerget-Raslain, B., Gluckman, J.C., Guétard, D., Montagnier, L. and Bahraoui, E. (1989). Role of *N*-linked glycans in the interaction between the envelope glycoprotein of human immunodeficiency virus and its CD4 cellular receptor. Structural enzymatic analysis. *J. Exp. Med.* **169**, 807–22.

Fisher, R.A., Bertonis, J.M., Meier, W. *et al.* (1988). HIV infection is blocked *in vitro* by recombinant soluble CD4. *Nature* **331**, 76–8.

Fleury, S., Lamarre, D., Meloche, S. *et al.* (1991). Mutational analysis of the interaction between CD4 and class II MHC: class II antigens contact CD4 on a surface opposite the gp120-binding site. *Cell* **66**, 1037–49.

Folks, T.M. (1991). Human immunodeficiency virus in bone marrow: still more questions than answers. *Blood* **77**, 1625–6.

Folks, T.M., Kessler, S.W., Orenstein, J.M., Justement, J.S., Jaffe, E.S. and Fauci, A.S. (1988). Infection and replication of HIV-1 in purified progenitor cells of normal human bone marrow. *Science* **242**, 919–22.

Folks, T.M., Clouse, K.A., Justement, J. *et al.* (1989). Tumor necrosis factor α induces expression of human immunodeficiency virus in a chronically infected T-cell clone. *Proc. Nat. Acad. Sci. (USA)* **86**, 2365–8.

Freed, E.O., Myers, D.J. and Risser R. (1990). Characterization of the fusion domain of the human immunodeficiency virus type 1 envelope glycoprotein gp41. *Proc. Nat. Acad. Sci. (USA)* **87**, 4650–4.

Fuchs, D., Hausen, A., Reihnegger, G., Werner, E.R., Dierich, M.P. and Wachter, H. (1988). Neopterin as a marker for activated cell-mediated immunity: application in HIV infection. *Immunol. Today* **9**, 150–5.

Gallo, R.C., Bolognesi, D.P. and Nerurkar, L.S. (1989). The immune response to human immunodeficiency virus infection. pp. 374–7. In Fauci, A.S., moderator. Development and evaluation of a vaccine for human immunodeficiency virus (HIV) infection. *Ann. Intern. Med.* **110**, 373–85.

Gardner, M.B. (1990). Vaccination against SIV infection and disease. *AIDS Res. Hum. Retroviruses* **6**, 835–46.

Gardner, M.B., Jennings, M., Carlson, J.R. *et al.* (1989). Postexposure immunotherapy of simian immunodeficiency virus (SIV) infected rhesus with an SIV immunogen. *J. Med. Primatol.* **18**, 321–8.

Gartner, S., Markovits, P., Markovitz, D.M., Kaplan, M.H., Gallo, R.C. and Popovic, M. (1986). The role of mononuclear phagocytes in HTLV-III/LAV infection. *Science* **233**, 215–19.

Gendelman, H.E., Baca, L.M., Turpin, J. *et al.* (1990). Regulation of HIV replication in infected monocytes by IFN-α mechanisms for viral restriction. *J. Immunol.* **145**, 2669–76.

Giorgi, J.V. and Detels, R. (1989). T cell subset alterations in HIV-infected homosexual men: NIAID multicenter AIDS cohort study. *Clin. Immunol. Immunopathol.* **52**, 10–18.

Girard, M.P. and Eichberg, J.W. (1990). Progress in the development of HIV vaccines. *AIDS* **4** (suppl. 1), S143–S150.

Girard, M.M., Fultz, P., Kieny, M.P. *et al.* (1989). Immune responses of chimpanzees to live recombinant, inactivated, subunit and synthetic prototype HIV vaccines. In *Quatrième Colloque des Cent Gardes: Retroviruses of Human AIDS and Related Animal Diseases*, ed. Girard and Valette, pp. 265–9.

Girard, M.M., Kieny, M.P., Pinter, A. *et al.* (1991). Immunization of chimpanzees confers protection against challenge with human immunodeficiency virus. *Proc. Nat. Acad. Sci. (USA)* **88**, 542–6.

Goedert, J.J., Biggar, R.J., Melbye, M. *et al.* (1987). Effect of T4 count and cofactors on the incidence of AIDS in homosexual men infected with human immunodeficiency virus *JAMA* **257**, 331–4.

Goedert, J.J., Mendez, H., Drummond, J.E. *et al.* (1989). Mother-to-infant transmission of human immunodeficiency virus type 1: association with prematurity or low anti-gp120. *Lancet* **ii**, 1351–4.

Golding, H., Shearer, G.M., Hillman, K. *et al.* (1989). Common epitope in human immunodeficiency virus (HIV) GP41 and HLA class II elicits immunosuppressive autoantibodies capable of contributing to immune dysfunction in HIV I-infected individuals. *J. Clin. Invest.* **83**, 1430–5.

Goudsmit, J., Lange, J.M.A., Paul, D.A. and Dawson, G.J. (1987). Antigenemia and antibody titers to core and envelope antigens in AIDS, AIDS-related complex, and subclinical human immunodeficiency virus infection. *J. Infect. Dis.* **155**, 558–60.

Goudsmit, J., Debouck, C., Meloen, R.H. *et al.* (1988). Human immunodeficiency virus type 1 neutralization epitope with conserved architecture elicits early type-specific antibodies in experimentally infected chimpanzees. *Proc. Nat. Acad. Sci. (USA)* **85**, 4478–82.

Goudsmit, J., Kuiken, C.L. and Nara, P.L. (1989). Linear versus conformational variation of V3 neutralization domains of HIV-1 during experimental and natural infection. *AIDS* **3** (suppl. 1), S119–S123.

Gowda, S.D., Stein, B.S., Mohagheghpour, N., Benike, C.J. and Engleman, E.G. (1989). Evidence that T cell activation is required for HIV-1 entry in $CD4^+$ lymphocytes. *J. Immunol.* **142**, 773–80.

Groopman, J.E., Caiazzo, T., Thomas, M.A. *et al.* (1988). Lack of evidence of prolonged human immunodeficiency virus infection before antibody seroconversion. *Blood* **71**, 1752–4.

Groux, H., Torpier, G., Monté, D., Mouton, Y., Capron, A. and Ameisen, J.C. (1992). Activation-induced death by apoptosis in CD4+ T cells from human immunodeficiency virus-infected asymptomatic individuals. *J. Exp. Med.* **175**, 331–40.

Gruters, R.A., Terpstra, F.G., De Jong, R., van Noesel, C.J.M., van Lier, R.A.W. and Miedema, F. (1990). Selective loss of T-cell functions in different stages of HIV infection. *Eur. J. Immunol.* **20**, 1039–44.

Gruters, R.A., Terpstra, F.G., De Goede, R.E. *et al.* (1991a). Immunological and virological markers in individuals progressing from seroconversion to AIDS. *AIDS* **5**, 837–44.

Gruters, R.A., Terpstra, F.G., Lange, J.M. *et al.* (1991b). Differences in clinical course in zidovudine-treated asymptomatic HIV-infected men associated with T-cell function at intake. *AIDS* **5**, 43–7.

Gupta, S. and Vayuvegula, B. (1987). Human immunodeficiency virus-associated changes in signal transduction. *J. Clin. Immunol.* **7**, 486–9.

Gurley, R.J., Ikeuchi, K., Byrn, R.A., Anderson, K. and Groopman, J.E. (1989). $CD4^+$ lymphocyte function with early human immunodeficiency virus infection. *Proc. Nat. Acad. Sci. (USA)* **86**, 1993–7.

Haase, A.T. (1986). Pathogenesis of lentivirus infections. *Nature* **322**, 130–6.

Haigwood, N.L., Shuster, J.R., Moore, G.K. *et al.* (1990). Importance of hypervariable regions of HIV-1 gp120 in the generation of virus neutralizing antibodies. *AIDS Res. Hum. Retroviruses.* **6**, 855–69.

Hammond, S.A., Obah, E., Stanhope, P. *et al.* (1991). Characterization of a conserved T-cell epitope in HIV-1 gp41 recognized by vaccine-induced human cytolytic T-cells. *J. Immunol.* **146**, 1470–7.

Harouse, J.M., Kunsch, C., Hartle, H.T. *et al.* (1989). CD4-independent infection of human neural cells by human immunodeficiency virus type 1. *J. Virol.* **63**, 2527–33.

Harouse, J.M., Bhat, S., Spitalnik, S.L. *et al.* (1991). Inhibition of entry of HIV-1 in neural cell lines by antibodies against galactosyl ceramide. *Science* **253**, 320–3.

Harper, M.E., Marselle, L.M., Gallo, R.C. and Wong-Staal, F. (1986). Detection of lymphocytes expressing human T-lymphotropic virus type III in lymph nodes and peripheral blood from infected individuals by *in situ* hybridization. *Proc. Nat. Acad. Sci. (USA)* **83**, 772–6.

Hart, M.K., Palker, T.J., Matthews, T.J. *et al.* (1990). Synthetic peptides containing T- and B-cell epitopes from human immunodeficiency virus envelope gp120 induce anti-HIV proliferative responses and high titres of neutralizing antibodies in Rhesus monkeys. *J. Immunol.* **145**, 2677–85.

Hart, M.K., Weinhold, K.J., Scearce, R.M. *et al.* (1991). Priming of anti-human immunodeficiency virus (HIV) CD8+ cytotoxic T cells *in vivo* by carrier-free HIV synthetic peptides. *Proc. Nat. Acad. Sci. (USA)* **88**, 9448–52.

Hattori, N., Michaels, F., Fargnoli, K., Marcon, L., Gallo, R.C. and Franchini, G. (1990). The human immunodeficiency virus type 2 *vpr* gene is essential for productive infection of human macrophages. *Proc. Nat. Acad. Sci. (USA)* **87**, 8080–4.

Healey, D., Dianda, L., Moore, J.P. *et al.* (1990). Novel anti-CD4 monoclonal antibodies separate human immunodeficiency virus infection and fusion of CD4+ cells from virus binding. *J. Exp. Med.* **172**, 1233–42.

Ho, D.D., Rota, T.R. and Hirsch, M.S. (1986). Infection of monocyte/macrophage by human T lymphotropic virus type III. *J. Clin. Invest.* **77**, 1712–15.

Ho, D.D., Kaplan, J.C., Rackauskas, I.E. and Gurney, M.E. (1988). Second conserved domain of gp120 is important for HIV infectivity and antibody neutralization. *Science* **239**, 1021–3.

Ho, D.D., Moudgil, T. and Alam, M. (1989). Quantitation of human immunodeficiency virus type 1 in the blood of infected persons. *N. Engl. J. Med.* **321**, 1621–5.

Ho, D.D., McKeating, J.A., Li, X.L. *et al.* (1991a). Conformational epitope on gp120 important in CD4 binding and human immunodeficiency virus type 1 neutralization identified by a human monoclonal antibody. *J. Virol.* **65**, 489–93.

Ho, D.D., Fung, M.S., Cao, T.Y. *et al.* (1991b). Another discontinuous epitope on glycoprotein gp120 that is important in human immunodeficiency virus type 1 neutralization is identified by a monoclonal antibody. *Proc. Nat. Acad. Sci.*

(*USA*) **88**, 8949–52.

Hoffenbach, A., Langlade-Demoyen, P., Dadaglio, G. *et al.* (1989). Unusually high frequencies of HIV-specific cytotoxic T lymphocytes in human. *J. Immunol.* **142**, 452–62.

Hoffmann, G.W., Kion, Y.A. and Grant, M.D. (1991). An idiotypic network model of AIDS immunopathogenesis. *Proc. Nat. Acad. Sci. (USA)* **88**, 3060–4.

Hofmann, B., Orskov Lindhardt, B., Gerstoft, J. *et al.* (1987). Lymphocyte transformation response to pokeweed mitogen as a marker for the development of AIDS and AIDS related symptoms in homosexual men with HIV antibodies. *Brit. Med. J.* **295**, 293–6.

Hofmann, B., Jakobsen, K.D., Odum, N. *et al.* (1989). HIV-induced immunodeficiency. Relatively preserved phytohemagglutinin as opposed to decreased pokeweed mitogen responses may be due to possibly preserved responses via CD2/phytohemagglutinin pathway. *J. Immunol.* **142**, 1874–80.

Homsy, J., Tateno, M. and Levy, J.A. (1988). Antibody-dependent enhancement of HIV infection. *Lancet* **i**, 1285–6.

Homsy, J., Meyer, M., Tateno, M., Clarkson, S. and Levy, J.A. (1989). The Fc and not CD4 receptor mediates antibody enhancement of HIV infection in human cells. *Science* **244**, 1357–60.

Homsi, J., Meyer, M. and Levy, J.A. (1990). Serum enhancement of human immunodeficiency virus (HIV) infection correlates with disease in HIV-infected individuals. *J. Virol.* **64**, 1437–40.

Horsburgh, C.R., Ou, C.Y., Jason, J. *et al.* (1989). Duration of human immunodeficiency virus infection before detection of antibody. *Lancet* **ii**, 637–40.

Hosmalin, A., Clerici, M., Houghten, R. *et al.* (1990). An epitope in human immunodeficiency virus 1 reverse transcriptase recognized by both mouse and human cytotoxic T lymphocytes. *Proc. Nat. Acad. Sci. (USA)* **87**, 2344–8.

Hoxie, J.A., Alpers, J.D., Rackowski, J.L. *et al.* (1986). Alterations in T4 (CD4) protein and mRNA synthesis in cells infected with HIV. *Science* **234**, 1123–7.

Hu, S.L., Abrams, K., Baber, G.N. *et al.* (1992). Protection against SIV infection by vaccinia recombinant virus priming followed by gp160 boosting. *Science* **255**, 456–9.

Hussey, R.E., Richardson, N.E., Kowalski, M. *et al.* (1988). A soluble CD4 protein selectively inhibits HIV replication and syncytium formation. *Nature* **331**, 78–81.

Hwang, S.S., Boyle, T.J., Lyerly, H.K. and Cullen, B.R. (1991). Identification of the envelope V3 loop as the primary determinant of cell tropism in HIV-1. *Science* **253**, 71–4.

Ibegbu, C.C., Kennedy, M.S., Maddon, P.J. *et al.* (1989). Structural features of CD4 required for binding to HIV. *J. Immunol.* **142**, 2250–6.

Imagawa, D. and Detels, R. (1991). HIV-1 in seronegative homosexual men. *N. Engl. J. Med.* **325**, 1250–1 (letter).

Imagawa, D.T., Lee, M.H., Wolinsky, S.M. *et al.* (1989). Human immunodeficiency virus type 1 infection in homosexual men who remain seronegative for prolonged periods. *N. Engl. J. Med.* **320**, 1458–62.

Imberti, L., Sottini, A., Bettinardi, A., Puoti, M. and Primi, D. (1991). Selective depletion in HIV infection of T cells that bear specific T cell receptor Vβ sequences. *Science* **254**, 860–2.

Itescu, S., Brancato, L.J. and Winchester, R. (1989). A sicca syndrome in HIV infection: association with HLA-DR5 and CD8 lymphocytosis. *Lancet* **ii**, 466–8.

Ivey-Hoyle, M., Culp, J.S., Chaikin, M.A. *et al.* (1991). Envelope glycoproteins from biologically diverse isolates of immunodeficiency viruses have widely different affinities for CD4. *Proc. Nat. Acad. Sci. (USA)* **88**, 512–16.

Jackson, G.G., Perkins, J.T., Rubenis, M. *et al.* (1988). Passive immunoneutralization of human immunodeficiency virus in patients with advanced AIDS. *Lancet* **ii**, 647–52.

Janeway, C.A. Jr. (1991). MLS: makes a little sense. *Nature* **349**, 459–61.

Javaherian, K., Langlois, A.J., McDanal, C. *et al.* (1989). Principal neutralizing domain of the human immunodeficiency virus type 1 envelope protein. *Proc. Nat. Acad. Sci. (USA)* **86**, 6768–72.

Jehuda-Cohen, T., Slade, B.A., Powell, J.D. *et al.* (1990). Polyclonal B-cell activation reveals antibodies against human immunodeficiency virus type 1 (HIV-1) in HIV-1-seronegative individuals. *Proc. Nat. Acad. Sci. (USA)* **87**, 3972–6.

Jiang, S., Lin, K. and Neurath, A.R. (1991). Enhancement of human immunodeficiency virus type 1 infection by antisera to peptides from the envelope glycoproteins gp120/gp41. *J. Exp. Med.* **174**, 1557–63.

Johnson, P.R., Trocha, A., Yang, L. *et al.* (1991). HIV-1 gag-specific cytotoxic T lymphocytes recognize multiple highly conserved epitopes. Fine specificity of the gag-specific response defined by using unstimulated peripheral blood mononuclear cells and cloned effector cells. *J. Immunol.* **147**, 1512–21.

Johnson, P.R., Montefiori, D.C., Chou, J. *et al.* (1992) Inactivated whole-virus vaccine derived from a proviral DNA clone of SIV confers protection against homologous and heterologous challenge. *Vaccines 92*, Cold Spring Harbor Laboratory, New York, (in press).

Joly, P., Guillon, J.M., Mayaud, C. *et al.* (1989). Cell-mediated suppression of HIV-specific cytotoxic T lymphocytes. *J. Immunol.* **143**, 2193–201.

Jouault, T., Chapuis, F., Olivier, R., Parravicini, C., Bahraoui, E. and Gluckman, J.C. (1989). HIV infection of monocytic cells: role of antibody-mediated virus binding to Fc-gamma receptors. *AIDS* **3**, 125–33.

Kahn, J.O., Allan, D.A., Hodges, T.L. *et al.* (1990). The safety and pharmacokinetics of recombinant soluble CD4 (rCD4) in subjects with the acquired immunodeficiency syndrome (AIDS) and AIDS-related complex. A phase 1 study. *Ann. Int. Med.* **112**, 254–61.

Kalbic, T., Kinter, A., Poli, G., Anderson, M.E., Meister, A. and Fauci, A.S. (1991). Suppression of human immunodeficiency virus expression in chronically infected monocytic cells by glutathione, glutathione ester, and N-acetylcysteine. *Proc. Nat. Acad. Sci. (USA)* **88**, 986–90.

Kalyanaraman, V.S., Rausch, D.M., Osborne, J. *et al.* (1990). Evidence by peptide mapping that the region CD4 (81–92) is involved in gp120/CD4 interaction leading to HIV infection and HIV-induced syncytium formation. *J. Immunol.* **145**, 4072–8.

Kang, C.Y., Nara, P., Chamat, S. *et al.* (1991). Evidence for non-V3-specific neutralizing antibodies that interfere with gp120/CD4 binding in human immunodeficiency virus 1-infected humans. *Proc. Nat. Acad. Sci. (USA)*. **88**, 6171–5.

Karpas, A., Hewlett, I.K., Hill, F. *et al.* (1990). Polymerase chain reaction evidence for human immunodeficiency virus 1 neutralization by passive immunization in patients with AIDS and AIDS-related complex. *Proc. Nat. Acad. Sci. (USA)* **87**, 7613–17.

Karpas, A., Hill, F., Youle, M. *et al.* (1988). Effects of passive immunization in patients with the acquired immunodeficiency syndrome-related complex and acquired immunodeficiency syndrome. *Proc. Nat. Acad. Sci. (USA)* **85**, 9234–7.

Karpatkin, S., Nardi, M., Lennette, E.T., Byrne, B. and Poiesz, B. (1988). Anti-human immunodeficiency virus type I antibody complexes on platelets of seropositive thrombocytopenic homosexuals and narcotic addicts. *Proc. Nat. Acad. Sci. (USA)* **85**, 9763–7.

Kaslow, R.A., Duquesnoy, R., VanRaden, M. *et al.* (1990). A1, Cw7, B8, DR3 HLA antigen combination associated with rapid decline of T-helper lymphocytes in HIV-1 infection. A report from the multicenter AIDS Cohort Study. Comment in *Lancet* **335**, 1591–2.

Kestler, H.W., III, Ringler, D.J., Mori, K. *et al.* (1991). Importance of the *nef* gene for maintenance of high virus loads and for development of AIDS. *Cell* **65**, 651–62.

Khalife, J., Guy, B., Capron, M. *et al.* (1988). Isotypic restriction of the antibody response to human immunodeficiency virus. *AIDS Res. Hum. Retroviruses* **4**, 3–9.

Kion, T.A. and Hoffmann, G.W. (1991). Anti-HIV and anti-anti MHC antibodies in alloimmune and autoimmune mice. *Science* **253**, 1138–40.

Klasse, P.J., Pipkorn, R. and Blomberg, J. (1988). Presence of antibodies to a putatively immunosuppressive part of human immunodeficiency virus (HIV) envelope glycoprotein gp41 is strongly associated with health among HIV-positive subjects. *Proc. Nat. Acad. Sci. (USA)* **85**, 5225–9.

Klatzmann, D. and Montagnier, L. (1986). Approaches to AIDS therapy. *Nature* **319**, 10–11.

Klatzmann, D., Champagne, E., Chamaret, S. *et al.* (1984). T-lymphocyte T4 molecule behaves as the receptor for human retrovirus LAV. *Nature* **312**, 767–8.

Koenig, S., Gendelmann, H.E., Orenstein, J.M. *et al.* (1986). Detection of AIDS virus in macrophages in brain tissue from AIDS patients with encephalopathy. *Science* **233**, 1089–93.

Koenig, S., Earl, P., Powell, D. *et al.* (1988). Group-specific, major histocompatibility complex class I-restricted cytotoxic responses to human immunodeficiency virus 1 (HIV-1) envelope proteins by cloned peripheral blood T cells from an HIV-1-infected individual. *Proc. Nat. Acad. Sci. (USA)* **85**, 8638–42.

Koenig, S., Fuerst, T.R., Wood, L.V. *et al.* (1990). Mapping the fine specificity of a cytolytic T-cell response to HIV-1 Nef protein. *J. Immunol.* **145**, 127–35.

Koff, W.C. and Schultz, A.M. (1990). AIDS vaccines 1990: a brief update. *AIDS* **4** (suppl. 1), S179–S184.

Kopelman, R.G. and Zolla-Pazner, S. (1988). Association of human immunodeficiency virus infection and autoimmune phenomena. *Am. J. Med.* **84**, 82–8.

Kowalski, M., Potz, J., Basiripour, L. *et al.* (1987). Functional regions of the envelope glycoprotein of human immunodeficiency virus type 1. *Science* **237**, 1351–5.

Kowalski, M., Ardman, B., Basiripour, L. *et al.* (1989). Antibodies to CD4 in individuals infected with human immunodeficiency virus type 1. *Proc. Nat. Acad. Sci. (USA)* **86**, 3346–50.

Krämer, A., Wiktor, S.Z., Fuchs, D. *et al.* (1989). Neopterin: a predictive marker of acquired immune deficiency syndrome in human immunodeficiency virus infection. *J. Acquired Immune Deficiency Syndr.* **2**, 291–6.

Krowka, J.F., Stites, D.P., Jain, S. *et al.* (1989). Lymphocyte proliferative responses to human immunodeficiency virus antigens *in vitro*. *J. Clin. Invest.* **83**, 1198–203.

Lahdevirta, J., Maury, C.P., Teppo, A.M. and Repo, H. (1988). Elevated levels of circulating cachectin/tumor necrosis factor in patients with acquired immunodeficiency syndrome. *Am. J. Med.* **85**, 289–91.

Lamarre, D., Ashkenazi, A., Fleury, S., Smith, D.H., Sekaly, R.P. and Capon, D.J. (1989a). The MHC-binding and gp120-binding functions of CD4 are separable. *Science* **245**, 743–6.

Lamarre, D., Capon, D.J., Karp, D.R., Gregory, T., Long, E.O. and Sekaly, R.P. (1989b). Class II MHC molecules and the HIV gp120 envelope protein interact with functionally distinct regions of the CD4 molecule. *EMBO J.* **8**, 3271–7.

Lane, H.C., Masur, H., Edgar, L.C., Whalen, G., Rook, A.H. and Fauci, A.S. (1983). Abnormalities of B-cell activation and immunoregulation in patients with the acquired immunodeficiency syndrome. *N. Engl. J. Med.* **309**, 453–8.

Lane, H.C., Masur, H., Gelman, E.P. *et al.* (1985a). Correlation between immunologic function and clinical subpopulations of patients with the acquired immune deficiency syndrome. *Am. J. Med.* **78**, 417–22.

Lane, H.C., Depper, J.M., Greene, W.C., Whalen, G., Waldmann, T.A. and Fauci, A.S. (1985b). Qualitative analysis of immune function in patients with the acquired immunodeficiency syndrome. Evidence for a selective defect in soluble antigen recognition. *N. Engl. J. Med.* **313**, 79–84.

Langhoff, E., McElrath, J., Bos, H.J. *et al.* (1989). Most $CD4^+$ T cells from human immunodeficiency virus-1 infected patients can undergo prolonged clonal expansion. *J. Clin. Invest.* **84**, 1637–43.

Langhoff, E., Terwilliger, E.F., Bost, H.J. *et al.* (1991). Replication of human immunodeficiency virus type 1 in primary dendritic cell cultures. *Proc. Nat. Acad. Sci. (USA)* **88**, 7998–8002.

Langlade-Demoyen, P., Michel, F., Hoffenbach, A. *et al.* (1988). Immune recognition of AIDS virus antigens by human and murine cytotoxic T lymphocytes. *J. Immunol.* **141**, 1949–57.

Lanzavecchia, A., Roosneck, E., Gregory, T., Berman, P. and Abrignani, S. (1988). T cells can present antigens such as HIV gp120 targeted to their own surface molecules. *Nature* **334**, 530–2.

LaRosa, G.J., Davide, J.P., Weinhold, K. *et al.* (1990). Conserved sequence and structural elements in the HIV-1 principal neutralizing determinant. *Science* **249**, 932–5.

Lasky, L.A., Nakamura, G., Smith, D.H. *et al.* (1987). Delineation of a region of the human immunodeficiency virus type 1 gp120 glycoprotein critical for interaction with the CD4 receptor. *Cell* **50**, 975–85.

Laure, F., Courgnaud, V., Rouzioux, C. *et al.* (1988). Detection of HIV1 DNA in infants and children by means of the polymerase chain reaction. *Lancet* **ii**, 538–41.

Laurence, J., Saunders, A. and Kulkosky, J. (1987). Characterization and clinical association of antibody inhibitory to HIV reverse transcriptase activity. *Science* **235**, 1501–4.

Laurence, J., Friedman, S.M., Chartash, E.K., Crow, M.K. and Posnett, D.N. (1989). Human immunodeficiency virus infection of helper T cell clones. Early proliferative defects despite intact antigen-specific recognition and interleukin 4 secretion. *J. Clin. Invest.* **83**, 1843–8.

Laurent-Crawford, A.G., Krust, B., Muller, S. *et al.* (1991). The cytopathic effect of HIV is associated with apoptosis. *Virology* **185**, 829–39.

Levine, A.M. (1991). Immunization of HIV-infected individuals with inactivated HIV immunogen. In *Quatrième Colloque des Cent Gardes: Retroviruses of Human AIDS and Related Animal Diseases*, ed. M. Girard and L. Valette, pp. 247–50.

Lifson, J.D., Reyes, G.R., McGrath, M.S., Stein, B.S. and Engleman, E.G. (1986). AIDS retrovirus induced cytopathology: giant cell formation and involvement of CD4 antigen. *Science* **232**, 1123–7.

Lifson, J.D., Rausch, D.M., Kalyanaraman, V.S., Hwang, K.M. and Eiden, L.E. (1991). Synthetic peptides allow discrimination of structural features of CD4 (81–92) important for HIV-1 infection virus HIV-1 induced syncytium formation. *AIDS Res. Hum. Retroviruses* **7**, 521–7.

Linette, G.P., Hartzman, R.J., Ledbetter, J.A. and June, C.H. (1988). HIV-1-infected T cells show a selective signaling defect after perturbation of CD3/antigen receptor. *Science* **241**, 573–6.

Liu, M.A. and Liu, T. (1988). Effect of recombinant soluble CD4 on human peripheral blood lymphocyte responses *in vitro*. *J. Clin. Invest.* **82**, 2176–80.

Ljunggren, K., Bottiger, B., Biberfeld, G., Karlson, A., Fenyo, E.M. and Jondal, M. (1987). Antibody-dependent cellular cytotoxicity-inducing antibodies against human immunodeficiency virus. Presence at different clinical stages. *J. Immunol.* **139**, 2263–7.

Ljunggren, K., Broliden, P.A., Morfeldt-Manson, L., Jondal, M. and Wahren, B. (1988). IgG subclass response to HIV in relation to antibody-dependent cellular cytotoxicity at different clinical stages. *Clin. Exp. Immunol.* **73**, 343–7.

Loche, M. and Mach, B. (1988). Identification of HIV-infected seronegative individuals by a direct diagnostic test based on hybridisation to amplified viral DNA. *Lancet* **ii**, 418–21.

Looney, D.J., Hayashi, S., Nicklas, M. *et al.* (1990). Differences in the interaction of HIV-1 and HIV-2 with CD4. *J. AIDS* **3**, 649–57.

Louache, F., Bettaieb, A., Henri, A. *et al.* (1991). Infection of megakaryocytes by human immunodeficiency virus in seropositive patients with immune thrombocytopenic purpura. *Blood* **78**, 1697–705.

Lui, K.J., Darrow, W.W. and Rutherford, G.W. (1988). A model-based estimate of the mean incubation period for AIDS in homosexual men. *Science* **240**, 1333–5.

Lusso, P., Markham, P.D., Ranki, A. *et al.* (1988). Cell-mediated immune response toward viral envelope and core antigens in gibbon apes (*Hylobates lar*) chronically infected with human immunodeficiency virus-1. *J. Immunol.* **141**, 2467–73.

Lusso, P., Ensoli, B., Markham, P.D. *et al.* (1989). Productive dual infection of human $CD4^+$ T lymphocytes by HIV-1 and HHV-6. *Nature* **337**, 370–3.

Lyerly, H.K., Matthews, T.J., Langlois, A.J., Bolognesi, D.P. and Weinhold, K.J. (1987a). Human T-cell lymphotropic virus IIIB glycoprotein (gp120) bound to CD4 determinants on normal lymphocytes and expressed by infected cells serves as target for immune attack. *Proc. Nat. Acad. Sci. (USA)* **84**, 4601–5.

Lyerly, H.K., Reed, D.L., Matthews, T.J. *et al.* (1987b). Anti-gp120 antibodies from HIV seropositive individuals mediate broadly reactive anti-HIV ADCC. *AIDS Res. Hum. Retroviruses* **3**, 409–22.

McChesney, M., Tanneau, F., Regnault, A. *et al.* (1990). Detection of primary cytotoxic T lymphocytes specific for the envelope glycoprotein of HIV-1 by deletion of the env-amino terminal signal sequence. *Eur. J. Immunol.* **20**, 215–20.

McDougal, J.S., Kennedy, M.S., Sligh, J.M., Cort, S.P., Mawle, A. and Nicholson, J.K.A. (1986a). Binding of HTLV III/LAV to T4+ T cells by a complex of the 110K viral protein and the T4 molecule. *Science* **231**, 382–5.

McDougal, J.S., Nicholson, J.K.A., Cross, G.D. *et al.* (1986b). Binding of the human retrovirus HTLV-III/LAV/ARV/HIV to the CD4 (T4) molecule: conformation dependence, epitope mapping, antibody inhibition and potential for idiotypic mimicry. *J. Immunol.* **137**, 2937–44.

McDougal, J.S., Kennedy, M.S., Nicholson, J.K.A. *et al.* (1987). Antibody response to human immunodeficiency virus in homosexual men. Relation of antibody specificity, titer and isotype to clinical status, severity of immunodeficiency and disease progression. *J. Clin. Invest.* **80**, 316–24.

McElrath, M.J., Pruett, J.E. and Cohn, Z.A. (1989). Mononuclear phagocytes of blood and bone marrow: comparative roles as viral reservoirs in human immunodeficiency virus type 1 infections. *Proc. Nat. Acad. Sci. (USA)* **86**, 675–9.

McElrath, M.J., Steinman, R.M. and Cohn, Z.A. (1991). Latent HIV-1 infection in enriched populations of blood monocytes and T cells from seropositive patients. *J. Clin. Invest.* **87**, 27–30.

McKeating, J.A. and Willey, R.L. (1989). Structure and function of the HIV envelope. *AIDS* **3** (suppl. 1), S35–S41.

McKeating, J.A., Griffiths, P.D. and Weiss, R.A. (1990). HIV susceptibility conferred to human fibroblasts by cytomegalovirus-induced Fc receptor. *Nature* **343**, 659–61.

Macatonia, S.E., Lau, R., Patterson, S., Pinching, A.J. and Knight, S.C. (1990). Dendritic cell infection, depletion and dysfunction in HIV-infected individuals. *Immunology* **71**, 38–45.

Machado, S.G., Gail, M.H. and Ellenberg, S.S. (1990). On the use of laboratory markers as surrogates for clinical endpoints in the evaluation of treatment for HIV infection. *J. Acquired Immune Deficiency Syndr.* **3**, 1065–73.

Mackewicz, C.E., Ortega, H.W. and Levy, J.A. (1991). CD8+ cell anti-HIV activity correlates with the clinical state of the infected individual. *J. Clin. Invest.* **87**, 1462–6.

Maddon, P.J., Dalgleish, A.G., McDougal, J.S., Clapham, P.R., Weiss, R.A. and Axel, R. (1986). The T4 gene encodes the AIDS virus receptor and is expressed in the immune system and the brain. *Cell* **47**, 333–48.

Maddon, P.J., McDougal, J.S., Clapham, P.R. *et al.* (1988). HIV infection does not require endocytosis of its receptor, CD4. *Cell* **54**, 865–74.

Malkovsky, M., Philpott, K., Dalgleish, A.G. *et al.* (1988). Infection of B lymphocytes by the human immunodeficiency virus and their susceptibility to cytotoxic cells. *Eur. J. Immunol.* **18**, 1315–21.

Mann, D.L., Gartner, S., Le Sane, F., Buchow, H. and Popovic, M. (1990). HIV-1 transmission and function of virus-infected monocytes/macrophages. *J. Immunol.* **144**, 2152–8.

Martinez, A.C., Marcos, M.A.R., De La Hera, A. *et al.* (1988). Immunological consequences of HIV infection: advantage of being low responder casts doubts on vaccine development. *Lancet* **i**, 454–7.

Massari, G.F., Poli, G., Schnittman, S.M., Psallidopoulos, M.C., Davey, V. and Fauci, A.S. (1990). *In vitro* T lymphocyte origin of macrophage-tropic strains of HIV. Role of monocytes during in vitro isolation and in vivo infection. *J. Immunol.* **144**, 4628–32.

Meyerhans, A., Cheynier, R., Albert, J. *et al.* (1989). Temporal fluctuations in HIV quasispecies *in vivo* are not reflected by sequential HIV isolations. *Cell* **58**, 901–10.

Michel, F., Hoffenbach, A., Langlade-Demoyen, P. *et al.* (1988). HIV-specific T-lymphocyte immunity in mice immunized with a recombinant vaccinia virus. *Eur. J. Immunol.* **18**, 1917–24.

Miedema, F. (1992). Immunological abnormalities in the natural history of HIV infection: mechanisms and clinical relevance. *Immunodef. Rev.* **3**, 173–93.

Miedema, F., Petit, A.J.C., Terpstra, F.G. *et al.* (1988). Immunological abnormalities in human immunodeficiency virus (HIV)-infected asymptomatic homosexual men: HIV affects the immune system before $CD4^+$ T helper cell depletion occurs. *J. Clin. Invest.* **82**, 1908–14.

Milich, D.R. (1988). T- and B-cell recognition of hepatitis B viral antigens. *Immunol. Today* **9**, 380–6.

Mills, K.H.G., Nixon, D.F. and McMichael, A.J. (1989). T-cell strategies in AIDS vaccines: MHC-restricted T-cell responses to HIV proteins. *AIDS* **3**, (suppl. 1), S101–S110.

Mills, K.H.G., Kitchin, P.A., Mahon, B.P. *et al.* (1990). HIV p24-specific helper T cell clones from immunized primates recognize highly conserved regions of HIV-1. *J. Immunol.* **144**, 1677–83.

Mittler, R.S. and Hoffmann, M.K. (1989). Synergism between HIV gp120 and gp120-specific antibody in blocking human T cell activation. *Science* **245**, 1380–2.

Mizukami, T., Fuerst, T.R., Berger, E.A. and Moss, B. (1988). Binding region for human immunodeficiency virus (HIV) and epitopes for HIV-blocking monoclonal antibodies of the CD4 molecule defined by site-directed mutagenesis. *Proc. Nat. Acad. Sci. (USA)* **85**, 9273–7.

Mizuma, H., Litwin, S. and Zolla-Pazner, S. (1988). B-cell activation in HIV infection: relationship of spontaneous immunoglobulin secretion to various immunological parameters. *Clin. Exp. Immunol.* **71**, 410–16.

Montagnier, L., Gruest, J., Chamaret, S. *et al.* (1984). Adaptation of lymphadenopathy associated virus (LAV) to replication in EBV-transformed B lymphoblastoid cell lines. *Science* **225**, 63–6.

Montefiori, D.C., Robinson, W.E., Jr., Hirsch, V.M., Modliszewski, A., Mitchell, W.M. and Johnson, P.R. (1990). Antibody-dependent enhancement of simian immunodeficiency virus (SIV) infection *in vitro* by plasma from SIV-infected rhesus macaques. *J. Virol.* **64**, 113–19.

Moore, J.P. (1990). Simple methods for monitoring HIV-1 and HIV-2 gp120 binding to soluble CD4 by enzyme-linked immunosorbant assay: HIV-2 has 25-fold lower affinity than HIV-1 for soluble CD4. *AIDS* **4**, 297–305.

Moore, J.P., McKeating, J.A., Weiss, R.A. and Sattentau, Q.J. (1990). Dissociation of gp120 from HIV-1 virions induced by soluble CD4. *Science* **250**, 1139–42.

Moore, J.P., McKeating, J.A., Norton, W.A. and Sattentau, Q.J. (1991). Direct measurement of soluble CD4 binding to human immunodeficiency virus type 1 virions: gp120 dissociation and its implications for virus-cell binding and fusion reactions and their neutralization by soluble CD4. *J. Virol.* **65**, 1133–40.

Moss, A.R., Bacchetti, P., Osmond, D. *et al.* (1988). Seropositivity for HIV and the development of AIDS or AIDS-related condition: three year follow up of the San Francisco General Hospital cohort. *Br. Med. J.* **296**, 745–50.

Murphey-Corb, M., Martin, L.N., Davison-Fairburn, B. *et al.* (1989). A formalin-inactivated whole SIV vaccine confers protection in macaques. *Science* **246**, 1293–7.

Murphey-Corb, M., Montelaro, R.C., Miller, M.A. *et al.* (1991). Efficacy of SIV/DeltaB670 glycoprotein-enriched and glycoprotein-depleted subunit vaccines in protecting against infection and disease in rhesus monkeys. *AIDS* **5**, 655–62.

Murray, H.W., Rubin, B.Y., Masur, H. and Roberts, R.B. (1984). Impaired production of lymphokines and immune gamma interferon in the acquired immunodeficiency syndrome. *N. Engl. J. Med.* **310**, 883–9.

Murray, H.W., Scavuzzo, D.A., Kelly, C.D., Rubin, B.Y. and Roberts, R.B. (1988). T4+ cell production of interferon gamma and the clinical spectrum of patients at risk for and with acquired immunodeficiency syndrome. *Arch. Int. Med.* **148**, 1613–16.

Nair, M.P.N., Pottathil, R., Heimer, E.P. and Schwartz, S.A. (1988). Immuno-regulatory activities of human immunodeficiency virus (HIV) proteins: effect of HIV recombinant and synthetic peptides on immunoglobulin synthesis and proliferative responses by normal lymphocytes. *Proc. Nat. Acad. Sci. (USA)* **85**, 6498–502.

Nakajima, K., Martinez-Maza, O., Hirano, T. *et al.* (1989). Induction of IL-6 (B cell stimulatory factor-2/IFN-β2) production by HIV. *J. Immunol.* **142**, 531–6.

Namikawa, R., Kaneshima, H., Lieberman, M., Weissman, I.L. and McCune, J.M. (1988). Infection of the SCID-hu mouse by HIV-1. *Science* **242**, 1684–6.

Neurath, A.R., Strick, N., Taylor, P., Rubinstein, P. and Stevens, C.E. (1990). Search for epitope-specific antibody responses to the human immunodeficiency virus (HIV-1) envelope glycoproteins signifying resistance to disease development. *AIDS Res. Hum. Retroviruses* **6**, 1183–92.

Neurath, A.R., Strick, N., Fields, R. and Jiang, S. (1991). Peptides mimicking selected disulfide loops in HIV-1 gp120, other than V3, do not elicit virus-neutralizing antibodies. *AIDS Res. Hum. Retroviruses* **7**, 657–62.

Ng, V.L., Chen, K.H., Hwang, K.M., Khayam-Bashi, H. and McGrath, M.S. (1989). The clinical significance of human immunodeficiency virus type 1-associated paraproteins. *Blood* **74**, 2471–5.

Nicholson, J.K.A., Cross, G.D., Callaway, C.S. and McDougal, J.S. (1986). *In vitro* infection of human monocytes with human T lymphotropic virus type III/lymphadenopathy-associated virus (HTLV-III/LAV). *J. Immunol.* **137**, 323–9.

Nishanian, P., Hofmann, B., Wang, Y., Jackson, A.L., Detels, R. and Fahey, J.L. (1991). Serum soluble CD8 molecule is a marker of CD8 T-cell activation in HIV-1 disease. *AIDS* **5**, 805–12.

Nixon, D.F. and McMichael, A.J. (1991). Cytotoxic T-cell recognition of HIV proteins and peptides. *AIDS* **5**, 1049–59.

Nixon, D.F., Townsend, A.R.M., Elvin, J.G., Rizza, C.R., Gallwey, J. and McMichael, A.J. (1988). HIV-1 gag-specific cytotoxic T lymphocytes defined with recombinant vaccinia virus and synthetic peptides. *Nature* **336**, 484–7.

Nye, K.E. and Pinching, A.J. (1990). HIV infection of H9 lymphoblastoid cells chronically activates the inositol polyphosphate pathway. *AIDS* **4**, 41–5.

O'Brien, W.A., Koyanagi, Y., Namazie, A. *et al.* (1990). HIV-1 tropism for mononuclear phagocytes can be determined by regions of gp120 outside the CD4-binding domain. *Nature* **348**, 69–73.

Ohno, T., Terada, M., Yoneda, Y. *et al.* (1991). A broadly neutralizing monoclonal antibody that recognizes the V3 region of human immunodeficiency virus type 1 glycoprotein gp120. *Proc. Nat. Acad. Sci. (USA)* **88**, 10726–9.

Oksenhendler, E. and Seligmann, M. (1990). HIV-related thrombocytopenia. *Immunodeficiency Rev.* **2**, 221–31.

Oksenhendler, E., Bierling, P., Ferchal, F., Clauvel, J.P. and Seligmann, M. (1989). Zidovudine for thrombocytopenic purpura related to human immunodeficiency virus (HIV) infection. *Ann. Intern. Med.* **110**, 365–8.

Olshevsky, U., Helseth, E., Furman, C., Li, J., Haseltine, W. and Sodroski, J. (1990). Identification of individual human immunodeficiency virus type 1 gp120 amino acids important for CD4 receptor binding. *J. Virol.* **64**, 5701–7.

Orentas, R.J., Hildreth, J.E., Obah, E. *et al.* (1990). Induction of CD4+ human cytolytic T cells specific for HIV-infected cells by a gp160 subunit vaccine. *Science* **248**, 1234–7.

Osborn, L., Kunkel, S. and Nabel, G.J. (1989). Tumor necrosis factor α and interleukin 1 stimulate the human immunodeficiency virus enhancer by activation of the nuclear factor κB. *Proc. Nat. Acad. Sci. (USA)* **86**, 2336–40.

Osmond, D.H., Shiboski, S., Bacchetti, P., Winger, E.E. and Moss, A.R. (1991). Immune activation markers and AIDS prognosis. *AIDS* **5**, 505–11.

Oyaizu, N., Chirmule, N., Kalyanaraman, V.S. *et al.* (1990). Human immunodeficiency virus type 1 envelope glycoprotein gp120 produces immune defects in $CD4^+$ T lymphocytes by inhibiting interleukin 2 mRNA. *Proc. Nat. Acad. Sci. (USA)* **87**, 2379–83.

Pahwa, S., Pahwa, R., Good, R.A. *et al.* (1986). Stimulatory and inhibitory influences of human immunodeficiency virus on normal B lymphocytes. *Proc. Nat. Acad. Sci. (USA)* **83**, 9124–8.

Palker, T.J., Clark, M.E., Langlois, A.J. *et al.* (1988). Type-specific neutralization of the human immunodeficiency virus with antibodies to *env*-encoded synthetic peptides. *Proc. Nat. Acad. Sci. (USA)* **85**, 1932–6.

Palker, T.J., Matthews, T.J., Langlois, A.J. *et al.* (1989). Polyvalent human immunodeficiency virus synthetic immunogen comprised of envelope gp120 T helper cell sites and B cell neutralization epitopes. *J. Immunol.* **142**, 3612–19.

Pan, L.Z., Shepard, H.W., Winkelstein, W. and Levy, J.A. (1991). Lack of detection of human immunodeficiency virus in persistently seronegative homosexual men with high or medium risks for infection. *J. Infect. Dis.* **164**, 962–4.

Pantaleo, G., Koenig, S., Baseler, M., Lane, H.C. and Fauci, A.S. (1990). Defective clonogenic potential of CD8+ T lymphocytes in patients with AIDS: expansion in vivo of a nonclonogenic CD3+ CD8+ CR+ CD25− T cell population. *J. Immunol.* **144**, 1696–704.

Pantaleo, G., Butini, L., Graziosi, C. *et al.* (1991). Human immunodeficiency virus (HIV) infection in CD4+ T lymphocytes genetically deficient in LFA-1: LFA-1 is required for HIV-mediated cell fusion but not for viral transmission. *J. Exp. Med.* **173**, 511–14.

Papadopoulos, N.M., Lane, H.C., Costello, R. *et al.* (1985). Oligoclonal immunoglobulins in patients with the acquired immunodeficiency syndrome. *Clin. Immunol. Immunopathol.* **35**, 43–6.

Papsidero, L.D., Sheu, M. and Ruscetti, F.W. (1989). Human immunodeficiency virus type 1-neutralizing monoclonal antibodies which react with p17 core protein: characterization and epitope mapping. *J. Virol.* **63**, 267–72.

Parekh, B.S., Schaffer, N., Pau, C.P. *et al.* (1991). Lack of correlation between maternal antibodies to V3 loop peptides of gp120 and perinatal HIV-1 transmission. *AIDS* **5**, 1179–84.

Parkin, J.M., Helbert, M., Hughes, C.L. and Pinching, A.J. (1989). Immunoglobulin G subclass deficiency and susceptibility to pyogenic infections in patients with AIDS-related complex and AIDS. *AIDS* **3**, 37–9.

Perno, C.F., Baseler, M.W., Broder, S. and Yarchoan, R. (1990). Infection of monocytes by human immunodeficiency virus type 1 blocked by inhibitors of CD4-gp120 binding, even in the presence of enhancing antibodies. *J. Exp. Med.* **171**, 1043–56.

Peterson, A. and Seed, B. (1988). Genetic analysis of monoclonal antibody and HIV binding sites on the human lymphocyte antigen CD4. *Cell* **54**, 65–72.

Phillips, A.N., Lee, C.A., Elford, J. *et al.* (1991). Serial CD4 lymphocyte counts and development of AIDS. *Lancet* **337**, 389–92.

Phillips, R.E., Rowland-Jones, S., Nixon, D.F. *et al.* (1991). Human immunodeficiency virus genetic variation that can escape cytotoxic T cell recognition. *Nature* **354**, 453–9.

Pinching, A.J. (1988). Factors affecting the natural history of human immunodeficiency virus infection. *Immunodeficiency Rev.* **1**, 23–38.

Pinching, A.J. (1991). Antibody responses in HIV infection. *Clin. Exp. Immunol.* **84**, 181–4.

Pinching, A.J. and Nye, K.E. (1990). Defective signal transduction – a common pathway for cellular dysfunction of HIV infection? *Immunol. Today* **11**, 256–9.

Plata, F., Autran, B., Martins, L.P. *et al.* (1987). AIDS virus-specific cytotoxic T lymphocytes in lung disorders. *Nature* **328**, 348–51.

Plata, F., Dadaglio, G., Chenciner, N. *et al.* (1989). Cytotoxic T lymphocytes in HIV-induced disease: implications for therapy and vaccination. *Immunodeficiency Rev.* **1**, 227–46.

Poli, G., Bottazzi, B., Acero, R. *et al.* (1985). Monocyte function in intravenous drug abusers with lymphadenopathy syndrome and in patients with acquired immunodeficiency syndrome: selective impairment of chemotaxis. *Clin. Exp. Immunol.* **62**, 136–42.

Poli, G., Orenstein, J.M., Kinter, A., Folks, T.M. and Fauci, A.S. (1989). Interferon-alpha but not AZT suppresses HIV expression in chronically infected cell lines. *Science* **244**, 575–7.

Poli, G., Bressler, P., Kinter, A. *et al.* (1990a). Interleukin-6 induces HIV expression in infected monocytic cells alone and in synergy with tumor necrosis factor alpha by transcriptional and post-transcriptional mechanisms. *J. Exp. Med.* **172**, 151–8.

Poli, G., Kinter, A., Justement, J.S. *et al.* (1990b). Tumor necrosis factor α functions in an autocrine manner in the induction of human immunodeficiency virus expression. *Proc. Nat. Acad. Sci. (USA)* **87**, 782–5.

Polk, B.F., Fox, R., Brookmeyer, R. *et al.* (1987). Predictors of the acquired immunodeficiency syndrome developing in a cohort of seropositive homosexual men. *N. Engl. J. Med.* **316**, 61–6.

Polsky, B., Gold, J.W.M., Whimbey, E. *et al.* (1986). Bacterial pneumonia in patients with the acquired immunodeficiency syndrome. *Ann. Intern. Med* **104**, 38–41.

Posner, M.R., Hideshima, T., Cannon, T., Mukherjee, M., Mayer, K.H. and Byrn, R.A. (1991). An IgG human monoclonal antibody that reacts with HIV-1 gp120, inhibits virus binding to cells, and neutralizes infection. *J. Immunol.* **146**, 4325–32.

Price, R.W., Brew, B., Sidtis, J., Rosenblum, M., Schleck, A.C. and Cleary, P. (1988). The brain in AIDS: central nervous system HIV-1 infection and AIDS dementia complex. *Science* **239**, 586–92.

Prince, A.M., Horowitz, B., Baker, L. *et al.* (1988). Failure of a human immunodeficiency virus (HIV) immune globulin to protect chimpanzees against experimental challenge with HIV. *Proc. Nat. Acad. Sci. (USA)* **85**, 6944–8.

Prince, A.M., Reesink, H., Pascual, D. *et al.* (1991). Prevention of HIV infection by passive immunization with HIV immunoglobulin. *AIDS Res. Hum. Retroviruses* **7**, 971–3.

Prince, H.E. and Jensen, E.R. (1991). HIV-related alterations in CD8 cell subsets defined by *in vitro* survival characteristics. *Cell. Immunol.* **134**, 276–86.

Pullian, L., Herndier, B.G., Tang, N.M. and McGrath, M.S. (1991). Human immunodeficiency virus-infected macrophages produce soluble factors that cause histological and neurochemical alterations in cultured human brains. *J. Clin. Invest.* **87**, 503–12.

Putkonen, P., Thorstensson, R., Ghavamzadeh, L. *et al.* (1991). Prevention of HIV-2 and SIVsm infection by passive immunization in cynomolgus monkeys. *Nature* **352**, 436–8.

Quinn, T.C., Piot, P., McCormick, J.B. *et al.* (1987). Serologic and immunologic studies in patients with AIDS in North America and Africa. The potential role of infectious agents as cofactors in human immunodeficiency virus infection. *JAMA* **257**, 2617–21.

Raffoux, C., David, V., Couderc, L.J. *et al.* (1987). HLA-A, B and DR antigen frequencies in patients with AIDS-related persistent generalized lymphadenopathy (PGL) and thrombocytopenia. *Tissue Antigens* **29**, 60–2.

Ranki, A., Valle, S.L., Krohn, M. *et al.* (1987a). Long latency precedes overt seroconversion in sexually transmitted human immunodeficiency-virus infection. *Lancet* **ii**, 589–93.

Ranki, A., Weiss, S.H., Valle, S.L. *et al.* (1987b). Neutralizing antibodies in HIV (HTLV-III) infection: correlation with clinical outcome and antibody response against different viral proteins. *Clin. Exp. Immunol.* **69**, 231–9.

Redfield, R.R., Birx, D.L., Ketter, N. *et al.* (1991). A phase I evaluation of the safety and immunogenicity of vaccination with recombinant gp160 in patients with early human immunodeficiency virus infection. *New Engl. J. Med.* **324**, 1733–5.

Reitz, M.S., Wilson, C., Naugle, C., Gallo, R.C. and Robert-Guroff, M. (1988). Generation of neutralization resistant variant of HIV1 is due to selection for a point mutation in the envelope gene. *Cell* **54**, 57–63.

Rich, E.A., Toossi, Z., Fujiwara, H., Hanigosky, R., Lederman, M.M. and Ellner, J.J. (1988). Defective accessory function of monocytes in human immunodeficiency virus-related disease syndromes. *J. Lab. Clin. Med.* **112**, 174–81.

Richardson, N.E., Brown, N.R., Hussey, R.E. *et al.* (1988). Binding site for human immunodeficiency virus coat protein gp120 is located in the NH_2-terminal region of T4 (CD4) and requires the intact variable-region-like domain. *Proc. Nat. Acad. Sci. (USA)* **85**, 6102–6.

Rieckmann, P., Poli, G., Kehrl, J.H. and Fauci, A.S. (1991). Activated B-lymphocytes from human immunodeficiency virus infected individuals induce virus expression in infected T cells and monocytes. *J. Exp. Med.* **173**, 1–5.

Rivière, Y., Tanneau-Salvadori, F., Regnault, A. *et al.* (1989a). Multiple cytotoxic effector cells are induced by infection with the human immunodeficiency virus. *Res. Immunol.* **140**, 110–15.

Rivière, Y., Tanneau-Salvadori, F., Regnault, A. *et al.* (1989b). HIV-specific cytotoxic responses of seropositive individuals: distinct types of effector cells mediate killing of targets expressing gag and env proteins. *J. Virol.* **63**, 2270–7.

Robert-Guroff, M., Brown, M. and Gallo, R.C. (1985). HTLV-III-neutralizing antibodies in patients with AIDS and AIDS-related complex. *Nature* **316**, 72–4.

Robert-Guroff, M., Reitz, M.S., Robey, W.G. and Gallo, R.C. (1986). *In vitro* generation of an HTLV-III variant by neutralizing antibody. *J. Immunol.* **137**, 3306–9.

Robert-Guroff, M., Goedert, J.J., Naugle, C.J., Jennings, A.M., Blattner, W.A. and Gallo, R.C. (1988). Spectrum of HIV-1 neutralizing antibodies in a cohort of homosexual men: results of a 6 year prospective study. *AIDS Res. Hum. Retroviruses* **4**, 343–50.

Robinson, W.E., Montefiori, D.C. and Mitchell, W.M. (1988). Antibody-dependent enhancement of human immunodeficiency virus type 1 infection. *Lancet* **i**, 790–4.

Robinson, W.E., Jr., Montefiori, D.C., Mitchell, W.M. *et al.* (1990a) Complement-mediated antibody-dependent enhancement of HIV-1 infection requires CD4 and complement receptors. *Virology* **175**, 600–4.

Robinson, W.E., Jr., Kawamura, T., Gorny, M.K. *et al.* (1990b). Human monoclonal antibodies to the human immunodeficiency virus type 1 (HIV-1) transmembrane glycoprotein gp41 enhance HIV-1 infection *in vitro*. *Proc. Nat. Acad. Sci. (USA)* **87**, 3185–9.

Robinson, W.E., Jr., Kawamura, T., Lake, D., Masuho, Y., Mitchell, W.M. and Hersh, E.M. (1990c). Antibodies to the primary immunodominant domain of human immunodeficiency virus type 1 (HIV-1) glycoprotein gp41 enhance HIV-1 infection *in vitro*. *J. Virol.* **64**, 5301–5.

Robinson, W.E., Jr., Gorny, M.K., Xu, J.Y., Mitchell, W.M. and Zolla-Pazner, S. (1991). Two immunodominant domains of gp41 bind antibodies which enhance human immunodeficiency virus type 1 infection *in vitro*. *J. Virol.* **65**, 4169–76.

Rook, A.H., Masur, H., Lane, H.C. *et al.* (1983). Interleukin-2 enhances the depressed natural killer and cytomegalovirus-specific cytotoxic activities of lymphocytes from patients with the acquired immune deficiency syndrome. *J. Clin. Invest.* **72**, 398–403.

Rook, A.H., Lane, H.C., Folks, T., McCoy, S., Alter, H. and Fauci, A.S. (1987). Sera from HTLV-III/LAV antibody-positive individuals mediate antibody-dependent cellular cytotoxicity against HTLV-III/LAV-infected T cells. *J. Immunol.* **138**, 1064–7.

Rosenberg, Z.F. and Fauci, A.S. (1990). HIV and the immune

system. Immunopathogenic mechanisms of HIV infection: cytokine induction of HIV expression. *Immunol. Today* **11**, 176–80.

Rossi, P., Moschese, V., Broliden, P.A. *et al.* (1989). Presence of maternal antibodies to human immunodeficiency virus 1 envelope glycoprotein gp120 epitopes correlates with the uninfected status of children born to seropositive mothers. *Proc. Nat. Acad. Sci. (USA)* **86**, 8055–8.

Roux-Lombard, P., Medoux, C., Cruchaud, A. and Dayer, J.M. (1989). Purified blood monocytes from HIV 1-infected patients produce high levels of TNFα and PL-1. *Clin. Immunol. Immunopathol.* **50**, 374–84.

Rusche, J.R., Javaherian, K., McDanal, C. *et al.* (1988). Antibodies that inhibit fusion of human immunodeficiency virus-infected cells bind a 24-aminoacid sequence of the viral envelope gp120. *Proc. Nat. Acad. Sci. (USA)* **85**, 3198–203.

Rutherford, G.W., Lifson, A.R., Hessol, N.A. *et al.* (1990). Course of HIV-1 infection in a cohort of homosexual and bisexual men: an 11 year follow up study. *Brit. Med. J.* **301**, 1183–8.

Ryu, S.E., Kwong, P.D., Truneh, A. *et al.* (1990). Crystal structure of an HIV-binding recombinant fragment of human CD4. *Nature* **348**, 419–26.

Saag, M.S., Hahn, B.H., Gibbons, J. *et al.* (1988). Extensive variation of human immunodeficiency virus type-1 *in vivo*. *Nature* **334**, 440–4.

Sadat-Sowti, B., Debré, P., Idziorek, T. *et al.* (1991). A lectin-binding soluble factor released by CD8+CD57+ lymphocytes from AIDS patients inhibits T cell cytotoxicity. *Eur. J. Immunol.* **21**, 737–41.

Salk, J. (1987). Prospects for the control of AIDS by immunizing seropositive individuals. *Nature* **327**, 473–6.

Salmon, P., Olivier, R., Rivière, Y. *et al.* (1988). Loss of CD4 membrane expression and CD4 mRNA during acute human immunodeficiency virus replication. *J. Exp. Med.* **168**, 1953–69.

Sattentau, Q.J., Dalgleish, A.G., Weiss, R.A. and Beverley, P.C. (1986). Epitopes of the CD4 antigen and HIV infection. *Science* **234**, 1120–3.

Sattentau, Q.J., Arthos, J., Deen, K. *et al.* (1989). Structural analysis of the human immunodeficiency virus-binding domain of CD4. Epitope mapping with site-directed mutants and anti-idiotypes. *J. Exp. Med.* **170**, 1319–34.

Scadden, D.T., Zon, L.I. and Groopman, J.E. (1989). Pathophysiology and management of HIV-associated hematologic disorders. *Blood* **74**, 1455–63.

Schechter, M.T., Neumann, P.W., Weaver, M.S. *et al.* (1991). Low HIV-1 proviral DNA burden detected by negative polymerase chain reaction in seropositive individuals correlates with slower disease progression. *AIDS* **5**, 373–9.

Schellekens, P.T., Roos, M.T., De Wolf, F., Lange, J.M. and Miedema, F. (1990). Low T-cell responsiveness to activation via CD3/TCR is a prognostic marker for AIDS in HIV-1 infected men. *J. Clin. Immunol.* **10**, 121–7.

Schnittman, S.M., Lane, H.C., Higgins, S.E., Folks, T. and Fauci, A.S. (1986). Direct polyclonal activation of human B lymphocytes by the acquired immune deficiency syndrome virus. *Science* **233**, 1084–6.

Schnittman, S.M., Lane, H.C., Greenhouse, J., Justement, J.S., Baseler, M. and Fauci, A.S. (1990). Preferential infection of CD4+ memory T cells by human immunodeficiency virus type 1: evidence for a role in the selective T-cell functional defects observed in infected individuals. *Proc. Nat. Acad. Sci. (USA)* **87**, 6058–62.

Schnittman, S.M., Psallidopoulos, M.C., Lane, H.C. *et al.* (1989). The reservoir for HIV 1 in human peripheral blood is a T cell that maintains expression of CD4. *Science* **245**, 305–8.

Schooley, R.T., Merigan, T.C., Gaut, P. *et al.* (1990). Recombinant soluble CD4 therapy in patients with the acquired immunodeficiency syndrome (AIDS) and AIDS-related complex. A phase I-II escalating dosage trial. *Ann. Int. Med.* **112**, 247–53.

Schols, D., Baba, M., Pauwels, R., Desmyter, J. and De Clercq, E. (1989). Specific interaction of aurintricarboxylic acid with the human immunodeficiency virus/CD4 cell receptor. *Proc. Nat. Acad. Sci. (USA)* **86**, 3322–6.

Schrier, R.D., Gnann, J.W., Langlois, A.J., Shriver, K., Nelson, J.A. and Oldstone, M.B. (1988). B- and T-lymphocyte responses to an immunodominant epitope of human immunodeficiency virus. *J. Virol.* **62**, 2531–6.

Schrier, R.D., Gnann, J.W., Landes, R. *et al.* (1989). T cell recognition of HIV synthetic peptides in a natural infection. *J. Immunol.* **142**, 1166–76.

Schwartz, S., Felber, B.K., Fenyö, E.M. and Pavlakis, G.N. (1989). Rapidly and slowly replicating human immunodeficiency virus type 1 isolates can be distinguished according to target-cell tropism in T-cell and monocyte cell lines. *Proc. Nat. Acad. Sci. (USA)* **86**, 7200–3.

Scott, G.B., Hutto, C., Makuch, R.W. *et al.* (1989). Survival in children with perinatally acquired human immunodeficiency virus type 1 infection. *N. Engl. J. Med.* **321**, 1791–6.

Seligmann, M., Pinching, A.J., Rosen, F.S. *et al.* (1987). Immunology of human immunodeficiency virus infection and the acquired immunodeficiency syndrome: an update. *Ann. Intern. Med.* **107**, 234–42.

Serigawa, I., Chamow, S.M., Groopman, J.E. and Byrn, R.A. (1990). CD4 immunoadhesin, but not recombinant soluble CD4, blocks syncytium formation by human immunodeficiency virus type 2-infected lymphoid cells. *J. Virol.* **64**, 5194–8.

Sethi, K.K., Näher, H. and Stroehmann, I. (1988). Phenotypic heterogeneity of cerebrospinal fluid-derived HIV-specific and HLA-restricted cytotoxic T-cell clones. *Nature* **335**, 178–81.

Shafferman, A., Jahrling, P.B., Benveniste, R.E. *et al.* (1991). Protection of macaques with a simian immunodeficiency virus envelope peptide vaccine based on conserved human immunodeficiency virus type 1 sequences. *Proc. Nat. Acad. Sci. (USA)* **88**, 7126–30.

Shalaby, M.R., Krowka, J.F., Gregory, T.J. *et al.* (1987). The effects of HIV recombinant envelope glycoprotein on immune cell functions *in vitro*. *Cell. Immunol.* **110**, 140–8.

Shaw, G.M., Hahn, B.H., Arya, S.K., Groopman, J.E., Gallo, R.C. and Wong-Staal, F. (1984). Molecular characterization of human T-cell leukemia (lymphotropic) virus type III in the acquired immune deficiency syndrome. *Science* **226**, 1165–71.

Shearer, G.M., Payne, S.M., Joseph, L.J. and Biddison, W.E. (1984). Functional T lymphocyte immune deficiency in a population of homosexual men who do not exhibit symptoms of acquired immune deficiency syndrome. *J. Clin. Invest.* **74**, 496–506.

Shen, L., Chen, Z.W., Miller, M.D. *et al.* (1991). Induction of simian immunodeficiency virus-specific CD8+ cytotoxic T lymphocytes following vaccination with a recombinant virus vaccine. *Science* **252**, 440–3.

Siekevitz, M., Josephs, S.F., Dukovich, M., Peffer, N., Wong-Taal, F. and Greene, W.C. (1987). Activation of the HIV-1 LTR by T cell mitogens and the trans-activator protein of HTLV-I. *Science* **238**, 1575–8.

Siliciano, R.F., Lawton, T., Knall, C. *et al.* (1988). Analysis of host–virus interactions in AIDS with anti-gp120 T cell clones: effect of HIV sequence variation and a mechanism for CD4+ cell depletion. *Cell* **54**, 561–75.

Skinner, M.A., Ting, R., Langlois, A.J. *et al.* (1988). Characteristics of a neutralizing monoclonal antibody to the HIV envelope glycoprotein. *AIDS Res. Hum. Retroviruses* **4**, 187–97.

Smith, D.H., Byrn, R.A., Marsters, S.A., Gregory, T., Groopman, J.E. and Capon, D.J. (1987). Blocking of HIV-1 infectivity by a soluble, secreted form of the CD4 antigen. *Science* **238**, 1704–7.

Smith, P.D., Ohura, K., Masur, H., Lane, H.C., Fauci, A.S. and Wahl, S.M. (1984). Monocyte function in the acquired immune deficiency syndrome. Defective chemotaxis. *J. Clin. Invest.* **74**, 2121–8.

Sodroski, J., Goh, W.C., Rosen, C., Campbell, K. and Haseltine, W.A. (1986). Role of the HTLV-III/LAV envelope in syncytium formation and cytopathicity. *Nature* **322**, 470–4.

Sonigo, P., Montagnier, L., Tiollais, P. and Girard, M. (1989). AIDS vaccines: concepts and first trials. *Immunodeficiency Rev.* **1**, 349–66.

Steel, C.M., Ludlam, C.A., Beatson, D. *et al.* (1988). HLA haplotype A1 B8 DR3 as a risk factor for HIV-related disease. *Lancet* **i**, 1185–8.

Steimer, K.S., Scandella, C.J., Skiles, P.V. and Haigwood, N.L. (1991). Neutralization of divergent HIV-1 isolates by conformation-dependent human antibodies to gp120. *Science* **254**, 105–8.

Stein, B.S., Gowda, S.O., Lifson, J.D., Penhallow, R.C., Bensch, K.G. and Engleman, E.G. (1987). pH-independent HIV entry into CD4-positive T cells via virus envelope fusion to the plasma membrane. *Cell* **49**, 659–68.

Stevenson, M., Stanwick, T.L., Dempsey, M.P. and Lamonica, C.A. (1990). HIV-1 replication is controlled at the level of T cell activation and proviral integration. *EMBO J.* **9**, 1551–60.

Stimmler, M.M., Quismorio, F.P. Jr., McGehee, W.G., Boylen, T. and Sharma, O.P. (1989). Anticardiolipin antibodies in acquired immunodeficiency syndrome. *Arch. Intern. Med.* **149**, 1833–5.

Stites, D.P., Moss, A.R., Bacchetti, P. *et al.* (1989). Lymphocyte subset analysis to predict progression to AIDS in a cohort of homosexual men in San Francisco. *Clin. Immunol. Immunopathol.* **52**, 96–103.

Stoot, E.J. (1991). Anti-cell antibody in macaques. *Nature* **353**, 393 (letter).

Stoot, E.J., Chan, W.L., Mills, K.H. *et al.* (1990). Protection of cynomolgus macaques against simian immunodeficiency virus by fixed infected-cell vaccine. *Lancet* **336**, 1538–41.

Sun, N.C., Ho, D.D., Sun, C.R. *et al.* (1989) Generation and characterization of monoclonal antibodies to the putative CD4-binding domain of human immunodeficiency virus type 1 gp120. *J. Virol.* **63**, 3579–85.

Syu, W., Jr., Huang, J.H., Essex, M. and Lee, T.H. (1990). The N-terminal region of the human immunodeficiency virus envelope glycoprotein gp120 contains potential binding sites for CD4. *Proc. Nat. Acad. Sci. (USA)* **87**, 3695–9.

Swiss Group for Clinical Studies on the Acquired Immunodeficiency Syndrome (AIDS) (1988). Zidovudine for the treatment of thrombocytopenia associated with human immunodeficiency virus (HIV). A prospective study. *Ann. Intern. Med.* **109**, 718–21.

Tagliabue, A., Nencioni, L., Mantovani, A. *et al.* (1988). Impairment of *in vitro* natural antibacterial activity in HIV-infected patients. *J. Immunol.* **141**, 2607–11.

Takahashi, H., Cohen, J., Hosmalin, A. *et al.* (1988). An immunodominant epitope of the human immunodeficiency virus envelope glycoprotein gp160 recognized by class I major histocompatibility complex molecule-restricted murine cytotoxic T lymphocytes. *Proc. Nat. Acad. Sci. (USA)* **85**, 3105–9.

Takahashi, H., Houghten, R., Putney, S.D. *et al.* (1989a). Structural requirements for class-I MHC molecule-mediated antigen presentation and cytotoxic T-cell recognition of an immunodominant determinant of the HIV envelope protein. *J. Exp. Med.* **170**, 2023–35.

Takahashi, H., Merli, S., Putney, S.D. *et al.* (1989b). A single amino acid interchange yields reciprocal CTL specificities for HIV gp160. *Science* **246**, 118–21.

Takahashi, H., Takeshita, T., Morein, B., Putney, S., Germain, R.N. and Berzofsky, J.A. (1990). Induction of CD8+ cytotoxic T cells by immunization with purified HIV-1 envelope protein in ISCOMs. *Nature* **344**, 873–5.

Takeda, A., Tuazon, C.U. and Ennis, F.A. (1988). Antibody-enhanced infection by HIV-1 via Fc receptor-mediated entry. *Science* **242**, 580–3.

Tateno, M., Gonzalez-Scarano, F. and Levy, J.A. (1989). Human immunodeficiency virus can infect CD4-negative human fibroblastoid cells. *Proc. Nat. Acad. Sci. (USA)* **86**, 4287–90.

Teeuwsen, V.J.P., Logtenberg, T., Siebelink, K.H.J. *et al.* (1987). Analysis of the antigen- and mitogen-induced differentiation of B lymphocytes from asymptomatic human immunodeficiency virus-seropositive male homosexuals. *J. Immunol.* **139**, 2929–35.

Tenner-Racz, K., Racz, P., Bofill, M. *et al.* (1986). HTLV III/LAV viral antigens in lymph nodes of homosexual men with persistent generalized lymphadenopathy and AIDS. *Am. J. Pathol.* **123**, 9–15.

Terai, C., Kornbluth, R.S., Pauza, C.D., Richman, D.D. and Carson, D.A. (1991). Apoptosis as a mechanism of cell death in cultured T lymphoblasts acutely infected with HIV-1. *J. Clin. Invest.* **87**, 1710–15.

Terpstra, F.G., Al, B.J.M., Roos, M.T.L. *et al.* (1989). Longitudinal study of leukocyte functions in homosexual men seroconverted for HIV: rapid and persistent loss of B cell function after HIV infection. *Eur. J. Immunol.* **19**, 667–73.

Tersmette, M. and Miedema, F. (1990). Interactions between HIV and the host immune system in the pathogenesis of AIDS. *AIDS* **4** (suppl. 1), S57–S66.

Tersmette, M., Lange, J.M.A., De Goede, R. *et al.* (1989). Association between biological properties of human immunodeficiency virus variants and risk for AIDS and AIDS mortality. *Lancet* **i**, 983–5.

The National Institute of Child Health and Human Development Intravenous Immunoglobulin Study Group. (1991).

Intravenous immune globulin for the prevention of bacterial infections in children with symptomatic human immunodeficiency virus infection. *N. Engl. J. Med.* **325**, 73–80.

Thiriart, C., Goudsmit, J., Schellenkens, P. *et al.* (1988). Antibodies to soluble CD4 in HIV-1 infected individuals. *AIDS* **2**, 345–51.

Thomas, E.K., Weber, J.N., McLure, J. *et al.* (1988). Neutralizing monoclonal antibodies to the AIDS virus. *AIDS* **2**, 25–9.

Till, M.A., Ghetie, V., Gregory, T. *et al.* (1988). HIV-infected cells are killed by rCD4-ricin A chain. *Science* **242**, 1166–8.

Toth, F.D., Szabo, B., Ujhelyi, E. *et al.* (1991). Neutralizing and complement-dependent enhancing antibodies in different stages of HIV infection. *AIDS* **5**, 263–8.

Traunecker, A., Lüke, W. and Karjalainen, K. (1988). Soluble CD4 molecules neutralize human immunodeficiency virus type 1. *Nature* **331**, 84–6.

Traunecker, A., Schneider, J., Kiefer, H. and Karjalainen, K. (1989). Highly efficient neutralization of HIV with recombinant CD4–immunoglobulin molecules. *Nature* **339**, 68–70.

Truneh, A., Buck, D., Cassatt, D.R. *et al.* (1991). A region in domain 1 of CD4 distinct from the primary gp120 binding site is involved in HIV infection and virus-mediated fusion. *J. Biol. Chem.* **266**, 5942–8.

Tschachler, E., Groh, V., Popovic, M. *et al.* (1987). Epidermal Langerhans cells — a target for HTLV-III/LAV infection. *J. Invest. Dermatol.* **88**, 233–7.

Tsubota, H., Ringler, D.J., Kannagi, M. *et al.* (1989a). $CD8^+$ $CD4^-$ lymphocyte lines can harbor the AIDS virus *in vitro*. *J. Immunol.* **143**, 858–63.

Tsubota, H., Lord, C.I., Watkins, D.I. *et al.* (1989b). A cytotoxic T lymphocyte inhibits acquired immunodeficiency syndrome virus replication in peripheral blood lymphocytes. *J. Exp. Med.* **169**, 1421–34.

Tsubota, H., Winkler, G., Meade, H.M., Jakubowski, A., Thomas, D.W. and Letvin, N.L. (1990). CD4-Pseudomonas exotoxin conjugates delay but do not fully inhibit human immunodeficiency virus replication in lymphocytes *in vitro*. *J. Clin. Invest.* **86**, 1684–9.

Tyler, D.S., Nastala, C.L., Stanley, S.D. *et al.* (1989a). GP120 specific cellular cytotoxicity in HIV-1 seropositive individuals: evidence for circulating CD16+ effector cells armed *in vivo* with cytophilic antibody. *J. Immunol.* **142**, 1177–82.

Tyler, D.S., Lyerly, H.K. and Weinhold, K.J. (1989b). Anti-HIV-1 ADCC. *AIDS Res. Hum. Retroviruses* **5**, 557–63.

Tyler, D.S., Stanley, S.D., Nastala, C.A. *et al.* (1990). Alterations in antibody-dependent cellular cytotoxicity during the course of HIV-1 infection: humoral and cellular defects. *J. Immunol.* **144**, 3375–84.

Vahlne, A., Horal, P., Eriksson, K. *et al.* (1991). Immunizations of monkeys with synthetic peptides disclose conserved areas on gp120 of human immunodeficiency virus type 1 associated with cross-neutralizing antibodies and T-cell recognition. *Proc. Nat. Acad. Sci. (USA)* **88**, 10744–8.

Valentine, F.T. and Jacobson, M.A. (1990). Immunological and virological surrogate markers in the evaluation of therapies for HIV infection. *AIDS* **4** (suppl. 1), S201–S207.

van Noesel, C.J.M., Gruters, R.A., Terpstra, F.G., Schellekens, P.Th., van Lier, R.A.W. and Miedema, F. (1990). Functional and phenotypic evidence for a selective loss of memory T cells in asymptomatic human immunodeficiency virus-infected men. *J. Clin. Invest.* **86**, 293–9.

Van der Lelie, J., Lange, J.M., Vos, J.J.E., Van Dalen, C.M., Danner, S.A. and von dem Borne, A.E. (1987). Autoimmunity against blood cells in human immunodeficiency-virus (HIV) infection. *Br. J. Haematol.* **67**, 109–14.

Vazeux, R.M., Brouss, N., Jarry, A. *et al.* (1987). AIDS subacute encephalitis: identification of HIV-infected cells. *Am. J. Pathol.* **126**, 403–10.

Via, C.S., Morse, H.C. III and Shearer, G.M. (1990). HIV and the immune system. Altered immunoregulation and autoimmune aspects of HIV infection: relevant murine models. *Immunol. Today* **11**, 250–5.

Wahl, S.M., Allen, J.B., Gartner, S. *et al.* (1989). HIV-1 and its envelope glycoprotein down-regulate chemotactic ligand receptors and chemotactic function of peripheral blood monocytes. *J. Immunol.* **142**, 3553–9.

Wahren, B., Rosen, J., Sandström, E., Mathiesen, T., Modrow, S. and Wigzell, H. (1989). HIV-1 peptides induce a proliferative response in lymphocytes from infected persons. *J. Acquired Immune Deficiency Synd.* **2**, 1166–76.

Walker, B.D., Chakrabarti, S., Moss, B. *et al.* (1987). HIV-specific cytotoxic T lymphocytes in seropositive individuals. *Nature* **328**, 345–8.

Walker, B.D., Flexner, C., Paradis, T.J. *et al.* (1988). HIV-1 reverse transcriptase is a target for cytotoxic T lymphocytes in infected individuals. *Science* **240**, 64–6.

Walker, B.D., Flexner, C., Birch-Limberger, K. *et al.* (1989). Long-term culture and fine specificity of human cytotoxic T-lymphocyte clones reactive with human immunodeficiency virus type 1. *Proc. Nat. Acad. Sci. (USA)* **86**, 9514–18.

Walker, C.M. (1989). How do CD8+ T lymphocytes control HIV replication *in vivo* ? *Res. Immunol.* **140**, 115–18.

Walker, C.M., Steimer, K.S., Rosenthal, K.L. and Levy, J.A. (1988). Identification of human immunodeficiency virus (HIV) envelope type-specific T helper cells in an HIV-infected individual. *J. Clin. Invest.* **82**, 2172–5.

Walsh, C.M., Nardi, M.A. and Karpatkin, S. (1984). On the mechanism of thrombocytopenic purpura in sexually active homosexual men. *N. Engl. J. Med.* **311**, 635–9.

Ward, R.H., Capon, D.J., Jett, C.M. *et al.* (1991). Prevention of HIV-1 IIIB infection in chimpanzees by CD4 immunoadhesin. *Nature* **352**, 434–6.

Watanabe, M., Reimann, K.A., DeLong, P.A., Liu, T., Fisher, R.A. and Letvin, N.L. (1989). Effect of recombinant soluble CD4 in rhesus monkeys infected with simian immunodeficiency virus of macaques. *Nature* **337**, 267–70.

Watanabe, M., Chen, Z.W., Tsubota, H., Lord, C.I., Levine, C.G. and Letvin, N.L. (1991). Soluble human CD4 elicits an antibody response in rhesus monkeys that inhibits simian immunodeficiency virus replication. *Proc. Nat. Acad. Sci. (USA)* **88**, 120–4.

Weber, J.N., Wadsworth, J., Rogers, L.A. *et al.* (1986). Three year prospective study of HTLV-III/LAV infection in homosexual men. *Lancet* **i**, 1179–82.

Weber, J.N., Clapham, P.R., Weiss, R.A. *et al.* (1987). Human immunodeficiency virus infection in two cohorts of homosexual men: neutralizing sera and association of anti-gag antibody with prognosis. *Lancet* **i**, 119–22.

Weinberg, J.B., Matthews, T.J., Cullen, B.R. and Malim, M.H. (1991). Productive human immunodeficiency virus type 1 (HIV-1) infection of nonproliferating human monocytes. *J. Exp. Med.* **174**, 1477–82.

Weinhold, K.J., Lyerly, H.K., Matthews, T.J. *et al.* (1988). Cellular anti-gp120 cytotoxic reactivities in HIV-1 seropositive individuals. *Lancet* **i**, 902–5.

Weinhold, K.J., Lyerly, H.K., Stanley, S.D., Austin, A.A., Matthews, T.J. and Bolognesi, D.P. (1989). HIV-1 gp120-mediated immune suppression and lymphocyte destruction in the absence of viral infection. *J. Immunol.* **142**, 3091–7.

Weiss, L., Haeffner-Cavaillon, N., Laude, M., Gilquin, J. and Kazatchkine, M.D. (1989). HIV infection is associated with the spontaneous production of interleukin-1 (IL-1) *in vivo* and with an abnormal release of IL-1α *in vitro*. *AIDS* **3**, 695–9.

Weiss, R.A., Clapham, P.R., Weber, J.N., Dalgleish, A.G., Lasky, L.A. and Berman, P.W. (1986). Variable and conserved neutralization antigens of human immunodeficiency virus. *Nature* **324**, 572–5.

Westervelt, P., Gendelman, H.E. and Ratner, L. (1991). Identification of a determinant within the human immunodeficiency virus 1 surface envelope glycoprotein critical for productive infection of primary monocytes. *Proc. Natl. Acad. Sci. (USA)* **88**, 3097–3101.

Wiley, C.A., Schrier, R.D., Nelson, J.A., Lampert, P.W. and Oldstone, M.B. (1986). Cellular localization of human immunodeficiency virus infection within the brains of AIDS patients. *Proc. Nat. Acad. Sci. (USA)* **83**, 7089–93.

Willey, R.L., Smith, D.H. and Lasky, L.A. (1988). *In vitro* mutagenesis identifies a region within the envelope gene of the human immunodeficiency virus that is critical for infectivity, *J. Virol.* **62**, 139–47.

Wolfs, T.F., De Jong, J.J., Van Den Berg, H., Tunagel, J.M., Krone, W.J. and Goudsmit, J. (1990). Evolution of sequences encoding the principal neutralization epitope of human immunodeficiency virus 1 is host dependent, rapid, and continuous. *Proc. Nat. Acad. Sci. (USA)* **87**, 9938–42.

Wolinsky, S.M., Rinaldo, C.R., Kwok, S. *et al.* (1989). Human immunodeficiency virus type 1 (HIV-1) infection a median of 18 months before a diagnostic western blot. Evidence from a cohort of homosexual men. *Ann. Intern. Med.* **111**, 961–72.

Yarchoan, R., Redfield, R.R. and Border, S. (1986). Mechanism of B cell activation in patients with acquired immunodeficiency syndrome and related disoders. *J. Clin. Invest.* **78**, 439–47.

Zack, J.A., Cann, A.J., Lugo, J.P. and Chen, I.S.Y. (1988). HIV-1 production from infected peripheral blood T cells after HTLV-I induced mitogenic stimulation. *Science* **240**, 1026–9.

Zack, J.A., Arrigo, S.J., Weitsman, S.R., Go, A.S., Haislip, A. and Chen, I.S.Y. (1990). HIV-1 entry into quiescent primary lymphocytes: molecular analysis reveals a labile, latent viral structure. *Cell* **61**, 213–22.

Zagury, D., Bernard, J., Cheynier, R. *et al.* (1988). A group specific anamnestic immune reaction against HIV induced by a candidate vaccine against AIDS. *Nature* **332**, 728–31.

Zeira, M., Byrn, R.A., Groopman, J.E. (1990). Inhibition of serum enhanced HIV-1 infection of U937 monocytoid cells by recombinant soluble CD4 and anti-CD4 monoclonal antibody. *AIDS Res. Hum. Retroviruses* **6**, 629–39.

Ziegler, J.L. and Stites, D.P. (1986). Hypothesis: AIDS is an autoimmune disease directed at the immune system and triggered by a lymphotropic retrovirus. *Clin. Immunol. Immunopathol.* **41**, 305–13.

Zinkernagel, R.M. (1988). Virus-triggered AIDS: a T-cell-mediated immunopathology? *Immunol. Today* **9**, 370–2.

Zucker-Franklin, D. and Cao, Y. (1989). Megakaryocytes of human immunodeficiency virus-infected individuals express viral RNA. *Proc. Nat. Acad. Sci. (USA)* **86**, 5595–9.

72: Clinical Aspects of Acquired Immune Deficiency Syndrome and Human Immunodeficiency Virus Infection

A.J. Pinching

Introduction

During the last decade, the pandemic of the acquired immune deficiency syndrome (AIDS) has revealed the diverse clinical consequences of a profound acquired cellular immunodeficiency. It has sharpened our concepts of the balance between host defence and microbial pathogenicity and of functional interactions within the immune system. The causative agent of AIDS, human immunodeficiency virus (HIV), has become a paradigm for viral immunopathogenesis and is the first human example of a cytopathic retrovirus.

This chapter will examine the clinical profile of HIV infection and of AIDS against the background of the characteristic biology of HIV, outlined in detail in previous chapters and summarized here. Because of the vast literature on AIDS, references have had to be selective and in many cases the reader is referred to recent reviews on specific areas, where more detailed referencing may be found.

The nature of the human immunodeficiency virus

The HIV envelope glycoprotein, gp120, has a binding site whereby it attaches to its target cell receptor, the CD4 molecule. This molecule determines the cellular tropism of HIV, in particular for CD4 lymphocytes and antigen-presenting cells of the macrophage lineage. Following binding, the membrane of HIV and that of the host cell fuse, leading to internalization. As a retrovirus, HIV has a ribonucleic acid (RNA) genome that is able to make a deoxyribonucleic acid (DNA) copy of itself, by virtue of its endogenous enzyme, reverse transcriptase. This DNA copy can then be spliced into the genome of infected host cells, thereby establishing latent or persistent infection. The net effects of the regulatory genes of HIV and the ability of activated host cell mediators to switch on HIV gene transcription seem to favour virus replication. The new virus particles can then infect more host cells, resulting in the pathogenic effects of HIV on the immune and nervous systems. Productive infection also enables HIV to pass from the infected host to others.

Transmission of the human immunodeficiency virus

Transmission routes for HIV infection have been established through extensive epidemiological and case studies (Des Jarlais and Friedman 1987; Friedland and Klein 1987; Curran *et al.* 1988; Johnson and Laga 1988; Piot *et al.* 1988, 1989). In essence, three routes apply: sexual, blood- or tissue-borne and maternofetal. Sexual transmission may occur through anal intercourse in homosexual men; HIV can pass from active to passive partner or vice versa. Heterosexual transmission may occur through vaginal or anal intercourse, passing either from male to female or from female to male. Spread through semen used in artificial insemination has been documented (Stewart *et al.* 1985).

Blood-borne infection has been documented through blood or blood product transfusion and notably though the sharing of equipment by injecting drug-users. Tissue transmission has occurred through organ or tissue transplantation. Infection through accidental inoculation injury or the contamination of broken skin or mucous membranes may also occur, though rarely (Centers for Disease Control 1989).

Maternofetal spread probably occurs predominantly through transplacental blood transfer, though additional spread may occur at parturition (Ryder and Hassig 1988). Breast-feeding has apparently led to HIV transmission where the mother had been infected postnatally, but its relevance where the mother was already infected during gestation has yet to be established. No other routes of transmission have been demonstrated.

An HIV-infected person can pass on infection at any stage of infection, though several recent studies have indicated that infectiousness is greater as disease supervenes and as disease markers appear, such as falling CD4 cell count in blood and rising HIV antigen in serum (Goedert *et al.* 1987b; Johnson and Laga 1988; Pinching 1988a). The latter in particular seems to serve as a surrogate marker for active virus replication, though it is probably relatively insensitive in this role. It is widely assumed that the rise in HIV antigen levels seen just before seroconversion may mark another peak of infectiousness (Anderson and Medley 1988). Other peaks may, in principle, be expected during intercurrent infection and may in part explain the association between sexually transmitted infections and sexual transmission of HIV. These factors influence inoculum size.

Factors in the recipient of HIV infection may influence infectibility, notably in sexual transmission. These include the possibility of genital trauma, though formal evidence of this as a major factor is limited, and genital infection or ulceration, for which there is evidence (Johnson and Laga 1988; Piot *et al.* 1989). Whether the latter acts by interrupting mucosal integrity, as has been widely assumed, or by increasing the number and accessibility of target cells for HIV infection is not known. Such factors could affect the inoculum threshold for infection.

Pathogenic aspects of the human immunodeficiency virus

The two major target cells for HIV, CD4 lymphocytes and antigen-presenting cells, are very differently affected by HIV infection (Ho *et al.* 1987; Daar and Ho 1989; Pinching 1990). CD4 cells are largely destroyed following infection, while macrophages and related cells are generally not, serving as important reservoirs of infection. The destruction of CD4 lymphocytes may result from a combination of several possible effects, including virus cytotoxicity and host-mediated effects. The human immunodeficiency virus may cause direct lysis or the formation of syncytia between both infected and uninfected cells. In addition, HIV-infected cells expressing HIV antigens may become targets for antibody-dependent or major histocompatibility complex (MHC)-restricted cytotoxic lymphocytes. Human immunodeficiency virus infection of antigen-presenting cells, although not typically leading to their destruction, may affect their function.

In addition to these effects, HIV may influence the function of cells that are not themselves infected. These effects may be consequential effects of the loss of critical cell types or their numbers, the loss of cytokine signals or the release of macrophage cell products, or they may be mediated by HIV products, such as the envelope glycoprotein, gp120. The latter has been shown to cause suppression of function in uninfected CD4 lymphocytes and to be a potent polyclonal activator of B cells. Some of these diverse functional effects may be due to a common defect in the inositol polyphosphate signal transduction pathway induced by HIV infection (Kornfeld *et al.* 1988; Nye and Pinching 1989; Pinching and Nye 1990).

In order to understand the clinical profile of disease caused by HIV, it is helpful to identify a number of key biological defects resulting from HIV infection. The loss of CD4 cells and their cytokine signals leads to failure of macrophage activation. This causes the susceptibility to infection by facultative intracellular pathogens and herpesviruses that is responsible for the opportunist infections characteristic of AIDS and AIDS-related complex (ARC) (Seligmann *et al.* 1987). Polyclonal B cell activation and the resulting dysglobulinaemia leads to susceptibility to infection by capsulated bacteria seen in some adults (Parkin *et al.* 1989) and most children (Wiznia and Rubinstein 1988) with symptomatic HIV infection. Both these defects may be compounded by defective antigen presentation. Natural killer cell production and function is impaired by the loss of their regulatory cytokines; these and related defects may account for the emergence of opportunist tumours such as Kaposi's sarcoma and lymphoma.

The pathogenesis of neurological disease due to HIV infection is more obscure (Ho *et al.* 1989; Pinching 1990). Human immunodeficiency virus encephalopathy may result from the functional or cytopathic effects mediated on neural cells by HIV proteins released from infected macrophages or microglia or from factors released by infected cells themselves. Effects of HIV on peripheral and autonomic nerves may be similarly mediated but there is little evidence on this. Direct infection of neural cells appears to be a rare event and is thus probably not responsible for most of the effects seen.

Natural history of the human immunodeficiency virus infection

Once HIV infection has been established, there follows a phase of symptomless infection. A substantial proportion of infected individuals go on to develop symptomatic disease — ARC, AIDS, HIV encephalopathy — in subsequent years (Goedert *et al.* 1986; Melbye *et al.* 1987a; Pinching 1988a). The ultimate attack rate cannot be known until infected individuals have been followed for many more years, but incubation periods have been calculated on the basis of studies so far (Medley *et al.* 1987, 1988; Anderson and Medley 1988; Lui *et al.* 1988). However, cohort studies of those infected early in the epidemic indicate that at 3 years 15–20% have developed AIDS, at 5 years 25–30% and at 10 years 50%. With further follow-up, more are likely to develop disease, since some of those remaining symptomless show markers suggestive of adverse prognosis. These estimates are based on minimum periods of infection and assume that the groups under long-term study are representative. An international study of seroconverters in whom the time of infection can be determined with some accuracy indicates a cumulative AIDS risk in adult homosexuals of 33% at 6 years with little variation by geographical area (Biggar and International Registry of Seroconverters 1990). Adult haemophiliacs showed 24% progression by 6 years, the difference being mainly due to lack of Kaposi's sarcoma; children with haemophilia had a lower rate of 13%. There is no formal direct evidence that all will progress in due course, though projections have been made that imply this. It is certainly possible in principle that a proportion will remain symptomless indefinitely, whether due to innate resistance to disease, to protective immunity, however mediated, or to lack of factors enhancing HIV replication *in vivo* (Pinching 1988a).

Among those cohorts and individuals studied to date, a number of factors seem to increase the risk of progression to symptomatic disease (Pinching 1988a). These include intercurrent sexually transmitted infections (and possibly other infections) (Weber *et al.* 1986a, b) and possibly having more than one HIV +ve pregnancy (Scott *et al.* 1985). Progression is also more rapid in very young children and possibly in adults over 50. Immunosuppressive drugs, notably high-dose corticosteroids given for long periods, and malnutrition are also associated with higher risk of progression. Major surgery may also adversely affect prognosis. Drug-users who continue to inject are at greater risk than those who abstain, whether due to the drugs themselves or to injection-associated infections (Des Jarlais and Freidman 1987; Des Jarlais *et al.* 1987). Two basic mechanisms seem likely to underlie these associations with increased progression of HIV infection: activation of infected host cells by antigenic challenge (infective, fetal or other exogenous antigens) or additional immunosuppressive influences acting on cell-mediated immunity.

Immunogenetic factors may also play a part in determining disease progression. Two studies have now shown that disease progression and/or increased rate of CD4 lymphocyte decline are associated with the human leucocyte antigen (HLA) haplotype A1, B8, Cw7, DR3 (Steele *et al.* 1988; Kaslow *et al.* 1990) and other genetic factors are also possible (Pinching 1988a).

A number of cohort studies have also shown that greater risk of progression is associated with a number of prognostic markers. Falling CD4 cell numbers in blood might have been expected to be a useful index of declining cell-mediated immunity and are indeed a feature of progression in studies on large patient numbers (Des Jarlais *et al.* 1987; Goedert *et al.* 1987a; Polk *et al.* 1987; Seligmann *et al.* 1987; Moss *et al.* 1988; Taylor *et al.* 1989; Fahey *et al.* 1990). However, it should be used with caution in individual patients. Single low values may be misleading, unless severely reduced, and trends may be more informative.

Serological tests for HIV p24 core antibody and p24 antigen are proving of considerable value (Lange *et al.* 1989; Weber and Jeffries 1989), though they too have significant shortcomings. In many patients due to progress, there is a progressive fall in p24 antibody followed by a rise in p24 antigen (Allain *et al.* 1987; de Wolf *et al.* 1987; Goudsmit *et al.* 1987; Lange *et al.* 1987; Pedersen *et al.* 1987; Weber *et al.* 1987a; Forster *et al.* 1988a). The p24 antibody fall is not, however, seen in patients in Africa. Also, some 20% of AIDS patients are not antigenaemic at presentation. Nevertheless, when abnormal, these two markers are of some value, with positive antigen tests being a good short-term marker (say, 1–2 years) and falling or absent p24 antibody indicative of rather more remote events (2–4 years).

Other studies have suggested that β-2-microglobulin (Moss *et al.* 1988; Fahey *et al.* 1990), acid-labile interferon-α (DeStefano *et al.* 1982) and neopterin (Fuchs *et al.* 1988; Fahey *et al.* 1990) have predictive value, perhaps most usefully in combination with other markers. These 'activation markers' may also reflect current clinical events, being associated on careful examination with clinical disease progression, such as features of ARC, which is itself the strongest predictive marker for progression to AIDS.

Clinical spectrum and classification of human immunodeficiency virus infection

As the full spectrum of clinical manifestations of HIV infection has emerged, so the terminology used to describe its constituent parts has had to be modified. So also have the biological implications of existing terms, some of which have had to be retained because they have become part of common parlance. Several classifications have been devised, alongside formal definitions of terms such as AIDS and ARC. Some classifications are simply descriptive, while others seek to identify prognostically different groups. The former have the advantage of robustness, while the latter are vulnerable to changing perceptions regarding the validity of prognostic markers. Perhaps the best approach is to use a basic descriptive classification and to superimpose the best available prognostic categories. In the following description, I will use the 1986 CDC classification (Centers for Disease Control 1986), relating it to commonly used terms (Fig. 72.1).

Although the initial infection is silent, a proportion of HIV-infected subjects, perhaps 10–15%,

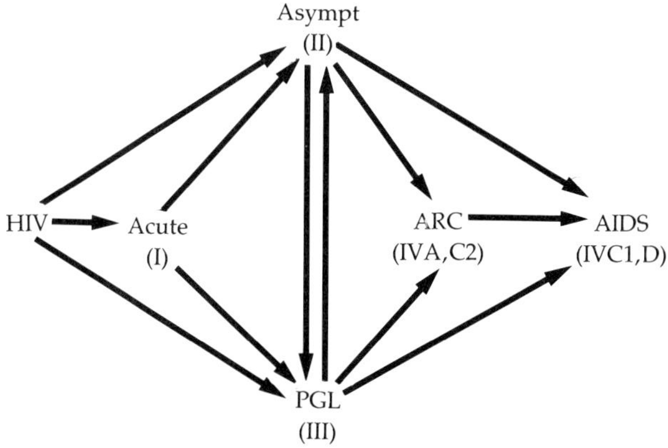

Fig. 72.1. Pathways of disease progression in HIV infection using main descriptors and numbering according to the classification of human immunodeficiency virus infection (Centers for Disease Control 1986).

develop an acute, self-limiting illness at the time of seroconversion (CDC group I). This typically occurs within 2–8 weeks of infection and lasts 2–4 weeks.

Whether or not an acute symptomatic seroconversion illness occurs, infected persons develop one of two possible asymptomatic states, asymptomatic infection without lymphadenopathy (CDC group II) and asymptomatic infection with lymphadenopathy, or persistent generalized lymphadenopathy (PGL; CDC group III). The latter has been defined as peripheral lymphadenopathy affecting two or more extrainguinal sites and lasting for more than 3 months, for which no cause other than HIV is apparent. These two forms of chronic asymptomatic HIV infection seem to have similar natural histories in terms of progression to symptomatic disease, but they do show some biological differences. Individuals may pass from one form to another, although most seem to remain stable in one. Group II and III infection may be subdivided according to the presence or absence of adverse prognostic markers, such as the absence of p24 antibody, the presence of p24 antigen and low or falling CD4 lymphocyte counts.

After some years in most instances, a proportion of patients with either form of chronic asymptomatic infection progress to develop symptomatic disease (CDC group IV), often but not always preceded by the acquisition of one or more adverse prognostic markers. Symptomatic HIV infection may take the form of ARC (CDC groups IVA and IVC2), AIDS itself (CDC groups IVC1 and IVD), HIV-related neurological disease (CDC group IVB) or various miscellaneous disorders (CDC group IVE). Individual patients may have more than one manifestation of group IV HIV infection.

The AIDS-related complex comprises a number of constitutional features such as unexplained weight loss, fever or diarrhoea (CDC group IVA) and/or minor opportunist infections, oral candidiasis, hairy oral leucoplakia or shingles (CDC group IVC2), infections that do not form part of the definition of AIDS itself. Individually and especially in combination, such features are strongly associated with progression to AIDS. However, some patients with ARC are themselves severely ill and may show biological evidence of a more profound immunodeficiency than some AIDS patients (such as those with cutaneous Kaposi's sarcoma).

The acquired immune deficiency syndrome is defined for epidemiological purposes by the presence of certain severe opportunist infections (CDC group IVC1) or tumours (CDC group IVD). The defining infections are *Pneumocystis carinii* pneumonia (PCP), *Toxoplasma* cerebral abscess, chronic cryptosporidiosis, isosporiasis, extra-intestinal strongyloidiasis, oesophageal or bronchial candidiasis, cryptococcosis, disseminated histoplasmosis, disseminated or chronic ulcerative herpes simplex, cytomegalovirus (CMV) infection, progressive multifocal leucoencephalopathy, disseminated *Mycobacterium tuberculosis* infection and atypical mycobacterial infection. Other less common infections, such as visceral leishmaniasis (Peters *et al.* 1990) and coccidiomycosis (Bronnimann *et al.* 1987), which are seen in particular geographical locations, are clearly also part of the biological spectrum of AIDS, though not formally included in the definition. Many clinicians would also include severe pulmonary tuberculosis and *Salmonella* bacteraemia as part of a clinical definition of AIDS, even if they are excluded from surveillance definitions. It is important in clinical management not to be hidebound by the surveillance definitions, which were designed for a somewhat different purpose. Another important consideration is that marked regional differences exist in the prevalence of opportunist pathogens, which will influence the local clinical profile. For example, *M. tuberculosis* is common and *Pneumocystis* infection rare in many tropical regions.

The opportunist tumours defining AIDS (CDC group IVD) are Kaposi's sarcoma, non-Hodgkin's lymphoma and primary cerebral lymphoma, though it is increasingly clear that HIV is also associated with cases of Hodgkin's lymphoma. Other tumours may in time prove to be associated, possibly including squamous carcinoma of the anus and seminoma.

Centers for Disease Control group IVE includes lymphocytic interstitial pneumonitis and other HIV-associated conditions not included elsewhere. Among these could be included thrombocytopenic purpura, although, unlike all other parts of the classification, such patients may show resolution and a return to group II or III (Abrams 1989).

Centers for Disease Control group IVB includes all HIV-associated neurological disease. This comprises chronic HIV encephalopathy (AIDS–dementia complex), myelopathy, peripheral or autonomic neuropathy and myopathy. Typically these are seen in conjunction with other symptomatic HIV infection but may less often be seen in isolation.

The definition of AIDS is dependent in most instances on the ability to conduct special investigations to define the presence of opportunist infections or tumours. In many developing countries, this may not be practicable, so the WHO have devised a definition for AIDS in Africa (World Health Organization 1986). The acquired immune deficiency syndrome is diagnosed if a person has at least one minor and two major signs from the following, in the absence of another defined cause:

1 Minor: weight loss (>10% body-weight), diarrhoea or fever for >1 month.

2 Major: persistent cough for >1 month, generalized pruritic dermatitis, recurrent herpes zoster, oropharyngeal candidiasis, chronic progressive or disseminated herpes simplex infection, generalized lymphadenopathy.

While it is apparent that this list includes features that would elsewhere be classified as ARC, the definition has proved to be useful and to compare well with stricter definitions. Further refinement may be possible with more extensive observation in such settings. However, it could be argued that the distinction between ARC and AIDS is arbitrary and unnecessarily rigid. Hence, a more pragmatic approach, having excluded other causes of symptoms or signs, would be simply to divide HIV infection into asymptomatic and symptomatic.

Clinical features of human immunodeficiency virus infection

Acute human immunodeficiency virus infection

Although the exact time of infection may be hard to pin-point in many cases, some patients develop an acute illness (group I) soon after (Cooper *et al.* 1985; Gaines *et al.* 1988; Pedersen *et al.* 1989). The manifestations are non-specific, ranging from a flu-like to a glandular fever-like illness. Some constitutional features are suggestive of a viraemic disorder while other features are more suggestive of an immune complex pathogenesis; this fits with the temporal association of the syndrome with seroconversion. In rare instances seroconversion and the associated acute illness have been seen many months after infection and appear to have been provoked by other intercurrent infection (Pinching and Parkin 1987).

Fever, malaise, sore throat, headache, myalgia, maculopapular rash, arthralgia and lymphadenopathy are common. Some patients have troublesome cough, nausea, vomiting or diarrhoea, and a transient encephalitis has been reported in some cases. Some patients have transient immunodeficiency as shown by oesophageal candidiasis (Pedersen *et al.* 1989), which may lead inappropriately to an AIDS diagnosis. Laboratory findings include leucopenia and an increase in banded neutrophils; CD4 cell counts may fall transiently. Many patients have HIV antigenaemia at the beginning of their illness. Antibodies to HIV usually become detectable within a week or two of the onset of the illness. As the symptoms resolve, lymphadenopathy may persist in some, leading to PGL, while in others it resolves. It remains unclear whether the development of this acute illness has any influence on subsequent outcome, but recent studies suggest that a prolonged seroconversion illness may be associated with increased progression rates (Pedersen *et al.* 1989).

Asymptomatic human immunodeficiency virus infection and persistent generalized lymphadenopathy

After infection most individuals, although chronically infected, remain symptomless for several years. Progression to symptomatic HIV infection rarely occurs before 1 year, but is seen in increasing numbers in succeeding years. It remains possible that some will not develop disease. Some individuals show no signs of infection, having totally asymptomatic HIV infection (group II). Some of these go on to develop PGL, while others progress to symptomatic disease without ever developing detectable lymphadenopathy.

Other subjects with chronic HIV infection develop PGL (group III), with enlarged, usually symmetrical, peripheral lymph nodes in anterior and posterior cervical, occipital, supraclavicular, epitrochlear, axillary and inguinal groups. The latter are excluded from the definition of PGL since persistently enlarged inguinal nodes are common in normal people, especially those with a history of sexually transmitted infections. Enlargement of tonsils, adenoids or other parts of Waldeyer's ring is sometimes apparent. Mediastinal, paratracheal, hilar, para-aortic, iliac and mesenteric nodes and spleen are rarely significantly enlarged. The nodes are typically between 1 and 2 cm in diameter, but occasionally are grossly enlarged. If nodes are asymmetrically or grossly enlarged or enlarging, or there are haematological or other systemic features, lymph node biopsy may be indicated to exclude other pathology, whether HIV-associated or not. Nodes may regress in the absence of other HIV-associated symptoms and the patients revert to group II HIV infection. However, the development of constitutional or other features of ARC is also often associated with regression of lymph nodes, as are AIDS-associated opportunist infections.

Apart from HIV antibody positivity, laboratory features of symptomless HIV infection are few. Increased CD8 lymphocytes and polyclonal hypergammaglobulinaemia are seen, especially in PGL. A proportion of patients show declining CD4 counts over time, a progressive loss of p24 antibody and the subsequent emergence of HIV antigen. These are associated with progression to symptomatic disease, as outlined above. Other more complex tests of immune function may show changes that resemble, but are less marked than, those seen in AIDS itself, though others such as aspects of macrophage and B cell function are distinctive in asymptomatic and PGL subjects (Seligmann *et al.* 1987; Pinching 1990). Histology of lymph nodes in PGL shows enlarged germinal centres with some infiltration of CD8 cells; the follicular dendritic reticulum cell structure remains intact (Janossy *et al.* 1985; Biberfeld *et al.* 1986).

Acquired-immune-deficiency-syndrome-related complex and miscellaneous conditions

For the purposes of this account, the individual manifestations that constitute ARC are described (Melbye *et al.* 1987a), although many clinicians tend to use the term for patients fulfilling more than one criterion. Nevertheless, even a single clinical feature that is unequivocally due to HIV should be regarded as a sign of symptomatic HIV infection, carrying a worse prognosis and meriting the consideration of treatment intervention appropriate to active chronic HIV infection.

Constitutional features (group IVA) are important features of ARC but they are also early manifestations of some of the presenting opportunist infections of AIDS, such as *Pneumocystis* pneumonia, *Mycobacterium tuberculosis* infection and cryptococcal meningitis, or of Addison's disease due to CMV adrenalitis. Many of the constitutional symptoms are also seen in patients with severe anxiety. Patients are often aware of ARC symptoms and similar symptoms due to anxiety can set up a vicious circle, increasing their conviction that they have ARC or AIDS. While it is unwise to try to explain away symptoms in the absence of anxiety, it must also be recognized that anxiety may itself have been provoked by the patient's awareness of symptoms. The clinician may need to exclude other causes of constitutional symptoms before attributing them to ARC, as well as continually reappraising the diagnosis. The features of ARC may be seen in AIDS patients; if they coexist with Kaposi's sarcoma, they are indicative of more severely compromised immunity than Kaposi's sarcoma without associated symptoms.

Unexplained weight loss is a strong marker of symptomatic HIV disease; loss of >10% bodyweight is used for formal definition, though any significant change from baseline should be regarded with suspicion. Diarrhoea persisting for more than 1 month and not due to any other cause is a not uncommon feature. It is typically mild, with loose rather than watery motions and a frequency of 2–5 times a day. There may be subtle malabsorption and partial villous atrophy seems to be present in such cases, often described as HIV enteropathy (Kotler *et al.* 1984; Miller *et al.* 1988). Symptoms may usually be controlled by loperamide.

Unexplained fever persisting for more than 1 month is frequently cited as a feature of ARC. While it certainly does occur, it is typically low-grade and only rarely causes symptoms; in many cases, persistent fever proves ultimately to have been due to an undiagnosed opportunist infection, such as *Pneumocystis* pneumonia. Other patients have recurrent bouts of otherwise unexplained high fever lasting for a few days or a week, rarely longer. Night sweats have gained considerable notoriety as ARC features. While in the clinician's mind they may be thought of as aspects of fever, HIV-associated night sweats are rarely associated with fever, are usually not drenching and may be curiously localized to one part of the body, such as the upper trunk or neck. However, the specificity of this symptom is very low, with night sweats being seen in anxiety and through changes in sleeping habits. In isolation they are not strongly associated with progression and may be best ignored in many cases.

Skin changes are very common in symptomatic HIV infection (Farthing 1986). Generalized dryness is a frequent complaint and may present as frank ichthyosis. Emollients or emulsifying ointment are valuable in controlling these symptoms. The commonest feature is seborrhoeic dermatitis; it usually affects the eyebrows and nasolabial folds, but is sometimes seen over the trunk or limbs. It may reflect low-grade fungal infection with *Pytisporium* and responds well to topical applications combining low-dose hydrocortisone with an antifungal. It may be associated with progression in some cases. Atopic subjects may develop exacerbation of atopic eczema, or other atopic features such as asthma, hay fever or rhinitis (Parkin *et al*. 1987). Non-specific pharyngitis or mouth ulcers are sometimes seen in ARC. Retinal examination may reveal cotton wool spots and these seem to be associated with progression.

Minor opportunist infections are important markers of ARC (group IVC2) (Melbye *et al*. 1987a) as well as being seen in AIDS itself. Probably the commonest and most significant is oral candidiasis (Klein *et al*. 1984). This presents with either white plaques or punctate lesions, which are detachable and have a varying amount of associated inflammatory change in the underlying mucous membrane; candidiasis may also take an erythematous form without plaques, which may be misdiagnosed. The tongue may be coated (though this may also be due to other causes) and there may also be angular cheilitis. Isolation of *Candida* from a normal mouth is common in normal subjects and cannot be used as a criterion of oral candidiasis. Treatment with topical nystatin, amphotericin or miconazole may alleviate symptoms but is often insufficient to control any but the mildest candidiasis. Oral ketoconazole, fluconazole or itraconazole are much more effective; maintenance is generally required to avoid relapse (Glatt *et al*. 1988; Gold 1988; Pinching 1988b).

If there is oesophageal involvement, which may or may not be associated with dysphagia, this is formally part of the AIDS case definition. However, some observers have suggested that oral candidiasis in HIV infection is always assoicated with some oesophageal involvement seen at endoscopy (Tavitian *et al*. 1986). This serves as a reminder that the boundary between ARC and AIDS is somewhat arbitrary. Many clinicians are inclined to diagnose oesophageal disease, and hence AIDS itself, only if there are symptoms or when oesophageal studies provoked by gross oral disease reveal extensive oesophageal plaques.

Hairy oral leucoplakia is another important ARC feature, consisting of characteristic corrugated whitish plaques on the lateral border and under-side of the tongue (Greenspan *et al*. 1984). It rarely causes symptoms and shows considerable spontaneous variation in extent, but it is a valuable disease marker associated with progression (Greenspan *et al*. 1987). It must be distinguished from candidiasis. Histology typically shows koilocytosis. Epstein–Barr virus has been implicated in its aetiology. No treatment is required and it has not been shown to lead to malignant change. It may occur on other buccal membranes and rarely a similar condition may be seen as ulceration in the middle third of the oesophagus (Kitchen *et al*. 1990).

Shingles, as in other clinical settings, is a striking marker of a degree of cellular immunodeficiency and hence of progression to AIDS (Melbye *et al*. 1987b). It is often multidermatomal and may recur in several sites over time. Dissemination and visceral disease are rare but cropping may continue for some time. Severe episodes may necessitate treatment with high-dose acyclovir (Glatt *et al*. 1988). Extensive scarring and secondary bacterial infection are common. Zoster seems more common in ARC than AIDS, but this may be due to the widespread use of prophylactic acyclovir for herpes simplex infection (Pinching 1988b).

Although pulmonary tuberculosis, nocardiosis and *Salmonella* bacteraemia are part of the formal definition of group IVC2 HIV infection, they are more conveniently discussed under AIDS itself, to which some clinicians feel they more properly belong. Bacterial infections with *Staphylococcus* and capsulated bacteria such as *Pneumococcus, Haemophilus* and *Branhamella* are also seen in both ARC and AIDS, probably due to dysglobulinaemia; they will also be discussed under AIDS.

Lymphocytic interstitial pneumonitis (group IVE) is a common manifestation of HIV infection in children (Rubinstein *et al*. 1986) but may occasionally affect adults with ARC or AIDS. It causes chronic, sometimes progressive, pulmonary impairment, usually manifested by dyspnoea on exertion; cough and chest pain are unusual. The course varies considerably, with some spontaneous fluctuation in symptoms and physiological disturbance. Some adults, like children, may have an associated parotitis, which appears to be due to a similar pathological process (Andiman *et al.* 1985). Chest X-ray typically shows reticulonodular or interstitial shadowing throughout the lung fields; this may be more marked than would be expected for the degree of physiological disturbance, the reverse of the situation in *Pneumocystis* infection. Lung volumes and gas transfer are reduced. Histology of lung shows variable interstitial infiltration with lymphocytes. Epstein–Barr virus and HIV itself have been separately implicated in the aetiology of this disorder (Andiman *et al.* 1985; Chayt *et al.* 1986). Its main importance is as part of the differential diagnosis of impaired lung function and abnormal chest radiology in ARC and AIDS.

Patients with HIV infection may develop inflammatory, non-erosive arthropathy of the Reiter's or psoriatic type, which may present for the first time with HIV disease or may be an exacerbation of pre-existing joint disease (Winchester *et al.* 1987; Forster *et al.* 1988b). Patients are typically HLA B27 +ve and may develop associated skin, conjunctival or urethral symptoms at the same time. Arthropathy usually appears as other HIV-related symptoms develop and may be resistant to non-steroidal anti-inflammatory drugs.

Human immunodeficiency virus infection has been associated with thrombocytopenic purpura (Walsh *et al.* 1984; Abrams *et al.* 1986; Abrams 1989). This may be seen at any stage of HIV infection, including otherwise symptomless infection. It may be viewed as the extreme end of the spectrum that includes the lesser degrees of thrombocytopenia commonly seen in HIV infection. While cutaneous purpura and epistaxis are common, severe internal bleeding seems rare, despite platelet counts of 10×10^9 or less. Bone marrow examination shows plentiful megakaryocytes. Untreated patients may show spontaneous remission of thrombocytopenia after months or a few years and some patients may remain symptomless (group II or III). Thrombocytopenic purpura does not of itself carry adverse prognostic implications for AIDS.

Although platelet autoantibodies have been described (Stricker *et al.* 1985), there is also evidence in favour of an immune complex pathogenesis (Walsh *et al.* 1984). The latter is supported by the favourable and early response to zidovudine therapy (Hymes *et al.* 1988). Prior to this, variable responses had been seen with corticosteriod therapy or splenectomy, but both are associated with increased risk of infection (Abrams *et al.* 1986). In view of this, the lack of severe bleeding in most patients and the likelihood of spontaneous remission, a conservative approach seems justified, with zidovudine seeming the most appropriate therapy (Abrams *et al.* 1986; Hymes *et al.* 1988; Abrams 1989). Benefit has also been obtained with intravenous gammaglobulin but, as its effects rarely last more than 2–3 weeks, it is best used to tide patients over acute bleeding episodes or operative interventions.

Acquired immune deficiency syndrome: opportunistic infections

PROTOZOA

Pneumocystis carinii has until recently been regarded as a protozoon and will be discussed as such here, despite recent genetic evidence suggesting that it is closer to the fungi (Edman *et al.* 1988). It has long been known as an organism that only causes disease, typically an interstitial pneumonia, in people with defective cell-mediated immunity. *Pneumocystis carinii* pneumonia (PCP) is one of the commonest opportunist infections in AIDS in temperate climates (Gottlieb *et al.* 1981; Masur *et al.* 1981; Kovacs *et al.* 1984; Murray *et al.* 1984, 1987; Hopewell and Luce 1986; Mills 1986), but it seems relatively uncommon in tropical regions. Serological evidence suggests that exposure to *Pneumocystis* occurs in early life without discernible illness. It is not clear whether the organism then remains latent, re-emerging to cause disease if cell-mediated immunity becomes seriously impaired, or whether this is due to reinfection.

In AIDS, PCP tends to present more insidiously than in other compromised hosts, developing over weeks or even months (Kovacs *et al.* 1984). Early symptoms are often constitutional, such as general malaise, weight loss and fever, resembling those of ARC. The typically pulmonary symptoms are a dry cough and gradually increasing shortness of breath on exertion; either may be present alone. Some patients produce sputum, notably if they also have bacterial infection. Patients often feel unable to take a full breath and may have mild pleuritic pain. Fever, tachycardia, tachypnoea and sometimes dry crackles on auscultation are the only signs.

Chest X-ray may show interstitial shadowing, especially in advanced disease, characteristically in a perihilar distribution, sparing the periphery, but it may be more localized (Cohen *et al*. 1984). Earlier, even in a patient with pulmonary symptoms, the X-ray may be normal. Some centres have found high-definition gallium scanning to be a sensitive indicator of PCP (Coleman *et al*. 1984). Early changes in pulmonary function include a fall in forced vital capacity (FVC) and carbon monoxide transfer (TLCO) (Shaw *et al*. 1988), while later the arterial $P\text{O}_2$ may be reduced.

Sputum is rarely obtainable, but may be induced by giving nebulized hypertonic saline (Bigby *et al*. 1986; Pitchenik *et al*. 1986). With experienced and assiduous cytological examination, *Pneumocystis* may be identified in such samples. However, in many cases the definitive diagnosis can only be made by bronchoscopy with bronchoalveolar lavage or transbronchial biopsy (Murray *et al*. 1984; Stover *et al*. 1984; Broaddus *et al*. 1985; Golden *et al*. 1986; Francis *et al*. 1987), on which pneumocysts can be seen with silver or other special stains, even after some days of therapy. The use of monoclonal antibodies or gene probes may facilitate diagnosis on induced sputum or lavage fluid. Histology shows characteristic foamy material in alveoli and, in advanced or prolonged disease, fibrosis may be seen.

Treatments include 3 weeks of high-dose cotrimoxazole, dapsone/trimethoprim or intravenous pentamidine (Fischl 1988; Glatt *et al*. 1988; Gold 1988; Klein 1989; Medina *et al*. 1990). Clinical response may take 3–7 days and radiological improvement may lag behind, even deteriorating initially. Adverse drug reactions are common, including allergic skin rashes, fevers, leucopenia, severe nausea and vomiting with cotrimoxazole and malaise, hypotension, hypoglycaemia and subsequent glucose intolerance with pentamidine; dapsone exacerbates the myelotoxicity of zidovudine. Pentamidine by inhalation has been used for treatment of mild cases (Montgomery *et al*. 1987), but its efficacy and tolerance are not yet established. Some patients show very rapid progression despite treatment and, in these, a short course of high-dose methylprednisolone for 3–4 days has proved a valuable adjunct (MacFadden *et al*. 1987; Feinberg and Mills 1990). As PCP is common and often recurs, prophylaxis is now widely used following a first episode and as primary prophylaxis in patients with low CD4 counts (Fischl 1988). Long-term studies of efficacy and toxicity (notably sulphonamide hypersensitivity reactions) are defining optimal approaches. Daily or alternate day low-dose cotrimoxazole or dapsone, weekly or twice weekly Fansidar or dapsone/pyrimethamine and fortnightly/monthly inhaled pentamidine are being explored (Fischl 1988; Fischl *et al*. 1988; Glatt *et al*. 1988; Pinching 1988b; Klein 1989: Leoung *et al*. 1990). Extrapulmonary pneumocystosis has emerged in some patients receiving nebulized pentamidine.

Toxoplasma gondii infection is common in AIDS, representing re-emergence from latency and presenting with cerebral abscess or focal encephalitis (Luft *et al*. 1983; Snider *et al*. 1983; Wong *et al*. 1984; Levy *et al*. 1985; Navia *et al*. 1986a; Luft and Remington 1988). About one-third of *Toxoplasma*-seropositive AIDS patients will develop this complication during their course. It usually presents initially with low-grade fever, headache and non-specific neurological symptoms and signs. Focal neurological features such as hemiplegia or dysphasia may develop according to the location of specific lesions. Fits may occur with acute disease or after successful treatment. Evidence of raised intracranial pressure is often absent, perhaps because of coexisting atrophy due to HIV encephalopathy.

The investigation of choice is CT scanning, which shows low attenuation areas often with ring enhancement; the lesions are often multiple (Levy *et al*. 1985; Navia *et al*. 1986a). Magnetic resonance imaging (MRI) scanning is reported to have a greater sensitivity but is not always readily available. Serological diagnosis by high or rising titres or IgM response is unreliable (Navia *et al*. 1986a; Glatt *et al*. 1988) due to the dysglobulinaemia of HIV infection, though most patients show sero-positivity, indicating prior and hence latent infection. Most centres give a therapeutic trial of high-dose sulphadiazine and pyrimethamine to confirm the diagnosis (Navia *et al*. 1986a; Glatt *et al*. 1988; Gold 1988); a response is typically seen between the first and second weeks of treatment. *Toxoplasma* infection is by far the commonest cause of such lesions; other infections rarely cause cerebral abscesses and the main differential diagnosis is cerebral lymphoma. Brain biopsy to establish an alternative diagnosis is usually performed after failure of a therapeutic trial. Alternative therapies, which may be required because of toxicity (Haverkos and TE Study Group 1987), have included dapsone and pyrimethamine, clindamycin and pyrimethamine. Maintenance therapy is essential to prevent early relapse (Glatt *et al.* 1988; Pinching 1988b). Because of the high incidence of fits after successful treatment, anticonvulsants are usually given prophylactically.

Cryptosporidium causes major gastrointestinal disease in AIDS, most commonly with severe watery diarrhoea and abdominal cramps, associated with marked weight loss and malabsorption (Pitlik *et al.* 1983a; Soave and Armstrong 1986; Sewankambo *et al.* 1987; Soave and Johnson 1988). The diarrhoea is hard to control with conventional antidiarrhoeal agents. Upper gastrointestinal infestation may present with intractable anorexia, nausea and vomiting. The cysts may be seen in stool or rectal or jejunal biopsy. Although previously associated with contact with infected farm of domestic animals, person-to-person spread seems to occur more often, probably by faecal–oral contact, although water-borne infection is documented. In normal hosts cryptosporidial infection is less severe and is also self-limiting; cryptosporidiosis in AIDS is persistent and, as no generally effective treatment exists, often ultimately leads to the death of the patient. Symptomatic measures including nutritional support may enable the patient to survive with a reasonable quality of life for some months, however.

Cryptosporidium may also cause chronic biliary disease with biliary pain and an obstructive pattern of liver enzymes (Pitlik *et al.* 1983b; Margulis *et al.* 1986). The major bile-ducts show marked irregularity with areas of constriction and dilatation on ultrasound or ERCP; bile samples may show the organisms. Biliary disease may occur in the absence of bowel wall involvement.

Secretory diarrhoea similar to that of *Cryptosporidium* is seen with *Isospora belli* infection (DeHovitz *et al.* 1986; Sewankambo *et al.* 1987; Soave and Johnson 1988; Pape *et al.* 1989). It is less common than cryptosporidiosis in temperate countries but may be as common in tropical regions. This protozoon may, however, be successfully treated with high-dose cotrimoxazole, though maintenance is required to prevent early relapse.

Some cases of visceral leishmaniasis have been described in AIDS (Peters *et al.* 1990). They present with constitutional features and evidence of disseminated infection; splenomegaly may be absent or slight and serological responses are unreliable for diagnosis. Although some response to conventional treatment is seen, it is limited and early relapse is usual. As HIV spreads increasingly to areas endemic for leishmaniasis this problem may become more common. Although some cases of AIDS have been associated with severe malaria, malarial parasites do not generally seem to behave as opportunist pathogens in AIDS.

FUNGI

Oral candidiasis is more common, more extensive and more inclined to recur in AIDS than in ARC, but shows the same clinical features as those described under ARC above (Klein *et al.* 1984; Tavitian *et al.* 1986). Significant oesophageal involvement is common and may be associated with dysphagia; bronchial infection is also described. Oral systemic therapy and secondary prophylaxis are required (Glatt *et al.* 1988; Gold 1988; Pinching 1988b). In severe cases, parenteral amphotericin is needed.

Cryptococcosis is a significant cause of disease in AIDS (Kovacs *et al.* 1985; Eng *et al.* 1986; Zuger *et al.* 1986; Dismukes 1988; Chuck and Sande 1989). It typically presents with a low-grade meningitis, though there may also be evidence of disseminated infection. Early features are fever, headache and mild central ataxia. Meningism is absent or minimal except in very advanced disease. There may be signs of impaired higher function such as short-term memory and concentration. After CT scan to exclude toxoplasmosis or other space-occupying lesions (whose clinical features may mimic those of cryptococcal meningitis), cerebrospinal fluid (CSF) should be obtained. Typically this shows few if any lymphocytes, but cryptococci are often abundant. They may be confirmed by culture and antigen tests and the latter may also be positive in serum. Serial antigen tests may be valuable in monitoring treatment and in evaluating possible relapse, which is common without prophylaxis.

Cryptococcal pneumonitis may be seen and may resemble early *Pneumocystis*; it is rarely severe. Conventional treatment is with parenteral amphotericin for 4–6 weeks (Glatt *et al*. 1988; Gold 1988; Chuck and Sande 1989; Larsen *et al*. 1990); although flucytosine is often combined with amphotericin, it appears to offer little discernible benefit and can cause significant toxicity. The better tolerated fluconazole (Larsen *et al*. 1990) or itraconazole show some promise as primary treatment and, as oral formulations, seem particularly well suited to long-term secondary prophylaxis. Late complications include fits, which merit prophylactic anticonvulsants, and secondary hydrocephalus.

Other systemic mycoses are uncommon or have strong regional distribution. These include disseminated histoplasmosis (Bonner *et al*. 1984; Wheat *et al*. 1985; Johnson *et al*. 1989) and coccidiomycosis (Bronnimann *et al*. 1987). Cutaneous mycotic infection, notably with *Trichophyton*, is, however, common and may be troublesome, as is the seborrhoeic dermatitis discussed under ARC, in which *Pytisporium* is implicated.

VIRUSES

Herpes simplex infection is a common problem in AIDS. Unlike the presentation in the normal host, in AIDS it presents with progressive mucocutaneous ulceration (Siegal *et al*. 1981; Quinnan *et al*. 1984). This is commonly perianal in homosexual men but oral or genital lesions are also common. Less commonly herpes simplex may present with extremely painful, multiple, shallow, oesophageal ulcers. Herpes simplex encephalitis is very rare. Herpes infection in AIDS represents reemergence from latency. Treatment with acyclovir is very effective but long-term maintenance with low doses is generally needed to prevent relapse as this is very common (Pinching 1988b). Herpes zoster is relatively uncommon in AIDS and is discussed above under ARC.

Cytomegalovirus is an important pathogen in AIDS, but its organ distribution is somewhat different from that in other compromised hosts (Jacobsen and Mills 1988). The commonest presentation is with retinitis, showing the characteristic appearances of a focal choroidoretinitis (Palestine *et al*. 1984; Teich and Orellana 1986; Henderly *et al*. 1987; Pepose 1989). Visual loss or scotoma may be evident in central lesions and 'floaters' are a not uncommon premonitory symptom. Cytomegalovirus colitis is next most common and presents with abdominal pain and distension and variable if any change in bowel habit (Meiselman *et al*. 1985; Weber *et al*. 1987b). Cytomegalovirus inclusions are seen in rectal biopsy. Cytomegalovirus may cause chronic lower oesophageal ulceration, with clinical and radiological appearances resembling malignant ulcers, and inclusion bodies are seen on biopsy (Weber *et al*. 1987b).

Cytomegalovirus pneumonitis appears much less commonly in AIDS than was expected, but when it does the symptoms resemble PCP. Radiological changes are usually in a reticular pattern and extend to the periphery of the lung. Transbronchial biopsy shows CMV inclusions but positive CMV culture alone does not necessarily indicate CMV disease of the lung. Cytomegalovirus encephalitis is a rare clinical complication of disseminated CMV infection (Morgello *et al*. 1987).

Treatment of CMV disease with ganciclovir or phosphonoformate is usually effective in leading to clinical resolution (Collaborative DHPG Treatment Study Group 1986; Masur *et al*. 1986; Chachoua *et al*. 1987; Henderly *et al*. 1987; Laskin *et al*. 1987; Weber *et al*. 1987b; Glatt *et al*. 1988; Walmsley *et al*. 1988), though retinal lesions leave residual scarring and scotomata and late retinal detachment may occur (Freeman *et al*. 1987) and oesophageal ulcers tend to show little response. Maintenance therapy is always required for retinitis to prevent further visual loss and may be needed for other manifestations (Glatt *et al*. 1988; Pinching 1988b).

Another complication, usually due to CMV infection, is the development of Addison's disease (Greene *et al*. 1984; Guenthner *et al*. 1984; Tapper *et al*. 1984). This presents insidiously with fatigue, malaise, postural hypotension and reduced skin turgor; pigmentation is a late feature. There are usually no other signs of CMV disease. It has been shown that the predominant initial defect is of mineralocorticoid production and cortisol levels and responses may be relatively preserved (Guy *et al*. 1989). It is readily treated with replacement therapy, which may be used as a therapeutic trial to establish the diagnosis. Treatment of CMV itself is not needed unless there is CMV disease elsewhere.

Progressive multifocal leucoencephalopathy (PML) due to the JC papovavirus is a rare but serious complication of AIDS (Miller *et al*. 1982; Bedri *et al*. 1983; Krupp *et al*. 1985; Berger *et al*. 1987). Presentations include generalized pyramidal weakness or cerebellar ataxia with variable abnormality of higher function. Characteristic lesions are seen in white matter on CT or, more readily in early disease, on MRI scanning. The course is progressive, although sometimes characterized by periods of stable impairment and episodes of progression. No treatment is available.

BACTERIA

Mycobacteria present common problems in AIDS. *Mycobacterium tuberculosis* generally re-emerges from latency in patients previously infected and typically presents early in AIDS; the epidemiology thus reflects the geographical and population prevalence of this infection, being especially common in tropical regions and among drug-users (Pitchenik *et al*. 1984; Goedert *et al*. 1985; Pitchenik and Rubinson 1985; Mann *et al*. 1986; Saltzman *et al*. 1986; Sunderam *et al*. 1986; Centers for Diseases Control 1987; Chaisson *et al*. 1987; Glatt *et al*. 1988; Pitchenik 1988). A common presentation is with fever and cough. Pleuritic pain and pleural effusions are common. Extensive pulmonary disease may be seen, with diffuse parenchymal disease more common than cavitary disease; miliary patterns may be seen. Lymph node disease is also common, with asymmetrical and progressive enlargement associated with constitutional symptoms. Abnormal liver function with an obstructive enzyme pattern is common. Ileocaecal involvement and tuberculous meningitis are sometimes seen.

Organisms are plentiful in biopsy material and serosal fluid but sputum positivity occurs late, probably due to the lack of cavitary disease. Granulomas may be seen on biopsy but may be relatively poorly formed and lymphocyte-depleted. Some patients may show positive skin test responses to purified protein derivative (PPD), but anergy due to disease may confound its diagnostic value. Conventional treatment is effective but longer courses than usual may be needed and maintenance therapy is required to avoid relapse (Glatt *et al*. 1988; Pinching 1988b; Klein 1989).

Atypical mycobacterial infection, notably with *M. avium intracellulare*, is common in late stages of AIDS, as would be expected with organisms of such low intrinsic pathogenicity (Greene *et al*. 1982; Macher *et al*. 1983; Pitchenik *et al*. 1984; Hawkins *et al*. 1986; Young *et al*. 1986; Pitchenik 1988). Gastrointestinal and visceral lymph node involvement are commonest but pulmonary and hepatic disease are also seen. Symptoms are relatively mild for the extent of disease, reflecting the lack of host response, and disease is usually slowly progressive until late stages. Bone marrow involvement is common, causing a variable degree of pancytopenia, and bone marrow aspirates often yield positive cultures; blood cultures may also be positive. Chronic low-grade fever may be the only feature and many symptomless patients with advanced AIDS may have some evidence of this infection.

Biopsy specimens typically show no granulomata but numerous macrophages filled with sheets of acid-fast mycobacteria. Small-bowel biopsy may show appearances that resemble Whipple's disease. Treatment is unsatisfactory, but useful palliation may be obtained with conventional antimycobacterial drugs. Some additional benefit has been obtained with rifabutin, clofazimine and/or amikacin in combination with conventional agents (Glatt *et al*. 1988; Gold 1988; Feinberg and Mills 1990). Eradication is not achieved but symptoms may be controlled for long periods with such regimes.

Salmonella infection with bacteraemia is not uncommon in AIDS/ARC (Glaser *et al*. 1985; Jacobs *et al*. 1985; Nadelman *et al*. 1985; Profeta *et al*. 1985; Fischl *et al*. 1986; Whimbey *et al*. 1986; Celum *et al*. 1987; Schrager 1988; Gilks *et al*. 1990). Gastrointestinal disturbance is mild or absent and the usual presentation is marked pyrexia. Organisms may be found on culture of stool and blood. Conventional treatment is effective but maintenance therapy is needed as relapse is the norm.

A significant proportion of patients with ARC or AIDS develop recurrent and severe pyogenic infections with *Staphylococcus aureus* and with the capsulated bacteria *Pneumococcus, Haemophilus* and *Branhamella* (Simberkoff *et al*. 1984; Polsky *et al*. 1986; Whimbey *et al*. 1986; Witt *et al*. 1987; Parkin *et al*. 1989; Schrager 1988; Gilks *et al*. 1990). These usually cause pulmonary disease and may be especially troublesome in patients with endobronchial Kaposi's sarcoma. Bacteraemia is also seen. This pattern of infection resembles that seen in patients with hypogammaglobulinaemia. It reflects the fact that underlying the hypergammaglobulinaemia of HIV infection there is dysglobulinaemia. Patients with such infections show low immunoglobulin G2 (IgG2) levels (Aucouturier *et al.* 1986; Parkin *et al.* 1989 and defective pneumococcal antibody production (Ballet *et al.* 1987), and neoantigen responses are generally defective due to B cell (Lane *et al.* 1983, 1985) and antigen-presenting cell (Macatonia *et al.* 1990) defects. Treatment with regular antibiotics is effective but antibiotic prophylaxis or immunoglobulin replacement may be required in some patients with recurrent infections.

Acquired immune deficiency syndrome: opportunistic tumours

KAPOSI'S SARCOMA

The unusual tumour Kaposi's sarcoma, which is more a multifocal proliferative disease of endothelial cells, has been one of the most characteristic disorders seen in AIDS (Hymes *et al.* 1981; Friedman-Kien *et al.* 1982; Kornfeld and Axelrod 1983; Bayley 1984; Bayley *et al.* 1985; Friedman *et al.* 1985; Ognibene *et al.* 1985; Mitsuyasu 1987; Krown 1988; Ziegler and Dorfman 1988; Volberding 1988). It is most commonly seen in homosexual men and in African patients with heterosexually acquired disease and is rare in other risk behaviours. This is thought to reflect the fact that the hitherto unidentified causative agent of Kaposi's sarcoma is a sexually transmitted infection, probably a virus (Beral *et al.* 1990). There is now some suggestion that, among homosexual men, Kaposi's sarcoma is becoming less common (Volberding 1988), probably reflecting changed sexual behaviour and the relatively higher prevalence of HIV than of many other sexually transmitted infections in this population. Kaposi's sarcoma, when it occurs alone, presents with the least severe immunodeficiency within the spectrum of AIDS and has a correspondingly better long-term prognosis. Fatalities result from visceral involvement or from the subsequent development of major opportunist infections; the former is becoming increasingly prevalent as the overall prognosis for people with AIDS improves.

The appearances of the lesions of Kaposi's sarcoma are very characteristic, being raised reddish purple plaques on skin or mucous membranes. They may be seen anywhere on skin, with more frequent involvement of the trunk and palate than with other forms. Symptoms are few, although lesions on the feet may become painful, especially if they enlarge rapidly; such lesions may ulcerate and become secondarily infected, as may large palatal lesions. Lymph node and lymphatic disease is common and may lead to lymphoedema; there may be associated splenomegaly. Visceral disease most commonly affects the gastrointestinal tract or lungs. Cerebral disease is extremely rare. The histological appearances are typical, with spindle-shaped cells and slit-like spaces, filled with red cells.

A number of treatment options are available (Krown 1988; Volberding 1988; Ziegler and Dorfman 1988; Stewart 1990). No treatment may be required for indolent disease. Localized cutaneous lesions, especially on the face, may merit treatment with fractionated low-dose radiotherapy. Intralesional injections of vinblastine may also be useful for small numbers of small lesions. Rapidly progressive cutaneous disease and severe lymphatic and visceral disease usually require systemic chemotherapy. For this, various regimes have been tried with some success, including vinblastine, vincristine, bleomycin, etoposide, actinomycin D and adriamycin, usually given in various combinations; our preferred regimen is monthly bleomycin and vincristine. Regimens least likely to cause further immunosuppression are preferable. Medium-term responses are good but relapse is common. Some success has been achieved with high-dose interferon-α, notably with cutaneous disease in patients with relatively well-preserved immunity (Krown 1988); unfortunately long-term side-effects limit the usefulness of this approach for patients who are typically well otherwise. Whatever the treatment, treated lesions show flattening and loss of induration and the colour darkens, leaving residual haemosiderin pigmentation.

LYMPHOMA

Primary cerebral lymphoma is sometimes seen in AIDS (Snider *et al.* 1983; Gill *et al.* 1985; So *et al.* 1986; Rosenblum *et al.* 1988), presenting with focal neurological signs according to location and usually single enhancing lesions on CT scanning.

Radiotherapy may stem progression temporarily but long-term results are poor.

Systemic lymphoma is usually of B cell, Burkitt-like type with severe histological grading (Ziegler *et al.* 1982, 1984; Levine *et al.* 1984, 1985); it commonly presents with extranodal disease, especially affecting the gastrointestinal tract and skin. Optimal treatment regimes are not fully developed (Volberding 1988; Stewart 1990). Some tumours show a good and sustained response with two-drug regimes, while others respond poorly to multi-drug regimes. Increasingly, cases of Hodgkin's disease are being seen in association with HIV infection and they respond fairly well to conventional therapies (Volberding 1988).

A few cases of squamous carcinoma of the anus and of testicular germ cell tumours and other tumours have been seen in homosexual men associated with HIV infection, but their relatedness to HIV infection is not clearly established (Volberding 1988; Monfardini *et al.* 1989).

Human-immunodeficiency-virus-related neurological disease

Apart from causing cerebral opportunist infections, it has become increasingly apparent that HIV can itself cause neurological disease, though its pathogenesis remains obscure (Snider *et al.* 1983; Shaw *et al.* 1985; Navia and Price 1986; Navia *et al.* 1986b, c; Asher *et al.* 1987; Rosenblum *et al.* 1987; Levy and Bredesen 1988; Price *et al.* 1988; Ho *et al.* 1989). It tends to arise after symptomatic disease due to immunodeficiency, and may not be clinically overt until AIDS is quite advanced. Human immunodeficiency virus encephalopathy, also known as the AIDS–dementia complex, causes progressive loss of higher function with impaired short-term memory and concentration and withdrawal. Mood or personality change is seen, with organic depression or frontal disinhibition, but frank psychosis is rare. Patients may show atypical reactions to neurotropic drugs, in some cases resembling those seen in children or the elderly. Some drugs, especially drugs of abuse, may provoke severe psychotic reactions. Fits, focal or generalized, may be seen and some patients show epilepsia partialis continuans, which may pose diagnostic problems because of its non-specific presentation. Motor signs usually occur later, first with central ataxia and later with limb ataxia of cerebellar type; pyramidal, or rarely extra-pyramidal, signs occur late. Incontinence, mutism and inanition are also seen in severe disease.

Human immunodeficiency virus encephalopathy is a diagnosis of exclusion since many of its features, especially the early ones, are common to cerebral opportunists such as toxoplasmosis, cryptococcosis, lymphoma or PML. Encephalopathy of some duration may be associated with some cerebral atrophy on CT scanning and with multiple focal abnormalities on MRI, but quantitative correlation between clinical evidence and these changes is poor. Cerebrospinal fluid examination may show increased protein and a few cells. Psychometric testing may reveal early changes in the absence of overt disease (Grant *et al.* 1987; Koralnik *et al.* 1990), though the role of HIV in this is controversial, as well as documenting more striking involvement in patients with symptomatic HIV disease. The specificity of these tests for the documentation of HIV encephalopathy in otherwise asymptomatic individuals is not clear. An electroencephalogram (EEG) may show diffuse abnormalities including delta rhythm, and ictal activity may be evident. Electrophysiological changes have been shown in a relatively high proportion of people with asymptomatic HIV infection (Koralnik *et al.* 1990). Human immunodeficiency virus encephalopathy appears to comprise neuronal functional impairment as well as neuronal loss, since some features may resolve on zidovudine therapy.

A myelopathy, usually described as a vacuolar myelopathy (Petito *et al.* 1985), may also be seen in HIV, causing subacute development of cord signs leading to paraplegia, usually at thoracic level. Some cases of Guillain–Barré syndrome have also been seen, often in association with early infection. Peripheral neuropathy is common, occasionally with mononeuritis multiplex, but more commonly with a symmetrical glove and stocking distribution, predominantly affecting the legs (Cornblath *et al.* 1988; Rance *et al.* 1988). There is often painful dysaesthesia, which may be disabling, as well as sensory loss. Nerve conduction studies and biopsy show evidence of axonal loss, especially in small fibres, but there is also variable demyelination. Associated autonomic neuropathy is common, with erectile failure, diarrhoea and postural hypotension. Myelopathy and peripheral/autonomic neuropathy show minimal if any improvement on zidovudine therapy. Less commonly patients may develop a proximal myopathy which is not usually painful and is variably associated with raised muscle enzymes (Bailey *et al.* 1987; Simpson and Bender 1988; Panegyres *et al.* 1990). An inflammatory polymyositis has also been described (Dalakas *et al.* 1986).

Treatment of human immunodeficiency virus infection and acquired immune deficiency syndrome

There are four basic strategies in treatment: general management, treatment and prophylaxis of specific opportunist events, antiretroviral therapy and immunorestorative therapy (Pinching 1989). General measures include nutrition, health maintenance, avoidance of a few specific opportunists, such as *Salmonella*, and provision of patient access to care and physical and psychological support. Treatment and prophylaxis have been covered in outline under specific pathogens above.

Antiretroviral therapy has become the main focus for treatment of the underlying disease. While many agents show promise *in vitro*, only one agent, zidovudine (azidothymidine (AZT)), has shown unequivocal benefit *in vivo*, in patients with ARC and AIDS (Mitsuya *et al.* 1985; Yarchoan *et al.* 1986, 1987, 1988a, 1989a; Fischl *et al.* 1987, 1990b; Richman *et al.* 1987, 1988; Dournon *et al.* 1988; Jackson *et al.* 1988; Fischl 1989; Mildvan and Richman 1989; Pinching *et al.* 1989). It is a reverse transcriptase inhibitor, also acting as a DNA chain terminator. It thus stems HIV replication, and treated patients show a fall in HIV antigen on treatment, though not always to undetectable levels, or if they do there may be a later gradual rise (Jackson *et al.* 1988). There is no clear evidence of restoration of cell-mediated immunity, but rather a slower rate of attrition. CD4 cell counts often show a rise at 1–2 months but soon return to baseline; these changes do not correlate temporally with clinical effect.

The main clinical benefit, which is most apparent in the first 6 months to 1 year of therapy, is a reduction in the frequency and severity of opportunist infections. However, they do still occur, though generally later in the course than would be expected in untreated patients. Thus there is an early reduction in, or deferral of, morbidity and mortality in these patient groups. Some patients with HIV encephalopathy, especially those of recent onset and those without motor signs, show some degree of improvement on zidovudine (Yarchoan *et al.* 1987, 1988a; Schmitt *et al.* 1988; Pinching *et al.* 1989). There is now evidence of a reduced incidence of HIV encephalopathy in zidovudine-treated patients (Portegies *et al.* 1989). Human immunodeficiency virus-associated thrombocytopenia may also benefit from this agent (Fischl *et al.* 1987; Hymes *et al.* 1988). Trials are currently in progress to determine whether treatment of asymptomatic infection, with or without lymphadenopathy, can defer or prevent disease development. The early results from one of these (Volberding *et al.* 1990) suggest that zidovudine can reduce progression to AIDS and ARC in asymptomatic subjects with CD4 counts below 500 per mm^3, although the follow-up is short and many issues remain uncertain (Anon 1990; Pinching 1991).

Zidovudine has serious toxicity, notably on bone marrow, causing anaemia and neutropenia and sometimes thrombocytopenia (Richman *et al.* 1987); these may be exacerbated by the concurrent use of some drugs, including paracetamol, dapsone and ganciclovir (Pinching *et al.* 1989). Neutropenia, if severe, is associated with a further range of infections including *Staphylococcus aureus*, *S. epidermidis*, Gram-negative bacteria, invasive aspergillosis and systemic candidiasis. Some patients on long-term treatment have also developed a severe proximal myopathy, often with pain, tenderness and raised muscle enzyme levels (Bessen *et al.* 1988; Gorard *et al.* 1988; Helbert *et al.* 1988b; Pinching *et al.* 1989; Dalakas *et al.* 1990; Panegyres *et al.* 1990; Peters *et al.* 1991). Dose reduction or cessation may be needed to reduce or eliminate these toxic effects. However, dose reduction, if precipitate, can provoke an acute meningoencephalitic syndrome, apparently due to a 'rebound' effect (Helbert *et al.* 1988a). The comparative efficacy and toxicity of lower doses of zidovudine are currently being explored in the light of better understanding of the pharmacokinetics of the drug (Yarchoan *et al.* 1989a). Recent studies suggest that lower doses of zidovudine may have similar efficacy in terms of progression of immunodeficiency disease with better tolerance (Fischl *et al.* 1990a).

A number of other nucleoside analogues are currently under evaluation including didanosine (2′,3′-dideoxyinosine (ddI)) (Yarchoan *et al.* 1989b, 1990; Cooley *et al.* 1990; Lambert *et al.* 1990; Yarchoan *et al.* 1990) and dideoxycytidine (ddC) (Yarchoan *et al.* 1988b), for which encouraging phase I trial data are available. Other promising compounds under study are protease inhibitors, soluble CD4, glycosidase inhibitors and trichosanthin.

Immunorestorative therapy, although a logical approach to the management of the immunodeficiency disease of AIDS, has proved disappointing so far, though there is much interest in its combination with antiretroviral therapy. Bone marrow transplantation has led to successful engraftment but limited if any clinical benefit (Lane *et al.* 1984). As this may be due to the infection of donor cells, the combination of this approach with zidovudine may be more effective, though its application on any scale may be impracticable. A recent report is more optimistic about combined bone marrow transplantation and antiretroviral therapy, though the early death of the patient due to secondary lymphoma limits the interpretation put on the study (Holland *et al.* 1989).

Cytokine therapy would seem a logical alternative to the replacement of cells. Single-agent therapy with interleukin 2 (IL-2), interferon-γ and granulocyte–macrophage colony-stimulating factor (GM-CSF) has shown very limited clinical benefit (Kern *et al.* 1986; Parkin *et al.* 1986; Groopman *et al.* 1987; Lane 1989; Heagy *et al.* 1990), though the former were associated in some studies with *in vitro* and *in vivo* signs of efficacy. Interleukin 2 may increase HIV replication in lymphocytes and GM-CSF in macrophages, so combination therapy is doubly appropriate. Gamma globulin therapy has proved of value in adults with pyogenic infection; improved outcome has been seen in children with or without such infections, probably due to their more limited B cell repertoire by the time symptomatic disease supervenes (Connor *et al.* 1987). Attempts to stimulate remaining cells have met with little success to date, though the effects of interferon-α in Kaposi's sarcoma may be due in part to such an effect. Results with a variety of 'immunostimulants' have been disappointing. However, some encouraging results have been reported with trials of inosine pranobex (isoprinosine) and Imuthiol (Lang *et al.* 1988; Kweder *et al.* 1990; Pedersen *et al.* 1990; Reisinger *et al.* 1990).

Conclusions

Human immunodeficiency virus and AIDS have revealed the extraordinary spectrum of disease seen in patients with a profound acquired defect in cell-mediated immunity. They have sharpened up our concepts of immunosuppression and have shown both the value and the limitations of current methods for diagnosing and monitoring immunodeficiency disease of this type. Treatment for opportunist infections and with antiretroviral agents has started to make a major impact on medium-term prognosis. The acquired immune deficiency syndrome also offers major opportunities for immunotherapy, notably with the increasing range of recombinant cytokines, though these expectations remain largely unfulfilled to date. The acquired immune deficiency syndrome has also reinforced the need for both breadth and depth of clinical immunological expertise in modern medical centres.

References

Abrams, D.I. (1989). The persistent lymphadenopathy syndrome and immune thrombocytopenic purpura in HIV-infected individuals. In *AIDS: Pathogenesis and Treatment*, ed. J.A. Levy, pp. 323–43, Marcel Dekker, New York.

Abrams, D.I., Kiprov, D.D., Goedert, J.J. *et al.* (1986). Antibodies to human T-lymphotropic virus type III and development of the acquired immunodeficiency syndrome in homosexual men presenting with immune thrombocytopenia. *Ann. Intern. Med.* **104**, 47–50.

Allain, J.-P., Laurian, Y., Paul, D. *et al.* (1987). Long-term evaluation of HIV antigen and antibodies to p24 and gp41 in patients with haemophilia. *N. Engl. J. Med.* **317**, 1114–21.

Anderson, R.M. and Medley, G.F. (1988). Epidemiology of HIV infection and AIDS: incubation and infectious periods, survival and vertical transmission. *AIDS* **2** (suppl. 1), S57–S63.

Andiman, W.A., Eastman, R., Martin, K. *et al.* (1985). Opportunistic lymphoproliferations associated with Epstein–Barr viral DNA in infants and children with AIDS. *Lancet* **ii**, 1390–3.

Anon. (1990). Zidovudine for symptomless HIV infection. *Lancet* **335**, 821–2.

Asher, D.M., Epstein, L.G. and Goudsmit, J. (1987). Human immunodeficiency virus in the central nervous system. In *Current Topics in AIDS*, ed. M.S. Gottlieb, D.J. Jeffries, D. Mildvan, A.J. Pinching, T.C. Quinn and R.A. Weiss, vol. I, pp. 225–46, John Wiley, Chichester.

Aucouturier, P., Couderc, L.J., Gouet, D. *et al.* (1986). Serum immunoglobulin G subclass dysbalances in the lymphadenopathy syndrome and acquired immune deficiency syndrome. *Clin. Exp. Immunol.* **63**, 234–40.

Bailey, R.O., Turok, D.I., Jaufmann, B.P. *et al.* (1987). Myositis and acquired immunodeficiency syndrome. *Hum. Pathol.* **18**, 749–51.

Ballet, J.-J., Sulcebe, G., Couderc, L.J. *et al.* (1987). Impaired anti-pneumococcal antibody response in patients with AIDS-related persistent generalised lymphadenopathy. *Clin. Exp. Immunol.* **68**, 479–87.

Bayley, A.C. (1984). Aggressive Kaposi's sarcoma in Zambia, 1983. *Lancet* **i**, 1318–20.

Bayley, A.C., Downing, R.G., Cheingsong-Popov, R. *et al.* (1985). HTLV-III distinguishes atypical and endemic Kaposi's sarcoma in Africa. *Lancet* **i**, 359–61.

Bedri, J., Weinstein, W. and deGregorio, P. (1983). Progressive multifocal leukoencephalopathy in acquired immunodeficiency syndrome. *N. Engl. J. Med.* **309**, 492–3.

Beral, V., Peterman, T.A., Berkelman, R.L. and Jaffe, H.W. (1990). Kaposi's sarcoma among persons with AIDS: a sexually transmitted infection? *Lancet* **335**, 123–8.

Berger, J.R., Kaszovitz, B., Post, J.D. and Dickinson, G. (1987). Progressive multifocal leukoencephalopathy associated with human immunodeficiency virus infection: a review of the literature with a report of sixteen cases. *Ann. Intern. Med.* **107**, 78–87.

Bessen, L.J., Greene, J.B., Louie, E., Seitzman, P. and Weinberg, H. (1988). Severe polymyositis-like syndrome associated with zidovudine therapy of AIDS and ARC. *N. Engl. J. Med.* **318**, 708.

Biberfeld, P., Chayt, K.J., Marselle, L.M. *et al.* (1986). HTLV-III expression in infected lymph nodes and relevance to pathogenesis of lymphadenopathy. *Am. J. Pathol.* **125**, 436–44.

Bigby, T., Morgolskee, D., Curtis, J. *et al.* (1986). The usefulness of induced sputum in the diagnosis of *Pneumocystis carinii* pneumonia in patients with the acquired immunodeficiency syndrome. *Am. Rev. Respir. Dis.* **133**, 515–18.

Biggar, R.J. and International Registry of Seroconverters (1990). Risk of AIDS among 1115 HIV-seroconverters from different risk groups. *AIDS* **4**, 1059–66.

Bonner, J.R., Alexander, W.J., Dismukes, W.E. *et al.* (1984). Disseminated histoplasmosis in patients with the acquired immune deficiency syndrome. *Arch. Intern. Med.* **144**, 2178–81.

Broaddus, V.C., Dake, M.D., Stulbarg, M.S. *et al.* (1985). Bronchoalveolar lavage and transbronchial biopsy for the diagnosis of pulmonary infections in patients with the acquired immunodeficiency syndrome. *Ann. Intern. Med.* **192**, 747–52.

Bronnimann, D.A., Adam, R.D., Galgiani, J.N. *et al.* (1987). Coccidiomycosis in the acquired immunodeficiency syndrome. *Ann. Intern. Med.* **106**, 372–9.

Celum, C.L., Chaisson, R.E., Rutherford, G.W. *et al.* (1987). Incidence of salmonellosis in patients with AIDS. *J. Infect. Dis.* **156**, 998–1002.

Centers for Disease Control (1986). Classification system for human T-lymphotropic virus type III/lymphadenopathy associated virus infections. *Morb. Mort. Weekly Rep.* **35**, 334–9.

Centers for Disease Control (1987). Diagnosis and management of mycobacterial infection and disease in persons with human immunodeficiency virus infection. *Ann. Intern. Med.* **106**, 254–6.

Centers for Disease Control (1989). Guidelines for prevention of transmission of human immunodeficiency virus and hepatitis B virus to health care and public safety workers. *Morb. Mort. Weekly Rep.* **38**, 1–37.

Chachoua, A., Dieterich, D., Krasinski, K. *et al.* (1987). 9-(1,3,-dihydroxy-2-propoxymethyl) guanine (ganciclovir) in the treatment of cytomegalovirus gastrointestinal disease with the acquired immunodeficiency syndrome. *Ann. Intern. Med.* **107**, 133–7.

Chaisson, R.E., Schecter, G.F., Theuer, C.P. *et al.* (1987). Tuberculosis in patients with the acquired immunodeficiency syndrome: clinical features, response to therapy and survival. *Am. Rev. Respir. Dis.* **136**, 570–4.

Chayt, K., Harper, M., Marselle, L. *et al.* (1986). Detection of HTLV-III RNA in lungs of patients with AIDS and pulmonary involvement. *JAMA* **256**, 2356–9.

Chuck, S.L. and Sande, M.A. (1989). Infections with *Cryptococcus neoformans* in the acquired immunodeficiency syndrome. *N. Engl. J. Med.* **321**, 794–9.

Cohen, B.A., Pomerantz, S., Rabinowitz, J.G. *et al.* (1984). Pulmonary complications of AIDS: radiologic features. *AJR* **143**, 115–22.

Coleman, D.L., Hattner, R.S., Luce, J.M. *et al.* (1984). Gallium lung scanning in patients with suspected pneumonia and the acquired immunodeficiency syndrome. *Am. Rev. Respir. Dis.* **130**, 1166–9.

Collaborative DHPG Treatment Study Group (1986). Treatment of serious cytomegalovirus infections with 9-(1,3,-dihydroxy-2-propoxymethyl) guanine in patients with AIDS and other immunodeficiencies. *N. Engl. J. Med.* **314**, 801–5.

Connor, E.M., Minnefor, A.B. and Oleske, J.M. (1987). Human immunodeficiency virus infection in infants and children. In *Current Topics in AIDS*, ed. M.S. Gottlieb *et al.*, vol. I, pp. 185–209, John Wiley, Chichester.

Cooley, T.P., Kunches, L.M., Saunders, C.A. *et al.* (1990). Once daily administration of 2′,3′-dideoxyinosine (ddI) in patients with the acquired immunodeficiency syndrome or AIDS-related complex. *N. Engl. J. Med.* **322**, 1430–5.

Cooper, D.A., Gold, J., Maclean, P. *et al.* (1985). Acute AIDS retrovirus infection: definition of a clinical illness associated with seroconversion. *Lancet* **i**, 537–40.

Cornblath, D.R., McArthur, J., Rance, N.E. and Griffin, J.W. (1988). Predominantly sensory neuropathy in patients with AIDS and AIDS-related complex. *Neurology* **38**, 794–5.

Curran, J.W., Jaffe, H.W., Hardy, A.M., Morgan, W.M., Selik, R.M. and Dondero, T.J. (1988). Epidemiology of HIV infection and AIDS in the United States. *Science* **239**, 610–16.

Daar, E.S. and Ho, D.D. (1989). Immunopathogenesis of HIV-1 infection. In *Current Topics in AIDS*, ed. M.S. Gottlieb *et al.*, vol. II, pp. 151–75, John Wiley, Chichester.

Dalakas, M.C., Pezeshkpour, G.H., Gravell, M. and Sever, J.L. (1986). Polymyositis associated with AIDS retrovirus. *JAMA* **256**, 2381–3.

Dalakas, M.C., Illa, I., Pezeshkpour, G.H. *et al.* (1990). Mitochondrial myopathy caused by long-term zidovudine therapy. *N. Engl. J. Med.* **322**, 1098–105.

DeHovitz, J.A., Pape, J.W., Boncy, M. and Johnson, W.D., Jr (1986). Clinical manifestations and therapy of *Isospora belli* infection in patients with acquired immunodeficiency syndrome. *N. Engl. J. Med.* **315**, 87–90.

Des Jarlais, D.C. and Friedman, S.R. (1987). HIV infection among intravenous drug users: epidemiology and risk reduction. *AIDS* **1**, 67–76.

Des Jarlais, D.C., Friedman, S.R., Marmor, M. *et al.* (1987). Development of AIDS, HIV seroconversion and potential cofactors for T4 cell loss in a cohort of intravenous drug users. *AIDS* **1**, 105–11.

DeStefano, E., Friedman, R.M., Friedman-Kien, A.E. *et al.* (1982). Acid-labile human leukocyte interferon in homosexual men with Kaposi's sarcoma and lymphadenopathy. *J. Infect. Dis.* **145**, 451–5.

de Wolf, F., Goudsmit, J., Paul, D.A. *et al.* (1987). Risk of AIDS-related complex and AIDS in homosexual men with persistent HIV antigenaemia. *Br. Med. J.* **295**, 569–72.

Dismukes, W.E. (1988). Cryptococcal meningitis in patients with AIDS. *J. Infect. Dis.* **157**, 624–8.

Dournon, E., Matheron, S., Rozenbaum, W. *et al.* (1988). Effects of zidovudine in 365 consecutive patients with AIDS or AIDS-related complex. *Lancet* **ii**, 1297–302.

Edman, J.C., Kovacs, J.A., Masur, H. *et al.* (1988). Ribosomal RNA sequence shows *Pneumocystis carinii* to be a member of the fungi. *Nature* **334**, 519–22.

Eng, R.H., Bishburg, E., Smith, S.M. and Kapila, R. (1986). Cryptococcal infections in patients with acquired immune deficiency syndrome. *Am. J. Med.* **81**, 19–23.

Fahey, J.L., Taylor, J.M.G., Detels, R. *et al.* (1990). The prognostic value of cellular and serologic markers in infection with human immunodeficiency virus type 1. *N. Engl. J. Med.* **322**, 166–72.

Farthing, C. (1986). Non-malignant cutaneous disease in AIDS and related conditions. *Clin. Immunol. Allergy* **6**, 559–67.

Feinberg, J. and Mills, J. (1990). New developments in the treatment of opportunistic infections. *AIDS* **4** (suppl. 1) S209–S215.

Fischl, M.A. (1988). Treatment and prophylaxis of *Pneumocystis carinii* pneumonia. *AIDS* **2** (suppl. 1), S143–S150.

Fischl, M.A. (1989). State of antiretroviral therapy with zidovudine. *AIDS* **3** (suppl. 1), S137–S143.

Fischl, M.A., Dickinson, G.M., Sinave, C., Pitchenik, A.E. and Cleary, T.J. (1986). *Salmonella* bacteraemia as manifestation of acquired immunodeficiency syndrome. *Arch. Intern. Med.* **146**, 113–15.

Fischl, M.A., Richman, D.D., Grieco, M.H. *et al.* (1987). The efficacy of azidothymidine (AZT) in the treatment of patients with AIDS and AIDS-related complex: a double blind placebo controlled trial. *N. Engl. J. Med.* **317**, 185–91.

Fischl, M.A., Dickinson, G.M. and LaVoie, L. (1988). Safety and efficacy of sulfamethoxazole and trimethoprim chemoprophylaxis for *Pneumocystis carinii* pneumonia in AIDS. *JAMA* **259**, 1185–9.

Fischl, M.A., Parker, C.B., Pettinelli, C. *et al.* (1990a). A randomised controlled trial of a reduced daily dose of zidovudine in patients with the acquired immunodeficiency syndrome. *N. Engl. J. Med.* **323**, 1009–14.

Fischl, M.A., Richman, D.D., Hansen, N. *et al.* (1990b). The safety and efficacy of zidovudine (AZT) in the treatment of subjects with mildly symptomatic human immunodeficiency virus type 1 (HIV) infection: a double-blind, placebo-controlled trial. *Ann. Intern. Med.* **112**, 727–37.

Forster, S.M., Osborne, L.M., Cheingsong-Popov, R. *et al.* (1988a). Decline of anti-p24 antibody precedes antigenaemia as correlate of prognosis in HIV-1 infection. *AIDS* **1**, 235–40.

Forster, S.M., Seifert, M.H., Keat, A.C. *et al.* (1988b). Inflammatory joint disease and human immunodeficiency virus infection. *Br. Med. J.* **296**, 1625–7.

Francis, N.D., Goldin, R.D., Forster, S.M. *et al.* (1987). Diagnosis of lung disease in AIDS: biopsy or cytology and implications for management. *J. Clin. Pathol.* **40**, 1269–73.

Freeman, W.R., Henderly, D.E., Wan, W.L. *et al.* (1987). Prevalence, pathophysiology and treatment of rhegmatogenous retinal detachment in treated cytomegalovirus retinitis. *Am. J. Ophthalmol.* **103**, 527–36.

Friedland, G.H. and Klein, R.S. (1987). Transmission of the human immunodeficiency virus. *N. Engl. J. Med.* **317**, 1125–35.

Friedman, S.L., Wright, T.L. and Altman, D.F. (1985). Gastrointestinal Kaposi's sarcoma in patients with acquired immune deficiency syndrome — endoscopic and autopsy findings. *Gastroenterology* **890**, 102–8.

Friedman-Kien, A.E., Laubenstein, L.J., Rubinstein, P. *et al.* (1982). Disseminated Kaposi's sarcoma in homosexual men. *Ann. Intern. Med.* **96**, 693–700.

Fuchs, D., Hausen, A., Reibnegger, G. *et al.* (1988). Neopterin as a marker for activated cell-mediated immunity: application in HIV infection. *Immunol. Today* **9**, 150–5.

Gaines, H., von Sydow, M., Pehrson, P.O. and Lundbergh, P. (1988). Clinical picture of primary HIV infection presenting as a glandular-fever-like illness. *Br. Med. J.* **297**, 1363–8.

Gilks, C., Brindle, R.J., Otieno, L.S. *et al.* (1990). Life-threatening bacteraemia in HIV-1 seropositive adults admitted to hospital in Nairobi, Kenya. *Lancet* **336**, 545–9.

Gill, P.S., Levine, A.M., Meyer, P.R. *et al.* (1985). Primary central nervous system lymphoma in homosexual men. *Am. J. Med.* **78**, 742–8.

Glaser, J.B., Morton-Kute, L., Berger, S.R. *et al.* (1985). *Salmonella typhimurium bacteraemium* associated with the acquired immunodeficiency syndrome. *Ann. Intern. Med.* **102**, 189–93.

Glatt, A.E., Chirgwin, K. and Landesman, S.H. (1988). Treatment of infections associated with human immunodeficiency virus. *N. Engl. J. Med.* **318**, 1439–48.

Goedert, J.J., Weiss, S.H., Biggar, R.J. *et al.* (1985). Lesser AIDS and tuberculosis. *Lancet* **ii**, 52.

Goedert, J.J., Biggar, R.J., Weiss, S.H. *et al.* (1986). Three-year incidence of AIDS in five cohorts of HTLV-III-infected risk group members. *Science* **231**, 992–5.

Goedert, J.J., Biggar, R.J., Melbye, M. *et al.* (1987a). Effect of T4 count and cofactors on the incidence of AIDS in homosexual men infected with human immunodeficiency virus. *JAMA* **257**, 331–4.

Goedert, J.J., Eyster, M.E., Biggar, R.J. and Blattner, W.A. (1987b). Heterosexual transmission of HIV: association with severe depletion of T-helper lymphocytes in men with haemophilia. *AIDS Res. Hum. Retroviruses* **3**, 355–61.

Gold, J.W.M. (1988). Infectious complications in patients with HIV infection. *AIDS* **2**, 327–34.

Golden, J.A., Hollander, H., Stulbarg, M.S. *et al.* (1986). Bronchoalveolar lavage as the exclusive diagnostic modality for *Pneumocystis carinii* pneumonia. *Chest* **90**, 18–26.

Gorard, D.A., Henry, K. and Guiloff, R.J. (1988). Necrotising myopathy and zidovudine. *Lancet* **i**, 1050.

Gottlieb, M.S., Schroff, R., Schanker, H.M. *et al.* (1981). *Pneumocystis carinii* pneumonia and mucosal candidiasis in previously healthy homosexual men. *N. Engl. J. Med.* **305**, 1425–31.

Goudsmit, J., Lange, J.M.A., Paul, D.A. and Dawson, G.J. (1987). Antigenaemia and antibody titres to core and envelope antigens in AIDS, AIDS-related complex and subclinical human immunodeficiency virus infection. *J. Infect. Dis.* **155**, 558–60.

Grant, I., Atkinson, J.H., Hesselink, J.R. *et al.* (1987). Evidence for early central nervous system involvement in the acquired immunodeficiency syndrome (AIDS) and other human immunodeficiency virus (HIV) infections: studies with neuropsychologic testing and magnetic resonance imaging. *Ann. Intern. Med.* **107**, 828–36.

Greene, J.B., Sidhu, G.S., Lewin, S. *et al.* (1982). *Mycobacterium avium-intracellulare*: a cause of disseminated life-threatening infection in homosexuals and drug abusers. *Ann. Intern. Med.* **97**, 539–46.

Greene, L.W., Cole, W., Greene, J.B. *et al.* (1984). Adrenal insufficiency as a complication of AIDS. *Ann. Intern. Med.* **101**, 497–8.

Greenspan, D., Greenspan, J.S., Conant, M. *et al.* (1984). Oral 'hairy' leucoplakia in male homosexuals: evidence of association with both papillomavirus and a herpes-group virus. *Lancet* **ii**, 831–4.

Greenspan, D., Greenspan, J.S., Hearst, N.G. *et al.* (1987). Relation of oral hairy leucoplakia to infection with the human immunodeficiency virus and the risk of developing AIDS. *J. Infect. Dis.* **155**, 475–81.

Groopman, J.E., Mitsuyasu, R.T., DeLeo, M.J. *et al.* (1987). Effect of recombinant human granulocyte-macrophage colony stimulating factor on myelopoeisis in the acquired immunodeficiency syndrome. *N. Engl. J. Med.* **317**, 593–8.

Guenthner, E.E., Rabinowe, S.L., van Niel, A. *et al.* (1984). Primary Addison's disease in a patient with AIDS. *Ann. Intern. Med.* **100**, 847–8.

Guy, R.J.C., Turberg, Y., Davidson, R.N. *et al.* (1989). Mineralocorticoid deficiency in HIV infection. *Br. Med. J.* **298**, 496–7.

Haverkos, H.W. and TE Study Group (1987). Assessment of therapy for *Toxoplasma* encephalitis. *Am. J. Med.* **82**, 907–14.

Hawkins, C.C., Gold, J.W.M., Whimbey, *et al.* (1986). *Mycobacterium avium* complex infections in patients with the acquired immunodeficiency syndrome. *Ann. Intern. Med.* **105**, 184–8.

Heagy, W., Groopman, J.E., Schindler, J. and Finberg, R. (1990). Use of IFN-gamma in patients with AIDS. *J. Acquired Immune Deficiency Syndr.* **3**, 584–90.

Helbert, M., Robinson, D., Peddle, B. *et al.* (1988a). Acute meningoencephalitis on dose-reduction of zidovudine. *Lancet* **i**, 1249–52.

Helbert, M., Fletcher, T., Peddle, B., Harris, J.R.W. and Pinching, A.J. (1988b). Zidovudine associated myopathy. *Lancet* **ii**, 689–90.

Henderly, E.E., Freeman, W.R., Causey, D.M. and Rao, N.A. (1987). Cytomegalovirus retinitis and response to therapy with ganciclovir. *Ophthalmology* **94**, 425–34.

Ho, D.D., Pomerantz, R.J. and Kaplan, J.C. (1987). Pathogenesis of infection with human immunodeficiency virus. *N. Engl. J. Med.* **317**, 278–86.

Ho, D.D., Breseden, D.E., Vinters, H.V. and Daar, E.S. (1989). The acquired immunodeficiency syndrome (AIDS) dementia complex. *Ann. Intern. Med.* **111**, 400–10.

Holland, H.K., Saral, R., Rossi, J.J. *et al.* (1989). Allogenic bone marrow transplantation, zidovudine and human immunodeficiency virus type 1 (HIV-1) infection: studies in a patient with non-Hodgkin's lymphoma. *Ann. Intern. Med.* **111**, 973–81.

Hopewell, P.C. and Luce, J.M. (1986). Pulmonary manifestations of the acquired immunodeficiency syndrome. *Clin. Immunol. Allergy* **6**, 489–518.

Hymes, K.B., Cheung, T.L., Greene, J.B. *et al.* (1981). Kaposi's sarcoma in homosexual men: a report of eight cases. *Lancet* **ii**, 598–600.

Hymes, K.B., Greene, J.B. and Karpatkin, S. (1988). The effect of azidothymidine on HIV-related thrombocytopenia. *N. Engl. J. Med.* **318**, 516–17.

Jackson, G.G., Paul, D.A. and Falk, L.A. (1988). Human immunodeficiency virus (HIV) antigenaemia (p24) in the acquired immunodeficiency syndrome (AIDS) and the effect of treatment with zidovudine (AZT). *Ann. Intern. Med.* **108**, 175–180.

Jacobs, J.L., Gold, J.W.M., Murray, H.W. *et al.* (1985). Salmonellosis infections in patients with the acquired immunodeficiency syndrome. *Ann. Intern. Med.* **102**, 186–8.

Jacobsen, M.A. and Mills, J. (1988). Serious cytomegalovirus disease in the acquired immunodeficiency syndrome (AIDS): clinical findings, diagnosis and treatment. *Ann. Intern. Med.* **108**, 585–94.

Janossy, G., Pinching, A.J., Bofill, M. *et al.* (1985). An immunohistological approach to persistent lymphadenopathy and its relevance to AIDS. *Clin. Exp. Immunol.* **59**, 257–66.

Johnson, A.M. and Laga, M. (1988). Heterosexual transmission of HIV. *AIDS* **2** (suppl. 1), S49–S56.

Johnson, P.C., Hamill, R.J. and Sarosi, G.A. (1989). Clinical review: progressive disseminated histoplasmosis in the AIDS patient. *Semin. Respir. Inf.* **4**, 139–46.

Kaslow, R.A., Duquesnoy, R., van Raden, M. *et al.* (1990). A1, Cw7, B8, DR3 HLA antigen combination associated with rapid decline of T-helper lymphocytes in HIV-1 infection. *Lancet* **335**, 927–30.

Kern, P., Ernst, M., Flad, H.D. *et al.* (1986). Experiences with recombinant interleukin-2 in AIDS/ARC patients. In *Clinical Aspects of AIDS and AIDS-related Complex*, ed. G. Hemmer and M. Staquet, pp. 175–81, Oxford University Press, Oxford.

Kitchen, V.S., Helbert, M.H., Francis, N.D. *et al.* (1990). EBV-associated oesophageal ulcer in AIDS. *Gut* **31**, 1223–6.

Klein, R.S. (1989). Prophylaxis of opportunist infections in individuals infected with HIV. *AIDS* **3** (suppl. 1), S161–S173.

Klein, R.S., Harris, C.A., Butkas Small, C. *et al.* (1984). Oral candidiasis in high-risk patients as the initial manifestation of AIDS. *N. Engl. J. Med.* **311**, 354–8.

Koralnik, I.J., Beaumanoir, A., Hausler, R. *et al.* (1990). A controlled study of early neurologic abnormalities in men with asymptomatic human immunodeficiency virus infection. *N. Engl. J. Med.* **323**, 864–70.

Kornfeld, H. and Axelrod, J.L. (1983). Pulmonary presentation of Kaposi's sarcoma in a homosexual patient. *Am. Rev. Respir. Dis.* **127**, 248–9.

Kornfeld, H., Cruikshank, W.W. and Pyle, S.W. (1988). Lymphocyte activation by HIV-1 glycoprotein. *Nature* **335**, 445–8.

Kotler, D.P., Gaetz, H.P., Lange, M. *et al.* (1984). Enteropathy associated with AIDS. *Ann. Intern. Med.* **101**, 421–8.

Kovacs, J.A., Hiemenz, J.W. Macher, A.M. *et al.* (1984). *Pneumocystis carinii* pneumonia: a comparison between patients with the acquired immunodeficiency syndrome and patients with other immunodeficiencies. *Ann. Intern. Med.* **100**, 663–71.

Kovacs, J.A., Kovacs, A.A., Polis, M. *et al.* (1985). Cryptococcosis in the acquired immunodeficiency syndrome. *Ann. Intern. Med.* **103**, 533–8.

Krown, S.E. (1988). AIDS-associated Kaposi's sarcoma: pathogenesis, clinical course and treatment. *AIDS* **2**, 71–80.

Krupp, L.B., Lipton, R.B., Swerdlow, M.L. *et al.* (1985). Progressive multifocal leukoencephalopathy: clinical and radiographic features. *Ann. Neurol.* **17**, 344–8.

Kweder, S.L., Schnur, R.A. and Cooper, E.C. (1990). Inosine pranobex — is a single positive trial enough? *N. Engl. J. Med.* **322**, 1807–9.

Lambert, J.S., Seidlin, M., Reichman, R.C. *et al.* (1990). 2',3'-dideoxyinosine (ddI) in patients with the acquired immunodeficiency syndrome or AIDS-related complex — a phase I trial. *N. Engl. J. Med.* **322**, 1333–40.

Lane, H.C. (1989). The role of immunomodulators in the treatment of patients with AIDS. *AIDS* **3** (suppl. 1), S181–S185.

Lane, H.C., Masur, H., Edgar, L.C. *et al.* (1983). Abnormalities of B-cell activation and immunoregulation in patients with the acquired immunodeficiency syndrome. *N. Engl. J. Med.* **309**, 453–8.

Lane, H.C., Masur, H., Longo, D. *et al.* (1984). Partial immune reconstitution in a patient with the acquired immunodeficiency syndrome. *N. Engl. J. Med.* **311**, 1099–103.

Lane, H.C., Depper, J.M., Greene, W.C. *et al.* (1985). Qualitative analysis of immune function in patients with the acquired immunodeficiency syndrome: evidence for a selective defect in soluble antigen recognition. *N. Engl. J. Med.* **313**, 79–84.

Lang, J.M., Touraine, J.L., Trepo, C. *et al.* (1988). A randomised, double-blind placebo controlled trial of dithiocarb sodium (Imuthiol) in human immunodeficiency virus infection. *Lancet* **ii**, 702–6.

Lange, J.M.A., Paul, D.A., de Wolf, F., Coutinho, R.A. and Goudsmit, J. (1987). Viral gene expression, antibody production and immune complex formation in human immunodeficiency virus infection. *AIDS* **1**, 15–20.

Lange, J.M.A., de Wolf, F. and Goudsmit, J. (1989). Markers for progression in HIV infection. *AIDS* **3** (suppl. 1), S153–S160.

Larsen, R.A., Leal, M.A.E. and Chan, L.S. (1990). Fluconazole compared with amphotericin B plus flucytosine for cryptococcal meninigitis in AIDS. *Ann. Intern. Med.* **113**, 183–7.

Laskin, O.L., Cederberg, D.M., Mills, J. *et al.* (1987). Ganciclovir for the treatment and suppression of serious infections caused by cytomegalovirus. *Am. J. Med.* **83**, 201–7.

Leoung, G.S., Feigal, D.W., Montgomery, A.B. *et al.* (1990). Aerosolised pentamidine for prophylaxis against *Pneumocystis carinii* pneumonia: the San Francisco community prophylaxis trial. *N. Engl. J. Med.* **323**, 769–75.

Levine, A.M., Meyer, P.R., Begandy, M.K. *et al.* (1984). Development of B-cell lymphoma in homosexual men. *Ann. Intern. Med.* **100**, 7–13.

Levine, A.M., Gill, P.S., Meyer, P.R. *et al.* (1985). Retrovirus and malignant lymphoma in homosexual men. *JAMA* **254**, 1921–5.

Levy, R.M. and Bredesen, D.E. (1988). Central nervous system dysfunction in acquired immunodeficiency syndrome. *J. Acquired Immune Deficiency Syndr.* **1**, 41–64.

Levy, R.M., Bredesen, D.E. and Rosenblum, M.L. (1985). Neurological manifestations of the acquired immunodeficiency syndrome (AIDS): experience at UCSF and review of the literature. *J. Neurosurg.* **62**, 475–95.

Luft, B.J. and Remington, J.S. (1988). Toxoplasmic encephalitis. *J. Infect. Dis.* **157**, 1–6.

Luft, B.J., Conley, F.K. and Remington, J.S. (1983). Outbreak of central nervous system toxoplasmosis in Western Europe and North America. *Lancet* **i**, 781–4.

Lui, K., Darrow, W.W. and Rutherford, G.W. (1988). A model-based estimate of the mean incubation period for AIDS in homosexual men. *Science* **240**, 1333–5.

Macatonia, S.E., Lau, R., Patterson, S., Pinching, A.J. and Knight, S.C. (1990). Dendritic cell depletion and dysfunction in HIV infection. *Immunology* **71**, 38–45.

MacFadden, D.K., Edelson, J.D., Hyland, R.H. *et al.* (1987). Corticosteroids as adjunctive therapy in treatment of *Pneumocystis carinii* pneumonia in patients with acquired immunodeficiency syndrome. *Lancet* **i**, 1477–9.

Macher, A.M., Kovacs, J.A., Gill, V. *et al.* (1983). Bacteraemia due to *Mycobacterium avium-intracellulare* in the acquired immunodeficiency syndrome. *Ann. Intern. Med.* **99**, 782–5.

Mann, J.M., Snider, D.E., Francis, H. *et al.* (1986). Association between HTLV-III/LAV infection and tuberculosis in Zaire. *JAMA* **256**, 346–9.

Margulis, S.J., Honig, C.L., Soave, R. *et al.* (1986). Biliary tract obstruction in the acquired immunodeficiency syndrome. *Ann. Intern. Med.* **105**, 207–10.

Masur, H., Michelis, M.A., Greene, J.B. *et al.* (1981). An outbreak of community-acquired *Pneumocystis carinii* pneumonia: initial manifestation of cellular immune dysfunction. *N. Engl. J. Med.* **305**, 1439–44.

Masur, H., Lane, H.C., Palestine, A. *et al.* (1986). Effect of 9-(1,3,-dihydroxy-2-propoxymethyl) guanine on serious cytomegalovirus disease in eight immunosuppressed homosexual men. *Ann. Intern. Med.* **104**, 41–4.

Medina, I., Mills, J., Leoung, G. *et al.* (1990). Oral therapy for *Pneumocystis carinii* pneumonia in the acquired immunodeficiency syndrome — a controlled trial of trimethoprim-sulfamethoxazole versus trimethoprim-dapsone. *N. Engl. J. Med.* **323**, 776–82.

Medley, G.F., Anderson, R.M., Cox, D.R. and Billard, L. (1987). Incubation period of AIDS in patients infected via blood transfusion. *Nature* **328**, 719–21.

Medley, G.F., Anderson, R.M., Cox, D.R. and Billard, L. (1988). Estimating the incubation period for AIDS patients. *Nature* **333**, 504–5.

Meiselman, M.S., Cello, J.P. and Margatten, W. (1985). Cytomegalovirus colitis: report of the clinical, endoscopic and pathologic findings in two patients with the acquired immunodeficiency syndrome. *Gastroenterology* **88**, 171–5.

Melbye, M., Goedert, J.J. and Blattner, W.A. (1987a). The natural history of human immunodeficiency virus infection. In *Current Topics in AIDS*, vol. I, ed. M.S. Gottlieb, D.J. Jeffries, D. Mildvan, A.J. Pinching, T.C. Quinn and R.A. Weiss, pp. 57–93, John Wiley, Chichester.

Melbye, M., Grossman, R.J., Goedert, J.J., Eyster, M.E. and

Biggar, R.J. (1987b). Risk of AIDS after herpes zoster. *Lancet* **i**, 728–31.

Mildvan, D. and Richman, D.D. (1989). Strategies for the treatment of human immunodeficiency virus infection. In *Current Topics in AIDS*, vol. II, ed. M.S. Gottlieb *et al.* pp. 235–62. John Wiley, Chichester.

Miller, A., Griffin, G., Batman, P. *et al.* (1988). Jejunal mucosal architecture and fat absorption in male homosexuals infected with human immunodeficiency virus. *Quart. J. Med.* **69**, 1009–20.

Miller, J.R., Barrett, R.E., Britton, C.B. *et al.* (1982). Progressive multifocal leukoencephalopathy in a male homosexual with T-cell immune deficiency. *N. Engl. J. Med.* **307**, 1436–8.

Mills, J. (1986). *Pneumocystis carinii* and *Toxoplasma gondii* infections in patients with AIDS. *Rev. Infect. Dis.* **8**, 1001–11.

Mitsuya, H., Weinhold, K.J., Furman, P.A. *et al.* (1985). 3'-azido-3'-deoxythymidine (BW A509U): an antiviral agent that inhibits the infectivity and cytopathic effect of human T-lymphotropic virus type III/lymphadenopathy-associated virus *in vitro*. *Proc. Nat. Acad. Sci. (USA)* **82**, 7096–100.

Mitsuyasu, R.T. (1987). Clinical variants and staging of Kaposi's sarcoma. *Semin. Oncol.* **14** (suppl. 3), 13–18.

Monfardini, S., Vaccher, E., Pizzocaro, G. *et al.* (1989). Unusual malignant tumours in 49 patients with HIV infection. *AIDS* **3**, 449–52.

Montgomery, A.B., Debs, R.J., Luce, J.M. *et al.* (1987). Aerosolised pentamidine as sole therapy for *Pneumocystis carinii* pneumonia in patients with acquired immunodeficiency syndrome. *Lancet* **ii**, 480–3.

Morgello, S., Cho, E.S., Nielsen, S. *et al.* (1987). Cytomegalovirus encephalitis in patients with acquired immunodeficiency syndrome. *Hum. Pathol.* **18**, 289–97.

Moss, A.R., Bacchetti, P., Osmond, D. *et al.* (1988). Seropositivity for HIV and the development of AIDS or AIDS-related condition: three year follow-up of the San Francisco General Hospital cohort. *Br. Med. J.* **296**. 745–50.

Murray, J.F., Felton, C.P., Garay, S.M. *et al.* (1984). Pulmonary complications of the acquired immunodeficiency syndrome: report of a National Heart, Lung and Blood Institute workshop. *N. Engl. J. Med.* **310**, 1682–8.

Murray, J.F., Garay, S.M., Hopewell, P.C. *et al.* (1987). Pulmonary complications of the acquired immunodeficiency syndrome: report of the second National Heart, Lung and Blood Institute workshop. *Am. Rev. Respir. Dis.* **135**, 504–9.

Nadelman, R.B., Mathur-Wagh, U., Yancovitz, S.R. *et al.* (1985). *Salmonella* bacteraemia associated with the acquired immunodeficiency syndrome (AIDS). *Arch. Intern. Med.* **145**, 1968–71.

Navia, B.A. and Price, R.W. (1986). Central and peripheral nervous system complications of AIDS. *Clin. Immunol. Allergy* **6**, 543–58.

Navia, B.A., Petito, C.K., Gold, J.W.M. *et al.* (1986a). Cerebral toxoplasmosis complicating the acquired immune deficiency syndrome: clinical and neuropathological findings in 27 patients. *Ann. Neurol.* **19**, 224–38.

Navia, B.A., Jordan, B.D. and Price, R.W. (1986b). The AIDS dementia complex. I. Clinical features. *Ann. Neurol.* **19**, 517–24.

Navia, B.A., Cho, E.-S., Petito, C.K. and Price, R.W. (1986c). The AIDS dementia complex: neuropathology. *Ann. Neurol.* **19**, 525–35.

Nye, K.E. and Pinching, A.J. (1989). HIV infection of H9 lymphoblastoid cells chronically activates the inositol polyphosphate pathway. *AIDS* **4**, 41–5.

Ognibene, F.P., Steis, R.G., Macher, A.M. *et al.* (1985). Kaposi's sarcoma causing pulmonary infiltrates and respiratory failure in the acquired immunodeficiency syndrome. *Ann. Intern. Med.* **102**, 471–5.

Palestine, A.G., Rodrigues, M.M., Macher, A.M. *et al.* (1984). Ophthalmic involvement in acquired immunodeficiency syndrome. *Ophthalmology* **91**, 1092–9.

Panegyres, P.K., Papadimitriou, J.M., Hollingsworth, P.N., Armstrong, J.A. and Kakulas, B.A. (1990). Vesicular changes in the myopathies of AIDS: ultrastructural observations and their relationship to zidovudine treatment. *J. Neurol. Neurosurg. Psychiatry* **53**, 649–55.

Pape, J.W., Verdier, R.I. and Johnson, W.D., Jr (1989). Treatment and prophylaxis of *Isospora belli* infection in patients with the acquired immunodeficiency syndrome. *N. Engl. J. Med.* **320**, 1044–7.

Parkin, J.M., Eales, L.-J., Moshtael, O., Galaska, A. and Pinching, A.J. (1986). Preliminary results of a trial of recombinant gamma interferon in AIDS patients. In *Clinical Aspects of AIDS*, ed. G. Hemmer and M. Staquet, pp. 167–74, Oxford University Press, Oxford.

Parkin, J.M., Eales, L.-J., Galazka, A. and Pinching, A.J. (1987). Atopic manifestations in AIDS: response to recombinant interferon-gamma. *Br. Med. J.* **294**, 1157–9.

Parkin, J.M., Helbert, M., Hughes, C.L. and Pinching, A.J. (1989). Immunoglobulin G subclass deficiency and susceptibility to pyogenic infections in patients with AIDS-related complex and AIDS. *AIDS* **3**, 37–9.

Pedersen, C., Moller Nielsen, C., Vestergaard, B.F. *et al.* (1987). Temporal relation of antigenaemia and loss of antibodies to core antigens to development of clinical disease in HIV infection. *Br. Med. J.* **295**, 567–9.

Pedersen, C., Lindhardt, B.O., Jensen, B.L. *et al.* (1989). Clinical course of primary HIV infection: consequences for subsequent course of infection. *Br. Med. J.* **299**, 154–7.

Pedersen, C., Petersen, C.S., Sandstrom, E. *et al.* (1990). The efficacy of inosine pranobex in preventing the acquired immunodeficiency syndrome in patients with human immunodeficiency virus infection. *N. Engl. J. Med.* **322**, 1757–63.

Pepose, J.S. (1989). Ophthalmic manifestations of HIV infection. In *Current Topics in AIDS*, vol. II, ed. M.S. Gottlieb, D.J. Jeffries, D. Mildvan, A.J. Pinching, T.C. Quinn and R.A. Weiss, pp. 191–206, John Wiley, Chichester.

Peters, B.S., Fish, D., Golden, R. *et al.* (1990a). Visceral leishmaniasis in HIV infection and AIDS: clinical features and response to therapy. *Quart. J. Med.* **77**, 1101–11.

Peters, B.S., Winer, J., Landon, D.N., Stotter, A. and Pinching, A.J. (1991). The long-term myopathic and systemic toxic effects of zidovudine — a prospective study. (Submitted).

Petito, C.K., Navia, B.A., Cho, E.-S. *et al.* (1985). Vacuolar myelopathy pathologically resembling subacute combined degeneration in patients with acquired immunodeficiency syndrome (AIDS). *N. Engl. J. Med.* **312**, 874–9.

Pinching, A.J. (1988a). Factors affecting the natural history of human immunodeficiency virus infection. *Immunodeficiency*

Rev. **1**, 23–38.

Pinching, A.J. (1988b). Prophylaxis and maintenance therapy for opportunist infections in AIDS. *AIDS* **2**, 335–43.

Pinching, A.J. (1989). Current issues in the management of AIDS patients. *J. Acquired Immune Deficiency Syndr.* **1**, 583–92.

Pinching, A.J. (1990). Immunological consequences of human immunodeficiency virus infection. *Rev. Med. Microbiol.* **1**, 83–91.

Pinching, A.J. (1991). Zidovudine in early HIV infection: knowledge and uncertainties. *Int. J. STD AIDS* **2**, 157–61.

Pinching, A.J. and Nye, K.E. (1990). Defective signal transduction — a common pathway for cellular dysfunction in HIV infection? *Immunol. Today* **11**, 256–9.

Pinching, A.J. and Parkin, J.M. (1987). Clinical snippets. In *Current Topics in AIDS*, vol. I, ed. M.S. Gottlieb, D.J. Jeffries, D. Mildvan, A.J. Pinching, T.C. Quinn and R.A. Weiss, pp. 247–60, John Wiley, Chichester.

Pinching, A.J., Helbert, M., Peddle, B. *et al.* (1989). Clinical experience with zidovudine in the treatment of patients with AIDS and ARC. *J. Infect.* **18** (suppl. 1), 33–40.

Piot, P., Plummer, F.A., Mhalu, F.S. *et al.* (1988). AIDS: an international perspective. *Science* **239**, 573–9.

Piot, P., Laga, M., Ryder, R.W. and Chamberland, M.E. (1989). Epidemiology of heterosexual spread of HIV. In *Current Topics in AIDS*, vol. II, ed. M.S. Gottlieb, D.J. Jeffries, D. Mildvan, A.J. Pinching, T.C. Quinn and R.A. Weiss, pp. 11–31. John Wiley, Chichester.

Pitchenik, A.E. (1988). The treatment and prevention of mycobacterial disease in patients with HIV infection. *AIDS* **2** (suppl. 1), S177–S182.

Pitchenik, A.E. and Rubinson, H.A. (1985). The radiographic appearance of tuberculosis in patients with the acquired immunodeficiency syndrome. *Am. Rev. Respir. Dis.* **131**, 393–6.

Pitchenik, A.E., Cole, C., Russell, B.W. *et al.* (1984). Tuberculosis, atypical mycobacteriosis and the acquired immunodeficiency syndrome among Haitian and non-Haitian patients in south Florida. *Ann. Intern. Med.* **101**, 641–5.

Pitchenik, A.E., Ganjei, P., Torres, A. *et al.* (1986). Sputum examination for the diagnosis of *Pneumocystis carinii* in the acquired immunodeficiency syndrome. *Am. Rev. Respir. Dis.* **133**, 226–9.

Pitlik, S.D., Fainstein, V., Garza, D. *et al.* (1983a). Human cryptosporidiosis: spectrum of disease. Report of six cases and review of the literature. *Arch. Intern. Med.* **143**, 2269–75.

Pitlik, S.D., Fainstein, V., Rios, A. *et al.* (1983b). Cryptosporidial cholecystitis. *N. Engl. J. Med.* **308**, 967.

Polk, B.F., Fox, R., Brookmeyer, R. *et al.* (1987). Predictors of the acquired immunodeficiency syndrome developing in a cohort of seropositive homosexual men. *N. Engl. J. Med.* **316**, 61–6.

Polsky, B., Gold, J.W.M., Whimbey, E. *et al.* (1986). Bacterial pneumonia in patients with the acquired immunodeficiency syndrome. *Ann. Intern. Med.* **104**, 38–41.

Portegies, P., de Gans, J., Lange, J.M.A. *et al.* (1989). Declining incidence of AIDS dementia complex after introduction of zidovudine treatment. *Br. Med. J.* **299**, 819–21.

Price, R.W., Brew, B., Sidtis, J. *et al.* (1988). The brain in AIDS: central nervous system HIV-1 infection and the AIDS dementia complex. *Science* **239**, 586–92.

Profeta, S., Forrester, C., Eng, R.H.K. *et al.* (1985). *Salmonella* infections in patients with the acquired immunodeficiency syndrome. *Arch. Intern. Med.* **145**, 670–2.

Quinnan, G.V., Masur, H., Rook, A.H. *et al.* (1984). Herpes simplex infections in the acquired immune deficiency syndrome. *JAMA* **252**, 72–7.

Rance, N.E., McArthur, J.C., Cornblath, D.R. *et al.* (1988). Gracile tract degeneration in patients with sensory neuropathy and AIDS. *Neurology* **38**, 265–71.

Reisinger, E.C., Kern, P., Ernst, M. *et al.* (1990). Inhibition of HIV progresssion by dithiocarb. *Lancet* **335**, 679–82.

Richman, D.D., Fischl, M.A., Grieco, M.H. *et al.* (1987). The toxicity of azidothymidine (AZT) in the treatment of patients with AIDS and AIDS-related complex. *N. Engl. J. Med.* **317**, 192–7.

Richman, D.D., Andrews, J. and the AZT Collaborative Working Group (1988). Results of continued monitoring of participants in the placebo-controlled trial of zidovudine for serious human immunodeficiency virus infection. *Ann. Intern. Med.* **89** (suppl. 24), 208–13.

Rosenblum, M.L., Levy, R.M. and Bredesen, D.E. (1987). *AIDS and the Nervous System*. Raven, New York. 424 pp.

Rosenblum, M.L., Levy, R.L., Bredesen, D.E. *et al.* (1988). Primary central nervous system lymphomas in patients with AIDS. *Ann. Neurol.* **23** (suppl. 1), S13–S16.

Rubinstein, A., Morecki, R., Silverman, B. *et al.* (1986). Pulmonary disease in children with AIDS and AIDS related complex. *J. Pediatr.* **108**, 498–503.

Ryder, R.W. and Hassig, S.E. (1988). The epidemiology of perinatal transmission of HIV. *AIDS* **2** (suppl. 1), S83–S89.

Saltzman, B.R., Motyl, M.R., Friedland, G.H., McKitrick, J.C. and Klein, R.S. (1986). *Mycobacterium tuberculosis* bacteraemia in the acquired immunodeficiency syndrome. *JAMA* **256**, 390–1.

Schmitt, F.A., Bigley, J.W., McKinnis, R. *et al.* (1988). Neuropsychological outcome of zidovudine (AZT) treatment of patients with AIDS and AIDS-related complex. *N. Engl. J. Med.* **319**, 1573–8.

Schrager, L.K. (1988). Bacterial infections in AIDS patients. *AIDS* **2** (suppl. 1), S183–S189.

Scott, G.B., Fischl, M. and Klimas, (1985). Mothers of infants with AIDS: evidence for both symptomatic and asymptomatic carriers. *JAMA* **253**, 363–6.

Seligmann, M., Pinching, A.J., Rosen, F.S. *et al.* (1987). Immunology of HIV infection and AIDS — an update. *Ann. Intern. Med.* **107**, 234–42.

Sewankambo, N.K., Mugerwa, R.D., Goodgame, R. *et al.* (1987). Enteropathic AIDS in Uganda: an endoscopic, histological and microbiological study. *AIDS* **1**, 9–13.

Shaw, G.M., Harper, M.E., Hahn, B.H. *et al.* (1985). HTLV-III infection in brains of children and adults with AIDS encephalopathy. *Science* **227**, 177–82.

Shaw, R.J., Roussak, C., Forster, S.M. *et al.* (1988). Lung function abnormalities in HIV infected patients, with and without overt pneumonitis. *Thorax* **43**, 436–40.

Siegal, F.P., Lopez, C., Hammer, B.S. *et al.* (1981). Severe acquired immunodeficiency in male homosexuals, manifested by chronic perianal ulcerative herpes simplex lesions. *N. Engl. J. Med.* **305**, 1439–44.

Simberkoff, M.S., El Sadr, W., Schiffman, G. and Raha, J.J., Jr (1984). *Streptococcus pneumoniae* infections and bacteraemia in patients with acquired immunodeficiency syndrome, with report of pneumococcal vaccine failure. *Am. Rev. Respir. Dis.* **130**, 1174–6.

Simpson, D.M. and Bender, A.N. (1988). Human immunodeficiency virus-associated myopathy: analysis of 11 patients. *Ann. Neurol.* **24**, 79–84.

Snider, W.D., Simpson, D.M., Nielsen, S. *et al.* (1983). Neurological complications of acquired immune deficiency syndrome: analysis of 50 patients. *Ann. Neurol.* **14**, 403–18.

So, Y.T., Beckstead, J.H. and Davis, R.L. (1986). Primary central nervous system lymphoma in acquired immune deficiency syndrome: a clinical and pathological study. *Ann. Neurol.* **20**, 566–72.

Soave, R. and Armstrong, D. (1986). *Cryptosporidium* and cryptosporidiosis. *Rev. Infect. Dis.* **8**, 1012–23.

Soave, R. and Johnson, W.D., Jr (1988). *Cryptosporidium* and *Isospora belli* infections. *J. Infect. Dis.* **157**, 225–9.

Steele, C.M., Beatson, D., Cuthbert, R.J.G. *et al.* (1988). HLA haplotype A1 B8 DR3 as a risk factor for HIV-related disease. *Lancet* **i**, 1185–8.

Stewart, G.J., Tylor, J.P.P., Cunningham, A.L. *et al.* (1985). Transmission of human lymphotropic virus type III (HTLV-III) by artificial insemination by donor. *Lancet* **ii**, 581–5.

Stewart, S. (1990). Treatment of tumours in AIDS. *AIDS* **4** (suppl. 1) S217–S221.

Stover, D.E., White, D.A., Romano, P.A. and Gellene, R.A. (1984). Diagnosis of pulmonary disease in acquired immune deficiency syndrome (AIDS): roles of bronchoscopy and bronchoalveolar lavage. *Am. Rev. Respir. Dis.* **130**, 659–62.

Stricker, R.B., Abrams, D.I., Corash, L. and Shuman, M.A. (1985). Target platelet antigen in homosexual men with immune thrombocytopenia. *N. Engl. J. Med.* **313**, 1375–80.

Sunderam, G., McDonald, R.J., Maniatis, T. *et al.* (1986). Tuberculosis as a manifestation of the acquired immunodeficiency syndrome (AIDS). *JAMA* **256**, 362–6.

Tapper, M.L., Rotterdam, H.Z., Lerner, C.W. *et al.* (1984). Adrenal necrosis in the acquired immunodeficiency syndrome. *Ann. Intern. Med.* **100**, 239–41.

Tavitian, A., Raufman, J.-P. and Rosenthal, L.E. (1986). Oral candidiasis as a marker for oesophageal candidiasis in AIDS. *Ann. Intern. Med.* **104**, 54–5.

Taylor, J.M.G., Fahey, J.L., Detels, R. and Giorgi, J.V. (1989). CD4 percentage, CD4 number and CD4:CD8 ratio in HIV infection: which to choose and how to use. *J. Acquired Immune Deficiency Syndr.* **2**, 114–23.

Teich, S. and Orellana, J. (1986). Retinal lesions in cytomegalovirus infection. *Ann. Intern. Med.* **104**, 132.

Volberding, P.A. (1988). Treatment of malignant disease in AIDS patients. *AIDS* **2** (suppl. 1), S169–S175.

Volberding, P.A., Lagakos, S.W., Koch, M.A. *et al.* (1990). Zidovudine in asymptomatic human immunodeficiency virus infection: a controlled trial in persons with fewer than 500 CD4-positive cells per cubic millimeter. *N. Engl. J. Med.* **322**, 941–9.

Walmsley, S.L., Chew, E., Read, S.E. *et al.* (1988). Treatment of cytomegalovirus retinitis with trisodium phosphonoformate hexahydrate (foscarnet). *J. Infect. Dis.* **157**, 569–72.

Walsh, C.M., Nardi, M.A. and Karpatkin, S. (1984). On the mechanism of thrombocytopenic purpura in sexually active homosexual men. *N. Engl. J. Med.* **311**, 635–6.

Weber, J.N. and Jeffries, D. (1989). Humoral immune responses to HIV-1. In *Current Topics in AIDS*, vol. II, ed. M.S. Gottlieb, D.J. Jeffries, D. Mildvan, A.J. Pinching, T.C. Quinn and R.A. Weiss, pp. 177–89, John Wiley, Chichester.

Weber, J.N., Wadsworth, J., Rogers, L.A. *et al.* (1986a). Three year prospective study of HTLV-III/LAV infection in homosexual men. *Lancet* **i**, 1179–82.

Weber, J.N., McCreaner, A., Berrie, E. *et al.* (1986b). Factors affecting seropositivity to HTLV-III and disease progression in sexual partners of patients with AIDS. *Genitourinary Med.* **62**, 177–80.

Weber, J.N., Clapham, P.R., Weiss, R.A. *et al.* (1987a). Human immunodeficiency virus infection in two cohorts of homosexual men: neutralising sera and association of anti-gag antibody with prognosis. *Lancet* **i**, 119–22.

Weber, J.N., Thom, S., Barrison, I. *et al.* (1987b). Cytomegalovirus colitis and oesophageal ulceration in the context of AIDS — clinical manifestations and preliminary report of treatment with Foscarnet (phosphonoformate). *Gut* **28**, 482–8.

Wheat, L.J., Slama, T.G. and Zeckel, M.L. (1985). Histoplasmosis in the acquired immune deficiency syndrome. *Am. J. Med.* **78**, 203–10.

Whimbey, E., Gold, J.W.M., Polsky, B. *et al.* (1986). Bacteraemia and fungaemia in patients with acquired immunodeficiency syndrome. *Ann. Intern. Med.* **104**, 511–14.

Winchester, R., Bernstein, D.H., Fischer, H.D. *et al.* (1987). The co-occurrence of Reiter's syndrome and acquired immunodeficiency. *Ann. Intern. Med.* **106**, 19–26.

Witt, D.J., Craven, D.E. and McCabe, W.R. (1987). Bacterial infections in adult patients with the acquired immunodeficiency syndrome (AIDS) and AIDS-related complex. *Am. J. Med.* **82**, 900–6.

Wiznia, A. and Rubinstein, A. (1988). Pediatric infections and therapy. *AIDS* **2** (suppl. 1), S195–S199.

Wong, B., Gold, J.W.M., Brown, A.E. *et al.* (1984). Central nervous system toxoplasmosis in homosexual men and parenteral drug abusers. *Ann. Intern. Med.* **100**, 36–42.

World Health Organization (1986). Acquired immunodeficiency syndrome (AIDS). *Weekly Epidemiol. Rec.* **61**, 69–73.

Yarchoan, R., Klecker, K.W., Weinhold, K.J. *et al.* (1986). Administration of 3′-azido-3′-deoxythymidine, an inhibitor of HTLV-III/LAV replication, to patients with AIDS or AIDS-related complex. *Lancet* **i**, 575–80.

Yarchoan, R., Berg, G., Brouwers, P. *et al.* (1987). Response of human immunodeficiency virus associated neurological disease to 3′-azido-3′-dideoxythymidine. *Lancet* **i**, 132–5.

Yarchoan, R., Thomas, R.V., Grafman, J. *et al.* (1988a). Long-term administration of 3′-azido-2′,3′-dideoxythymidine to patients with AIDS related neurological disease. *Ann. Neurol.* **23** (suppl.), S82–S87.

Yarchoan, R., Perno, C.F., Thomas, R.V. *et al.* (1988b). Phase I studies of 2′,3′-dideoxycytidine in severe human immunodeficiency virus infection as a single agent and alternating with zidovudine (AZT). *Lancet* **i**, 76–81.

Yarchoan, R., Mitsuya, H., Myers, C.E. and Broder, S. (1989a). Clinical pharmacology of 3′-azido-2′,3′-dideoxythymidine (zidovudine) and related dideoxynucleosides. *N. Engl. J. Med.*

321, 726–38.

Yarchoan, R., Mitsuya, H., Thomas, R.V. *et al.* (1989b). *In vivo* activity against HIV and favourable toxicity profile of 2',3'-dideoxyinosine. *Science* **245**, 412–15.

Yarchoan, R., Pluda, J.M., Thomas, R.V. *et al.* (1990). Long-term toxicity/activity profile of 2',3'-dideoxyinosine in AIDS or AIDS-related complex. *Lancet* **336**, 526–9.

Young, L.S., Inderlied, C.B., Nerlin, O.G. and Gottlieb, M.S. (1986). Mycobacterial infections in AIDS patients, with an emphasis on the *Mycobacterium avium* complex. *Rev. Infect. Dis.* **8**, 1024–33.

Ziegler, J.L. and Dorfman, R.F. (1988). *Kaposi's Sarcoma: Pathophysiology and Clinical Management*. Marcel Dekker, New York. 266 pp.

Ziegler, J.L., Drew, W.L., Miner, R.C. *et al.* (1982). Outbreak of Burkitt's-like lymphoma in homosexual men. *Lancet* **ii**, 631–3.

Ziegler, J.L., Beckstead, J.A., Volberding, P.A. *et al.* (1984). Non-Hodgkin's lymphoma in 90 homosexual men — relation to generalised lymphadenopathy and the acquired immunodeficiency syndrome. *N. Engl. J. Med.* **311**, 565–70.

Zuger, A., Louie, E., Holzman, R.S., Simberkoff, M.S. and Rahal, J.J. (1986). Cryptococcal disease in patients with the acquired immunodeficiency syndrome: diagnostic features and outcome of treatment. *Ann. Intern. Med.* **104**, 234–40.

Index